VOLUME 2

JOHN F. CONNOLLY, M.D., F.A.C.S.
Professor and Chairman
Department of Orthopedic Surgery
and Rehabilitation, The University of
Nebraska Medical Center, Omaha, Nebraska
and Chief of Orthopedic Surgery
Omaha Veterans' Administration Hospital,
Omaha, Nebraska

Illustrations by
Steven McCoy, Barbara B. Finnerson and William Osburn

Third Edition

DePalma's
THE MANAGEMENT OF FRACTURES AND DISLOCATIONS
an atlas

Edited by
JOHN F. CONNOLLY, M.D., F.A.C.S.

W. B. SAUNDERS COMPANY
Philadelphia   London   Toronto   Mexico City   Rio de Janeiro   Sydney   Tokyo

W. B. Saunders Company: West Washington Square
Philadelphia, PA 19105

1 St. Anne's Road
Eastbourne, East Sussex BN21 3UN, England

1 Goldthorne Avenue
Toronto, Ontario M8Z 5T9, Canada

Apartado 26370 – Cedro 512
Mexico 4, D.F., Mexico

Rua Coronel Cabrita, 8
Sao Cristovao Caixa Postal 21176
Rio de Janeiro, Brazil

9 Waltham Street
Artarmon, N.S.W. 2064, Australia

Ichibancho, Central Bldg., 22-1 Ichibancho
Chiyoda-Ku, Tokyo 102, Japan

Library of Congress Cataloging in Publication Data

De Palma, Anthony F.
De Palma's The management of fractures and dislocations.

Second ed. published in 1970 under title: The management of fractures and dislocations.

1. Fractures – Atlases.   2. Dislocations – Atlases.
   I. Connolly, John F.   II. Title.   III. Title: The management of fractures and dislocations.

RD101.D29 1980   617'.15   79-64588

ISBN 0-7216-2666-1

Listed here is the latest translated edition of this book
together with the language of the translation and the publisher.

Italian (*3rd Edition*) (4 Volumes)—Verduci Editore, Rome, Italy

Spanish (*3rd Edition*) (2 Volumes)—Editorial Medica Panamericana, Buenos Aires, Argentina

Japanese (*3rd Edition*) (2 Volumes)—Hirokawa Publishing Co., Tokyo, Japan

De Palma's the Management of Fractures
and Dislocations

Volume 1: ISBN 0-7216-2702-1
Volume 2: ISBN 0-7216-2703-X
Complete Set: ISBN 0-7216-2666-1

© 1981 by W. B. Saunders Company. Copyright 1970 and 1959 by W. B. Saunders Company. Copyright under the Uniform Copyright Convention. Simultaneously published in Canada. All rights reserved. This book is protected by copyright. No part of it may be reproduced, stored in a retrieval system, or transmitted in any form or by any means, electronic, mechanical, photocopying, recording, or otherwise, without written permission from the publisher. Made in the United States of America. Press of W. B. Saunders Company. Library of Congress catalog card number 79-64588.

Last digit is the print number: 9   8   7   6

CONTENTS

VOLUME 1

Principles

DEFINITIONS AND CAUSES	2
TYPES OF FRACTURES	8
REPAIR OF FRACTURES	13
CONDITIONS INFLUENCING RATE OF HEALING	21
COMPLICATIONS OF FRACTURES	26
CLINICAL AND RADIOGRAPHIC FEATURES OF FRACTURES	100
GENERAL PRINCIPLES OF FRACTURE MANAGEMENT	106
REDUCTION OF FRACTURES	110
IMMOBILIZATION	115
MANAGEMENT OF OPEN FRACTURES	125
FUNCTIONAL REHABILITATION DURING AND AFTER FRACTURE HEALING	135

Injuries to Physes and Epiphyses

ANATOMIC FEATURES	144
MECHANISMS OF INJURIES (AFTER BRIGHT, BURSTEIN AND ELMORE)	149
SEPARATION OF THE UPPER EPIPHYSIS OF THE HUMERUS	156
FRACTURE OF THE EPIPHYSIS OF THE LATERAL CONDYLE OF THE HUMERUS (CAPITELLUM)	163
APOPHYSEAL SEPARATION OF THE MEDIAL EPICONDYLE OF THE HUMERUS	169
AVULSION OF THE LATERAL EPICONDYLE OF THE HUMERUS	179
EPIPHYSEAL SEPARATION OF THE LOWER END OF THE HUMERUS	184

Separation of the Upper Radial Epiphysis	186
Separation of the Lower Radial Epiphysis	190
Separation of the Phalangeal Epiphysis	193
Avulsion of Traction Apophyses of the Pelvis	197
Separation of the Upper Femoral Epiphysis	199
Slipped Capital Femoral Epiphysis	207
Malunited Upper Femoral Epiphyseal Slips Greater Than 60 Degrees	213
Separation of the Epiphysis of the Lesser Trochanter	217
Separation of the Distal Femoral Epiphysis	219
Fractures of the Tibial Spine	234
Separation of the Proximal Tibial Epiphysis	237
Complete Avulsion of the Tibial Tubercle	243
Injuries of the Distal Tibial Epiphysis	246
Summary: Pitfalls in Managing Epiphyseal Fractures	257

Injuries of the Cervical Spine

Epidemiology	260
Pertinent Anatomic Features	261
Mechanisms of Injury	267
Emergency Treatment of Cervical Spine Injuries	290
Management of Subluxations, Dislocations, and Fracture-Dislocations	303
Occipito-Atlantal Dislocations	306
Fracture of the Atlas (Bursting or Jefferson's Fracture)	310
Fracture of the Neural Arch of C2 (Hangman's Fracture)	312
Unilateral Atlanto-Axial Subluxation	315
Traumatic Forward Dislocation of the Atlas	319
Traumatic Posterior Dislocation of the Atlas	323
Lesions of the Odontoid Process	326
Superior Subluxation of Odontoid	328

Unilateral and Bilateral Dislocation of a Cervical Vertebra	334
Management of Flexion Injuries	345
Management of Extension Injuries	363
Posterior Fusion for Instability Following Laminectomies (Robinson and Southwick)	370
Management of Injuries of the Cervical Discs and Soft Tissues	373
Rehabilitative Management of the Patient with Spinal Cord Injury	393
Summary: The Pitfalls of Cervical Spine Fractures and Dislocations	397

Dislocations, Fractures, and Fracture-Dislocations of the Thoracic and Lumbar Spine

Anatomic Features and Mechanisms of Injuries	400
Evaluation and Management of Injuries to the Thoracic and Lumbar Spine	416
Rehabilitation of the Patient with Traumatic Paraplegia	453

Fractures and Dislocations of the Pelvis

Pertinent Anatomic Features and Mechanisms of Injury	460
General Principles of Treatment for Pelvic Injuries	468
Management of Minor Pelvic Fractures	471
Management of Major Pelvic Fractures and Dislocations	478
Summary: Pitfalls in Managing Pelvic Fractures and Dislocations	496

Injuries to the Thoracic Cage

General Considerations	500
Fractures and Dislocations of the Ribs	502
Fractures and Dislocations of Costal Cartilages	506
Emergency Management of Complications From Rib Fractures	509
Double Fractures of the Ribs (Steering Wheel Injury, Flail Chest, Stove-In Chest)	513

FRACTURES OF THE STERNUM	519
SUMMARY: PITFALLS OF MANAGING INJURIES TO THE THORACIC CAGE	522

Fractures and Dislocations of the Shoulder Girdle

FRACTURES OF THE CLAVICLE	524
LIGAMENTOUS INJURIES OF THE ARTICULATIONS OF THE CLAVICLE	545
FRACTURES OF THE SCAPULA	566
FRACTURES OF THE GLENOID	570
DISLOCATION OF THE SCAPULA	583
SUMMARY: THE PITFALLS OF FRACTURES AND DISLOCATIONS OF THE SHOULDER GIRDLE	585

Injuries of the Ligaments and Capsule of the Glenohumeral Joint (Subluxations and Dislocations)

ANATOMIC FEATURES AND MECHANISMS OF INJURY	588
MANAGEMENT OF SPRAINS AND SUBLUXATIONS OF THE GLENOHUMERAL JOINT	602
MANAGEMENT OF GLENOHUMERAL DISLOCATIONS	616
MANAGEMENT OF COMPLICATIONS OF GLENOHUMERAL DISLOCATION	642
SUMMARY: PITFALLS OF MANAGING SUBLUXATIONS AND DISLOCATIONS OF THE SHOULDER	682

Fractures of the Humerus

FRACTURES OF THE UPPER END OF THE HUMERUS	686
FRACTURES OF THE SHAFT OF THE HUMERUS	718
SUMMARY: COMPLICATIONS AND PITFALLS OF FRACTURES OF THE HUMERUS	737

Fractures and Dislocations in the Region of the Elbow

FRACTURES OF THE LOWER END OF THE HUMERUS	740
DISLOCATIONS OF THE ELBOW JOINT	791
FRACTURES ASSOCIATED WITH DISLOCATION OF THE ELBOW JOINT	806
VASCULAR AND NEURAL COMPLICATIONS ASSOCIATED WITH FRACTURES AND DISLOCATIONS OF THE ELBOW JOINT	826
RECURRENT DISLOCATION OF THE ELBOW JOINT	837
OLD UNREDUCED DISLOCATIONS OF THE ELBOW JOINT	839

Traumatic Myositis Ossificans	848
Other Fractures, Dislocations, and Injuries about the Elbow	851
Summary: Complications and Pitfalls of Fractures and Dislocations of the Elbow	883

Fractures of the Shafts of the Bones of the Forearm

Anatomic Considerations	888
General Considerations in Treatment	901
Closed Reduction and Functional Treatment of Forearm Fractures (Sarmiento)	910
Operative Management of Forearm Fractures	918
Management of Open Fractures of the Bones of the Forearm	954
Fracture of the Ulna with Dislocation of the Radial Head (Monteggia Fracture)	959
Fractures of the Bones of the Forearm in Children	979
Summary: Complications and Pitfalls of Forearm Fractures	1003
Index	i–xxxiii

Volume 2

Fractures and Dislocations in the Region of the Wrist

Fractures of the Lower End of the Radius: Colles', Smith's and Barton's Fractures	1008
Fracture of the Radial Styloid Process	1033
Traumatic Dislocation and Subluxation of the Distal End of the Ulna (With and Without Fracture)	1036
Complications of Distal Radial Fractures	1043
Fractures and Dislocations of the Carpal Bones: General Principles	1052
Fractures of the Scaphoid	1059
Lunate and Perilunate Dislocations and Subluxations	1084
Other Dislocations and Subluxations of the Carpus	1103
Fractures of the Carpal Bones	1115
Neurologic Complications of Carpal Injuries	1130
Summary: Complications and Pitfalls of Fractures and Dislocations of the Wrist	1134

Fractures and Dislocations of the Hand

Applied Anatomy 1138

Common Mechanisms of Injury to Extrinsic and Intrinsic
Tendon and Joint Function—The "Jammed" Finger or Thumb 1148

Basic Principles in Managing Hand Injuries 1153

Dislocations and Fracture-Dislocations of the Thumb 1158

Fractures, Dislocations, and Fracture-Dislocations
of the Fingers 1190

Summary: Pitfalls of Fractures and Dislocations of the Hand 1258

Dislocations and Fracture-Dislocations of the Hip and Acetabulum

Anatomic Features and Classification of Injuries 1262

Posterior Dislocations of the Hip 1268

Anterior Dislocations of the Hip 1315

Traumatic Dislocation of the Hip in Children 1331

Fractures of the Acetabulum 1335

Summary: Complications and Pitfalls in Managing Hip
Dislocations and Fracture of the Acetabulum 1361

Fractures of the Femur

Fractures of the Upper End of the Femur 1366

Fractures of the Neck of the Femur 1407

Fractures of the Femoral Shaft 1456

Fractures of the Lower End of the Femur 1511

Summary: Pitfalls of Managing Femoral Fractures 1537

Injuries of the Soft Tissues and Bony Elements of the Knee Joint

Anatomic Features 1542

Injuries to the Ligaments of the Knee Joint 1548

Disclocations and Fracture-Dislocations of the Knee Joint 1620

Fractures of the Patella 1631

Rupture of the Extensor Apparatus of the Knee Joint 1649

Dislocations of the Patella 1663

Subluxation and Dislocation of the Proximal
Tibiofibular Joint 1688

Acute Traumatic Hemarthrosis 1691

Open Joint Injuries 1693

Fractures of the Condyles of the Tibia 1696

Summary: Pitfalls and Complications of Knee Injuries 1719

Fractures of the Tibia and Fibula

Fractures of the Shaft of the Tibia 1724

Open Tibial Fractures 1749

Other Problems in Tibial Fracture 1767

Fractures of the Shaft of the Fibula Alone 1797

Summary: Complications and Pitfalls of Managing
Tibial Fractures 1798

Injuries of the Ankle: Sprains, Dislocations, and Fractures

Anatomic Features and Mechanisms of Injuries 1802

Evaluation and Management of Acute Ankle Sprains 1809

Fractures of the Ankle 1835

Posterior Dislocation of the Foot with Posterior Marginal
Fracture of the Tibia 1887

Pronation-Dorsiflexion Injuries 1898

Dislocations of the Ankle Joint 1916

Open Fractures and Fracture-Dislocations of the
Ankle Joint 1931

Malunited Fracture–Dislocations of the Ankle 1939

Summary: Pitfalls in Managing Ankle Injuries 1947

Fractures and Fracture-Dislocations of the Bones of the Foot

Fractures and Dislocations of the Talus 1952

Complications of Fractures and Fracture-Dislocations
of the Talus 1993

FRACTURES OF THE CALCANEUS 2005

FRACTURES AND FRACTURE-DISLOCATIONS OF THE
TARSAL NAVICULAR 2031

FRACTURES OF THE CUBOID AND CUNEIFORM BONES 2039

DISLOCATIONS AND FRACTURE-DISLOCATIONS OF THE
MIDTARSAL JOINT 2045

DISLOCATIONS AND FRACTURE-DISLOCATIONS OF THE
TARSOMETATARSAL JOINT 2051

FRACTURES OF THE METATARSAL BONES 2058

DISLOCATIONS OF THE METATARSOPHALANGEAL JOINTS 2070

FRACTURES OF THE TOES 2073

SUMMARY: PITFALLS AND COMPLICATIONS OF FRACTURES AND
DISLOCATIONS OF THE FOOT 2078

Birth Fractures and Pathologic Fractures

BIRTH FRACTURES OF LONG BONES 2083

PATHOLOGIC FRACTURES 2088

SUMMARY: PITFALLS AND COMPLICATIONS OF BIRTH FRACTURES
AND PATHOLOGIC FRACTURES 2134

Appendix

MULTIPLE TRAUMA: EARLY MANAGEMENT IN THE
EMERGENCY DEPARTMENT 2138

TREATMENT PROTOCOL FOR PREHOSPITAL MANAGEMENT OF THE
TRAUMA PATIENT 2140

PNEUMATIC COUNTER-PRESSURE DEVICE 2146

Index .... i–xxxiii

FRACTURES AND DISLOCATIONS IN THE REGION OF THE WRIST

FRACTURES OF THE LOWER END OF THE RADIUS: COLLES', SMITH'S AND BARTON'S FRACTURES

REMARKS

Like most fractures of the upper limb, these eponymic fractures result from a fall on the outstretched hand. Varying force vectors produced by the fall, the position of the wrist, and the differing structural properties of bones account for the differences in fracture types.

Forceful hyperextension with the forearm and wrist pronated drives the carpals into the distal radius and produces a bending and compressive failure of the cancellous subchondral bone.

Colles' fracture is a typical fracture of weakened osteoporotic bone; 60 to 70 per cent of these fractures occur in postmenopausal women.

The same hyperextension mechanism in the young adult male is more likely to produce a fracture of the scaphoid.

The hyperextension injury to the child's wrist usually results in failure through the physis or produces a distal greenstick fracture.

Occasionally, the force vector of the injury drives the carpal bones in a volar direction. This results in a fracture that angulates volarly instead of dorsally, i.e., Smith's fracture.

The same force vectors with volar direction in a young adult male shear off the articular surface of the distal radius and produce a Barton's fracture with volar dislocation of the carpus.

Each of these fracture types carries different implications regarding stability of reduction and prognosis; however, each is managed with the same ultimate objective — restoration of painless function.

Colles' Fracture

REMARKS

Colles' fracture with its dinner-fork deformity is among the most common fractures seen in emergency rooms.

The force vectors of injury produce the characteristic fork deformity of the patient's wrist. This consists of three components: radial shortening, dorsal tilt, and radial deviation of the distal radial fragment.

Correcting the dinner-fork deformity is done by pulling the radius out to length and then restoring the normal volar and radial tilt of its distal end.

The reduction must be maintained until the weak subchondral bone heals sufficiently to prevent redisplacement. This is the difficult aspect. In actual practice, recurrence of deformity, particularly radial shortening, is common because of the eggshell structural properties of the fractured bone in this region.

A good reduction is important for the patient's subjective opinion about the result, which is based primarily on the appearance of the wrist and the range of rotation after healing.

Avoid overtreating these injuries in the elderly patient. Particularly avoid extreme positions of forced flexion, pronation, and ulnar deviation (Cotton-Loder position), which add to the likelihood of postreduction neuropathy and disuse hand-shoulder syndrome.

The deformity may actually be worsened by forced pronation, which accentuates the deforming pull of the brachioradialis on the distal fragment.

For unstable fractures use pin fixation through the distal radius. This technique is particularly useful to correct the disruption of the radioulnar joint and radial shortening that commonly cause the unsatisfactory appearance and rotational limitation after Colles' fracture.

Avoid pins through the hand, which can produce extremely recalcitrant disuse hand-shoulder or ocular-palmar syndrome. The latter syndrome occurs in the patient who has become so intimidated by the injury or, more often, by its treatment that whenever he looks at the hand it hurts.

The hand-shoulder disuse syndrome after fracture can be virtually eliminated by treating the fracture with emphasis on early active range of motion to the fingers and shoulder, and by avoiding the use of a support sling.

COLLES' FRACTURE WITHOUT COMMINUTION

Dinner-Fork Deformity

1. Abrupt dorsal prominence.
2. Gently rounded volar prominence.
3. The wrist is broadened.
4. The hand is deviated radially.

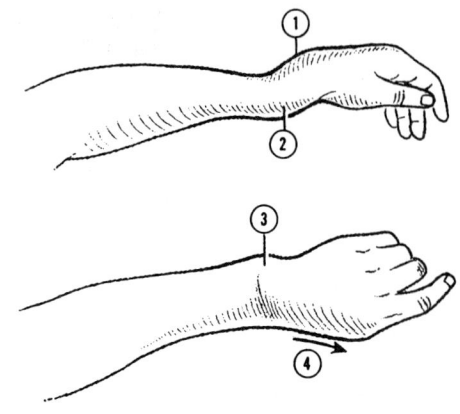

Appearance on X-Ray

NORMAL WRIST

1. The styloid process of the radius extends 1 cm beyond that of the ulna.
2. The articular surface of the radius projects toward the ulna 15 to 30 degrees (average 23 degrees).
3. The plane of the radial articular surface slopes downward and forward 1 to 23 degrees (average 11 degrees).

Note: Compare these anatomic features with those seen in a Colles' fracture.

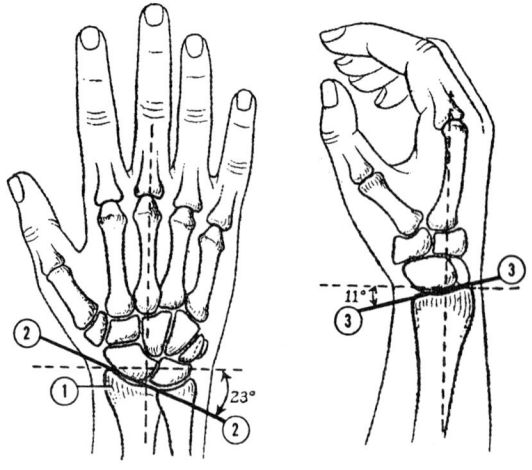

COLLES' FRACTURE

1. The distal radial fragment is displaced proximally. (The radial styloid may be on the same plane as the ulnar styloid or proximal to it.)
2. The distal radial fragment displaces dorsally and proximally.
3. The plane of the articular surface of the radial fragment tilts dorsally. (This angle varies greatly in different patients.)
4. The carpus and the hand deviate toward the radius.
5. The ulnar styloid may or may not be fractured.

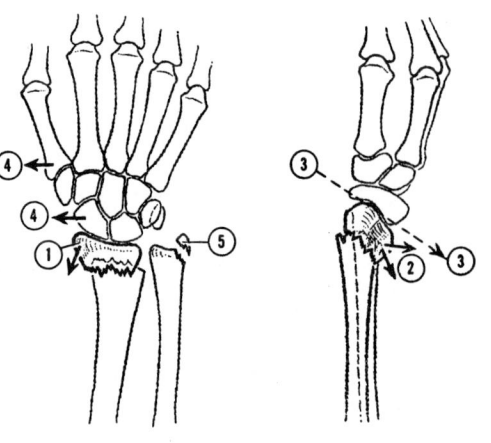

FRACTURES OF THE RADIUS: COLLES', SMITH'S AND BARTON'S FRACTURES

Preferred Method of Anesthesia: Regional Intravenous Anesthetic

1. Mix 15 cc. of 1% lidocaine and 30 cc. of normal saline to make a 0.33% solution. The dosage should be 0.5 cc. of this solution per kg. of body weight.
2. Insert a small butterfly needle into the hand on the fractured side, which is immobilized in a splint.
3. Elevate the limb for at least 3 minutes to diminish edema.
4. Using a pretested and securely taped blood pressure cuff, stop circulation by rapid inflation to at least 210 mm Hg.

Note: Specially designed double tourniquets may also be used.

5. Lower the arm and inject the lidocaine solution in appropriate dose.

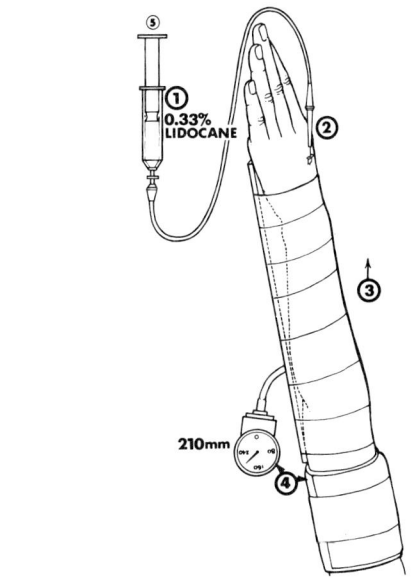

1. The needle is removed, and after 10 minutes the fracture is reduced. Always keep the cuff inflated for at least 15 minutes.

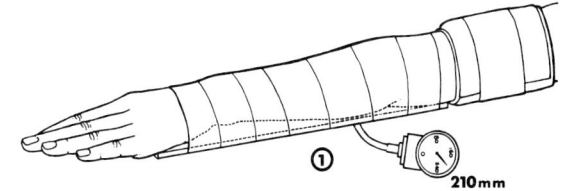

Reduction by Traction and Manipulation

The patient assumes the supine position on the fracture table.
1. Finger traction is applied.
2. The elbow is flexed to a right angle.
3. The forearm is in neutral rotation.
4. Counter traction is made using a muslin sling with a water bucket for traction.
5. Traction is maintained for approximately 5 minutes to pull the radial styloid distal to the ulnar styloid.

Note: The tourniquet for intravenous anesthesia is maintained during reduction.

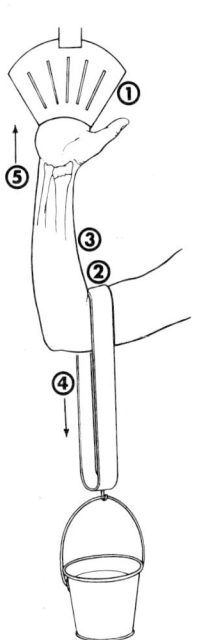

Reduction by Traction and Manipulation (Continued)

1. With the fingers of both hands on the volar side of the forearm, use both thumbs to push the distal fragment forward and toward the ulna.

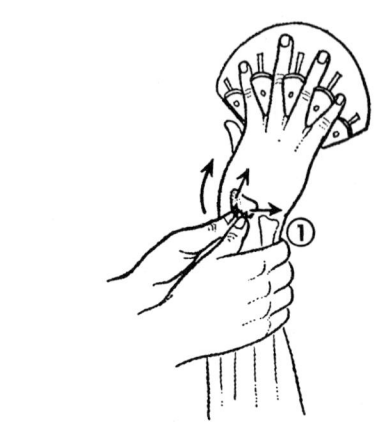

Application of Sugar-Tong Splint (Miller Method)

1. Apply cast padding from the metacarpal heads to above the elbow.
2. Add a felt pad to the volar surface of the proximal fragment.
3. Wrap a 10-cm sugar-tong plaster splint with circumferential gauze bandage.
4. The dorsal half of the splint ends at the metacarpal heads and is molded over the distal fragments.
5. The volar half ends 1 to 2 cm proximal to the fracture.

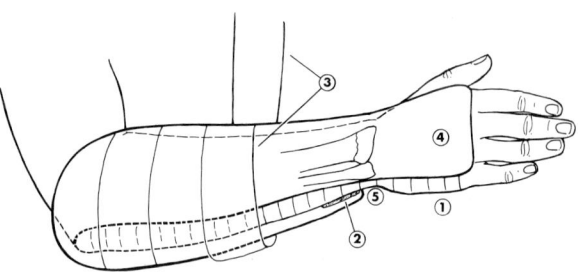

1. The wrist is in neutral rotation and slight flexion. Forced flexion or pronation accentuates the deforming pull of the brachioradialis and should be avoided.
2. The sugar tong splint allows slight wrist flexion and
3. Limited elbow motion without forearm rotation.

Note: If reduction is satisfactory, deflate the tourniquet for intravenous anesthetic to 80 mm Hg and after 10 seconds reinflate it to 210 mm Hg. Monitor vital signs and mental status; if they are unchanged, remove the tourniquet completely. Continue monitoring vital signs and mental status for 10 minutes following release of tourniquet. The entire procedure requires two assistants, one to monitor the pressure of the cuff during the block and the other to assist in reduction. Minimum tourniquet time should always exceed 15 minutes. Resuscitation equipment should be immediately available when administering anesthetic of any type.

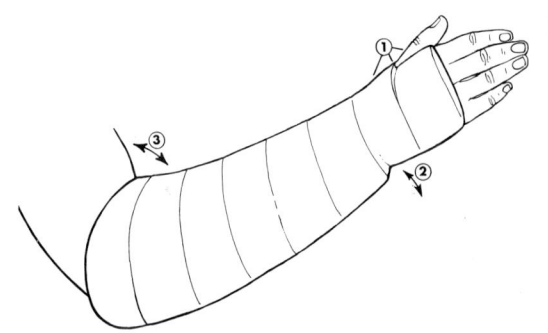

Alternate Method of Reduction

Local anesthesia may be used.

To reduce a fracture of the right radius:

1. Grasp the distal fragment with the right hand.
2. Grasp the wrist above the level of the fracture with the left hand.
3. Make steady traction in the angle of displacement of the distal fragment.

While traction is maintained,

4. Flex and pronate the distal fragment with the right hand, using
5. The index finger of the left hand on the volar surface, which acts as the fulcrum; at the same time,
6. Push the distal fragment forward and downward with the thumb of the left hand.
7. Take a new grip on the wrist with the right hand. The thenar eminence is placed against the radial styloid.
8. Grasp the forearm with the left hand.
9. With the right hand, push the distal fragment toward the ulna.

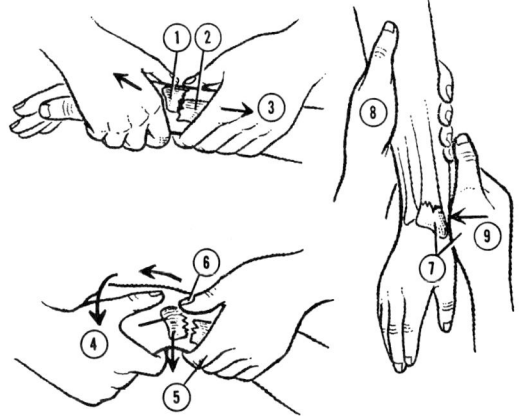

IMMOBILIZATION

1. A sugar tong splint is applied to allow room for swelling after reduction (see page 1012).
2. Limited wrist flexion permits volar angulation of the distal fragment.
3. Limited elbow flexion is possible without forearm rotation.

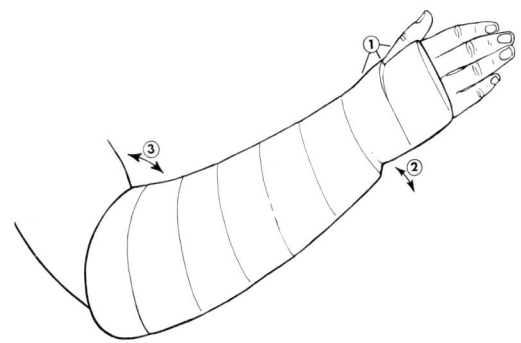

Postreduction X-Ray

1. The normal length of the radius has been restored. The radial styloid is distal to the ulnar styloid.
2. The articular plane of the radius is now directed toward the ulna.
3. The articular surface of the radius is directed downward, forward, and inward.

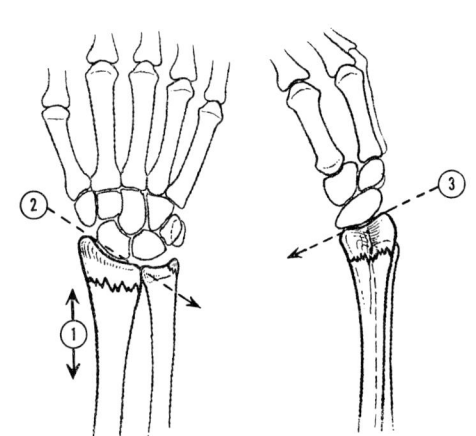

Postreduction Management

Take x-rays after applying the sugar tong splint. If reduction is not complete perform a second reduction, but do not manipulate repeatedly.

The splint should allow room for swelling without compromising circulation. If there is any evidence of circulatory embarrassment, the splint may be cut through the padding down to the skin.

The arm should be elevated with the fingers pointing toward the ceiling for the first 24 hours, and ice should be applied.

Check the patient within 24 to 48 hours and begin hourly active range-of-motion exercises of the fingers and shoulder. Avoid the use of an arm sling for support, which inhibits active exercise.

Take more x-rays within 5 to 10 days to evaluate fracture position.

If the splint becomes loose after 10 days, it should be rewrapped with new circumferential gauze roll, or a short arm cast should be applied.

After one month, remove the splint and evaluate healing clinically and radiographically.

If the patient still has pain and tenderness at the fracture site, reapply the cast for two weeks; otherwise, permit active range of wrist motion without the cast.

COLLES' FRACTURES WITH COMMINUTION

REMARKS

Comminuted Colles' fracture may occur in any group but is most common in the elderly. Usually the distal ulna or the ulnar styloid is fractured and the distal radioulnar joint is disrupted.

Dorsal redisplacement and shortening of the radius is the rule following reduction of these comminuted fractures. This can be prevented by transfixing the fragments with a distal pin inserted through the radial styloid process.

Since the wrist ligaments remain intact with these injuries, they can be used to maintain tension on the fracture fragments, which they surround.

A pin inserted through the distal radius maintains ligamentous tension much as a tent pole supports the roof of a pyramidal tent. Pin fixation thereby minimizes radial shortening and maintains reduction of the distal radio-ulnar joint.

While the pin is in place, the patient can actively exercise the fingers and the shoulder joint to minimize the effects of disuse. This is in contrast to pin fixation methods in the hand metacarpals, which quite frequently inhibit active exercises.

Prereduction X-Rays of Some of the Types of Fractures Encountered

1. The distal radial fragments are severely comminuted.
2. The radial fragments are displaced dorsally and proximally.
3. The length of the radius is decreased; the tip of the ulnar styloid is almost on the same plane as the radial styloid.
4. The plane of the articular surface of the radial fragments projects dorsally.
5. The tip of the ulnar styloid is pulled off.

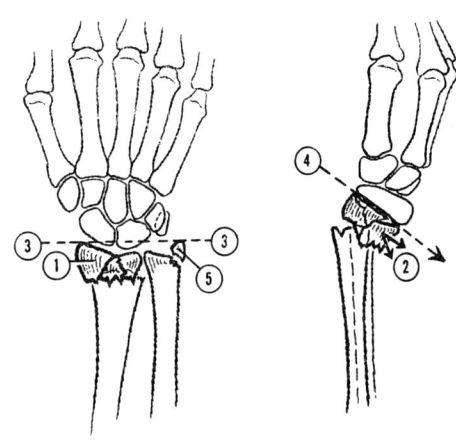

1. There is severe comminution of the distal radial fragment with impaction.
2. The distal radial fragments are displaced directly volarly (and not dorsally).
3. The length of the radius is shortened.

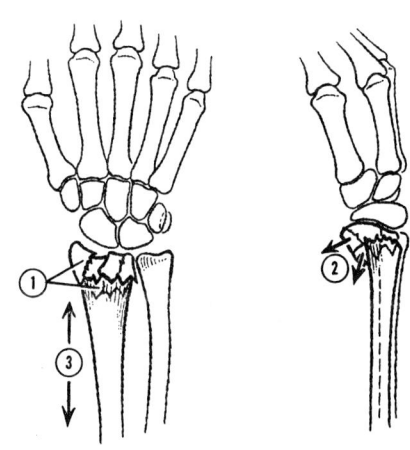

1. There is comminution of the distal radial fragment.
2. Moderate dorsal displacement of the radial fragments has occurred.
3. The radial and ulnar styloid are almost on the same plane.
4. There is fracture with comminution of the distal end of the ulna.

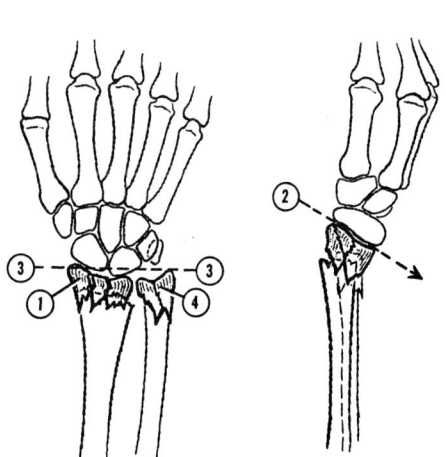

1015

FRACTURES OF THE RADIUS: COLLES', SMITH'S AND BARTON'S FRACTURES

Preferred Method of Management (Rowland Fixation Technique)

Reduction by traction, manipulation, and transfixion pin is accomplished under either general or regional intravenous anesthetic (see page 1011).

The patient assumes a supine position on the fracture table. Ideally, image-intensified fluoroscopy should be used if available.

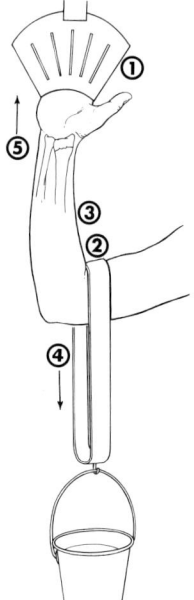

TRACTION

1. The fingers are supported with a finger traction apparatus.
2. The elbow is flexed 90 degrees.
3. The forearm is in neutral rotation to relax the brachioradialis.
4. Counter traction is applied using the weight of a water bucket.
5. Traction is continued until the radial styloid is pulled distal to the ulnar styloid.

Note: A tourniquet is maintained for intravenous anesthetic during traction maneuvers (page 1011).

MANIPULATION

1. Place the fingers of both hands on the volar side of the forearm and
2. Use the thumbs on the dorsal aspect of the wrist to push the distal fragment volarly and distally.

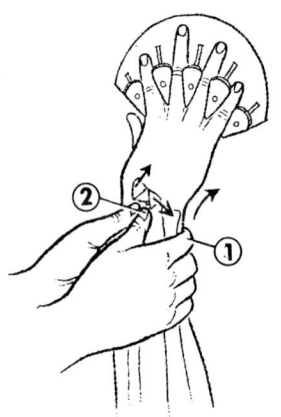

FRACTURES OF THE RADIUS: COLLES', SMITH'S AND BARTON'S FRACTURES

INSERTION OF TRANSFIXION PIN

1. Confirm the reduction by fluoroscopy and then prepare the distal forearm for surgery.
2. While traction and the position of the wrist are maintained by an assistant,
3. Pass a threaded Steinmann pin 2.0 mm in diameter from the radial styloid across the fracture and into the opposite radial cortex. The pin is directed from the radial styloid at approximately a 45-degree angle. Confirm the position of the pin by fluorosopy.

Note: The pin should be heavy enough so that it does not break and should be threaded so that it does not loosen.

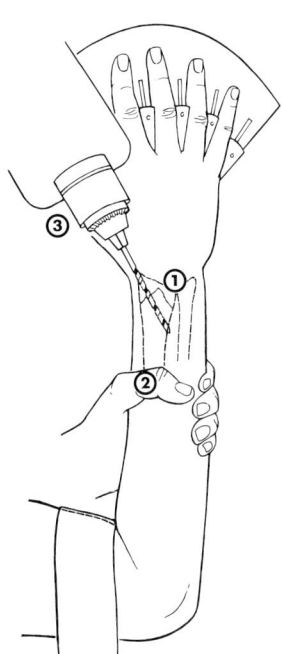

Application of Sugar Tong Splint

1. Apply a sugar tong splint.
2. The pin is cut off outside the skin but is not incorporated in the plaster.

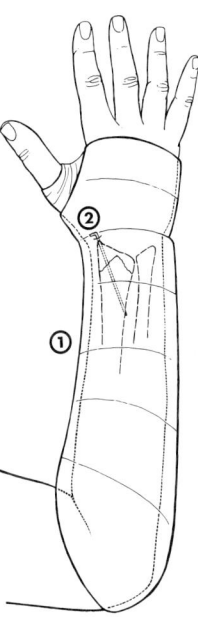

Postreduction X-Ray

In all three instances:

1. The pin from the radial styloid crosses the fracture site and holds the comminuted fragments out to length much as a tent pole holds a pyramidal tent.
2. The pin is fixed on the opposite radial cortex.
3. Reduction of the radial shortening also corrects the distal radioulnar joint relationships.

Note: Always check the median, ulnar, and radial nerve function before and after reduction and pin fixation.

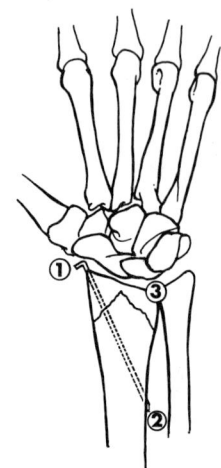

Postreduction Management

If fluoroscopy is not available, take an x-ray immediately after insertion of the Steinmann pin. If reduction is not satisfactory, repeat the procedure. This is rarely necessary.

The splint should be applied firmly but without impairing circulation. Loosen the splint through the padding if swelling occurs or if the patient complains that it is tight.

Elevate the arm with the fingers pointing toward the ceiling for 24 hours and apply ice bags.

Avoid the use of a sling support and insist on active exercises to the fingers and shoulder.

Take x-rays again within 5 to 10 days and at the end of 4 to 6 weeks to confirm position.

If the splint loosens, apply a new splint.

During the healing period, the patient must actively exercise the fingers and thumb as well as the shoulder.

At the end of 8 weeks, remove the splint and, using local anesthetic, take out the Steinmann pin. Occasionally in older patients with osteoporotic bone, internal fixation for 10 weeks may be required.

Following removal of the pin, start active range-of-motion exercises of the fingers, wrist, elbow, and shoulder.

Note: The worst complications of a Colles' fracture, the hand-shoulder and ocular-palmar syndromes, can be prevented by not using a sling support and by insisting on active functional exercises from the first day after injury.

The major complication from the transfixion pin method relates to poor pin placement. Use image-intensified fluoroscopy if possible and insert pins that are heavy enough (2.0 mm) not to break.

FRACTURES OF THE RADIUS: COLLES', SMITH'S AND BARTON'S FRACTURES

If the pin is removed before 8 weeks, recurrence of the deformity is possible.

Although anatomic and functional results do not always correlate, this method maximizes anatomic restoration. It also gives the patient the best chance for functional recovery when combined with early exercises of the fingers and shoulder.

COMPLICATIONS OF COLLES' FRACTURE

The most common complication of Colles' fracture is loss of finger motion and grip strength due to the edema of injury and secondary weakness from disuse. This can be minimized by active range of finger and shoulder motion.

If the syndrome persists it will occasionally respond to cervical sympathetic blocking by 1% procaine every 4 to 5 days to relieve pain.

The complications that most often concern the patient, wrist deformity and limitation of rotation, can be mitigated by the use of the radial pin fixation. This prevents radial shortening and disruption of the radioulnar joint.

Approximately 3 per cent of Colles' fractures cause injury to the median nerve. Median neuropathy is usually transient provided that the wrist is not forced and held in the Cotton-Loder flexion position.

Rarely, the median nerve may be compressed by callus or by bone spicules from the fracture and may require surgical decompression.

Always check for median, radial, and ulnar nerve function before and after reduction either with or without pin fixation.

Sometimes (in less than 1 per cent of cases), the extensor pollicis longus tendon may rupture over the fracture. Its function should be evaluated regularly during follow-up examinations.

Because of the swelling that frequently follows distal radial fractures, constrictive dressings can aggravate hand edema and may even result in compartmental syndromes. A sugar tong splint rather than a circumferential cast is ideal in the immediate management of the Colles' fracture.

Malunion, or at least recurrence of the fracture deformity, is a common complication, particularly if an unstable fracture is not held by pin transfixion. The major cause of symptomatic deformity is disruption of the distal radioulnar joint, which can be corrected by resecting the distal ulna.

Rarely, osteotomy of the radius will also be necessary to correct persistent dorsal angulation (see page 1045).

About 5 per cent of Colles' fractures are complicated by fracture of the scaphoid or other carpal bones. This is especially likely in younger patients or in men without osteoporotic bone. Evaluate the initial and subsequent x-rays carefully, because the symptoms of scaphoid fracture may be masked by those of the more obvious radial fracture.

Colles' Fracture Complicated by Fracture of the Carpal Scaphoid

Appearance on X-Ray

1. Fractured carpal scaphoid.
2. Comminuted Colles' fracture.

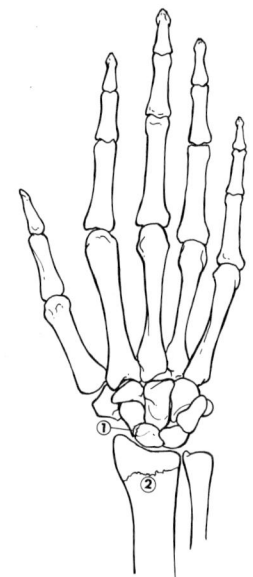

Most of these combined injuries can be treated primarily for the scaphoid fracture.

Immobilization

1. The wrist is held in 25 degrees of extension and 20 degrees of radial deviation.
2. The cast includes the thumb, with the first metacarpal aligned along the long axis of the radius.
3. The forearm is in neutral rotation.
4. The cast extends above the elbow to immobilize both the distal radial and the scaphoid fractures.

Note: If the Colles' fracture is unstable insert a pin across the fracture from the radial styloid (see page 1017). Then apply the cast for the scaphoid fracture with the wrist extended and in radial deviation.

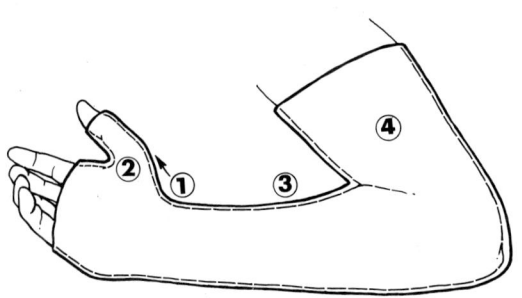

Smith's Fracture

REMARKS

Robert Smith like Abraham Colles was an 18th-century Dublin surgeon who described the clinical manifestations of distal radial fractures. In contrast to the dorsally displaced Colles' fracture, the less common Smith's fracture displaces volarly. Smith's fracture occurs about one tenth as often as Colles' fracture. It frequently is extremely unstable and may cause significant disability if mistaken for and treated as a Colles' fracture.

The usually described mechanism that produces Smith's fracture is a fall backward on the supinated wrist.

A motorcyclist is especially susceptible to Smith's fracture during an accident, because his wrists are hyperextended as he is being thrown over his grip on the handlebars.

The force vectors from this injury displace the carpus and the distal radius in a volar rather than a dorsal direction. Extension of the wrist accentuates the displacement, and wrist function may be seriously impaired by recurrence of the deformity.

Usually this unstable fracture can be reduced by supinating the wrist to tighten the pronator quadratus muscle and the volar capsule of the wrist.

For extremely unstable Smith's fracture the distal radius can be fixed by pins.

Smith's fracture, which occurs 1 to 2 cm above the articular surface of the metaphyseal bone, must be distinguished from Barton's fracture-dislocation, which occurs through the volar articular surface. Smith's fracture can usually be managed by closed methods. Open reduction and buttress plate fixation are necessary for the unstable Barton's fracture-dislocation.

Garden-Spade Deformity

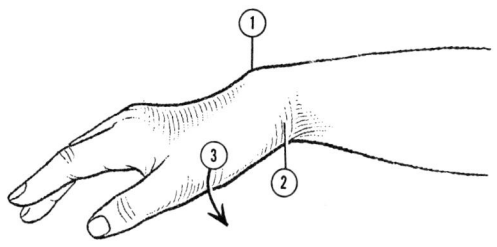

1. Dorsal prominence of the distal end of the proximal fragment.
2. Fullness of the wrist on the volar side due to the displaced distal fragment.
3. Deviation of the hand toward the radial side.

FRACTURES OF THE RADIUS: COLLES', SMITH'S AND BARTON'S FRACTURES

Prereduction X-ray

1. The distal fragment displaces volarly and proximally.
2. The fracture lines runs obliquely through the metaphyseal bone approximately 1 to 2 cm proximal to the articular surface.
3. The fracture runs through the full width of the metaphysis.
4. The hand and the distal fragment displace radially.

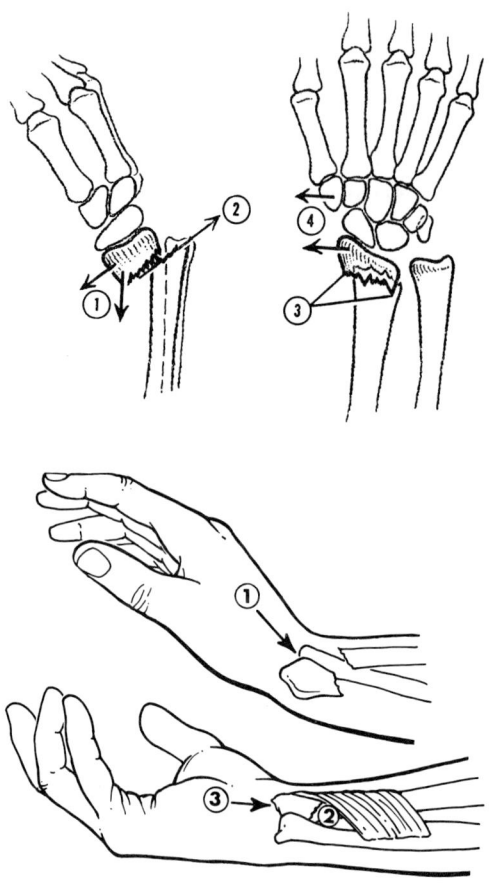

Mechanics of Reduction

1. Wrist extension usually reproduces the force vectors of injury and displaces the fracture volarly.
2. Supination tightens the pronator quadratus as a buttress against volar displacement.
3. Neutral or slightly flexed position of the wrist eliminates shear across the fracture.

Reduction by Traction and Manipulation

The patient is under regional intravenous anesthesia (see page 1011).

Traction

1. Apply finger traction apparatus.
2. Flex the elbow at a right angle.
3. Supinate the forearm.
4. Apply counter traction with muslin bandage and a water bucket for weight.
5. Maintain traction for at least 5 minutes, until the radial styloid is distal to the ulnar styloid.

Note: Keep the tourniquet inflated during manipulation to maintain intravenous anesthesia.

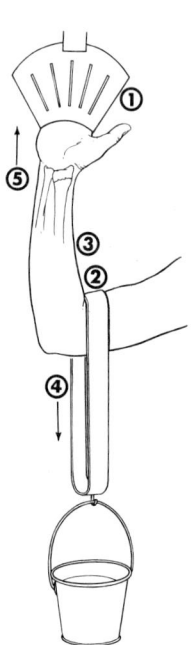

1022

Manipulation

While traction is maintained,

1. The fingers of both hands support the dorsal surface of the proximal fragment.
2. Both thumbs push the distal fragment dorsally.
3. The wrist is directed into slight flexion and ulnar deviation.

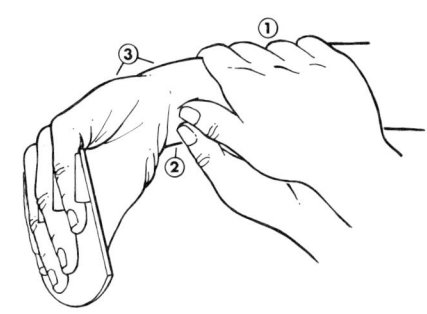

Application of Cast

1. While the position of slight flexion and ulnar deviation is maintained by an assistant, apply a circular cast from the middle of the arm to metacarpal heads; the elbow is flexed 90 degrees and the arm is fully supinated.
2. Hold the wrist in slight flexion and ulnar deviation and supination.
3. Mold firmly over the volar surface of the distal end of the radius and the carpus.

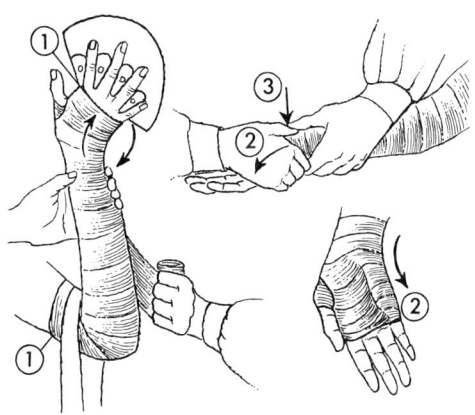

Postreduction X-Ray

1. The radial styloid is distal to the ulnar styloid.
2. The distal fragment is restored to its normal relationship with the proximal fragment. The wrist is slightly flexed to impact the fracture.
3. Radial deviation of the lower fragment and hand has been corrected.

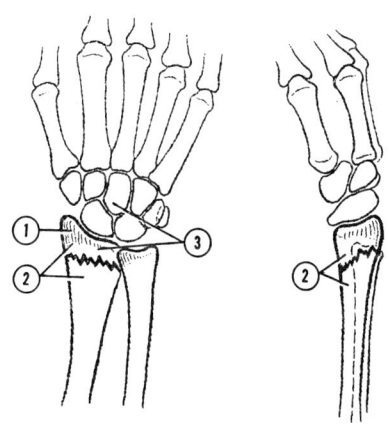

Note: If reduction is satisfactory, deflate the tourniquet for intravenous anesthetic to 80 mm Hg, and after 10 seconds reinflate it to 210 mm Hg. Monitor vital signs and mental status; if these are unchanged, remove the tourniquet completely. Continue monitoring vital signs and mental status for 10 minutes following release of the tourniquet. The entire procedure requires two assistants, one to monitor the pressure of the cuff during the block and the other to assist in reduction. Minimum tourniquet time should always exceed 15 minutes.

Postreduction Management

Evaluate reduction by means of image-intensified fluoroscopy or standard x-rays. If reduction is unsatisfactory, repeat manipulation to achieve accurate alignment of the fracture. If the fracture remains unstable, employ pin fixation technique.

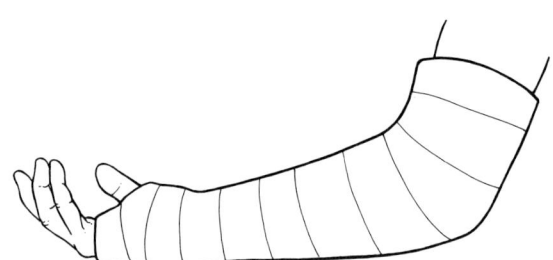

The cast should be applied firmly so as to prevent loss of position but not so tightly as to cause circulatory embarrassment. Elevate the arm with the fingers pointed toward the ceiling for the first 24 hours, and apply ice bags.

If the patient complains that the cast is too tight, bivalve the cast down through the padding.

After 24 to 48 hours encourage active exercises of the fingers and shoulder.

Take x-rays again within 5 to 10 days to evaluate position.

After 2 to 3 weeks a new cast that allows some elbow flexion but prevents wrist extension and forearm rotation may be applied.

During the healing period, supervise active finger and shoulder motion exercises.

Avoid the use of a support sling, which discourages shoulder and finger exercises.

Remove the plaster cast after 6 weeks and allow the patient to begin active wrist exercises.

UNSTABLE SMITH FRACTURE OF THE LOWER END OF THE RADIUS WITH COMMINUTION

REMARKS

In a number of Smith's fractures, because of fracture obliquity or comminution, redisplacement frequently occurs.

Volar displacement of Smith's fracture causes significantly more functional disability than does dorsal displacement of Colles' fracture.

The fracture deformity and instability can be prevented by distal-radial pin fixation.

FRACTURES OF THE RADIUS: COLLES', SMITH'S AND BARTON'S FRACTURES

Prereduction X-Ray

1. The distal radial fragment is comminuted.
2. Displacement is volar and proximal.
3. The distal fragments are deviated radially.
4. The styloid process of the ulna is avulsed and is more distal than the radial styloid.

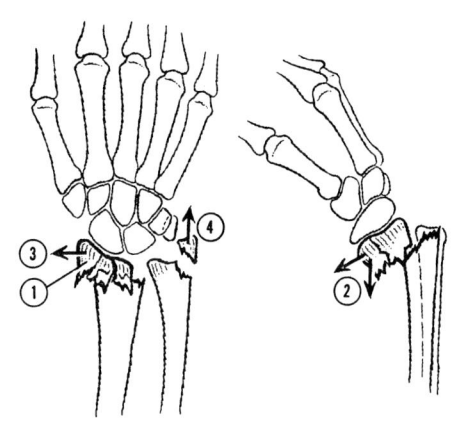

Reduction by Traction, Manipulation, and Transfixion Pin

The patient is under general or regional intravenous anesthesia (see page 1011).

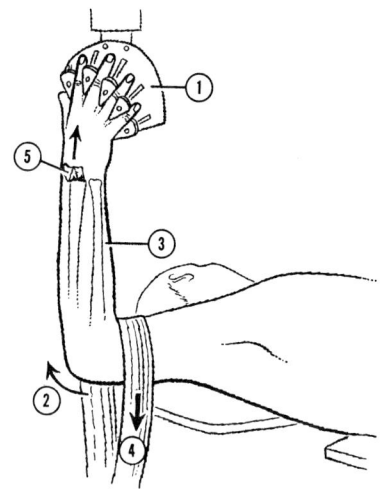

TRACTION

1. Apply a finger traction apparatus.
2. The elbow is flexed 90 degrees.
3. The forearm is supinated fully.
4. Make counter traction using a muslin bandage and water bucket for weight.
5. While maintaining forearm supination, continue traction until the radial styloid is distal to the ulnar styloid.

Reduction by Traction, Manipulation, and Transfixion Pin (Continued)

MANIPULATION

1. Place the fingers of both hands on the dorsum of the wrist.
2. Place the thumbs just proximal to the distal fragments on the volar aspect of the wrist.

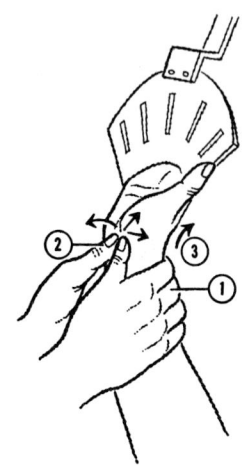

3. Dorsiflex the wrist, and at the same time push the distal fragment upward, backward, and toward the ulna with both thumbs.
4. While maintaining direct thumb pressure upward on the distal fragment, bring the wrist down into slight flexion and ulnar deviation.

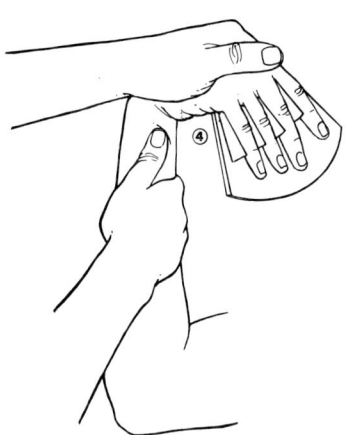

Insertion of Transfixion Pin

1. Confirm the reduction by fluoroscopy and then prepare the distal forearm for surgery.
2. While traction and the position of the wrist are maintained by an assistant,
3. Pass a threaded Steinmann pin, 2.0 mm in diameter, from the radial styloid across the fracture and into the opposite radial cortex. The pin is directed from the radial styloid at approximately a 45 degree angle. Confirm the position of the pin by fluoroscopy.

Note: The pin should be heavy enough so that it does not break and should be threaded so it does not loosen.

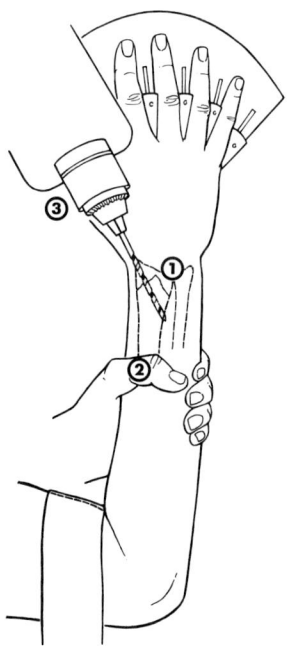

Application of Sugar-Tong Splint

1. Apply a sugar-tong splint.
2. The pin is cut off outside the skin but is not incorporated in the plaster.

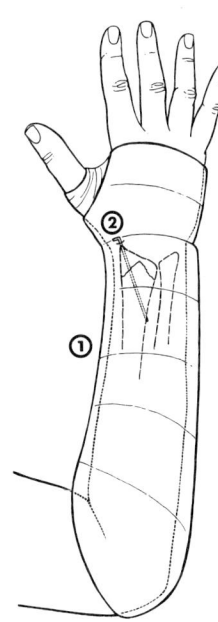

Postreduction X-Rays

1. The pin from the radial styloid crosses the fracture site and holds the comminuted fragments out to length much as a tentpole holds a pyramidal tent.
2. The pin is fixed on the opposite radial cortex.
3. Reduction of the radial shortening also corrects the distal radioulnar joint relationships.

Note: Always check the median, ulnar, and radial nerve function before and after the reduction and pin fixation.

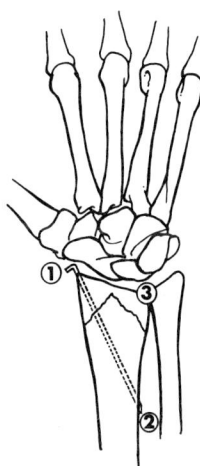

Postreduction Management

Ascertain the position of the pin and the reduction of the fracture by means of image-intensified fluoroscopy or standard x-ray. If reduction is not satisfactory, repeat the procedure. This is rarely necessary.

The splint should not be applied so tightly as to cause circulatory embarrassment. If at any time the patient complains that the splint is too tight or his hand is swollen, loosen the splint and padding.

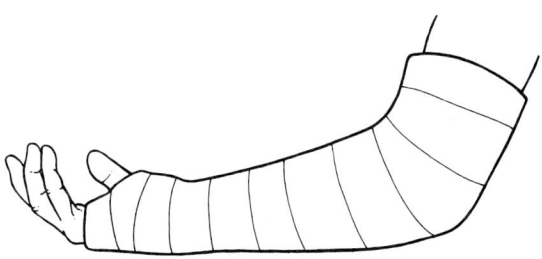

Elevate the arm with fingers pointing toward the ceiling for the first 24 hours, and apply ice bags.

Avoid the use of a sling and insist on active finger and shoulder exercise from the start.

By 2 to 3 weeks the cast may become loose and may have to be changed. Keep the forearm in the supinated position for at least 6 to 8 weeks.

Remove the cast at the end of 6 to 8 weeks, depending on the status of the healing, and, using local anesthetic, remove the pin fixation.

Continue active range-of-motion exercises to the wrist after the cast and pin are removed.

Barton's Fracture

John Rhea Barton in 1838 described posterior and anterior marginal fractures of the distal radial articular surface. Barton's posterior marginal fracture is best classified as a Colles' fracture.

The term *Barton's fracture* should be confined to describing an anterior fracture-dislocation in which a wedge-shaped articular fragment shears off the volar surface of the radius and displaces with the carpus forward and proximally.

In contrast to the Colles' fracture, Barton's fracture is produced by a violent direct injury to the carpus and wrist. Seventy per cent of Barton's fractures occur in young male laborers or motorcyclists.

Usually the dislocated fragment includes all of the anterior portion of the lower metaphysis. The radial styloid may occasionally be separated as well.

Because of the extreme instability of this injury, it is best managed by prompt open reduction and buttress plate fixation. Screws are not inserted in the distal fragment in order to avoid comminuting it further.

If the radial styloid is fractured and separated, it is held with a Kirschner wire or screw fixation.

Prereduction X-rays

SIMPLE BARTON'S FRACTURE-DISLOCATION

1. A large fragment of the anterior articular surface of the radius is displaced anteriorly and proximally.
2. The carpus follows the radial fragment.
3. Some comminution of the radial fragment exists.

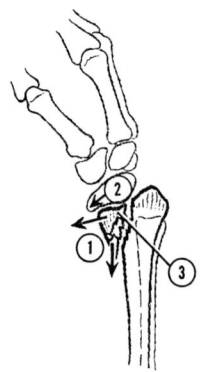

FRACTURES OF THE RADIUS: COLLES', SMITH'S AND BARTON'S FRACTURES

COMMINUTED BARTON'S FRACTURE-DISLOCATION

1. The comminuted fracture of the volar articular surface is associated with
2. Volar dislocation of the carpus.
3. Occasionally, the radial styloid process is also fractured.

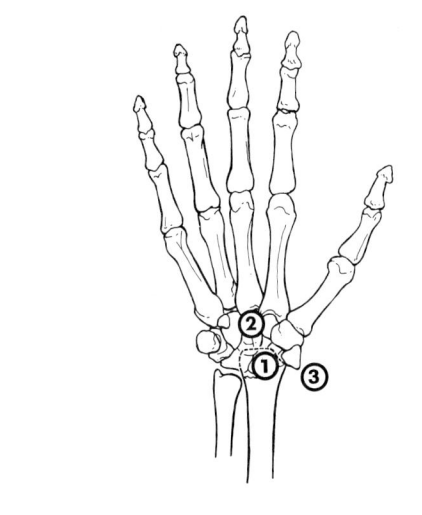

Open Reduction and Buttress Plate Fixation (Technique of Cauchoix and De Oliveira)

INCISION AND EXPOSURE

1. Approach the fracture from the volar aspect via a longitudinal radial incision.

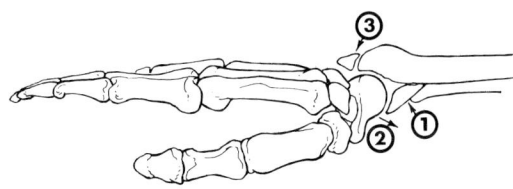

2. After incising the aponeurosis, retract the flexor carpi radialis and the finger flexors medially and the radial vessels laterally.
3. Expose the fracture by dividing the external fibers of the pronator quadratus.

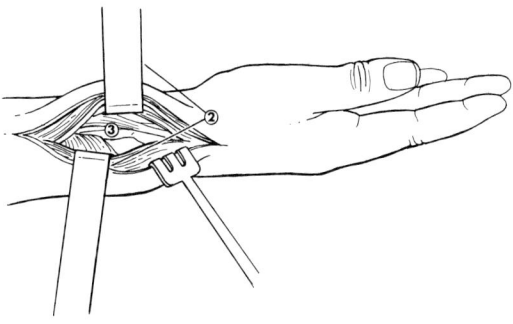

Open Reduction and Buttress Plate Fixation (Technique of Cauchoix and De Oliveira) *(Continued)*

REDUCTION AND FIXATION

1. Remove fragments from the joint and reduce the detached cortical fragments into the metaphysis. Usually they are entirely detached and rotated.

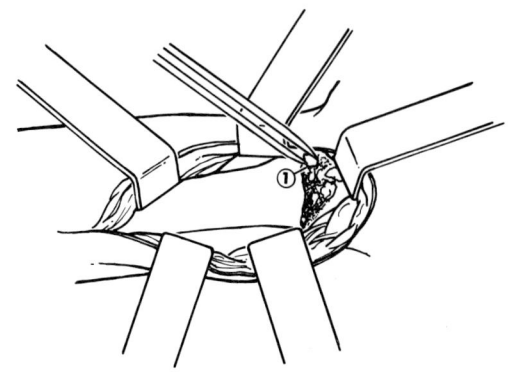

2. A small angled plate is fixed to the intact shaft with screws.
3. The pressure of the lower end of the plate over the distal fragment reduces and holds the articular surfaces.

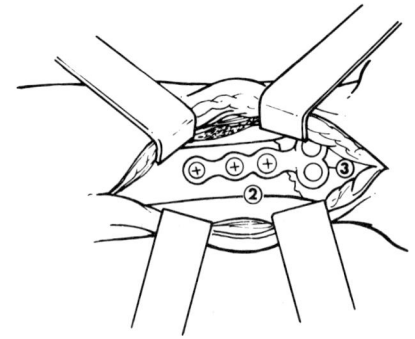

4. If the radial styloid process is detached, fix it with a Kirschner wire.

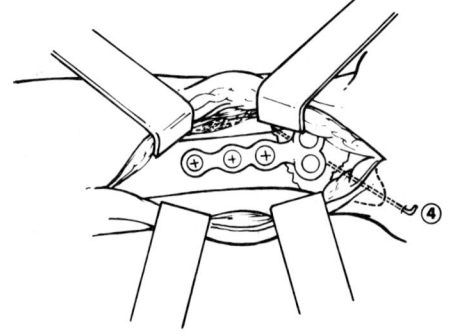

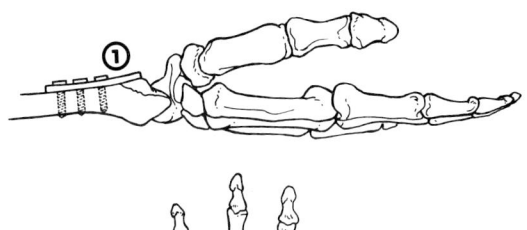

Postreduction X-Ray

1. Reduction is held by a buttress plate without a screw in the distal fragment.

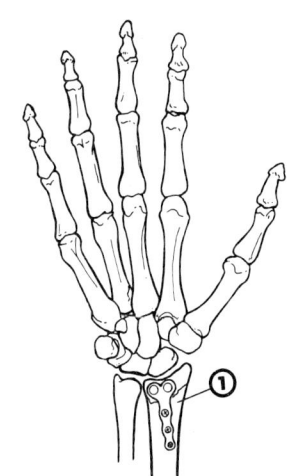

2. The radial styloid fracture is held by Kirschner wire.

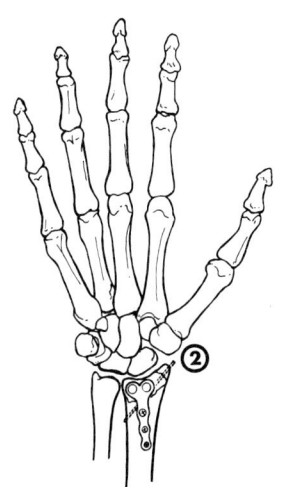

Postreduction Management

Release the tourniquet and obtain hemostasis prior to skin closure.

Apply a postoperative hand compression dressing to immobilize the finger and wrist and to minimize edema (see page 1072).

After postoperative swelling has subsided (3 to 5 days), the patient may begin active assisted range-of-motion exercises to the fingers and wrist.

If the fracture was extremely unstable or if the radial styloid was fixed with a Kirschner wire, a cast should be applied for 4 weeks. Remove the cast and Kirschner wires at 4 to 6 weeks.

Insist that the patient mobilize the fingers immediately after the operation.

Follow the status of the fracture-dislocation by means of frequent x-rays.

The average time to complete healing is sixteen weeks, after which time the patient is usually able to return to work if the fracture was treated by operative fixation.

Reverse Barton's Fracture

1. Occasionally the displaced articular fragment may come from the dorsal surface.

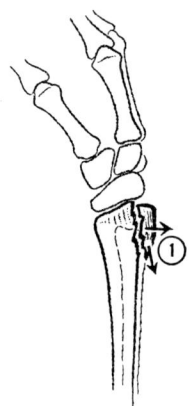

The reverse Barton's fracture, or a fracture of the dorsal articular surface, is best classified as a Colles' fracture. It must, however, be treated with the wrist in extension rather than in flexion, which is the normal position for immobilization of the Colles' fracture.

1. Dorsiflexion of the wrist reduces the dorsal radial fracture and aligns the lunate against the volar surface of the radius.

2. The articular surface of the radius shows no incongruity.

Note: If reduction of the articular fragment is not accurate, open reduction and internal fixation should be carried out as with the Barton's fracture and volar dislocation.

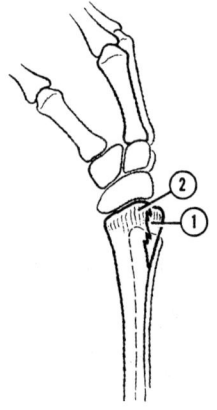

FRACTURE OF THE RADIAL STYLOID PROCESS

REMARKS

This lesion is important because it implicates the articular surface of the radius.

In most instances there is no displacement of the radial fragment; hence simple immobilization in a plaster cast for four to six weeks is all that is required.

If there is displacement and reduction fails to restore perfect anatomic congruity of the articular surface, open reduction and fixation with a screw are indicated.

Occasionally a styloid fracture may be associated with a significant carpal injury such as a perilunate dislocation. Always evaluate thoroughly for any associated injuries.

Prereduction X-Ray

1. The fracture line is directed upward and outward.
2. The articular surface of the radius is involved.
3. The carpus is shifted slightly to the radial side along with the radial fragment.

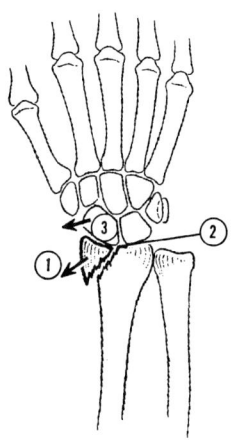

FRACTURE OF THE RADIAL STYLOID PROCESS

Reduction Technique for Styloid Fracture

The procedure is performed with the patient under general or regional intravenous anesthesia (see page 1011).

TRACTION

1. Apply finger traction apparatus.
2. The elbow is flexed 90 degrees.
3. The forearm is in neutral rotation.
4. Make counter traction by using a muslin sling and a water bucket for weight.
5. Continue the strong traction upward until the radial styloid is pulled out to length.

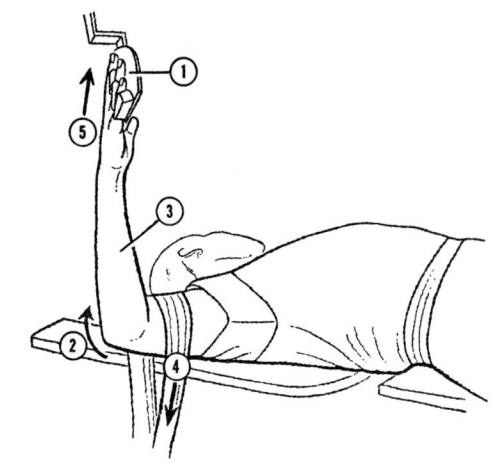

MANIPULATION

While traction is maintained:
1. Compress the fragment firmly with the heels of both hands; first compress the fragment laterally, and then
2. Compress the volar and dorsal surfaces.

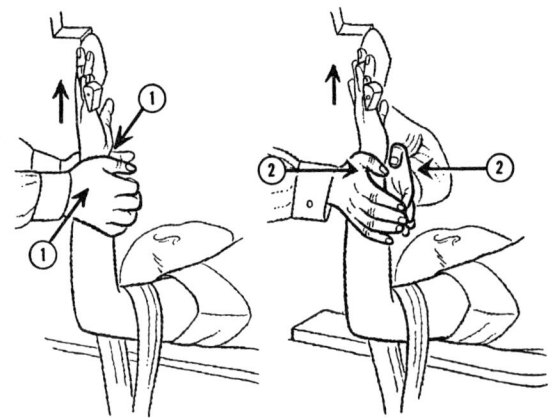

APPLICATION OF CAST

While an assistant holds the forearm in midposition and the wrist in ulnar deviation, apply a plaster cast.
1. The cast extends from below the elbow to just proximal to the metacarpal heads.
2. The forearm is in midposition.
3. The hand is deviated toward the ulna.

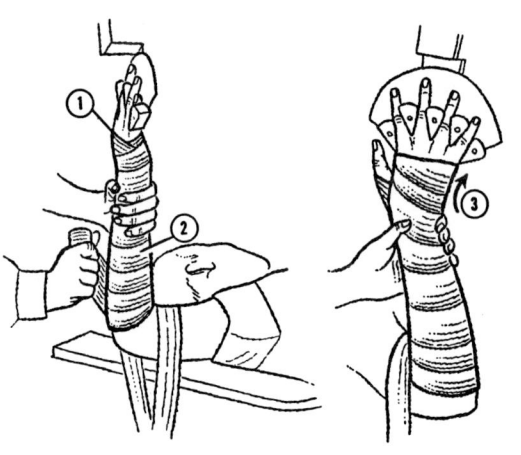

Postreduction X-Ray

1. The radial fragment is restored to its anatomic position.
2. The articular surface of the radius is congruous.
3. The radial shift of the carpus is corrected.

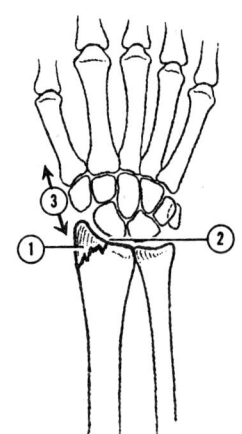

Postreduction Management

Take x-rays immediately after application of the cast. If the reduction is not satisfactory, another attempt to achieve accurate reduction of the fracture should be made.

The cast should be applied tightly enough to prevent loss of position of the fragments but not so tightly as to cause circulatory embarrassment. If there is any evidence of circulatory embarrassment, split the cast along the dorsum for its entire length. (Be sure to cut any constricting padding beneath the cast.)

Elevate the arm with the fingers pointing toward the ceiling for the first 24 hours and apply ice bags.

After the first 24 to 48 hours, allow free use of the arm, elbow, and fingers.

In 5 to 10 days, take x-rays again to evaluate position.

Change the cast if it becomes loose by 10 days.

Instruct the patient in active range-of-motion exercises to the fingers and shoulder during healing. Avoid the use of a sling for support of the arm, which inhibits finger and shoulder exercises.

Remove the plaster cast after 6 weeks. Allow the patient to begin active range-of-motion exercises for the wrist at that time.

Alternate Method: Screw Fixation

(This method should be employed for the most part with displaced radial styloid fractures, which are difficult to reduce anatomically.)

1. The articular surfaces are congruous.
2. Fixation is maintained with a screw.

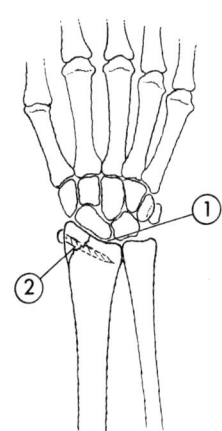

TRAUMATIC DISLOCATION AND SUBLUXATION OF THE DISTAL END OF THE ULNA (WITH AND WITHOUT FRACTURE)

REMARKS

Dislocation of the distal ulna must be recognized promptly when it is associated with a fracture of either the radius or ulna.

Dislocation or subluxation of the joint can occur as an acute injury without fracture. The most serious problem associated with this type of injury is making the correct diagnosis. In about half of these isolated injuries, the diagnosis is overlooked clinically and radiographically.

In some instances the deformity may be strikingly obvious, with narrowing of the transverse diameter of the wrist, dorsal or volar prominence of the distal ulna, and inability to pronate or supinate the wrist.

If the wrist has become swollen after injury, the clinical deformity may not be apparent, and the diagnosis depends on radiographic interpretation. The wide variation of possible radioulnar relationships on x-ray causes both the surgeon and the radiologist to ignore inconsistencies in this region.

To visualize the distal radioulnar joint adequately, the x-ray beam must be centered over the wrist rather than the forearm, and the elbow must be flexed so as to prevent compensatory shoulder rotation.

The diagnosis of an ulnar subluxation depends on a characteristic x-ray showing a lateral shift of the ulnar styloid with forearm pronation.

Forceful pronation of the wrist can also produce subluxation rather than complete dislocation of the ulna. This is a unique condition in that there is pain without clinical deformity.

Ulnar subluxation can also result from forceful pronation imposed on the wrist as treatment for a distal radial fracture. Changing the position of the forearm from pronation to supination corrects this condition.

Pathomechanics of Injury (Snook and Coworkers)

The three structures that support the distal radioulnar joint are:

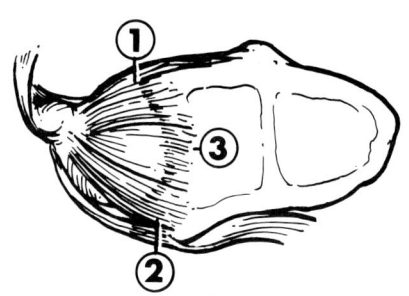

1. Dorsal radioulnar ligament.
2. Volar radioulnar ligament.
3. Triangular fibrocartilage ligament.

Note: Disruption of either the dorsal or the volar ligament must occur along with partial disruption of the triangular fibrocartilage in order for the joint to be dislocated.

Relationship of Distal Ulna and Radius

1. The ulnar head is round for the usual 140 degrees of rotation. Beyond this range it is irregular.
2. Forceful supination displaces the ulna volarly if the dorsal radioulnar ligament is torn.
3. Pronation displaces the ulna dorsally if the volar radioulnar ligament is torn.
4. If the ligaments remain intact, the radius locks on the incongruent surface of the ulna, causing the ulna to remain subluxed.

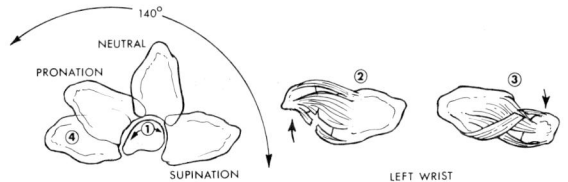

CLINICAL APPEARANCE OF DISLOCATIONS

Dorsal Dislocation

1. The wrist and hand are forcefully extended and
2. Pronated.
3. Dorsal dislocation results if the ligament supports are ruptured.

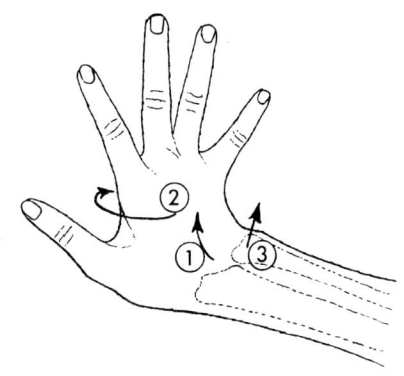

TRAUMATIC DISLOCATION AND SUBLUXATION OF THE DISTAL END OF THE ULNA

Dorsal Dislocation (Continued)

CLINICAL FEATURES

Marked prominence of the head of the ulna on the dorsum of the wrist.

The hand is locked in pronation.

The transverse diameter of the wrist appears to be narrower than normal.

Any attempt to supinate the hand elicits severe pain.

Note: In half of cases, extreme swelling after injury obscures the position of the ulna.

Volar Dislocation

1. The wrist and hand are forcefully extended and
2. Supinated.
3. Volar dislocation results if the ligament supports are ruptured.

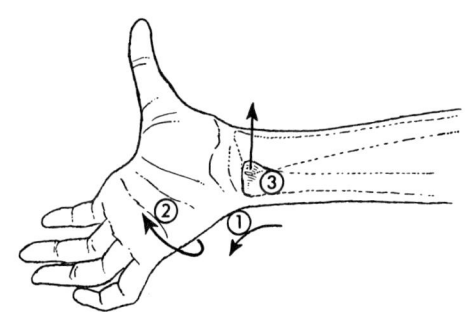

CLINICAL FEATURES

The normal prominence of the head of the ulna on the dorsum of the wrist is absent.

The hand is locked in supination.

The prominence of the head of the ulna is on the volar aspect of the wrist.

The transverse diameter of the wrist is narrower than normal.

Any attempt to pronate the hand is painful.

Subluxation

1. Hyperpronation applied to the wrist is insufficient to rupture the ligaments.
2. The radius locks on the incongruent surface of the ulna.

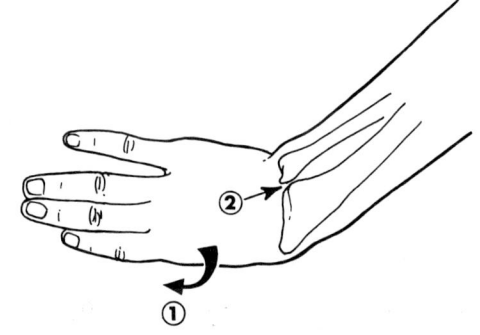

CLINICAL FEATURES

If there is no fracture of the radius, ulnar subluxation has no presenting deformity.

Symptoms include extreme pain and tenderness with marked reluctance to move the wrist out of the pronated position.

RADIOGRAPHIC APPEARANCE OF DISLOCATIONS

Note: Radiographic interpretation may be erroneous if it is made on the basis of anteroposterior and oblique views that are not properly centered on the wrist.

Volar Dislocation

On the anteroposterior view,
1. The head of the ulna has shifted radially.
2. A true lateral view centered on the wrist will demonstrate the dislocation and volar displacement of the ulna, particularly when compared with the opposite wrist.

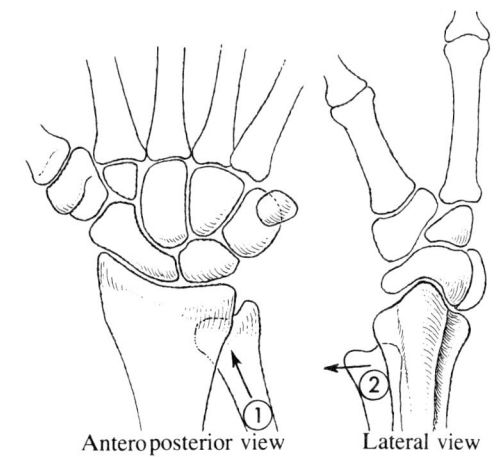
Anteroposterior view   Lateral view

Dorsal Dislocation

1. The anteroposterior view shows some lateral shift of the ulna.
2. A true lateral view demonstrates dorsal displacement of the ulna, particularly when compared with the opposite wrist.

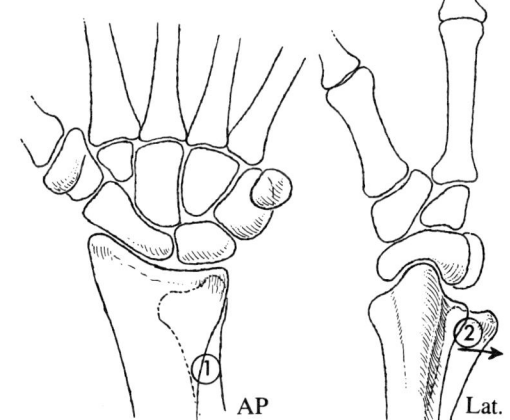
AP   Lat.

Subluxation from Hyperpronation

The diagnosis of a subluxated ulna is entirely dependent on anteroposterior and oblique views of the pronated wrist taken with the elbow flexed so as to prevent compensatory motion of the shoulder.
1. Pronated view of normal wrist shows the ulnar styloid positioned on the lateral aspect of the ulna.
2. In the pronated view of a subluxated wrist, the ulnar styloid is displaced to the center of the bone or sometimes to the radial side.

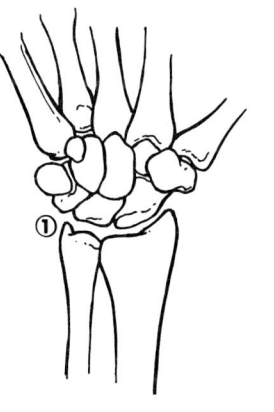
NORMAL

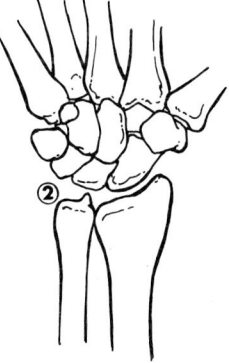
SUBLUXED

TRAUMATIC DISLOCATION AND SUBLUXATION OF THE DISTAL END OF THE ULNA

Ulnar Subluxation with Radial Fracture

1. Hyperpronated immobilization of a distal radial fracture can be associated with
2. Subluxation of the ulna, as indicated by displacement of the ulnar styloid.

Note: This should be corrected by changing the position of the wrist to supination.

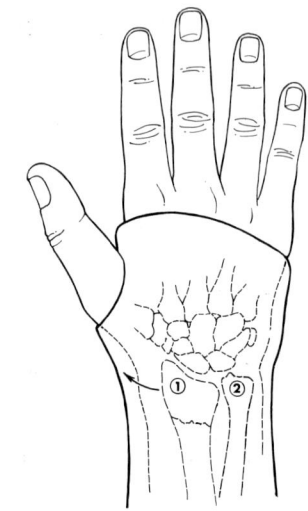

Subluxation in Children

In children subluxation from forceful pronation cannot be diagnosed by x-ray if the distal ulna epiphysis has not ossified.

This injury is analogous to a pulled elbow and should be treated, on the basis of clinical findings, by firm supination.

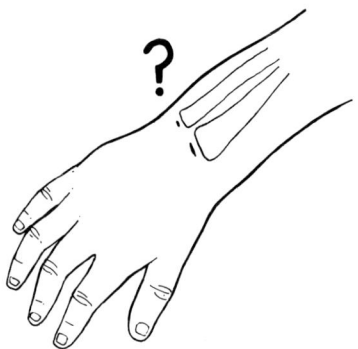

MANIPULATIVE REDUCTION

The patient is given general or regional intravenous anesthetic.

Volar Dislocation of Right Wrist

1. Grasp and steady the patient's supinated forearm with your left hand.
2. With the right hand, grasp the patient's hand and place your thumb over the prominence of the head of the ulna.
3. While making firm backward pressure on the head of the ulna,
4. Forcefully pronate the hand and wrist.

Note: Reduction is accompanied by a definite snap.

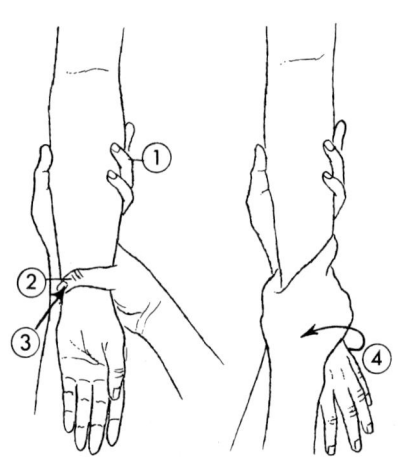

TRAUMATIC DISLOCATION AND SUBLUXATION OF THE DISTAL END OF THE ULNA

Dorsal Dislocation or Subluxation of Right Wrist

1. Grasp and steady the patient's pronated forearm with your left hand.
2. With your right hand grasp the patient's hand and place your thumb over the prominence of the head of the ulna.
3. While making steady and firm forward pressure on the head of the ulna,
4. Forcefully supinate the hand and wrist.

Note: Reduction is accompanied by a definite snap.

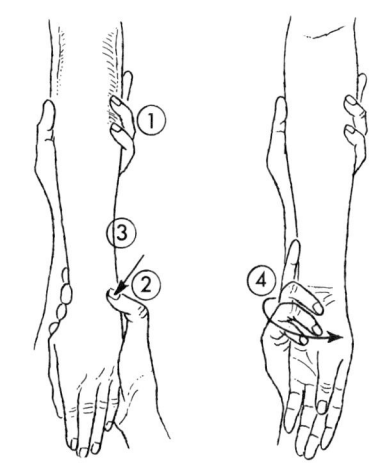

Immobilization

VOLAR DISLOCATION

Apply a plaster cast from the middle of the arm to just proximal to the metacarpal joints.
1. The elbow is flexed 90 degrees.
2. The forearm is fully pronated.

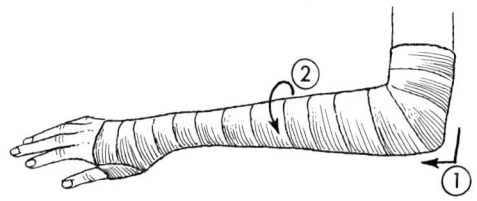

DORSAL DISLOCATION OR SUBLUXATION

1. The elbow is flexed 90 degrees.
2. The forearm is fully supinated.

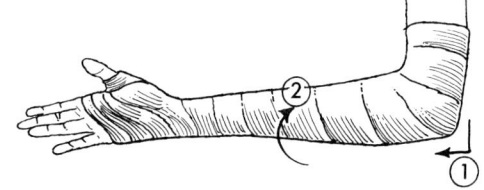

Postreduction Management

The cast is maintained for four weeks.

After removal of the cast allow free use of the limb within the patient's tolerance.

Avoid any forceful rotation of the hand and wrist, especially against resistance.

Habitual or Recurrent Subluxation of the Inferior Radioulnar Joint

REMARKS

This disorder follows inadequately treated acute traumatic dislocations of the head of the ulna.

There is always a history of an acute traumatic injury.

In the reduced state the joint exhibits pronounced anteroposterior laxity.

A click accompanies the subluxation.

The disorder may be very disabling because of the associated pain and weakness of the wrist. In anterior habitual dislocations supination is weakened, whereas in posterior dislocations pronation is weakened.

Occasionally the disorders produce no significant impairment of function; these cases should not be treated.

Excision of the head of the ulna is the procedure of choice for painful and disabling lesions.

Reconstruction procedures designed to repair the ligaments of the joint generally fail.

For excision of the head of the ulna, see page 1044 for technique and postoperative management.

COMPLICATIONS OF DISTAL RADIAL FRACTURES

Disruption of the Radioulnar Joint from Shortening in Adults or Growth Arrest in Children

REMARKS

Disruption of the radioulnar joint is the most common cause of persistent pain and limitation of rotation after distal radial fracture.

It frequently is the result of shortening at the fracture site in the adult Colles' fracture. It may also follow a growth arrest after injury to the distal physis in a child; advise the patient and the patient's parents of this possibility during and after treatment.

If the pain from radioulnar disruption is significant, it can be managed by resection of the distal ulna in the adult.

In the young patient with radioulnar asymmetry from growth arrest, realignment and better cosmetic appearance can be achieved by shortening of the ulna.

Ulnar shortening can be done by epiphysiodesis if the bone is still growing. Usually, however, osteotomy and direct bone resection are necessary.

Preoperative X-Ray

1. Radius has impacted on itself owing to fracture or physeal growth arrest.
2. Radial shortening is significant because it causes
3. The ulna to extend distally and
4. The radioulnar joint to dislocate.
5. The hand is pushed into radial deviation

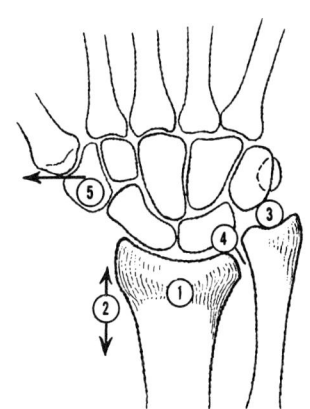

RESECTION OF THE ULNA IN THE OLDER ADULT

Operative Procedure

1. Make a 5 cm incision along the medial aspect of the ulna, beginning at the tip of the styloid and extending upward.
2. Expose the distal end of the ulna by subperiosteal dissection.
3. 2.5 cm above the tip of the styloid, make several drill holes in the ulna and divide the bone obliquely at this level.
4. Preserve the ulnar collateral ligament.
5. Reef the periosteal sleeve and ligament to make a continuous structure.

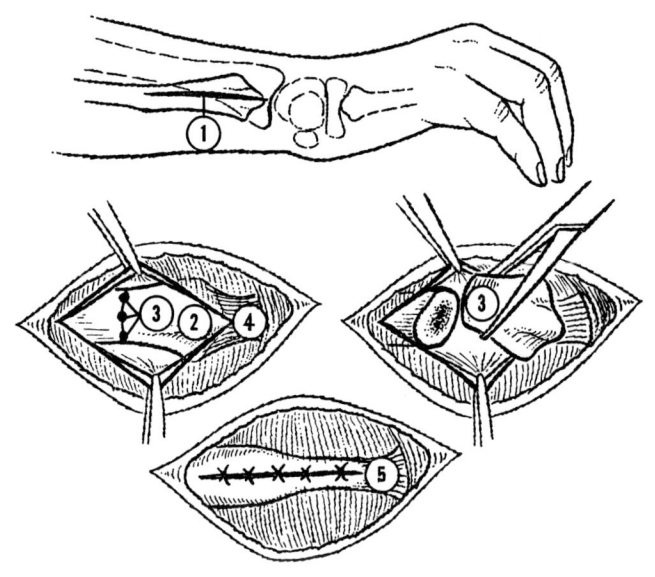

Postoperative X-Ray

1. The distal end of the ulna has been resected.
2. The hand is now in neutral position.

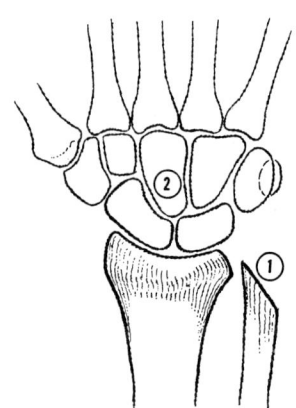

SHORTENING OF THE ULNA IN THE YOUNGER PATIENT

Operative Procedure

The incision and exposure are the same as for operative excision in the older patient. The bone is then shortened 2.5 cm above the tip of the styloid so that the radioulnar joint can be reduced. The osteotomized ulna is fixed with pins or screws, and the periosteal sleeve and the ulnar ligament are reefed as above.

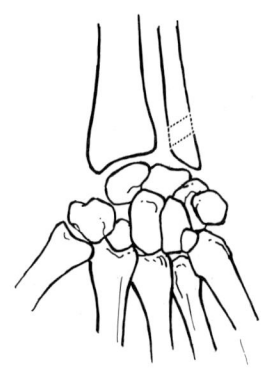

COMPLICATIONS OF DISTAL RADIAL FRACTURES

Postoperative X-Ray

1. The oblique osteotomy and shortening has reduced
2. The distal radioulnar joint.
3. The shortened ulna is fixed with a lag screw.

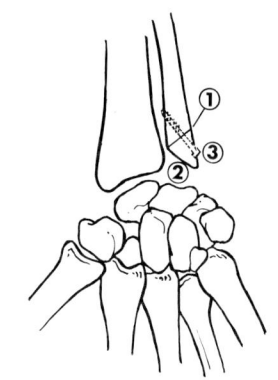

IMMOBILIZATION

Apply an anterior plaster slab to the forearm and wrist that extends distally as far as the proximal palmar crease.

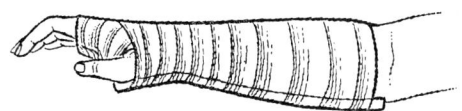

POSTOPERATIVE MANAGEMENT

Following ulna resection, remove the plaster splint at five to seven days and begin active exercises to restore normal wrist and finger function.

Following ulna shortening continue plaster immobilization for six to eight weeks, until union of the osteotomy is complete. Then remove the external support and supervise active range-of-motion exercises to the fingers and wrist.

Malunited Fracture of the Distal End of the Radius

REMARKS

Numerous gradations of malunited fractures are encountered.

Many cases with only minor deformity give rise to no dysfunction; the deformity should be accepted and requires no surgical intervention.

In cases with marked deformity and dysfunction, incongruity of the distal radioulnar joint is always present in varying degrees and is the prime source of pain.

Simple osteotomy of the radius without excision of the distal 2.5 cm of the ulna is justified only in those cases with a residual dorsal tilt of the radius, with little or no loss of length of the radius, and with minimal or no implication of the distal radioulnar joint.

Malunion with gross deformity and marked implication of the radioulnar joint is best treated by osteotomy of the distal end of the radius and excision of the distal 2.5 cm of the ulna.

In cases that are associated with Sudeck's atrophy, avoid surgical intervention until symptoms have subsided.

Manipulative maneuvers with forceful traction as previously described may be attempted in cases of malposition up to two or three weeks following injury. After this period, conservative measures invariably will fail and operative intervention is indicated.

Osteotomy of the radius or osteotomy of the radius and excision of the ulna are applicable to malunion in both the Colles' and Smith's fractures.

Osteotomy usually may be carried out through the recently healed malunion. Occasionally, a wedge osteotomy may be necessary to correct the deformity.

Preoperative X-Ray

COLLES' FRACTURE

1. The radius is shortened.
2. Relations of the radio-ulnar joint are disturbed.
3. The articular surface of the radius is directed upward and backward.

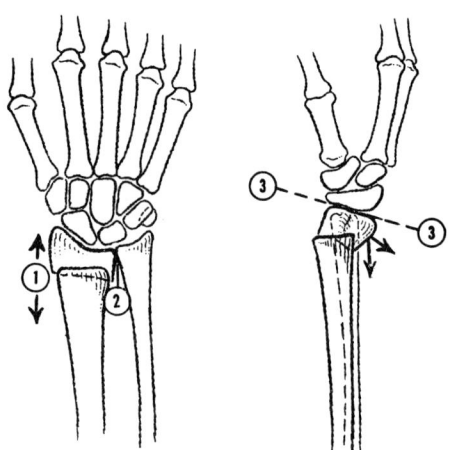

SMITH'S FRACTURE

1. The radius is shortened.
2. The distal fragment is displaced anteriorly.
3. The normal relations of the radio-ulnar joint are altered.

Note: Persistent malunion of the Smith's fracture is especially likely to impair nerve and tendon function.

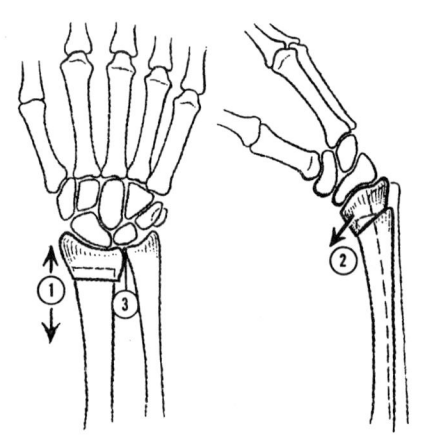

Operative Procedure: Osteotomy Through the Malunion

1. Make a 7.5-cm incision extending upward in the midline of the dorsal aspect of the radius beginning at the level of the wrist joint.
2. Divide the deep fascia and expose the tendons of the extensor carpi radialis longus and the extensor carpi radialis brevis as they emerge from under the extensor pollicis brevis on the lateral side of the wound and the extensor pollicis longus on the medial side.
3. Make a longitudinal incision in the periosteum of the radius in the interval between the extensor carpi radialis brevis and the extensor pollicis longus.

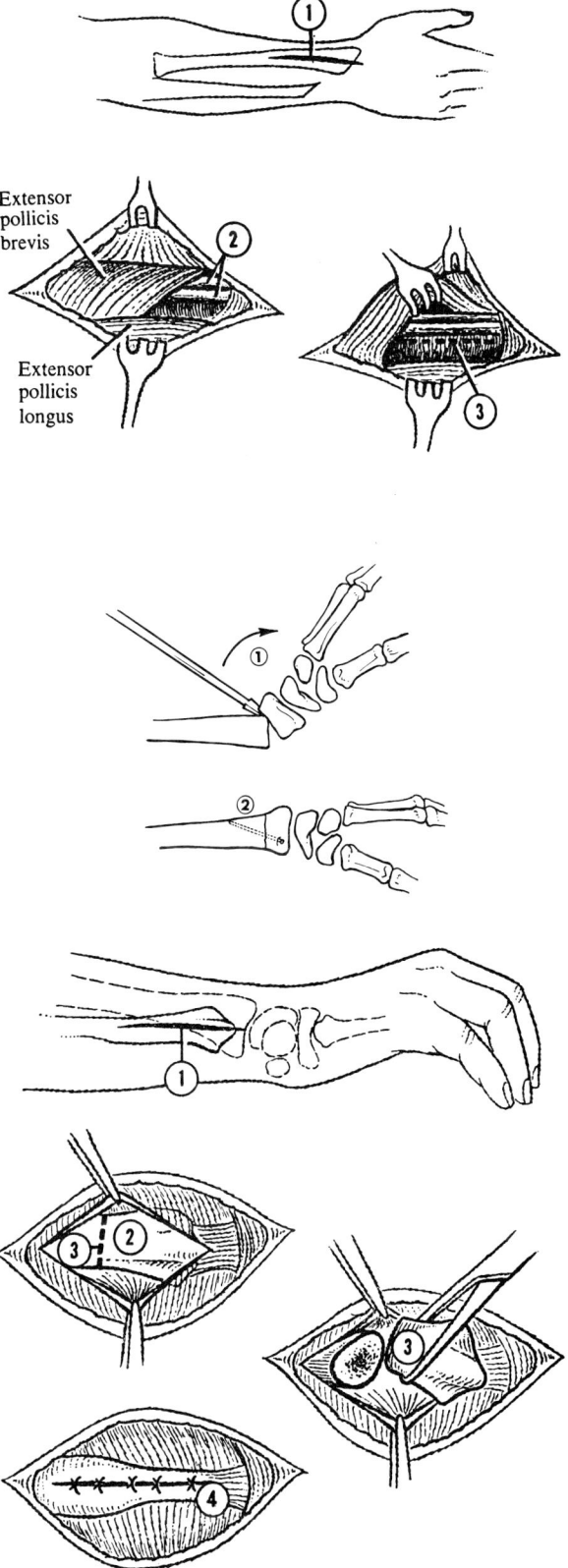

1. With a sharp osteotome, cut through the site of the malunion and direct the articular surface of the radius distally and volarly.
2. Fix the distal fragment in the corrected position with a radioulnar pin.

1. Next make a 5-cm incision along the medial aspect of the ulna, beginning at the tip of its styloid process and extending upward.
2. Expose the distal end of the ulna by subperiosteal dissection.
3. Divide the ulna 2.5 cm above the tip of the styloid process and remove it by sharp dissection, leaving the ulnar collateral ligament intact.
4. On closure, the periosteal tube of the ulna should be continuous with the collateral ligament.

Postoperative X-Ray

1. The distal end of the ulna is resected.
2. The articular surface of the radius is restored to its normal plane as a result of the osteotomy.
3. The length of the radius has increased beyond the ulna.

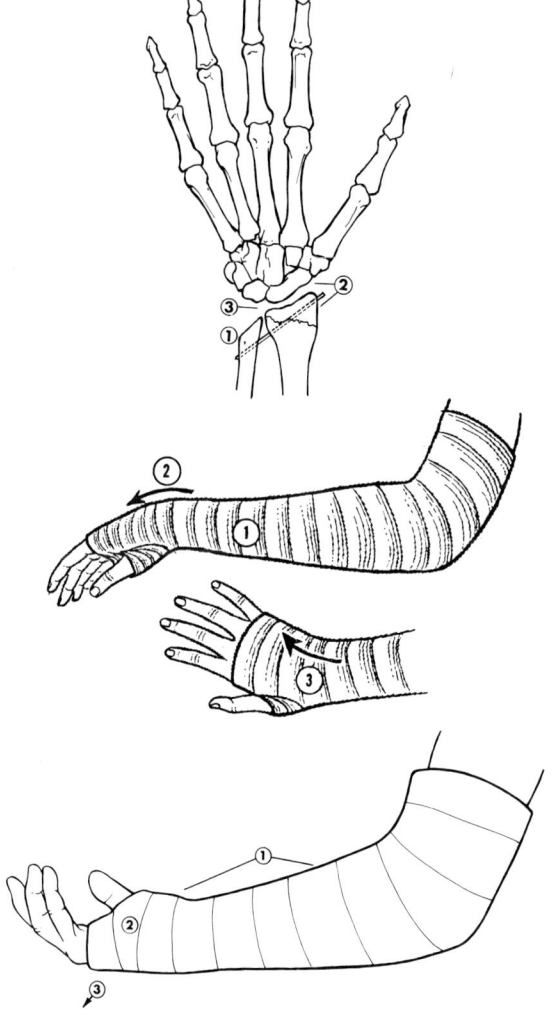

Immobilization

FOR COLLES' FRACTURE

Apply a circular cast from the metacarpophalangeal joints to below the axilla.
1. The forearm is in midposition.
2. The wrist is slightly flexed.
3. The hand is deviated toward the ulna.

FOR SMITH'S FRACTURE

1. The forearm is supinated.
2. The wrist is slightly flexed.
3. The hand is deviated slightly toward the ulna.

Postoperative Management

Take x-rays after the first and second weeks and check for maintenance of position of the fragments.

If after 10 to 14 days the plaster cast becomes loose, apply a new cast.

Usually at the end of 6 to 8 weeks, healing is advanced enough to permit removal of the threaded wire.

Immobilize for 2 more weeks after the removal of the wire. Immobilization should be continued until there is radiographic and clinical evidence of bony union, perhaps 10 to 16 weeks.

After removal of the cast, institute physical therapy and exercises to restore motion in all joints.

During immobilization, the fingers and shoulder should be exercised continuously.

Nonunion of the Distal End of the Radius

REMARKS

This is a rare complication following Colles' or Smith's fractures.

There is always shortening of the radius and malalignment at the distal radioulnar joint.

The treatment of choice is resection of the distal 2.5 cm of the ulna, realignment of the radial fragment, internal fixation by a transfixion wire, and bone grafting.

Preoperative X-Ray

1. Radial deviation of the wrist and hand.
2. The radius is shortened.
3. The distal end of the ulna extends beyond the styloid of the radius.

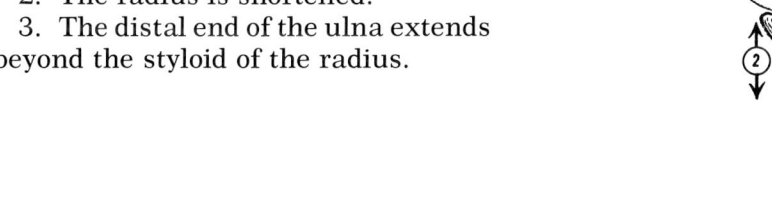

Operative Management

1. Make a 5-cm incision along the medial aspect of the ulna, beginning at the tip of the styloid and extending upward.
2. Expose the distal end of the ulna by subperiosteal dissection.
3. Divide the ulna obliquely 2.5 cm above the tip of the styloid process and remove the distal segment by sharp dissection, preserving the ulnar collateral ligament.
4. On closure of the wound, the periosteal tube of the ulna should be continuous with the ulnar collateral ligament.

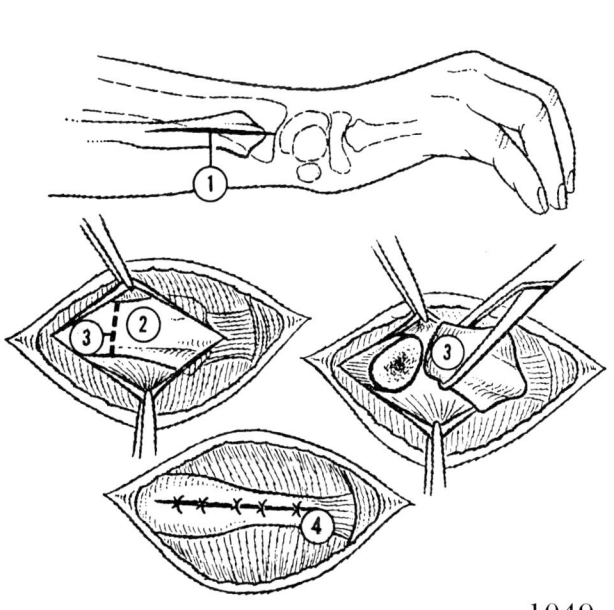

Operative Management
(Continued)

1. Make a 7-cm incision extending upward in the midline of the dorsal aspect of the radius, beginning at the level of the wrist joint.
2. Divide the deep fascia and expose the tendons of the extensor carpi radialis longus and the extensor carpi radialis brevis as they emerge from under the extensor pollicis brevis on the lateral side of the wound and the extensor pollicis longus on the medial side.
3. Make a longitudinal incision in the periosteum of the radius in the interval between the extensor carpi radialis brevis and the extensor pollicis longus.
4. Cut out the fibrous tissue between the fragments, freshen the ends of the fragments, and realign the distal fragment with the proximal fragment.

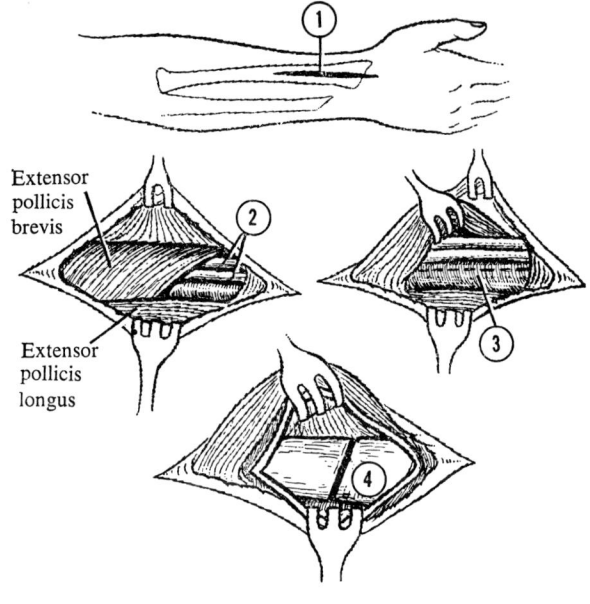

1. With the hand in ulnar deviation and the fragments in the corrected position, transfix the fragments with a 4-mm threaded wire.
2. Cut the wire below the level of the skin.
3. Surround the fracture site with cancellous bone.

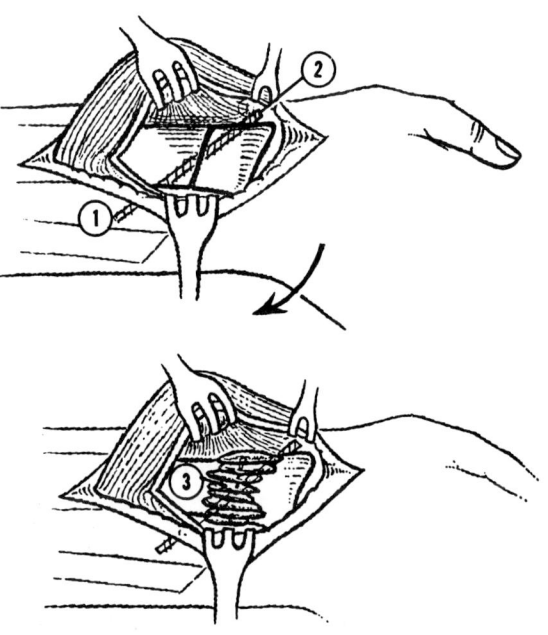

Immobilization

For Colles' Fracture

Apply a circular cast from the metacarpophalangeal joints to below the axilla.
1. The forearm is in midposition.
2. The wrist is slightly flexed.
3. The hand is deviated toward the ulna.

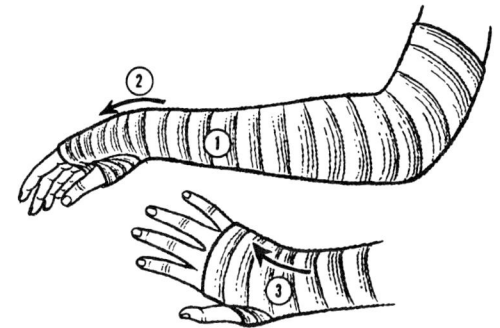

For Smith's Fracture

1. The forearm is supinated.
2. The wrist is slightly flexed.
3. The hand is deviated slightly toward the ulna.

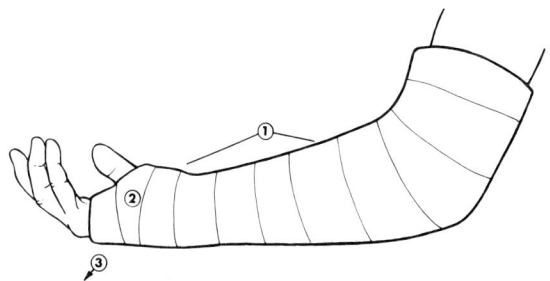

Postoperative Management

Take x-rays after the first and second weeks. Check for maintenance of the position of the fragments.

If after 10 to 14 days the plaster cast becomes loose, apply another cast.

Usually at the end of 6 to 8 weeks healing is advanced enough to permit removal of the threaded wire.

Immobilize for 2 more weeks after the removal of the wire. Immobilization should be continued until there is radiographic and clinical evidence of bony union, which may take 10 to 16 weeks.

After removal of the cast, institute physical therapy and exercises to restore motion in all joints.

During immobilization, the fingers and shoulder should be exercised continuously.

FRACTURES AND DISLOCATIONS OF THE CARPAL BONES: GENERAL PRINCIPLES

Injuries to the wrist implicating the carpal bones are common lesions in all age groups, particularly in young adults.

Knowledge of the anatomic features of the wrist is important in understanding the mechanisms of injury and the rationale of treatment.

Anatomic Considerations

REMARKS

The wrist consists of the interval between the distal ends of the radius and ulna and the proximal ends of the metacarpal bones. Within this area is a linkage system of articulations that work in unison to provide an almost global range of motion.

There are eight carpal bones of different sizes and shapes. They are arranged in two rows: the distal row articulates with the proximal surface of the metacarpal bones. The bones in the proximal row are arranged in a smooth arch and articulate with the radius and the fibrocartilage joining the ulna and radius. The ulna does not articulate with the carpus.

The proximal row moves freely in relation to the forearm. The distal row moves on the proximal row. The second and third carpometacarpal joints are practically immobile so as to create the fixed keystone of the arching hand. The saddle shape of the first carpometacarpal joint permits thumb mobility. The hinge shape of the fourth and fifth carpometacarpal joints permits slight flexion and extension during grip.

Spanning the proximal and distal carpal rows is the long scaphoid bone, which acts as a linking bar to support the carpus. This position also makes the scaphoid most vulnerable to injury.

Volar and Dorsal Aspects of the Wrist

1. The scaphoid is the boat-shaped bone spanning the proximal and distal rows.
2. The lunate is crescent shaped; the convex surface articulates with the radius and the concave surface articulates with the capitate.
3. The triquetrum is pyramidal with its base proximal and lateral and its apex distal and medial.
4. The pisiform, or pea-shaped, bone articulates only with the triquetrum.
5. The trapezium has a saddle-shaped articulation to allow divergence of the first metacarpal in relationship with other metacarpals.
6. The wedge-shaped trapezoid helps stabilize the second metacarpal.
7. The capitate is the largest carpal bone and stabilizes the third metacarpal.
8. The hamate is wedge shaped with a hooklike process; its base is directed distally.
9. The radioulnar fibrocartilage articulates with the carpus, but the ulna does not.

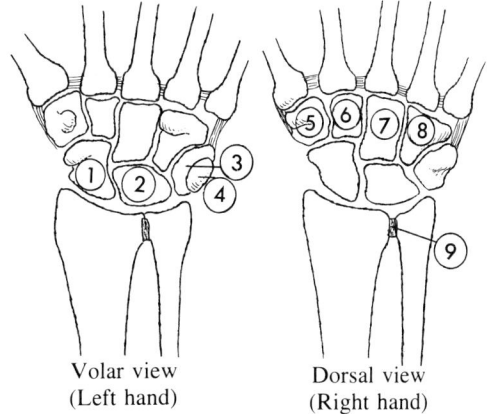

Volar view
(Left hand)

Dorsal view
(Right hand)

The proximal row forms a smooth arc; its convex side articulates with the radius and the fibrocartilage of the ulna, and the capitate and hamate fit snugly into the concave side of the arc. Although the carpal bones are of different sizes and shapes they fit together into a strong compact unit.

Longitudinal and Transverse Arches of the Hand

The hand is composed of five longitudinal and two transverse arches. Disruption of these arches frequently produces rotational deformities of the fingers.

1. The longitudinal arches are composed of carpals, metacarpals, and phalanges.
2. The mobile distal transverse arch is composed of the intermetacarpal (intervolar plate) ligaments with the interposed metacarpal heads.
3. The proximal transverse arch is a rigid semicircular structure made up of the distal row of carpal bones and the intercarpal ligaments with the keystone of the arch at the capitate bone.

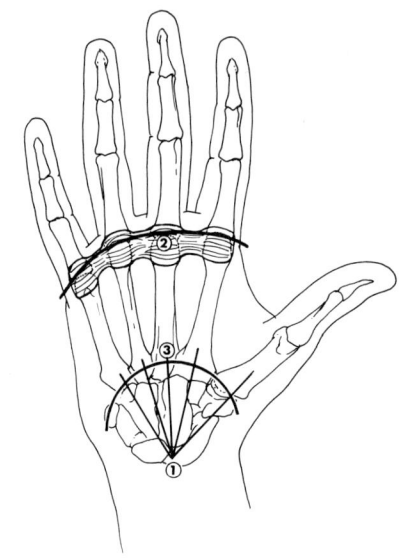

1. The proximal transverse arch, combined with the heads of the second and third metacarpals to which it firmly attaches, is the fixed unit of the hand.
2. The mobile proximal and distal structures rotate about the rigid unit.

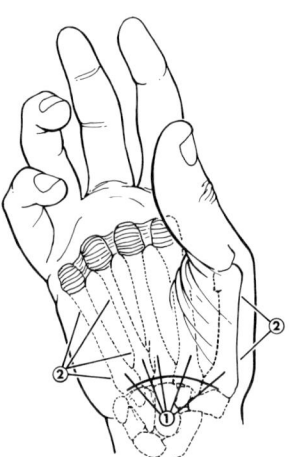

The Mechanics of Wrist Motion

REMARKS

Rotation does not occur through the radiocarpal and carpal joints. Only flexion-extension and abduction-adduction are possible. The absence of rotation is compensated for by pronation and supination movements of the forearm.

Although the exact measurement of wrist motion varies, depending on the subject and the observer, approximately 40 per cent of wrist palmar flexion takes place in the radiocarpal joint and 60 per cent in the carpal joint.

The proximal and distal rows move simultaneously but in opposite directions. When the wrist is extended, the proximal row glides volarly and the distal row rotates dorsally.

When the wrist is flexed, the proximal row of carpal bones glides dorsally and abuts against the dorsal lip of the distal articular surface of the radius; the distal row shifts volarly.

When the hand is deviated toward the radius, the proximal row shifts toward the ulna while the distal row and the metacarpal bones move toward the radius. Conversely, when the hand deviates toward the ulna, the proximal row moves toward the radius while the distal row and metacarpals move toward the ulna.

Radial abduction of the wrist is slight, usually not more than 15 degrees, whereas ulnar abduction may reach up to 40 degrees.

Owing to its connecting and supporting function for the synchronous motion between proximal and distal carpal rows, the scaphoid is subjected to the greatest shear forces and the highest incidence of injury of all the carpal bones.

Radial Deviation of the Wrist

1. The proximal row glides toward the ulna.
2. The distal row with the metacarpals moves toward the radius.

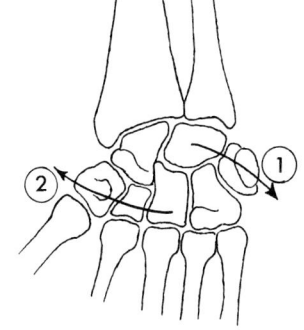

Ulnar Deviation of the Wrist

1. The proximal row glides toward the radius.
2. The distal row and the metacarpals move toward the ulna.

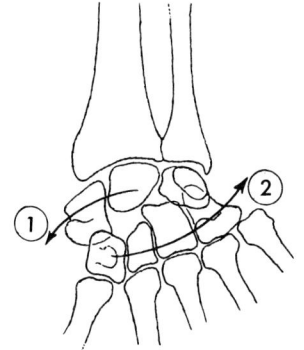

FRACTURES AND DISLOCATIONS OF THE CARPAL BONES: GENERAL PRINCIPLES

Extension of the Wrist

1. The proximal row moves volarly. The slope of the distal radius allows greater motion in the radiocarpal joint.
2. The distal row moves dorsally.

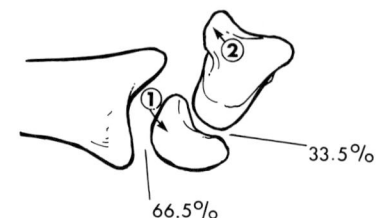

Flexion of the Wrist

1. The proximal row moves dorsally. The slope of the distal radius limits motion in the radiocarpal joint.
2. The distal row moves anteriorly.

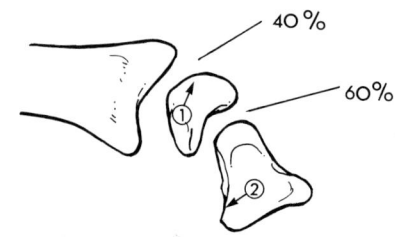

Carpal Ligaments

The strength of the wrist depends on the numerous strong bands that encircle it and also upon a tough intricate complex of ligaments of which the volar component is the strongest. The strong ligaments anchor the bones in place and to each other, to the radius, and to the metacarpal bones; this is especially true on the volar surface of the bones. The pisiform bone actually lies within the tendon of the flexor carpi ulnaris, which in turn continues onto the carpus and metacarpals and hamate through strong ligaments extending from the pisiform to these bones.

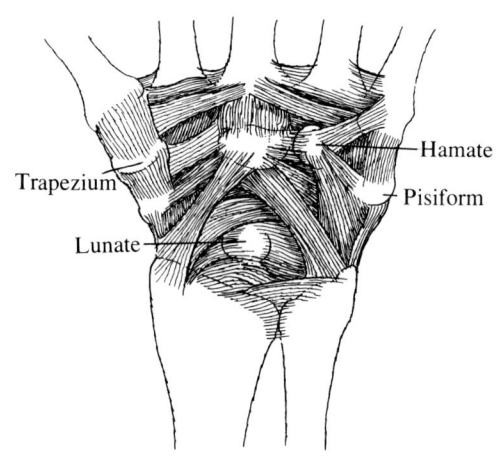

Carpal Tunnel

The carpal bones arch to form the floor of the carpal tunnel, through which the median nerve and the finger flexor tendons enter the wrist. The roof of the tunnel is formed by the transverse carpal ligament, which attaches out to the trapezium and the hook of the hamate. Swelling within this tightly enclosed space commonly results in median nerve compression (carpal tunnel syndrome).

1. Bony sides of the tunnel.
2. Transverse carpal ligament.
3. Flexor tendons of the fingers.
4. Median nerve.

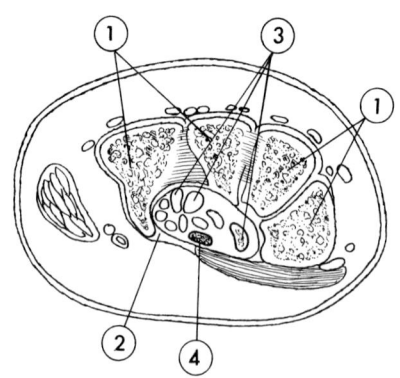

FRACTURES AND DISLOCATIONS OF THE CARPAL BONES: GENERAL PRINCIPLES

Carpal Stability

1. The scaphoid acts as a mechanical shaft that stabilizes the intercarpal area by its oblique position between the proximal and distal rows.

2. The strong scapholunate and scaphocapitate ligaments permit synchronous carpal motion in flexion, extension, and radial and ulnar deviation.

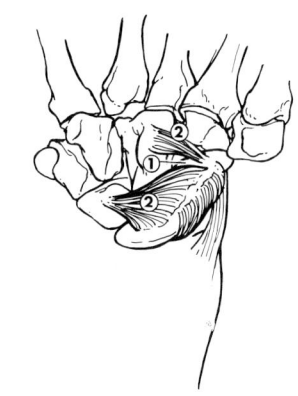

Note: Carpal instability may result from either displaced fracture of the scaphoid or disruption of the scaphocarpal ligaments.

Radiographic Diagnosis of Fractures and Dislocations of Carpal Bones

REMARKS

Adequate x-ray technique is critical for prompt diagnosis and proper treatment of these common injuries. Injuries to the carpal bones are among the most likely to be missed or to be subject to delayed diagnosis.

Occasionally the fracture may be so subtle that it becomes radiographically apparent only after two to four weeks of vascular response and osteolysis.

Complete dislocation may not be recognized if an incomplete radiographic study is relied on.

Radiographic evaluation of the injured wrist should include anteroposterior views with the wrist in neutral, maximal ulnar deviation, and maximal radial deviation. In addition, a true lateral view and lateral views with the wrist in flexion and extension should also be obtained.

If pain symptoms are located on the volar aspect, a carpal tunnel view is necessary to rule out such injuries as fracture of the hook of the hamate (see page 1125).

Standard X-Ray Views of the Injured Wrist

1. Anteroposterior views with the wrist in neutral, ulnar deviation, and radial deviation.

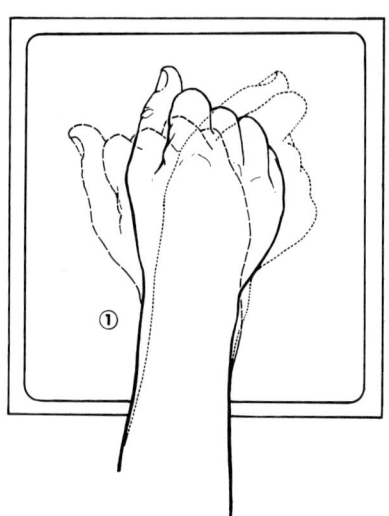

2. True lateral views with the wrist in neutral, flexion, and extension.

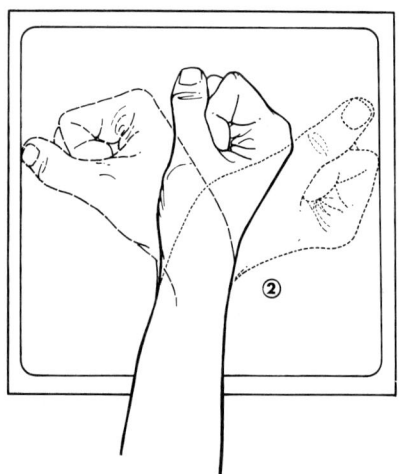

3. A view of the supinated wrist is also necessary if carpal dislocation or subluxation is suspected.

Note: Even if standard x-rays are normal, treat the patient with acute wrist pain after injury by protective immobilization. Undisplaced fractures or subluxations of the carpal bones may not become evident radiographically for several weeks after injury.

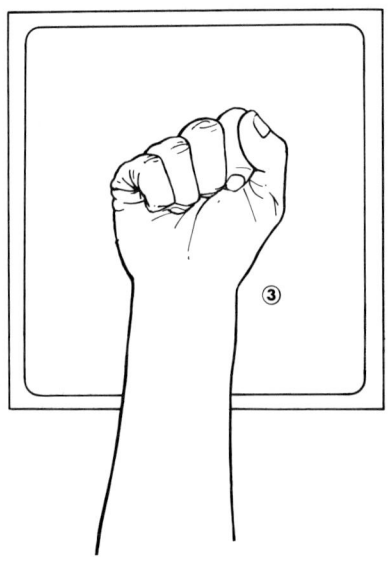

FRACTURES OF THE SCAPHOID

REMARKS

Of all the carpal bones, the scaphoid is the most frequently fractured. Its relationship to the radius and its linkage to both proximal and distal carpal rows render it vulnerable to injury. During dorsiflexion the scaphoid is sheared, as its proximal half is locked against the distal radius and its distal half is forced into further dorsiflexion because of its linkage with the distal carpal row. This results most frequently in a fracture through the midscaphoid.

With sufficient violence, the scaphoid may fracture and dislocate with the distal carpal row.

The rapidity of scaphoid fracture healing depends on the degree of circulatory damage as well as the displacement and instability of the fracture.

The scaphoid circulation enters the bone for the most part through the distal half, on both dorsal and volar surfaces. Fractures through the proximal third tend to cause loss of circulation and are slower to heal.

Fracture lines that run transversely or slightly obliquely across the long axis of the scaphoid tend to be compressed by finger muscle forces and to heal quickly. The vertical, oblique fracture, which is uncommon, is sheared by finger muscle forces and heals more slowly.

Fractures in which a longer than normal healing period can be anticipated include fractures in the proximal third with poor blood supply, oblique fractures that are unstable, and fractures that are displaced initially in either an axial or a transverse direction.

FRACTURES OF THE SCAPHOID

Blood Supply of the Scaphoid (Taleisnik and Kelly)

Extraosseous arteries originate from the radial artery and its superficial palmar branch. They enter through the distal half of the scaphoid.

1. The laterovolar group makes the largest contribution to intraosseous circulation.
2. The dorsal group penetrates a narrow groove on the dorsal surface.
3. The distal supply is limited to the tuberosity region.

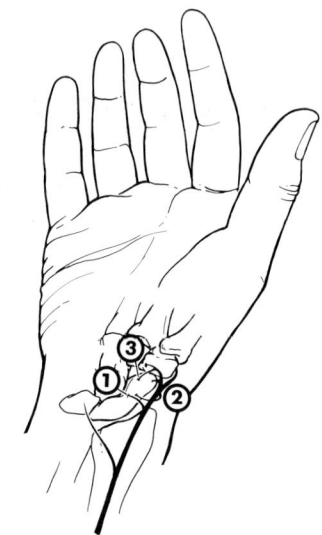

Mechanism of Injury

The scaphoid is fractured during forceful hyperextension of the wrist by a fall on the outstretched hand. It is sheared by the radius and by its attachment to surrounding carpal bones. The type of fracture sustained depends on the position of the wrist at the time of impact and in general can be categorized into one of four groups.

1. Fracture of the distal third or fracture of the tuberosity.
2. Transverse fracture of the middle third; this is the usual stable fracture.
3. Vertical oblique fracture; this is an unstable fracture.
4. Fracture of the proximal third; this is slow to heal because of impaired blood supply.

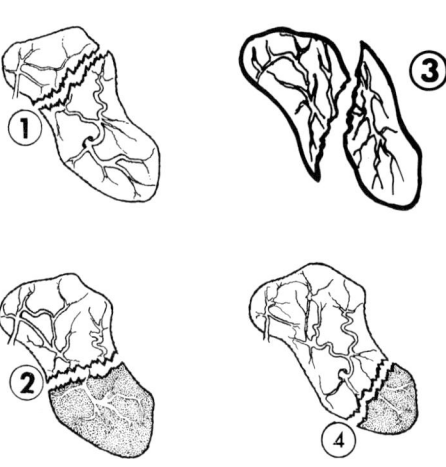

Approximately 85 per cent of all fractures of the scaphoid occur through the middle third, 5 per cent through the proximal third, and 5 to 7 per cent through the distal third. Most scaphoid fractures (85 per cent) are isolated injuries; however, there may also be injuries to adjacent structures, such as:

1. Transcaphoid perilunate dislocation (see page 1099).
2. Fractured scaphoid with a scapholunate dissociation (see page 1087).
3. A scaphoid fracture with Colles' fracture (see page 1020).

Epidemiology

The fracture occurs in all age groups but the highest incidence is in young adult males. Approximately 50 per cent occur in patients less than 30 years of age.

It occurs in children more generally than appreciated.

Approximately 85 per cent of scaphoid fractures occur in men.

The right hand is involved more frequently than the left (70 per cent).

Bilateral involvement occurs in 2 to 3 per cent of cases.

Recent Fractures of the Scaphoid (Less Than Four Weeks Old)

REMARKS

Scaphoid fractures are frequently underdiagnosed or completely overlooked. Suspect a fracture of the scaphoid in every case of "acutely sprained wrist."

Insist on adequate x-rays of any painful wrist after injury (see page 1058). In fresh injuries the x-ray may fail to show a fracture despite pain localized to the region of the snuffbox. If this is the case, treat the patient with cast immobilization and take another x-ray in two weeks. By that time the vascular reaction to the fracture will demonstrate the fracture line fairly consistently. If no fracture line is evident, consider the possibility of a scapholunate dissociation (see page 1103).

Fracture of the scaphoid may remain unrecognized, untreated, and asymptomatic. The patient then may present many years after the injury with "bipartite scaphoid." This chronic fracture is characterized by smooth margins rather than the usual irregular lines of recent fractures. In addition, the demineralization generally associated with a recent fracture is not evident.

A chronic but asymptomatic ununited scaphoid fracture may become painful when it is subjected to acute injury. In this instance it can be treated as an acute fracture by cast immobilization.

The best principle for wrist injuries and recent or old scaphoid fractures is to treat on the basis of the wrist symptoms rather than the radiographic appearance.

PROGNOSIS

Ninety-five per cent of acute fractures of the scaphoid, including those not treated for 3 to 4 weeks after injury, heal with plaster immobilization for 6 to 10 weeks. In fact, 70 to 75 per cent of fractures in which diagnosis is delayed and treatment is not instituted for several months will heal with adequate immobilization.

Fractures that require longer than normal immobilization include those in the proximal third, those with an oblique fracture line that is unstable, and those with initial axial or transverse displacement.

In general, treatment should be based on the patient's freedom from pain and his ability to grip without discomfort. Clinical evidence of union frequently precedes radiographic evidence by several months.

MANAGEMENT OF SCAPHOID FRACTURES THAT HEAL RAPIDLY

The majority of scaphoid fractures are undisplaced and should heal within eight weeks. These include:

Prereduction X-Rays

Fracture through the mid third.

Fracture through the distal third.

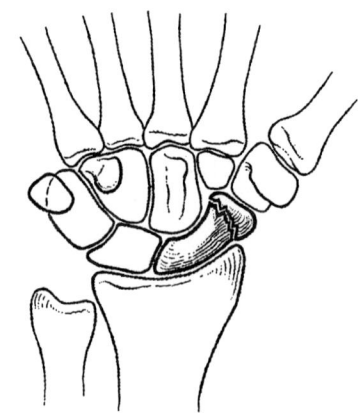

FRACTURES OF THE SCAPHOID

Fracture through the tubercle.

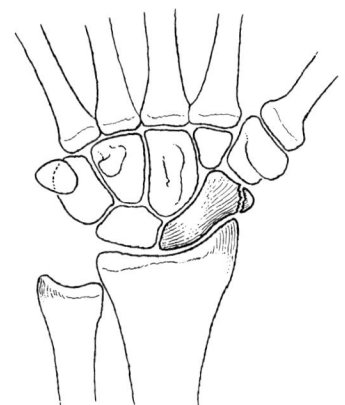

Initial Immobilization

If the patient is seen immediately after injury and has considerable swelling, apply an anterior and posterior splint.

1. The splint extends from below the elbow to the metacarpophalangeal joints.
2. The thumb is in a grasp position and is included in the plaster beyond the interphalangeal joint.
3. The wrist is in slight extension and slight radial deviation.

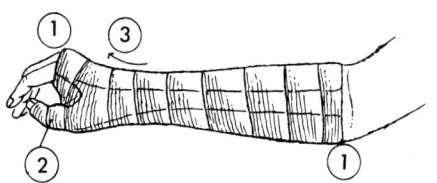

Subsequent Immobilization for Stable Fracture

After all the swelling has subsided, usually within five to seven days, apply a circular cast over stockinette without padding.

1. The cast extends from just below the elbow to the metacarpophalangeal joints.
2. The wrist is slightly dorsiflexed and in radial deviation.
3. The thumb is in the grasp position and is
4. Included in the cast as far as the base of the thumbnail.
5. The plaster is well molded in the palm.
6. The cast extends to the distal palmar crease.

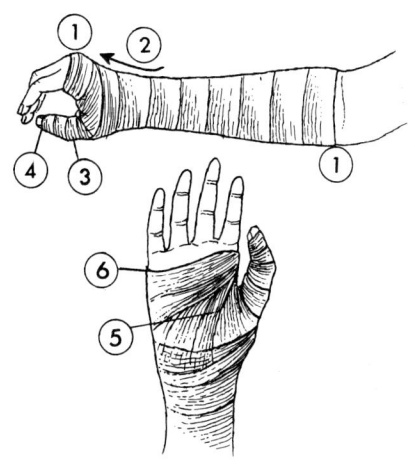

Symptomatic Follow-up Management (After London)

Remember that 95 per cent of scaphoid fractures should heal if treated by adequate immobilization and rational appreciation of the patient's needs.

Immobilization must be complete, although the patient should be encouraged to use the nonimmobilized fingers.

Inspect the cast every two weeks, and when it becomes loose apply a new cast.

Emphasize treatment of the wrist on the basis of symptoms rather than its radiographic appearance. Maintain cast immobilization for eight weeks; at the end of that time, if the patient has a comfortable wrist and a reasonable range of motion and is able to grip with little or no local tenderness, discard the plaster cast irrespective of radiographic appearance. The patient should protect the wrist with a splint and should avoid contact sports or heavy use until complete union is evident on x-ray.

If the patient still has discomfort, weakness, pain, or tenderness, reapply a complete plaster cast for 4 to 6 more weeks. Discard the plaster in 3 months, and if the fracture is still clinically symptomatic, consider bone grafting.

Indications for operation should be purely clinical and should be based on the patient's symptoms. There is no conclusive evidence that prolonged immobilization prevents nonunion. Bony union can occur without it.

Even when a fracture line is visible after discarding the plaster, it may frequently become obliterated over the subsequent 6 to 12 months.

Established nonunions most often cause disability from reinjury. These recurrent symptoms can be relieved quite frequently by a short time in plaster.

The unstable or slowly healing scaphoid fracture, which is uncommon (5 to 8 per cent), requires critical analysis of reduction and a more prolonged immobilization or early operative treatment.

MANAGEMENT OF UNSTABLE DISPLACED, OR SLOWLY HEALING FRACTURES

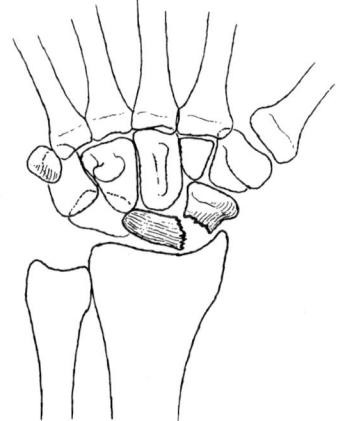

Types

A fracture with horizontal displacement and a fracture gap, which takes longer to fill in.

An oblique fracture, which is displaced by intrinsic and extrinsic muscle pull.

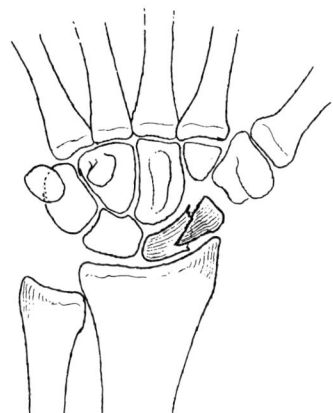

A fracture of the proximal third. This heals more slowly owing to deprivation of blood supply, which must enter from the distal fragment.

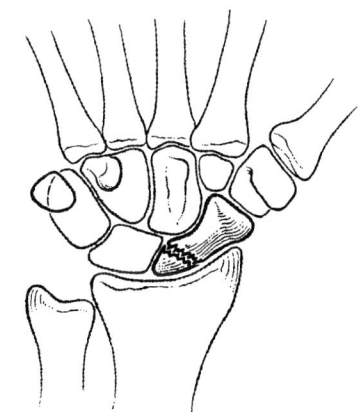

A scaphoid fracture associated with a perilunate dislocation. Unless anatomic reduction is achieved by closed manipulation of this unstable injury, it should be opened and the scaphoid should be fixed and stabilized internally.

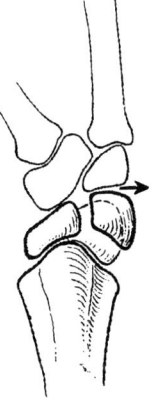

FRACTURES OF THE SCAPHOID

AN EXAMPLE OF A FRACTURE WITH DISPLACEMENT OF THE FRAGMENTS

Prereduction X-Ray

1. Fracture of the mid third of the scaphoid.
2. The normal relationship of the fragments to the surrounding carpal bones is disturbed.
3. The fragments are angulated.

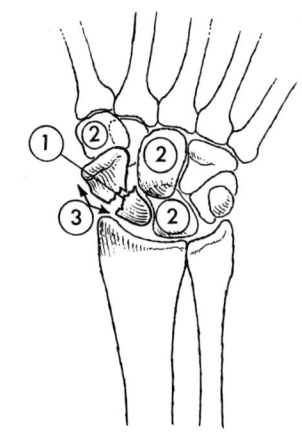

Reduction

Fluoroscopic study revealed that a position of moderate radial deviation of the hand realigned the fragments.

1. The hand is deviated toward the radius.
2. The fragments are in normal alignment.

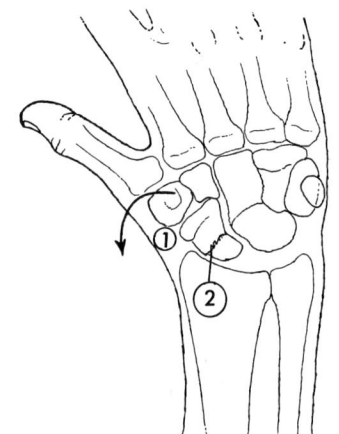

Immobilization Following Reduction

Apply a circular cast over a stockinette without padding.

1. Hold the wrist slightly dorsiflexed and
2. In moderate radial deviation.

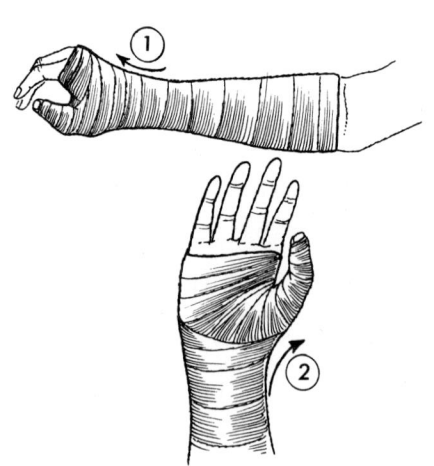

1066

Symptomatic Follow-up Management

If the reduction has closed the fracture gap, continue the cast immobilization and encourage the patient to use the nonimmobilized fingers.

Inspect the cast every two weeks and if it becomes loose apply a new cast.

Emphasize treatment of the wrist based on clinical symptoms rather than radiographic appearance.

Unstable, slowly healing fractures generally require at least 10 to 12 weeks of cast immobilization. At the end of this time, if the patient has a comfortable wrist and a reasonable range of motion and is able to grip with little or no local tenderness, discard the plaster irrespective of radiographic appearance.

The patient should use a protective splint for an additional 4 to 6 weeks and should refrain from contact sports or heavy lifting until there is radiographic evidence that the fracture has consolidated.

If the patient is still clinically symptomatic at the end of 3 to 4 months, consider bone grafting.

Operative intervention for a fracture that is symptomatic is of more benefit to the patient, in general, than is persistent closed treatment.

Subacute Fractures of the Scaphoid (Diagnosed Three or More Months After Injury)

REMARKS

Many of these fractures are initially unrecognized or are treated as wrist sprains.

By the time the correct diagnosis is made, bone absorption may have occurred or cysts may have formed in the fracture fragments. There may also be evidence of avascular necrosis or sclerosis of the fracture fragments.

Bone changes of a more advanced nature do not preclude bony union with closed treatment. At least 75 per cent of these unrecognized fractures will heal with closed reduction and cast immobilization.

The prognosis for a satisfactory fracture union is especially good if there is no evidence of arthritis and little displacement of the fragment.

Treat the clinical symptoms rather than the radiographic appearance.

Appearance on X-Ray

1. Cysts have developed in the proximal and distal fragments.
2. The proximal fragment appears dense.

Note: These radiographic changes are very commonly seen and do not contraindicate closed treatment.

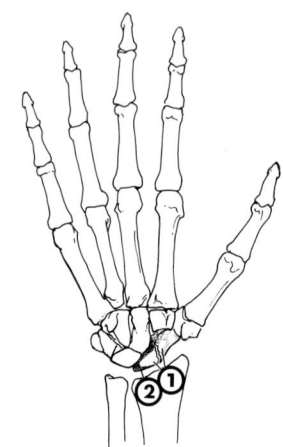

Symptomatic Management

Reduce and immobilize subacute scaphoid fracture by continuous plaster immobilization, as used for acute fracture (see page 1066).

Remove the cast at the end of four months regardless of the state of repair evidenced by x-ray.

If the patient is free of pain, and has a reasonable range of motion and a satisfactory grip strength without discomfort, no further treatment is needed. Radiographic evidence of union may follow clinical evidence by many months.

The management of patients who develop established nonunion is governed by the intensity of symptoms, if present, and the degree of functional impairment of the wrist.

Nonunion of the Scaphoid

REMARKS

Established nonunion of the scaphoid may exist without symptoms or significant functional impairment. The wrist may become symptomatic only when subjected to stress or trauma.

Among the changes associated with chronic nonunion are avascular necrosis and cyst formation in the fragments. Traumatic arthritis may also occur, particularly between the radius and the scaphoid.

Frequently, arthritic changes or fibrous union may diminish motion sufficiently at the fracture site to relieve the pain symptoms.

Many elderly patients or patients with sedentary occupations are capable of adjusting their activities to the tolerance of the wrist and need no treatment other than occasional rest and anti-inflammatory medication for the arthritis.

FRACTURES OF THE SCAPHOID

NONOPERATIVE MANAGEMENT

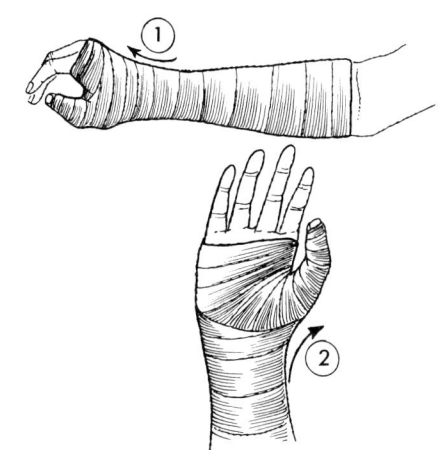

Apply a circular cast over stockinette without padding.
1. Hold the wrist slightly dorsiflexed and
2. In moderate radial deviation. (Evaluate the ideal position for fracture reduction under image-intensified fluoroscopy.)

SURGICAL MANAGEMENT

REMARKS

The usual candidate for operative treatment is the young working adult less than 30 years of age with pain, loss of grip strength, and limitation of wrist motion. A trial of nonoperative treatment should always be employed before deciding on operative methods.

The duration of nonunion does not affect the prognosis for union or relief of pain. However, prolonged nonunion will limit recovery of wrist motion despite successful bone grafting.

The surgical procedure most often employed for scaphoid nonunion is bone graft with or without radial styloidectomy.

Internal fixation in conjunction with bone graft may also be needed for unstable fractures.

Arthroplasty is indicated for symptomatic, long-standing nonunion in the older patient in whom arthritis of the radiocarpal joint is evident. Use either a Silastic scaphoid or a total wrist joint replacement, depending on the degree of arthritis.

An arthrodesis may rarely be necessary for the patient who does heavy work and is not a suitable candidate for arthroplasty. In most instances arthroplasty should be chosen prior to arthrodesis.

BONE GRAFTING WITH RADIAL STYLOIDECTOMY

REMARKS

This is the procedure of first choice for the majority of symptomatic nonunions in young patients.

The presence of cystic changes or radiographic signs of avascular necrosis in the fragments does not contraindicate this procedure.

Radial styloidectomy is valuable to aid in surgical approach, particularly if there is evidence of arthritis in the radioscaphoid articulation.

Occasionally, for the unstable fracture, internal fixation should supplement the bone grafting.

Note: If arthritis is severe or the scaphoid is fragmented, consider a silastic arthroplasty. For far-advanced radiocarpal arthritis, a total wrist arthroplasty is preferable to arthrodesis in most patients.

Appearance on X-Ray

1. Old ununited fracture through the body.
2. Fractured surfaces are smooth and sclerotic.
3. Sclerosis of fragments does not alter prognosis for healing.

Note: There is slight evidence of arthritis in the radiocarpal joint adjacent to the fracture.

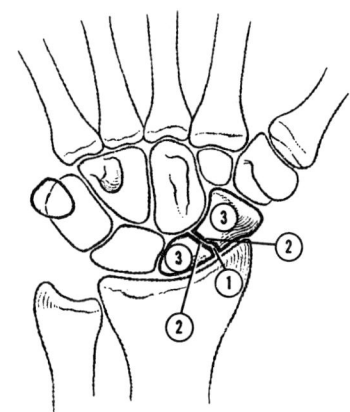

Operative Procedure

Bone Grafting

1. Make a 6-cm incision centered over the anatomic snuffbox; it begins at the base of the first metacarpal and is directed upward and proximally.
2. Divide the fascia between the extensor pollicis longus dorsally and the extensor pollicis brevis ventrally. Identify and protect the sensory branch of the radial nerve and the radial artery.
3. Expose the dorsal carpal ligament proximally.
4. Mobilize the tendons of the extensor pollicis longus and the extensor carpi radialis from the joint capsule and retract them dorsally.
5. Make a linear incision in the joint capsule and divide the dorsal carpal ligament.

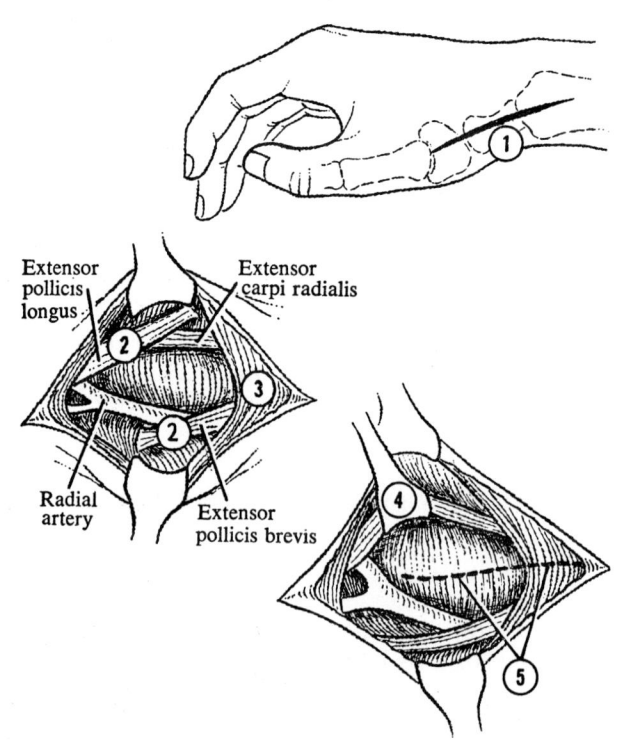

FRACTURES OF THE SCAPHOID

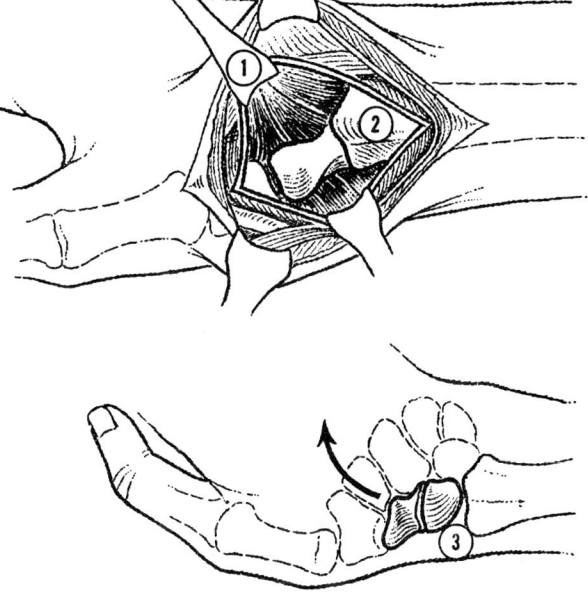

1. Retract the margins of the capsule.
2. Strip the periosteum and capsule from the radius for 2 cm.

3. Deviate the wrist toward the ulna; the scaphoid is now clearly visualized.

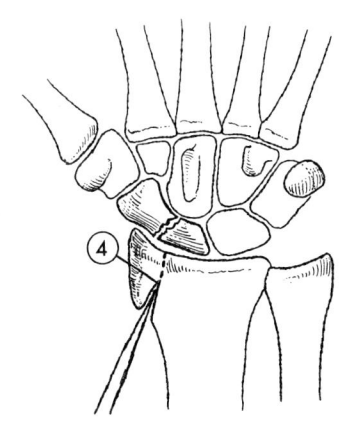

4. With a fine osteotome resect the styloid process just proximal to the fracture line and perpendicular to the long axis of the scaphoid.

Note: Always obtain an intraoperative x-ray at this point to be sure of the nonunion site. Otherwise you might bone graft the distal scaphoid fragment to the multangulum.

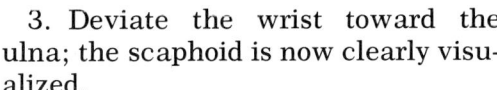

1. With a small gouge, freshen the sclerotic bone ends and form a cavity extending well into the adjacent fragments.
2. Fill cavity with an oblong graft, 2 × 1 × 1 cm, taken from the radial styloid.
3. Pack cancellous chips taken from the distal radius in the cyst around the graft.

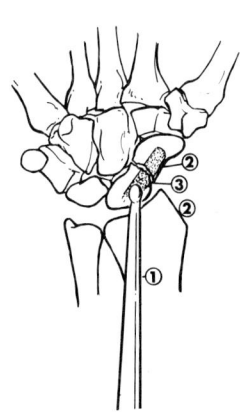

FRACTURES OF THE SCAPHOID

Operative Procedure (Continued)

INTRAOPERATIVE X-RAY

1. The bone graft traverses the fracture line, stabilizing both fragments.
2. If the fracture is not stabilized by the graft, supplement with a transarticular Kirschner wire passed through the greater multangulum and scaphoid. This is rarely necessary.

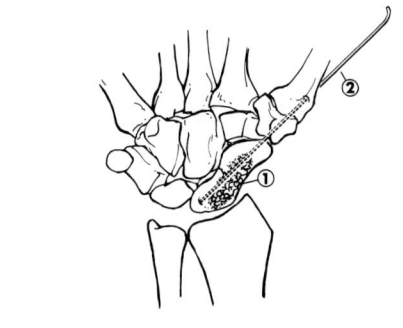

Postoperative Care

After confirming the position of the fracture and the graft by intraoperative x-ray, release the tourniquet and close the capsule and skin.

Apply a postoperative hand dressing.

1. The wrist is slightly extended. The metacarpophalangeal joints are flexed and the interphangeal joints are extended.
2. The thumb is in apposition with the fingers.
3. Soft tissue fluffs are applied liberally in the palm and between the fingers.
4. Rolled gauze is wrapped around the soft tissue fluffs from the elbow to the fingertips.
5. Plaster is applied over the rolled gauze.

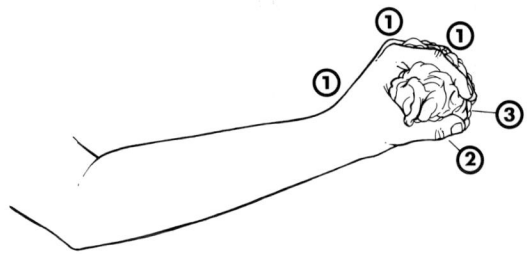

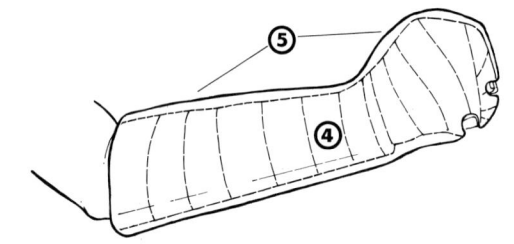

6. Elevate the limb postoperatively on arm rest.

When swelling has subsided, usually by five to seven days, remove the postoperative dressing and sutures. Apply a snug, short arm cast.

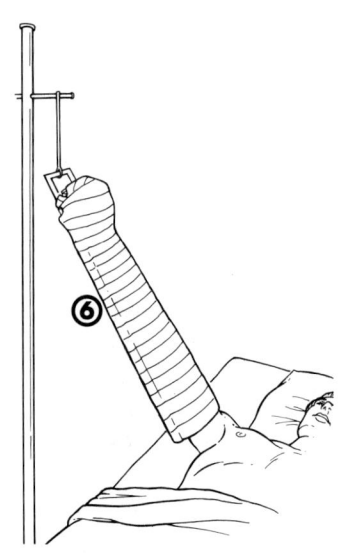

Cast Immobilization

1. The cast extends from just below the elbow to the metacarpophalangeal joints.
2. The wrist is slightly dorsiflexed and in the neutral position.
3. The base of the thumb is in a position of abduction and its metacarpophalangeal and interphalangeal joints are slightly flexed.
4. The cast incorporates the thumb to the middle of the nail.
5. The plaster is well molded in the palm of the hand.
6. The cast extends to the distal palmar crease of the hand.

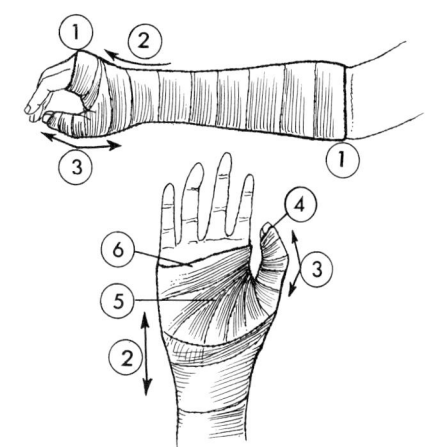

Follow-up Management

As with fresh fractures, immobilization must be rigid and complete.

Check the cast every 2 weeks, and apply a new cast when the original becomes loose.

If a transarticular Kirschner wire was used for additional fixation, remove it by 4 to 6 weeks.

Maintain immobilization until union is demonstrated clinically and radiographically; this usually takes 3 to 5 months.

Even if union is not complete by the end of 6 months, remove the cast and allow the patient free use of the limb.

Some residual stiffness may be anticipated, but pain relief and fracture union may be anticipated in 90 to 95 per cent of cases treated by this method.

SWANSON SILASTIC REPLACEMENT ARTHROPLASTY

REMARKS

This procedure is indicated if there is significant fragmentation and avascular necrosis of the scaphoid, especially in older patients.

It is particularly useful for ununited fractures in the proximal third, which would be difficult to treat by bone graft.

A silastic replacement may also be used when bone grafting procedures have failed. It can be inserted in the presence of mild radiocarpal arthritis, but generalized arthritis is an indication for total wrist joint replacement or arthrodesis.

If radial stylectomy has been performed previously, a silastic prosthesis will be unstable and its use is contraindicated.

FRACTURES OF THE SCAPHOID

Preoperative X-Rays

1. The proximal fragment is a third of the scaphoid.
2. The fragment is dense and
3. Comminuted.

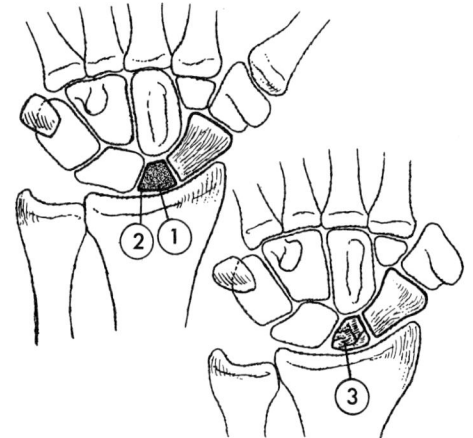

SYMPTOMATIC NONUNION

1. Cystic fragmentation persists despite previous attempt at bone grafting.
2. There is slight radiocarpal arthritis but not generalized involvement.

Note: The radial styloid has not been extensively resected and will serve to stabilize a Silastic prosthesis.

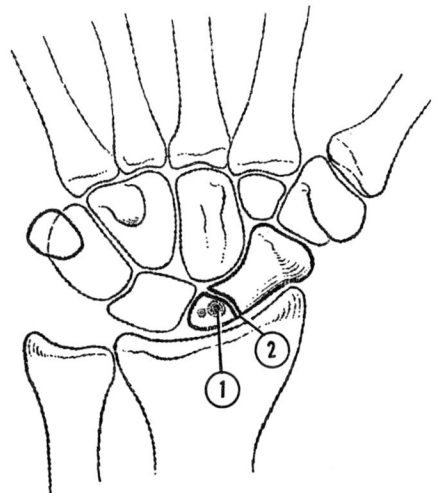

FRACTURES OF THE SCAPHOID

Operative Procedure

1. Make a 6-cm incision centered over the anatomic snuffbox; it begins at the base of the first metacarpal and extends upward and proximally.
2. Divide the fascia between the extensor pollicis longus dorsally and the extensor pollicis brevis ventrally.
3. Expose the dorsal carpal ligament proximally.
4. Retract the tendons of the extensor pollicis longus and the extensor carpi radialis upward.
5. Make a linear incision in the joint capsule and divide the dorsal carpal ligament.

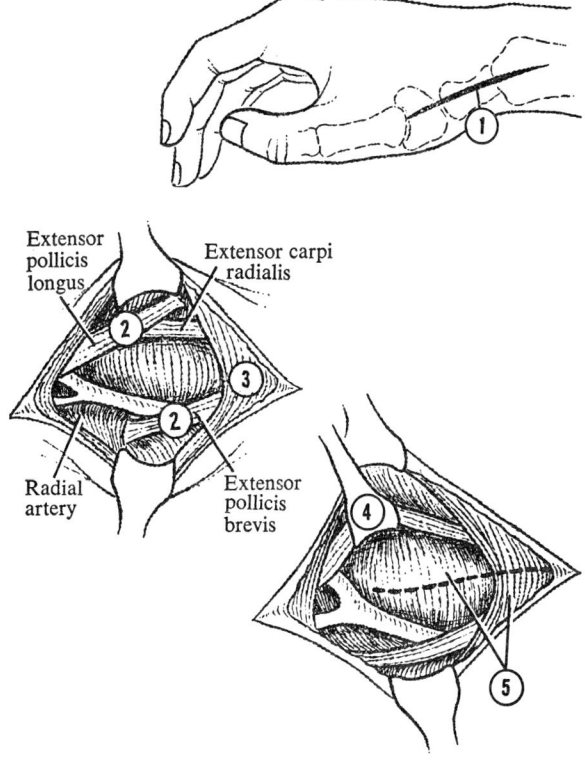

1. Retract the margins of the capsule.
2. Strip the periosteum and the capsule from the radius for 2 cm.
3. Turn the wrist toward the ulna.

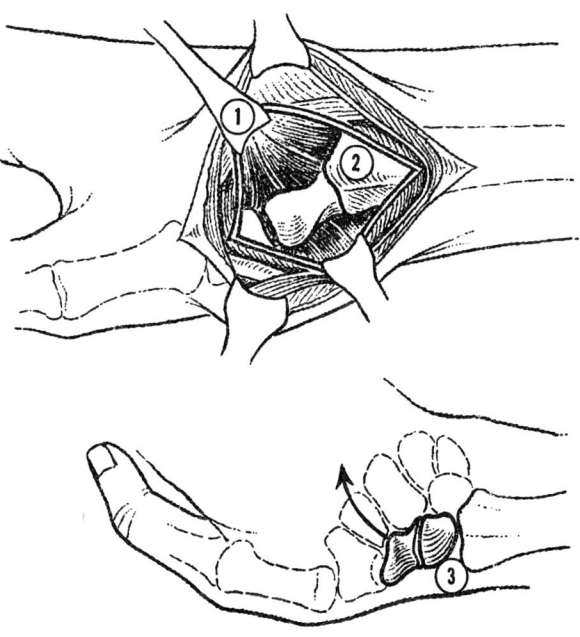

FRACTURES OF THE SCAPHOID

Operative Procedure (Continued)

1. Obtain an intraoperative x-ray to identify the carpal structures.
2. Rongeur the entire scaphoid, including proximal and distal fragments. Take another intraoperative x-ray to ascertain the completeness of the excision.

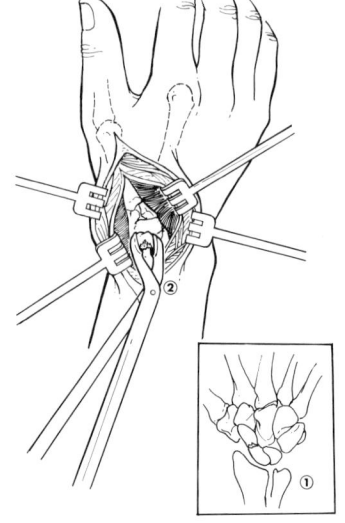

1. After confirming the correct size with a trial prosthesis, insert the Silastic prosthesis, which fills the gap and is stable.
2. Occasionally a transcarpal Kirschner wire may be needed to insure stability.

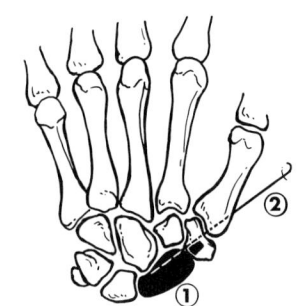

Postoperative Immobilization

Apply postoperative hand dressing.
1. The wrist is slightly extended. The metacarpophalangeal joints are flexed and the interphalangeal joints are extended.
2. The thumb is in apposition with the fingers.
3. Soft tissue fluffs are applied liberally in the palm and between the fingers.
4. Rolled gauze is wrapped around the soft tissue fluffs from the elbow to the fingertips.
5. Plaster is applied over the rolled gauze.

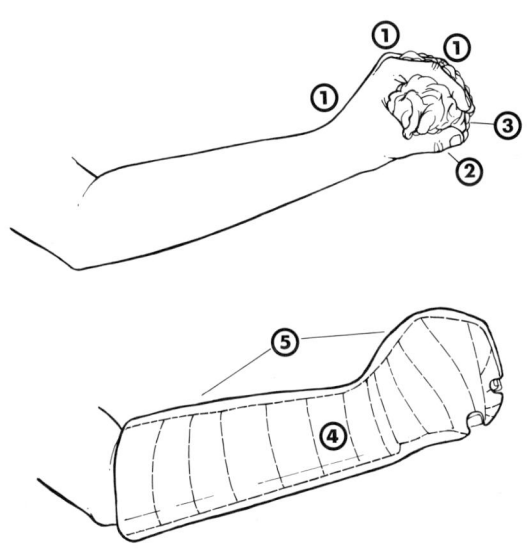

6. The limb is elevated postoperatively on an arm rest.

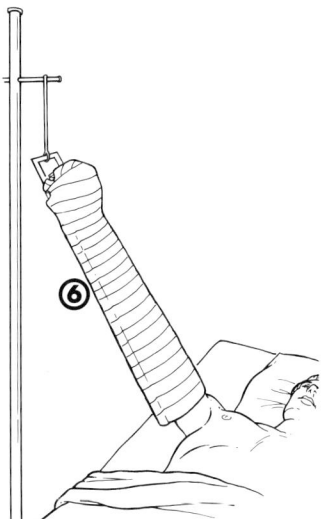

Subsequent Management

Remove the postoperative hand dressing by 4 to 6 days and apply a scaphoid cast (see page 1073).

Continue cast immobilization for 4 to 6 weeks, depending on the stability of the prosthesis.

If a Kirschner wire was inserted, remove it by 4 to 6 weeks.

Allow the patient to begin active range-of-motion exercises when the cast is removed.

Full use of the wrist is usually possible by 10 to 12 weeks.

MANAGEMENT OF CHRONIC POST-TRAUMATIC ARTHRITIS — ARTHROPLASTY OR ARTHRODESIS

REMARKS

Occasionally, nonunion of the scaphoid fracture will produce severe symptomatic arthritis years later. This is especially likely if carpal instability and dorsiflexion collapse have resulted from the loss of scaphoid stability.

The majority of patients with generalized carpal arthritis are older.

Frequently, the symptoms are intermittent and are the result of overuse. Local intra-articular cortisone injection, splint immobilization, and systemic anti-inflammatory agents will relieve periodic symptoms for many years.

Should the wrist pain and functional loss cause significant disability despite nonoperative measures, total wrist arthroplasty is indicated for most patients. If the patient does heavy work, arthrodesis may be indicated primarily, but most patients will be better aided by arthroplasty, which still leaves the option for arthrodesis.

Appearance on X-Ray I

1. Nonunion of the fracture of the scaphoid.
2. The ulnar fragment is dense and sclerotic.
3. The radial fragment shows cystic changes.
4. The joint space is narrowed, indicative of degeneration of articular cartilage.
5. Bony spurs are consistent with osteoarthritis.

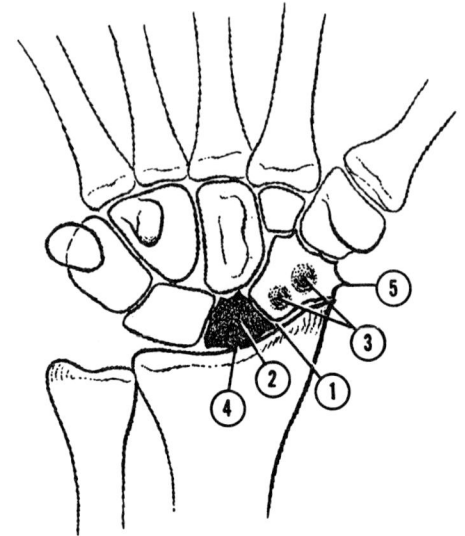

Appearance on X-Ray II

Anteroposterior View

1. Persistent nonunion of the scaphoid.
2. The scaphoid is cystic and irregular with osteophytes.
3. The radiocarpal joint space is narrowed.
4. The palmar horn of the lunate has shifted distally on the neck of the capitate, and the scapho-lunate space is widened.

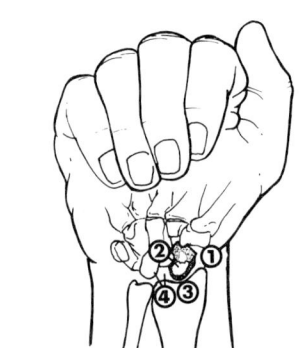

Lateral View

1. The lunate has dorsiflexed as the result of loss of scaphoid stability.
2. The capitate has shifted proximally and dorsally.

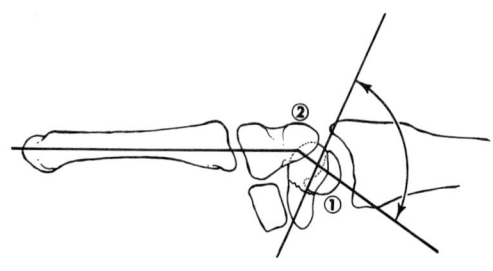

Voltz–University of Arizona Wrist Arthroplasty

1. Make a straight longitudinal incision beginning just proximal to the base of the third metacarpal and extending 6 cm above the wrist joint.

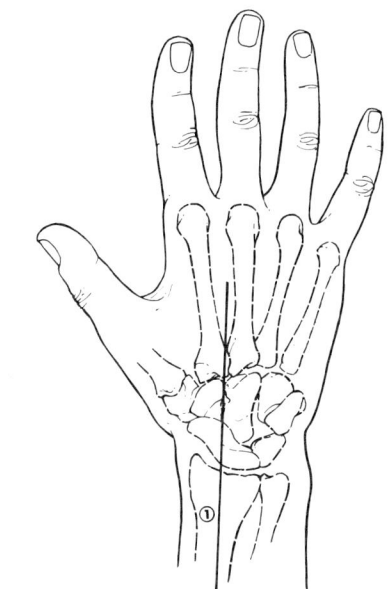

2. Incise the dorsal carpal ligament and deep fascia. (Tag with a suture for later closure.)
3. Develop the interval between the extensor pollicis longus and the extensor digitorum communis tendon of the index finger, and expose the radius.
4. Incise the periosteum, and by subperiosteal dissection expose the dorsal surface of the radius.
5. Retract the extensor pollicis longus and its fascial canal together with the tendons of the extensor carpi radialis longus and the extensor carpi radialis brevis to the radial side of the wound.
6. Extend the radial incision into the capsule as far as the base of the third metacarpal bone, and reflect the capsule from the margin of the radius, from the adjacent carpal bones, and from the base of the third metacarpal bone. (Tag the capsule with a suture for later closure.)

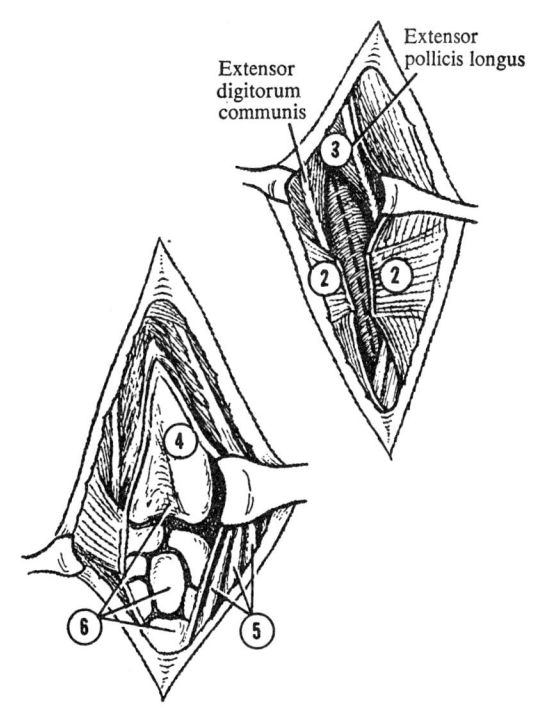

Voltz-University of Arizona Wrist Arthroplasty (Continued)

1. Excise the scaphoid, the lunate, and the base of the capitate with a rongeur to provide space for the carpal component.
2. Excise approximately 5 mm of the distal end of the radius to fit the radial component of the prosthesis. (The ulna also should be removed distal to the radius.)

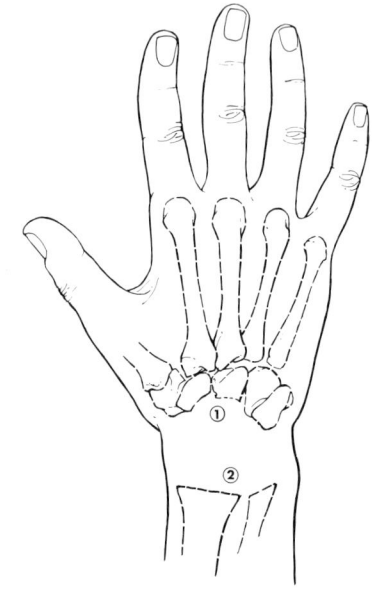

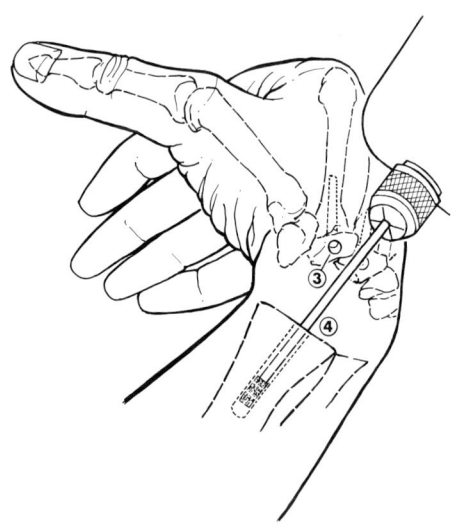

3. Ream the medullary canal of the second and third metacarpal sufficiently to seat the stems of the prosthesis.
4. Ream the distal end of the radius to seat the radial component.

1. After trial reduction, cement the carpal and radial components in the properly reamed canals.

Note: A stable range of 15 to 20 degrees of extension and 40 to 45 degrees of flexion should be possible; otherwise, further bone resection or release of flexor capsule may be necessary.

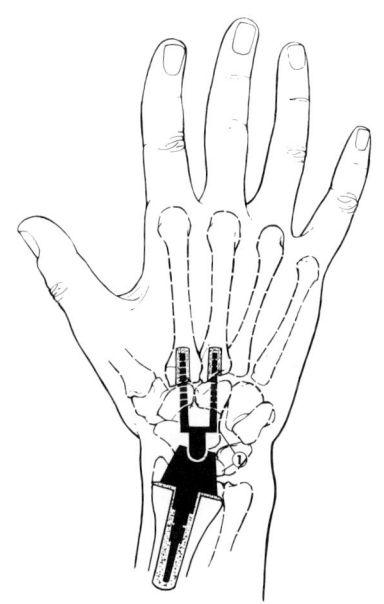

Fractures of the Scaphoid

Postoperative Management

Immobilize the patient's hand in a postoperative hand dressing.

1. The wrist is slightly extended. The metacarpophalangeal joints are flexed and the interphalangeal joints are extended.
2. The thumb is in apposition to the fingers.
3. Soft tissue fluffs are applied liberally in the palm and between the fingers.

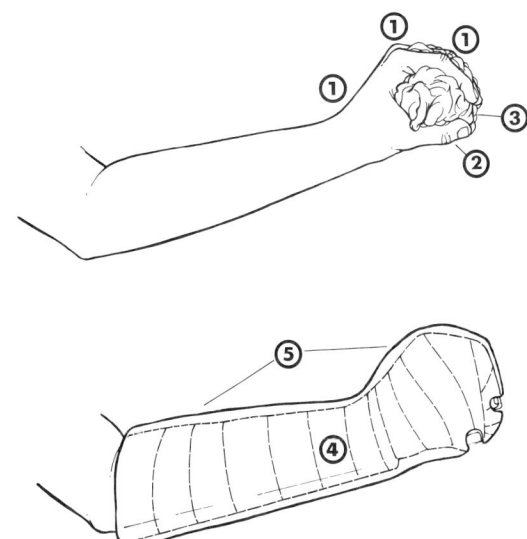

4. Rolled gauze is wrapped around the soft tissue fluffs and from the elbow to the fingertips.
5. Plaster is applied over the rolled gauze.

6. The limb is elevated postoperatively on an arm rest.

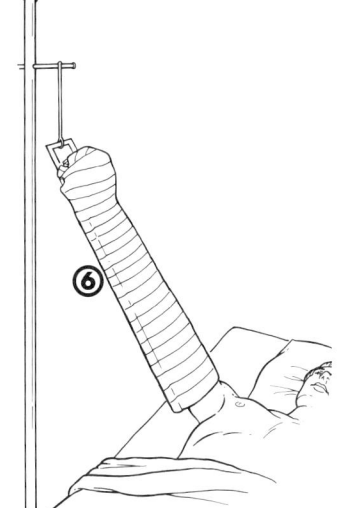

Subsequent Management

When swelling has subsided and the soft tissue has healed satisfactorily, remove the stitches and begin active range of motion. This is usually possible by seven to ten days.

Occasionally, if motion is limited, a temporary period of splinting may be necessary to prevent flexion contracture.

Full active use of the wrist is usually possible by two to three months after the operation.

Alternate Procedure: Arthrodesis

If arthrodesis is chosen for chronic traumatic arthritis, approach the wrist by the surgical exposure used for arthroplasty (see page 1079).

1. With a sharp, thin osteotome, cut out a trough 2 cm wide in the dorsum of the carpus connecting the distal end of the radius with the base of the third metacarpal.

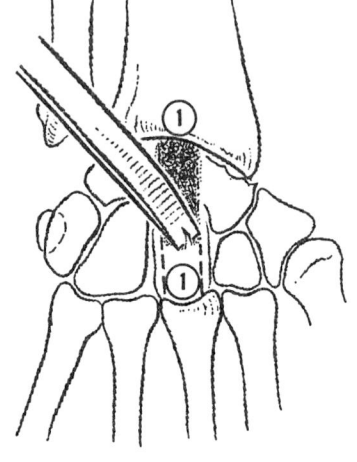

2. With sharp curettes, open the medullary canal in the radius and the base of the third metacarpal.

A cortical graft 2 cm wide and 5 cm longer than the prepared bed is obtained from the tibia.

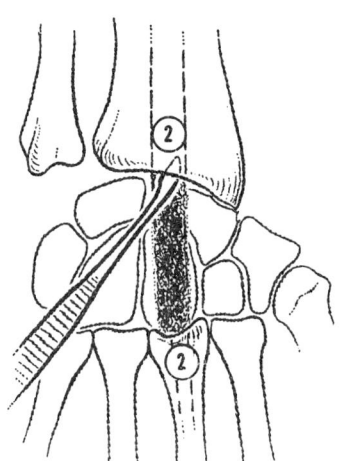

1. The open end of the graft is shaped to fit tightly in the medullary canal of the third metacarpal.
2. The other end is driven into the medullary canal of the radius.
3. While traction is made on the hand, the distal end of the graft is tapped into the medullary canal of the third metacarpal bone.

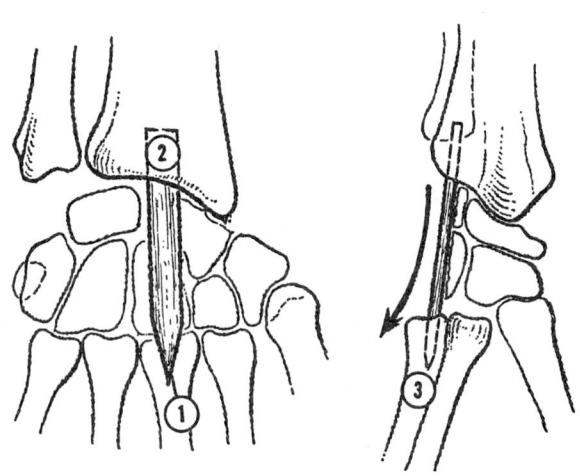

Postoperative X-Ray

1. The tibial graft is well seated in the medullary canal of the radius and third metacarpal bone.
2. The wrist is dorsiflexed 15 to 20 degrees.

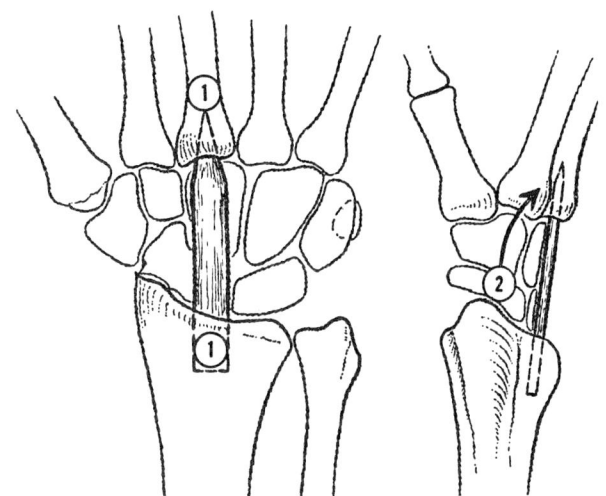

Immobilization

Apply a circular cast from the upper arm down to the metacarpophalangeal joints; include the base of the thumb.
1. The elbow is at a right angle.
2. The forearm is in midposition.
3. The wrist is dorsiflexed 15 to 20 degrees.

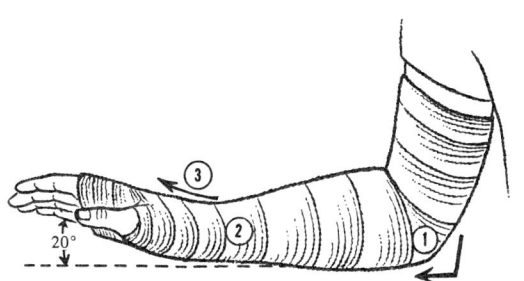

Postoperative Management

Watch for swelling and evidence of circulatory embarrassment.
Elevate the arm and apply ice bags.
If the swelling is excessive, split the cast throughout its entire length and cut all padding beneath the cast.
After 3 weeks, remove the long arm cast and apply a short cast extending from below the elbow to the metacarpophalangeal joints.
Continue immobilization until union is firm (10 to 14 weeks).

LUNATE AND PERILUNATE DISLOCATIONS AND SUBLUXATIONS

REMARKS

In addition to fracturing the scaphoid, hyperextension force vectors may also disrupt the strong scapholunate and perilunate ligaments. The result can be either dislocation or subluxation of the carpal bones.

Critical analysis of the carpal relationships, which are visualized by adequate x-ray, is necessary for correct diagnosis. Uncritical acceptance of inadequate x-rays will lead to misdiagnosis and inappropriate treatment of seriously disabling injuries.

Dislocations or subluxations of the carpal bones are not uncommon injuries, and failure to recognize carpal disruption or dissociation is common.

Complete dislocation of the wrist has occasionally been missed because true lateral x-rays were not obtained. Be sure that the x-ray demonstrates the proper relationships in two planes and in varying wrist positions (see page 1058).

The degree of carpal instability may vary from a complete dislocation to a subluxation or carpal dissociation.

Reduction of a complete dislocation must be anatomic; partial restoration is unacceptable. Frequently, open reduction and internal fixation are required.

Carpal subluxation is a different manifestation of the mechanism of injury that produces a scaphoid fracture. Scaphoid fracture and carpal subluxation are similar in a number of ways, and both conditions are frequently missed or dismissed as "wrist sprain." As with undisplaced scaphoid fracture, definitive radiographic changes may not be apparent for some time in lesser degrees of ligamentous disruption. Disability from chronic scapholunate subluxation or dissociation may, like the ununited scaphoid fracture, range from minimal limitation of motion to extremely painful, traumatic arthritis.

Awareness of the normal and abnormal relationships of the carpal bones is essential to avoid dismissing a significant injury as a sprained wrist.

Normal Carpal Relationships

On a true lateral view,
1. The axes of the radius, lunate, and capitate form a straight line.
2. The axis of the scaphoid intersects the radius-lunate-capitate axis at an angle of 30 to 60 degrees.

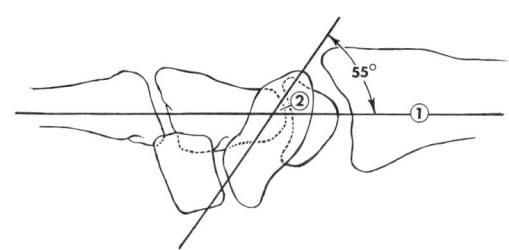

Abnormal Carpal Relationships: Carpal Subluxation or Dislocation (Dorsiflexion Instability)

This is best seen on a posteroanterior view taken with the wrist supinated and the fist clenched.
1. The space between the scaphoid and lunate exceeds 2 mm.
2. The height of the scaphoid is decreased.

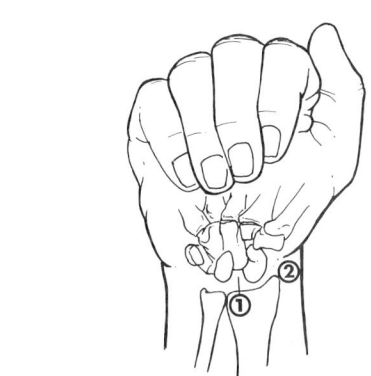

Lateral X-Ray

1. The lunate is dorsiflexed and the radial-lunate-capitate axis is no longer a straight line.
2. The scapholunate angle exceeds 70 degrees.

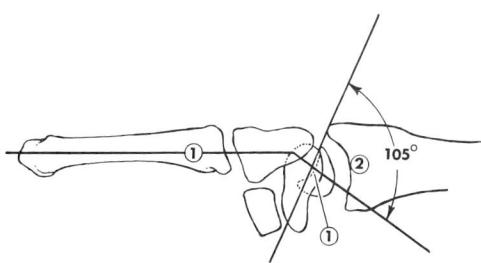

MECHANISMS OF INJURY

Dislocations and subluxations of the carpal bones result generally from extension injuries to the wrist. A variety of lesions may occur, depending on the direction and intensity of force vectors and the position of the hand in relation to the forearm at the time of impact.

When the wrist is forced into extension, most commonly by a fall on the outstretched hand, a lunate, or perilunate dislocation or a transcaphoid fracture-dislocation may occur.

Scapholunate subluxation or dissocation may result as a primary lesion from hyperextension mechanisms. It also persists after incomplete reduction of a complete carpal dislocation and after nonunion of a scaphoid fracture.

Mechanism of Lunate Dislocation

The hand and carpus are severely hyperextended by:
1. The force acting upward on the fingers and metacarpal heads and
2. The force acting downward in the line of the radius.
3. The capitate rotates dorsally on the lunate.
4. The lunate is squeezed out of the wrist joint.
5. The rotated lunate lies anterior to the wrist joint.

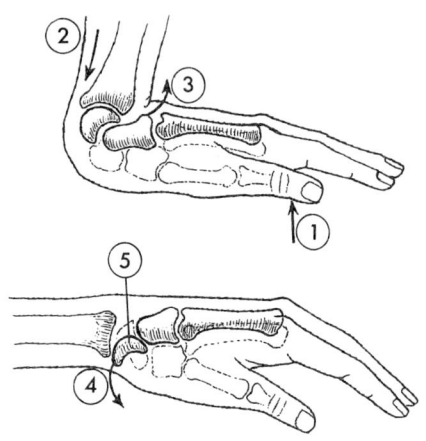

Mechanism of Dorsal Perilunate Dislocation

This lesion occurs when the hand is only moderately hyperextended, as in a fall on the outstretched hand away from the body.

The main point of impact is on the palm of the hand. The force thus generated, together with the oblique downward force traveling along the radius, disrupts the lunate-capitate articulation and drives the carpal bones dorsally behind the lunate.

The hand and carpus are not severely extended.
1. The force acts upward on the palm of the hand.
2. A second force acts obliquely downward along the shaft of the radius.
3. The lunate-capitate articulation is disrupted.
4. The carpal bones (except the lunate) are driven dorsally and behind the lunate.
5. Perilunar dislocation.
6. The radiolunate relationship is preserved.

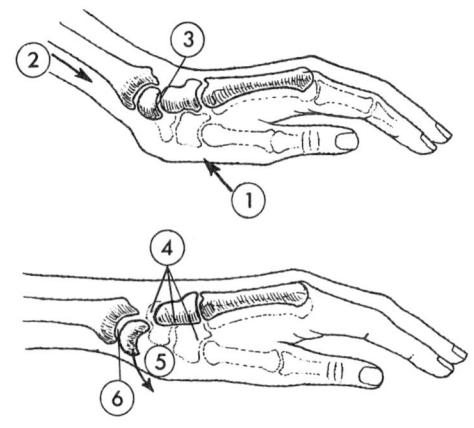

Mechanisms of Scapholunate Subluxation or Dissociation

This lesion occurs as a secondary effect on an incompletely reduced transcaphoid-perilunate or perilunate dislocation. It may also be a residuum of a chronic scaphoid nonunion.

1. A chronic nonunion has eliminated the scaphoid support to the proximal and distal carpal rows.
2. The scapholunate space is widened more than 2 mm as a result of chronic loss of support to the joint space.
3. The scaphoid has displaced volarly, and dorsiflexion instability is evidenced by the capitate's migrating into the widened scapholunate gap.

Note: Scapholunate subluxation may also follow an incomplete reduction of lunate or perilunate dislocation (see pages 1091 and 1097). Reduction must be carefully evaluated for scapholunate dissociation in order to determine whether internal fixation is necessary.

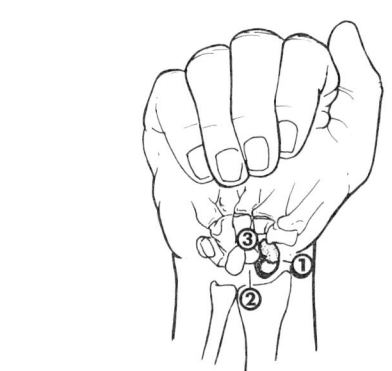

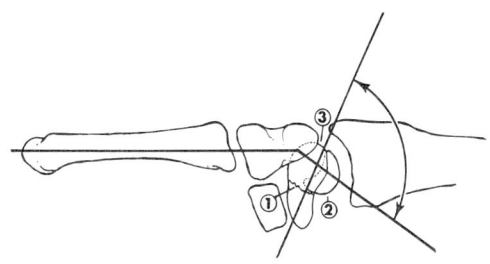

Volar Dislocation of the Lunate Bone

REMARKS

Replacement of the lunate by closed methods is generally achieved if the reduction is performed early; in rare instances closed methods fail even in fresh lesions, making open reduction necessary.

After two weeks, closed methods rarely achieve a reduction; therefore when the dislocation is more than two weeks old, an open reduction through the posterior approach should be performed.

Excision of the lunate is not indicated because reduction gives a much more satisfactory result. Avascular necrosis of this bone after dislocation is rare, and poor wrist function often follows excision of the lunate.

There is often an initial perilunar displacement of the carpal bones associated with volar dislocation of the lunate. Reduction of the dislocation may have been spontaneous, but the scaphoid may remain rotated. The posterior approach permits correction and reduction of the scapholunate relationship and fixation by transcarpal Kirschner wire between the scaphoid and the lunate.

Occasionally, an additional anterior incision may be required if the lunate has displaced greatly or the median nerve requires decompression.

Prereduction X-Ray

1. The lunate lies in front of the wrist and its articular surface tilts forward.
2. The capitate articulates with the articular surface of the radius.
3. In the anteroposterior view, the lunate appears to be triangular instead of quadrilateral and the scapholunate joint space is widened.

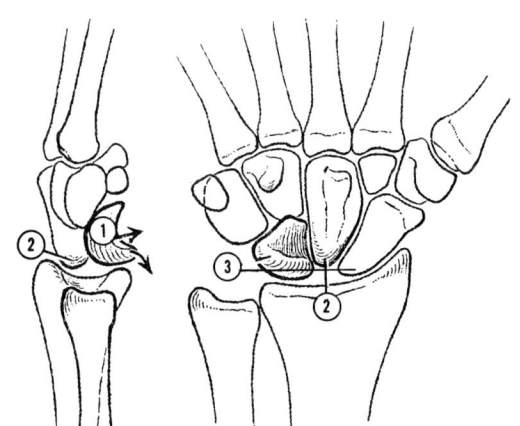

Reduction by Traction and Manipulation

1. Apply finger traction.
2. The elbow is flexed at a right angle.
3. The forearm is supinated.
4. Counter traction is applied with a muslin bandage and a water pail for weight.
5. Traction is maintained for approximately five minutes.

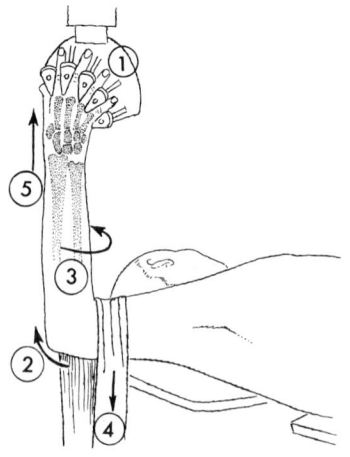

While traction is maintained:

1. Place both thumbs against the front of the lunate and make strong pressure directly backward while
2. The wrist is dorsiflexed.

Note: Check the position of the lunate by x-ray before applying the plaster slabs.

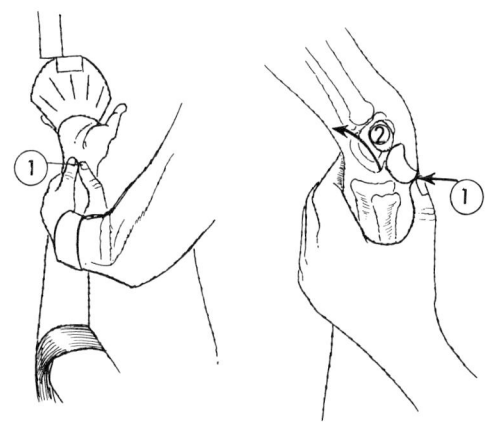

Postreduction X-Ray

1. The lunate is in its normal anatomic position and articulates with the radius.
2. Its concave articular surface articulates with the capitate.
3. In the anteroposterior view, the profile of the lunate is quadrilateral and the scapholunate joint space has been restored to normal.

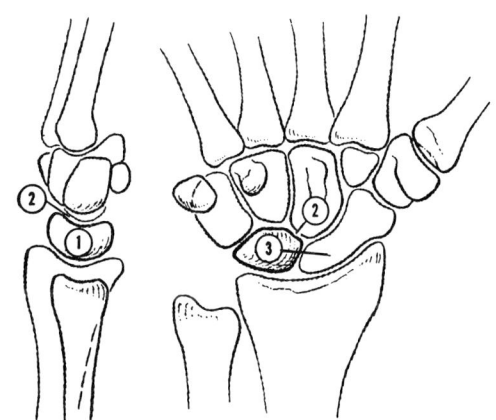

Immobilization

1. Apply anterior and posterior plaster slabs from just below the elbow to just proximal to the metacarpophalangeal joints.
2. The wrist is flexed 45 degrees.

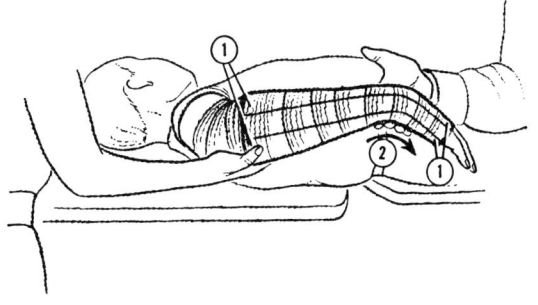

Postreduction Management

After 1 week, remove the plaster slabs, bring the wrist to a neutral position, and again immobilize with anterior and posterior plaster slabs.

Continue immobilization, insist on a program of active finger exercises.

After removal of the plaster slabs, institute a program of active wrist and finger exercises.

The prognosis is good in cases of recent dislocation; recovery should be complete in 8 to 12 weeks.

Note: Rarely the lunate is dislocated posteriorly; the treatment is the same as for forward dislocation, except that the wrist is immobilized in slight dorsiflexion.

Open Reduction

REMARKS

Open reduction is indicated if closed reduction fails in a fresh injury or if the dislocation is more than two weeks old.

A dorsal approach is most applicable. The relationship of the scaphoid to the reduced lunate must be carefully evaluated and must be corrected if there is rotational malalignment of the scaphoid (scapholunate subluxation).

A dorsal approach is also applicable to fix fracture of the scaphoid associated with transcaphoid-perilunate dislocation.

In all these instances, carefully evaluate the reduction achieved by means of intraoperative x-rays.

1. Make a longitudinal skin incision running between the extensor pollicis longus and the extensor digitorum communis tendons.
2. Open the dorsal carpal ligament and continue dissection between the tendons. Preserve the ligament for closure.
3. Apply traction to the hand.
4. Locate the defects in the dorsum of the carpus.

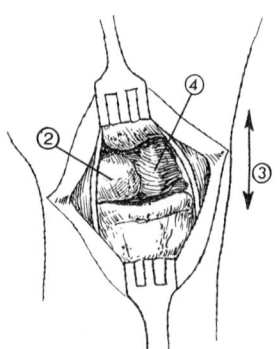

1. By sharp dissection clean out the scar tissue occupying the space of the lunate bone.
2. Identify the capitate distally and the articular surface of the radius proximally.
3. While traction and slight dorsiflexion are maintained, lever the lunate into its normal position.

Note: Obtain intraoperative x-rays to insure that complete reduction of the lunate and scapholunate joint has been achieved.

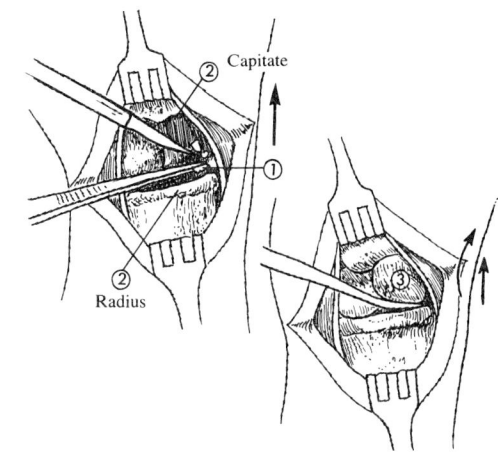

Postoperative Management

If this is an uncomplicated volar dislocation, repair the scapholunate ligament and approximate the edges of the dorsal radiocarpal ligament. The forearm, wrist, and hand are immobilized by:
1. Anterior and posterior splints.
2. The wrist is flexed slightly.

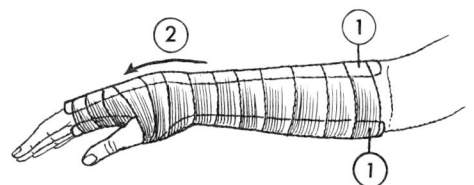

Encourage full use of the fingers and elbow.
After three weeks remove the plaster splints.
Institute a program of physical therapy and active exercises to restore finger and wrist motion.
Avascular necrosis is unlikely, but the case should be followed for 12 to 18 months for evaluation of the viability of the lunate.

VOLAR DISLOCATION OF THE LUNATE WITH SUBLUXATION OF THE SCAPHOLUNATE JOINT

REMARKS

After closed or open reduction of the lunate there may be persistent subluxation or dissociation of the scaphoid and lunate.
The subluxation should be corrected and fixed by open reduction.
Failure to correct this dissociation may result in dorsal instability and poor function.

Intraoperative X-ray of Scapholunate Subluxation After Reduction of the Lunate Dislocation

1. The lunate has been restored to normal.
2. The scaphoid is rotated volarly and appears to be beneath the trapezoid and trapezium.
3. The scapholunate space is greater than 2 mm.

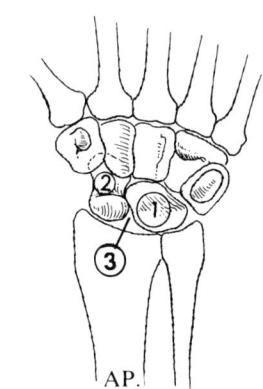

To reduce the scaphoid properly during open reduction, apply traction to the slightly dorsiflexed wrist:

1. Lever the scaphoid into its normal anatomic position with a blunt dissector or periosteal elevator.
2. Transfix the lunate and the scaphoid with a 2-mm threaded Kirschner wire, which enters the scaphoid on the radial side of the tendon of the extensor pollicis longus. Cut the wire below the level of the skin and repair the scapholunate ligament.

Note: While the wire is being inserted, take care in maintaining at all times the normal relationship between the lunate and scaphoid. The wire should be removed at the end of three weeks.

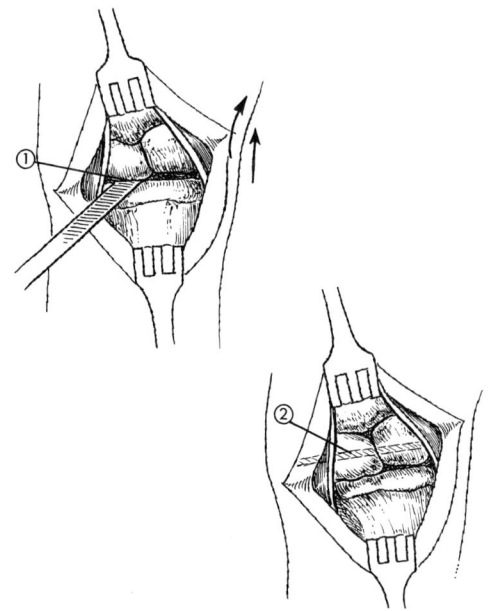

Scaphoid Fracture With Lunate Dislocation

STABILIZATION OF DISPLACED FRAGMENTS OF FRACTURED SCAPHOID

After closed or open reduction of the lunate, displacement of the fragments from associated fracture of the scaphoid generally persists.

Internal fixation is necessary to hold this unstable injury. Use either a lag screw (McLaughlin technique) or a threaded Kirschner wire.

Appearance on X-Ray

1. The lunate is in normal alignment with the capitate and radius.
2. Displaced fragments of the scaphoid.

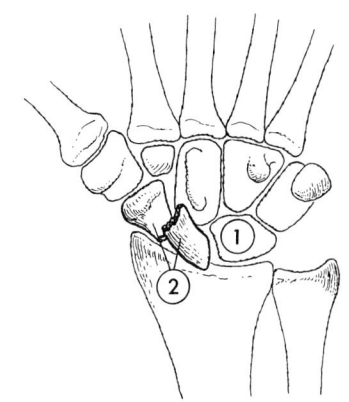

Operative Procedure

1. The scaphoid fragment is realigned and is fixed temporarily by a Kirschner wire drilled through a double-barreled guide.
2. After the second barrel of the guide is drilled through, a lag screw is inserted while fracture fixation is maintained with a Kirschner wire. Following lag screw fixation, the wire is removed.

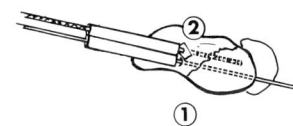

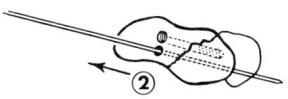

Note: Occasionally the fragment will be too small for lag screw fixation and transcarpal Kirschner wire fixation can be used.

Postoperative Immobilization

Apply a postoperative hand dressing.

1. The wrist is slightly extended. The metacarpophalangeal joints are flexed and the interphalangeal joints are extended.
2. The thumb is in apposition with the fingers.
3. Soft tissue fluffs are applied liberally in the palm and between the fingers.

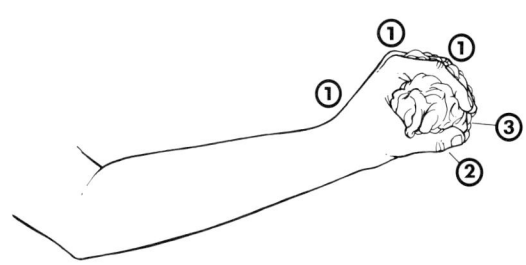

4. Rolled gauze is wrapped around the soft tissue fluffs from the elbow to the fingertips.
5. Plaster is applied over the rolled gauze.

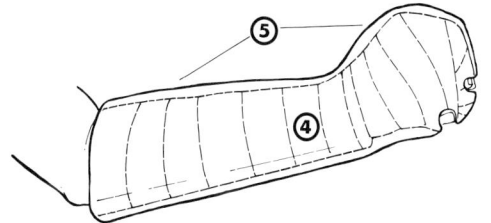

LUNATE AND PERILUNATE DISLOCATIONS AND SUBLUXATIONS

Postoperative Immobilization (Continued)

6. Elevate the limb postoperatively on an arm rest.

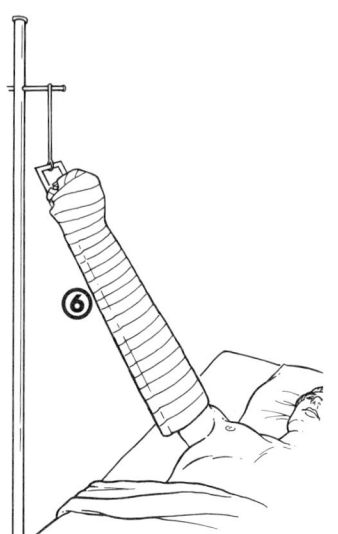

Subsequent Management

1. After five to seven days, apply a circular cast from below the elbow to the metacarpophalangeal joints.
2. The thumb is in the grasp position and is included in the cast to the base of the thumbnail.
3. The wrist is slightly dorsiflexed; otherwise it is in the neutral position.

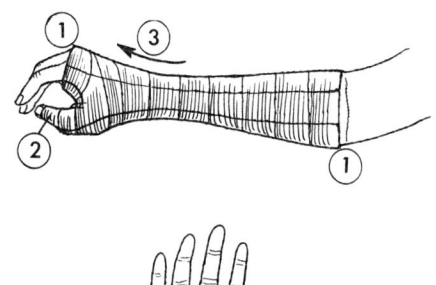

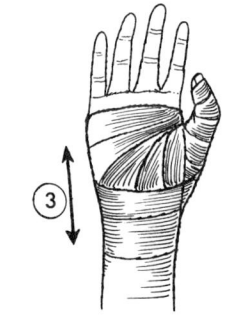

If a transcarpal wire has been used for fixation, remove it at the end of six to eight weeks, depending on the state of healing at the fracture site.

Continue immobilization in a plaster cast until bony union is achieved, usually by four months. If bony union is not attained at the end of six months, take the cast off and mobilize the wrist.

Chronic Lunate Dislocation with Avascular Necrosis

REMARKS

Open reduction through the posterior approach, as previously described, should be performed for chronic dislocation of the lunate, provided that the bone is not destroyed.

If avascular necrosis develops either prior or subsequent to reduction of the lunate, excision with Silastic replacement arthroplasty is a useful reconstructive procedure.

Excision of the lunate along generally does not permit satisfactory wrist function.

Preoperative X-Ray

Dislocation of the lunate is eight months old.

1. The lunate is in front of the wrist.
2. The capitate is in line with the radius.
3. The lunate is dense and sclerotic, indicative of aseptic necrosis.

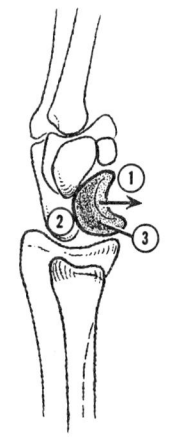

Operative Procedure: Swanson Silastic Arthroplasty

1. Make an S-shaped incision on the volar aspect of the wrist beginning at the base of the thenar eminence.
2. Divide the fascia and the transverse carpal ligament.

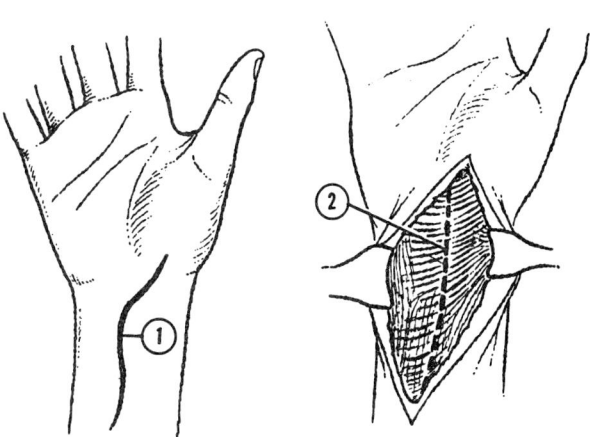

Operative Procedure: Swanson Silastic Arthroplasty (Continued)

1. Retract the median nerve, the palmaris longus, and the tendon of the flexor pollicis longus to the radial side.
2. Retract the tendons of the flexor digitorum sublimis and the profundus to the ulnar side.
3. Incise the capsule of the joint.
4. Remove the lunate with a rongeur or with sharp dissection. Take care to preserve the palmar radiocarpal and ulnocarpal ligaments.

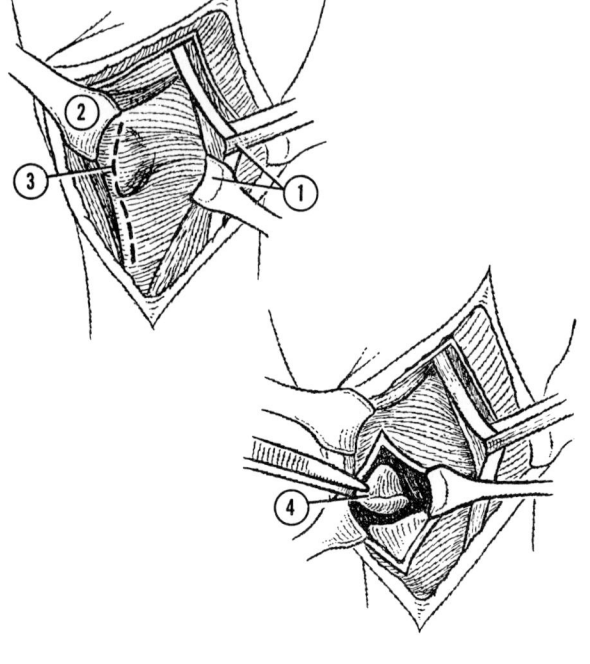

1. After using a trial prosthesis to determine size, the Silastic implant is fitted snuggly into the space of the resected lunate.
2. A small curette or drill is used to make a hole in the triquetrum to accept the stem of the implant.

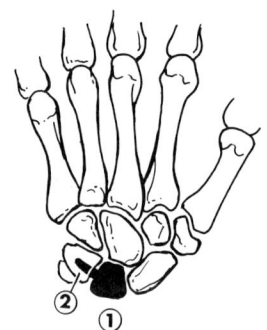

Immobilization

After the position of the implant is determined by intraoperative x-rays, close the capsule carefully.

Immobilize the wrist in a postoperative hand dressing.

Postoperative Management

Remove the postoperative dressing after one week and apply a short arm cast.

The cast is worn for 4 to 6 weeks. Full wrist activity is usually possible after 12 weeks.

If silastic replacement arthroplasty cannot be successfully accomplished, consider either resection of the proximal carpal row or total wrist arthroplasty (see page 1079).

Uncomplicated Dorsal Perilunate Dislocations

REMARKS

This lesion is relatively common.

The lunate is the focal point around which the dislocation of the remaining carpus occurs.

The lunate maintains its normal anatomic position in relation to the radius; the rest of the carpus is displaced upward, backward, and outward.

Open reduction is rarely indicated in fresh lesions; it may be necessary in old lesions that cannot be reduced by closed methods.

Clinical Deformity

1. The injured wrist is always swollen after these injuries.
2. There is a distal dinner-folk deformity as a result of the dorsal displacement of the distal carpal row.

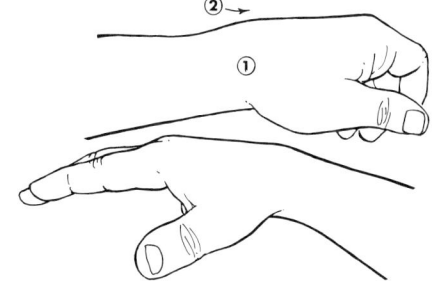

Prereduction X-Ray

1. The normal relationship of the lunate to the remaining carpal bones is lost; the carpus is displaced to the radial side.
2. The lunate is in normal relation with the radius.
3. The remaining carpus is displaced upward and backward.

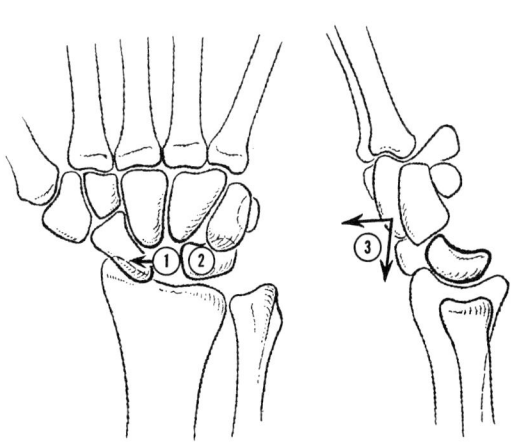

Reduction by Traction and Manipulation

Traction

1. Apply finger traction.
2. The elbow is flexed at a right angle.
3. The forearm is fully supinated.
4. Counter traction is accomplished by a muslin bandage attached to a water bucket.
5. Traction is maintained for at least five to ten minutes to overcome carpal shortening.

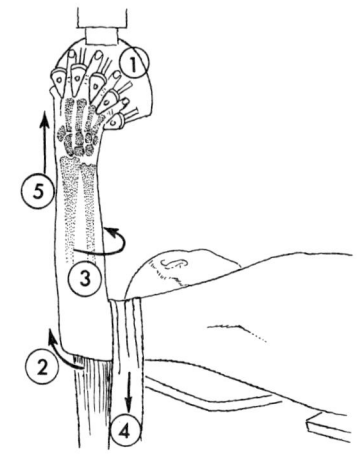

Manipulation

While traction is maintained:

1. Place both thumbs against the posterior aspect of the carpus and make strong pressure forward and outward, and at the same time flex the wrist.

Note: Check the position of the carpus by x-ray before applying the plaster cast.

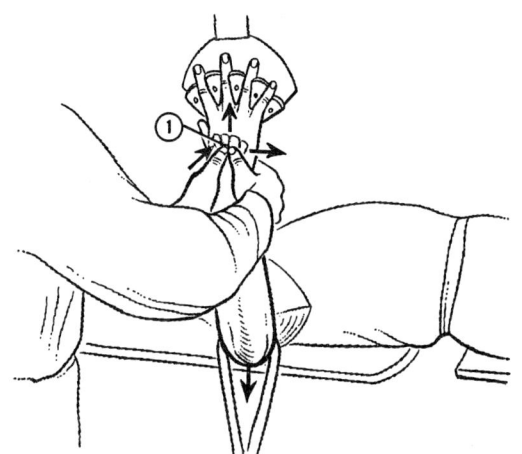

Postreduction X-Ray

The carpus is in normal anatomic alignment and the scapholunate space is less than 2 mm.

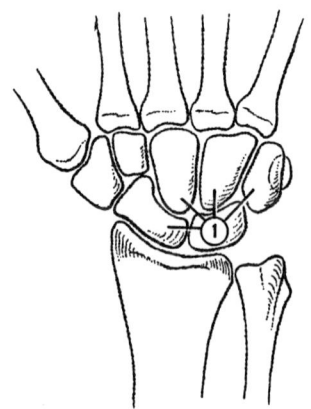

Immobilization

1. Apply anterior and posterior plaster slabs from just below the elbow to just proximal to the metacarpophalangeal joints.
2. The wrist is flexed 45 degrees.

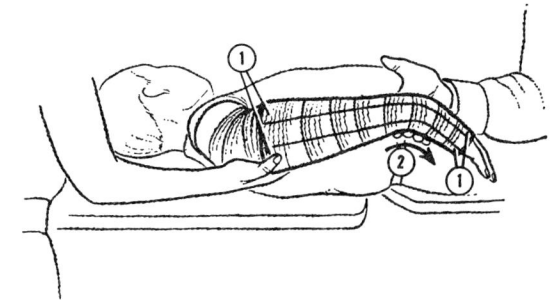

Postreduction Management

Remove the plaster slabs after one week, bring the wrist to a neutral position, and again immobilize with anterior and posterior plaster slabs.

Continue immobilization for 2 more weeks.

During immobilization, insist on a program of active finger exercises.

After removal of the plaster slabs, institute a regimen of physical therapy and active exercises for the wrist and fingers.

Prognosis in fresh dislocation is good; recovery should be complete in 8 to 12 weeks.

Note: The aforementioned method may be employed in old unreduced dislocation of several weeks' duration. As a rule, if this method fails, operative reduction is indicated.

Dorsal Perilunate Dislocation Complicated by Fracture or Dislocation of Other Carpal Bones

Dorsal perilunate dislocation is frequently complicated by lesions of the other carpal bones; the scaphoid is most frequently involved.

DORSAL PERILUNATE DISLOCATION WITH FRACTURE OF THE SCAPHOID WITHOUT DISPLACEMENT OF THE FRAGMENTS

REMARKS

Lack of displacement of the scaphoid fragments indicates that there is still continuity of the fragments through the articular cartilage. The prognosis is good.

Clinical Deformity

1. The injured wrist is always swollen after these injuries.
2. There is a distal dinner-fork deformity as a result of the dorsal displacement of the distal carpal row.

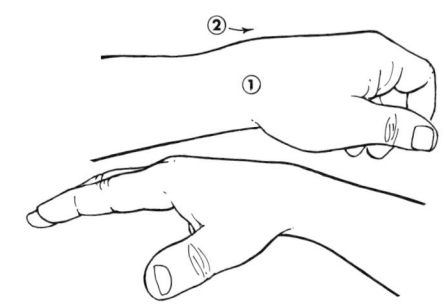

Appearance on X-Ray

1. Normal relationship of the lunate to the remaining carpal bones is lost; the carpus is displaced to the radial side.
2. The lunate is in normal relationship to the radius.
3. The remaining carpus is displaced upward and backward.
4. Fracture of the scaphoid with no displacement of the fragments.

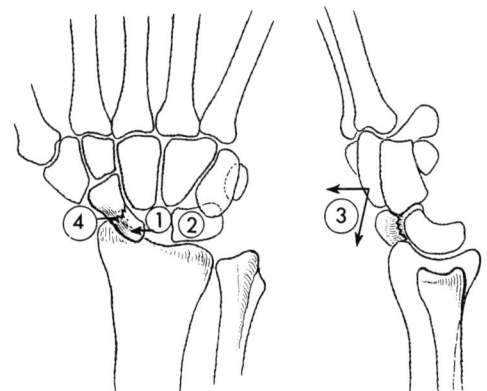

Management

Reduce the perilunate dislocation by traction and manipulation as described on page 1098.

Then treat the fracture of the scaphoid by continuous plaster fixation as described on page 1063.

DORSAL PERILUNATE DISLOCATION WITH FRACTURE OF THE SCAPHOID WITH DISPLACEMENT OF THE FRAGMENTS

REMARKS

The proximal fragment remains with the lunate and the distal fragment is displaced dorsally with the rest of the carpus. This is the usual occurrence with these fracture-dislocations.

Appearance on X-Ray

1. Fracture through the waist of the scaphoid.
2. Normal relationship of the carpal bones is disturbed; note the wide gap between the lunate and the capitate.
3. The lunate and the proximal half of the scaphoid are in normal relationship to the radius.
4. The carpus and the distal half of the scaphoid are displaced backward.
5. The carpus distal to the lunate and the proximal half of the scaphoid are displaced radially.

Note: Scaphoid fracture with this much displacement and instability of the carpus is best managed by primary internal fixation.

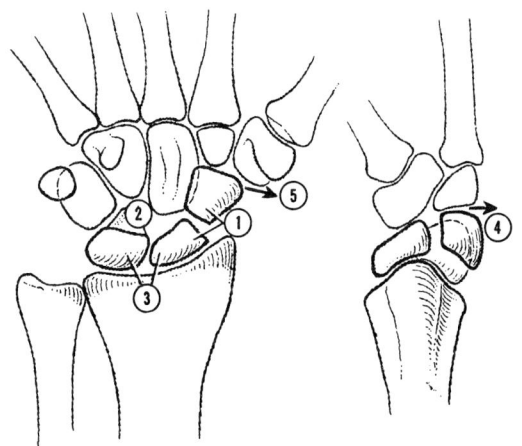

Management

Reduce the perilunate dislocation by traction and manipulation, as described on page 1098.

Then expose the scaphoid through a dorsal approach.

Realign the fragments and fix them internally with a lag screw or Kirschner wire, as described on page 1093.

DORSAL PERILUNATE DISLOCATION WITH FRACTURE OF THE CAPITATE

REMARKS

After reduction of the dislocation, the proximal fragment of the capitate may remain displaced.

Closed reduction usually fails; open operation is usually necessary to replace the fragment.

Results are poor if the fragment remains displaced.

If the fragment is small, remove it; if it is large, realign it with the distal fragment of the capitate and fix it with a threaded wire.

This fracture may also be associated with a displaced fracture of the scaphoid.

Appearance on X-Ray

1. Fracture of the capitate.
2. Fracture of the scaphoid with displacement.
3. Dorsal displacement of the carpus distal to the lunate.

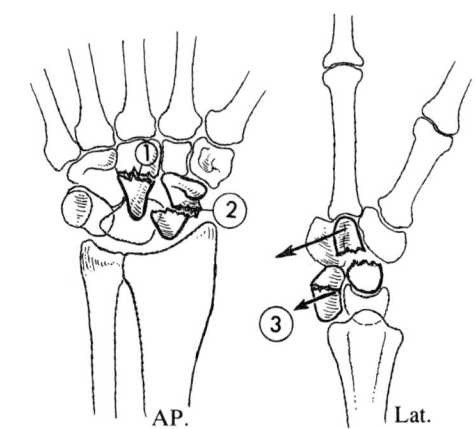

Management

Reduce the perilunar dislocation by traction and manipulation as described on page 1098.

Through a dorsal incision expose the capitate, scaphoid, and lunate bones.

With a blunt dissector, level the fragments of the capitate into normal position and transfix them with a threaded wire.

Note: If there is a displaced fracture of the scaphoid, realign the fragments and transfix them as described on page 1093.

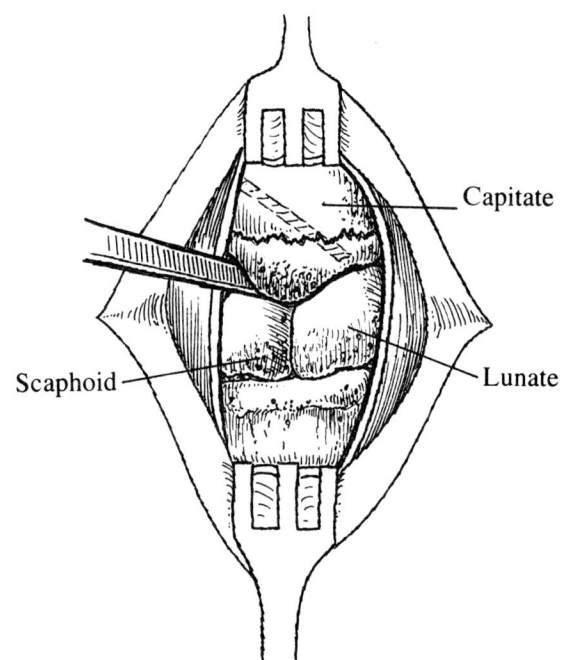

OTHER DISLOCATIONS AND SUBLUXATIONS OF THE CARPUS

Rotatory Subluxation of the Scaphoid-Scapholunate Dissociation

Rotatory subluxation of the scaphoid with its proximal pole displaced dorsally and its distal pole volarly may persist after incomplete reduction of carpal dislocation (see page 1091).

Rotatory subluxation can also occur independent of a carpal dislocation in individuals, such as carpenters, who use their wrists frequently in heavy labor.

The diagnosis can be recognized if it is specifically sought.

The patient characteristically has:
1. Pain in the radioscaphoid region, particularly on wrist extension.
2. A palpable click on extension of the wrist.
3. Loss of grip strength and decreased wrist motion.

For the gap between the scaphoid and lunate to be produced, the dorsal and palmar radiocarpal ligaments as well as the scapholunate interosseous ligaments must have ruptured. Reconstruction of these ligamentous structures is difficult, and results are generally less satisfactory than with early treatment.

When recognized early after injury, the subluxation can be treated by closed methods.

Occasionally, open reduction and Kirschner wire fixation of the scapholunate joint are necessary.

OTHER DISLOCATIONS AND SUBLUXATIONS OF THE CARPUS

Appearance on X-Ray

On the anteroposterior view of the supinated wrist,
1. The scapholunate space is widened more than 2 mm.

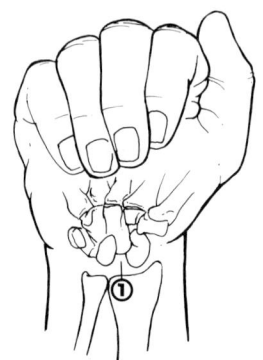

On the lateral view,
2. The scapholunate angle exceeds 70 degrees.
3. The capitate is subluxating proximally through the space between the scaphoid and the lunate.
4. The lunate is dorsiflexed and is not aligned with the long axis of the radius.

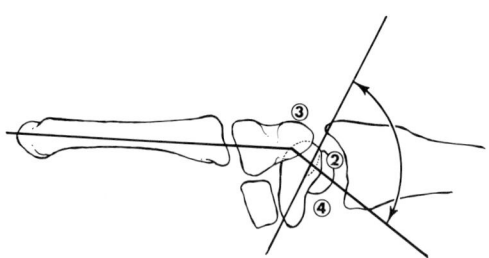

Pathomechanics

1. Disruption of the scapholunate ligaments on the dorsal and volar surface and
2. Rupture of the radioscaphoid ligaments allow rotatory displacement of the scaphoid and dorsiflexion collapse.

Note: Dorsiflexion collapse may also occur with a nonunion of the scaphoid (see page 1078).

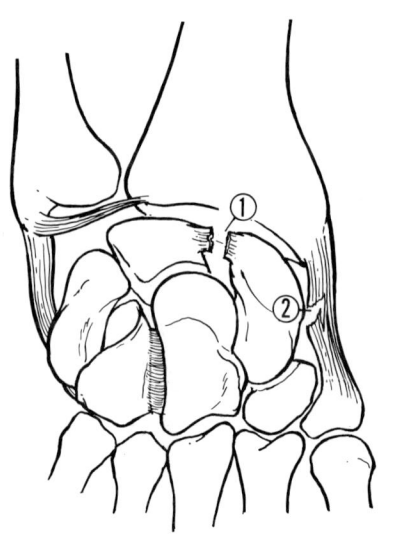

Closed Treatment

Reduction of the unstable scaphoid may be difficult but it is not impossible.

The reversal of the mechanism by which the injury was sustained helps to achieve alignment. If the injury occurred with the wrist in ulnar deviation, reduce it by radial deviation.

Alignment of the capitate with the lunate is best achieved by wrist extension.

Reduction must be confirmed on fluoroscopy. The alignment is then best maintained by two smooth Kirschner wires through the scaphoid into the capitate and the lunate.

1. The wrist is held in extension or radial deviation to close its scapholunate space.
2. A smooth Kirschner wire is inserted percutaneously through the scaphoid into the capitate and the lunate to maintain alignment.

Note: The best position for closed reduction should be determined by fluoroscopy. If closed reduction does not restore normal carpal relationships, open reduction and internal fixation are necessary.

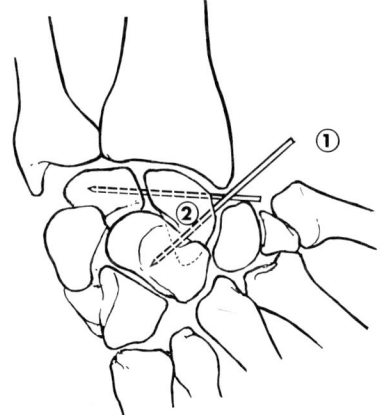

Subsequent Management

The hand and wrist are supported in a long arm cast.

The pins are left protruding slightly through the skin and are not buried in the plaster.

The cast and pins are removed after six weeks and the patient is allowed to begin range-of-motion exercises to the wrist.

Dorsal Periscapholunate Dislocation

REMARKS

In this lesion the lunate and scaphoid remain articulated with the radius while the remaining carpus displaces dorsally. The scaphoid may be forced into a volar position as the carpus is shortened.

After reduction always check for any malposition of the scaphoid. Usually realignment is achieved by closed reduction. Open reduction is rarely indicated except in old fracture-dislocations.

Appearance on X-Ray

1. The scaphoid and lunate articulate with the radius.
2. The remaining carpus is displaced dorsally and proximally.

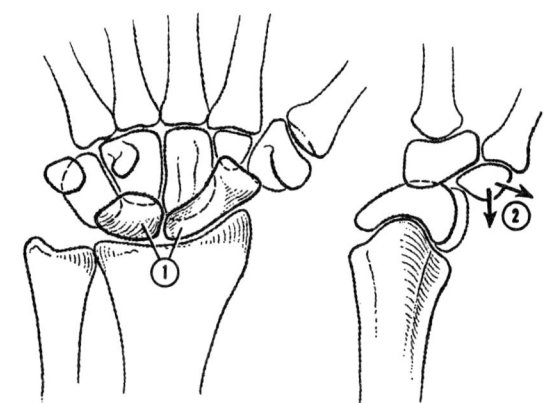

Management

Reduce the dislocation by traction and manipulation as described for perilunate dislocation (page 1098).

Dislocation of the Lunate and the Proximal Half of the Scaphoid

Appearance on X-Ray

1. The lunate and the proximal half of the scaphoid do not articulate with the radius but are in an anterior position.
2. The capitate articulates with the radius.

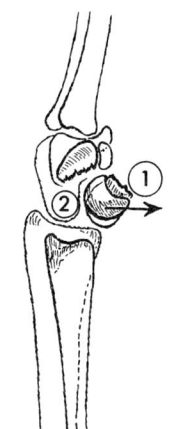

After reduction the fragments of the scaphoid usually remain displaced. Open reduction and internal fixation are generally needed as described on page 1093.

Dislocation of the Lunate and Entire Scaphoid

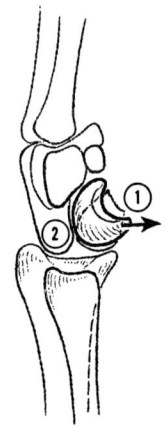

Appearance on X-Ray

1. The lunate and the entire scaphoid are displaced anteriorly.
2. The capitate articulates with the radius.

Management

Reduce the dislocation by traction and manipulation as described for dislocation of the lunate (page 1088).

Dislocation of the Metacarpal Bones on the Carpus

Appearance on X-Ray

1. The metacarpal bones together with
2. The trapezium are displaced anterior to the remaining carpus.
3. The trapezoid is displaced to the dorsum of the wrist on the ulnar side. (In this instance this bone was excised.)

Note: This degree of disruption is likely to damage the motor branch of the ulnar nerve. Check ulnar nerve function carefully before and after reduction. If the nerve is involved, perform open reduction and pin fixation (page 1194).

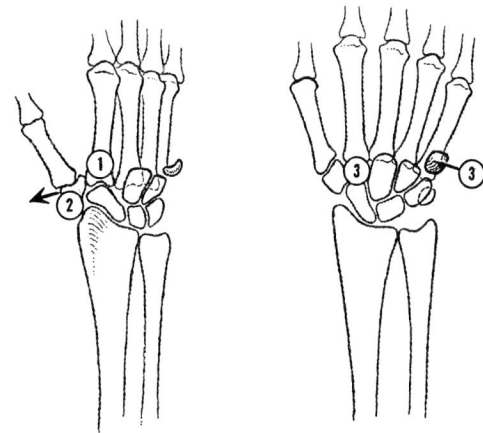

Reduction by Traction and Manipulation

Note: This method applies to most carpal dislocations. The direction of manipulation varies with the direction of displacement.

Traction

1. Apply finger traction.
2. The elbow is flexed at a right angle.
3. The forearm is fully supinated.
4. Counter traction is made by a muslin bandage with a weight attached.
5. Make strong traction directly upward for at least five minutes.

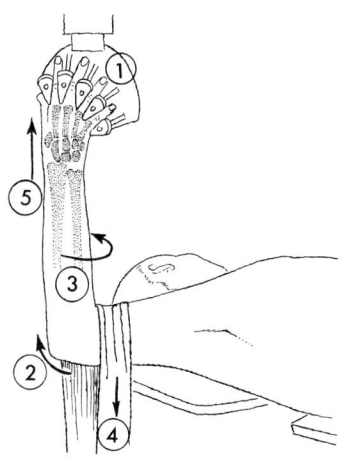

1109

Reduction by Traction and Manipulation (Continued)

Manipulation

While traction is maintained, pressure is made on the displaced elements.

1. If one or two metacarpal bones are displaced anteriorly, pressure is made directly backward, and at the same time.
2. The wrist is dorsiflexed.
3. If these elements are displaced posteriorly, pressure is made directly forward and
4. The wrist is flexed in a palmar direction.

Note: If lateral displacement is present, pressure is directed in the opposite direction to correct it.

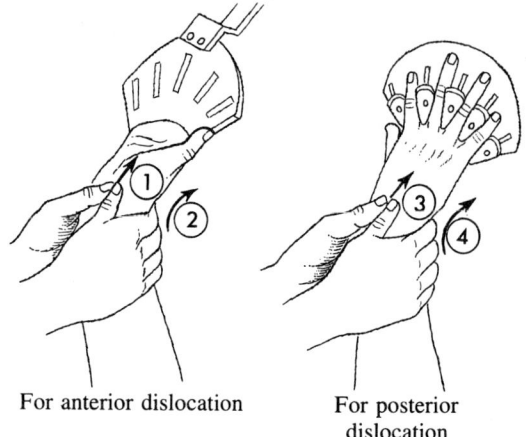

For anterior dislocation   For posterior dislocation

Immobilization

1. Apply anterior and posterior plaster slabs; flex the wrist for anterior dislocation.

Frequently, transcutaneous pin fixation is necessary in order to stabilize the carpometacarpal joint (see page 1113).

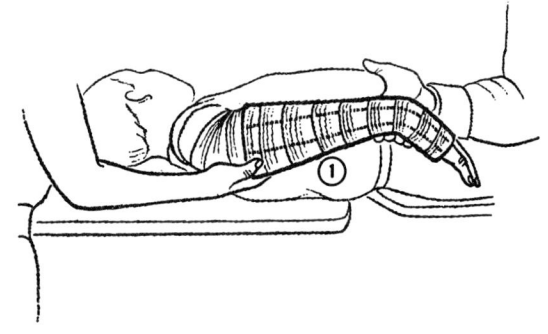

Postreduction Management

Carefully evaluate the postreduction x-ray to insure that an anatomic reduction has been achieved. If the carpus has not been completely reduced, open reduction is indicated.

Following adequate closed reduction, change the plaster splints to a long arm cast when the swelling subsides, usually by five to seven days.

For dislocations without fracture, the cast may usually be removed by the end of four weeks. Fracture-dislocations require immobilization until bony union of the fractured carpal bone is complete.

Dislocation of the Trapezoid (Lesser Multangular)

REMARKS

This is a rare lesion. It may occur as an isolated injury or with other lesions of the carpal bones.
The dislocation is usually dorsal, but in rare instances it is volar.
Aseptic necrosis of the bone is a common sequela.

Management

Closed reduction rarely is successful.
Excision of the bone is the procedure of choice, whether dislocation has occurred as an isolated lesion or with other carpal injuries.

Disruption of the Proximal Row of the Carpus

REMARKS

Occasionally, as a result of severe violence, the proximal carpal row can be completely disrupted and the scaphoid and lunate can be fractured and dislocated.
Because of the multiplicity of injury and the likelihood of persistent traumatic arthritis, particularly from the lunate fracture, excision of the proximal carpal row may be justified rarely as a primary procedure.
This means excision of the lunate, scaphoid, and triquetrum. Although the result is usually not an excellent one, the patient generally has a painless wrist with varying degrees of restriction of motion. This procedure is preferable to primary arthrodesis of the wrist.
Wrist immobilization should be maintained for six weeks to achieve a fibrous ankylosis. Should the patient suffer persistent pain with motion after a proximal row resection, a total wrist arthroplasty or arthrodesis may be employed as a secondary procedure.

Appearance on X-Ray

1. Dorsal perilunar dislocation of the carpus.
2. The lunate is fractured.
3. The scaphoid is fractured and its distal fragment is dislocated on the radius.

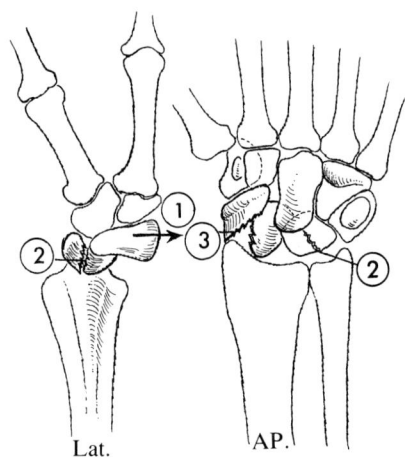

Postoperative X-Ray

1. The proximal row of carpal bones (except the pisiform) has been excised.

Note: Immobilize the wrist for at least six weeks to achieve a fibrous ankylosis. If the patient has persistent pain on wrist motion, a total wrist arthroplasty or arthrodesis may be used as a secondary procedure (see page 1079).

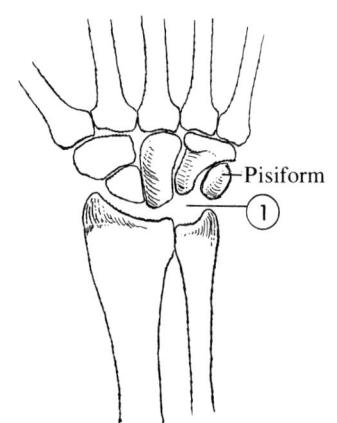

Disruption of the Distal Row of the Carpus (Proximal Carpal Arch)

REMARKS

Crush injuries to the hand can disrupt the stabilizing transverse arch, which includes the distal carpal row (see page 1054).

Damage to the bony and ligamentous support that is provided by the capitate and hamate is particularly likely to disrupt the stability of the arch. This is reflected clinically as rotational finger deformities and flattening of the palm, which should be corrected by restoring the continuity between the capitate and hamate.

Since the distal carpal row also forms the floor of the carpal tunnel, decompression of the median nerve is also necessary with these injuries.

Preoperative X-Ray

1. Crush injury to the hand leaves the patient with a widening of the capitate-hamate articulation.
2. Clinical malrotation of the ring and small fingers may go unexplained if there is no fracture of the metacarpal bones or phalanx.

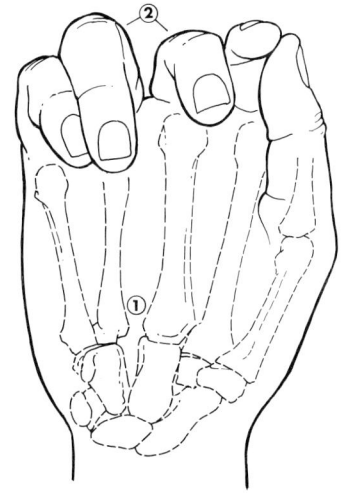

After Open Reduction of the Distal Carpal Row

1. The capitate-hamate articulation has been reduced and fixed with Kirschner wire.
2. There is normal convergence with finger flexion.

Note: Decompression of the median nerve in the carpal tunnel is also necessary.

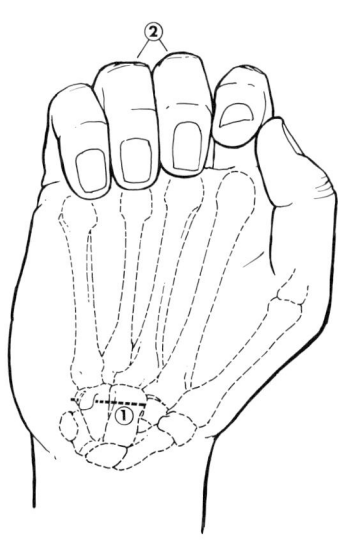

Volar Perilunate Dislocation and Fracture-Dislocation

REMARKS

These are indeed rare lesions. Volar perilunate dislocation may be complicated by fracture or fracture-dislocation of the scaphoid just as the dorsal lesion.

Volar Perilunate Dislocation

1. The lunate is in normal relation to the radius.
2. The remaining carpus is displaced anterior to the lunate.

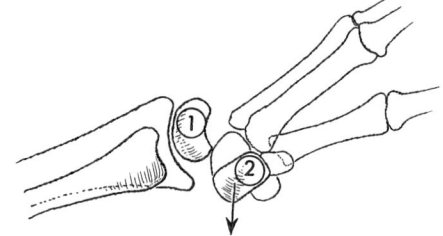

The principles of management are the same as for dorsal dislocation with or without associated fractures of other carpal bones.

FRACTURES OF THE CARPAL BONES

Fracture of the Capitate

Anatomic Considerations

Its size and relationships to the other carpal bones make the capitate vulnerable to injury; it is the largest of all the carpal bones and articulates with seven bones: the scaphoid and the lunate proximally, the lesser multangular on the radial side, the hamate on the ulnar side, and the second, third, and fourth metacarpals distally.

The capitate receives its blood supply from vessels penetrating the dorsal surface of the neck and waist of the bone, so that trauma may sever a portion of the bone from an adequate blood supply, thus causing aseptic necrosis of the affected segment.

It is firmly anchored to the bases of the second, third, and fourth metacarpal bones by an intricate system of tough intercarpal ligaments.

The capitate is intimately related to the axial motion of the third metacarpal bone.

1. The capitate, the largest bone, occupies a central position in the carpus.
2. Distally it articulates with the second, third, and fourth metacarpals.
3. Proximally it articulates with the scaphoid and lunate.
4. It is related to the axial movements of the third metacarpal.

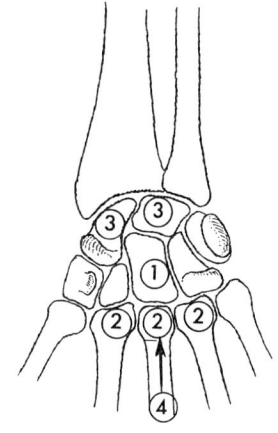

FRACTURES OF THE CARPAL BONES

Mechanism of Fracture

Fractures of the capitate are produced either as the result of direct or indirect violence:

1. Direct violence causes injury to other carpal bones.
2. Indirect violence due to a fall on the outstretched hand is by far the most common mechanism. The type of lesion produced depends on the direction of the hand and wrist.
   a. If the hand and wrist are dorsiflexed and are deviated toward the ulna, the lunate is caught between the radius and the capitate and is squeezed volarly out of the wrist joint. This lesion may be associated with a fracture of the distal tip of the radius or the capitate.
   b. If the hand and wrist are dorsiflexed and are deviated toward the radius, the styloid process of the radius digs into the waist of the scaphoid, producing a fracture; with continuance of the force the capitate is also fractured through its waist and the proximal fragments may rotate as much as 180 degrees.

Also, trauma to the radial side of the dorsum of the hand with the wrist flexed in a palmar direction may result in a fracture of the capitate.

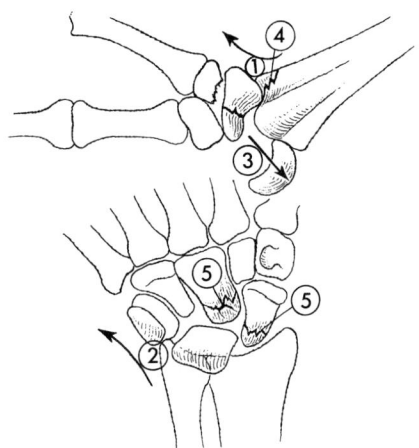

1. Wrist is in extreme dorsiflexion.
2. The wrist and the hand are deviated toward the ulna.
3. Lunate is forced volarly out of the wrist joint.
4. The distal tip of the radius may fracture.
5. The capitate may fracture; also, a fracture may occur through the proximal head of the scaphoid.

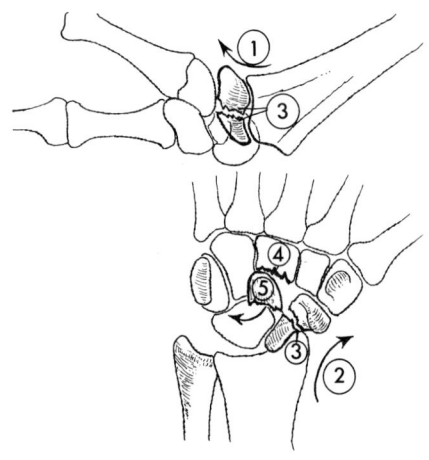

1. The wrist is in extreme dorsiflexion.
2. The wrist and the hand are deviated toward the radius.
3. The styloid process of the radius digs into the waist of the scaphoid, producing a fracture. With continuance of the force
4. The capitate fractures through the waist and
5. Its proximal fragment rotates (almost 180 degrees).

Many fractures of the capitate are missed; take oblique x-rays and laminograms to establish the diagnosis, especially if symptoms localized to the region of the capitate persist.

The fractures may be transverse (the most common), oblique, vertical, and incomplete.

Most of the fractures are isolated lesions, although many are associated with other carpal injuries.

When the scaphoid and capitate bones alone are involved, the combination is referred to as the "scaphoid-capitate fracture syndrome."

MANAGEMENT OF ISOLATED FRACTURE OF THE CAPITATE

REMARKS

Most of these lesions are the result of a fall on the palm of the hand.
Most fractures are transverse and show little or no displacement.
Simple plaster fixation for eight weeks is adequate treatment.
Bony union is the rule.
If fibrous union or avascular necrosis of a fragment occurs and produces painful disability, the fragment should be excised.

Immobilization

1. Apply a plaster cast from below the elbow to the metacarpophalangeal joints.
2. The thumb is in the grasp position and is included in the cast up to the base of the thumbnail.
3. The wrist is only slightly dorsiflexed; otherwise it is in the neutral position.

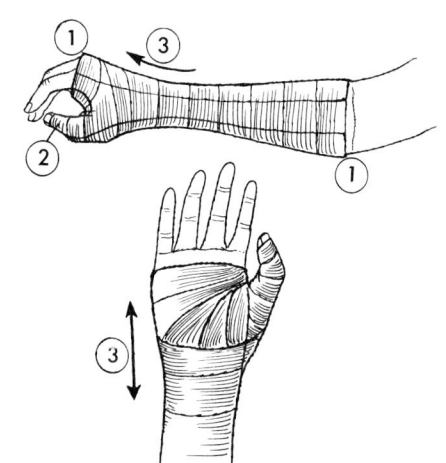

Subsequent Management

Maintain immobilization for six weeks.
Reapply the cast every two or three weeks if it should get loose.
After six weeks remove the cast and
Institute a program of physical therapy to restore finger and wrist motion.

Note: If fibrous union or aseptic necrosis of the proximal fragment occurs and produces a painful wrist, excise the fragment through a dorsal incision.

MANAGEMENT OF "SCAPHOID-CAPITATE FRACTURE SYNDROME"

REMARKS

As a rule, the fracture of the capitate is transverse and the proximal fracture is rotated up to 180 degrees.

This lesion may have been produced in association with a dorsal perilunate dislocation that reduced spontaneously. In these instances the proximal capitate fragment may remain in a displaced position on the dorsum of the wrist.

In most instances the fracture of the capitate should be fixed internally, but very small displaced fragments may be excised.

The incidence of traumatic arthritis when the fragments are unreduced, particularly if the proximal fragment is rotated, is very high. Operative reduction gives the best chance for a satisfactory result.

Operative Procedure

1. Make a transverse incision on the dorsum of the wrist at a level just proximal to the base of the third metacarpal.
2. Divide the deep fascia longitudinally in line with the shaft of the third metacarpal.
3. Deepen the incision between the extensor tendons of the fourth and fifth fingers.

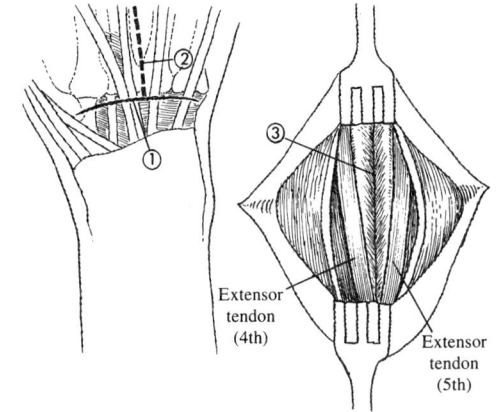

1. By sharp dissection, expose the fragments of the capitate. (Do not strip them of soft tissue attachment any more than is necessary.)
2. With a blunt dissector pry the proximal fragment into its normal position and transfix the fragments with a 2-mm threaded wire. Cut the wire below the level of the skin.

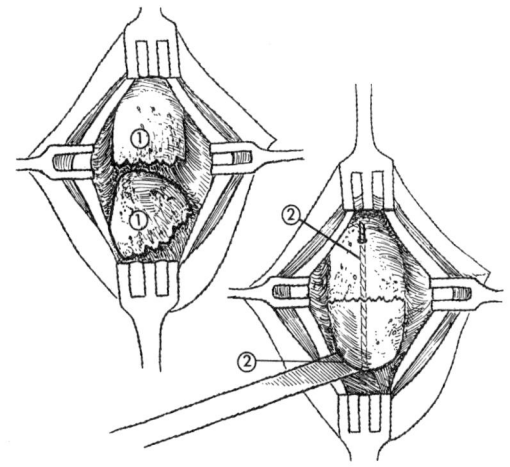

If there is an unstable fracture of the scaphoid:
1. Expose the styloid process of the radius.
2. Divide the dorsal carpal ligament and deep fascia longitudinally between the extensor pollicis longus and the extensor tendon of the index finger; open the capsule to expose the scaphoid.
3. Make traction on the hand toward the ulna to bring into view both fragments of the scaphoid.

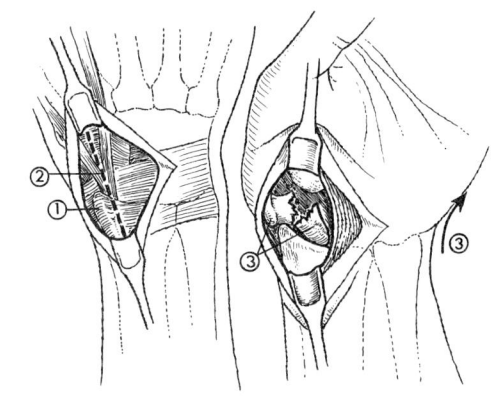

1. Lever the fragments into normal position.
2. Transfix them with a threaded 2-mm wire or a lag screw (see page 1093).

Note: If necessary, run the wire through the lunate for further stability.

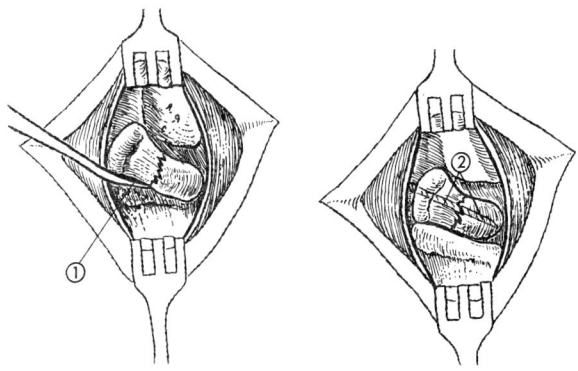

Postoperative Immobilization

Apply anterior and posterior plaster splints holding the wrist slightly dorsiflexed and otherwise in the neutral position. After 10 to 14 days apply a circular cast.
1. The cast extends from below the elbow to the metacarpophalangeal joints.
2. The thumb is in the grasp position and is included in the cast to the base of the thumbnail.
3. The wrist is slightly dorsiflexed; otherwise it is in the neutral position.

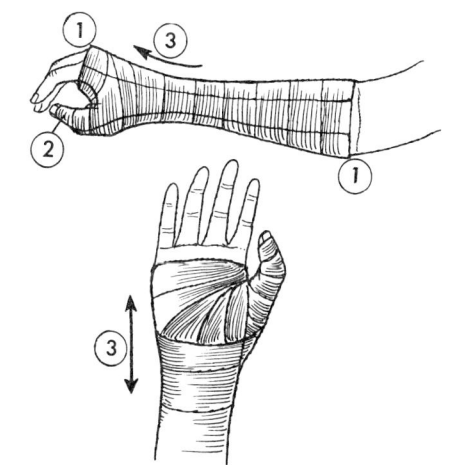

Remove the wires at the end of 6 to 8 weeks.

Continue immobilization in plaster until bony union is achieved (usually 3 to 4 months).

If bony union is not obtained in 6 months, take the cast off and mobilize the wrist.

Note: Some cases of radiographically apparent nonunion will eventually achieve bony union after the cast is removed. Also, avascular necrosis of the proximal fragments of the capitate or of the scaphoid does not preclude achievement of a painless wrist with good function.

MANAGEMENT OF CAPITATE FRACTURE ASSOCIATED WITH OTHER CARPAL INJURIES

In general, treatment of these injuries is the same as that described for isolated capitate fracture and scaphoid-capitate fracture, except that the treatment is also directed to the other associated injuries, which in some instances may be more severe than the fracture of the capitate; for example, a fracture of the distal end of the radius.

If the principles of the treatment of capitate fracture just described are adhered to when the fracture is associated with other carpal injuries, a plan of adequate management should readily evolve.

Fractures of the Triquetrum

REMARKS

The triquetrum is frequently fractured, but it is rarely displaced because of its strong ligamentous support.

These fractures may frequently be overlooked on x-ray unless an oblique projection is obtained.

Mechanism of Fracture

By direct violence to the dorsum of the hand.

Extreme dorsiflexion, as in a fall on the outstretched hand (this is the most common mechanism), or extreme palmar flexion due to a fall on the flexed hand.

Twisting movements against resistance.

The type of fracture may be a chip fracture, varying in size, of the dorsum of the bone with some separation of the fragments or a fracture of the body which may also be comminuted.

Separation of fragments is never marked; bony union is the rule; fibrous union occurs rarely. Aseptic necrosis does not occur.

The lesions may be isolated or associated with other injuries, such as fractures of the scaphoid or of the distal end of the radius.

Untreated cases frequently masquerade as chronic sprains of the wrist.

Appearance on X-Ray

LATERAL VIEW

1. Chip fracture from dorsum of the bone.

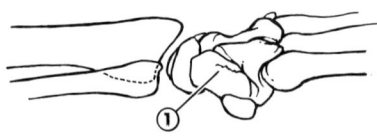

OBLIQUE VIEW

1. Fracture through the body of the bone.

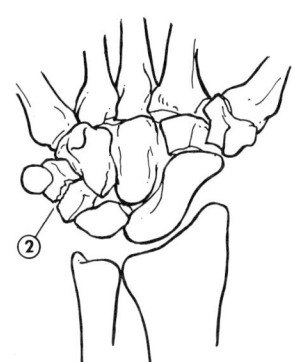

MANAGEMENT OF ISOLATED FRACTURES

Immobilization

1. Apply a well-molded short arm cast from below the elbow to the metacarpal joints. The wrist is slightly dorsiflexed.
2. The thumb is free.
3. The fingers are free to flex and extend fully.

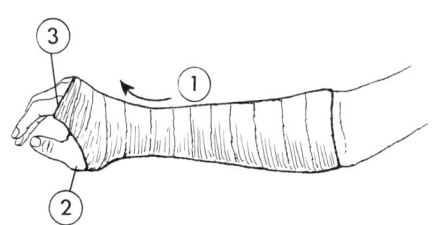

Subsequent Management

Remove the cast after six to eight weeks, regardless of what the status of union may be as interpreted on x-ray.

The wearing of a wrist support for several weeks after the cast is removed may be helpful in some instances.

Institute a program of physical therapy and exercises to restore normal motion of the fingers and wrist.

Note: Union may be delayed, especially in fractures with separation of the fragments. Bony union may not occur for many weeks after the cast is removed; fibrous union or delayed union does not preclude achievement of good wrist function without pain.

MANAGEMENT OF FRACTURES OF THE TRIQUETRUM ASSOCIATED WITH OTHER INJURIES

When triquetrum fracture is associated with other injuries, attention should be directed to the treatment of the other injuries, because they are usually more serious.

The most common associated fractures are fracture of the scaphoid and fracture of the distal end of the radius.

Fractures of the Pisiform

REMARKS

The anatomic features of this bone render it vulnerable to injury.

Its volar surface is attached to the volar ligament and the tendon of the flexor carpi ulnaris, which sends fibrous strands to the hamate and metacarpal bones, forming the pisohamate and pisometacarpal ligaments.

The dorsal surface of the pisiform articulates with the triquetrum, forming the pisotriquetrum joint, which is enclosed in a tough fibrous capsule.

Mechanism of Injury

The bone may be fractured by direct trauma (the most common mechanism) or by forceful hyperextension, as in a fall on the outstretched hand, or with forceful dorsiflexion of the wrist against resistance.

The types of fracture produced are:
  Avulsion fracture by the action of the flexor carpi ulnaris.
  Transverse or linear fracture of the body of the pisiform.
  Comminuted fracture.

Because the capsule and ligaments are attached to the bone, separation of the fragments is never marked.

The fractures may be isolated lesions or may be associated with other carpal injuries.

The diagnosis is often missed; oblique x-ray projections are necessary to show the lesions.

Appearance on X-Ray

1. Fracture of pisiform involving the articular surface.

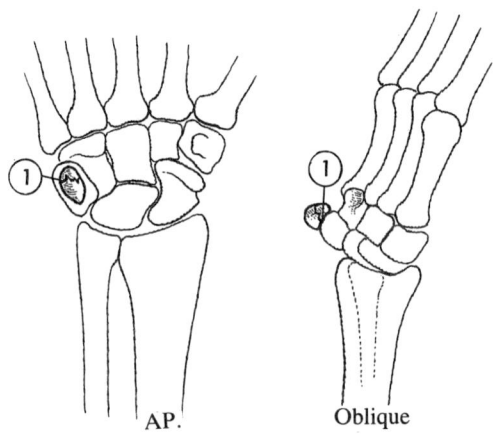

1. Comminuted fracture of pisiform can be seen on oblique view.
Nonunion is rare but may occur; bony union is nearly always achieved and recovery is usually complete.

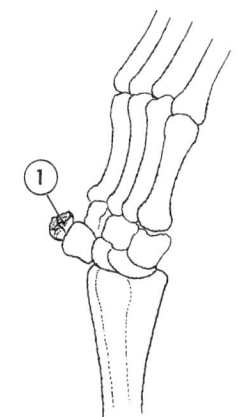

MANAGEMENT OF AN ISOLATED LESION

Immobilization

1. Apply a well-molded short arm cast from below the elbow to the metacarpophalangeal joints.
2. The thumb is free.
3. The fingers are free to flex and extend fully.

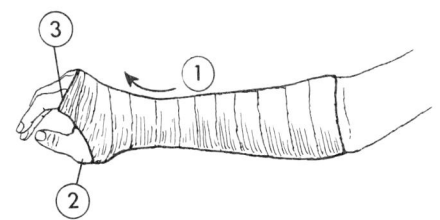

Subsequent Management

Remove the cast after four weeks.
Institute a program of physical therapy and exercises to restore normal finger and wrist motion.

MANAGEMENT OF FRACTURE OF THE PISIFORM ASSOCIATED WITH OTHER CARPAL INJURIES

When pisiform fracture is associated with other injuries, attention should be directed to treatment of the other injuries, because they are usually more serious.

The most common associated fractures are fractures of the triquetrum, of the hamate, and of the distal end of the radius.

CHRONIC SPRAIN OF THE PISOTRIQUETRAL JOINT

Persistent pain localized over the pisiform and aggravated by radial deviation of the wrist may be caused by a chronic sprain of the pisotriquetral joint, usually seen in women. Pain may be referred to the fourth and fifth fingers.

Treat this lesion as a strain.
Injection of a steroid into the joint may be effective.
If symptoms persist, excise the pisiform bone.
Do not traumatize the ulnar nerve.

Calcification, such as is seen in the supraspinatus tendon, may occur in the tendon of the flexor carpi ulnaris, producing an acute or chronic syndrome. Treat this lesion as you would a calcific deposit causing pain in the supraspinatus tendon.

Fracture of the Hook of the Hamate

REMARKS

Fracture of the hook of the hamate may be caused by a fall or a crushing injury.

It is most often a diagnostic problem in athletes who sustain a direct blow against the hamate by the handle of a tennis racquet, golf club, or bat during an unbalanced swing.

The hamate hook is not fractured by indirect forces of attached ligaments or muscle, but these structures interfere with bone healing by exerting intermittent forces on the hamate.

Characteristically, the diagnosis is delayed one or more months because the x-ray views usually taken of the wrist do not demonstrate the lesion.

Occasionally, rupture of the finger flexor tendons, secondary either to the fracture or to cortisone injections, may occur.

Typically, the patient has pain localized to the dorsal ulnar aspect of the wrist rather than over the hamate, because the fracture is usually at the base of the hook.

Diagnosis depends on a suspicion from the history and the physical examination and particularly on adequate carpal tunnel x-rays.

Although this fracture may unite if the hand and wrist are immobilized in plaster after the acute injury, in most instances excision of the fracture fragment is necessary.

Mechanism of Injury

1. The fracture always occurs in the hand that grasps the end of the club, bat, or racquet.
2. The butt end of the club strikes the hook of the hamate when the patient loses control of his swing.

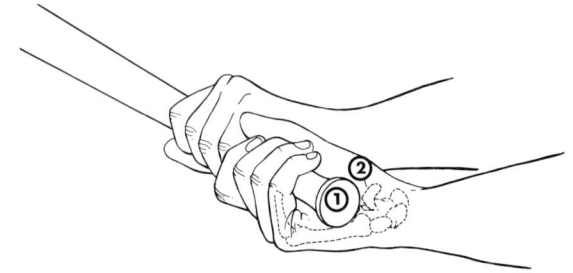

X-Ray Technique for Carpal Tunnel View

1. Place a radiolucent pad 2 cm thick between the wrist and the casette.
2. Have the patient hold the wrist in maximum dorsiflexion by pulling the fingers dorsally with the opposite hand.
3. Direct the central ray to a point approximately 2.5 cm distal to the base of the fourth metacarpal.
4. Angle the tube 25 degrees toward the horizontal from the long axis of the hand.

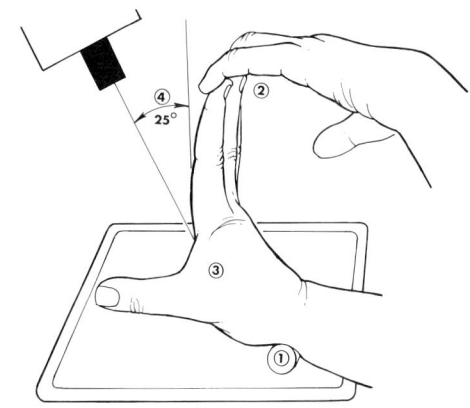

Preoperative X-Ray

1. The carpal tunnel view shows a one-month-old fracture of the hook of the left hamate in a baseball player.

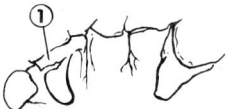

Operative Treatment: Excision of the Fractured Fragment

1. Use Henry's medial approach to avoid scarring in the palmar skin.

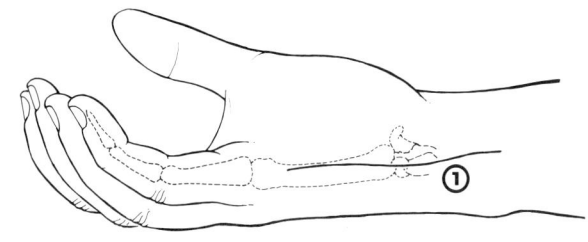

2. The superficial and
3. The deep branches of the ulnar nerve are identified and protected.
4. After the periosteum is stripped, the hamate fragment is removed, the base of the hamate is smoothed, and the wound is closed.

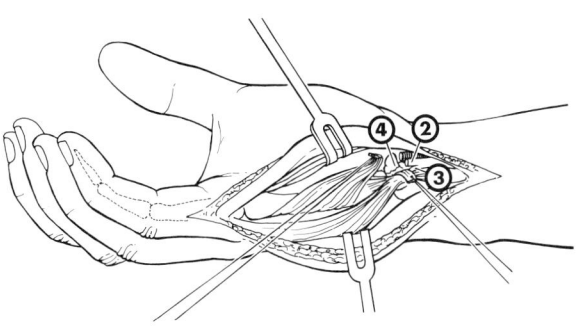

Postoperative Management

Apply a plaster cast with the wrist in neutral position.

Maintain plaster immobilization for two to three weeks, and remove the cast.

The patient may be allowed to use the hand for all activities as soon as the local tenderness has subsided.

Fracture of the Trapezium (Greater Multangular)

Mechanism of Injury

Fracture of the trapezium is produced by direct trauma to the radiodorsal aspect of the joint or by extreme dorsiflexion of the wrist, as occurs in a fall on the outstretched hand. The bone is caught between the styloid process of the radius and the base of the first metacarpal bone.

The fracture may be an isolated lesion or may be associated with other carpal lesions, the most common being fracture of the first metacarpal and fracture of the distal end of the radius.

Anatomic Features

The trapezium (greater multangular) is trapezoid in shape and articulates with the first and second metacarpals, the scaphoid, and the trapezoid (lesser multangular).

The articulation with the first metacarpal is saddle-shaped and is enveloped in a loose capsule, permitting a wide range of motion.

Fractures may be of various types: vertical, comminuted, or avulsion fractures. The vertical type is by far the most common and is invariably associated with dislocation of the first metacarpal bone.

Management

Accurate restoration of the fragments is most essential for normal function of the thumb; therefore, open reduction and internal fixation, unless contraindicated, are the treatment of choice.

Appearance on X-Ray

1. Fracture of the trapezium.
2. The outer fragment is displaced proximally.
3. The articular surface of the first metacarpal is subluxated.

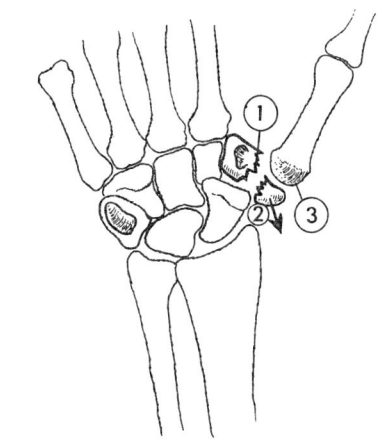

Operative Procedure

1. Make a 5-cm transverse incision proximal to the base of the first metacarpal.
2. Identify the cutaneous branch of the radial nerve and retract it ulnarward.
3. Retract the abductor pollicis longus and the extensor pollicis brevis volarward.
4. Retract the extensor pollicis longus together with the radial artery dorsally.
5. Divide longitudinally for 2 cm the dorsal carpal ligament.

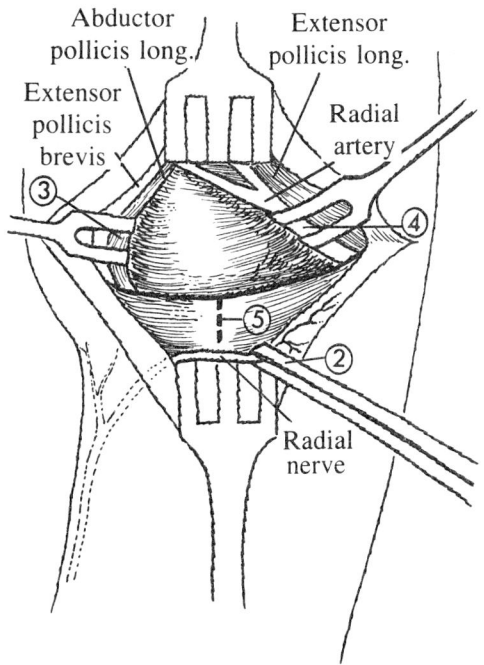

Operative Procedure (Continued)

1. Open the capsule with a transverse incision.
2. Make traction on the thumb and bring the fracture into view.
3. Approximate the fragments and hold them with a towel clip.
4. Transfix the fragments with a 2-mm threaded wire.
5. Cut the wire below the level of the skin.

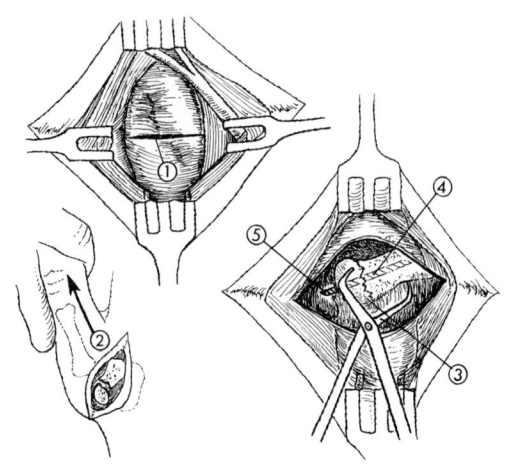

Postoperative Immobilization

1. Apply a plaster cast from below the elbow to the metacarpophalangeal joints, including the thumb to the base of the thumbnail.
2. The thumb is in the grasp position.
3. The wrist is slightly dorsiflexed; otherwise it is in the neutral position.

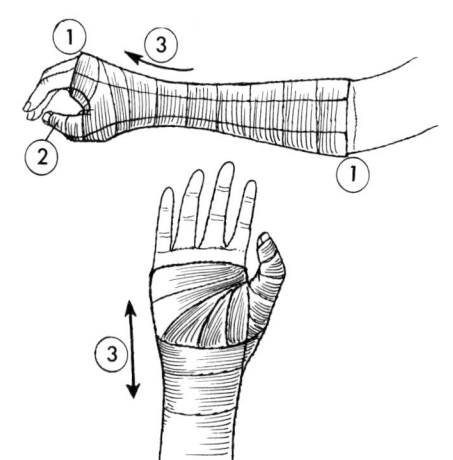

Subsequent Management

Remove the cast after six weeks.
Institute a program of physical therapy and exercises to restore motion of the fingers, thumb, and wrist.

MANAGEMENT OF SEVERELY COMMINUTED FRACTURES OF THE TRAPEZIUM

REMARKS

In this instance, excision of the bone fragments is preferable. The thumb is immobilized in the position of function for six weeks to allow for soft tissue healing and stability. Subsequent circumduction of the thumb should then be pain free.

Preoperative X-Ray

1. Severe comminution of the trapezium.
2. Proximal displacement of the first metacarpal.

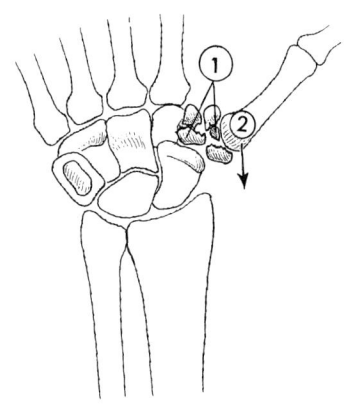

Postoperative X-Ray

1. The comminuted fracture fragments have been surgically excised.
2. The thumb and first metacarpal are stabilized externally in a position of function using a cast for six weeks.

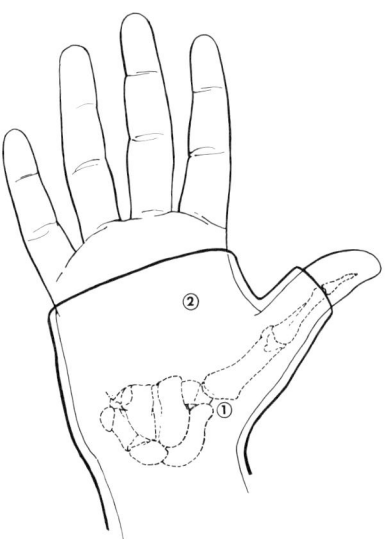

NEUROLOGIC COMPLICATIONS OF CARPAL INJURIES

Ulnar Nerve Involvement

REMARKS

In closed fractures of the pisiform, hamate, triquetrum, and fourth and fifth metacarpals, the motor branch of the ulnar nerve, which is the chief motor nerve of the hand, may be injured; the sensory branch is rarely affected.

Blunt trauma to the hypothenar eminence of the hand may also contuse the ulnar nerve.

Following fracture or soft tissue injuries, the nerve may be compressed by edema or hemorrhage. Intraneural fibrosis may result, as indicated by delayed or progressive paralysis of the intrinsic muscles of the hand.

Management

If there is a large hematoma it should be evacuated. Generally, spontaneous recovery occurs; however, if there is no recovery after six to eight weeks the ulnar nerve should be explored.

If the nerve is being compressed, excise the tight ligament.

If a neuroma is present, excise it.

Decompression and neurolysis of the nerve may be necessary, particularly with injuries to the hamate or to the bases of the fourth and fifth metacarpals. Approach the ulnar nerve via a lateral exposure around the pisiform (see page 1125).

Median Nerve Involvement

CARPAL TUNNEL SYNDROME

REMARKS

This disorder is characterized by sensory disturbances in the index and middle fingers such as tingling. Pressure over the volar ligament accentuates pain and paresthesia along the course of the median nerve.

Late in the disorder the thenar eminence exhibits muscular atrophy.

Implication of the median nerve is the result of compression due to (1) constriction of the osseofibrous tunnel containing the flexor tendons of the fingers and the median nerve or (2) swelling of the structures within the tunnel, as in tenosynovitis of the flexor tendons. Direct trauma to the volar aspect of the wrist may cause swelling of the volar ligament.

Occasionally the syndrome is associated with Colles' fracture, fracture of one of the carpal bones, or perilunar dislocation.

During the early stages of the disorder, simple rest of the limb in a plaster splint for several weeks will permit subsidence of any reactive process of the structure within the tunnel or of the walls of the tunnel and hence decompression of the median nerve ensues. If conservative measures fail, either in recent lesions or in old established syndromes, resection of a portion of the volar ligament is the treatment of choice.

Appearance on X-Ray

RECENT LESION

1. Perilunar dislocation.
2. Fracture of the scaphoid.

This patient had an acute compression of the median nerve.

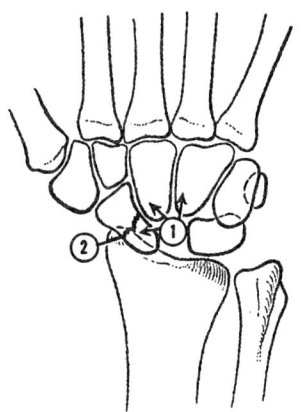

Appearance on X-Ray (Continued)

OLD LESION

1. Old nonunion of fractured scaphoid.
2. The ulnar fragment is dense and sclerotic.
3. The radiocarpal joint is thin.
4. Osteophytes indicative of advanced osteoarthritis.

Note: This lesion was six years old and was complicated by compression of the median nerve.

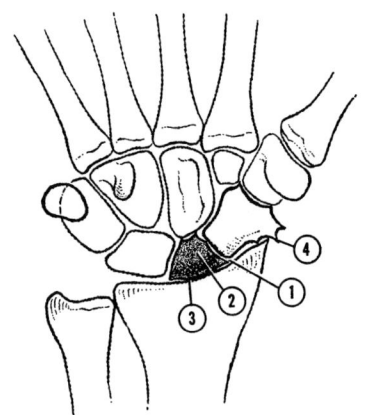

Operative Procedure

1. Make a curved incision distal to the thenar eminence and avoiding the superficial branch of the median nerve, which lies just above the tuberosity of the scaphoid.

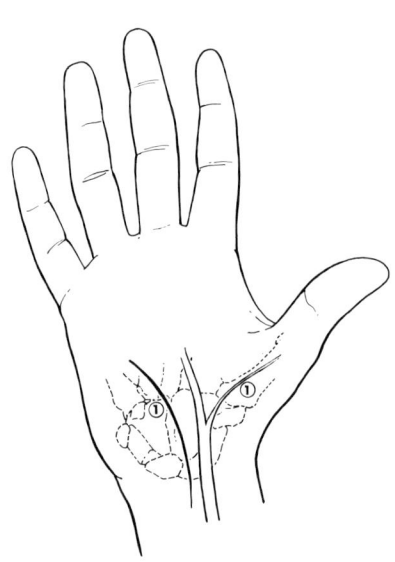

2. Make a longitudinal incision in the transverse carpal ligament; retract its margins.

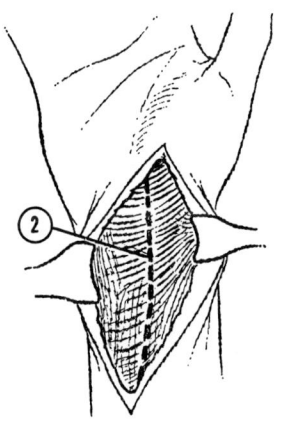

1. Expose the median nerve; it is compressed.

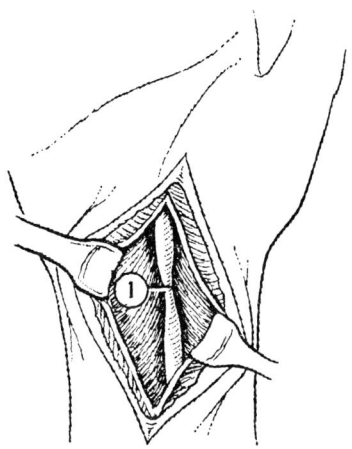

2. Excise a portion of the transverse carpal ligament from each margin.

Note: If the contracture of the median nerve is severe, perform a neurolysis by injecting saline with a fine needle into the nerve sheath to stretch the sheath and decompress the nerve.

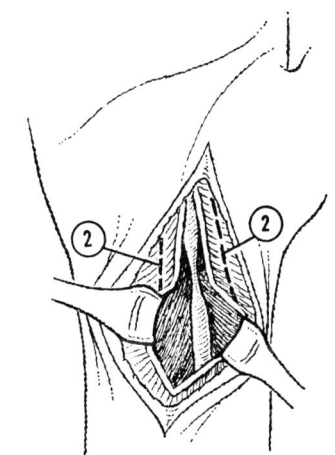

Immobilization

1. Apply an anterior plaster slab holding the wrist in the neutral position.

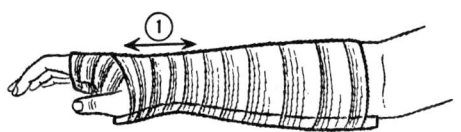

Postoperative Management

Remove the plaster slab after seven days.
Institute physical therapy and active exercises to restore function in the wrist and fingers.

SUMMARY: COMPLICATIONS AND PITFALLS OF FRACTURES AND DISLOCATIONS OF THE WRIST

The common complications from Colles' fracture result most often from failure of reduction leading to an unsightly wrist deformity and symptomatic disruption of the distal radioulnar joint. Inadequate anesthesia in reducing these fractures frequently leads to the pitfall of inadequate reduction. Intravenous regional anesthesia is ideal for emergency treatment, provided that the technique is followed closely and adequate equipment and assistants are available. Use of percutaneous fixation pins inserted through the radial styloid maintains reduction and minimizes the frequency of unsatisfactory results. Complications from hand swelling after cast immobilization can be avoided by the use of a sugar-tong splint. This provides excellent immobilization without constricting the wrist or causing edema of the hand. The use of a sling should be avoided so as to encourage rather than inhibit functional exercises after reduction of the Colles' fracture.

The malunited Smith's fracture is especially likely to impair tendon and nerve function of the hand. Reduction of the Smith's fracture should correct the volar displacement of the distal fragment and should hold it corrected either by supinated position to tighten the pronator quadratus or by pin fixation.

Barton's fracture is essentially a volar dislocation of the carpus, which is best treated by open reduction and internal fixation. Attempted closed reduction of these unstable fractures is likely to produce unsatisfactory wrist function.

Fractures of the carpal scaphoid tend to heal satisfactorily but are frequently subject to the complication of overtreatment. Clinical union precedes radiographic union since the fracture heals without periosteal callus. Avoid the pitfall of treating the radiographic evidence rather than the clinical problem. If, in rare instances, after an adequate period of immobilization (three to four months), the fracture remains clinically ununited, proceed with bone grafting and internal fixation rather than prolonging immobilization. Recognizing the five to ten per cent of these fractures that are unstable and likely to lead to nonunion also aids in the selection of appropriate treatment.

An additional pitfall in radiographic evaluation of a wrist injury is initial reliance on inadequate studies. Carpal fractures and dislocations may go unrecognized or incompletely diagnosed if one relies merely on anteroposterior and oblique views in the emergency room. Within the diagnosis of "wrist sprain" lurks a number of diagnostic pitfalls, including scapholunate dissociation and radioulnar subluxation, that can be diagnosed readily if they are only considered. Insist that the x-rays show the carpal relationships and include true lateral and supinated views to assess for dislocations and subluxations of the carpal bones as well as fractures.

Fracture-dislocations of the carpus, such as a transcaphoid perilunate dislocation, are unstable injuries and are generally best treated with open reduction and internal fixation. Attempted closed reduction of these combined injuries to bone and ligamentous structures usually proves to be a pitfall that in itself should be avoided.

Isolated fractures of carpal bones may lead to surprisingly frequent failures of diagnosis. Fractures of the hamate are notorious for going unrecognized and causing persistent pain symptoms, particularly in athletes or individuals requiring a strong grip.

A high index of suspicion alerts the physician to the pitfalls of the common and uncommon injuries to the wrist and leads to appropriate and effective treatment.

References

Chrisman, O. D., and Shortell, J. H.: Fractures of the distal end of the radius complicated by fractures of the carpal scaphoid. N. Engl. J. Med., 241:58, 1949.

Dameron, T. B., Jr.: Traumatic dislocation of the distal radio-ulnar joint. Clin. Orthop., 83:55, 1972.

DeOliveira, J. C.: Barton's fractures. J. Bone and Joint Surg., 55-A:586, 1973.

Dowling, J. J., and Blackwell, S., Jr.: Comminuted Colles' fractures. J. Bone and Joint Surg., 43-A:657, 1961.

Frykman, G.: Fractures of the distal radius including sequelae — shoulder-hand-finger syndrome, disturbance in the distal radio-ulnar joint and impairment of nerve function. Acta Orthop. Scand., 108:3, 1967.

Henry, A.: Extensile Exposure. 2nd edition. Baltimore, The Williams & Wilkins Company, 1962, pp. 120–124.

Linscheid, R. L., Dobyns, J. H., Beabout, J. W., et al.: Traumatic instability of the wrist. J. Bone and Joint Surg., 54-A:1612, 1972.

London, P. S.: The broken scaphoid bone, the case against pessimism. J. Bone and Joint Surg., 43-B:237, 1961.

McLaughlin, H. L.: Fracture of the carpal navicular (scaphoid) bone. J. Bone and Joint Surg., 36-A:765, 1954.

Miller, W. E.: Colles' fracture. S. Med. J., 53:1382, 1960.

Primiano, G. A., and Reef, T. C.: Disruption of the proximal carpal arch of the hand. J. Bone and Joint Surg. 56-A:328, 1974.

Rask, M. R.: Carponavicular subluxation: Report of a case treated by percutaneous pins. Orthopaedics, 2:133, 1979.

Russe, O.: Fracture of the carpal navicular. J. Bone and Joint Surg., 42-A:759, 1960.

Sarrafian, S. K., Melamed, J. L., and Goshgarian, G. M.: Study of wrist motion in flexion and extension. Clin. Orthop., 126:153, 1977.

REFERENCES

Schiller, M. G.: Intravenous regional anesthesia for closed treatment of fractures and dislocations of the upper extremities. Clin. Orthop. 118:25, 1976.

Snook, G. A., Chrisman, O. D., Wilson, T. C., et al.: Subluxation of the distal radio-ulnar joint by hyperpronation. J. Bone and Joint Surg., 51-A:1315, 1969.

Stark, H. H., Jobe, F. W., Boyes, M. J. H., et al.: Fracture of the hook of the hamate in athletes. J. Bone and Joint Surg., 59-A:575, 1977.

Stein, F., and Siegel, M. W.: Naviculocapitate fracture syndrome. J. Bone and Joint Surg., 51-A:391, 1969.

Swanson, A. B.: Flexible Implant Resection Arthroplasty in the Hand and Extremities. St. Louis, The C. V. Mosby Company, 1973, pp. 240–253.

Taleisnik, J., and Kelly, P. J.: The extraosseous and intraosseous blood supply of the scaphoid bone. J. Bone and Joint Surg., 48-A:1125, 1966.

Thomas, F. B.: Reduction of Smith's fracture. J. Bone and Joint Surg., 39-B:463, 1957.

Volz, R. G.: Total wrist arthroplasty. Clin. Orthop., 128:180, 1977.

FRACTURES AND DISLOCATIONS OF THE HAND

APPLIED ANATOMY

REMARKS

The great versatility of the hand, which permits actions ranging from precision pinch to power grip, depends on a well-tuned interplay of intrinsic and extrinsic muscle function.

Normal mobility of joint and skeletal support is critical for hand function.

Thorough knowledge of applied anatomy is essential in managing all injuries, major or minor, that disrupt the delicate balance that is hand function.

Osseous Components of the Hand from the Volar Aspect

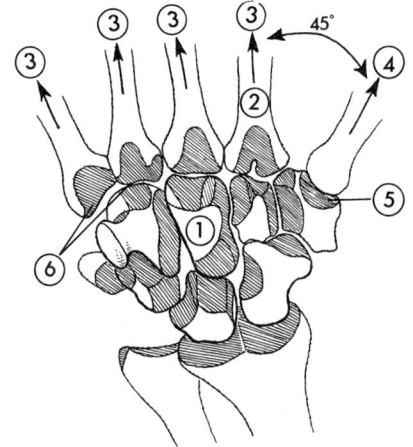

1. Capitate articulates with second, third, and fourth metacarpals.
2. Second metacarpal articulates with the trapezium, trapezoid, and capitate.
3. The metacarpals of the fingers are parallel to one another.
4. The metacarpal of the thumb is 45 degrees to the metacarpal of the index finger.
5. The carpometacarpal articulation of the thumb is saddle-shaped.
6. The carpometacarpal articulations of the fourth and fifth carpometacarpal joints are hinge-shaped.

LIGAMENTS OF THE HAND

Metacarpal Ligaments

The metacarpals of the fingers are bound together by the intermetacarpal ligaments, which span the intervals between them.

At the distal end of the metacarpal region the intermetacarpal ligaments thicken to form the deep transverse carpal ligaments, which loosely bind together the heads of the metacarpal bones.

APPLIED ANATOMY

This arrangement permits considerable volar and dorsal mobility of the distal ends of the metacarpal bones but very little lateral mobility.

The deep transverse ligaments are intimately related to the capsular ligaments and to the palmar ligaments, or the fibrocartilaginous plate on the volar aspects of the metacarpophalangeal joints.

The lumbricalis muscles pass in front of these ligaments, whereas the interossei pass behind.

Relationship of Deep Transverse Ligaments

1. Palmar ligaments (fibrocartilaginous portion of the anterior capsule).
2. Deep transverse metacarpal ligaments.
3. Attachment of palmar aponeurosis to the palmar ligament.
4. Lumbrical muscles are in front of the ligament.
5. Interossei are behind the ligament.

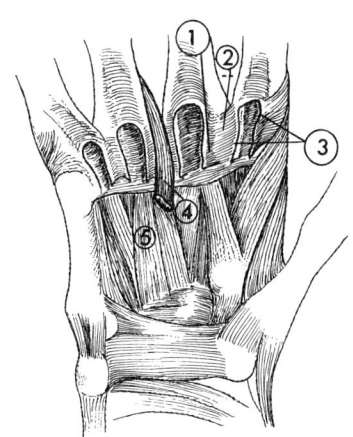

LONGITUDINAL AND TRANSVERSE ARCHES OF THE HAND

The hand is composed of five longitudinal and two transverse arches. Disruption of these arches frequently produces rotational deformities of the fingers.

1. The longitudinal arches are composed of carpals, metacarpals, and phalanges.
2. The mobile distal transverse arch is composed of the intermetacarpal ligaments (intervolar plate) with the interposed metacarpal heads.
3. The proximal transverse arch is a rigid semicircular structure consisting of the distal row of carpal bones and the intercarpal ligaments with the keystone of the arch at the capitate bone.

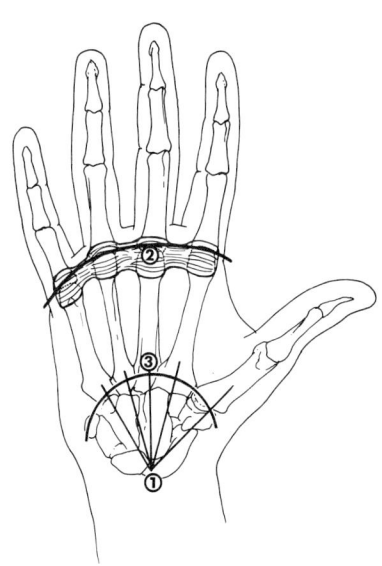

1139

1. The proximal transverse arch combined with the heads of the second and third metacarpals to which it firmly attaches is the fixed unit of the hand.

2. The mobile proximal and distal structures rotate about the rigid unit.

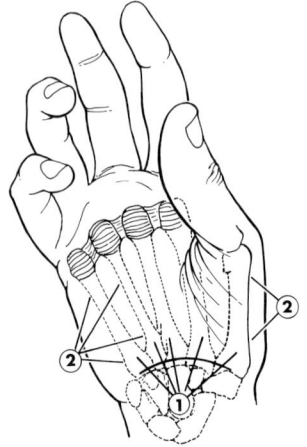

METACARPOPHALANGEAL JOINTS OF THE FINGERS

REMARKS

Each metacarpophalangeal (MP) joint is so fashioned that upon flexion of the corresponding digit the distal phalanx points to the tubercle of the scaphoid and the fingers do not overlap. This is a very important anatomic arrangement and must always be borne in mind when treating fractures of the phalanges of the fingers.

Malunion with rotation of a phalanx produces overlapping of the finger when the hand makes a fist.

The sphericity of the metacarpal head is slightly eccentric, so that the capsular structures tighten with full flexion. This is important for adduction-abduction motion of the joint.

Normal position of finger on flexion
1. The distal phalanges all point to the tubercle of the scaphoid.
2. The fingers do not overlap.

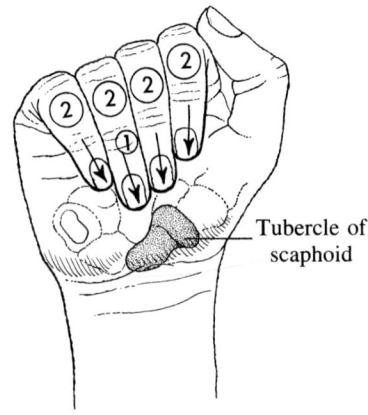

APPLIED ANATOMY

Abnormal position due to malrotation
1. Fracture of a phalanx or metacarpal.

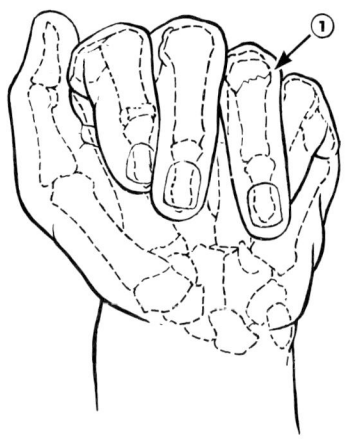

2. Disruption of the distal carpal row.

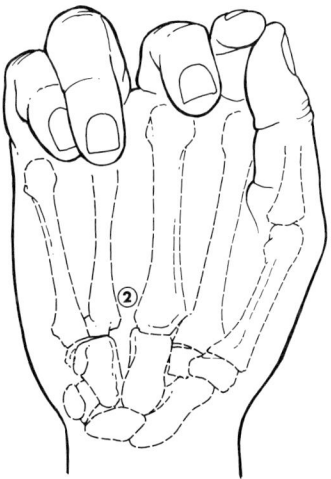

The MP joint also permits abduction of the finger away from the midline and some circumduction. This motion is greater in the index and little fingers than in the long and ring fingers.

The stability of the MP joint depends largely on its capsular ligaments and collateral structures.

The eccentric shape of the metacarpal head makes these ligaments tight in flexion and loose in extension.

APPLIED ANATOMY

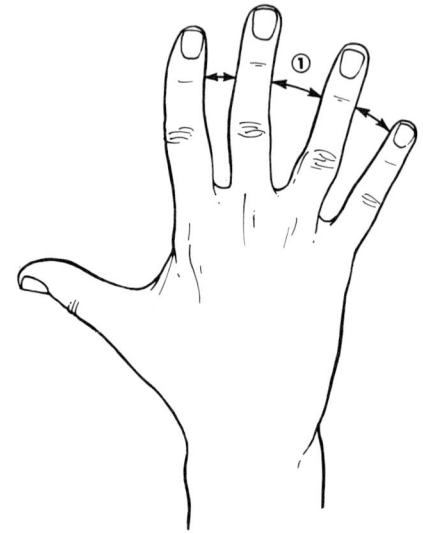

Test the stability in your own fingers:

1. In extension, 40 degrees of lateral (abduction, adduction) motion is present at the MP joint.

2. With the MP joint flexed 70 degrees, lateral motion is eliminated.

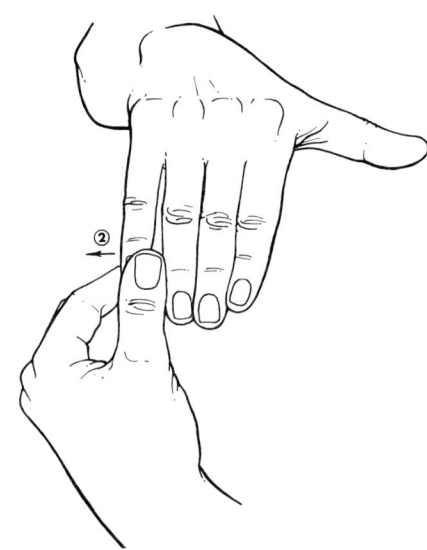

METACARPOPHALANGEAL JOINT OF THE THUMB

REMARKS

The MP joint of the thumb must be stable for the important pinch mechanism. Consequently the joint has more of the characteristics of a hinge joint and functions like an interphalangeal joint of the finger.

APPLIED ANATOMY

1. The MP joint of the thumb is stable in extension.
2. Disruption of the thumb support ligaments causes considerable loss of pinch strength.

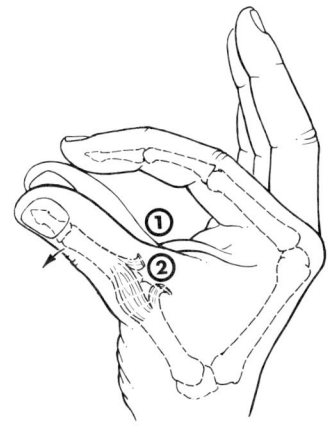

INTERPHALANGEAL JOINTS

REMARKS

The shape of the interphalangeal (IP) joints permits motion in only one plane, flexion and extension.

The IP joints have the same capsular structure, collateral ligaments, and volar plates, as do the metacarpophalangeal joints.

Owing to their different shapes, the MP joint support structures are stretched to their fullest, in full flexion, while the IP joint support structures are tightest, in very slight flexion. This is essentially the intrinsic-plus position.

Capsule and Collateral Ligaments of Metacarpophalangeal and Interphalangeal Joints

1. Capsule.
2. Collateral ligaments.
3. Palmar ligament (volar plate).
4. Deep transverse metacarpal ligaments.

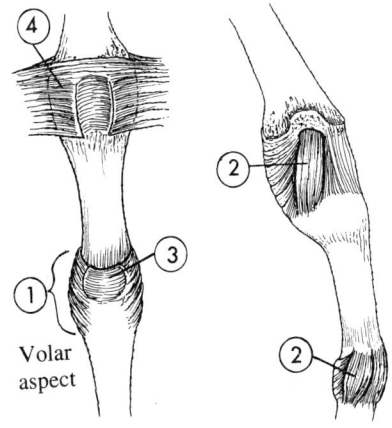

1143

Capsule and Collateral Ligaments of Metacarpophalangeal and Interphalangeal Joints (Continued)

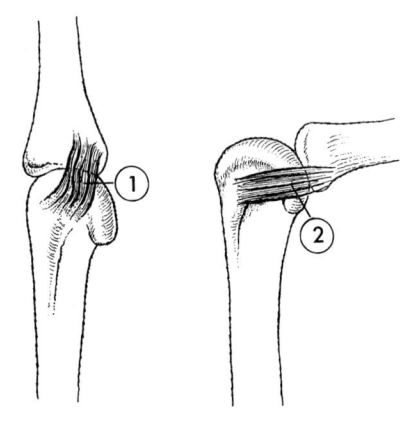

The shape of the articular surfaces has the following effect on the joint capsule.
1. Collateral ligament of the MP joint is slack in extension but
2. Tight in flexion.
3. Collateral ligament of the IP joint is tight in slight flexion.

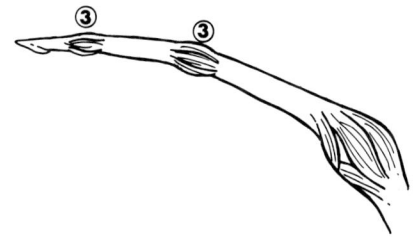

The Intrinsic-Plus Position for Immobilization

To minimize stiffening of the joints, never immobilize the MP joint in full extension or the IP joint in full flexion for even a short time after injury.

In the position of function or the safe position for immobilization of the injured hand,
1. MP joints are flexed as near 70 degrees as possible.
2. IP joints are in slight (15 degrees) flexion.
3. The thumb is abducted and apposed to the fingers.

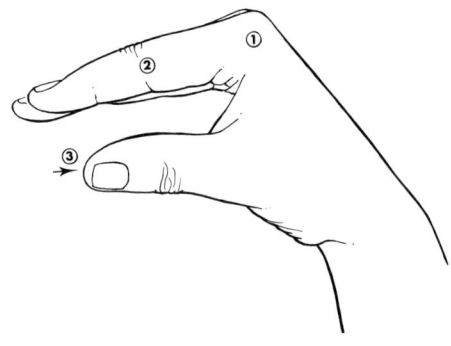

Muscles of the Hand

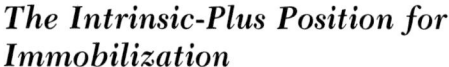

Intrinsic muscles of the hand include the thenar and hypothenar or intrinsic muscles of the thumb and small finger, and the seven interossei and four lumbricals that serve the central three fingers.

The four lumbricals arise from the tendons of the flexor digitorum profundus, pass distally on the radial side of the fingers beneath the axis of the MP joint, and then blend with the dorsal fibrous expansion of the extensor digitorum communis.

The four dorsal and three volar interossei arise from and occupy the interval between the metacarpals. They pass distally close to the axis of motion of the MP joint and for the most part attach to the base of the proximal phalanx and the dorsal expansion of the extensor digitorum communis. The primary function of the intrinsics is to flex the MP and extend the proximal and distal IP joints.

Both the intrinsic and the extrinsic muscles must work in synchrony for hand function to be effective.

Thenar and Hypothenar Muscles

1. Opponens pollicis.
2. Abductor pollicis brevis.
3. Flexor pollicis brevis.
4. Adductor pollicis.
5. Palmaris brevis.
6. Abductor digiti quinti.
7. Flexor brevis digiti quinti.
8. Opponens digiti quinti.

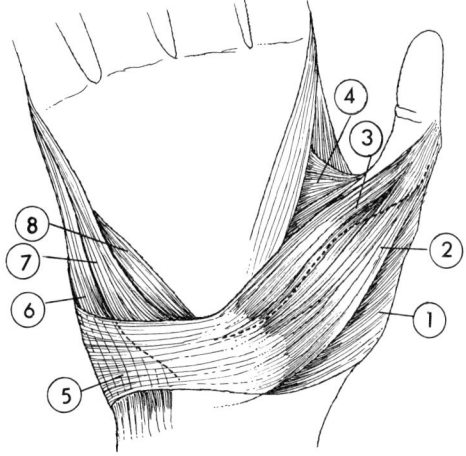

Lumbrical Muscles

Observe:

1. Lumbricals arise from the tendons of the flexor digitorum profundus and
2. Insert on the radial side of the expansion of the extensor digitorum communis.

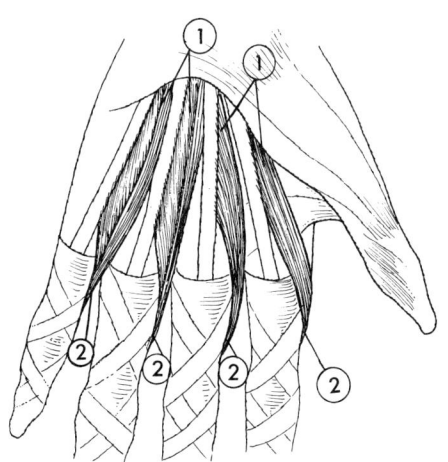

APPLIED ANATOMY

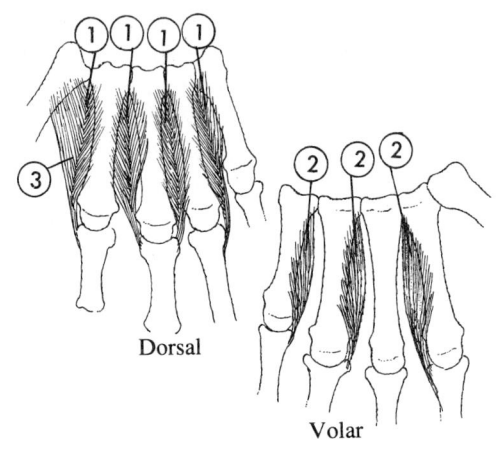

Interossei Muscles

Observe:
1. There are four dorsal and
2. Three volar interossei.
3. The first dorsal is the largest.

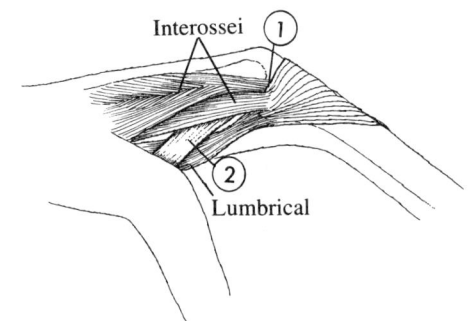

1. The dorsal interosseous inserts into the proximal phalanx and the fibrous expansion of the extensor communis.
2. The interosseous and lumbrical tendons are separated by the deep transverse carpal ligament, allowing the lumbrical to be a more effective MP flexor.

Dorsal Expansion of the Digitorum Communis

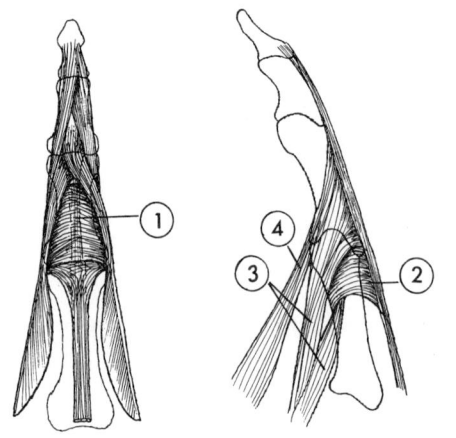

Observe:
1. Expansion of the extensor tendon forms a sleeve over the metacarpophalangeal joint.
2. Concentration of the transverse fibers form the mobile hood (this is anchored to the fibrocartilaginous volar plate).
3. Two heads of the dorsal interossei; one inserts into the proximal phalanx, the other in the fibrous dorsal expansion.
4. Lumbrical muscle inserts into the fibrous expansion distal to the insertion of the interossei.

1146

Shift of the Dorsal Expansion

On flexion, the middle slip of the extensor tendon pulls the dorsal expansion distally in front of the proximal phalanx.

On extension, the extensor tendon pulls the dorsal expansion over the joint and stabilizes it; the lumbrical and interossei muscles extend the distal joint by pulling on the lateral band.

Normal Finger Flexion

The synchrony between intrinsic and extrinsic muscle function allows normal finger flexion consisting of:
1. 70 to 80 degrees of MP flexion.
2. 110 to 120 degrees of proximal IP flexion.
3. 90 degrees of distal IP flexion.

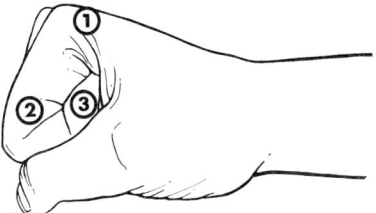

Abnormal Finger Flexion– Intrinsic-Minus Position

Absence of intrinsic function, as with median and ulnar nerve palsy, produces grossly inefficient flexion or clawing of the hand.

Intrinsic-minus hand flexion consists of:
1. Hyperextension of the MP joint and
2. Inability to flex the fingertips into the palm for grasp.

Note: The intrinsic-plus position is the same as the position for immobilization (See page 1144).

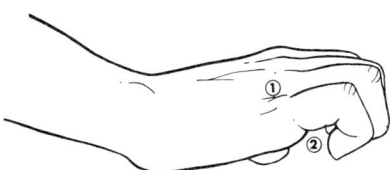

COMMON MECHANISMS OF INJURY TO EXTRINSIC AND INTRINSIC TENDON AND JOINT FUNCTION — THE "JAMMED" FINGER OR THUMB

Normal Finger

1. The common extensor tendons form the central slip, which inserts at the base of the middle phalanx and extends the proximal interphalangeal (PIP) joint.
2. The intrinsic tendons pass beneath the axis of the MP joint as flexors.
3. Lateral bands pass slightly dorsal to the PIP joint to insert on the base of the distal phalanx. They supplement the central slip for extension of the PIP joint and also extend the distal interphalangeal (DIP) joint.

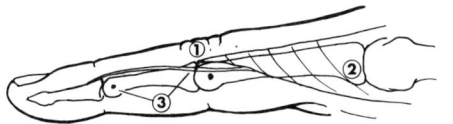

Mallet Finger Deformity

1. Rupture of the extensor tendon inserting into the distal phalanx, causing flexion deformity of the DIP joint.
2. Contracture of lateral bands, producing hyperextension of the PIP joint.

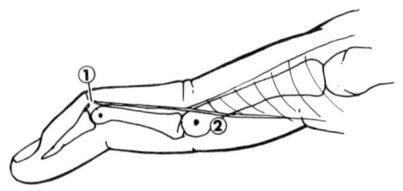

Avulsion of the Flexor Profundus

1. Forceful hyperextension of the ring or long finger occurs while grasping a lunging individual.
2. Resultant loss of active DIP flexion from disruption of the flexor profundus may not be initially detected.

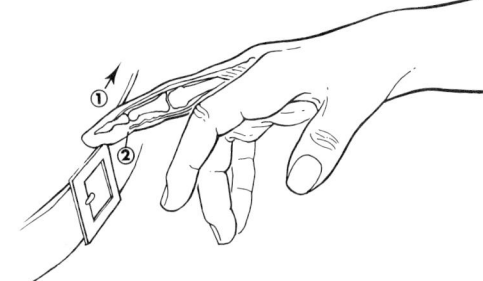

Boutonniere Deformity

1. Central slip rupture causes loss of extension of the PIP joint.
2. Gradual displacement of the lateral bands volar to the axis of the PIP joint may occur after several weeks. The result is flexion deformity of the PIP joint and
3. Hyperextension of the DIP joint.

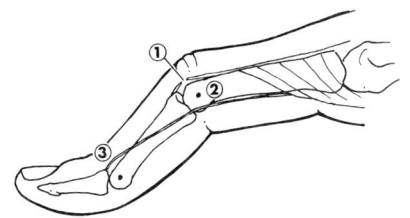

Boutonniere Deformity from Anterior Dislocation of the PIP Joint

1. Anterior displacement of the PIP joint ruptures the central slip and
2. Tears the volar plate.
3. Usually the collateral ligament is torn as well.

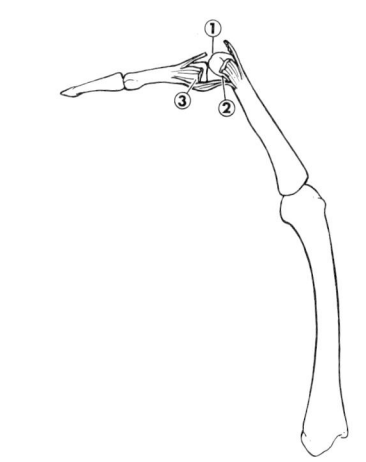

Pseudoboutonniere Deformity

1. Hyperextension injury to the PIP joint disrupts the
2. Proximal attachment of the volar capsule and volar plate to proximal phalanx.

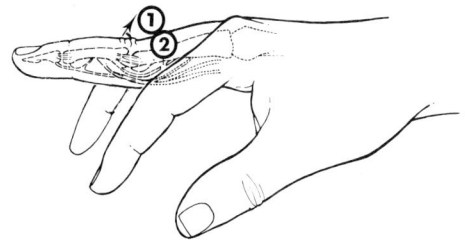

THE "JAMMED" FINGER OR THUMB

Pseudoboutonniere Deformity (Continued)

This results gradually in
  1. Bone spur formation at the capsular attachment.
  2. And fixed flexion contracture of the PIP joint from scarring in the capsule and at least one lateral band.
  3. Slight hyperextension of the DIP joint is not as marked or as fixed as a true boutonniere deformity because only one lateral band is usually contracted.

  Note: This most often occurs in athletic injuries, particularly football injuries to the little finger.

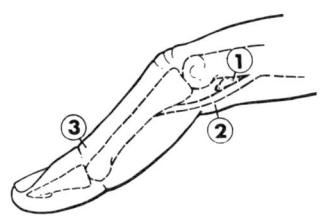

Reverse Boutonniere or Swan-neck Deformity — Volar Plate Injury with Hyperextension Deformity

Hyperextension of the PIP joint results from:
  1. Disruption of the volar plate attachment to the middle phalanx or fracture of the middle phalanx.
  2. Relaxation of the extensor mechanism permits the unapposed flexor profundus pull to draw the distal phalanx into slight flexion.

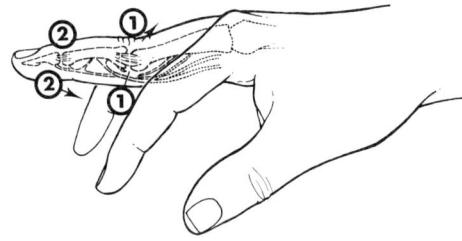

Lateral Instability of the PIP Joint

Most often this results from acute or chronic disruption of the radial collateral ligament after a lateral dislocation. Always check for collateral instability after reduction of an IP joint dislocation, particularly one that does not reduce with a definite "click."
  1. Disruption of the radial collateral ligament from dislocation produces
  2. Gross clinical and radiographic instability.

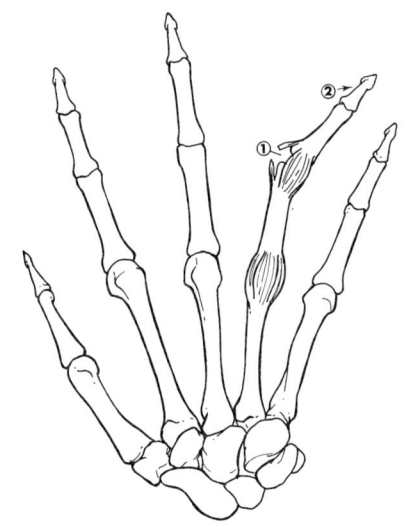

Mechanisms of Injuries to the Metacarpophalangeal Joints

LATERAL INSTABILITY OF THE MP JOINT OF THE THUMB

REMARKS

The MP joint of the thumb is analogous to the PIP joint of other fingers.

It is subject to frequent strain; most commonly this is a ski injury that occurs when a skier falls into a hard-packed bank of snow and jams his thumb.

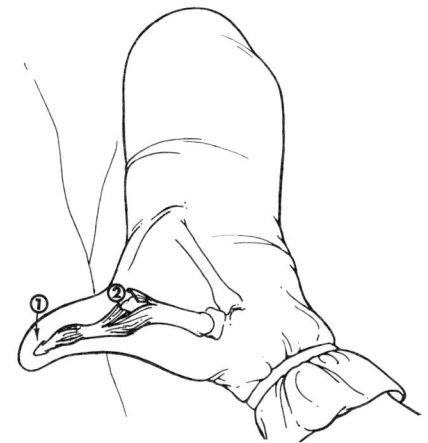

1. Valgus strain to MP joint of thumb results in disruption of the ulnar collateral ligament.
2. Instability, particularly of the pinch mechanism, results.

DISLOCATION OF THE MP JOINT

REMARKS

Hyperextension injuries to the MP joints can tear the attachment of the volar plate from the metacarpal and permit dislocation.

This serious dislocation, which may present as "a jammed finger," may be either simple or complex.

Simple Dislocation

1. In a simple dislocation the volar plate tears from its looser attachment to the metacarpal head but is not entrapped in the joint.
2. The proximal phalanx remains at right angles to the metacarpal head.

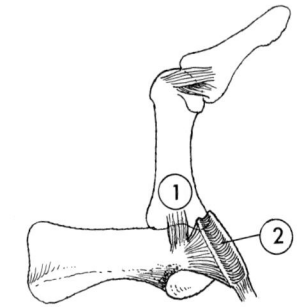

Complex Dislocation

1. The palmar plate is interposed between the proximal phalanx and metacarpal head.
2. The proximal phalanx is parallel to the metacarpal head.

Note: A complex dislocation is impossible to reduce by closed methods.

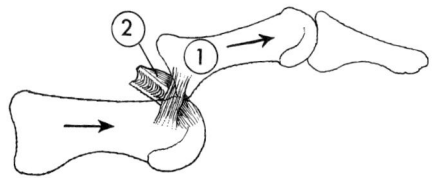

BASIC PRINCIPLES IN MANAGING HAND INJURIES

REMARKS

In addition to damaging the gliding mechanism of tendon and joint systems directly, hand injuries may disrupt finger mechanisms indirectly by sepsis, by stiffness from prolonged (more than three weeks) immobilization, or by edema.

The basic aim of management should be to prevent sepsis, to eliminate edema, and to reduce fractures and dislocations by closed or open methods that permit early functional exercise.

Any open hand injury, fracture or dislocation must be treated by thorough wound cleansing and meticulous excision of the wound edges. Particularly beware of "minor" wounds over joints. Some of the worst finger infections develop from human bites over knuckles.

Extensive open injury requires staged wound management consisting of thorough primary excision with delayed closure three to five days later.

Stabilization of fractures and joint injuries is most important for the extremely swollen hand in order to permit active motion and thereby allow "pumping out" of the swollen soft tissues.

Permanent joint stiffness is especially likely to ensue from immobilization longer than three weeks. Closed or open treatment should be designed to permit active functional exercise of the fingers and joints within the first one to two weeks after injury.

The majority of common finger fractures and dislocations tend to be minor injuries. However, by dismissing all these injuries as minor, the physician will fail to recognize significant injuries such as the locked MP joint dislocation, the anterior fracture dislocation of the PIP joint, and the angulated fracture of the proximal phalanx. These three injuries can frequently produce permanent and total loss of function of the involved finger.

It is extremely important to recognize potentially troublesome injuries by careful examination of all "trivial" injuries. Familiarity with the many types of injuries to the hand and their effects on the delicate balance of function helps avoid pitfalls in management.

By far the majority of fractures and dislocations are best treated by simple closed methods. However, the more complicated or complex the external support necessary to hold the fracture in reduction, the greater is the indication for internal fixation.

Unstable fractures, irreducible dislocations, angulated fractures of the proximal or middle phalanx, and multiple fractures in the same hand are, as a rule, more effectively treated by prompt operative reduction and fixation.

OPEN WOUNDS OF THE HAND

All open wounds of the hand require complete wound excision and cleansing. Be particularly wary of:

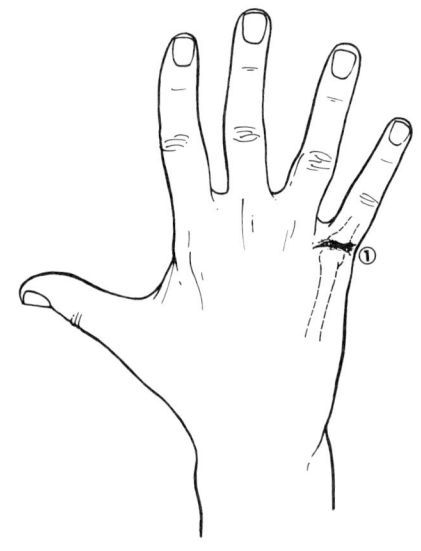

1. Open wounds over MP knuckles sustained from a human bite, which inevitably become infected if closed primarily. These are extremely contaminated and must be thoroughly excised, cleansed, and left open.

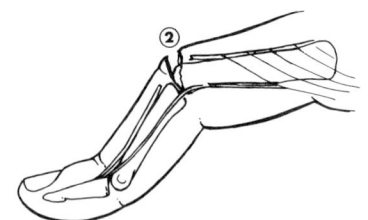

2. Laceration over PIP joint that detaches the extensor central slip insertion and leads to boutonniere deformity.

MANAGEMENT OF CRUSHING, OPEN WOUNDS

Open fractures from high-velocity wounds or crushing injuries are best treated by staged wound management. Initial debridement should be thorough and antibiotics should be used. Frequently, it is necessary also to:

1. Release tight carpal ligaments.
2. Free intermetacarpal fascia compartments by dorsal fasciotomy.

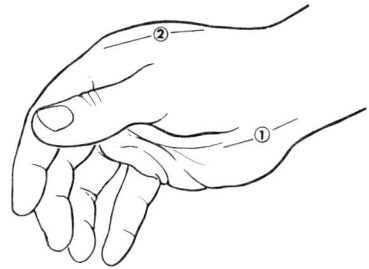

3. Fix multiple fractures with Kirschner wires.

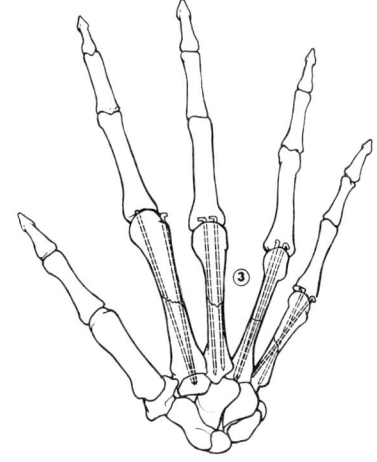

Secondary wound excision and closure is performed in three to five days with assurance that the wound is clean. To eliminate edema before closure:

1. Elevate the limb in a hand compression dressing and maintain constantly until closure.

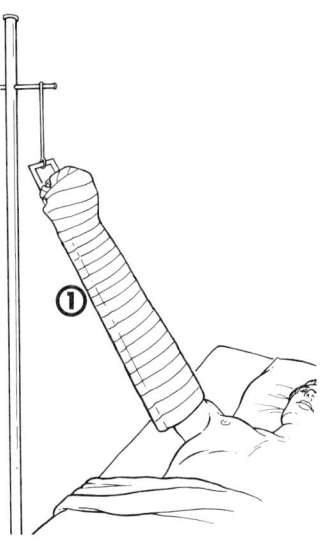

Methods of Closed Fracture Management

Splint For Mallet Finger

1. DIP joint is in slight hyperextension.
2. PIP joint is free.

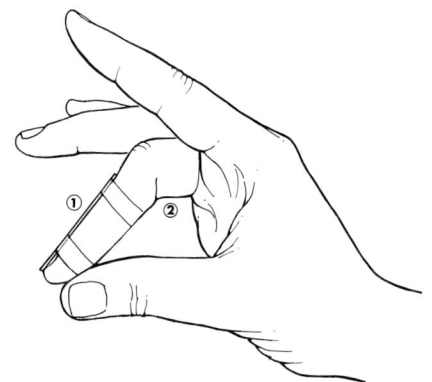

For Boutonniere Deformity

1. PIP joint is extended.
2. DIP joint is free.

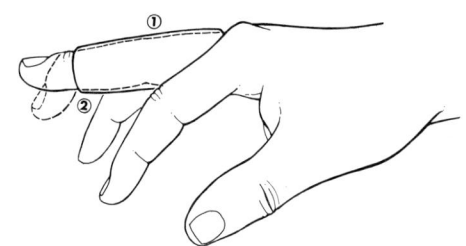

For Stable Phalangeal Fractures

1. The fractured finger is taped to the adjacent finger.
2. The tips of both fingers point to the scaphoid tuberosity in flexion.

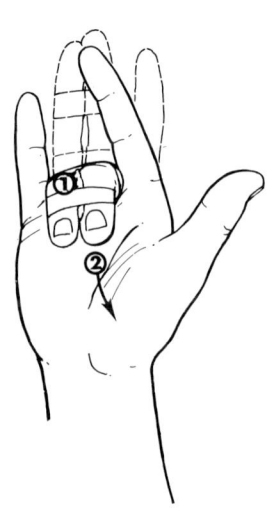

Cast-Splint Immobilization after Reduction of Phalangeal or Metacarpal Fracture

The fractured finger and adjacent finger are immobilized together.
1. Incorporate the fractured and the adjacent unfractured finger.
2. The MP joints are flexed 70 degrees.
3. The IP joints are in slight flexion.
4. The tips of the fingers are aligned to point toward the scaphoid tuberosity for correct rotational alignment.

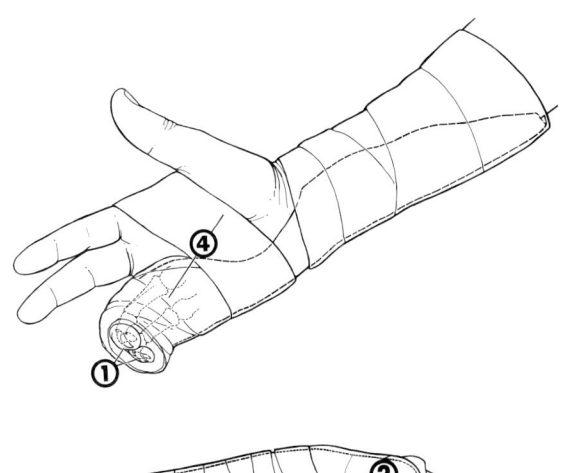

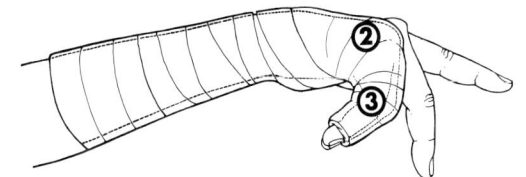

Methods of Internal Fixation

Closed treatment is not always the most "conservative" method. Operative fixation of unstable injuries permits early restoration of hand and finger function.

Kirschner wire fixation is used for
1. Avulsion fracture of the distal phalanx,
2. Fracture-dislocation of the PIP joint, or
3. Shortened oblique fracture of the middle phalanx.
4. Transverse Kirschner wires are used for multiple metacarpal fractures.

Small fragment screw is used for
5. Condylar fractures.
6. Angulated fractures of the proximal phalanx, or
7. Bennett's fracture-dislocation.

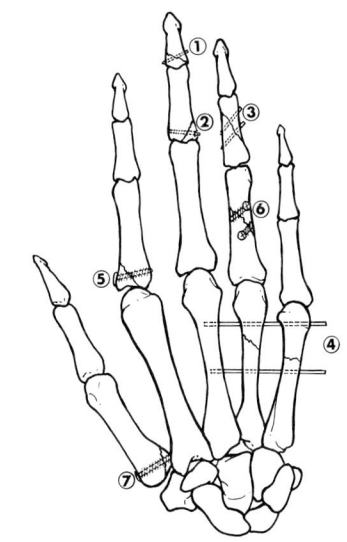

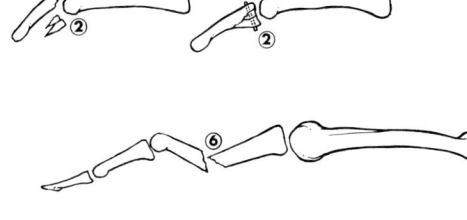

DISLOCATIONS AND FRACTURE-DISLOCATIONS OF THE THUMB

REMARKS

The thumb is the most mobile component of the hand. Through the carpometacarpal (CM) joint, which may be considered the thumb's MP joint, the thumb is capable of almost universal motion. This great range of mobility is necessary for the hand to function effectively in prehension. Complete loss of thumb function is equivalent to the loss of at least 50 per cent of hand function.

The bony architecture of the CM joint provides little stability. The stability of this joint is chiefly derived from its capsule and collateral ligaments.

The very nature of the thumb's position and function renders it vulnerable to injury varying from sprains to complete disruption of its linkage system.

The most common injuries to the thumb's linkage system include:
1. Bennett's fracture — fracture-dislocation of the CM joint.
2. Rolando's fracture — fracture comminuted into the CM joint.
3. Transverse fracture of the first metacarpal.
4. Dislocation of the MP joint.
5. Skier's thumb — subluxation of the MP joint from ulnar collateral tear.
6. Fracture of the phalanges and dislocation of the IP joint.

Fracture-Dislocation of the Carpometacarpal (CM) Joint of the Thumb (Bennett's Fracture)

REMARKS

Essentially this is an oblique fracture through the base of the first metacarpal with dislocation of the radial portion of its articular surface. The medial portion of the articular surface, which is triangular in shape and smaller than the radial shaft fragment, remains attached by its ligaments to the trapezium.

Bennett's fracture is usually produced by direct violence applied to the end of the metacarpal, driving the shaft proximally and dorsally.

The dislocated portion of the metacarpal disrupts the dorsal capsular structures.

It is essential to restore the fragments to their normal intra-articular relationships and to maintain this position until bone healing is complete.

Incomplete reduction and inadequate immobilization can cause malunion and secondary traumatic arthritis.

Closed reduction is usually possible using Kirschner wire fixation to hold the large, unstable shaft to the small but stable ulnar fragment.

If closed reduction does not restore the joint surface satisfactorily, use an open method to insure reduction of the joint continuity.

For Bennett's fracture-dislocation with a single large ulnar fragment comprising more than one third of the articular surface, use small fragment-screw fixation. Otherwise use small Kirschner wires to fix smaller fragments.

Prereduction X-ray

1. The shaft fragment is displaced radially and dorsally.
2. The triangular ulnar fragment maintains its normal relationship to the trapezium.

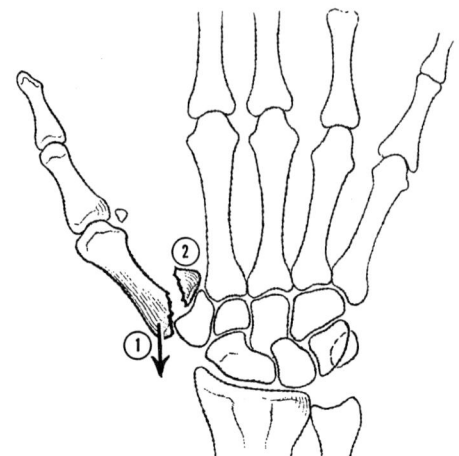

Closed Reduction and Kirschner Wire Fixation

This procedure is performed with the patient under intravenous block or general anesthesia (see page 909).

1. Abduct the thumb metacarpal to align the radial shaft fracture with the intra-articular fragment. Check alignment by image-intensified fluoroscopy.
2. Insert a smooth Kirschner wire through the shaft fragment into the trapezium. Do not attempt to fix the ulnar fragment with a pin, but rather to restore the continuity of the joint surface.

Note: If attempted closed reduction does not reduce joint surface, open the fracture and fix the fragments internally.

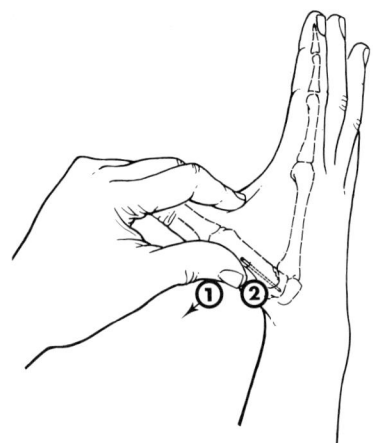

Postreduction X-Ray (After Closed Kirschner Wire Fixation)

1. The relationship between the radial and ulnar fragments and the articular surface is restored.
2. The pin through the metacarpal shaft fragment crosses the articular surface into the trapezium.

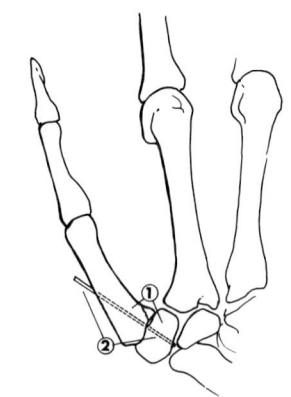

Note: If closed reduction and Kirschner wire fixation do not restore the joint surface satisfactorily, open the fracture and fix the fragments internally.

Operative Procedure: Internal Fixation

INCISION AND EXPOSURE

1. Make a 5-cm incision centered over the dorsum of the first metacarpal. It extends from the juncture of the distal and middle thirds of the metacarpal to the distal limits of the anatomic snuffbox.
2. Divide the periosteum longitudinally between the abductor pollicis brevis and the extensor pollicis brevis and expose the bone by subperiosteal dissection.
3. At the proximal end of the wound, divide the capsule of the carpometacarpal joint and expose the interior of the joint. Part of the abductor pollicis longus insertion may also be reflected.

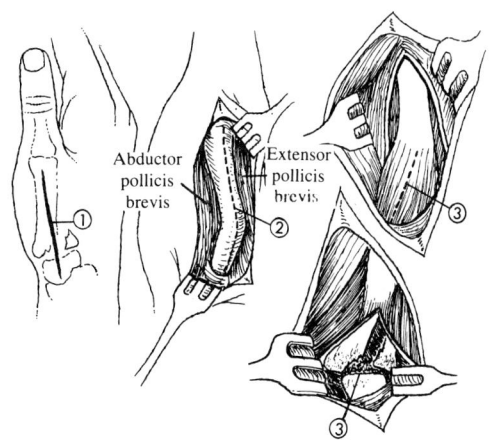

REDUCTION AND FIXATION

1. Abduct the thumb to approximate the shaft to the fracture fragment.

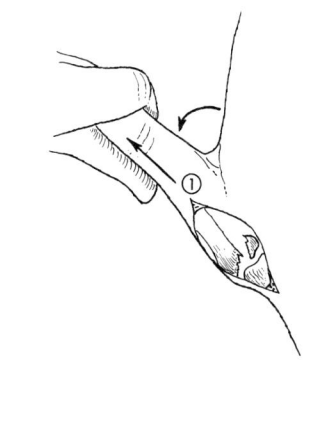

2. Hold the fragments in apposition with a towel clip.
3. Power drill both cortices using a 2-mm bit and drill guide.

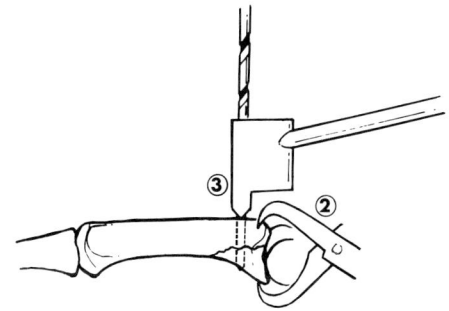

Operative Procedure: Internal Fixation (Continued)

4. Tap both cortices with 2.7-mm bit.

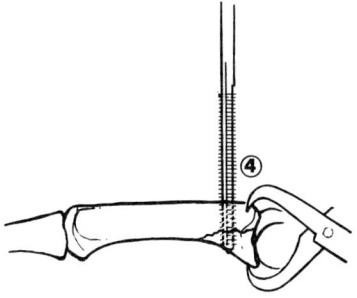

5. Power drill near the cortex with 2.7-mm bit to provide a gliding hole.

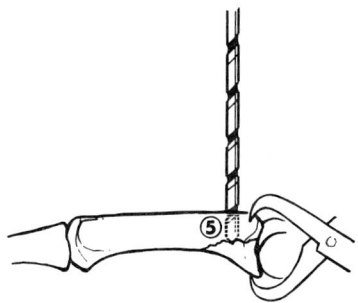

6. Insert a 2.7-mm screw of the correct length to compress the fracture.

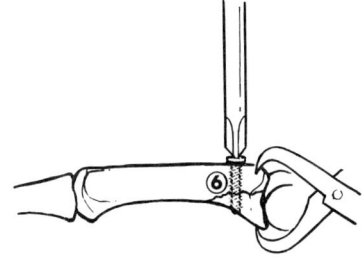

Postoperative X-Ray (After Open Reduction)

1. The fracture-dislocation is adequately reduced.
2. The small fragment screw stabilizes the fracture in anatomic position.

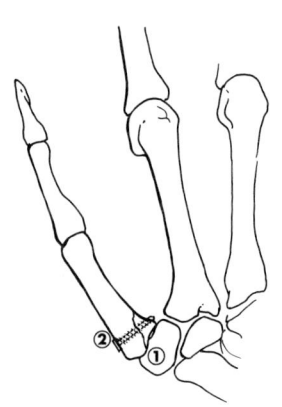

Immobilization

1. Apply a cast from below the elbow.
2. The thumb is abducted and plaster is molded over the CM joint.
3. The IP joint of the thumb is free.
4. The uninjured fingers are free to exercise.

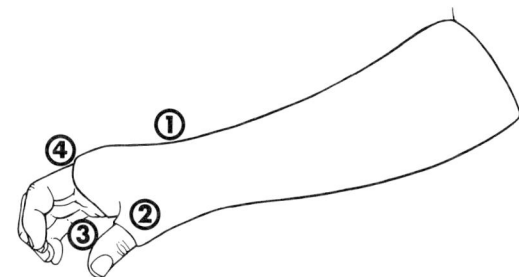

Postoperative Management

If Kirschner wire fixation has been used, remove the wire at three weeks and permit the patient active exercises. If the fracture is still tender, use a protective splint for two more weeks.

If small fragment-screw fixation has been used, immobilize for three weeks and then remove the plaster. The screw need not be removed unless it causes local tenderness.

Rolando's Intra-Articular Fracture

REMARKS

In contrast to a Bennett's fracture, Rolando's fracture consists of multiple intra-articular fragments. Anatomic reduction is frequently impossible.

Provided that the metacarpal shaft can be realigned with the trapezium, the comminution of the joint surface may be accepted. Attempted operative reduction of the fragments usually only worsens the joint disruption.

Preoperative X-ray

1. The metacarpal fragment has displaced radially and dorsally.
2. The base of the metacarpal is shattered.

X-Ray After Closed Reduction and Kirschner Wire Fixation

1. The metacarpal shaft fragment is realigned with the trapezium.
2. The comminuted articular surface remains incompletely reduced.

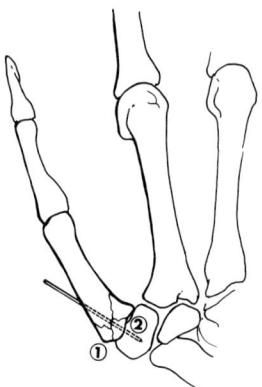

Postoperative Management

Immobilize the hand in a thumb spica for three weeks and then remove the cast and pin.

Evaluate the degree of healing clinically and radiographically.

If the shaft fragment is stable, begin guarded range-of-motion exercises to regain as much circumduction as possible in the thumb.

Traumatic arthritis of varying degrees is likely to follow this injury.

Subluxation of the Carpometacarpal Joint of the Thumb

Like most highly mobile joints, the CM joint of the thumb is subject to a number of strains and capsular injuries.

This joint is a common site for osteoarthritis in later years because of its susceptibility to "wear and tear."

Acute injuries of the CM joint without fracture-dislocation can be treated by rest with cast immobilization for two to three weeks.

DISLOCATIONS AND FRACTURE-DISLOCATIONS OF THE THUMB

Prereduction X-Ray

1. The metacarpal has subluxated radially and dorsally.

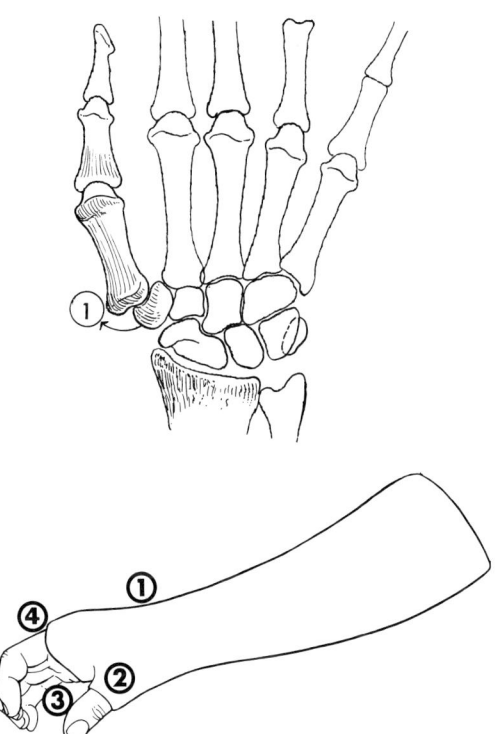

Closed Treatment

Apply a short arm cast.
1. The cast extends above the wrist.
2. The thumb is apposed to the fingers and the cast is molded over the CM joint.
3. The IP joint of the thumb is free to move.
4. The unaffected fingers are free to move.

Maintain the thumb in the plaster cast for three weeks.

Encourage free use of the unaffected fingers.

After three weeks remove the cast and permit active range of motion.

The patient should avoid heavy usage or contact sports, which are likely to reinjure the thumb, for three to four weeks longer.

Unstable Subluxations or Dislocations of the Carpometacarpal Joint of the Thumb

REMARKS

If the capsular tissues are severely disrupted the joint is very unstable and may subluxate even in plaster.

It is essential that the tissues heal with the articular surfaces of the joint in the normal anatomic position.

DISLOCATIONS AND FRACTURE-DISLOCATIONS OF THE THUMB

Incongruity of the joint surfaces predisposes to chronic subluxation with marked impairment of function; secondary osteoarthritic changes may develop subsequently, necessitating an arthrodesis of the joint.

Treat unstable injuries by Kirschner wire fixation.

Prereduction X-Ray

1. The metacarpal is displaced upward and backward.
2. The metacarpal rests on the posterior aspect of the trapezium.

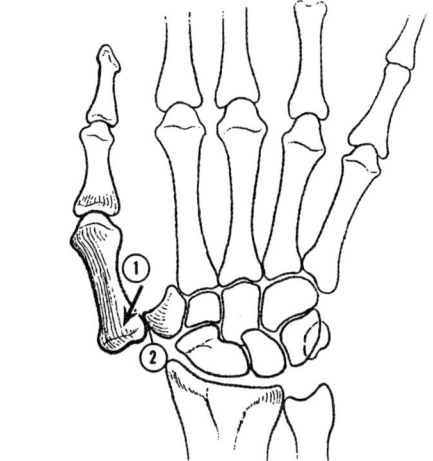

Manipulative Reduction

1. A bandage is looped first around the patient's thumb and then around the operator's hand.
2. While traction is made in the long axis of the thumb, the thumb is gradually abducted and, at the same time,
3. Direct pressure is exerted against the head of the metacarpal bone.
4. As the thumb is pulled downward and outward,
5. The head of the metacarpal is pushed forward and inward.

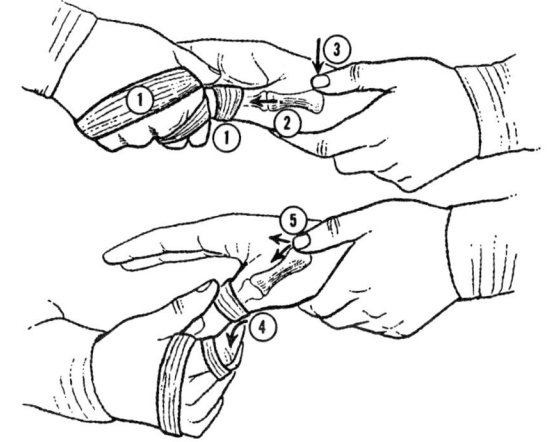

Postreduction X-Ray

1. The head of the metacarpal is in normal relationship to the trapezium.

Note: If the reduction is unstable, use Kirschner wire fixation (see page 1167).

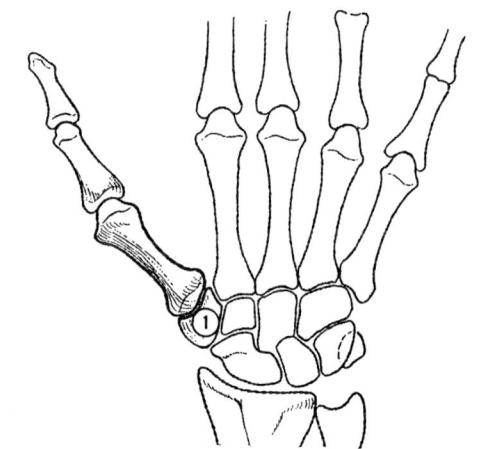

DISLOCATIONS AND FRACTURE-DISLOCATIONS OF THE THUMB

Immobilization

1. Apply a cast from below the elbow.
2. The thumb is abducted and plaster is molded over the CM joint.
3. The IP joint of the thumb is free.
4. The unaffected joints are allowed to move freely.

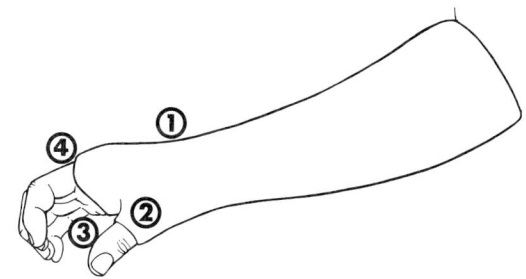

Postreduction Management

Take x-rays on the fifth and tenth days. Check the position of the articular surfaces of the joint.

Encourage active exercises of the unaffected fingers.

Remove the cast at the end of three weeks and have the patient begin active exercise to the joint.

If the dislocation or subluxation recurs in plaster use Kirschner wire fixation through the joint.

Closed Reduction with Internal Fixation

If the carpometacarpal joint proves unstable or displaces while in plaster, internal fixation becomes necessary.

Persistent subluxation of the joint is likely to result in traumatic arthritis and impairment of thumb function.

Operative Procedure

1. An assistant makes traction on the abducted thumb and, at the same time,
2. Makes inward pressure on the metacarpal with his thumb.
3. While this position is maintained, pass a smooth Kirschner wire through the base of the metacarpal into the trapezium. Cut the wire off below the level of the skin.

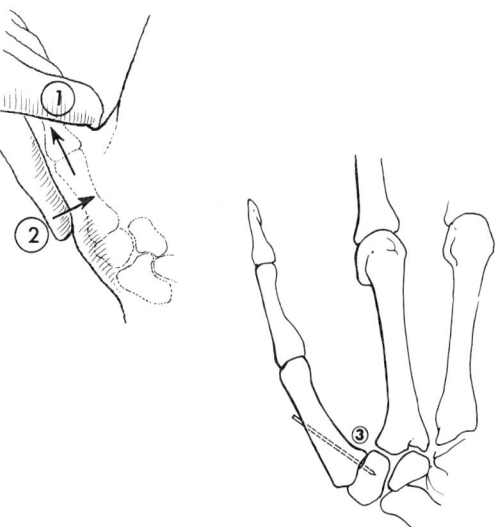

1167

Immobilization

1. Apply a cast from below the elbow.
2. The thumb is abducted and plaster is molded over the CM joint.
3. The IP joint of the thumb is free.
4. The unaffected joints are allowed to move freely.

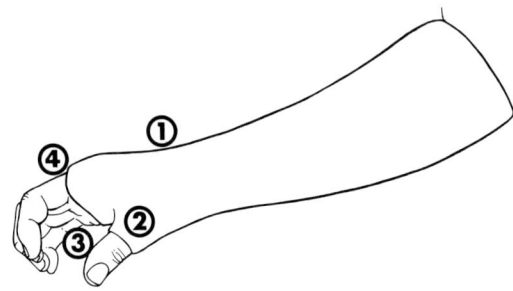

Subsequent Management

Remove the cast after three weeks and permit active motion of the thumb.

If Kirschner wire fixation was necessary, remove the wire after three weeks and begin protected active motion.

If the patient is going to use the thumb in heavy labor or sports, a protective bandage should be applied for three more weeks.

Fractures at the Base of the Metacarpal of the Thumb

REMARKS

Fractures at the base of the thumb metacarpal may be transverse, oblique, or comminuted.

Generally they occur in men. In children the lesion is essentially an epiphyseal separation with a triangular fragment of the diaphysis displaced with the epiphysis.

Usually the deformity is posterior with outward bowing.

Most lesions are readily reduced by traction and manipulative maneuvers and are stable; they can be treated by immobilizing the thumb in abduction.

Unstable fractures should be treated by open reduction and fixation by small fragment screw.

STABLE FRACTURES

Prereduction X-Ray

A. IN ADULT MALE

1. Fracture through the base of the metacarpal.
2. The distal fragment is displaced upward and backward.
3. The usual deformity is posterior with outward bowing.

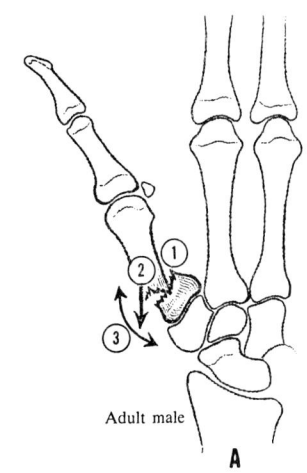

Adult male

A

B. IN 13-YEAR-OLD CHILD

1. Epiphyseal fracture with detachment of the triangular portion of the diaphysis.
2. The deformity is posterior with outward bowing.

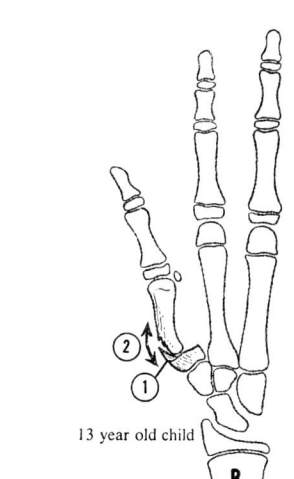

13 year old child

B

Manipulative Reduction

1. Apply strong traction to the abducted thumb.
2. The surgeon places the thumb of his other hand at the base of the metacarpal.
3. While traction is maintained,
4. Firm pressure is made over the proximal end of the distal fragment.
5. The thumb is hyperabducted.

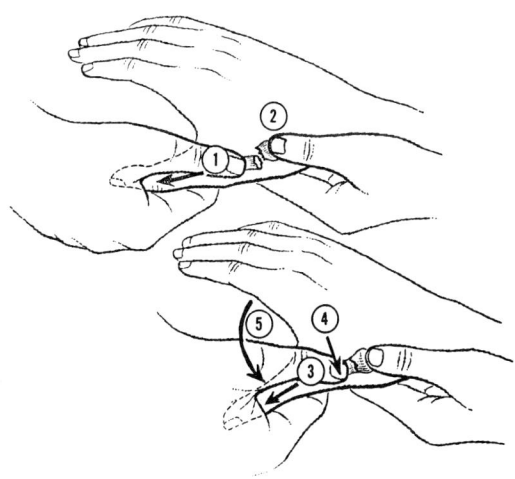

Postreduction X-Ray

1. The fragments are engaged and in normal alignment.
2. The posterior and outward bowing is corrected.

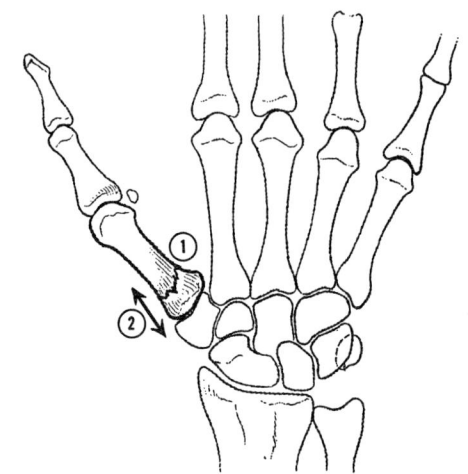

Immobilization

1. Apply a cast from below the elbow.
2. The thumb is abducted and plaster is molded over the MP joint.
3. The IP joint of the thumb is free.
4. The unaffected joints are allowed to move freely.

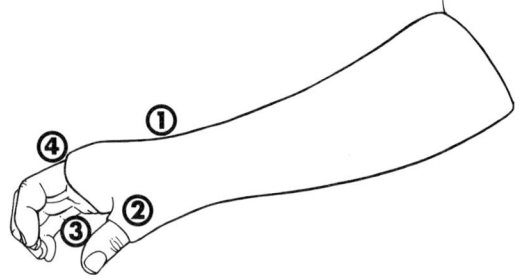

Postreduction Management

Check the position by x-ray within 1 week.

Encourage the patient to use the uninjured fingers of the hand during immobilization.

Reapply a new cast at the end of 10 to 14 days if the original cast becomes loose.

The patient should actively exercise all the joints of the fingers that are not immobilized on a regular daily basis.

Remove the cast at the end of 3 weeks and evaluate healing of the fracture clinically and radiographically.

Usually the fracture is sufficiently stable clinically by 3 weeks that active, protected motion is possible. If the fracture site is still tender, apply a light finger splint that can be removed for regular exercises of the thumb.

Do not wait for complete radiographic union to permit some active exercises. Clinical union precedes radiographic evidence of healing by several weeks.

UNSTABLE FRACTURES OF THE BASE OF THE METACARPAL OF THE THUMB

Prereduction X-Ray

1. Oblique fracture through the base of the metacarpal.
2. The carpometacarpal joint is not involved. This is in contrast to Bennett's or Rolando's fracture.

Note: If plaster fixation fails to hold this fracture, operative reduction with screw fixation is necessary.

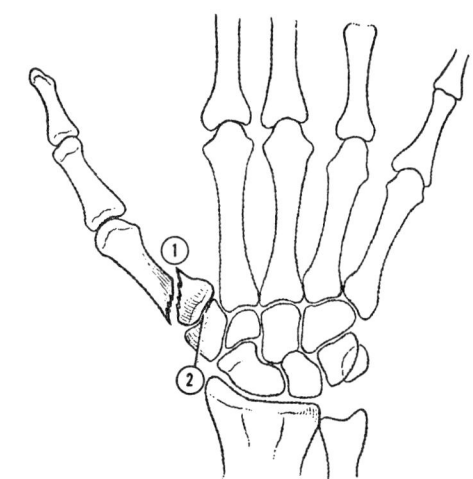

Operative Reduction: Fixation by Small Fragment Screw

1. Make a 5-cm incision centered over the radial aspect of the first metacarpal.
2. Divide the periosteum longitudinally between the abductor pollicis brevis and the extensor pollicis brevis to expose the bone and fracture.
3. If it is necessary to visualize the carpometacarpal joint, divide the capsule of the joint proximal to the end of the incision.

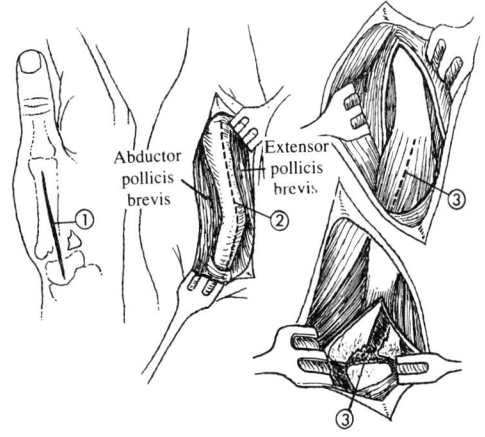

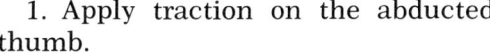

1. Apply traction on the abducted thumb.

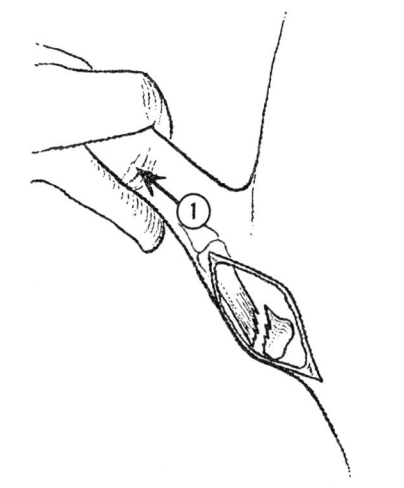

Operative Reduction: Fixation by Small Fragment Screw (Continued)

2. Approximate the proximal and distal fragments and hold them in normal position with a towel clip.

3. After drilling and tapping the fragments, fix them with a small fragment screw (see page 1161).

Note: For long oblique fractures, two small screws may be necessary.

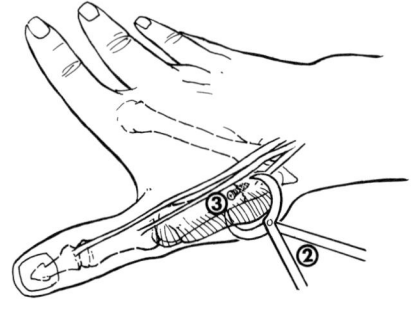

Postoperative X-Ray

1. The fracture is reduced and is held by two small fragment screws, which stabilize the fragment sufficiently to permit early exercises of the hand.

Immobilization

1. Apply a compression hand dressing and elevate the limb for several days until edema subsides.

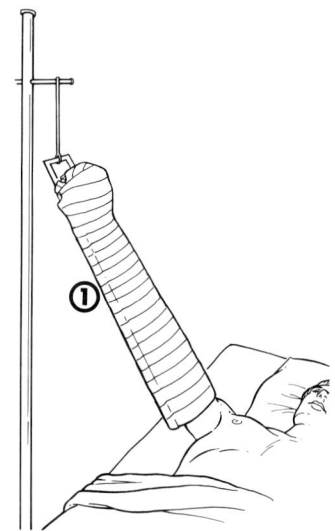

Subsequent Management

By three to five days remove the compression hand dressing and permit the patient guarded active exercises.

When the patient is not exercising the hand, have him wear a protective splint.

The fixation must be secure to permit this early exercise program. If there has been any comminution of the fracture, cast immobilization must be continued for at least three weeks.

Fractures of the Shaft of the Metacarpal of the Thumb

REMARKS

In general what has been noted for fractures of the base of the first metacarpal is applicable to the entire metacarpal shaft. The fractures can be grouped into stable and unstable types.

Stable fractures are treated by plaster immobilization with the thumb in abduction.

Unstable fractures should be treated by open reduction with fixation by small fragment screw.

STABLE FRACTURES OF THE SHAFT OF THE METACARPAL OF THE THUMB

Prereduction X-Rays

1. Fracture of the shaft of the thumb metacarpal with no displacement.

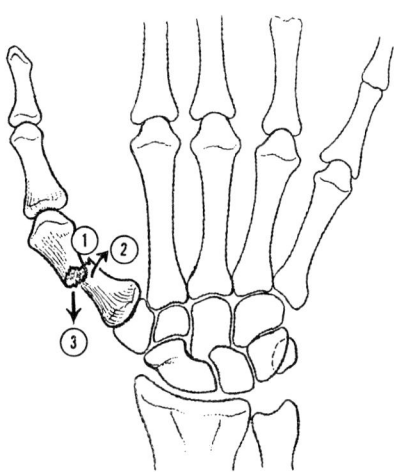

1. Fracture of the shaft of the thumb metacarpal with backward displacement.

2. The proximal fragment is tilted forward.

3. The distal fragment is displaced upward and backward.

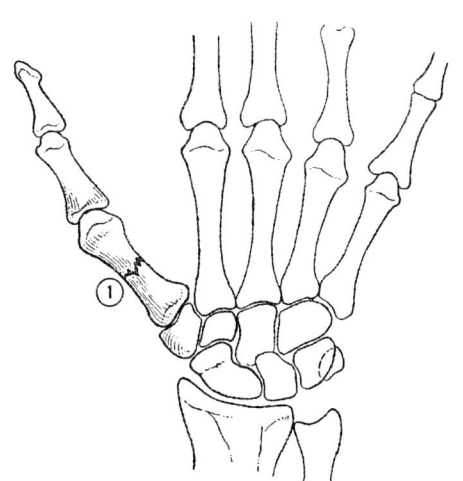

Manipulative Reduction (For Displaced Fractures)

1. Apply strong traction on the abducted thumb.
2. Place the thumb of your other hand over the end of the proximal fragment.
3. While traction is maintained,
4. Make firm pressure on the proximal end of the distal fragment and
5. Hyperabduct the thumb.

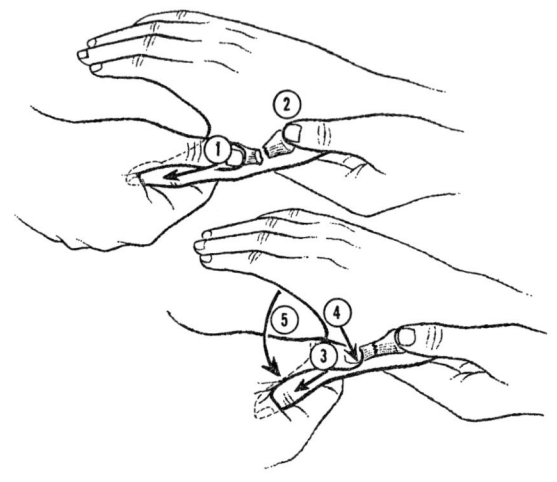

Postreduction X-Ray

1. The fragments are engaged and in normal alignment.
2. The posterior angulation is corrected.
3. The length of the shaft is restored.

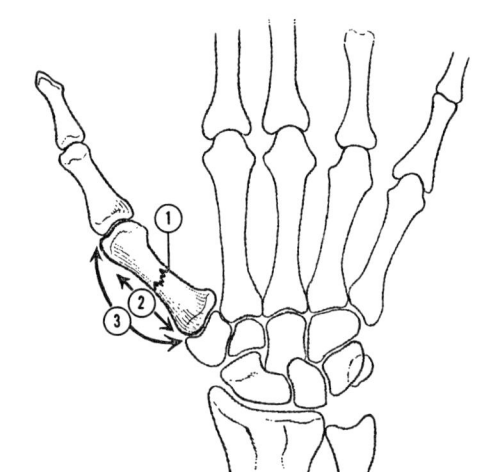

Immobilization

1. Apply a cast from below the elbow.
2. The thumb is abducted and plaster is molded over the CM joint.
3. The IP joint of the thumb is free.
4. The uninjured fingers are free to exercise.

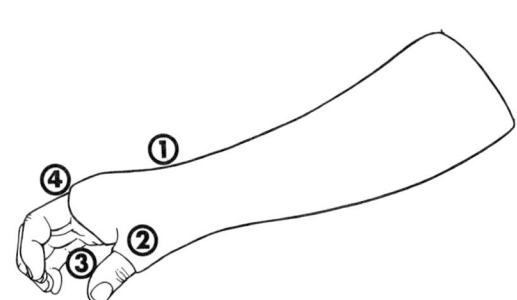

Postreduction Management

Check the fracture position by x-ray within one week.
Encourage the patient to use the nonimmobilized fingers actively during immobilization.
The cast may be removed at three weeks and fracture healing may be evaluated clinically and radiographically.

DISLOCATIONS AND FRACTURE-DISLOCATIONS OF THE THUMB

If there is still localized tenderness at the fracture site, apply a protective splint; otherwise encourage the patient to begin active exercises out of the plaster.

The patient should avoid contact sports or activities that are likely to reinjure the hand for three weeks after the cast is removed.

Clinical union usually precedes radiographic union of these metacarpal fractures by several weeks or a month. Do not wait for complete radiographic union of the fracture to permit active, protected range-of-motion exercises to the thumb.

OPEN REDUCTION AND FIXATION BY SMALL FRAGMENT SCREW

REMARKS

Open reduction using internal fixation with small fragment screw is the procedure of choice for the unstable thumb metacarpal fracture.

Most often a closed reduction is possible, but fixation is necessary to maintain alignment.

If closed reduction proves impossible, carry out open reduction with internal fixation as described on page 1161 for fractures of the base of the metacarpal.

Prereduction X-Ray

1. Oblique fracture of the shaft of the metacarpal.
2. The metacarpal is shortened.
3. The distal fragment is displaced upward and backward.

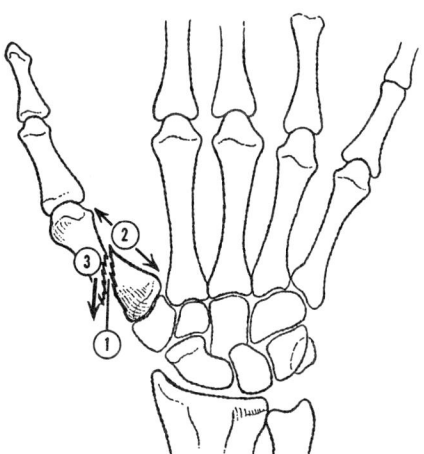

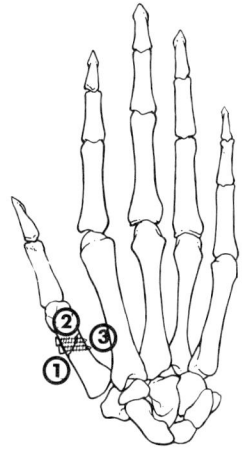

X-Ray after Closed Reduction and Screw Fixation

1. The shortening of the metacarpal has been corrected.
2. The displacement and rotation malalignment of the fracture have been reduced, and
3. The fracture is compressed with two small fragment screws applied perpendicular to the fracture line.

Postreduction Management

Apply a compression hand dressing and elevate the limb for several days until the edema subsides (see page 1172).

By three to five days remove the compression hand dressing and permit guarded active exercises.

The fixation must be secure to permit this early, active exercise program. If there has been any comminution of the fracture, cast immobilization should be continued for at least three weeks.

The screw need not be removed unless it causes local tenderness.

Injuries to the Metacarpophalangeal Joint of the Thumb

REMARKS

Dislocations and disruptions occur as frequently in the MP joint of the thumb as in the CM joint.

The mechanism of injury may be either a hyperextension force, which produces an anterior dislocation, or a lateral strain, which disrupts the collateral ligament.

Lateral strain with instability is frequently known as "skier's thumb," because it most often results from a skier's jamming the thumb while falling into a bank of hard-packed snow.

Because of the importance of the MP joint for pinch, any significant lateral instability should generally be treated by operative repair of the torn capsular ligament.

Complete anterior dislocation of the MP joint has been classified by McLaughlin as either simple or complex, depending on whether the volar plate is blocking reduction.

Simple MP dislocation may be recognized by the perpendicular relationship of the proximal phalanx to the first metacarpal. Reduction of a simple dislocation can be done by closed means provided that the surgeon avoids entrapping the volar plate in the MP joint by direct traction.

A complex MP dislocation is recognized clinically by the relationship of the proximal phalanx, parallel to the metacarpal. Dimpling of the skin directly over the metacarpal head also indicates that the volar plate has become trapped within the joint. Radiographically, a complex dislocation can be diagnosed by the fact that the sesamoid bone in the volar plate can be seen within the joint.

A complex MP dislocation requires open reduction via a volar approach so as to remove the volar plate, which has become entrapped within the joint and is preventing reduction.

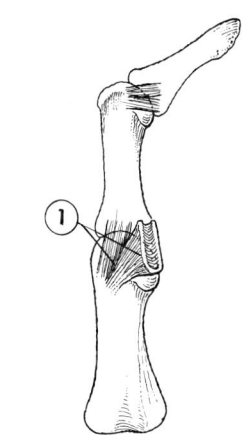

Normal Joint

1. Normal arrangement of the collateral ligaments and volar plate of the MP joint.

Simple Dislocation

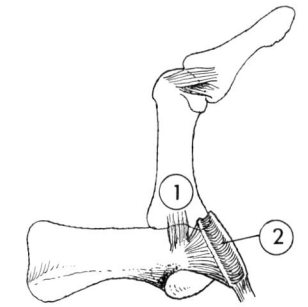

1. The phalanx sits on the back of the metacarpal in a vertical position.
2. The volar plate hangs in front of the metacarpal head but has not become entrapped within the joint. Note that the plate is always detached from its weaker metacarpal insertion.

Conversion of a Simple Dislocation to a Complex Dislocation by Traction

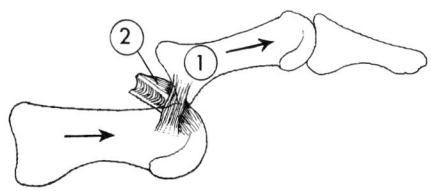

If traction is applied directly to a simple dislocation, the volar plate frequently becomes entrapped in the joint and produces an irreducible or complex dislocation.
1. The proximal phalanx is now parallel to the metacarpal.
2. The volar plate has become interposed in the joint.

The intrinsic muscles of the thumb may also obstruct reduction.
1. Proximal phalanx.
2. Protruding head of the metacarpal.
3. Intrinsic muscles of the thumb.

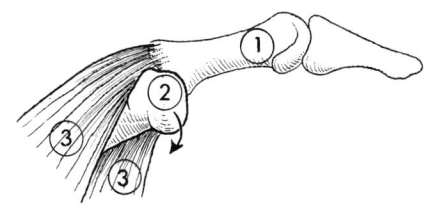

REDUCING A SIMPLE DISLOCATION OF THE METACARPOPHALANGEAL JOINT OF THE THUMB

REMARKS

The technique of reduction is to push rather than pull the dislocated phalanx into the MP joint.

If this reduction is not possible after one or two attempts, open reduction is indicated.

Do not inflict more damage on the thumb by repeated and futile attempts at closed reduction when the probability is that the volar plate is interposed in the joint.

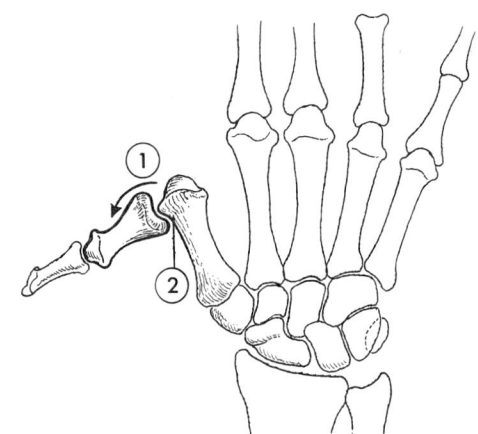

Prereduction X-Ray

1. The phalanx is hyperextended and is displaced upward and backward.
2. The base of the phalanx rests on the head of the metacarpal at a right angle.

Manipulative Reduction (Using Intravenous or General Anesthesia)

1. A bandage is looped around the patient's thumb and then around the operator's hand.
2. Grasp the patient's thumb and hyperextend the dislocated phalanx about 90 degrees on the metacarpal.
3. Push the dorsal surface of the dislocated phalanx to reduce the dislocation. Avoid reducing this dislocation by traction alone.
4. While continuing to push against the dorsal surface of the phalanx, flex the thumb, and reduction should be accomplished.

Note: If this simple dislocation is manipulated by traction alone, a complex or irreducible dislocation is likely to result.

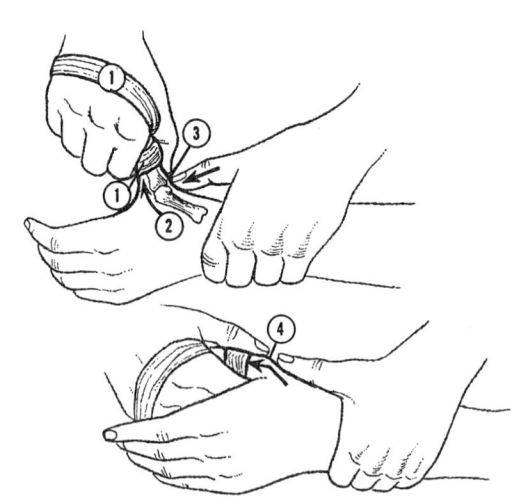

Postreduction X-Ray

1. The base of the phalanx is in normal relationship to the head of the metacarpal.

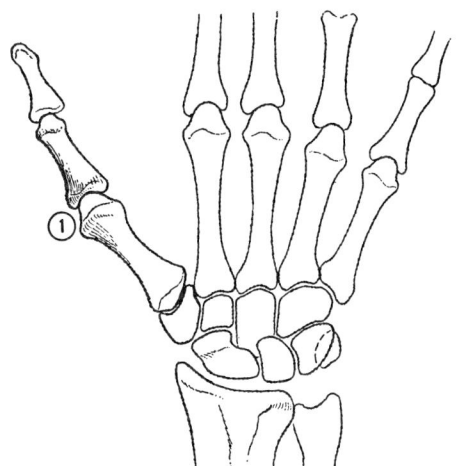

Immobilization

Always test stability and motion following reduction. Usually the joint is quite stable after closed reduction. A minimum amount of external support is necessary. Avoid immobilizing the injury for longer than ten days, because this is likely to produce a stiff MP joint.

Apply 1-cm strips of adhesive.
1. The strapping encircles the MP joint.
2. The IP joint is left free.
3. The basket weave extends above the wrist.
4. Anchor the strips of adhesive encircling the thumb by strips encircling the wrist.
5. The thumb is strapped in the grasp position for 5 to 7 days.

Note: Allow the patient to use the hand actively, and after 5 to 7 days remove the strapping and permit full active exercises.

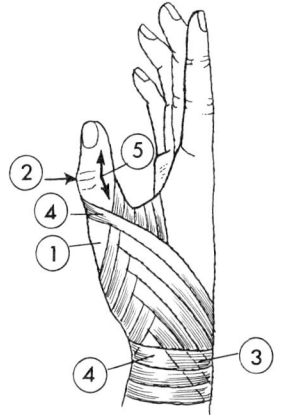

OPEN REDUCTION OF COMPLEX DISLOCATION OF THE METACARPOPHALANGEAL JOINT OF THE THUMB

REMARKS

An entrapped volar plate is always the major obstacle to reduction. Occasionally the flexor pollicis brevis or flexus pollicis longus may also block relocation.

A volar incision with radial extension is essential in order to visualize the pathologic process.

Carefully identify the digital neurovascular structures, which are always displaced close to the skin owing to the metacarpal head dislocation.

1. Make a curved volar incision centered over the MP joint.

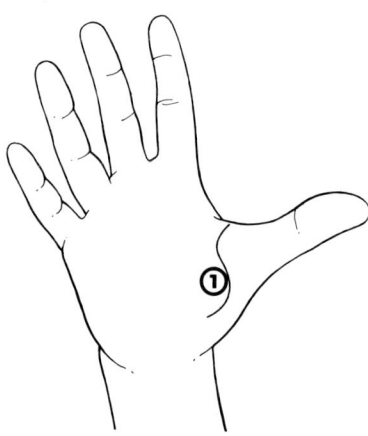

2. Identify and protect the neurovascular structures, which are displaced immediately beneath the skin.

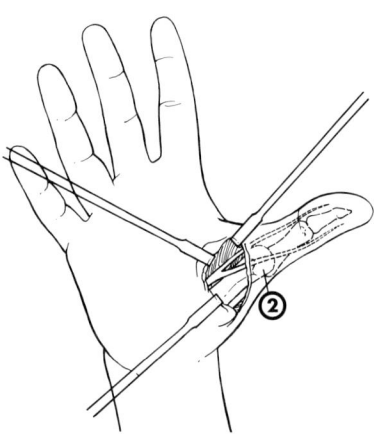

3. The short thenar muscles may envelop the metacarpal head, and they should be released by hyperextending the thumb.

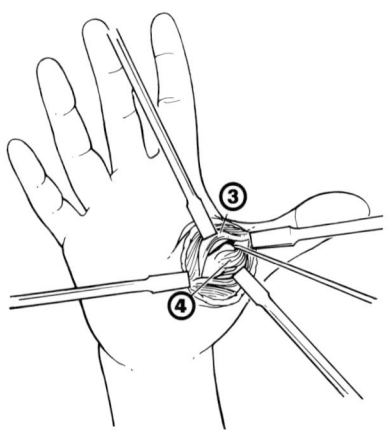

4. Make longitudinal incisions in the capsular attachment to the volar plate and then pull the plate out of the joint with a skin hook.

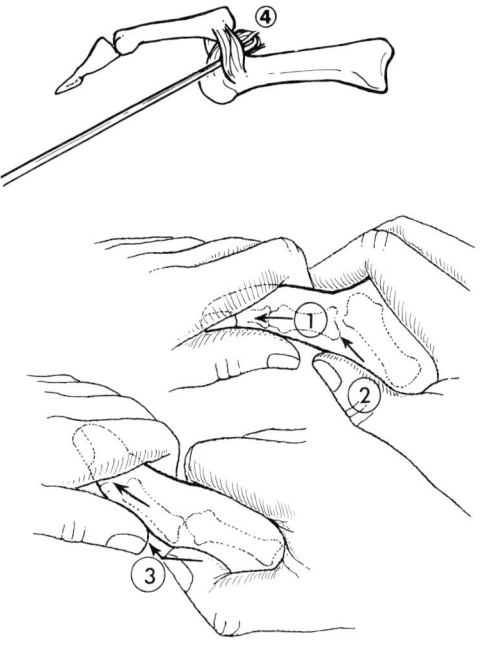

After the volar plate has been released from the joint, reduction can be accomplished as with a simple dislocation by pushing the phalanx forward.
1. The phalanx is hyperextended at least 90 degrees.
2. Reduce the dislocated phalanx by pushing it forward over the metacarpal head.
3. While continuing to push the phalanx, complete the reduction by flexing the MP joint.

Postreduction Management

Reduction should be stable and cast immobilization is usually unnecessary. Always check for instability after reduction to make sure that the collateral ligaments of the joint have not been disrupted sufficiently to require repair.
1. Elevate the limb in a postoperative hand dressing and begin active range-of-motion exercises to the thumb within three days, or as soon as the swelling subsides.

Note: Immobilization of the thumb for more than ten days will cause residual restriction of motion.

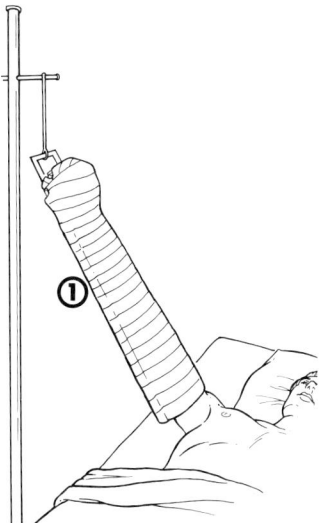

SKIER'S THUMB — COLLATERAL LIGAMENT DISRUPTION

REMARKS

Acute abduction injury to the MP joint of the thumb occurs most frequently when a skier falls and jams the thumb into hard-packed snow. This may cause either partial or complete rupture of the ulnar collateral ligament.

Occasionally the radial collateral ligament may be injured instead.

Clinically the joint is swollen and the thumb is tender in the region of the ulnar collateral ligament. Injecting local anesthesia into the painful region permits adequate clinical and radiographic evaluation of joint stability with stress testing.

For the most part these injuries may be treated by immobilization in a thumb spica cast for four weeks, which permits healing with adequate stability for pinch. Should the joint be completely unstable on stress x-ray, primary surgical repair is advisable, because the disrupted ligament usually folds back on itself and winds up beneath the proximal end of the adductor tendon insertion.

Radiographic evidence of an avulsion fracture at the base of the phalanx is also an indication for operative fixation.

Mechanism of Injury

1. Abduction strain to the thumb may cause either partial or complete disruption of the ulnar collateral ligament.

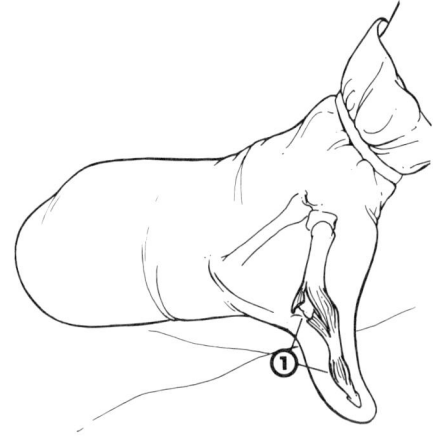

2. Avulsion fracture of the phalanx may also occur.

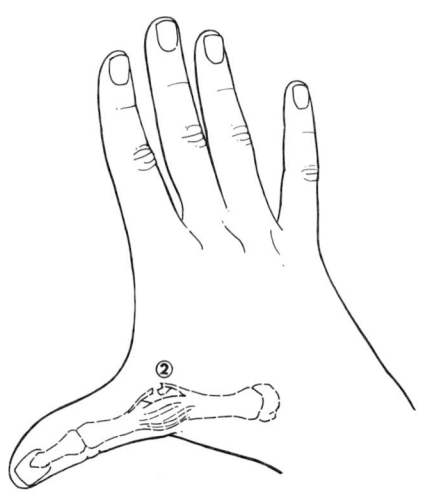

Clinical Appearance

Evaluate stability with stress testing under local anesthesia. The injury may cause:
1. Partial instability when compared with the uninjured side or
2. Complete disruption.

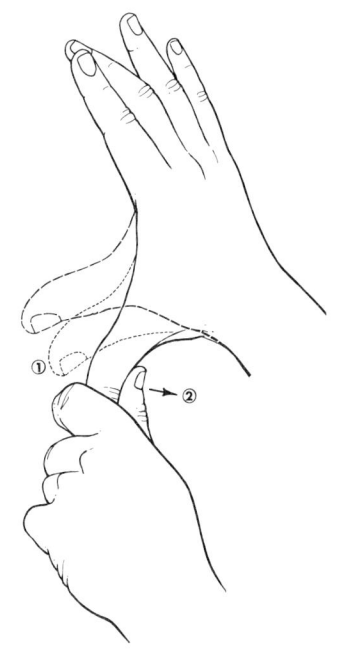

Closed Treatment for Partial Tear

1. Apply a thumb spica that includes the wrist and forearm.
2. The MP joint of the thumb is in slight flexion to relax the collateral ligament and the thumb is apposed to the other fingers.
3. The IP joint is immobilized in slight flexion.

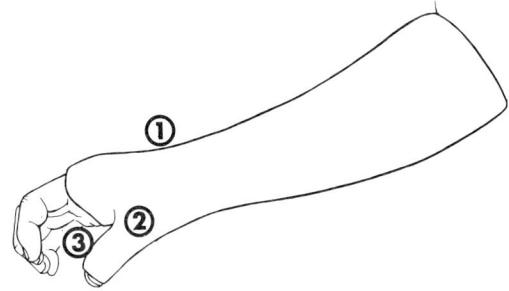

Subsequent Management

Continue cast immobilization for a minimum of four weeks and then evaluate stability of the MP joint.

If the joint is still significantly unstable, offer the patient operative repair. Otherwise allow active exercises with protection against abduction reinjury for four more weeks.

OPERATIVE REPAIR FOR COMPLETE DISRUPTION OR AVULSION FRACTURE

For treatment of a complete tear or an avulsion fracture,

1. Normal pinch requires stability of the MP joint's ulnar collateral ligament.
2. Complete disruption of the ligament impairs key pinch significantly and should be corrected surgically.

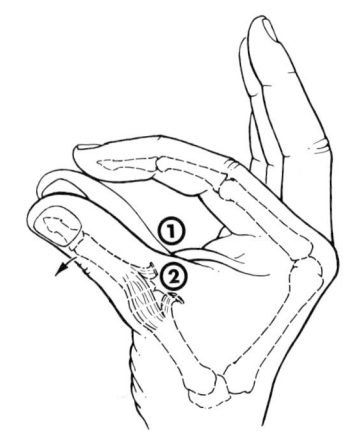

Surgical Procedure for Complete Disruption

1. The ulnar collateral ligament is usually turned outward and separated from its attachment by the adductor tendon.
2. Repair is accomplished after the adductor tendon is opened transversely.
3. Small, loose avulsion fractures may be removed. Fix larger fragments with a screw.

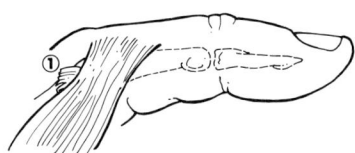

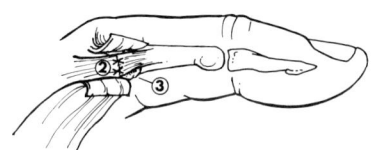

Avulsion Fracture

PREOPERATIVE X-RAY

1. A large triangular fracture avulsed from the proximal phalanx.
2. Radial deviation of the finger.

Note: This is best repaired by open reduction and screw fixation (see page 1161).

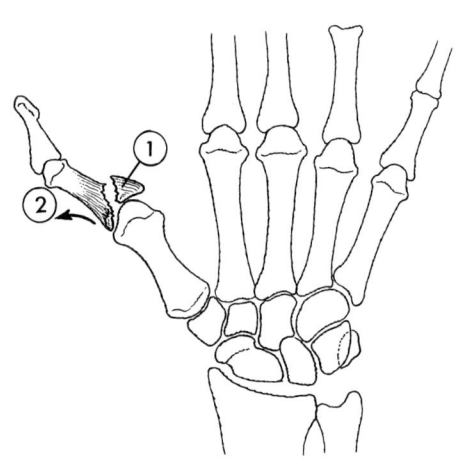

POSTOPERATIVE X-RAY

1. Radial deviation of the finger is corrected.

2. The fragment is fixed by a small fragment screw.

Note: The screw may be removed at the end of three weeks under local anesthesia if it is palpable beneath the skin.

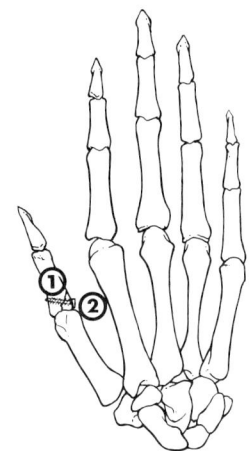

INJURY TO THE RADIAL COLLATERAL LIGAMENT OF THE METACARPOPHALANGEAL JOINT OF THE THUMB

This injury is less common than disruption of the ulnar collateral ligament because the other metacarpals protect the thumb against extreme adduction.

As with ulnar collateral ligament injury, indications for closed or open treatment depend on the degree of instability.

Occasionally an avulsed fragment from the phalanx may require operative fixation.

Preoperative X-Ray

1. Small fragment avulsed from the dorsoradial margin of the proximal phalanx.

2. Ulnar deviation of the proximal phalanx.

Note: Remove this fragment and repair the ligament; then treat as a severe sprain (see page 1183).

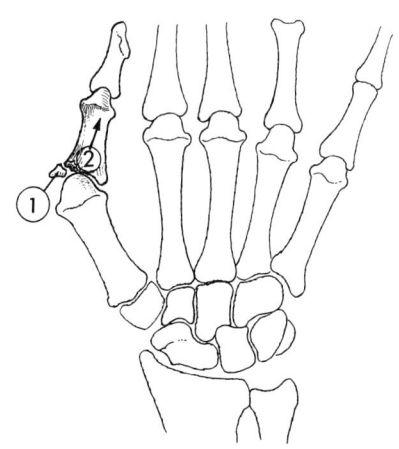

Postoperative X-Ray

1. Defect after removal of the fragment.
2. Phalanx is in normal alignment with the head of the metacarpal.

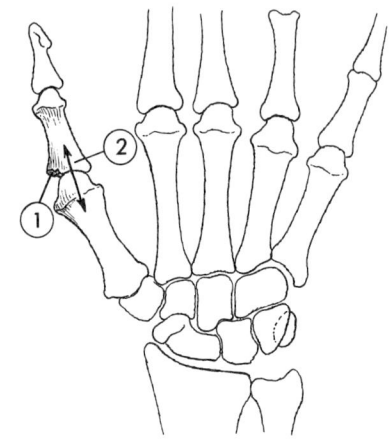

Preoperative X-Ray

1. Large triangular fragment avulsed from the proximal phalanx.
2. Ulnar deviation of the proximal fragment.

Note: Reduce this fragment and fix it with a small fragment screw set (see page 1161).

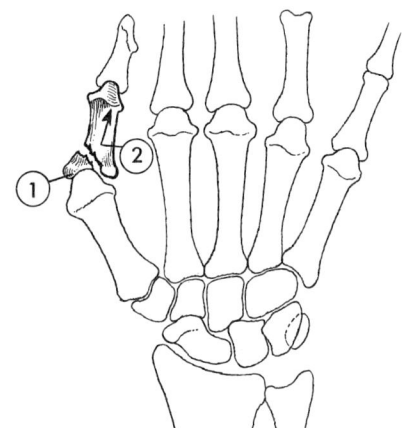

Postoperative X-Ray

1. The fragment has been reduced and fixed with a small fragment screw. The alignment between the proximal phalanx and metacarpal is restored.

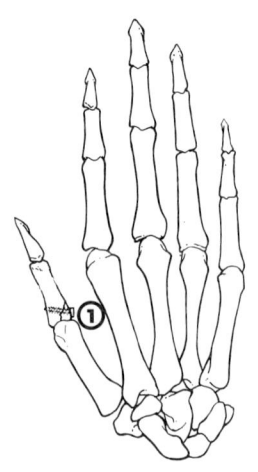

Injuries to the Interphalangeal Joint of the Thumb

REMARKS

Because of the stability that is provided by the insertions of the flexor and extensor tendons and by the strong collateral ligaments, dislocation of the IP joint is rare.

Occasionally, such a dislocation may be irreducible because of an interposition of the volar plate or the flexor pollicis longus tendon.

A dislocation or subluxation may be unstable because of a fracture of the phalanx.

Indications for closed or open treatment depend on the degree of instability and the reducibility of the injury.

Frequently these dislocations are open injuries and require thorough wound excision and appropriate fixation.

SUBLUXATION OF THE INTERPHALANGEAL JOINT OF THE THUMB

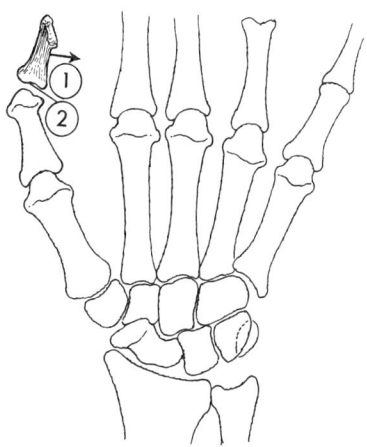

Appearance on X-Ray

RUPTURE OF ONE OF THE COLLATERAL LIGAMENTS

1. Lateral deviation of the distal phalanx.
2. Widening of the interphalangeal joint.

1187

Appearance on X-Ray (Continued)

FRACTURE WITHOUT DISPLACEMENT

1. Marginal fracture without displacement.

Immobilization with Thumb Spica

1. Apply a cast from below the elbow.
2. The thumb is abducted and the plaster is molded over the arches of the hand.
3. The IP joint of the thumb is immobilized in slight flexion and the thumb is apposed to the fingers.

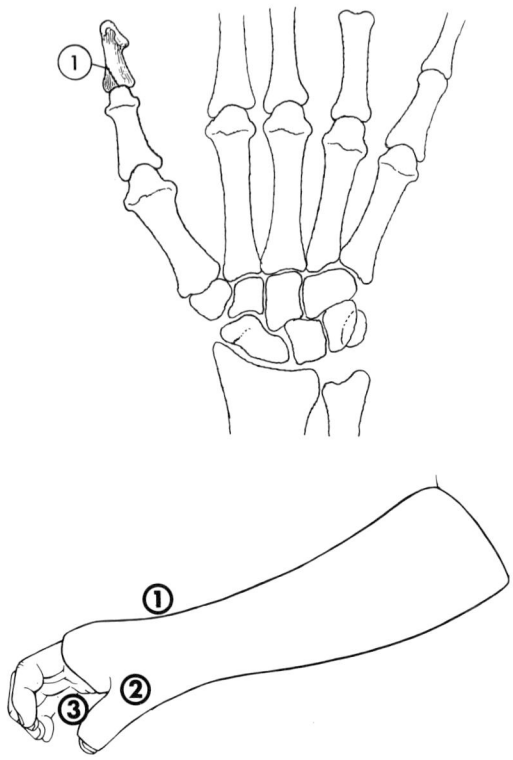

Subsequent Management

Remove the cast at the end of ten days and evaluate the joint stability clinically and radiographically.

If the joint is stable, allow the patient to begin guarded active range-of-motion exercises.

Immobilization for longer than ten days tends to produce stiffness of these joints and, if at all possible, should be avoided.

DISLOCATION OF THE INTERPHALANGEAL JOINT OF THE THUMB

Prereduction X-Ray

1. On the anteroposterior view, the distal phalanx is displaced laterally.
2. On the lateral view, the distal phalanx sits on the dorsum of the proximal phalanx.

Note: This relationship is analogous to complex dislocation of the MP joint and may indicate volar plate interposition in the joint.

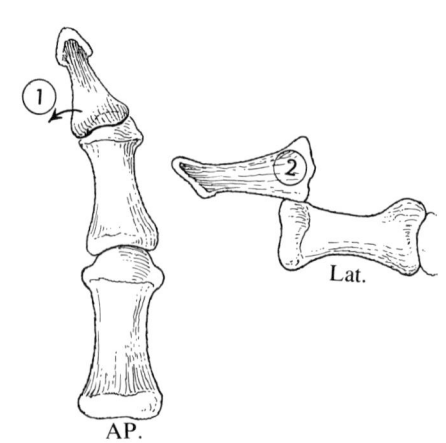

Reduction

1. Grasp the patient's thumb with your thumb and index finger.
2. Make steady traction in the line of deformity of the distal phalanx.
3. While traction is maintained flex the interphalangeal joint.

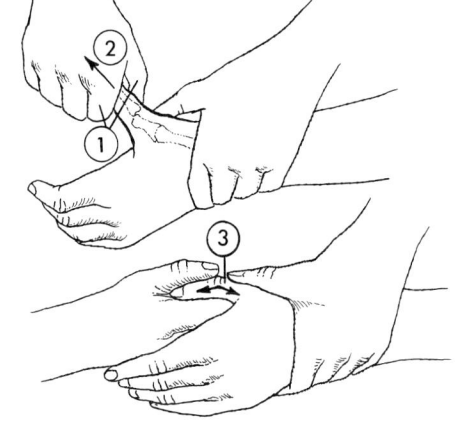

Reduction should be relatively simple. If the joint does not reduce with this maneuver there is either:

1. Entrapment of the volar plate in the joint or
2. Entrapment of the flexor pollicis longus, which is wrapped around the ulnar condyle of the proximal phalanx.

Note: Both of these situations require open reduction to remove the obstacle.

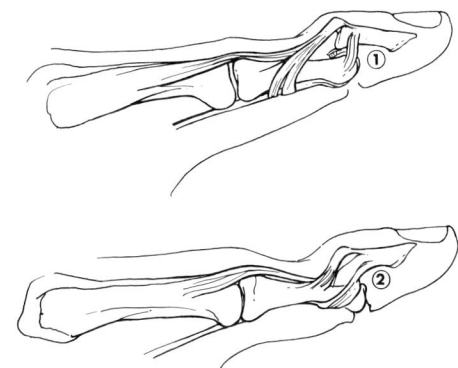

Immobilization

Following reduction the joint is usually stable.

If there is evidence of instability or if there is a small fracture, immobilize the thumb in a spica cast:

1. Apply a cast from below the elbow.
2. The thumb is abducted and the plaster is molded over the arches of the hand.
3. The IP joint of the thumb is immobilized in slight flexion and the thumb is apposed to the fingers.

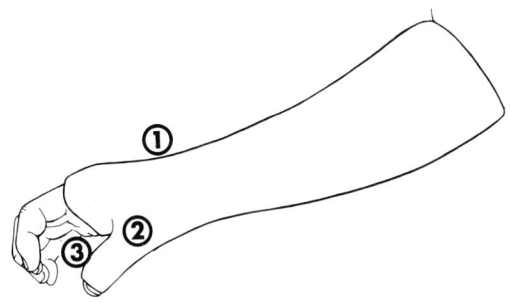

Remove the cast after ten days and evaluate the joint for instability.
Healing is usually satisfactory by ten days. Prolonging immobilization of the joint tends to produce joint stiffness and should be avoided if at all possible.

FRACTURES, DISLOCATIONS, AND FRACTURE-DISLOCATIONS OF THE FINGERS

Carpometacarpal Joints

REMARKS

Dislocation of the carpometacarpal joint is extremely rare because of the strong ligamentous support in this region.

The injury frequently is associated with extensive soft tissue damage, and the dislocation may go unrecognized unless true lateral x-rays visualize the carpometacarpal relationships.

Severe hyperextension or hyperflexion of the carpus may cause a rupture of the ligaments and may produce either dorsal or volar dislocation. The former is more common than the latter.

Generally, all the metacarpals are dislocated. Isolated dislocations can occur at either the fourth or the fifth carpometacarpal joint, because these joints are more mobile than the middle two.

Most commonly, dislocation of a single metacarpal is associated with a fracture of its base. Oblique fractures at the base of the metacarpal must be carefully assessed for the possibility of an associated dislocation.

Fracture-dislocations of the fifth metacarpal with volar displacement very commonly involve the motor branch of the ulnar nerve, which should be decompressed.

Dislocations of the carpometacarpal joint usually are unstable and require Kirschner wire fixation to maintain reduction.

DISLOCATIONS OF THE CARPOMETACARPAL JOINT

Prereduction X-Rays

DORSAL DISLOCATION

1. The four metacarpals are displaced dorsally en masse.
2. The bases of the metacarpals lie on the dorsum of the distal row of carpal bones.

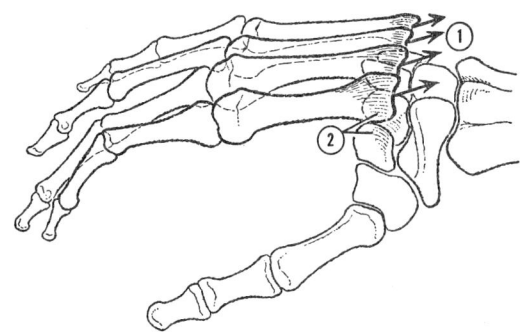

VOLAR DISLOCATION

1. The four metacarpals are displaced volarly.
2. The bases of the metacarpals are in the palm.

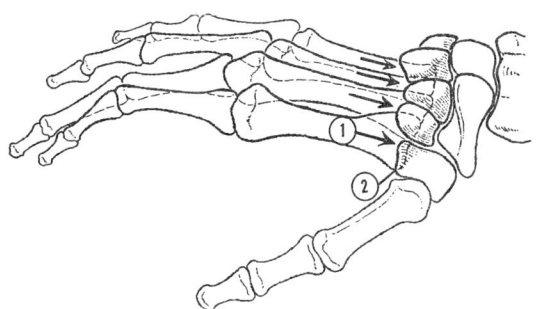

Reduction by Traction and Manipulation For Dorsal Dislocation

1. One hand of the operator encircles the wrist while the other encircles the hand.
2. The wrist is slightly dorsiflexed.
3. The fingers are flexed.
4. While counter traction is made on the wrist, make strong traction on the hand.
5. While the thumb of the proximal hand makes first downward pressure over the bases of the metacarpal bones, the fingers of the distal hand make upward pressure on the shafts of the metacarpals, and at the same time,
6. The wrist is dorsiflexed further.

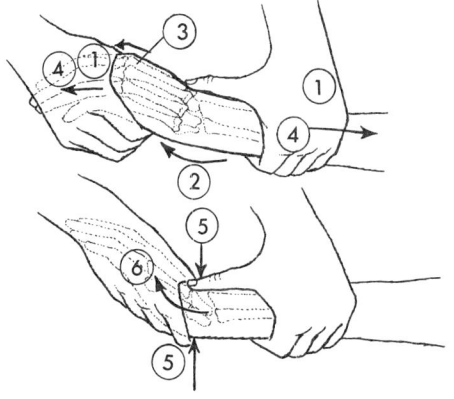

Note: For volar dislocation, the manipulative maneuvers are reversed and the wrist is immobilized in slight flexion.

Postreduction X-Ray

1. The bases of the metacarpals are now in normal relationship with the distal row of carpal bones.

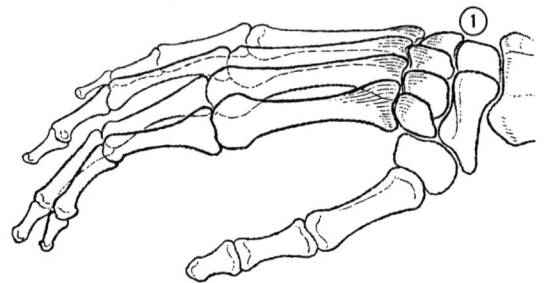

Stabilization with Kirschner Wires

1. A smooth Kirschner wire is inserted from the fifth metacarpal into the carpal bones to prevent redislocation.
2. Occasionally, a second pin through the fourth metacarpal into the carpus is necessary.

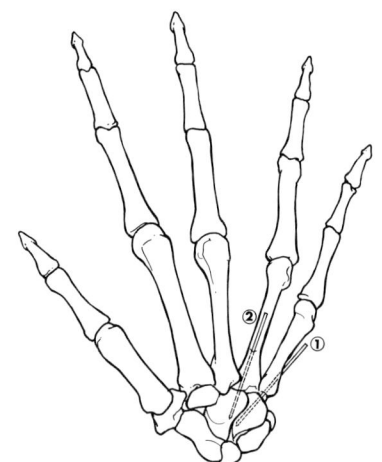

Immobilization

1. Apply a postoperative hand dressing and elevate the limb for several days to diminish edema. Monitor the circulation to the fingertips closely.

Note: If the injury is the result of a crushing trauma to the hand, surgical decompression of the intrinsic compartments may be necessary.

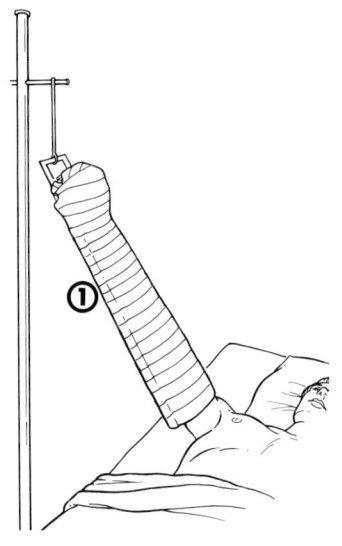

Subsequent Management

After the edema has subsided, apply a short arm cast with the hand in dorsiflexion.

Remove the pins at the end of three weeks and evaluate stability. If the injured carpometacarpal joint is stable allow the patient to begin guarded active range-of-motion exercises. Have the patient avoid hyperextension of the hand for at least six weeks.

FRACTURE-DISLOCATIONS OF THE CARPOMETACARPAL JOINTS

REMARKS

Carpometacarpal dislocation may be accompanied by a marginal fracture of the base of the metacarpal.

The dislocation may not be recognized unless true lateral views of the hand are scrutinized for the altered metacarpal-carpal relationships.

These are usually unstable injuries and require internal fixation with Kirschner wires.

Fractures with volar displacement of the fourth or fifth metacarpal frequently impinge on the motor branch of the ulnar nerve and cause intrinsic paralysis. Evaluate these fractures carefully for nerve injury and reduce them anatomically.

FRACTURE-DISLOCATION OF FOURTH METACARPAL

Prereduction X-Ray

1. Fracture of the base of the fourth metacarpal.
2. Dorsal displacement of the shaft of the metacarpal.

Note: This displacement may not be recognized unless a true lateral x-ray is obtained and is scrutinized for the altered carpometacarpal relationships.

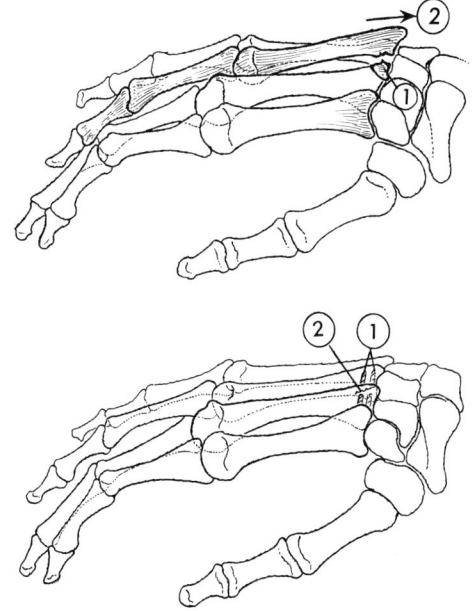

Postreduction X-Ray

1. The base of the fourth metacarpal is fixed to the adjacent metacarpals by Kirschner wires.
2. The fracture-dislocation is reduced.

Note: This procedure does not require exposing the fracture site (see page 1191).

FRACTURE-DISLOCATION OF FIFTH METACARPAL

Prereduction X-Ray

1. A fracture-dislocation of the base of the fifth metacarpal with volar displacement.
2. The motor branch of the ulnar nerve is involved by the injury.

Note: Always test for ulnar nerve function with this type of injury. Surgical decompression of the nerve is necessary to stabilize the fracture and prevent permanent intrinsic paralysis.

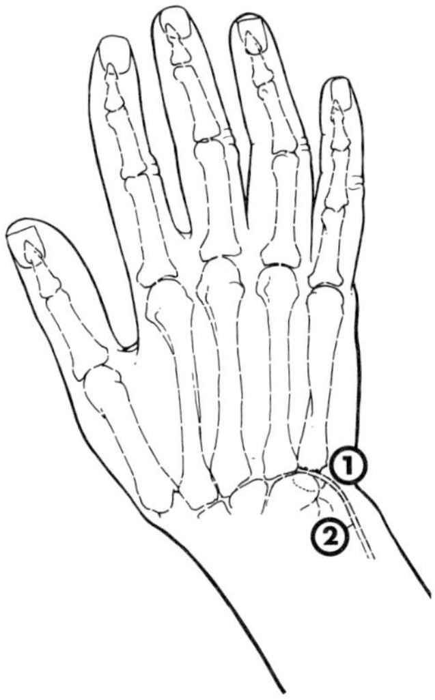

Operative Procedure

1. Use Henry's medial approach to avoid scarring in the palmar skin.
2. The motor branch of the ulnar nerve is identified and is freed from the fracture site.
3. The fracture-dislocation of the metacarpal is reduced and is fixed with a threaded Kirschner wire.

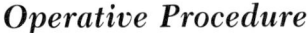

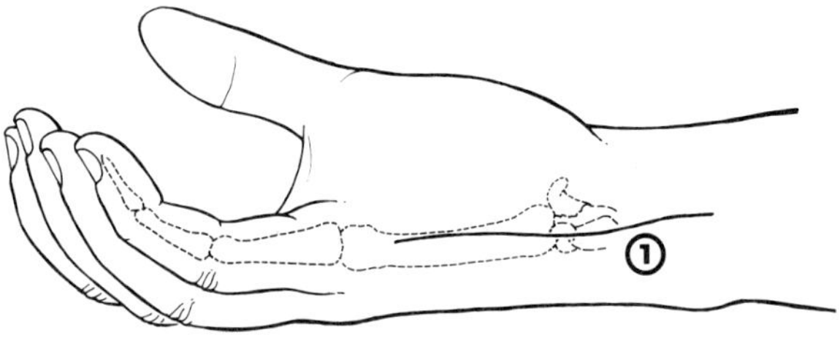

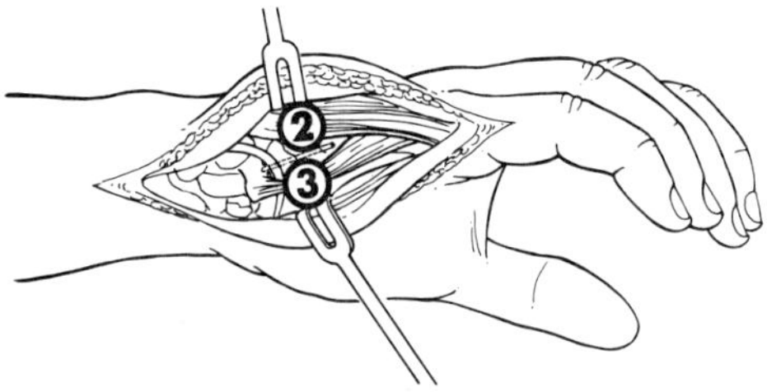

Postreduction X-Ray

1. The volar displacement of the fifth metacarpal is corrected.
2. The fragments are stabilized by a smooth Kirschner wire.

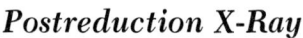

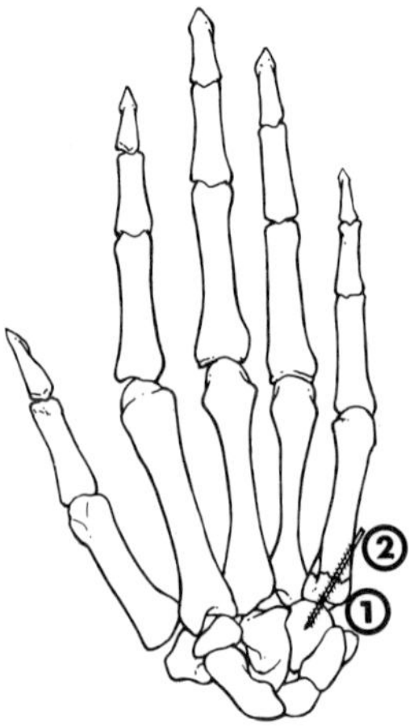

Immobilization

Apply a padded cast or hand dressing from the forearm to just proximal to the MP joints.
1. The wirst is slightly dorsiflexed.
2. The thumb is free.
3. The fingers are free.

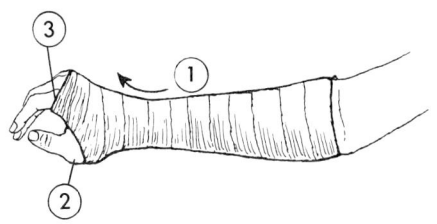

Postreduction Management

Remove the cast and wires at the end of four weeks. During immobilization allow free use of all the fingers.

Injuries of the Metacarpophalangeal Joints of the Fingers

REMARKS

Dislocations of the MP joints may be surprisingly difficult to recognize unless adequate true lateral x-ray views are obtained.

The injury usually occurs in either the index or the small finger. Visual examination of the finger can be deceiving in that it merely appears short and deviated slightly to the ulnar side.

A lateral x-ray will show the hyperextended position of the MP joint.

Like dislocations of the MP joint of the thumb, these injuries may be either simple or complex depending on whether or not the volar plate has become entrapped in the joint.

Reduction is possible by closed methods when the dislocation is simple, but open reduction is always necessary for complex dislocation.

Repeated attempts at reduction inflict further damage to joint structures. Do not make more than two attempts at closed reduction.

Surgical exposure is best done via a volar approach. The key to reduction is to release the transverse metacarpal ligament attachment to the volar plate to allow it to be removed from the joint.

Occasionally with a chronic dislocation, a dorsal extension of the incision is necessary to free the lateral capsular structures as well.

FRACTURES, DISLOCATIONS, AND FRACTURE-DISLOCATIONS OF THE FINGERS

SIMPLE DISLOCATION

Prereduction X-Ray

1. The base of the phalanx sits on the dorsum of the head of the metacarpal at a right angle.

Note: When the phalanx is in this position it can be assumed that the anterior capsule is not interposed between the bones. This is far less common than a complex dislocation with capsular interposition.

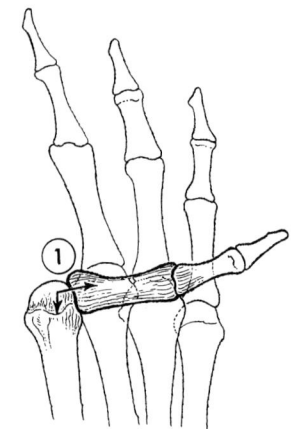

Manipulative Reduction

1. A bandage is first looped around the patient's finger and then around the operator's hand.
2. Grasp the finger with your thumb and index finger and make traction along the axis of the hyperextended phalanx (not along the axis of the metacarpal).
3. While traction is maintained push the base of the dislocated phalanx distalward to a position opposite the head of the metacarpal.
4. Flex the metacarpophalangeal joints.

Note: The key to reduction is to *push* the hyperextended dislocated phalanx volarly over the metacarpal head. Trying to reduce the dislocation by pulling the finger will entrap the volar plate in the joint and produce a complex dislocation.

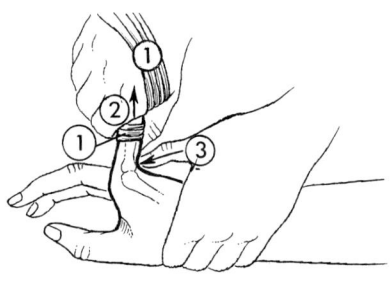

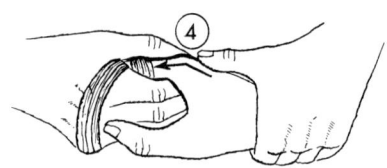

1196

FRACTURES, DISLOCATIONS, AND FRACTURE-DISLOCATIONS OF THE FINGERS

COMPLEX DISLOCATION

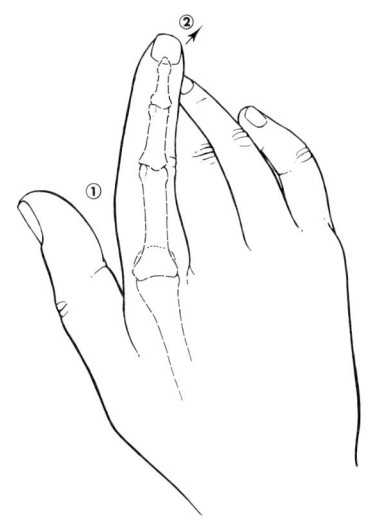

Clinical Appearance

Clinical appearance can be deceiving about the extent of injury.
1. The finger looks a little short.
2. There is slight ulnar deviation.

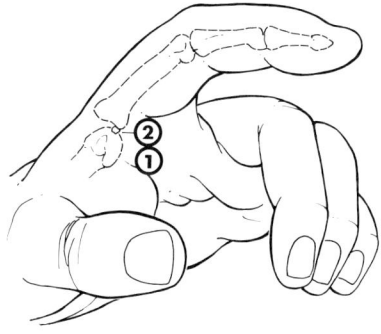

Clues to a complex dislocation:
1. Dimpling in the palm.
2. Inclusion of a sesamoid bone in the joint on x-ray.
Do not mistake this for a chip fracture.

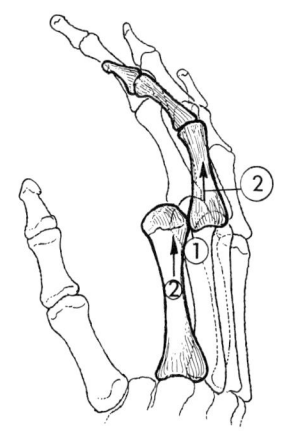

Prereduction X-Ray

1. The base of the phalanx lies on the dorsal surface of the head of the metacarpal.
2. The axis of the phalanx is almost parallel to that of the metacarpal.

Note: When the phalanx lies in this position it can be assumed that the anterior palmar ligament is interposed between the bones.

FRACTURES, DISLOCATIONS, AND FRACTURE-DISLOCATIONS OF THE FINGERS

Surgical Reduction of a Complex MP Dislocation of the Index or Small Finger

1. The dislocation is exposed through a curved palmar skin incision.
2. The metacarpal head is directly beneath the skin.
3. The flexor tendon and neurovascular structures are displaced as a result of the metacarpal head dislocation and must be carefully protected.

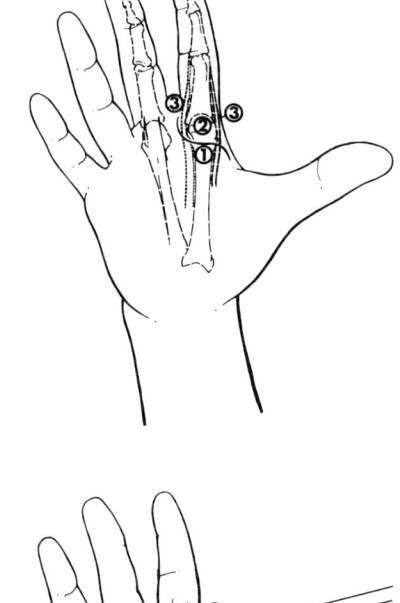

4. The major obstacle to reduction is the transverse metacarpal ligament, which is wedged between the metacarpal head and the proximal phalanx. This is divided longitudinally and
5. The volar capsule is then removed from the joint with a small hook.

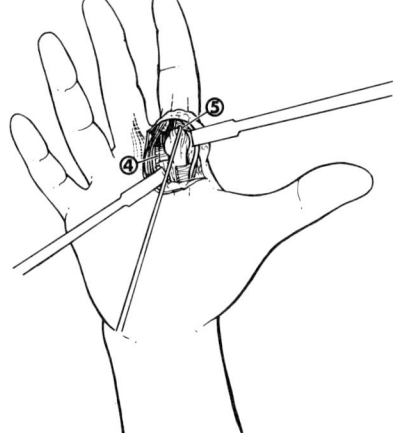

Immobilization

A simple MP dislocation treated by closed reduction can be splinted with buddy taping of the finger to the adjacent, uninjured finger. The patient is allowed to begin active exercises and the tape is removed after ten days (see page 1156).

If open reduction of a complex dislocation has been carried out, the joint is usually stable.

Stability of the joint should be confirmed at the time of surgery by passively moving the finger through a full range of motion.

Following open reduction of the MP dislocation, the hand is immobilized and elevated for three days to diminish edema and active exercise is permitted when the edema has subsided, usually by three to five days.

Immobilization of the hand after these injuries for longer than ten days contributes nothing except further stiffening of the joint.

FRACTURES, DISLOCATIONS, AND FRACTURE-DISLOCATIONS OF THE FINGERS

FRACTURE-DISLOCATIONS OF THE METACARPOPHALANGEAL JOINT

Appearance on X-Ray

SMALL DISPLACED FRAGMENT

1. Small avulsed fragment from the base of the phalanx.
2. Fragment is displaced.

Note: Remove this fragment and repair the torn ligament.

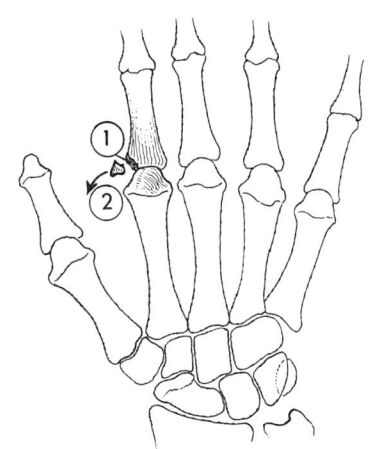

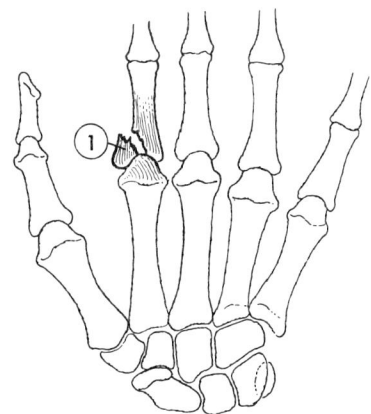

LARGE DISPLACED FRAGMENT

1. Large triangular fragment from volar aspect of the base of the phalanx.

Note: Reduce this fragment, which involves more than one third of the articular surface, and fix it with a small fragment screw (see page 1161).

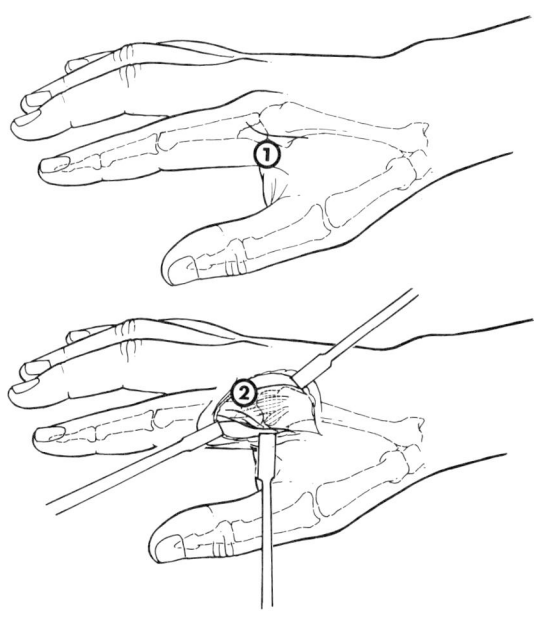

Surgical Approach

1. A curved dorsal incision is preferable.
2. A longitudinal incision between the lateral band and the extensor tendon permits excellent exposure of the fracture.

1199

Postreduction X-ray

1. The fragment is fixed in its normal position with a small fragment screw.

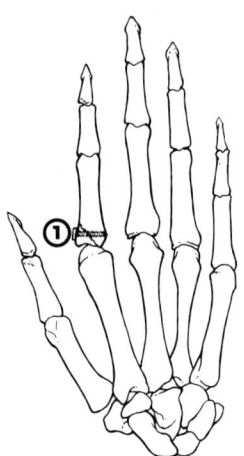

Postreduction Management

Motion is permitted when the postoperative edema has subsided, usually by three to five days.

After five to eight weeks, when the fracture is healed clinically and radiographically, the screw may be removed under local anesthesia.

Injuries to the Interphalangeal Joints of the Fingers

REMARKS

Dislocations and fracture-dislocations of the IP joints are common injuries and usually are produced by lateral or hyperextension overload of the joint structures.

Injury to the proximal interphalangeal (PIP) joint is particularly treacherous in that what is initially considered a "jammed finger" can cause significant and permanent impairment.

Since the PIP joint moves through the greatest range (100 to 110 degrees of flexion), loss of this joint's motion can impair finger function significantly.

The major source of disability is stiffness of the PIP joint, not instability. Treatment should be designed to permit prompt resumption of finger motion.

After any injury that causes swelling or tenderness of the joint, obtain a true lateral view of the finger (not the hand) to determine if bone fracture or joint instability has occurred.

Evaluate the patient's ability to move the finger actively through a full range. If necessary, use local digital anesthetic to relieve pain.

Should a joint deformity recur with active motions, there is significant instability that requires adequate splinting. If the joint is functionally stable and the patient is able to flex fully and extend without redisplacement, splinting may be minimized.

If redisplacement of the joint occurs in an anterior (palmar) direction, the disrupted dorsal capsule and central slip require splinting in extension to prevent boutonniere deformity. If anterior displacement is associated with a dorsal chip fracture from the midphalanx, operative repair is usually indicated primarily.

If the joint is unstable and displaces dorsally, treatment with an extension block splint is generally indicated. If a fracture involving more than 40 per cent of the joint's surface is causing the dorsal instability, operative repair is necessary.

Chronic disruption of the volar capsule from the middle phalanx will produce a swan-neck deformity, which requires treatment by surgical advancement of the volar capsule.

Chronic disruption of the volar capsule from its attachment on the proximal phalanx leads to scarring and a pseudo-boutonniere deformity.

The injured or swollen joint should also be stressed in a lateral direction to determine if disruption of the collateral ligament has occurred. Lateral instability of the IP joint can generally be treated by closed splinting methods, provided that the instability is recognized soon after injury.

Early recognition of dorsal, volar, or lateral instability offers enormous advantage because it generally permits closed treatment and satisfactory functional healing. Delay in recognition for longer than three weeks usually necessitates open treatment with variable prognosis for functional return.

Be suspicious of any "jammed finger." Evaluate it thoroughly by palpation, by active and passive stress testing, and by adequate anteroposterior and lateral x-rays centered on the finger, not the hand.

EVALUATION OF THE "JAMMED FINGER": SPRAIN, FRACTURE, DISLOCATION, OR TENDON AVULSION?

REMARKS

Only careful assessment will detect injuries likely to cause significant impairment of finger function.

Evaluation of the "jammed finger" should include careful direct palpation of areas of tenderness, adequate x-rays to show small fractures or signs of instability, and active and passive stress testing of joint stability.

FRACTURES, DISLOCATIONS, AND FRACTURE-DISLOCATIONS OF THE FINGERS

Palpation

Palpate the entire swollen finger for the precise areas of tenderness to identify common injuries, such as:
1. Collateral ligament injury.
2. Volar plate disruption.
3. Injury to the central slip.
4. Avulsion of extensor tendon insertion on distal phalanx.
5. Avulsion of flexor profundus tendon. This is tender at the point to which the tendon has retracted, either in the sheath or up in the palm.
6. Fracture or fracture-dislocation of the MP joint.

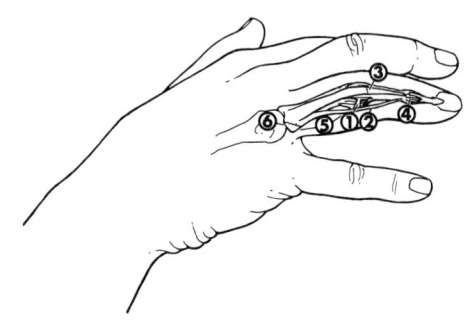

Radiographic Evaluation

X-ray view should be centered on the finger and not the hand in order to detect subtle changes such as:

1. Small fractures associated with PIP dislocation.

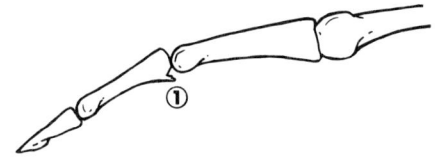

2. Avulsed bone fragments from hyperextension injury.

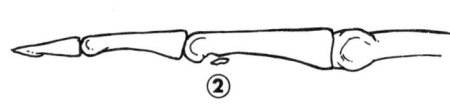

3. Avulsed bone fragments from mallet finger.

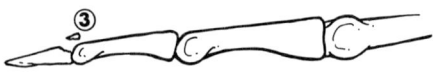

4. Avulsion of flexor profundus tendon.

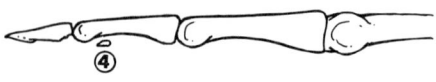

Active Testing of Functional Stability

PIP JOINT

Have the patient move the injured point actively through a full range to evaluate stability. This may require digital nerve block to determine if the PIP joint is unstable:

1. Dorsally from volar plate injury or

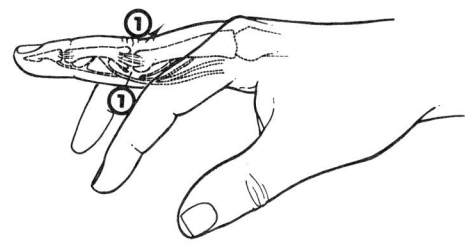

2. Anteriorly from central slip or capsular tear.

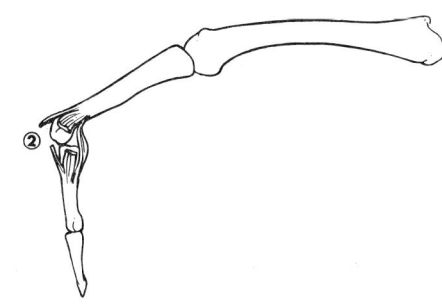

DIP JOINT

Evaluate motion of the DIP joint for

1. Loss of full extension due to mallet finger.

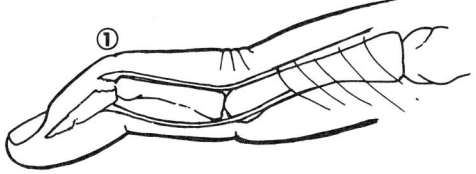

2. Loss of flexion due to avulsion of the flexor profundus.

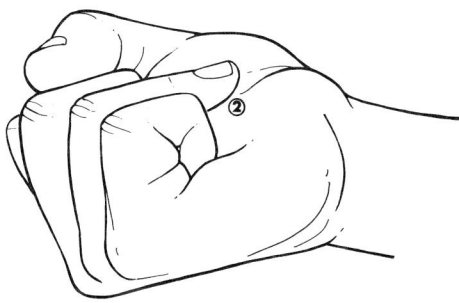

Passive Stress Testing

After the patient has carried out active functional testing, evaluate the joints for collateral stability by passive stress testing.
1. Finger is extended.
2. Lateral instability may be evident with gentle stressing.

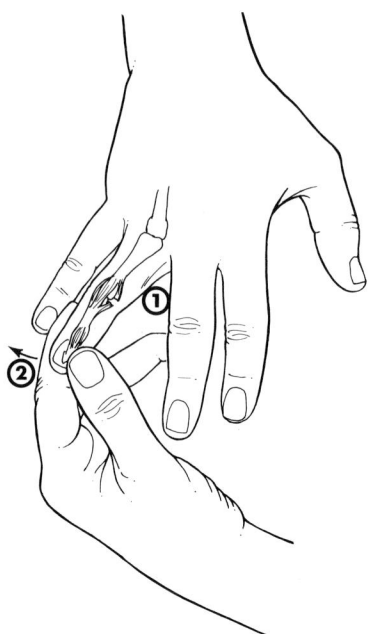

Note: Signs of acute injury or instability of joints do not necessarily indicate the need for immediate surgical reconstruction. They do indicate the need for appropriate external splinting of adequate duration.

LATERAL DISLOCATIONS OF THE INTERPHALANGEAL JOINTS

REMARKS

In lateral dislocation of the interphalangeal joint the collateral ligament is generally ruptured on the side to which the force was applied.

Dislocation usually is reduced by the patient or a bystander soon after injury.

Be wary of a joint that is unusually swollen or tender. This frequently indicates extensive damage to the collateral ligament and requires immobilization until the pain and swelling subside.

Evaluate the injury carefully to determine precisely the extent of the damage (see page 1201).

FRACTURES, DISLOCATIONS, AND FRACTURE-DISLOCATIONS OF THE FINGERS

Prereduction X-Ray

1. X-ray views should include true anteroposterior and lateral views of the finger and not just the hand so as to rule out small fractures.
2. A lateral dislocation of the PIP joint has occurred without anterior or posterior displacement.

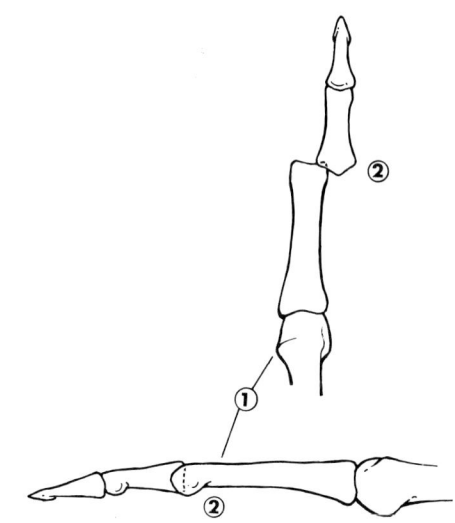

Manipulative Reduction

1. Loop a gauze bandage around the end of the injured finger and around the operator's hand.
2. Grasp the end of the finger with your thumb and index finger.
3. Make steady traction in the axis of the finger.
4. While traction is being maintained, bring the distal phalanx in line with the proximal phalanx.
5. Squeeze the sides of the joint to correct any residual lateral displacement.

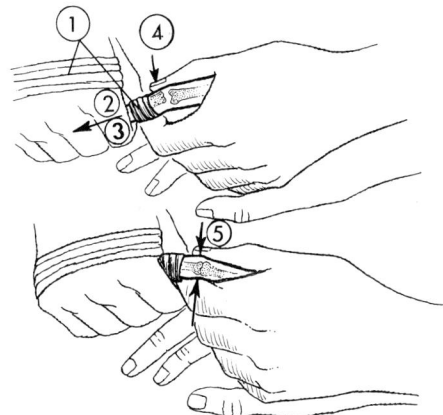

Postreduction Management

Evaluate functional stability and stress stability as described on page 1203.

If the joint is swollen, tender, or unstable, the finger should be immobilized in a finger cast-splint.

1. Apply anterior and posterior splints designed to accommodate for swelling.
2. The plaster extends from the MP joint to the base of the nail.
3. The IP joints are in almost full extension so as to keep the ligaments out to length (see page 1143).

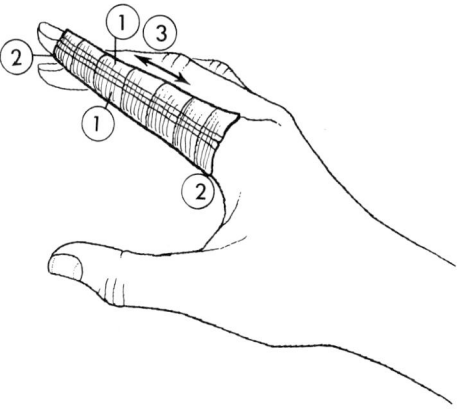

Postreduction Management (Continued)

In most instances the dislocated joint requires only brief support by buddy taping to the adjacent finger.
1. Apply tape to the fingers with the interdigital area padded.
2. Allow active flexion and extension.

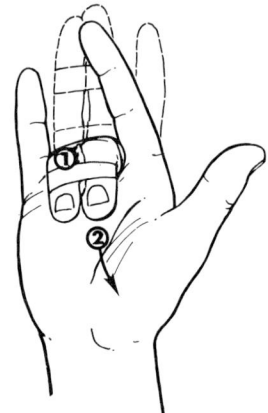

Subsequent Management

Avoid prolonging immobilization for more than one week.

If a finger cast is necessary because of swelling or edema, remove it at one week and use buddy taping to permit joint motion.

By far the more common problem with PIP joint injury is stiffness, not instability. Keep this in mind in applying treatment to an individual injury.

HYPEREXTENSION DISLOCATION OF THE INTERPHALANGEAL JOINTS OF THE FINGERS

REMARKS

Hyperextension dislocation is common, particularly of the PIP joint, and it frequently produces disability far out of proportion to the magnitude of the initial injury.

Usually it presents as a "jammed finger," particularly from football or other sports.

If the magnitude of the initial injury is not assessed properly (as described on page 1201), the treatment may be entirely inappropriate and may result in stiffness or instability, which makes the finger awkward to use.

Initial assessment includes direct palpation of the area of swelling and injury, adequate x-rays of the finger, evaluation of functional stability, and stress testing of the joint.

If the x-ray shows a fracture fragment involving more than 40 per cent of the joint surface, operative repair is indicated.

If functional testing demonstrates instability on active flexion or extension, several possibilities must be considered. Anterior displacement of the mid phalanx with motion indicates that at least the central slip has torn dorsally. This requires immobilization of the joint in extension for five to six weeks to prevent boutonniere deformity.

FRACTURES, DISLOCATIONS, AND FRACTURE-DISLOCATIONS OF THE FINGERS

Injury to the volar capsular attachment can cause recurrent instability in extension, or a swan-neck deformity. This results in a chronic problem whereby the middle phalanx catches in hyperextension. The patient then is unable to initiate flexion and grasp becomes awkward. If dorsal instability is evident on functional testing, the joint is splinted in 30 degrees of flexion by means of a dorsal block splint. This permits the volar plate attachment to heal to the middle phalanx and still allows active joint motion during the healing process.

Occasionally a hyperextension injury tears the volar plate from the proximal phalanx. The resultant scarring causes a contracture of the PIP joint or a pseudo-boutonniere deformity. This problem may be identified by an x-ray showing a small fragment of bone avulsed from the proximal phalanx. In this instance the PIP joint is best treated by immobilization in extension as for a true boutonniere deformity (see page 1149).

Prereduction X-Ray

1. X-ray view should be centered on the injured finger, not the hand.
2. Lateral view shows PIP joint has dislocated dorsally. A small avulsion fracture is evidence for damage to the volar plate attachment.

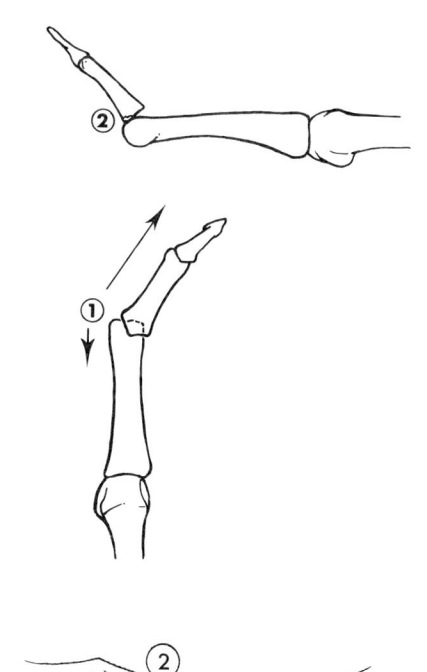

Manipulative Reduction

This is performed after injection of local anesthetic.

1. A bandage is first looped around the end of the injured finger and then around the operator's hand.
2. Grasp the dislocated finger with your thumb and index finger and make gentle traction along the axis of the dislocated phalanx; at the same time,
3. Bring the phalanx into the hyperextended position.
4. While traction is being maintained,
5. Slide the base of the phalanx distalward to a position opposite the head of the proximal phalanx; then,
6. Flex the interphalangeal joint.

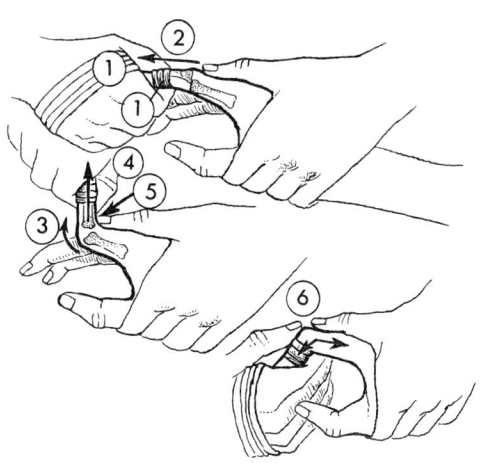

FRACTURES, DISLOCATIONS, AND FRACTURE-DISLOCATIONS OF THE FINGERS

Postreduction X-Ray

After reduction by the patient or the physician.

Evaluate carefully for functional stability. Look particularly for:

1. Dorsal instability due to avulsion of the volar plate from the middle phalanx.

2. Anterior instability as a result of central slip and capsular damage.

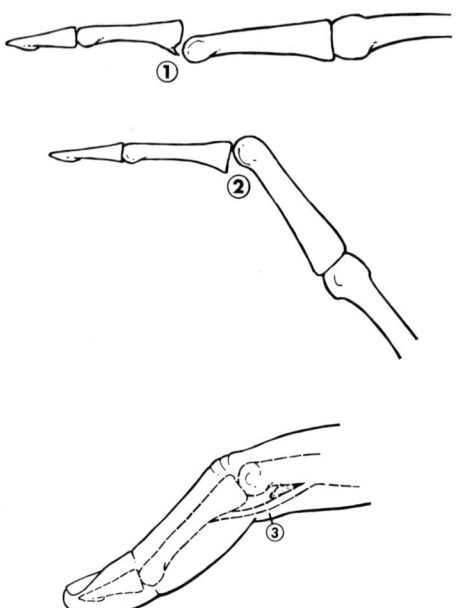

3. Avulsion of the volar capsule from the proximal phalanx causing pseudo-boutonniere deformity.

MANAGEMENT OF ACUTE DORSAL INSTABILITY BY EXTENSION BLOCK SPLINT

1. Apply a plaster gauntlet cast with a dorsal splint.
2. Maintain the MP joint in the position of full flexion.
3. Splint blocks extension of the PIP joint 10 to 15 degrees short of the point where subluxation occurs.
4. The proximal phalanx is taped to the splint.
5. Full flexion of the PIP joint is allowed from the beginning.

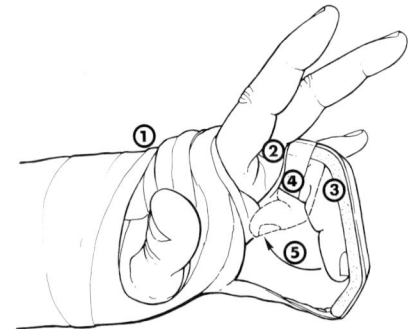

Note: If more than 40 per cent of the proximal phalangeal articular surface is fractured, open reduction and internal fixation are necessary. This procedure may be followed by postoperative use of the dorsal extension block splint.

Subsequent Management

Decrease the angle of the extension block 25 per cent each week.

The patient should be able to flex the joint 70 to 90 degrees by the third week.

Continue to block full extension for 6 to 12 weeks, depending on the degree of initial instability.

MANAGEMENT OF CHRONIC DORSAL INSTABILITY OF THE PROXIMAL INTERPHALANGEAL JOINT (SWAN-NECK DEFORMITY)

REMARKS

A chronic dorsal subluxation of the PIP joint may develop after a "sprain" treated by taping the finger to a tongue depressor.

If the torn volar capsule is allowed to heal in a lengthened position, it will permit dorsal displacement of the middle phalanx.

Treatment of the chronic condition requires excision of the volar plate and reconstruction by means of a strip from the collateral ligament (Kleinert procedure).

1. Rupture of the volar plate from the middle phalanx produces
2. Hyperextension deformity of the PIP joint.

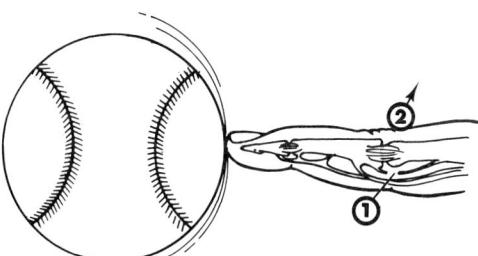

1. Chronic dorsal instability will impair function of the entire finger. It should be corrected by surgical reconstruction done by a skilled hand surgeon.

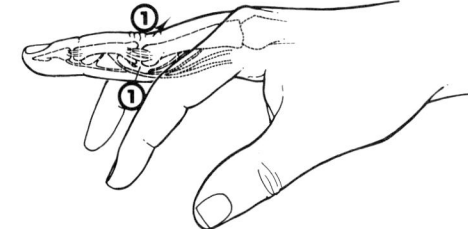

Kleinert Procedure for Chronic Dorsal Subluxation

1. The scarred and lengthened volar capsule is excised.
2. The proximal and volar portion of the collateral ligament is shifted volarly to stabilize the joint.

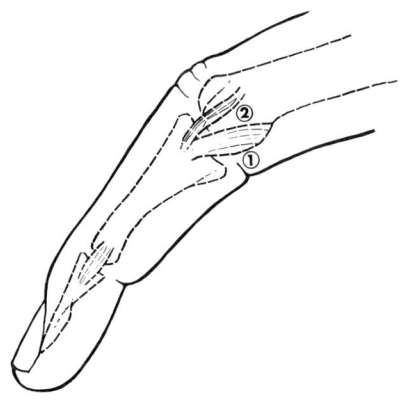

MANAGEMENT OF ACUTE ANTERIOR INSTABILITY OR DISLOCATION

1. Anterior dislocation of the PIP joint is unusual and indicates significant disruption of the central slip attachment. Capsular and collateral ligament structures are also frequently damaged.

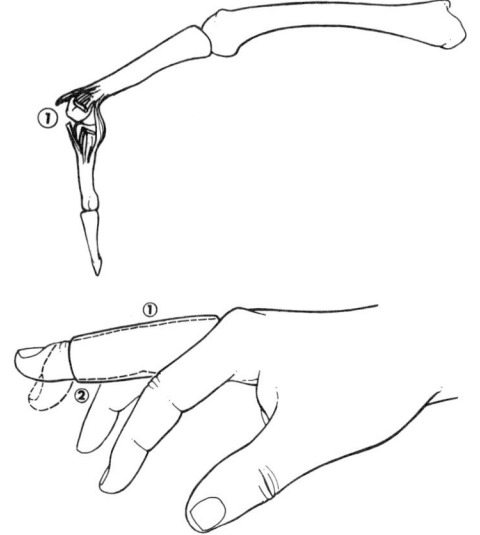

The complication of boutonniere deformity after this injury should be anticipated and prevented.
1. The PIP joint is immobilized in a finger cast or splint.
2. The DIP joint flexes actively.

Subsequent Management

Six weeks of continuous immobilization in extension are usually sufficient.

If the patient desires to return to sports or vigorous activities, protect the PIP joint with a dorsal splint for 4 to 6 weeks longer.

Note: For acute injuries with extreme instability, large fracture fragments, or open injuries, early operative repair is indicated (see page 1217).

PSEUDOBOUTONNIERE DEFORMITY

REMARKS

A pseudoboutonniere deformity develops as a chronic residual problem after acute disruption of the volar capsular attachment to the proximal phalanx. This can be prevented by anticipating the complication and treating it with adequate immobilization.

1. Hyperextension injury to the PIP joint may occasionally
2. Disrupt the capsular attachment from the proximal phalanx, eventually producing flexion contracture of the joint.

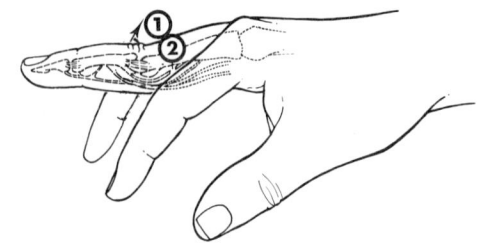

1. A small avulsed fragment of bone from the proximal phalanx may be a clue to the site of injury.
2. Chronic flexion contracture of the capsule produces pseudoboutonniere deformity.
3. The DIP joint is usually not fixed in extension, since both lateral bands are usually not involved. This is in contrast to a true boutonniere deformity (see pages 1210 and 1217).

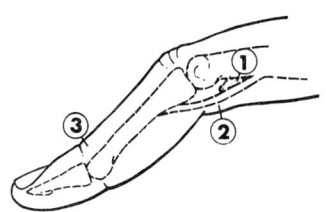

If you suspect, on the basis of tenderness or of an avulsion fracture from the proximal phalanx, that the hyperextension injury is likely to progress to a pseudoboutonniere deformity, immobilize the finger as for a true boutonniere deformity.

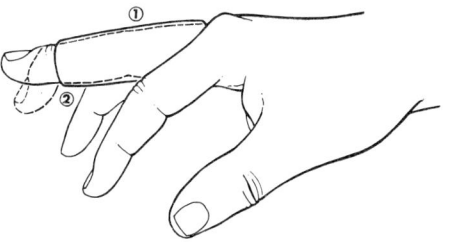

1. The PIP joint is immobilized in a finger cast or splint in extension.
2. The DIP joint is allowed to flex actively.

FRACTURE-DISLOCATIONS OF THE INTERPHALANGEAL JOINTS

REMARKS

Dislocation of the interphalangeal joints may be complicated by marginal avulsion fractures of the dislocated phalanx. These lesions are similar to fracture-dislocations of the metacarpophalangeal joints and are treated in a similar manner.

Undisplaced fractures are ignored and the treatment is directed to the dislocation.

Small displaced fragments should be removed and the ligament repaired.

Large displaced fragments should be replaced and fixed with a fine Kirschner wire or screw.

Following the operative stabilization, functional exercises may be permitted using an extension block splint (see page 1208).

FRACTURES, DISLOCATIONS, AND FRACTURE-DISLOCATIONS OF THE FINGERS

Appearance on X-Ray

UNDISPLACED FRACTURE

1. Small undisplaced fracture of the palmar aspect of the base of the middle phalanx.

Note: Evaluate stability carefully by palpation, x-ray, functional testing, and stress testing. If there is any evidence of dorsal instability, treat with an extension block splint.

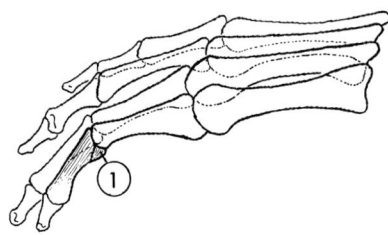

SMALL DISPLACED FRACTURE WITH SUBLUXATION

1. Small marginal fracture of the ulnar aspect of the base of the middle phalanx.

Note: This fragment should be removed and the volar plate should be reattached to the middle phalanx, permitting immobilization with a dorsal extension block splint.

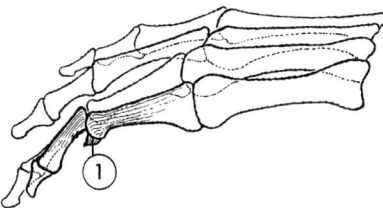

LARGE DISPLACED FRAGMENT

1. Large triangular fragment from the palmar aspect of the base of the middle phalanx with marked displacement.

Note: This is a very unstable fracture; the fragment should be replaced and fixed with a fine Kirschner wire.

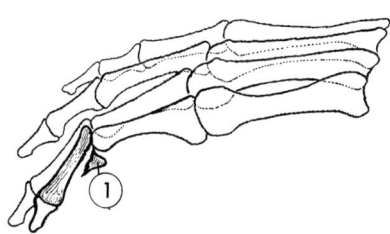

Postoperative X-Ray

1. Fragment is reduced and fixed with a Kirschner wire or with a small fragment screw.

Note: Stabilizing this articular fracture is necessary to permit treatment with active joint motion using a dorsal extension block splint (see page 1208).

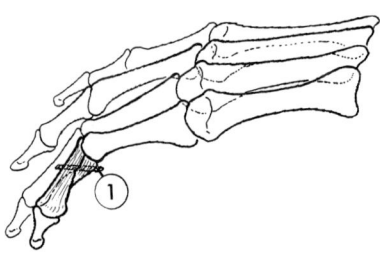

FRACTURES, DISLOCATIONS, AND FRACTURE-DISLOCATIONS OF THE FINGERS

TENDON AVULSIONS WITH OR WITHOUT FRACTURE

MALLET FINGER DEFORMITY

REMARKS

A mallet finger is among the most common injuries to the tendon structures of the digit.

Generally, the patient sustains a blow to the end of the finger and presents with pain, swelling, and a variable degree of deformity.

The injury disrupts the extensor tendon insertion at the base of the terminal phalanx, with or without fracture.

Prompt recognition of the tendon avulsion permits closed treatment using a dorsal splint continuously for five to six weeks. Closed treatment should be attempted for most mallet finger injuries, even those seen three to six weeks after injury.

Mallet fingers associated with fractures that cannot be anatomically reduced demand open reduction. Internal fixation with Kirschner wires or wire sutures permit healing of the tendon without lengthening.

For open mallet finger injuries, internal support with a transarticular Riordan pin may be necessary.

Clinical Appearance

1. A blow to the tip of the finger causes hyperflexion and avulsion of the extensor tendon.
2. Swelling and pain over the extensor insertion.
3. The deformity of the DIP joint varies but the patient cannot actively extend the distal phalanx.

Note: All injuries of this type to the distal phalanx should be suspected of and treated for tendon avulsion.

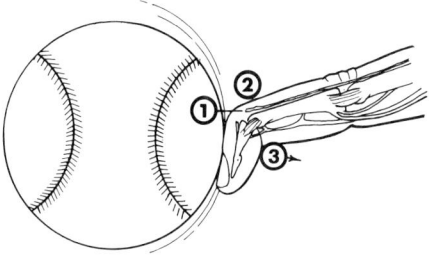

Management of a Mallet Finger Without Fracture

1. Apply dorsal splint with the DIP joint extended but not hyperextended.
2. Leave the PIP joint free and encourage active motion.

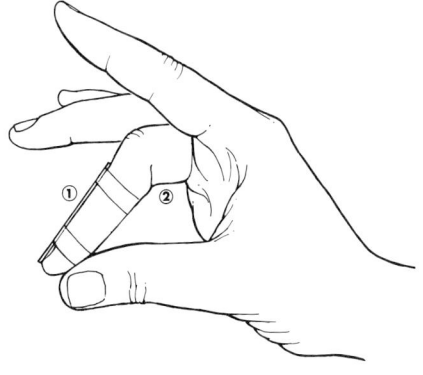

Subsequent Management

Continue splint immobilization for 4 to 5 weeks.

The splint tape may be changed carefully during this time to prevent skin maceration, but the patient must maintain extension of the joint.

After 4 to 5 weeks the patient may remove one strip of tape to allow active, gentle flexion of the joint. He reapplies the tape when not exercising.

When active joint motion reaches 40 degrees of flexion and full extension, the splint may be discarded.

MANAGEMENT OF A MALLET FINGER DEFORMITY WITH AVULSION FRACTURE

Prereduction X-Ray

1. Large fragment of bone is avulsed from the dorsum of the base of the distal phalanx.

Note: A closed reduction of this fracture can often be done within the first day of injury before the clot and scar develop in the fracture interface.

If the avulsion fracture cannot be restored anatomically, open reduction with internal fixation is necessary.

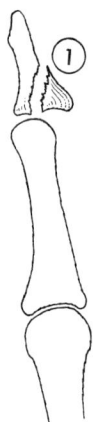

Operative Reduction

1. Make an L-shaped incision crossing the dorsum of the finger just distal to the distal interphalangeal joint.

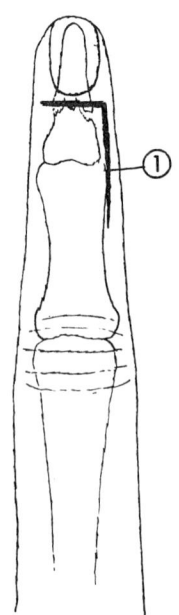

FRACTURES, DISLOCATIONS, AND FRACTURE-DISLOCATIONS OF THE FINGERS

2. Expose the fracture site and identify the loose fragment.

3. Using a small drill, make a transverse hole through the base of the phalanx.

1. Pass a 3-0 wire suture through the tendon and circumferentially around the avulsed tendon.

2. Pass the wire through the small holes made in the phalanx.

3. Tighten the wire suture to reduce the fracture.

Note: If the distal phalangeal reattachment is tenuous, use a transarticular Riordan pin for additional support.

Riordan Pin* Fixation for Open Mallet Finger Deformity

A useful way for managing the occasional mallet finger that is unstable or associated with a dorsal wound is by transarticular pin fixation.

External splint support is still needed to prevent breakage or pin migration.

1. A dorsal laceration involves the extensor tendon and DIP joint.

2. After thorough wound cleansing, a Riordan pin is inserted transarticularly to support the tendon reattachment.

3. The tendon is reattached and the skin laceration is closed by a figure-of-eight suture through both skin and tendon.

---

*Available from Zimmer–U.S.A., Warsaw, Indiana 46580.

Subsequent Management

Additional external support via dorsal splint is necessary during the healing phase.

Remove the pin at 5 to 6 weeks.

Continue external splinting but allow the patient to begin active exercises of the DIP joint.

When active flexion has reached 40 degrees and the patient has maintained active extension, the splint may be discarded.

AVULSION OF FLEXOR PROFUNDUS INSERTION WITH OR WITHOUT FRACTURE

REMARKS

Another frequently unrecognized injury that presents as a swollen, "jammed finger" is avulsion of the flexor profundus tendon insertion. This commonly results from the act of grasping the shirt of an individual, such as a football player, as he lunges forward. The injury may also occur in older individuals who avulse the tendon while lifting heavy objects.

The resultant complete disruption of the flexor insertion, which is most commonly from the ring finger or small finger, usually is inappropriately treated as a jammed finger.

If the injury is unrecognized, the tendon will retract proximally in its sheath or completely up into the palm.

Be alert to this commonly missed but significant problem in any individual who sustains a grasping injury.

The diagnosis can be made easily by the loss of active flexion of the DIP joint. Always check DIP as well as PIP joint motion.

Occasionally, the position of the tendon will be indicated on x-ray by a small fragment of bone avulsed with it.

Consistently, the point of tenderness is at the end of the retracted tendon, usually over the PIP joint but occasionally in the palm.

Repair of this injury should be performed only by a surgeon experienced in flexor tendon surgery including tendon graft.

Unsuccessful surgery will impair function of the uninjured flexor sublimis tendon.

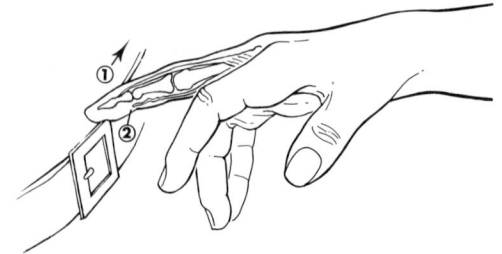

1. Avulsion of the flexor profundus is most commonly produced by forceful grasping.
2. Occasionally a small fragment of bone is seen on x-ray to be displaced within the tendon.

The area of tenderness is localized directly to the tendon either
1. Adjacent to the PIP joint or

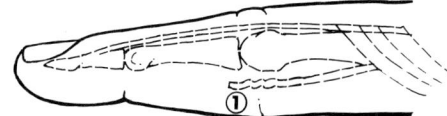

2. In the palm.

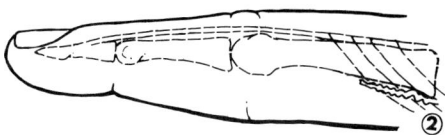

The diagnosis can be readily made on the basis of
1. Loss of active flexion of the DIP joint.

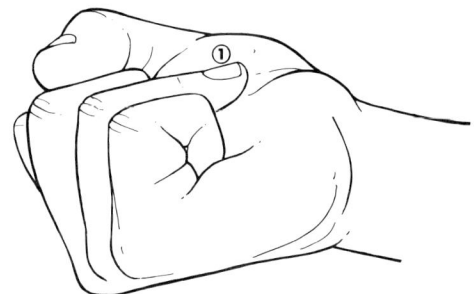

Note: If the diagnosis of flexor profundus avulsion is made immediately after injury, immobilize the finger to prevent further tendon retraction. Prompt repair should be carried out by an individual skilled in tendon surgery.

BOUTONNIERE DEFORMITY

REMARKS

Commonly a direct laceration over the PIP joint produces a rupture of the central slip attachment to the middle phalanx. Another common cause of this injury is a closed crushing injury that forces the joint into passive flexion while it is being actively extended.

Quite frequently the significance of injury to the extensor mechanism goes unrecognized or is treated with brief immobilization of the joint in flexion until the soft tissue wound heals.

The flexion immobilization permits the apex of the joint to prolapse through the "buttonhole" defect created by the disrupted central slip.

The disruption between the central slip and the lateral bands permits the lateral tendons to fall gradually beneath the axis of PIP motion. The result is that the intrinsics become flexors of the joint rather than extensors (see page 1149).

The typical boutonniere deformity may develop only gradually several weeks or months after the initial injury.

To avoid the difficulties of treating a chronic PIP deformity, all lacerations and direct injuries to the PIP knuckle must be carefully evaluated. A laceration through the tendon can usually be repaired by

FRACTURES, DISLOCATIONS, AND FRACTURE-DISLOCATIONS OF THE FINGERS

a simple figure-of-eight removable stitch of stainless steel wire that closes both the tendon and the skin.

The joint should be immobilized after an injury in the extension position for four to six weeks to insure adequate healing of the tendon. This also prevents flexion displacement of the lateral bands.

Even if seen six to twelve weeks after initial injury, closed treatment should be used.

The major indications for operative repair of a boutonniere deformity are avulsion fractures of the middle phalanx, long-standing deformities in young persons, or anterior dislocation with gross instability of the joint (see page 1210).

1. Laceration through the middle slip of the long extensor.
2. Apex of the joint buttonholes through the defect created by the laceration.
3. Longitudinal tearing allows the lateral bands to become flexors of the PIP joint and hyperextensors of DIP joint.

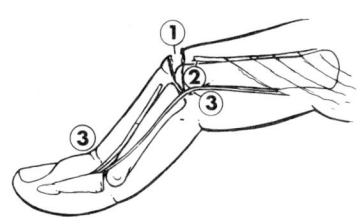

Treatment

1. Both the tendon and
2. The skin laceration may be repaired by a simple figure-of-eight wire.

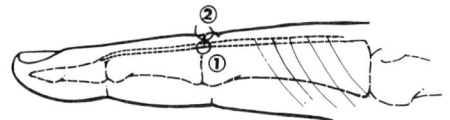

Immobilization in Extension

1. A finger cast is applied from the MP joint while keeping the PIP joint in extension.
2. The DIP joint is allowed free motion.

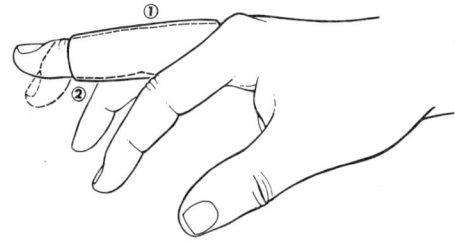

Subsequent Management

The cast is maintained for six weeks and then is removed.

A protective dorsal splint should be used if the patient is going to use the finger vigorously.

Apply another extension cast for three more weeks if the flexion deformity of the PIP joint recurs.

Occasionally with chronic boutonniere deformities, a preliminary period of dynamic extension splinting is necessary to correct flexion contractures and permit closed treatment.

Fractures of the Metacarpals of the Fingers

REMARKS

Of all hand fractures, metacarpal fractures are second in frequency only to phalangeal fractures. They result commonly from direct blows, as when a clenched fist hits a firm object and the fifth metacarpal head fractures. A crushing injury to the dorsum of the hand frequently causes multiple metacarpal fractures.

In a hand with severe swelling after fracture, a compression hand dressing and continuous elevation for two to three days are necessary to eliminate edema.

The major factors influencing the final result are the degree of the initial injury and the method of treatment.

The majority of metacarpal fractures are stable because of the support from surrounding intraosseous muscles. These fractures can be readily treated with closed reduction and plaster cast-splint support.

The aim of treatment is to provide sufficient stability by either external or internal fixation to allow early movement. There is no justification for immobilizing these fractures longer than three weeks. Significant loss of hand function, even with relatively minor fractures, is likely to follow longer immobilization.

Rotational realignment is critical and should be insured during the early phase of treatment by careful observation and by splinting the injured finger to the adjacent uninjured one.

Only rarely are metacarpal fractures sufficiently unstable to warrant internal fixation. The types that are likely to be unstable result from direct crushing injury that fractures more than one metacarpal and causes comminution or bone loss.

The most common fracture involves the head and neck of the fifth metacarpal. Dorsal angulation of this bone may usually be accepted. Vigorous operative or nonoperative treatment of this common injury frequently produces greater disability than does the fracture itself.

Dorsal angulation of the stable second and third metacarpals is less readily acceptable since these bones provide power grip, which can be impaired by displacement of the metacarpal heads into the palm.

FRACTURES, DISLOCATIONS, AND FRACTURE-DISLOCATIONS OF THE FINGERS

Mechanisms of Fracture

Fractures are produced by one of two mechanisms:

1. A direct blow to the end of the knuckle, fracturing the head and neck of the fifth metacarpal.

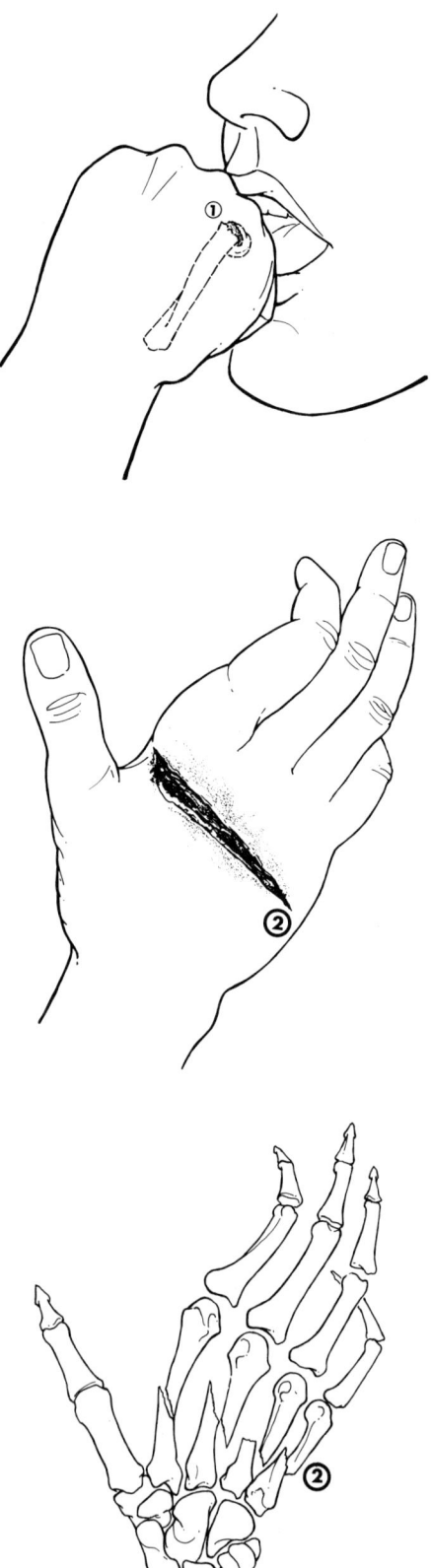

2. A crushing injury producing soft tissue damage and multiple metacarpal fractures with or without comminution.

FRACTURES, DISLOCATIONS, AND FRACTURE-DISLOCATIONS OF THE FINGERS

Normal Anatomic Relationships

1. Lumbrical and
2. Interossei muscles inserting into the dorsal expansion.
3. Extensor digitorum communis.
4. Flexor digitorum profundus.
5. Flexor digitorum sublimis.

Note: All these muscles function in perfect balance.

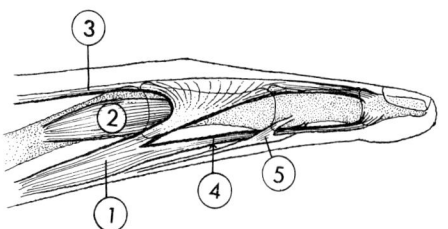

Mechanism of Deformity

1. A fracture of the metacarpal neck or shaft produces
2. A tightening of the extensor communis tendon, causing hyperextension of the MP joint.
3. The pull of the lumbricals accentuates the volar displacement of the distal fragment.

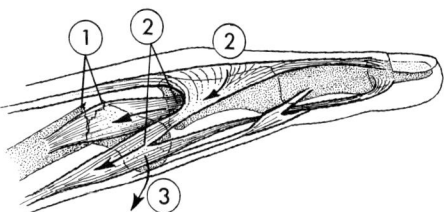

Reduction

1. Flexion of the MP joint relaxes the lumbrical and permits
2. Correction of the deformity by upward redirection of the metacarpal head.
3. Flexion of the MP joint and correction of the deformity permits the extensor to stabilize the fracture.

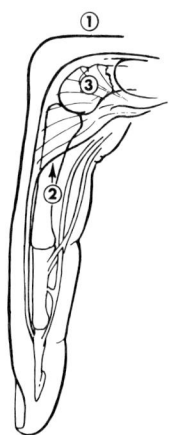

STABLE FRACTURE OF THE NECK OF THE METACARPAL OF THE FINGER

Prereduction X-Ray

1. Fracture of the fourth metacarpal.
2. The head of the metacarpal is tilted volarly into the palm.
3. The fracture is angulated dorsally.

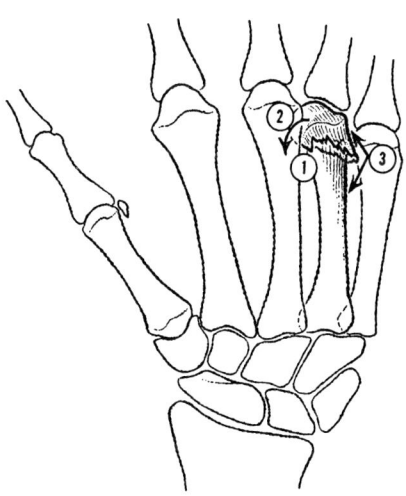

FRACTURES, DISLOCATIONS, AND FRACTURE-DISLOCATIONS OF THE FINGERS

Reduction

This procedure is performed with the patient under intravenous general or local anesthesia.

1. Flex the MP joint to a right angle.

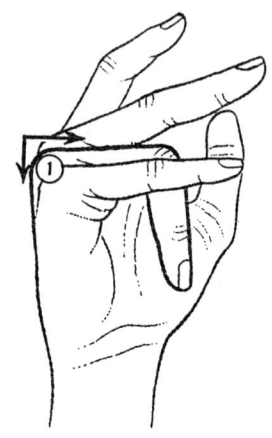

2. With the MP joint flexed, push the proximal phalanx upward so as to redirect the distal metacarpal head.

3. Push the proximal fragment down by direct pressure.

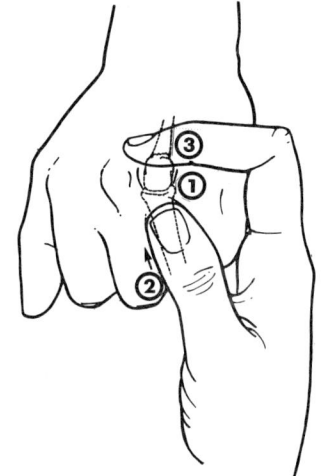

Postreduction X-Ray

1. The dorsal angulation is corrected.

2. The head of the metacarpal is directed in the long axis of the finger.

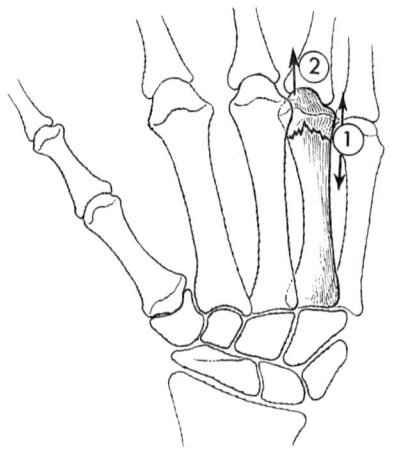

1222

FRACTURES, DISLOCATIONS, AND FRACTURE-DISLOCATIONS OF THE FINGERS

Immobilization

Apply a plaster cast-splint.
1. Incorporate the fracture and the adjacent, unfractured metacarpal.
2. The MP joint is flexed 70 degrees.

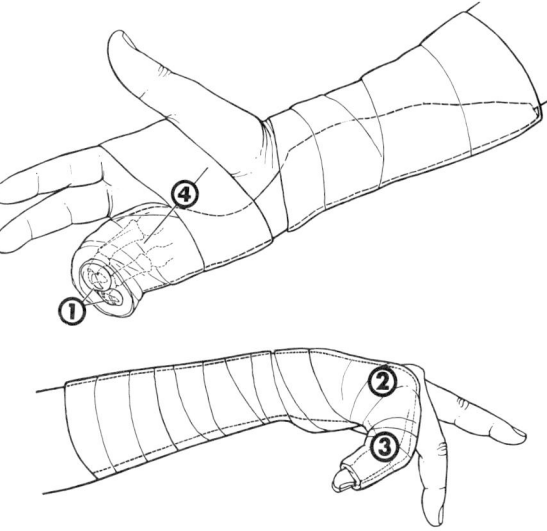

3. The IP joints are in slight flexion.
4. The tips of the fingers are aligned to point toward the scaphoid tuberosity for correct rotational alignment.

Note: The key to holding reduction is to maintain maximal flexion of the MP joints in order to tighten the extensor hood around the fracture.

Postreduction Management

Encourage the patient to exercise the nonimmobilized fingers actively.

Remove the splint at 10 days and have the patient begin active exercises in warm water 3 times a day.

Reapply the splint if the fracture is still tender and the patient is likely to injure his hand.

Some redisplacement, up to 40 degrees, may be accepted without remanipulation.

Discard the splint no later than 3 weeks. Immobilization longer than 3 weeks is likely to cause prolonged stiffness.

Angulation of these fractures causes very little clinical deformity and does not interfere with normal use of the hand.

Rotational malalignment, however, should not be accepted because it produces overlapping fingers in flexion.

UNSTABLE FRACTURES OF THE NECK OF THE METACARPAL OF THE FINGER

REMARKS

Rarely, dorsal angulation of the metacarpals cannot be satisfactorily corrected by closed means. This is particularly true with multiple fractures.

Persistent displacement of metacarpal heads into the palm is likely to impair grip. Internal fixation may be necessary to reduce and hold the fracture.

X-Ray after Unsuccessful Closed Reduction

1. Fracture of the neck of the fourth metacarpal.
2. The head of the metacarpal remains tilted into the palm.
3. The fracture is angulated dorsally.

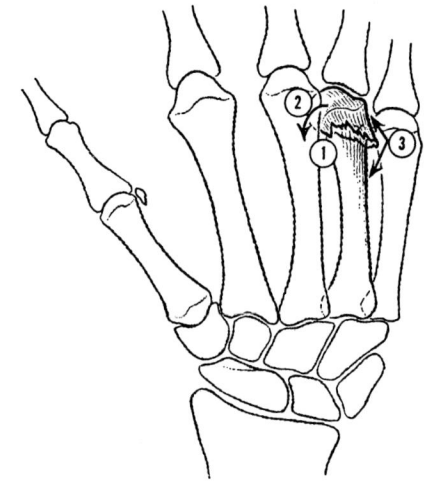

Reduction and Fixation

1. Flex the MP joint maximally.

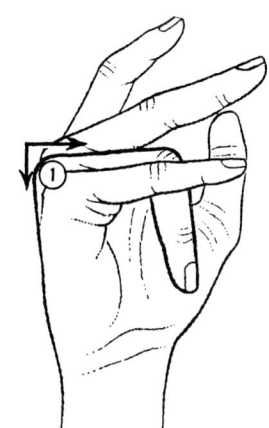

2. Reduce the fracture by direct upward pressure on the distal fragment and
3. Downward pressure on the proximal phalanx.

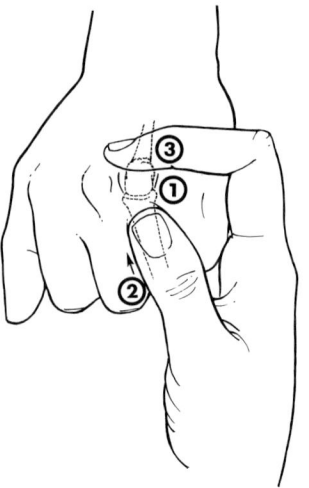

FRACTURES, DISLOCATIONS, AND FRACTURE-DISLOCATIONS OF THE FINGERS

1. While an assistant maintains flexion of the MP joint and reduction of the fracture,
2. Pass a fine threaded pin through the lateral condyle of the metacarpal head and across the fracture.
Cut the wire 1 cm from the skin.

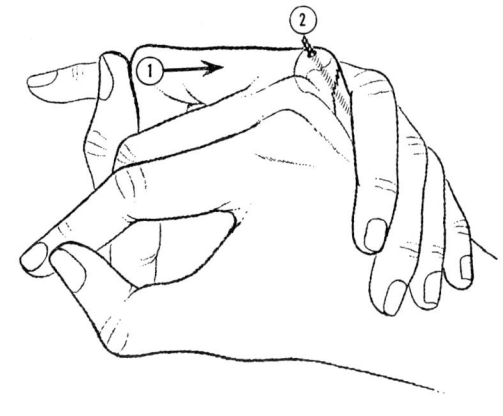

Postreduction X-Ray

1. The dorsal angulation is corrected.
2. The head of the metacarpal is redirected along the long axis of the finger.
3. The wire passes lateral to the MP joint.

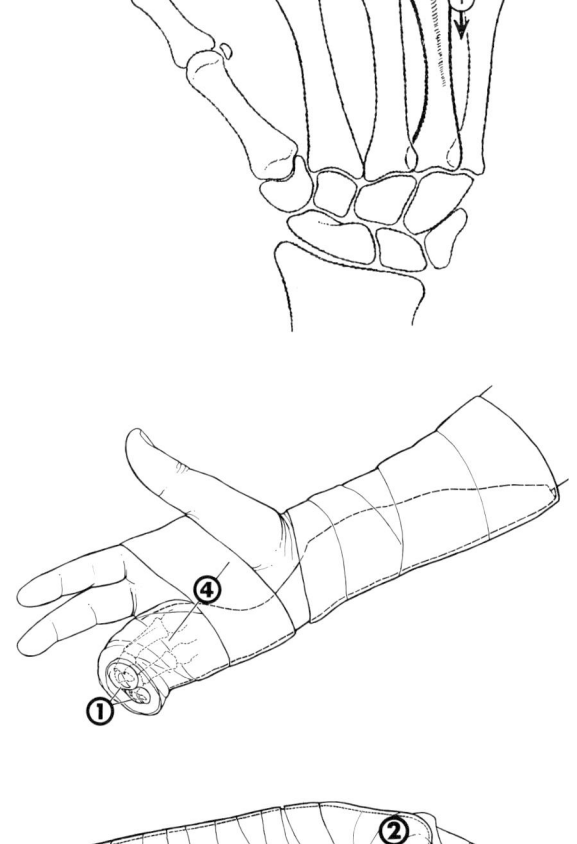

Immobilization

Apply a plaster cast-splint.
1. Incorporate the fractured metacarpal and the adjacent, uninjured metacarpal.
2. The MP joint is flexed 70 degrees.

3. The PIP joints are in slight flexion.
4. The tips of the fingers are aligned to point toward the scaphoid tuberosity for correct rotational alignment.

Postreduction Management

Remove the wire by ten days to two weeks. The patient may then begin active range of motion two to three times a day in warm water.

When the patient is not exercising, he should wear the gutter splint. Discard the splint completely by the end of three weeks, since immobilization for longer than this time is likely to cause permanent stiffness.

FRACTURE OF THE SHAFT OF THE METACARPAL OF THE FINGER

REMARKS

The majority of shaft fractures are injuries of one metacarpal. Splinting by the surrounding intraosseous muscles and adjacent metacarpals prevents significant displacement except for malrotation.

Single metacarpal fractures can be reduced and held in a functional position, and a guarded exercise program can be begun at 10 to 14 days.

Multiple metacarpal shaft fractures are usually produced by direct crushing trauma to the dorsum of the hand. These tend to be unstable.

With multiple metacarpal fractures the first priority is to eliminate edema by a hand compression dressing and elevation.

Internal fixation with Kirschner wire then should provide stability to permit early functional exercise.

STABLE FRACTURE OF THE SHAFT OF THE METACARPALS

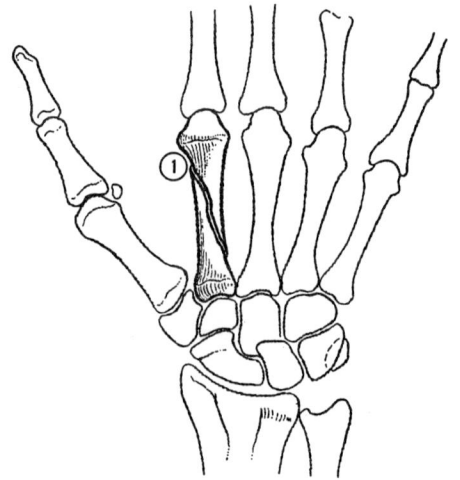

Appearance on X-Ray

NO DISPLACEMENT

1. Spiral fracture of the second metacarpal with no displacement.

FRACTURES, DISLOCATIONS, AND FRACTURE-DISLOCATIONS OF THE FINGERS

MINIMAL DISPLACEMENT

1. Spiral fracture of the third and fourth metacarpal with minimal displacement and shortening.

Note: This amount of shortening is acceptable.

MINIMAL DISPLACEMENT

1. Fracture of the fifth metacarpal with slight posterior angulation.

Note: This degree of angulation is acceptable. It causes only mild clinical deformity that does not interfere with use of the hand or cause patient dissatisfaction.

Immobilization

Apply a plaster cast-splint immobilizing the fractured metacarpal.

1. Incorporate the fracture and the adjacent metacarpal.
2. The MP joint is flexed 70 degrees.
3. The IP joints are in slight flexion.
4. The fingertips are directed toward the scaphoid tuberosity to prevent malrotation.

Note: If the hand is swollen as a result of the initial injury, elevate the limb for 2 to 3 days in a hand dressing prior to applying the cast-splint.

The key to reducing and holding the fracture is to keep the MP joint in maximum flexion so as to tighten the extensor apparatus.

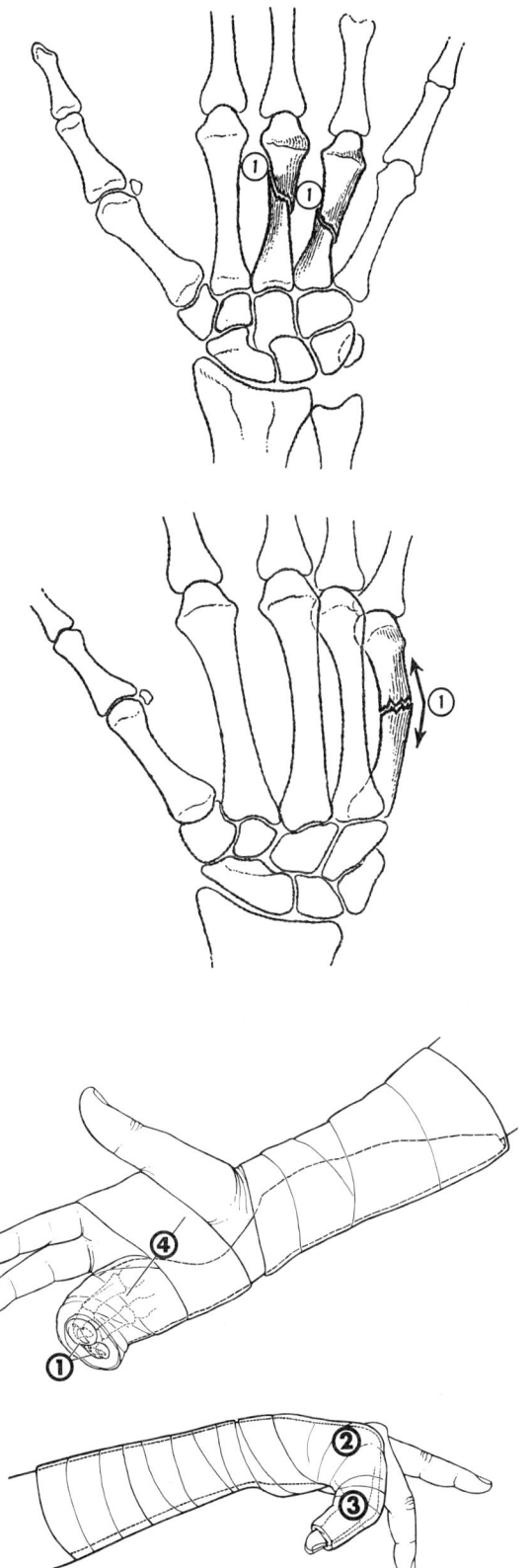

Subsequent Management

Encourage the patient to exercise the non immobilized fingers actively.

Remove the cast-splint by the end of 10 to 14 days and permit the patient to begin active exercises of the hand in warm water 3 times a day.

Reapply the splint if the fracture is still tender or if the patient is likely to reinjure the hand.

Discard the splint entirely by 3 weeks. Longer immobilization is likely to cause prolonged stiffness.

UNSTABLE FRACTURES OF FINGER METACARPALS

CLOSED TREATMENT

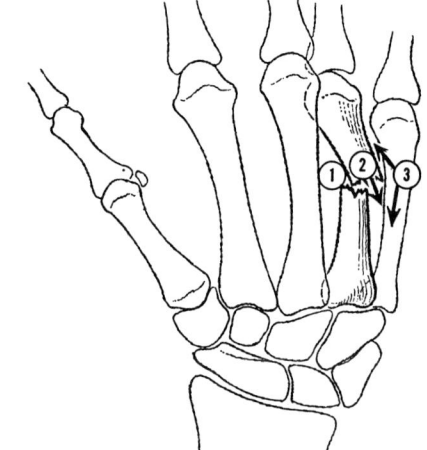

Prereduction X-Ray: Unacceptable Displacement

1. Transverse fracture of the fourth metacarpal.
2. The head of the metacarpal is displaced volarly.
3. Posterior angular deformity is marked.

Note: This much shortening and angulation is liable to impair intrinsic hand function or cause rotational malalignment.

Reduction

1. One hand of the operator encircles the wrist while the other hand grasps the finger of the fractured metacarpal.
2. The wrist is dorsiflexed and the MP joint is flexed 70 degrees.
3. Apply traction to the injured finger to restore the metacarpal length.
4. Apply direct pressure to the apex of the deformity.
5. With the MP joint flexed, push the distal fragment dorsally.

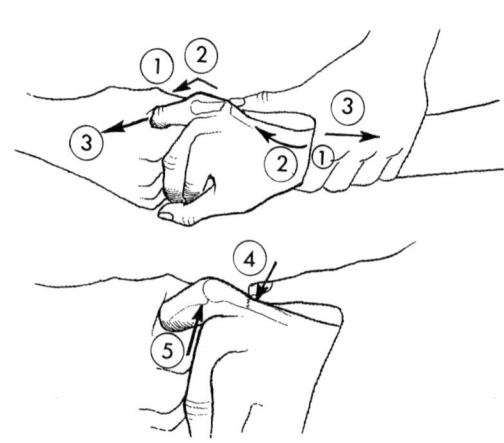

Immobilization

Note: For extensive swelling, apply a compression hand dressing for 2 to 3 days and elevate the limb. When swelling subsides, apply a plaster cast-splint.

1. Incorporate the fractured finger and the adjacent, uninjured finger.
2. The MP joint is flexed 70 degrees.

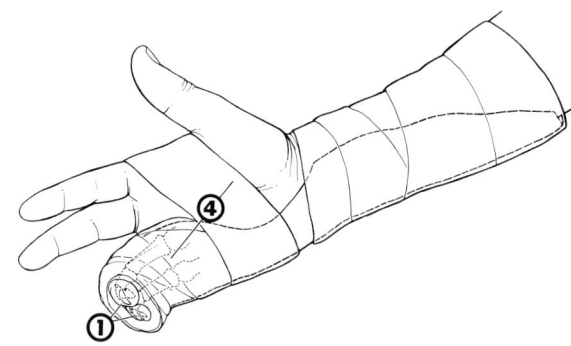

3. The IP joint is in slight flexion.
4. The fingertips are directed toward the scaphoid tuberosity to insure rotational realignment.

Note: The key to achieving and maintaining reduction is to hold the MP joint in maximum flexion so as to tighten the extensor apparatus.

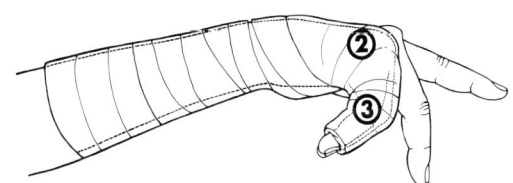

Postreduction Management

Have the patient actively exercise the nonimmobilized fingers.

Recheck the position of the metacarpals by x-ray at 5 to 7 days.

Remove the cast-splint by no later than 3 weeks and allow the patient to begin active exercises in warm water 2 to 3 times a day.

If the patient is likely to reinjure the hand, apply a temporary protective splint for 7 days.

Note: If reduction cannot be achieved by this closed method and shortening with angulation persists, use internal fixation.

INTERNAL FIXATION OF UNSTABLE FRACTURES OF THE FINGER METACARPALS

REMARKS

Internal fixation is especially applicable to displaced metacarpal fractures that cannot be reduced and held by plaster immobilization as previously described.

The fracture site need not be opened except when reduction is impossible by closed methods.

If the hand is extremely swollen, elevate the limb for two to three days in a hand compression dressing prior to internal fixation.

Prereduction X-Rays

FOURTH METACARPAL FRACTURE

1. Transverse fracture of the fourth metacarpal.
2. The distal fragment is displaced volarly and proximally, forming
3. A posterior angular deformity.

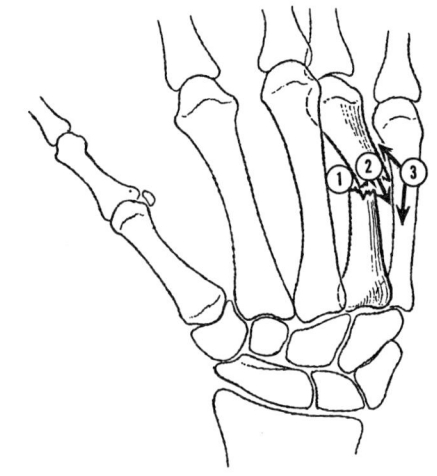

THIRD METACARPAL FRACTURE

1. Oblique fracture of the third metacarpal with posterior bowing.
2. The shaft of the metacarpal is shortened.

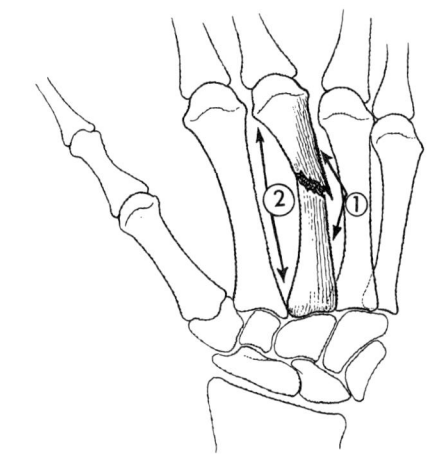

Reduction and Fixation of the Fracture

1. An assistant grasps the wrist in one hand and the affected finger in the other.
2. The wrist is held in dorsiflexion and the finger in flexion.
3. While the operator's proximal hand makes counter traction on the wrist, the distal hand makes longitudinal traction on the finger.
4. While traction is maintained, the operator's proximal thumb makes firm downward pressure over the apex of the deformity and the distal thumb and fingers push upward on the metacarpal head.

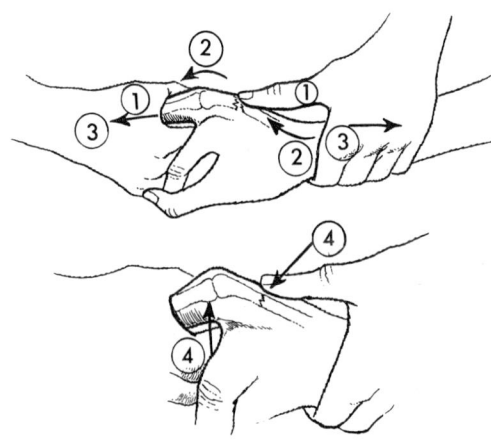

FRACTURES, DISLOCATIONS, AND FRACTURE-DISLOCATIONS OF THE FINGERS

1. While this position is maintained.
2. Transfix the fractured metacarpal to the adjacent metacarpals with Kirschner wires.

Note: One wire passes through the bones above the level of the fracture and one wire passes below.

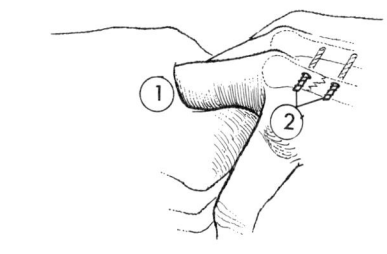

Postreduction X-Rays

FOURTH METACARPAL FRACTURE

1. The fracture of the fourth metacarpal is reduced.
2. The wires pass through the metacarpals above and below the fracture site.

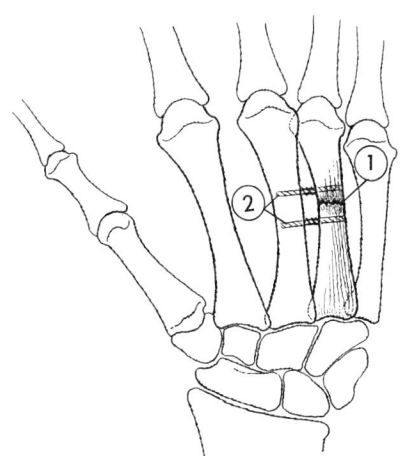

THIRD METACARDAL FRACTURE

1. Fracture of the third metacarpal is reduced.
2. Length of the third metacarpal is restored.
3. Wires pass through the bones above and below the fracture site.

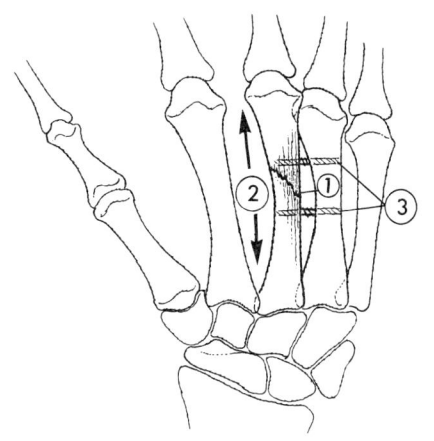

ALTERNATE METHOD FOR DISPLACED FRACTURES OF THE SHAFTS OF MULTIPLE METACARPALS

REMARKS

Fractures of more than one metacarpal may require intermedullary stabilization rather than transfixion to the adjacent metacarpal. To do this use an intramedullary Kirschner wire drilled from the lateral aspect of the metacarpal head across the reduced fracture.

Rarely, open reduction may be necessary for these unstable injuries.

Intramedullary fixation is especially useful in managing multiple metacarpal fractures with open wounds.

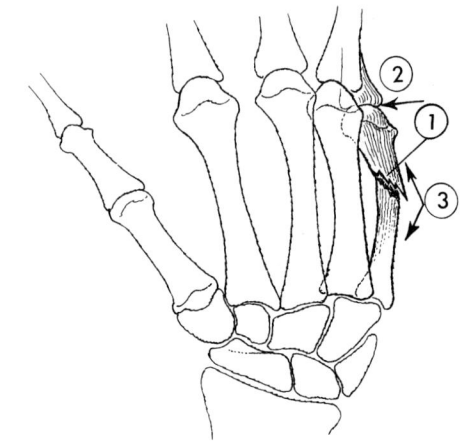

Prereduction X-Ray

Displaced fracture

1. Oblique fracture of the fifth metacarpal.
2. Volar displacement of the head.
3. Posterior angulation of the fragments.

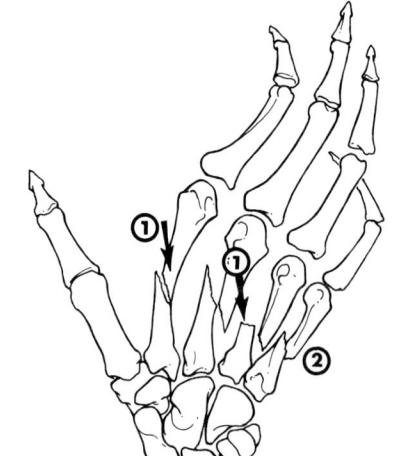

Multiple fractures with open wound

1. Crush injury to the dorsum of the hand has produced an open wound.
2. Multiple metacarpal fractures cause the injury to be extremely unstable.

Reduction and Transfixion

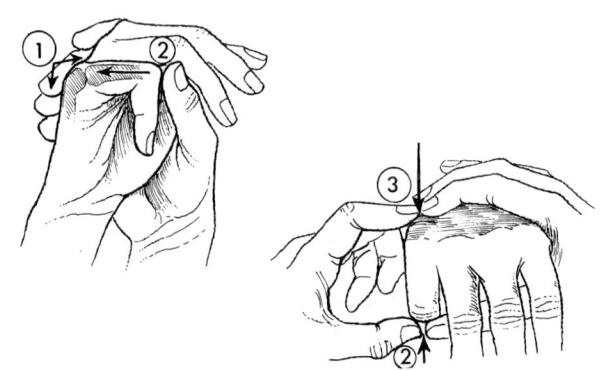

1. An assistant flexes the metacarpophalangeal joint to a right angle and
2. With the finger flexed makes direct pressure upward on the metacarpal head in the long axis of the proximal phalanx.
3. At the same time strong downward pressure is made over the apex of the deformity.

1232

While this position is maintained,

1. Pass a fine threaded wire through the metacarpal head and into the distal fragment — cut the wire 0.5 cm from the skin.

Note: With multiple unstable fractures, two intramedullary pins may be necessary.

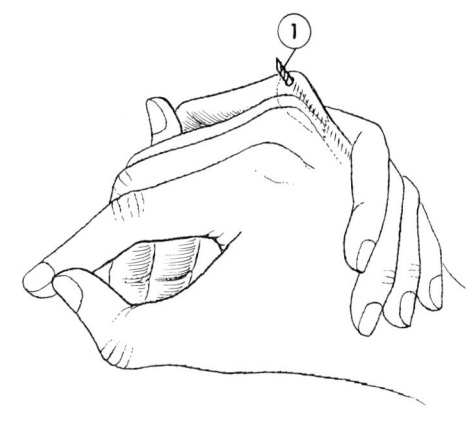

Postreduction X-Rays

Displaced fracture

1. The dorsal angulation of the fracture is corrected.

2. The intramedullary wire has restored length to the metacarpal.

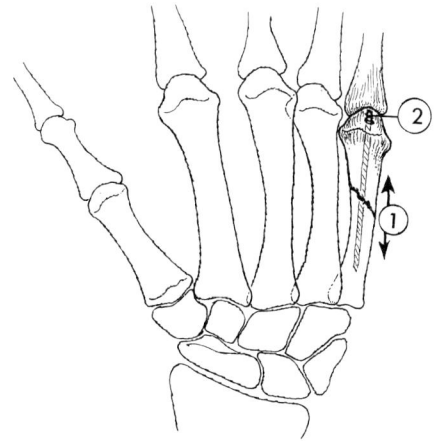

Multiple fractures with open wound

1. Two Kirschner wires in each metacarpal were necessary to stabilize the fracture.

2. Stabilization of the skeletal injury aids significantly in the management of the soft tissue wound.

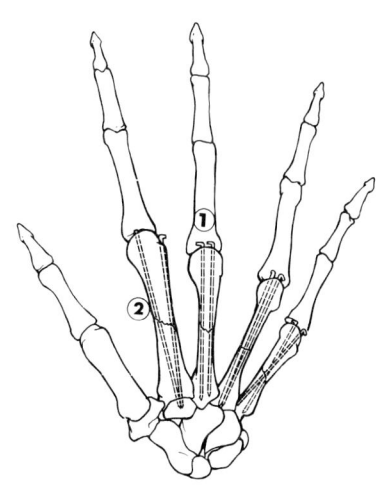

FRACTURES, DISLOCATIONS, AND FRACTURE-DISLOCATIONS OF THE FINGERS

Immobilizatiion

Apply a plaster cast-splint.
1. The two injured fingers are incorporated in the cast-splint.
2. The MP joints are flexed maximally.

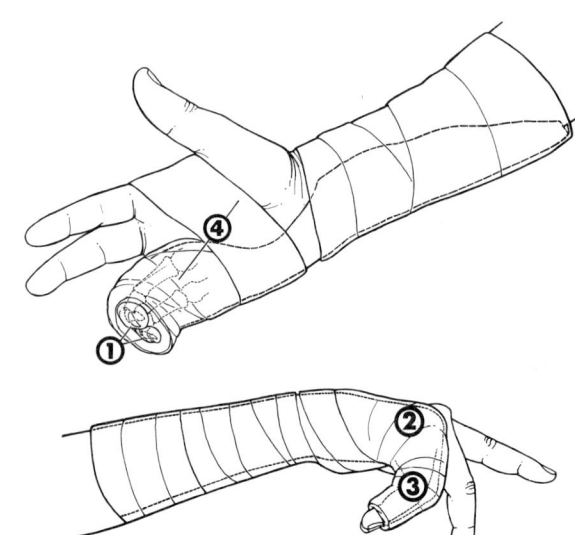

3. The IP joints are slightly flexed.
4. The fingertips are directed towards the scaphoid tuberosity to insure rotational realignment.

Postreduction Management

Remove the cast and wires at the end of three weeks.
During immobilization encourage active use of the unaffected fingers.

Open Reduction: Small Fragment Screw Fixation

Note: This is most often necessary for fractures that have healed in a malunited position.

1. Make a 3-cm longitudinal incision centered over the dorsum of the fractured metacarpal.
2. Displace the extensor tendon to one side and expose the fracture site by subperiosteal dissection.

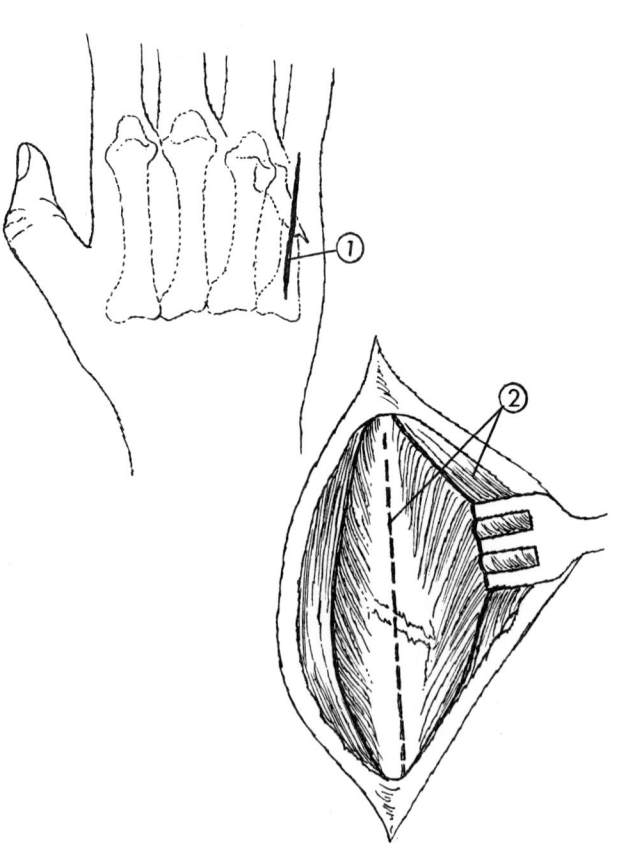

1234

1. Release any callus that has formed at the fracture site and correct the angulation with a small curette.

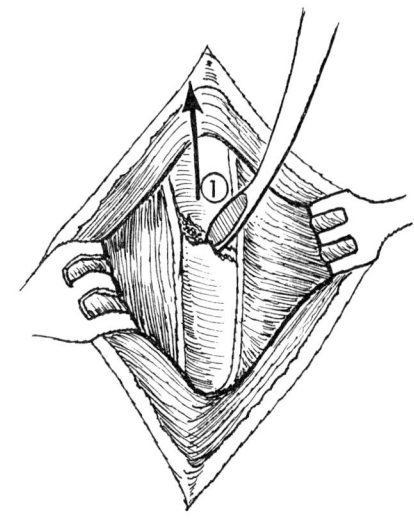

2. Hold the fragments corrected with a tenaculum.
3. Transfix the fragments with two small fragment screws as described on page 1161.

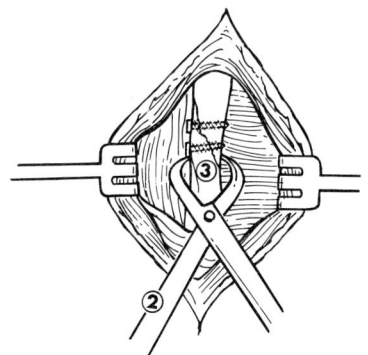

Postreduction X-Ray

Two screws stabilize the metacarpal fragments.

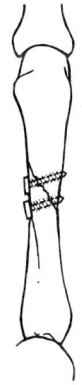

Immobilization

Apply a plaster cast-splint.
1. The two injured fingers are incorporated in the cast-splint.
2. The MP joints are flexed maximally.

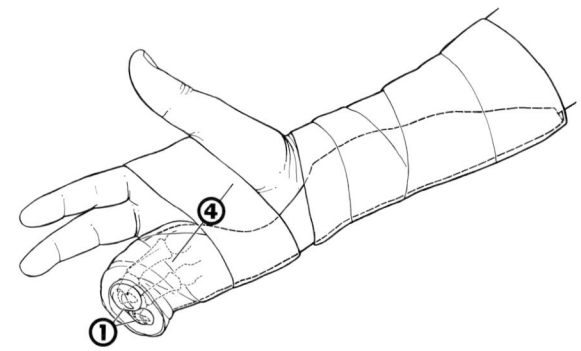

3. The IP joints are slightly flexed.
4. The fingertips are directed towards the scaphoid tuberosity to insure rotational realignment.

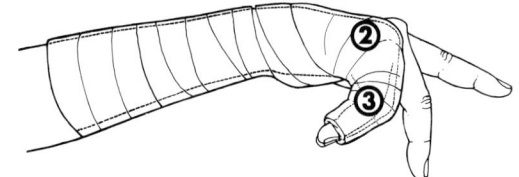

Postreduction Management

Remove the cast after three weeks.
Encourage active exercises of all the fingers while in the plaster.
After the wires and cast are removed the patient should actively exercise the fingers in warm water at least three to four times a day.
If the fracture is still tender, apply a protective splint for ten more days while the patient is regaining function.
The screws may be removed if they are palpable subcutaneously, otherwise they may be left in place.

FRACTURE OF THE BASE OF THE METACARPAL OF THE FINGER

REMARKS

The bases of the metacarpals are firmly bound together by the palmar and dorsal ligaments so that displacement of the fragments rarely occurs — except when the fracture is associated with a carpometacarpal dislocation.

Many of these fractures are impacted, so x-ray visualization may be very difficult; the fractures are frequently missed.

FRACTURES, DISLOCATIONS, AND FRACTURE-DISLOCATIONS OF THE FINGERS

Appearance on X-Ray

1. Comminuted fracture of the fourth metacarpal.

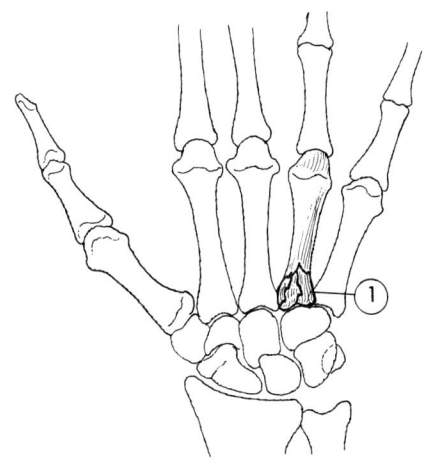

1. Undisplaced fractures of the third and fourth metacarpals.

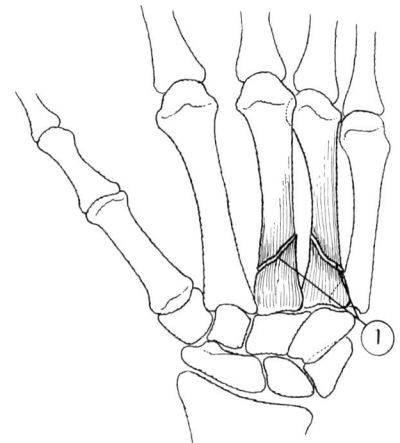

Note: Evaluate these fractures carefully on x-ray for any dissociation of the carpometacarpal joint. Volar displacement of the fracture may involve the motor branch of the ulnar nerve and may require open reduction with internal fixation (see page 1194).

Immobilization

If the hand is swollen, apply a compressive hand dressing for several days.

Most of these undisplaced fractures can be treated by immobilization in a short arm cast for two to three weeks.

1. The fingers are free.
2. The patient is able to actively exercise the MP joints.
3. The wrist is slightly dorsiflexed.

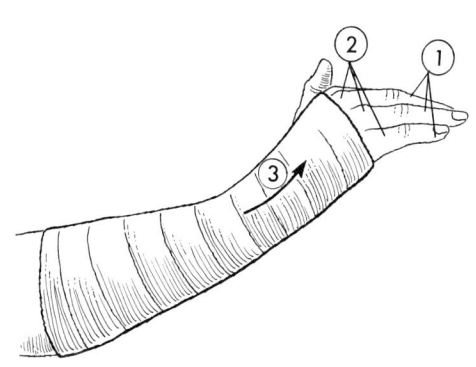

Postreduction Management

Remove the cast at no later than three weeks.
During immobilization insist that the patient actively exercise the fingers to maintain grip strength.

Fractures of the Phalanges

REMARKS

Phalangeal fractures, which can range from minor to severe, are the most common of all hand fractures.

The disability they cause depends on the degree of initial injury as well as the treatment.

Direct injury to the finger frequently produces open comminuted fractures. All open fractures must be thoroughly cleansed and the fracture must be immobilized by either internal or external means.

The objective of fracture treatment should be to provide sufficient stability by either external or internal fixation to permit early movement of the finger's joints and muscles.

Fracture reduction should be as close to anatomic as possible, with particular attention given to rotational realignment.

The majority of phalangeal shaft fractures are stable injuries that can be effectively managed by "buddy taping" to the adjacent finger. This stabilizes the fracture and insures correct rotational alignment while permitting joint and tendon motion.

Splinting the fractured finger alone is likely to accentuate rotational malalignment. Displaced, unstable phalangeal fractures can frequently be successfully treated by closed reduction and cast-splint immobilization with the finger in the intrinsic-plus position.

The reduction of unstable phalangeal fractures must be critically analyzed with true anteroposterior and lateral x-rays of the finger. Be alert to the deformities likely to follow certain types of fractures:

1. Impacted fractures of the proximal phalanx that angulate more than 25 degrees will significantly impair finger function.
2. Oblique fractures of the middle phalanx that shorten will also impair tendon gliding and generally require Kirschner wire fixation. The same type of oblique fracture in the proximal phalanx is better fixed internally with a small fragment screw.
3. T-condylar fractures with joint involvement that require internal fixation can be held by either a Kirschner wire or a small fragment screw.

FRACTURES, DISLOCATIONS, AND FRACTURE-DISLOCATIONS OF THE FINGERS

4. Multiple phalangeal fractures or open comminuted injuries are generally candidates for internal fixation using either a small fragment screw or Kirschner wires.

Although the majority of phalangeal fractures can be very effectively treated by closed means, knowledge of the deformities common with these injuries is important so as to select the most appropriate means of treatment.

ANATOMIC CONSIDERATIONS

Fractures of the shaft of the proximal phalanx are characterized by volar angulation of the fragments. Such angulation is due to the action of the extrinsic and intrinsic muscles, which buckle the fragments.

1. Fracture of the middle of the shaft of the proximal phalanx.
2. The pull of the intrinsic muscles flexes the proximal fragment while the central slip attachment to the PIP joint hyperextends the distal fragment.

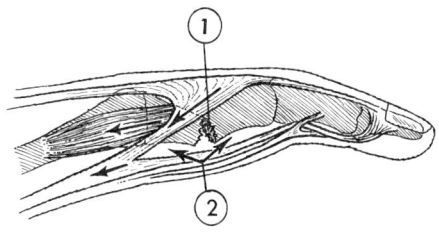

The type of deformity produced by fracture of the middle phalanx depends upon the relationship of the site of the fracture to the insertion of the tendon of the flexor digitorum sublimis.

If the fracture site is proximal to the insertion of the tendon, the action of the extensor slip on the proximal fragment and the action of the flexor digitorum sublimis on the distal fragment produce a dorsal angulation of the fragments.

1. Fracture of the middle phalanx.
2. The central slip of the extensor tendon extends the proximal fragment.
3. The flexor digitorum sublimis flexes the distal fragment, producing
4. Dorsal angulation of the fragments.

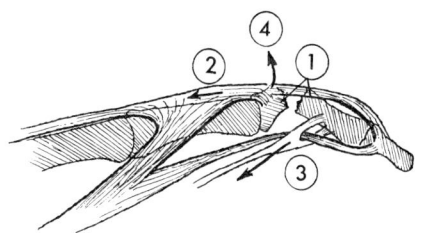

If the fracture site is distal to the insertion of the flexor sublimis tendon, the extensor tendon extends the distal fragment, and the flexor digitorum sublimis flexes the proximal fragment, producing a volar angulation of the fragments.

1239

FRACTURES, DISLOCATIONS, AND FRACTURE-DISLOCATIONS OF THE FINGERS

1. Fracture of the middle phalanx distal to the insertion of the flexor digitorum sublimis tendon.
2. The proximal fragment is flexed.
3. The distal fragment is extended, producing
4. Volar angulation of the fragments.

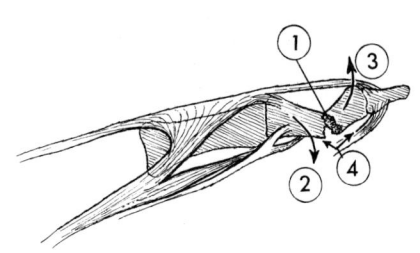

UNDISPLACED FRACTURES OF THE PROXIMAL PHALANX

REMARKS

These fractures need only immobilization by "buddy taping" to the adjacent, uninjured finger.

This method permits correct rotational alignment while allowing the patient to actively exercise the joints and tendons of the injured finger.

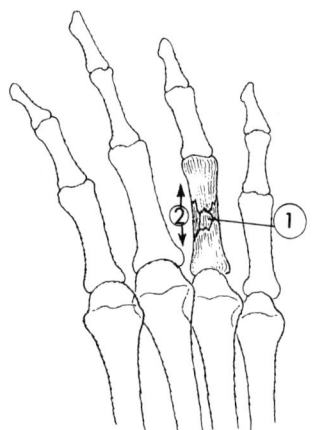

Appearance on X-Ray

1. Comminuted fracture of the proximal phalanx.
2. There is no displacement of the fragments.

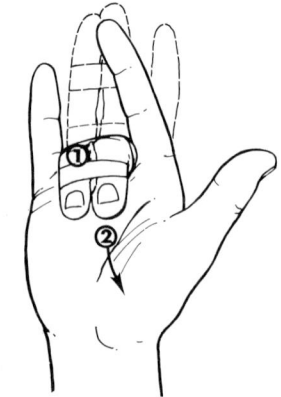

Immobilization

1. Tape the injured finger to the adjacent, uninjured one using a small amount of cast padding applied between the fingers.
2. Insure correct rotational alignment by directing the fingertips toward the scaphoid tuberosity.

1240

FRACTURES, DISLOCATIONS, AND FRACTURE-DISLOCATIONS OF THE FINGERS

Subsequent Management

Allow the patient to actively exercise the taped fingers.

The taping may be removed by 10 to 14 days, and active exercises should be continued.

Avoid prolonging immobilization beyond 3 weeks, as this adds significantly to the likelihood of impaired finger function.

DISPLACED FRACTURE OF THE PROXIMAL PHALANX

REMARKS

These fractures are usually the result of hyperextension injury, which causes either a transverse, an oblique, or a spiral type of fracture. In children, impacted fractures of the base of the proximal phalanx are epiphyseal injuries that must be reduced to restore rotational alignment.

Impacted fractures of the proximal phalanx may be deceptive and may heal with excessive volar angulation of more than 25 degrees which impairs finger function.

The two major errors in treating these fractures are:

1. Accepting an oblique view rather than a true lateral x-ray to evaluate reduction.
2. Failure to immobilize the MP joint in complete flexion.

Complete flexion of the MP joint is important to relax the intrinsic muscles and also to tighten the extensor hood about the fracture.

Prereduction X-Ray

1. Fracture of the proximal phalanx of the fourth finger.
2. Typical anterior angulation at the fracture site.

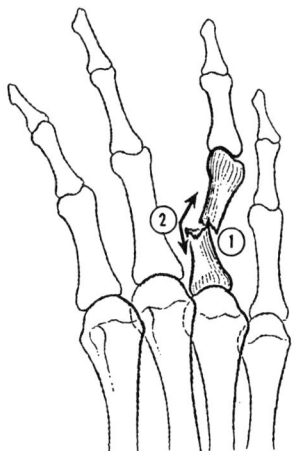

FRACTURES, DISLOCATIONS, AND FRACTURE-DISLOCATIONS OF THE FINGERS

Manipulative Reduction

1. Loop a gauze bandage around the end of the finger and around your hand.
2. Grasp the finger between your thumb and index finger.
3. Make steady traction in the line of the finger.
4. While traction is maintained,
5. Flex the finger over
6. The index finger of your other hand, which pushes upward at the apex of the angular deformity.

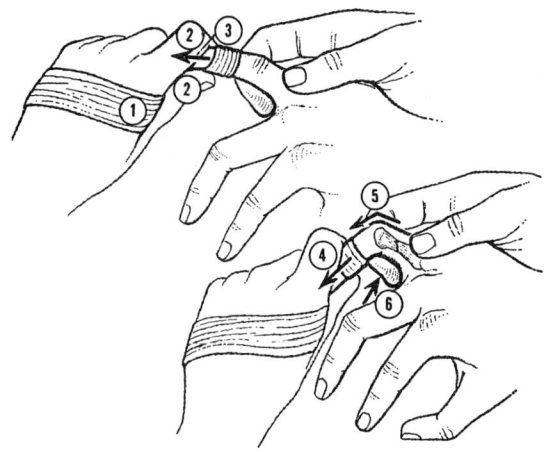

Postreduction X-Ray

1. The fragments of the proximal phalanx are engaged and in normal alignment.

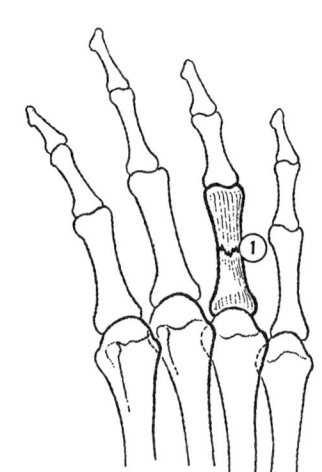

2. A true lateral x-ray shows that volar angulation has been completely corrected.

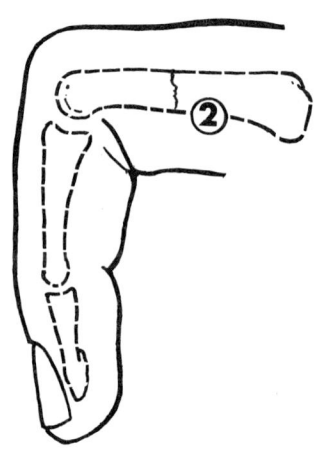

Immobilization

Apply a plaster cast-splint with the fingers in the intrinsic-plus position.

1. The injured finger and the adjacent uninjured finger are immobilized.
2. The MP joint is in 70 degrees of flexion.

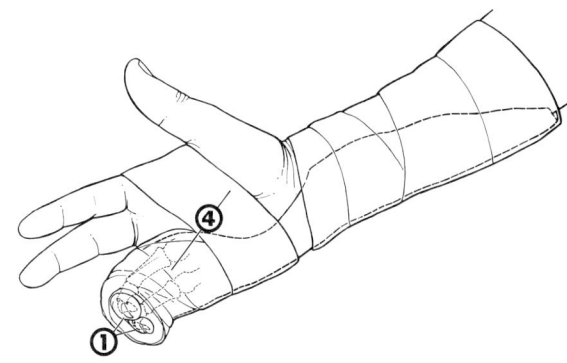

3. The PIP joints are slightly flexed.
4. The rotational realignment is assured by the fingertips pointing toward the tuberosity of the scaphoid.

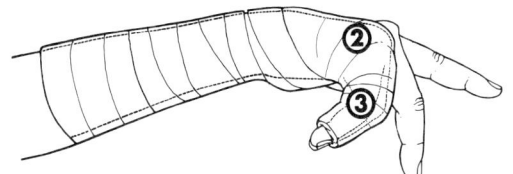

Postreduction Management

Take x-rays again on the fifth and tenth days; check for position.

During immobilization, encourage active exercises of all uninvolved fingers.

Remove the plaster cast-splint at the end of three weeks.

Institute physical therapy and active exercises to restore normal function.

IMPACTED FRACTURE OF THE PROXIMAL PHALANX IN CHILDREN

REMARKS

Fractures of the base of the phalanx in children are epiphyseal injuries that should be reduced.

The volar angulation may be difficult to estimate unless true lateral x-rays are obtained. To achieve reduction, a pencil or similar object is placed between the fingers to stabilize the proximal epiphysis while the phalanx is brought back into proper alignment.

FRACTURES, DISLOCATIONS, AND FRACTURE-DISLOCATIONS OF THE FINGERS

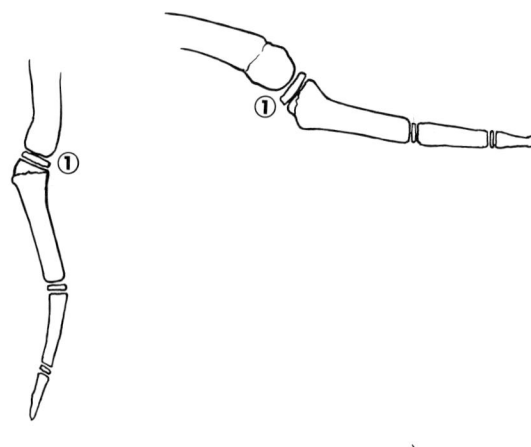

1. An impacted proximal epiphyseal fracture causes rotational malalignment of the finger.

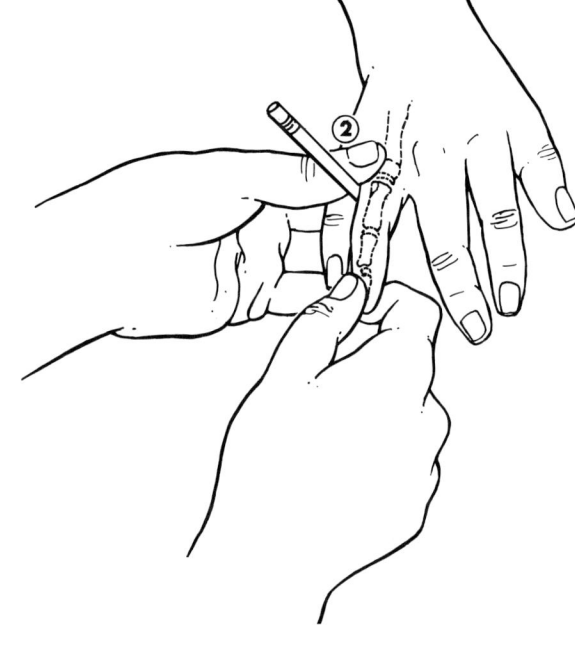

2. Reduction is achieved by inserting a pencil between the fingers and realigning the distal phalanx with the proximal epiphysis.

Immobilization

When the fracture is reduced, it may be immobilized by "buddy taping."

1. The injured finger is strapped to the adjacent, uninjured finger with cast padding between the fingers.
2. Rotational realignment is assured by direction of the fingertips toward the scaphoid tuberosity.

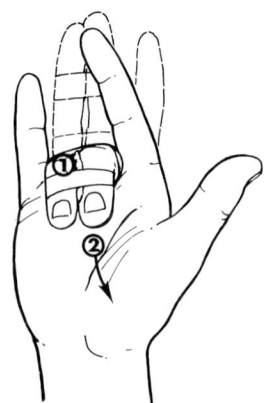

1244

FRACTURES, DISLOCATIONS, AND FRACTURE-DISLOCATIONS OF THE FINGERS

Postreduction Management

Allow the patient to actively exercise the fingers with "buddy taping" for 7 to 10 days.

Remove the taping by 10 to 14 days and allow active exercise without the support.

In active young people likely to reinjure the finger, use protective taping for an additional week.

OBLIQUE FRACTURES OF THE PROXIMAL PHALANX

REMARKS

These fractures are generally the result of direct injury and may be considerably displaced. To insure maximum functional recovery, operative reduction and screw fixation are generally indicated.

Prereduction X-Ray

1. A fracture has involved the entire proximal phalanx in the longitudinal axis.
2. The displacement of the fragments could not be reduced by closed means.

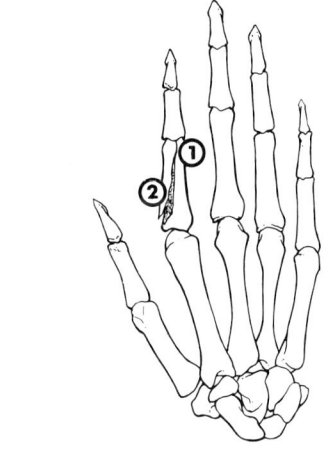

Operative Procedure

1. Approach the fracture site via a curved longitudinal incision through the dorsal extensor apparatus or
2. Between the dorsal apparatus and the lateral bands.

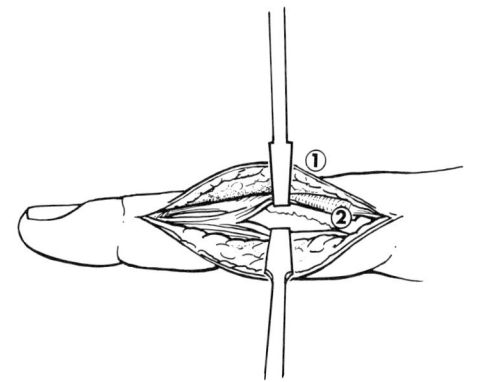

FRACTURES, DISLOCATIONS, AND FRACTURE-DISLOCATIONS OF THE FINGERS

Operative Procedure (Continued)

3. Reduce and hold the fracture with a tenaculum and then power drill both cortices using a 2-mm bit and drill guide.

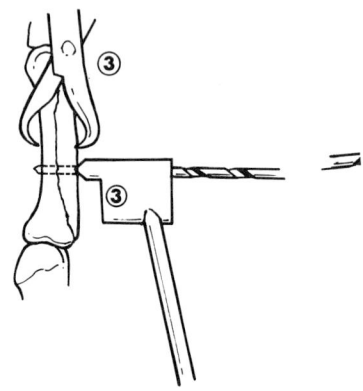

4. Tap both cortices with a 2.7-mm tap.

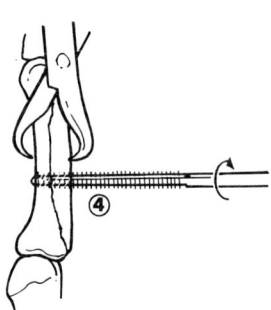

5. Power drill near cortex with a 2.7-mm drill to provide a gliding hole.

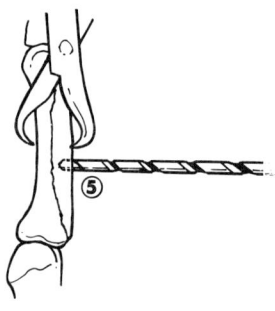

6. Insert a 2.7-mm screw, which compresses the fracture.

Note: A second screw may be necessary for longer oblique fractures.

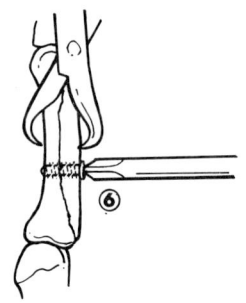

Postreduction X-Ray

1. The spiral oblique fracture has been stabilized adequately with the two screws to permit early range-of-motion exercises.

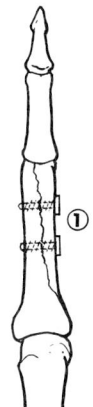

Postoperative Management

Immobilize the hand in a compression dressing for several days until the swelling subsides.

Allow guarded range-of-motion exercises by three to five days after the swelling has subsided.

The screws may be removed at eight to twelve weeks using local anesthetic when the fracture has consolidated.

T-CONDYLAR FRACTURE OF THE DISTAL END OF THE PROXIMAL PHALANX

REMARKS

The complete congruity of the articular surface must be restored; this is achieved by open reduction.

Failure to restore the fragments to their normal position results in a painful stiff joint with lateral deviation of the middle phalanx.

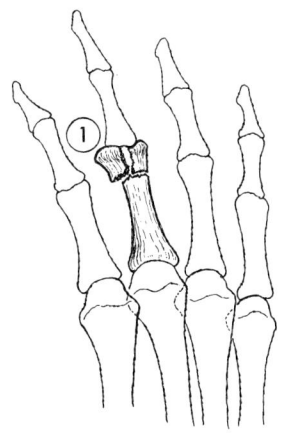

Prereduction X-Ray

1. T fracture of the end of the proximal phalanx of the third finger.

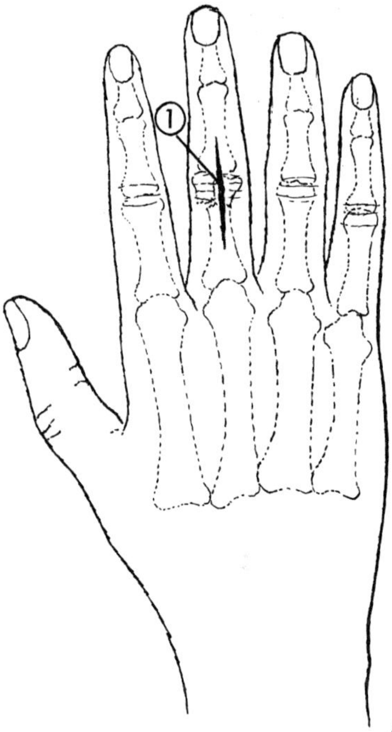

FRACTURES, DISLOCATIONS, AND FRACTURE-DISLOCATIONS OF THE FINGERS

Operative Reduction

1. Make a 4-cm incision over the fracture site.
2. By sharp subperiosteal dissection expose the fracture site.

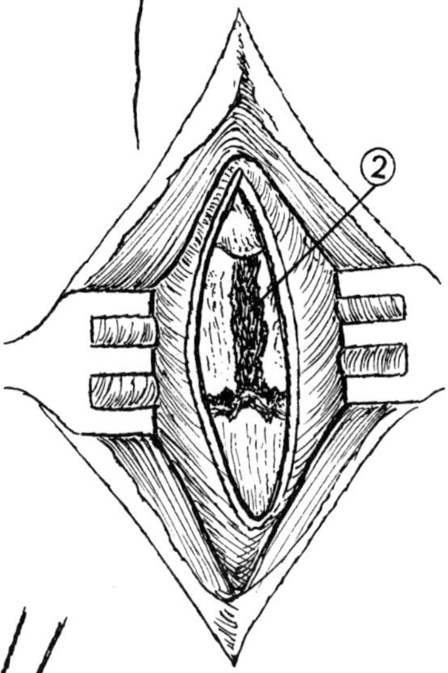

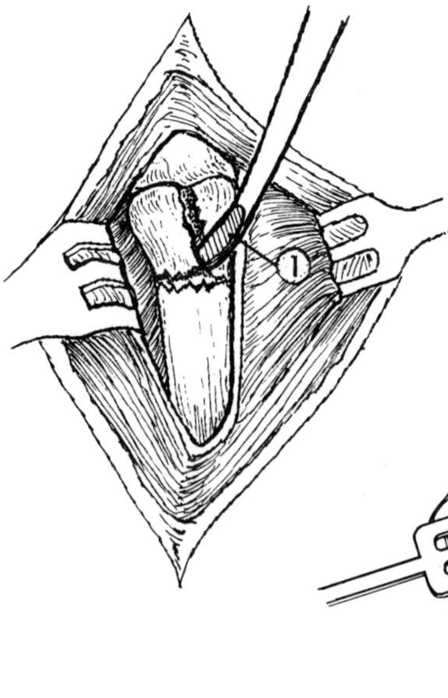

1. With a small curette, lever the fragments into normal position.
2. Fix the fragments in the desired position with a towel clip.
3. Transfix the fragments with a small fragment screw and plate.

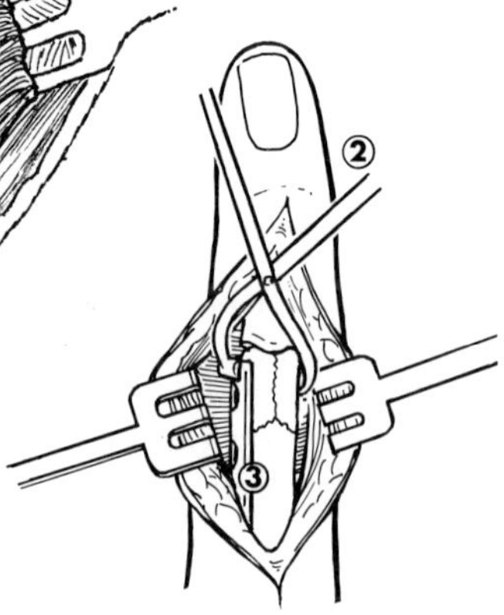

Postreduction X-Ray

1. The articular fragments are reduced by the screw.
2. The plate holds the articular fragments to the shaft of the phalanx.

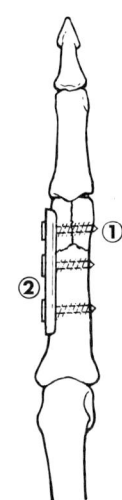

Immobilization

After swelling has subsided, use external support by means of "buddy taping" or a plaster cast-splint.

1. The injured finger is taped to the adjacent, uninjured finger and cast padding is applied between the fingers.
2. The fingertips are aligned to point toward the scaphoid tuberosity.

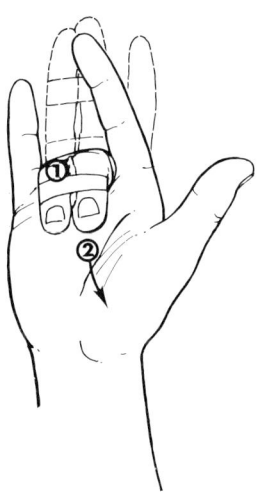

Subsequent Management

Encourage the patient to actively exercise the injured finger as soon as the swelling subsides.

Discard the taping by the end of three weeks.

When the fracture has consolidated, by eight to ten weeks, the screws and plate may be removed under local anesthetic.

FRACTURES OF THE SHAFT OF THE MIDDLE PHALANX

REMARKS

Transverse fractures of the middle phalanx are displaced in the direction of the pull of the flexor sublimis.

Angulation of the fracture may be in either a volar or dorsal direction, depending on whether the fracture is proximal or distal to the sublimis insertion.

In either instance, the fracture can be reduced by flexing the MP joint of the finger to a maximal degree, thereby relaxing the sublimis pull and tightening the extensor hood.

Oblique, longitudinal fractures of the middle phalanx may cause difficulty by shortening and impinging on tendinous structures. These fractures are frequently best stabilized with percutaneous Kirschner wires.

Prereduction X-Ray

VOLAR AUGULATION

1. Fracture of the middle phalanx distal to the insertion of the sublimis.
2. Volar angulation results from pull of the sublimis on the proximal fragment.

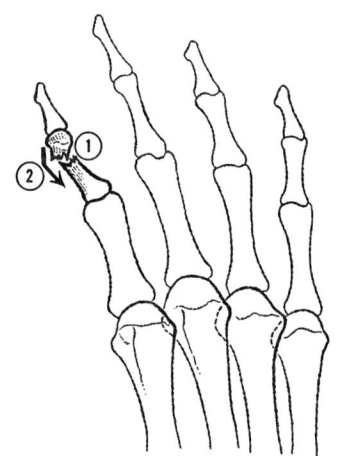

DORSAL ANGULATION

1. Fracture of the middle phalanx proximal to the sublimis insertion.
2. Dorsal angulation results from pull of the sublimis on the distal fragment.

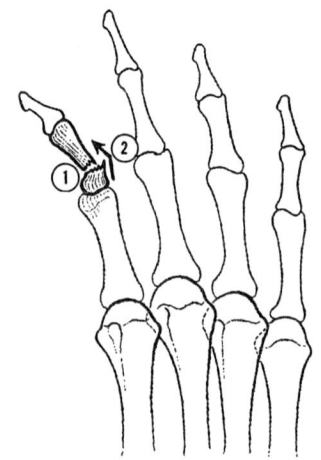

Reduction and Immobilization

Both of these fractures may be reduced by immobilizing the finger in the intrinsic-plus position.

1. The fractured finger is immobilized with the adjacent, uninjured finger.
2. The MP joint is flexed maximally to 70 degrees.
3. The PIP joints are in slight flexion.
4. The tips of the fingers are directed towards the scaphoid tuberosity.

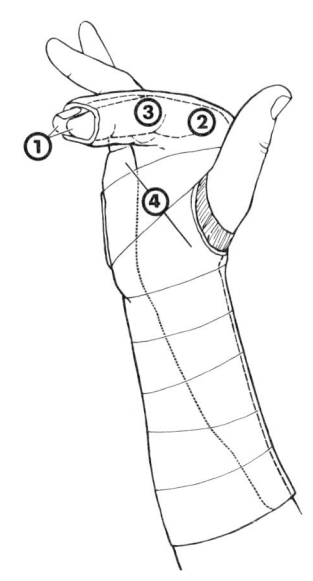

Postreduction X-Ray

1. The fracture distal to the sublimis insertion has been reduced by relaxing the tendon pull on the proximal fragment.

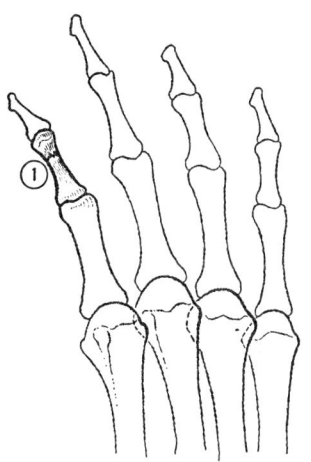

2. The fracture proximal to the sublimis insertion has been reduced by relaxing the tendon pull on the distal fragment.

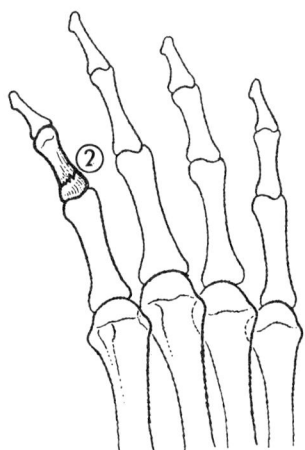

OBLIQUE FRACTURE OF THE MIDDLE PHALANX

REMARKS

Oblique fractures in this area must be reduced anatomically so as to avoid impingement on the surrounding tendon and capsule.

Appearance on X-Ray

1. An oblique fracture of the middle phalanx has shortened and angulated.
2. Unreduced fracture prominence will impale intrinsic and extrinsic tendons.

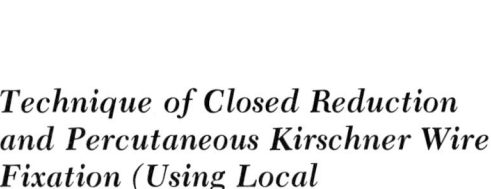

Technique of Closed Reduction and Percutaneous Kirschner Wire Fixation (Using Local Anesthesia)

1. Traction is maintained by an assistant to keep the fracture reduced.
2. A padded clamp is used to compress the spiral fracture fragments together.
3. Two fine Kirschner wires are drilled percutaneously through the fracture fragments and are bent outside of the skin.

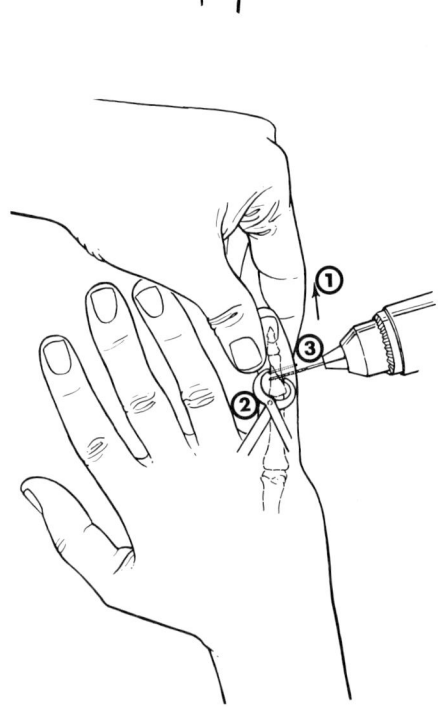

Postreduction Management

Remove the Kirschner wires no later than three weeks and permit active exercise.

STABLE FRACTURE OF THE DISTAL PHALANX

REMARKS

Comminution of the distal phalanx occurs quite frequently if the fingertip is crushed or caught in a door. Usually there is minimal or no displacement of the fragments.

In children and adolescents, the distal phalangeal epiphysis becomes separated and requires reduction.

The nail over the injury should be left in place if at all possible because it serves as a very effective splint for the displaced epiphysis.

Occasionally fractures of the distal phalanx will be so displaced that internal fixation with a Kirschner wire or Riordan pin may be necessary (see page 1215).

Frequently, the tip of the finger is amputated and the fractured bone is exposed. The most effective method of management for the majority of these tip amputations is simple continuous cast protection. Local skin grafting or flaps are usually not necessary, particularly in children.

Appearance on X-Ray

1. Severe comminution of the distal phalanx with minimal displacement of fragments.

Note: This fracture requires no reduction.

2. Fracture of the terminal phalanx with upward, backward, and lateral displacement of the distal fragment.

Note: This fracture should be reduced.

3. Epiphyseal separation of the terminal phalanx of the index finger.

Note: This epiphyseal fracture should be reduced. The nail bed serves as a very effective splint after the fracture is reduced.

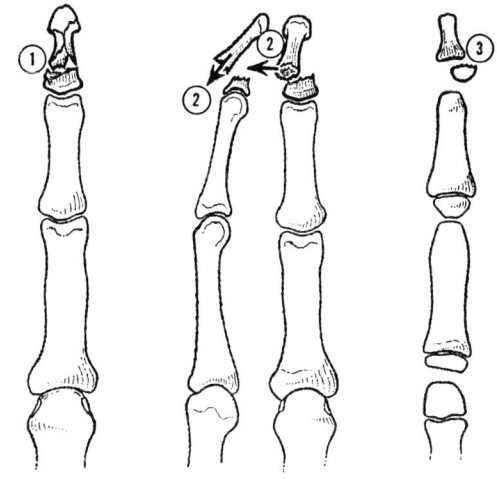

Manipulative Reduction

1. Make traction and mold the fragments by squeezing the end of the finger between your thumb and index finger.

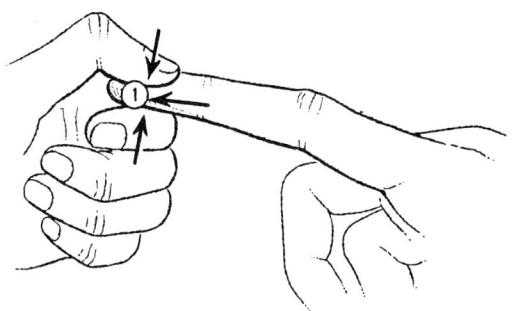

Manipulative Reduction (Continued)

2. Correct the lateral displacement by compressing the lateral borders of the terminal phalanx between your index finger and thumb.

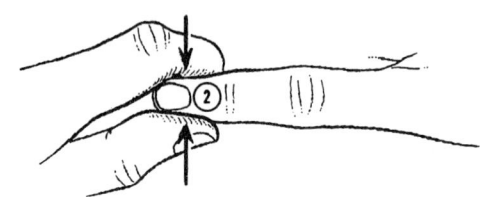

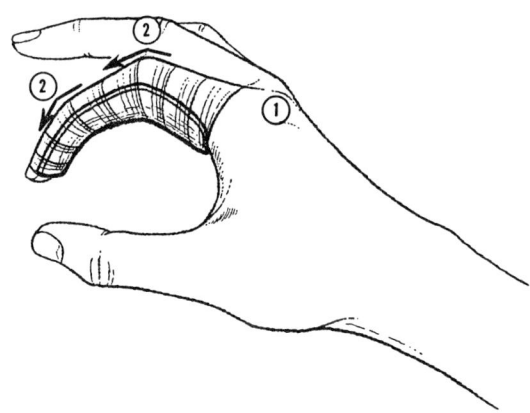

Immobilization

Apply an anterior plaster slab directly to the skin.
1. The metacarpophalangeal joint is free.
2. The interphalangeal joints are slightly flexed.

Postreduction Management

Allow free, active use of the uninvolved fingers. Remove the plaster cast at the end of two weeks. Institute active exercises to restore joint function.

UNSTABLE FRACTURE OF THE SHAFT OF THE DISTAL PHALANX

WITH LATERAL DISPLACEMENT OF THE FRAGMENT

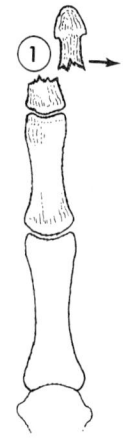

Prereduction X-Rays

1. Fracture of the shaft with lateral displacement of the distal fragment.

FRACTURES, DISLOCATIONS, AND FRACTURE-DISLOCATIONS OF THE FINGERS

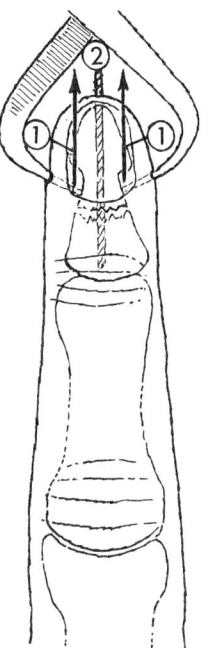

Reduction

1. Grasp the distal fragment with a towel clip and make straight traction — this realigns the fragments.
2. Pass a threaded wire through the distal end of the finger into the proximal fragment.

WITH LATERAL DEVIATION OF THE DISTAL FRAGMENT

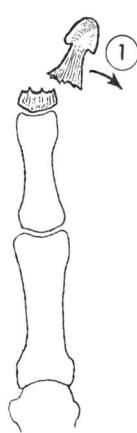

Prereduction X-Ray

1. Fracture through the base of the phalanx with lateral deviation of the distal fragment.

FRACTURES, DISLOCATIONS, AND FRACTURE-DISLOCATIONS OF THE FINGERS

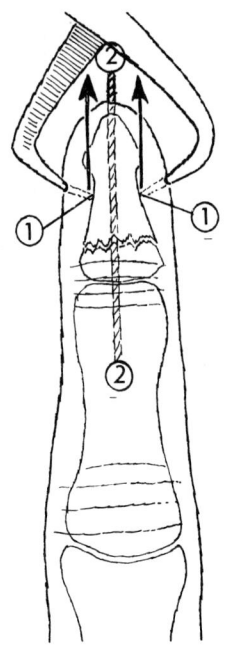

Reduction

1. Grasp the distal fragment with a towel clip and make straight traction.
2. Pass a threaded wire through both fragments, across the distal joint, and into the middle phalanx.

FINGERTIP AMPUTATION

REMARKS

This injury is seen very commonly in the emergency room, particularly in young children. Treatment should consist of thorough cleansing of the injury and cast immobilization.

In general, grafts or local flaps are not indicated and in fact give a poorer eschar than simple cast immobilization for three weeks.

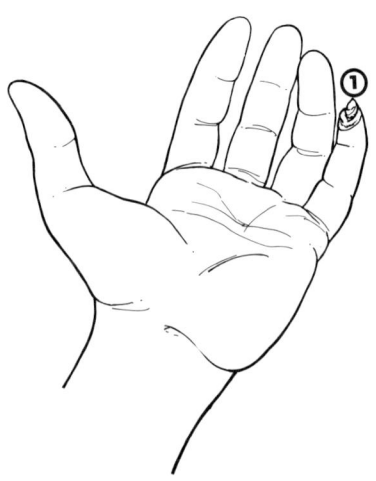

1. A typical amputation of the fingertip with exposed, fractured bone in a young patient.

2. After thorough cleansing of the wound, the fingertip is immobilized in a finger cast.

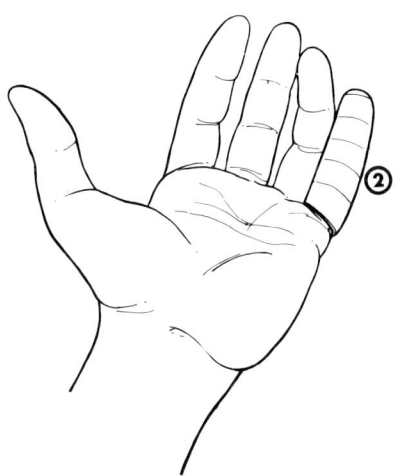

3. The cast is changed at ten days, and by three weeks the amputated fingertip has healed by granulation tissue and re-epithelialization.

Note: This continuous cast immobilization provides an occlusive dressing that allows natural wound intussusception to shrink the scar down to minimum size. Full-thickness skin graft or flaps inhibit this type of wound shrinkage.

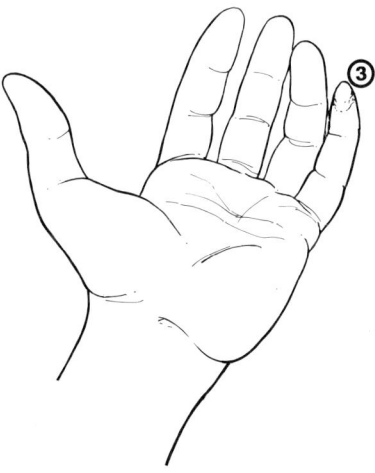

SUMMARY: PITFALLS OF FRACTURES AND DISLOCATIONS OF THE HAND

Fractures and dislocations of the fingers and metacarpals are common injuries with many common pitfalls. Careful assessment will anticipate these complications in the process of selecting appropriate treatment.

Failure to appreciate the three dimensions of fracture alignment leads frequently to rotational malunion and overlapping finger deformities from what might be considered minor fractures.

Most of these injuries can be immobilized by taping or splinting, which allows finger motion but maintains three-dimensional alignment.

Immobilization of more than ten days is usually too long for the majority of hand fractures and dislocations. When immobilized, the fingers should be maintained in the intrinsic-plus position to prevent shortening of capsular ligaments.

Closed reduction is not always the "conservative" approach to unstable fractures or complex dislocations. The physician should be aware of the types of injuries that are best treated by open reduction and internal fixation. He should also be critical of closed reduction, which does not permit early restoration of function. In general, the more complex and prolonged the external immobilization needed for closed reduction, the stronger is the indication for open reduction and internal fixation.

Dislocations of the carpometacarpal joints are usually unstable injuries requiring internal fixation with transcutaneous pins after closed reduction. Ulnar nerve function should be carefully assessed after these injuries to determine the need for operative decompression and reduction of the fracture.

Fractures of the metacarpals, particularly the common "boxer's" fracture of the fifth, tend to be overtreated. Emphasis is best placed on early functional exercise rather than on exact reduction. In contrast to the "boxer's" fracture, multiple metacarpal fractures produced by open or crushing injuries are frequently unstable and require internal fixation to maximize functional recovery.

Metacarpophalangeal dislocations occur in the thumb, and in index and small fingers. They can present problems if the simple and complex types are not distinguished. Prompt differentiation based on physical manifestations should lead to appropriate reduction by either closed or open techniques.

Fractures of the phalanges can be most effectively treated by taping to the adjacent fingers so as to allow joint motion and still maintain three-dimensional fracture alignment. Certain phalangeal fractures, particularly angulated fractures of the proximal phalanx, oblique fractures of the middle phalanx, and any fracture causing functional joint instability, frequently require internal fixation.

The "jammed" finger is a common problem concealing many potential pitfalls. These include tendon and capsular, as well as bony injuries. Mallet finger, boutonniere and pseudoboutonniere deformities, and flexor profundus avulsion can be effectively and simply treated if one only considers them to be potential complications in a "jammed" finger. The finger should be carefully and systematically assessed by palpation, by active and passive stress testing, and by x-ray of the finger in two views. Failure to appreciate instability or tendon disruption can result in more disability than is necessary after these common injuries.

Injuries to the distal phalanx or fingertip tend to lead to the pitfall of overtreatment. Simple finger cast immobilization, particularly for the most common patient, the young child with a fingertip injury, utilizes the biologic healing response most effectively.

Recognizing and appreciating the common types of injuries that need the least, as well as the most, therapeutic help is critical to minimizing complications and avoiding pitfalls.

References

Burkhalter, W. E., Butler, B., Metz, W., et al.: Experience with delayed primary closure of war wounds of the hand in Viet Nam. J. Bone and Joint Surg. 50-A:945, 1968.

Carroll, R. E., and Match, R. M.: Avulsion of the flexor profundus tendon insertion. J. Trauma 10:1109, 1970.

Coonrad, R. W., and Goldner, J. L.: A study of the pathological findings and treatment in soft-tissue injury of the thumb metacarpophalangeal joint. J. Bone and Joint Surg. 50-A:439, 1968.

Coonrad, R. W., and Pohlman, M. H.: Impacted fractures in the proximal portion of the proximal phalanx of the finger. J. Bone and Joint Surg. 51-A:1291, 1969.

Crawford, G. P.: Screw fixation for certain fractures of the phalanges and metecarpals. J. Bone and Joint Surg. 58-A:487, 1976.

Fox, J. W., Golden, G. T., and Rodeheaver, G., et al.: Nonoperative management of fingertip pulp amputation by occlusive dressings. Am. J. Surg. 133:255, 1977.

Green, D. P., and Terry, G. C.: Complex dislocation of the metacarpophalangeal joint. J. Bone and Joint Surg. 55-A:1480, 1973.

Green, D. P., and Anderson, J. R.: Closed reduction and percutaneous pin fixation of fractured phalanges. J. Bone and Joint Surg. 55-A:1651, 1973.

Henry, A. K.: Extensile Exposure, 2nd edition. Baltimore, The Williams & Wilkins Company 1962, p. 123.

Holm, A., and Zachariae, L.: Fingertip lesions. An evaluation of conservative treatment versus free skin grafting. Acta Orthop. Scand. 45:382, 1974.

Hsu, J. D., and Curtis, R. M.: Carpometacarpal dislocations on the ulnar side of the hand. J. Bone and Joint Surg. 52-A:927, 1970.

Hunter, J. M., and Cowen, N. J.: Fifth metacarpal fractures in a compensation clinic population. J. Bone and Joint Surg. 52-A:1159, 1970.

James, J. I. P.: Fractures of the proximal and middle phalanges of the fingers. Acta Orthop. Scand. 32:401, 1962.

REFERENCES

Kleinert, H. E., and Kasdan, M. L.: Reconstruction of chronically subluxated proximal interphalangeal finger joint. J. Bone and Joint Surg. 47-A:958, 1965.

McCue, F. C., Honner, R., Johnson, M. C., et al.: Athletic injuries of the proximal interphalangeal joint requiring surgical treatment. J. Bone and Joint Surg. 52-A:937, 1970.

McElfresh, E. C., Dobyns, J. H., and O'Brien, E. T.: Management of fracture-dislocation of the proximal interphalangeal joints by extension-lock splinting. J. Bone and Joint Surg. 54-A:1705, 1972.

McLaughlin, H. L.: Complex "locked" dislocation of the metacarpophalangeal joints. J. Trauma 5:683, 1965.

Salamon, P. B., and Gelberman, R. H.: Irreducible dislocation of the interphalangeal joint of the thumb. J. Bone and Joint Surg. 60-A:400, 1978.

Spinner, M., and Choi, B. Y.: Anterior dislocation of the proximal interphalangeal joint. J. Bone and Joint Surg. 152-A:1329, 1970.

Stark, H. H.: Troublesome fractures and dislocations of the hand. In Instructional Course Lectures, American Academy of Orthopaedic Surgeons, 19:130, 1970.

Wright, T. A.: Early mobilization in fractures of the metacarpals and phalanges. Can. J. Surg..11:491, 1968.

DISLOCATIONS AND FRACTURE-DISLOCATIONS OF THE HIP AND ACETABULUM

ANATOMIC FEATURES AND CLASSIFICATION OF INJURIES

REMARKS

Knowledge of the anatomy of the hip is essential in order to comprehend the tissues involved as the result of the different mechanisms capable of producing fractures and dislocations of the hip.

ANATOMY OF THE HIP JOINT

Anterior Superficial Structures

1. Iliacus.
2. Psoas major.
3. Pectineus.
4. Femoral nerve, artery, vein.
5. Adductor longus.

Note: The proximity of the femoral vessels to the hip joint exposes them to injury from anterior dislocation.

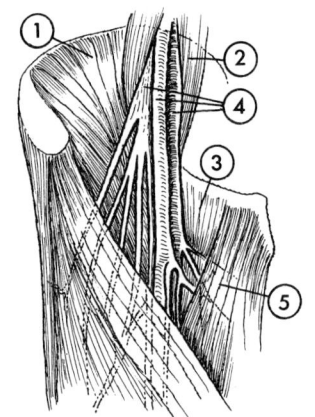

Anterior Deep Structures

1. Iliofemoral (Y) ligament.
2. Rectus femoris.
3. Iliopsoas tendon.
4. Thin or defective portion of the anterior capsule.
5. Obturator externus.
6. Obturator nerve (anterior and posterior divisions).

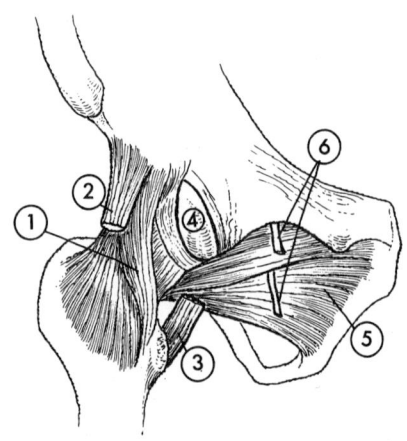

ANATOMIC FEATURES AND CLASSIFICATION OF INJURIES

Posterior Superficial Structures

1. Superior gluteal artery.
2. Inferior gluteal artery.
3. Piriformis.
4. Sciatic nerve.
5. Obturator internus and gemelli.
6. Quadratus femoris.

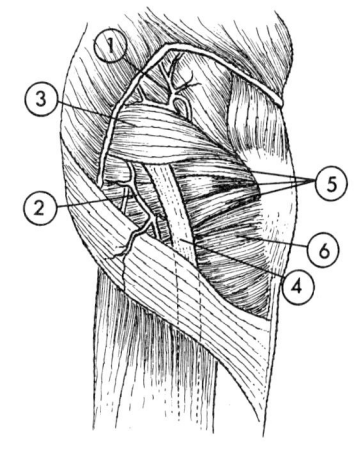

Posterior Deep Structures

1. Piriformis.
2. Gemelli.
3. Obturator internus.
4. Obturator externus.
5. Sciatic nerve.
6. Spiral fibers of posterior capsule and acetabular labrum.

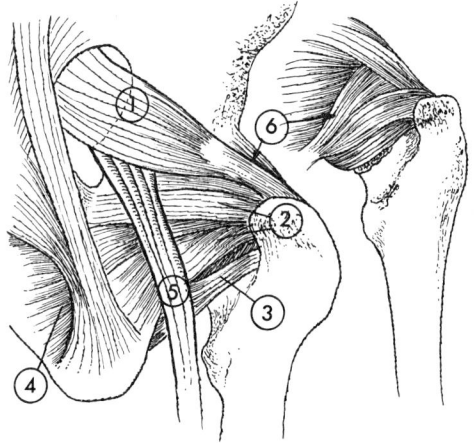

BLOOD SUPPLY OF THE FEMORAL HEAD AND NECK (AFTER OGDEN)

The femoral head, because of its unique growth pattern in the first three years of life, develops a circulatory system that is liable to damage by fracture or dislocation. The risk of vascular damage is considerably higher with a displaced fracture of the neck than with a dislocation for the reasons shown below.

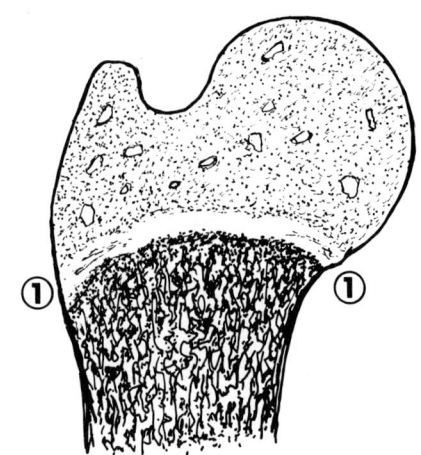

At Birth

1. The femoral growth plate or physis is mainly extra-articular and
2. Outside the capsular attachment, where blood vessels enter bone.

Note: This is in contrast to most physeal vascular rings such as the ring of the knee, which enters through the capsular insertion directly at the physis.

3. The lateral circumflex branch of the profunda femoris artery supplies the anterolateral growth plate, most of the greater trochanter, and the anteromedial femoral head.
4. The medial circumflex branch of the profunda femoris supplies the posteromedial chondroepiphysis, the posterior growth plate, and the posterior greater trochanter.
5. The artery of the ligamentum teres supplies the small medial portion of the femoral head.

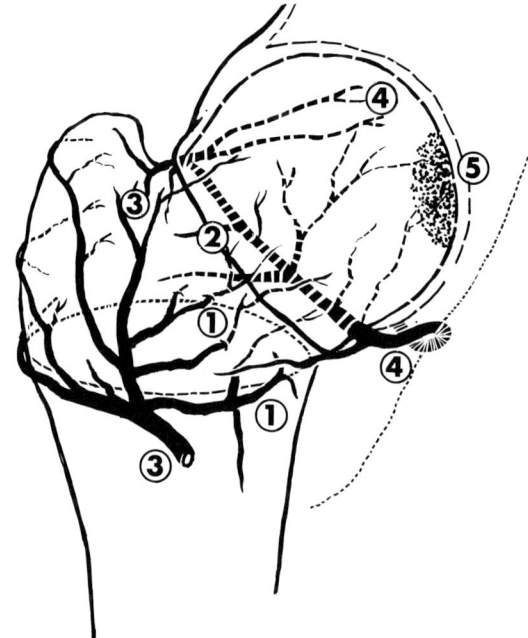

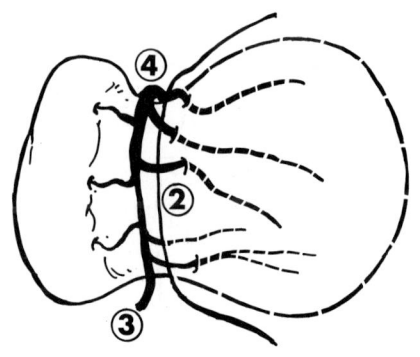

SUPERIOR VIEW

ANATOMIC FEATURES AND CLASSIFICATION OF INJURIES

At Three Years

1. The femoral neck elongates in its central portion.

2. The medial portion grows faster than the lateral (greater trochanteric) portion.

3. The major portion of the physis, which was extra-articular at birth, becomes intra-articular and superior to the capsular insertion and vascular ring at about three years.

4. The entire capital femoral epiphysis and physis are supplied by the medial circumflex via two retinacular (intracapsular) systems, namely,

5. The posterior superior branch and

6. The posterior inferior branch.

7. The lateral circumflex supplies the greater trochanter, part of the proximal femoral physis, and the anteromedial metaphysis. The elongation of the femoral neck has eliminated the contribution of the lateral circumflex to the capital femoral epiphysis.

Note: The transition from a blood supply of multiple small vessels to two large systems, the posterior superior and posterior inferior, predisposes the proximal end of the femur to vascular insult throughout life. Dislocation that disrupts ligamentum teres circulation is less likely to produce avascular necrosis than is a displaced femoral neck fracture that disrupts both posterior superior and posterior inferior blood supplies.

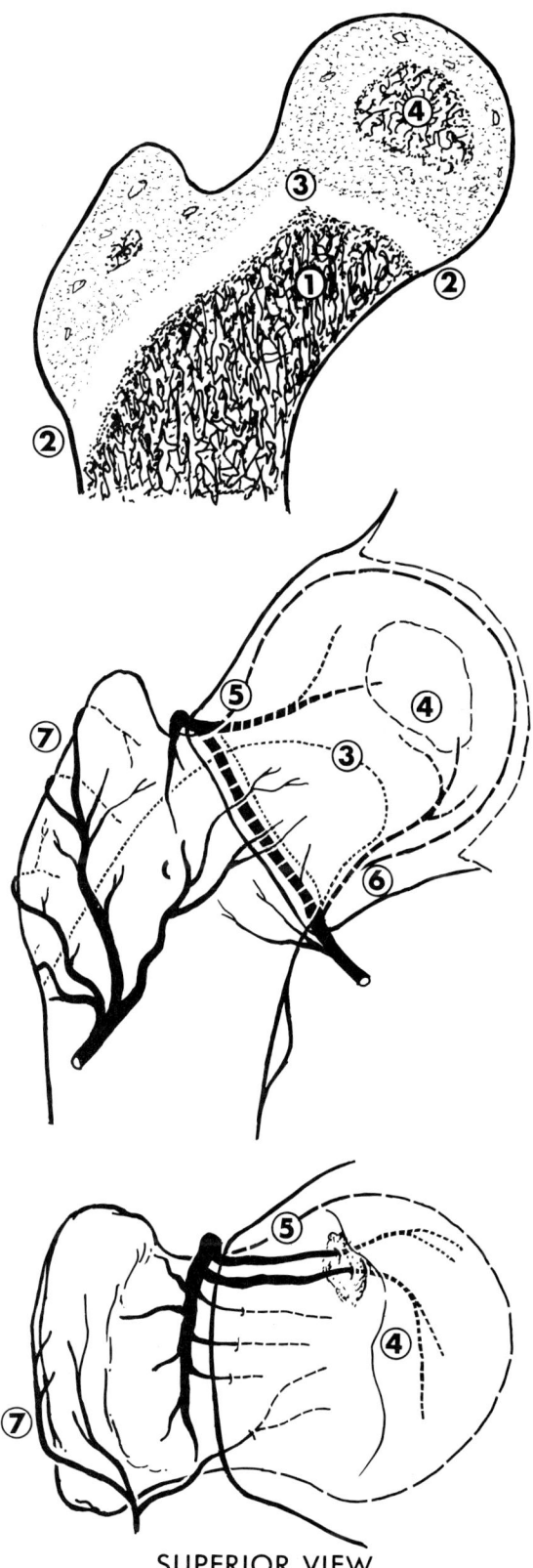

SUPERIOR VIEW

ANATOMIC FEATURES AND CLASSIFICATION OF INJURIES

CLASSIFICATION OF TRAUMATIC DISLOCATIONS OF THE HIP WITH AND WITHOUT FRACTURE

Dislocations are most often posterior.

Posterior dislocations are best classified according to Thompson and Epstein as:

Type I, with or without minor fracture.

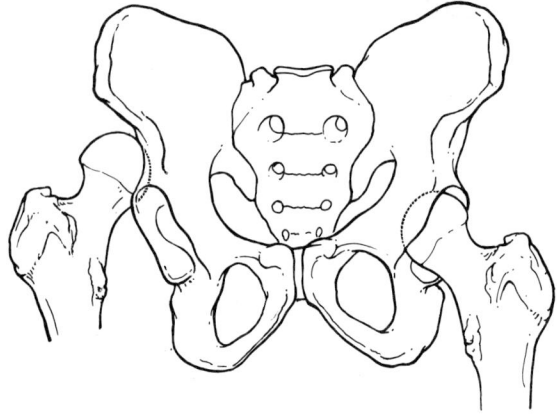

Type II, with a large single fracture of the posterior acetabular rim.

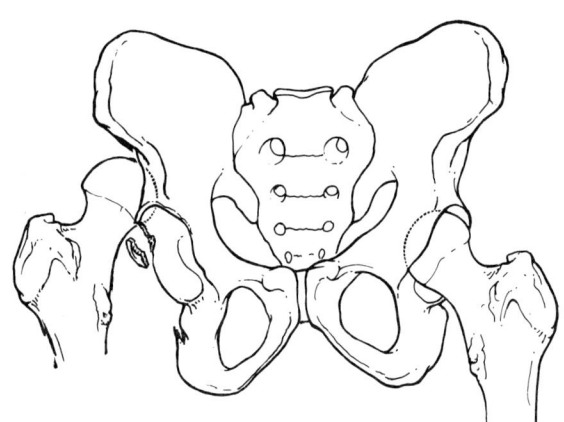

Type III, with a comminuted fracture of the rim of the acetabulum with or without a major fragment.

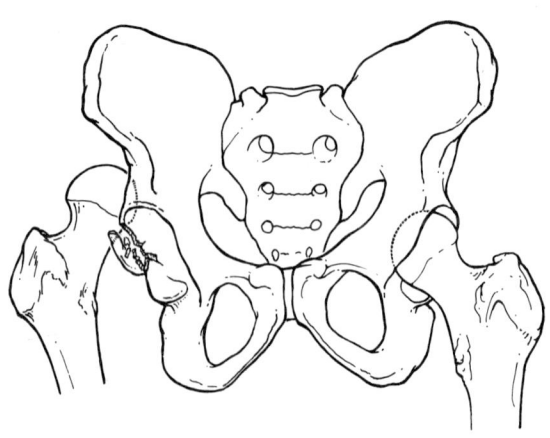

Type IV, with fracture of the acetabular rim and floor.

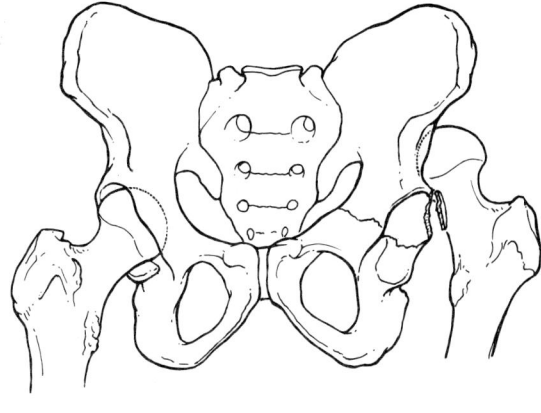

Type V, with fracture of the femoral head.

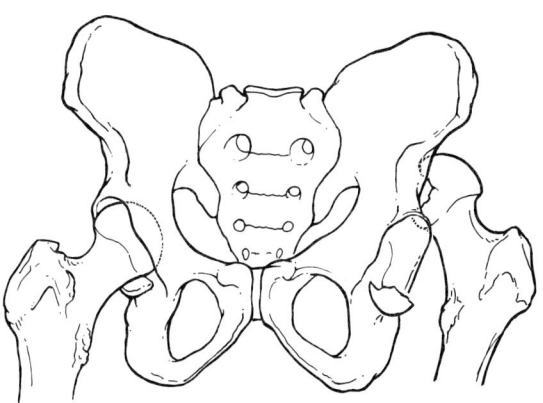

About 10 per cent of dislocations are anterior and may be either:

Obturator (common)

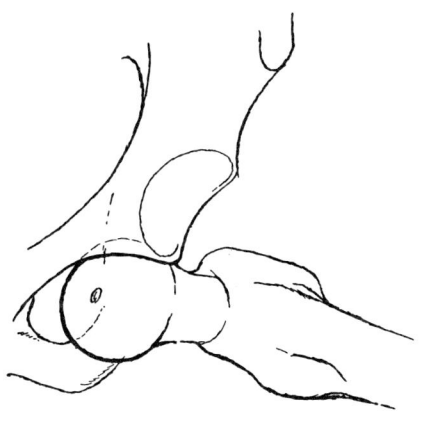

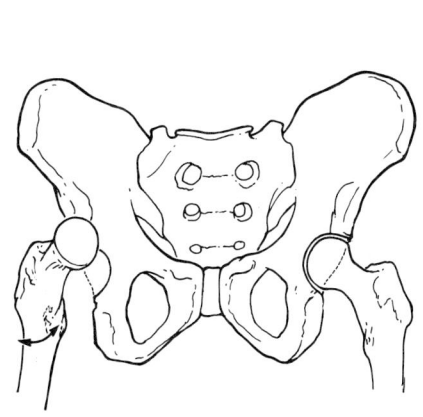

or
Pubic (rare).

POSTERIOR DISLOCATIONS OF THE HIP

GENERAL CONCEPTS

In contrast to the shoulder, the hip is a relatively stable articulation.

Dislocation and fracture-dislocations of the adult's hip result from violent injury, most often caused by motor vehicle accidents. In a child younger than six years, dislocation may result from a considerably less violent mechanism owing to the hip's greater mobility.

A direct blow of the knee against the dashboard forcefully adducts and flexes the victim's hip to produce most posterior dislocations. (Consistent use of a seatbelt would prevent the victim from becoming a flying object with the crashing car and would thereby eliminate most hip dislocations.)

In more than 50 per cent of these injuries the dislocating mechanism also produces a fracture of the acetabulum or the femoral head.

Dislocation associated with large single or comminuted acetabular fractures (Type III or Type IV) and any dislocation associated with a femoral head fracture (Type V) usually require primary open reduction to remove intra-articular fracture fragments.

Any dislocation that does not reduce anatomically after one or at the most two attempts by a competent surgeon should be opened to remove the usual soft tissue or osteocartilaginous obstruction to reduction.

Prior to reduction, the surgeon should evaluate the patient carefully for knee injury (30 per cent of cases), sciatic nerve injury (10 to 15 per cent), and the occasional injury to the spine and abdomen.

The most treacherous associated injury is an ipsilateral femoral shaft fracture, which occurs in about 3 per cent of hip dislocations and frequently delays recognition of the serious hip injury. Any patient with a femoral shaft fracture or with serious injury should have an x-ray of the pelvis to avoid this surprisingly frequent diagnostic lapse.

Before carrying out the reduction the surgeon should inform the patient of the indications for closed as well as open treatment and should obtain consent for both.

Open reduction should not be considered an admission of defeat of one's manipulative skills but rather as a realistic comprehension of all possible complications. If open reduction is indicated, it is best done as a primary procedure rather than secondary to closed reduction. This has been demonstrated convincingly by Epstein's long-term studies indicating that traumatic arthritis, which is considerably more common than avascular necrosis after hip dislocation, can be diminished considerably by precise operative reduction and joint irrigation via a posterior approach.

The dislocation that has been "reduced" by closed methods must be carefully assessed by postreduction x-ray. A widened joint space or abnormal position of the lesser trochanter indicates that the reduction has been incomplete, usually because of capsular interposition. The patient's persistent complaint of buttock pain for several days following a closed reduction should also raise suspicion regarding soft tissue entrapment in the joint.

Injury to the sciatic nerve is most often a stretch type involving the common peroneal nerve. This usually resolves spontaneously.

Nerve deficit that involves the tibial as well as the peroneal branches or that comes on several days after reduction indicates that entrapment neuropathy has occurred and operative exploration is wise. Occasionally the nerve injury may result from complete avulsion of the lumbar nerve root. The differential diagnosis of these lesions can only be made by careful assessment of the patient's muscle weakness.

Hip dislocations may go unrecognized in a patient with multiple injuries almost as frequently as do cervical spine injuries (see page 101).

All patients with serious injuries, particularly from motor vehicle accidents, should have x-rays of the pelvis as well as the cervical spine.

Delay in reducing the hip dislocation of more than 24 hours does compromise outcome, although not as significantly as previously thought. Satisfactory results may be obtained with closed or open reduction of a dislocation of less than 3 months' duration. For hip dislocation or fracture-dislocation that goes unrecognized and untreated for longer than 3 months, total hip arthroplasty appears to be the reconstructive procedure of choice.

Recurrent posterior dislocation is an infrequent complication but it does occur. Approximately 6 per cent of childhood dislocations can recur while at the most 1 to 2 per cent of adult dislocations are subject to recurrence. The most common factor associated with recurrent dislocation appears to be immobilization of only a few days following closed reduction of the posterior dislocation.

The best results for both dislocation and fracture-dislocation follow adequate assessment of the patient's entire injury and complete reduction of the hip by closed or open methods as soon as possible. The hip must then be protected after reduction for a sufficient period of time to permit healing of the disrupted soft tissues and articular structures.

MECHANISM OF INJURY

Posterior dislocation of the hip is usually the result of a force driving the femur backward while the thigh is flexed and adducted, such as when the knee strikes the dashboard of an automobile.

The femoral head is thrust through the capsule onto the dorsum of the ilium.

The external rotators of the hip (the piriformis, gemelli, and obturator internus) are usually disrupted.

The femoral head may assume a high (iliac) or low (ischial) position, depending on the degree of flexion of the thigh at the time of dislocation.

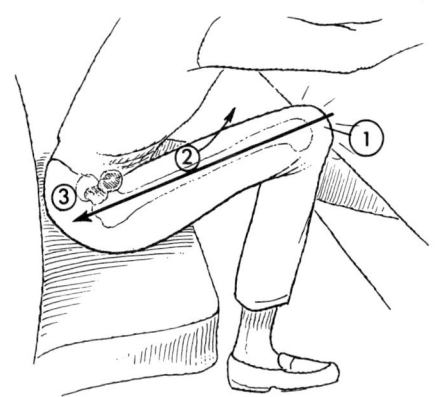

1. Knee strikes the dashboard.
2. The thigh is flexed and adducted.
3. The femoral head is driven backward out of the acetabulum.

Iliac Dislocation

Typical Deformity

1. Hip is flexed.
2. Hip is adducted.
3. Hip is internally rotated.
4. Affected extremity appears shortened.
5. Greater trochanter and buttock on affected side are unusually prominent.
6. Knee of the affected extremity rests on the opposite thigh.

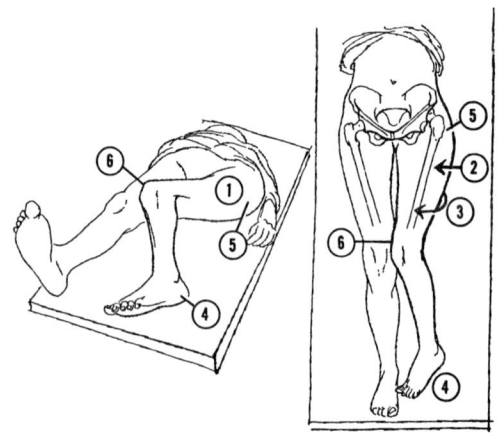

POSTERIOR DISLOCATIONS OF THE HIP

Prereduction X-Ray

This is a Type I (no fracture).
1. Femoral head is displaced upward and back.
2. Head lies on dorsum of the ilium.
3. Head lies above and posterior to the acetabulum.
4. Femur is adducted and internally rotated.

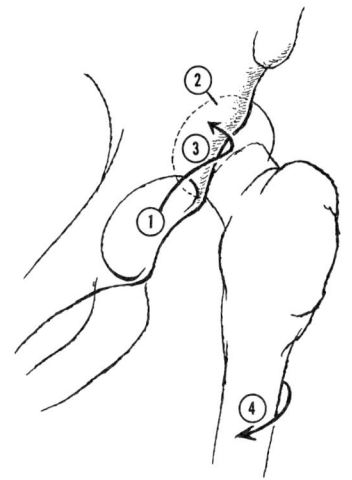

ISCHIAL DISLOCATION

Typical Deformity

1. The hip is flexed.
2. The hip is markedly adducted so that the knee of the affected limb lies on the opposite thigh.
3. The limb is in extreme internal rotation.
4. The greater trochanter and buttock on the affected side are unusually prominent.

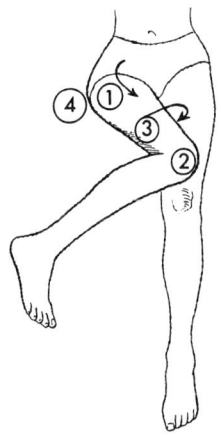

Prereduction X-Ray

This is a Type I (no fracture).
1. The femoral head lies inferior to, lateral to, and behind the acetabulum.
2. The lesser trochanter is not seen.
3. The femoral shaft is in extreme adduction; the findings resemble those of coxa vara.

Note: This type of dislocation may actually be missed despite x-ray if the quality of the x-ray is poor and the abnormal position of the lesser trochanter and adduction of femur are not recognized.

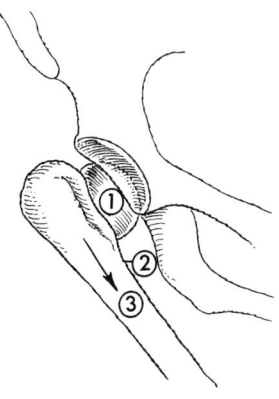

RADIOGRAPHIC ASSESSMENT OF DISLOCATION OF THE HIP AND FRACTURE OF THE ACETABULUM

Any seriously injured or comatose patient or any patient with a femoral shaft fracture should have an anteroposterior x-ray of the pelvis. Never order an anteroposterior view of just one hip; inevitably the injury will be in the hip not radiographed.

Assess all dislocated hips by oblique x-ray views as well as anteroposterior views in order to visualize any associated fractures.

Critically review x-rays after reduction of hip dislocation or fracture-dislocation to determine the adequacy of reduction. Persistent joint space widening, lateral displacement of the femoral head, or interruption of Shenton's line indicates incomplete reduction.

Technique of Oblique X-Ray

1. Oblique x-rays may be obtained without moving the patient.
2. Obtain a right oblique view of the hip from an angle of 45 degrees and
3. Also a left oblique view to ascertain the status of the femoral head and acetabulum.

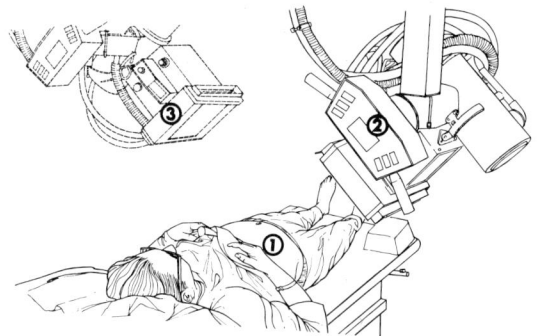

1. An anteroposterior view of the dislocated hip shows no acetabular disruption owing to supraimposition of the femoral head.

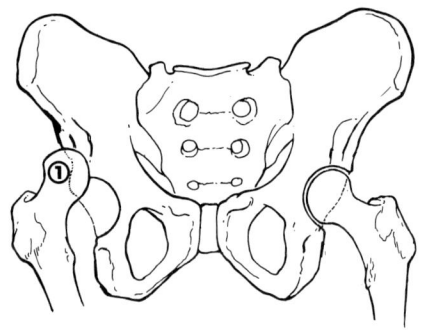

2. An oblique x-ray shows a sizable fragment that would probably contribute to instability and should be reduced.

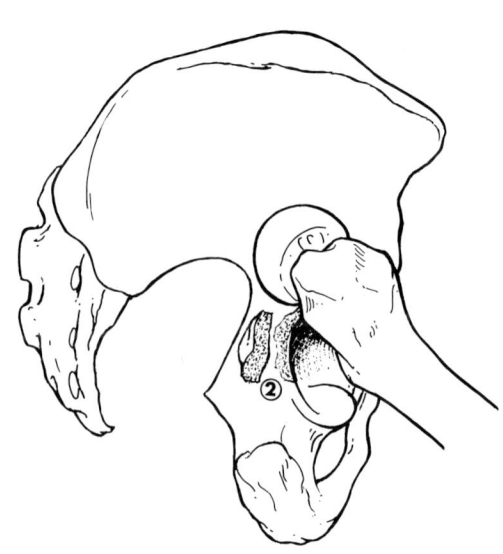

POSTERIOR DISLOCATIONS OF THE HIP

TECHNIQUE OF CLOSED REDUCTION

Preferred Method for Type I Dislocation or Minor Fracture-Dislocation (Stimson Technique)

This method uses the weight of the limb and the force of gravity to reduce the dislocation.

It is nontraumatic and should be employed first to attempt closed reduction.

This method may occasionally be successful without general anesthesia in a child or in a patient with multiple facial fractures or a full stomach for whom anesthesia is hazardous. Ideally, however, general anesthesia is necessary, and repeated manipulation should be avoided.

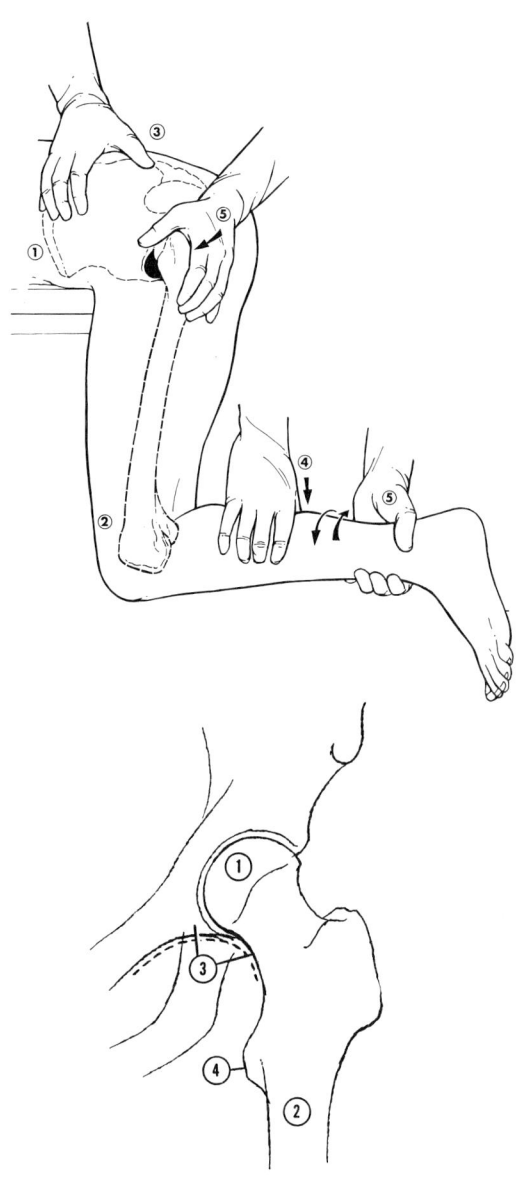

REDUCTION

1. The patient is placed on a table face downward.
2. The affected thigh hangs directly downward; the knee is flexed at a right angle.
3. The assistant supports the pelvis.
4. The operator makes steady downward traction at the flexed knee for several minutes.
5. While maintaining downward traction, the femoral head is gently rotated and an assistant pushes the greater trochanter forward toward the acetabulum. Avoid forceful rotation, which can fracture the femoral neck.

POSTREDUCTION X-RAY

1. The head of the femur is in the acetabulum.
2. The shaft of the femur is in a neutral position.
3. Shenton's line is intact.
4. The lesser trochanter is well visualized.

Note: If Shenton's line is broken or the lesser trochanter is not visualized, the femoral head lies behind the acetabulum.

1273

Alternate Method of Manipulative Reduction

The patient is under general anesthesia.

Note: With rare exception, reduction should always be done with complete muscle relaxation under general anesthesia. Attempts at forceful manipulation can readily fracture the femoral neck and damage circulation.

1. The assistant makes downward pressure on the anterior superior iliac spine.
2. With the knee flexed, the operator pulls on the limb in the line of deformity.

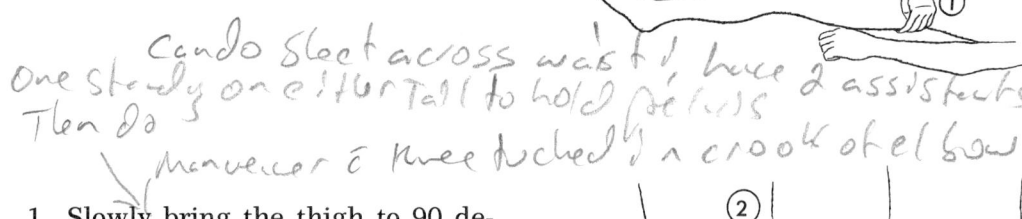

1. Slowly bring the thigh to 90 degrees of flexion.
2. Gently rotate internally and externally and rock the thigh gently backward and forward to disengage the head from the external rotator muscles and the posterior capsule.
3. Relocate the femoral head by (a) further internal rotation and extension of the thigh or (b) external rotation and extension of the thigh.

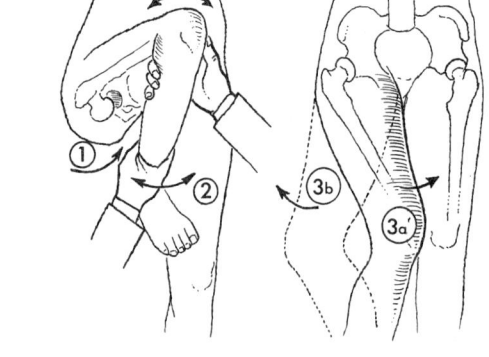

4. The assistant pushes firmly on the trochanter to direct the femoral head into the acetabulum while the limb is rotated and extended.

Note: Avoid forceful rotation, as it can readily fracture the femoral neck. If you do not accomplish the reduction with two adequate attempts, open reduction is indicated.

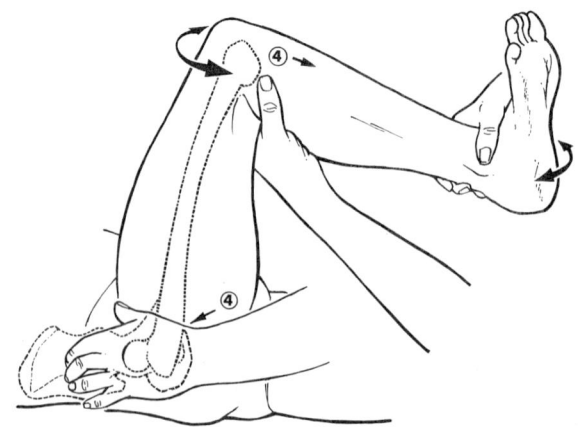

IMMOBILIZATION

Apply skin traction to the lower leg. The hip is extended and the extremity is slightly abducted.

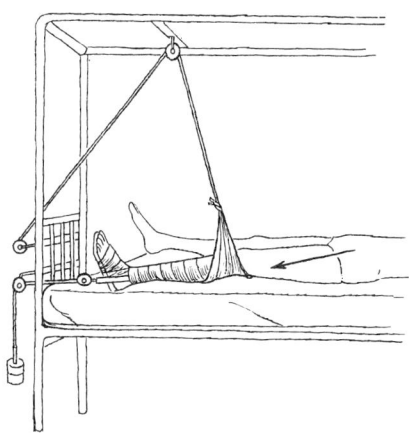

POSTREDUCTION MANAGEMENT

Maintain the skin traction for 3 weeks so as to permit healing of the disrupted soft tissue structures or minor fractures of the acetabulum.

Within a few days the patient may begin range-of-motion exercises to the hip, but hip flexion should be avoided.

During the recovery period give the patient aspirin, 3 grams daily in divided doses, which has been shown to protect against degenerative arthritis. Aspirin also appears to diminish the incidence of thromboembolism after hip procedures.

Continue the aspirin for 4 to 6 weeks, until the patient is walking without crutches.

The patient may begin weight bearing with crutches and may gradually increase the amount of weight borne until he can eliminate crutches. There is no evidence to indicate that early weight bearing increases the incidence of avascular necrosis or traumatic arthritis, provided that the joint reduction has been anatomic and there are no loose bodies persisting in the joint.

Follow-up of the patient with a dislocated hip should be a minimum of 2 years, but most significant complications will be manifested within the first year. Patients should be warned that symptoms such as aching or stiffness in the hip or knee or occasional "giving way" may indicate the beginning of traumatic arthritis or avascular necrosis.

Unreducible or Incompletely Reduced Posterior Dislocation of The Hip

REMARKS

In as many as 16 per cent of traumatic dislocations in which closed reduction is attempted, open reduction may become necessary either because the "reduction" is nonconcentric or because it cannot be achieved after two adequate attempts.

Closed reduction may frequently be blocked by buttonholing of the femoral head through the capsule or by the piriformis muscle, which is displaced across the acetabulum.

Concentric reduction may be prevented by an inverted labrum or an osteocartilaginous loose body in the acetabulum.

Persistent asymmetry of the hip joint from an inverted labrum can cause symptomatic degenerative arthritis. An incompletely reduced hip should be explored and redislocated so as to clear the joint of all entrapped debris.

X-Ray of an Irreducible Dislocation

1. After two attempts the femoral head remains superior, posterior, and lateral to the acetabulum.

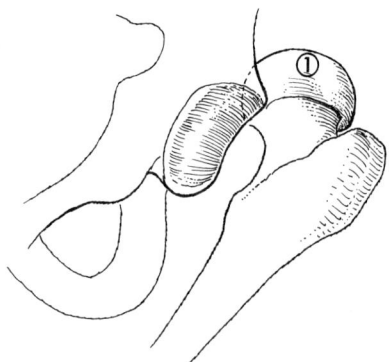

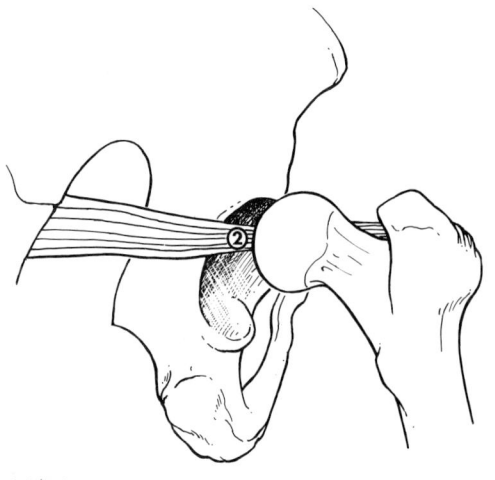

2. The anatomic cause of an irreducible dislocation is displacement of the piriformis across the acetabulum or a buttonhole defect in the capsule.

POSTERIOR DISLOCATIONS OF THE HIP

X-Ray of an Incomplete Reduction

1. The femoral head is not concentrically seated.
2. The femoral head is slightly below and lateral in the acetabulum.
3. Shenton's line is broken.
4. The interval between the femoral head and the acetabulum is greater than normal.

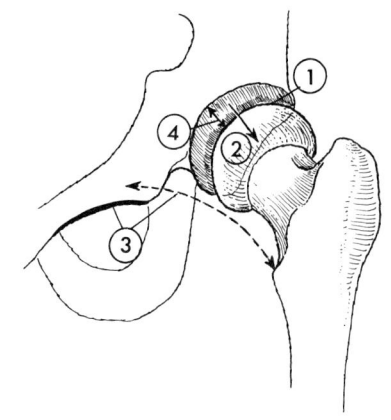

1. The anatomic cause of the incomplete reduction is usually an inverted acetabular labrum or
2. Multiple osteocartilaginous loose bodies in the joint space.

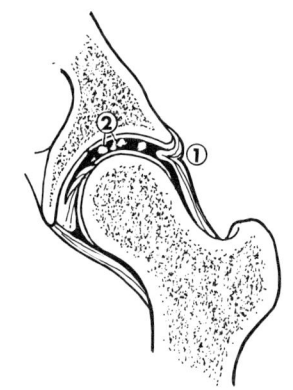

OPERATIVE REDUCTION OF IRREDUCIBLE DISLOCATION

Posterior Exposure of the Hip Joint

1. With the patient positioned on the uninjured side, make an incision beginning 5 cm distal to the posterior superior iliac spine and continue it lateral and distal, paralleling the fibers of the gluteus maximus muscle to the posterior aspect of the greater trochanter. Continue the incision distally in line with the posterior border of the trochanter for 10 cm.

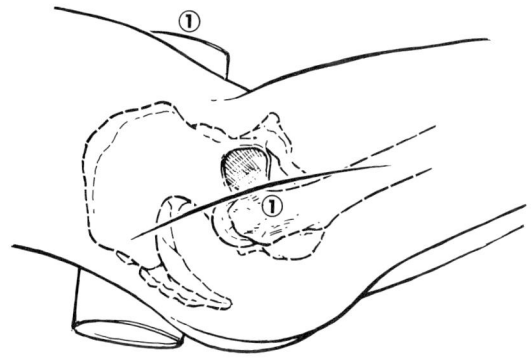

POSTERIOR DISLOCATIONS OF THE HIP

Posterior Exposure of the Hip Joint (Continued)

2. Deepen the incision through the gluteus maximus by separating its fibers parallel to the skin incision.

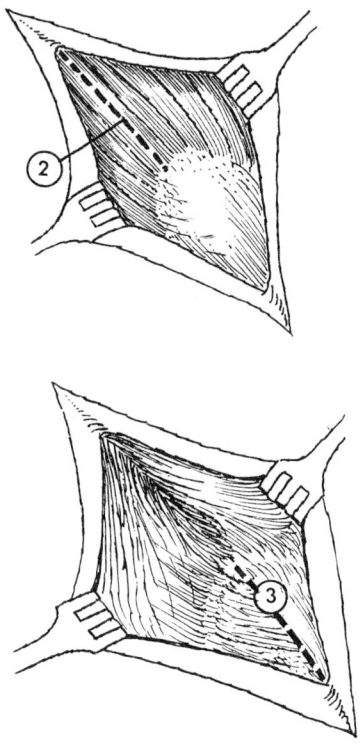

3. Divide the insertion of the gluteus maximus into the fasciae latae for 5 cm in line with the vertical limb of the skin incision.

Note: At this stage of the operation, if the rotator muscles are intact, a prominence made by the femoral head can be seen and felt under the muscles; if the muscles have been penetrated by the femoral head, the head is clearly visible.

1. Visualize the sciatic nerve.
2. Sever the tendons of the piriformis, gemelli, and obturator internus muscles at their line of insertion into the greater trochanter. Release of these muscles often relieves the obstruction.

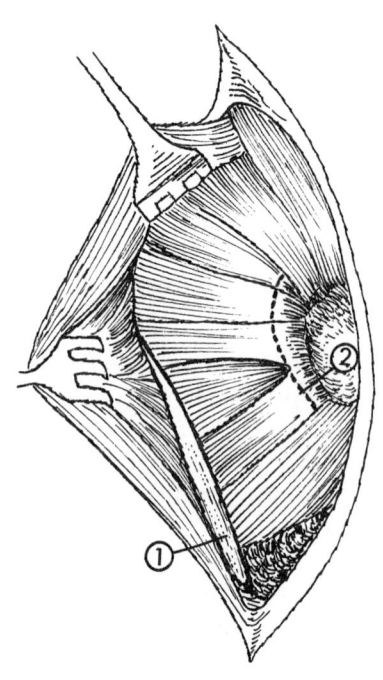

3. Retract the rotator muscles posteriorly together with the sciatic nerve.

4. Identify the capsule surrounding the femoral neck and, if necessary, enlarge the tear proximally and distally in order to free the neck and head of the femur.

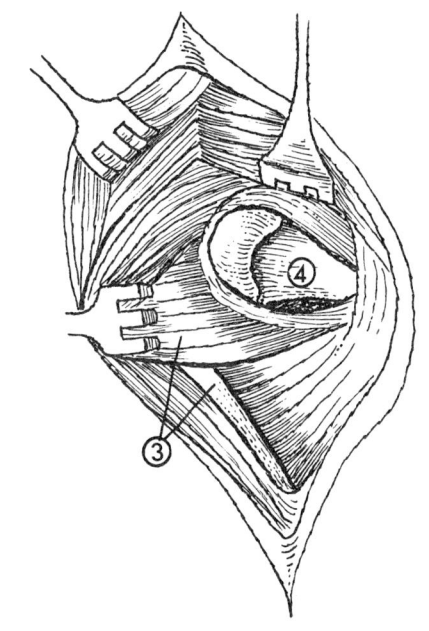

Examination and Irrigation

1. Thoroughly inspect the joint and irrigate out any loose cartilaginous bodies.

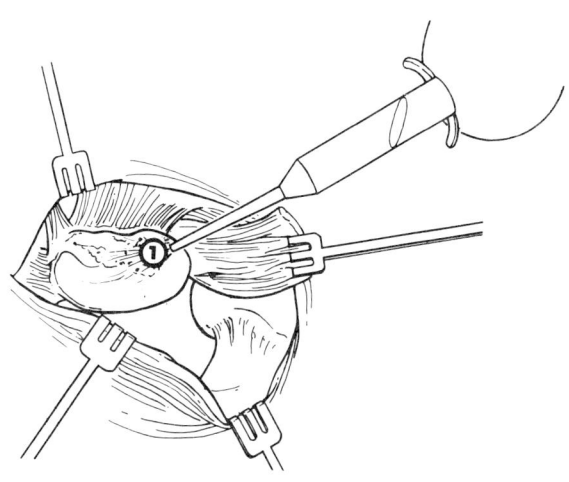

2. Frequently, if there has been a fracture of the acetabular rim, numerous osteocartilaginous bodies may be removed.

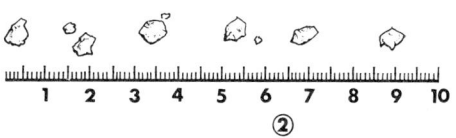

Redislocation and Reduction

Note: For cases in which concentric reduction is not achieved, the hip must be completely dislocated to allow visualization of the entire joint.

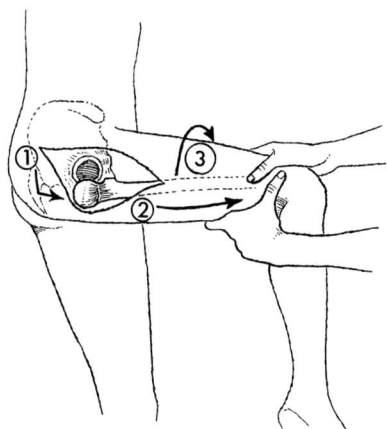

1. Flex the hip 90 degrees.
2. Adduct the hip.
3. Dislocate the head posteriorly by internal rotation of the thigh.

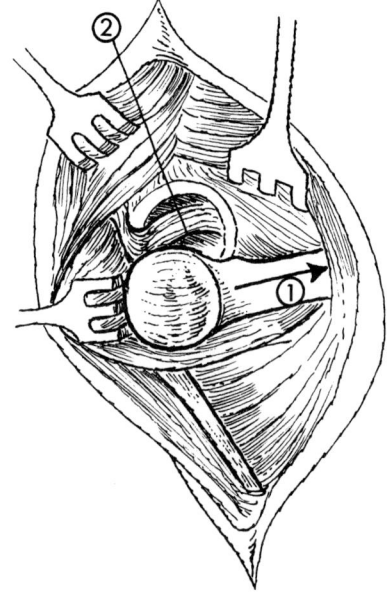

1. Make strong longitudinal traction on the femur.
2. Visualize the cartilaginous labrum inside the acetabulum.

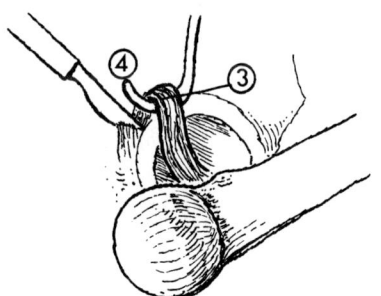

3. Pull the labrum out of the acetabulum with a blunt hook.
4. Excise the detached portion of the labrum.

POSTERIOR DISLOCATIONS OF THE HIP

5. Thoroughly explore and irrigate the joint to remove any loose osteocartilaginous bodies, particularly if there has been a fracture of the acetabular rim.

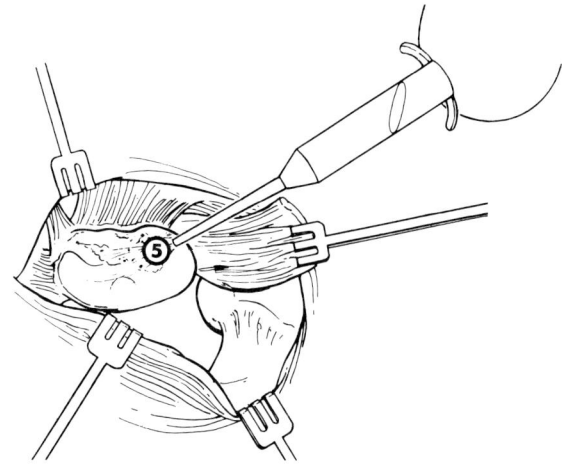

6. Reduce the femoral head by longitudinal traction on the flexed, adducted femur.

Note: Always obtain intraoperative x-rays to insure that the joint is reduced symmetrically.

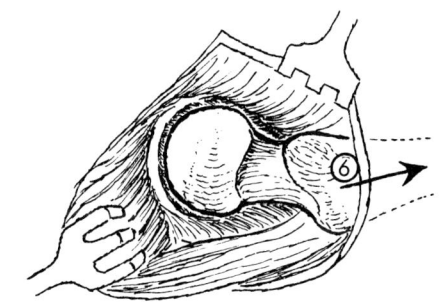

INTRAOPERATIVE X-RAY

1. The femoral head is in concentric relationship with the acetabulum.
2. The shaft of the femur is in a neutral position.
3. Shenton's line is intact.
4. The lesser trochanter is well visualized.

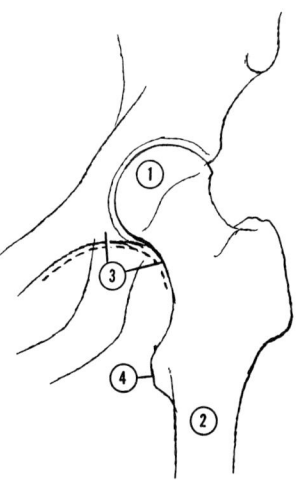

Immobilization

Apply skin traction to the lower leg. The hip is extended and the extremity is slightly abducted.

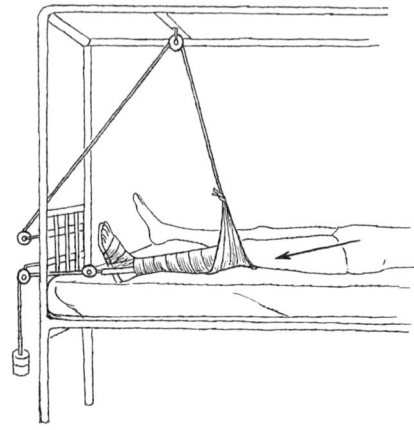

Postreduction Management

Maintain the skin traction for 3 weeks so as to permit healing of the disrupted soft tissue structures or minor fractures of the acetabulum.

Within a few days the patient may begin range-of-motion exercises to the hip, but hip flexion should be avoided.

During the recovery period give the patient aspirin, 3 grams daily in divided doses, which has been shown to protect against degenerative arthritis and appears to diminish the incidence of thromboembolism after hip procedures.

Continue the aspirin for 2 to 3 months, until the patient is walking independently.

After 3 to 4 weeks, the patient may begin weight bearing with crutches, gradually increasing the amount of weight borne until he can eliminate crutches. There is no evidence to indicate that early weight bearing increases the incidence of avascular necrosis or traumatic arthritis, provided that the joint reduction has been anatomic and there are no loose bodies persisting in the joint.

Follow-up of the patient with a dislocated hip should be a minimum of two years, but most significant complications will be manifested within the first year. Patients should be warned that symptoms such as aching or stiffness in the hip or knee or occasional "giving way" may indicate the beginning of traumatic arthritis or avascular necrosis.

Posterior Fracture-Dislocation

REMARKS

The majority of posterior dislocations are fracture-dislocations. Management depends on the nature of the fracture, but in many instances primary open reduction is necessary.

POSTERIOR DISLOCATIONS OF THE HIP

Closed reduction of a fracture-dislocation only inflicts further trauma to the hip, especially when open redislocation and exploration of the joint is necessary.

EPSTEIN TYPE II DISLOCATION (DISLOCATION WITH SMALL RIM FRACTURE)

Rim fractures usually occur through the posterior portion of the acetabulum. The size of the fragment depends on the degree of abduction of the flexed femur when the femoral head is driven backwards against the acetabulum. The more the femur is adducted, the greater is the tendency to dislocate without fracture. If the femur is in an abducted position, the fragment tends to be large and may be comminuted.

Small linear fractures of the acetabular rim can generally be treated by closed manipulation.

Stability of the joint should be evaluated by flexing the hip after manipulation. Anteroposterior and oblique x-rays are necessary to evaluate the size of the rim fragment and the need for open reduction (see page 1272).

Operative treatment is necessary only if (1) there are large fragments, (2) the head does not reduce symmetrically, or (3) the sciatic nerve is involved in the fracture.

Displacement of a small acetabular rim fracture after reduction can be disregarded provided that the hip is stable on flexion and the sciatic nerve is not injured.

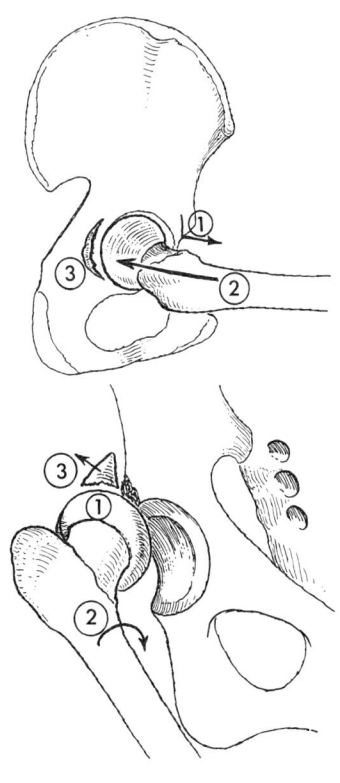

Mechanism of Injury

1. The femur is flexed.
2. A force applied to the knee is transmitted to the femoral head via the femur (as in a dashboard injury).
3. Posterior portion of the acetabulum is sheared off.

X-Ray (Oblique View)

1. The femoral head is out of the acetabulum and lies posterior to it.
2. The lesser trochanter is not visible, indicating internal rotation of the femur.
3. A small fragment of the posterior rim is displaced upward and backward.

Note: An oblique view is essential to assess the size of the rim fragment adequately.

POSTERIOR DISLOCATIONS OF THE HIP

Reduction

Reduce the hip by the same manipulative maneuvers employed for uncomplicated posterior dislocation (see page 1273).

Postreduction X-Ray (Oblique View)

1. The femoral head is seated concentrically in the acetabulum.
2. The posterior fragment is reduced satisfactorily.

Note: Slight displacement of the rim fracture is acceptable provided that the hip is stable on flexion and the sciatic nerve is not injured.

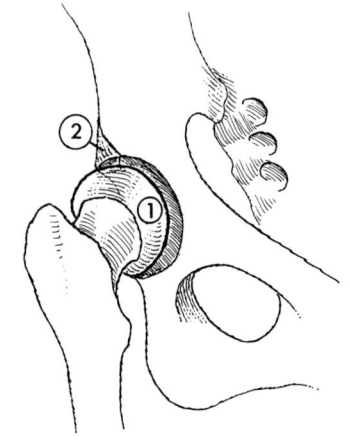

Immobilization

Apply skin traction to the lower leg. The hip is extended and the limb is slightly abducted.

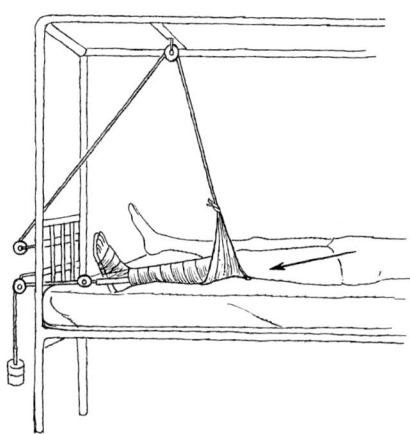

Postreduction Management (For Stable Hip with a Small Posterior Rim Fracture)

Maintain the skin traction for 3 weeks so as to permit healing of the disrupted soft tissue structures or minor fractures of the acetabulum.

Within a few days the patient should begin range-of-motion exercises to the hip, but hip flexion should be avoided.

During the recovery period give the patient aspirin, 3 grams daily in divided doses, which has been shown to protect against degenerative arthritis and appears to diminish the incidence of thromboembolism after hip procedures. Continue the aspirin for 2 to 3 months, until the patient is walking independently.

After 3 to 4 weeks, the patient may begin weight bearing with crutches and gradually increase the amount of weight borne until he can eliminate the crutches. There is no evidence to indicate that early weight bearing increases the incidence of avascular necrosis or traumatic arthritis, provided that the joint reduction has been anatomic and there are no loose bodies persisting in the joint.

Follow-up of the patient with a dislocated hip should be a minimum of 2 years, but most significant complications will be manifested within the first year. Patients should be warned that symptoms such as aching or stiffness in the hip or knee or occasional "giving way" may indicate the beginning of traumatic arthritis or avascular necrosis.

OPERATIVE MANAGEMENT OF EPSTEIN TYPES II, III, AND IV FRACTURE-DISLOCATIONS

Primary operative exploration of the hip with reduction of the fracture-dislocation is indicated for many of these fairly common injuries. The reason for this recommendation is that loose fragments frequently lodge in the hip after reduction and become abrasive agents on the femoral head.

Traumatic arthritis is twice as common as avascular necrosis following fracture-dislocations of the hip. It is to diminish this common and significant complication that primary open reduction is necessary.

Surgical approach must be posterior, through the area of capsular and soft tissue damage, so as to avoid inflicting further insult on the femoral head circulation.

Prereduction X-Ray

TYPE II FRACTURE-DISLOCATION

1. Posterior dislocation of the femoral head.
2. Large tilted acetabular fragment will cause instability of the hip unless stabilized. There are also likely to be intra-articular fragments, which will cause traumatic arthritis.

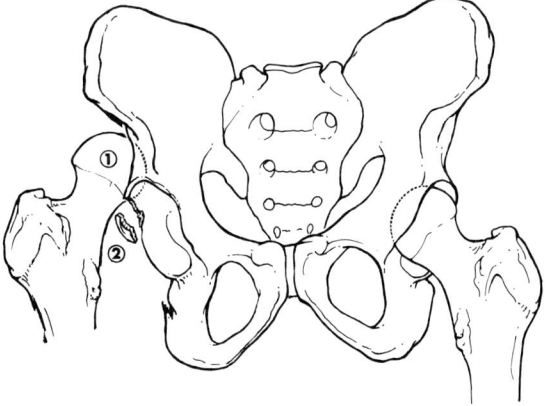

POSTERIOR DISLOCATIONS OF THE HIP

Prereduction X-Ray (Continued)

TYPE III FRACTURE-DISLOCATION

1. Posterior dislocation of the femoral head.
2. Large acetabular fragment will cause instability.

Note: With the degree of comminution, the likelihood is quite high that multiple fragments will be found in the hip joint.

The benefits of primary open reduction are particularly evident with this type of injury.

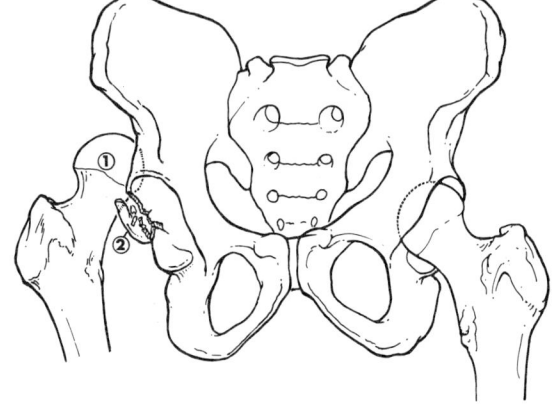

TYPE IV FRACTURE-DISLOCATION

1. Posterior dislocation of the femoral head.
2. Fracture of the acetabular rim and acetabular floor.

Note: The extent of injury with this fracture-dislocation makes a poor result fairly common with either open or closed treatment. The outcome depends on the degree of damage inflicted on the femoral head at the time of dislocation, which generally is severe to produce this much joint comminution. Surgical reduction is necessary to remove loose fragments, to reduce the dislocation, and to fix the posterior lip of the acetabulum for stability. Fixation of the inner acetabular wall is not necessary.

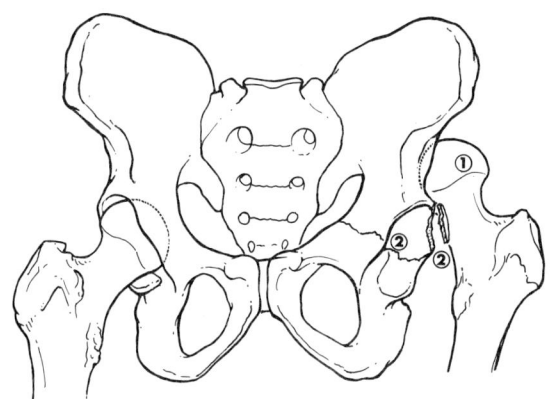

Operative Technique

Always use a posterior approach to the dislocated hip joint to avoid inflicting further damage to the circulation.

1. With the patient positioned on the uninjured side, make an incision beginning 5 cm distal to the posterior superior iliac spine, and continue it lateral and distal, paralleling the fibers of the gluteus maximus muscle to the greater trochanter. Continue the incision distal along the posterior border of the greater trochanter for 5 cm.

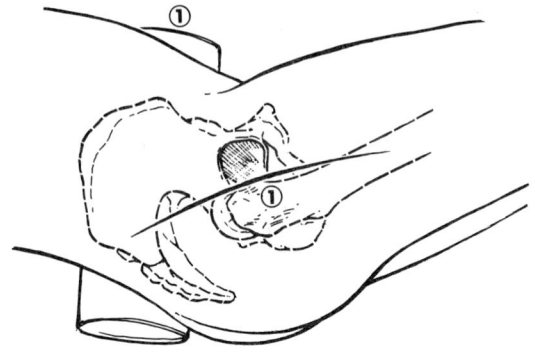

2. Continue the approach through the fascia lata to expose the gluteus maximus fibers.

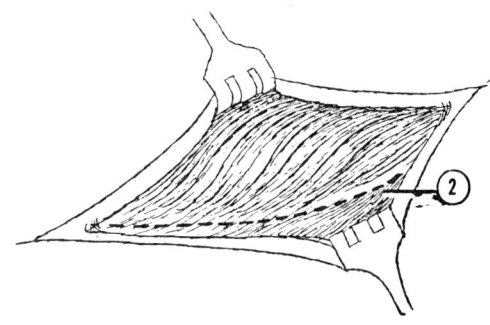

1. Separate the fibers of the gluteus maximus in line with the incision. The insertion of the gluteus maximus into the fascia lata may also be divided for additional exposure.
2. Visualize the sciatic nerve and examine it for any injury.
3. Divide the tendons of the piriformis, superior gemellus, internal obturator, and inferior gemellus muscles.

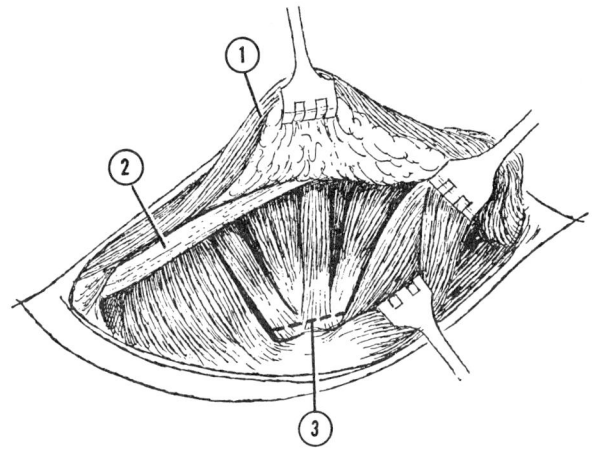

1. Retract the detached external rotators of the hip joint and the sciatic nerve posteriorly.
2. Locate the detached acetabular fragment.
3. Grasp the acetabular fragment with a towel clip to assess the degree of fragmentation.

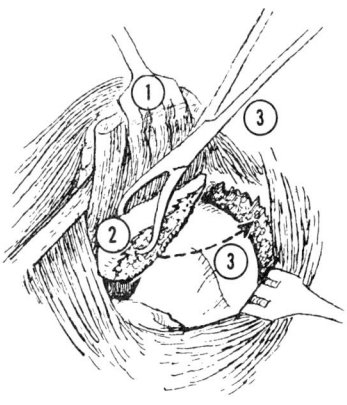

4. Dislocate the femoral head if it has been reduced, and thoroughly explore the joint for any loose fragments.

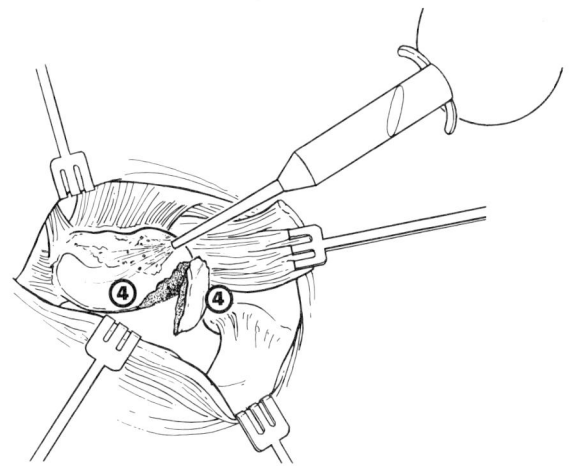

1287

Operative Technique (Continued)

5. Frequently there are numerous osteocartilaginous fragments not evident on x-ray.

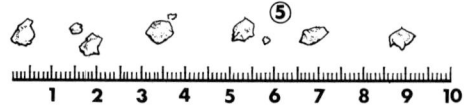

1. After reducing the hip, fix the acetabular rim fragment with one or two screws. Always assess position of screws by testing range of motion of the hip and also by intraoperative x-ray.

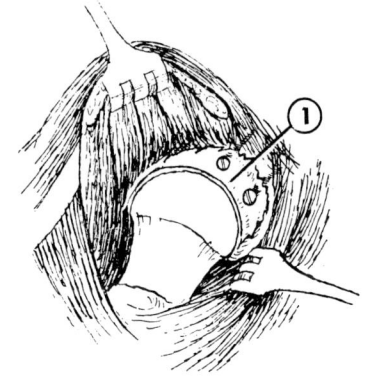

Intraoperative X-Rays

TYPE II AND TYPE III FRACTURE-DISLOCATIONS

1. The fracture-dislocation is reduced.
2. The fragment is fixed by two screws directed away from the hip joint.

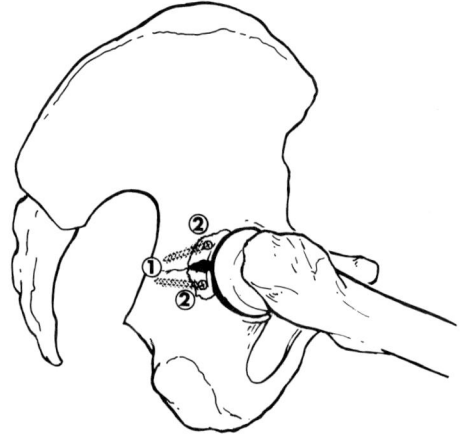

Type IV Fracture-Dislocation

1. A major portion of the rim fracture has been fixed for stability.
2. The central acetabular fracture does not ordinarily require fixation once the rim fracture is stabilized.

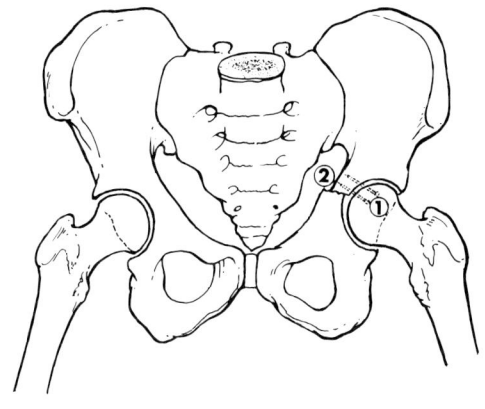

Immobilization

Apply skin traction to the leg.
The hip is extended and the leg is slightly abducted.

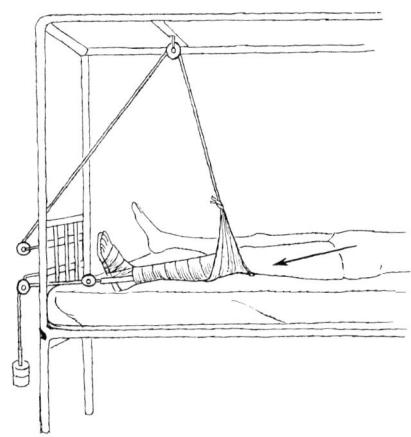

Postreduction Management

Maintain traction for 6 to 8 weeks to permit healing of the acetabular fracture.

The degree of stability achieved at surgery as well as radiographic evidence of healing should determine the ultimate length of time for traction. During the period of traction, give the patient aspirin, 3 grams daily in divided doses, since this has been shown to protect against degenerative arthritis and appears to diminish the risk of thromboembolism after hip procedures.

Continue aspirin until the patient is fully ambulatory.

Within the first few days the patient may begin range-of-motion exercises to the hip and muscles of the thigh but hip flexion should be avoided.

By 6 to 8 weeks, depending on the rate of healing of the fracture, the patient may start weight bearing with crutches and may gradually increase weight borne until the crutches can be eliminated. The speed with which the patient is allowed to become fully ambulatory depends on the degree of comminution of the acetabulum.

There is no evidence to indicate that early weight bearing increases avascular necrosis or traumatic arthritis, provided that the joint reduction has been anatomic and there are no loose bodies persisting in the joint.

Follow-up of patients with fracture-dislocations of the hip should be a minimum of 2 years. Most significant complications will be manifested within the first year. The patient should be warned that symptoms such as aching or stiffness in the hip or knee or occasional "giving way" may indicate the beginning of traumatic arthritis or avascular necrosis.

Associated Nerve Injuries

REMARKS

Ten to 15 per cent of all hip dislocations produce sciatic nerve injury, but the frequency may be as high as 35 per cent following Type II or Type III fracture-dislocation.

The majority of these injuries are due to stretching at the time of dislocation, but it is important to distinguish between peripheral nerve stretch and a compression injury.

Rarely, nerve roots may be avulsed in the lumbosacral region.

A differential diagnosis of these nerve injuries can only be made by careful assessment of the patient's neurologic deficit and muscle weakness.

Nerve Stretch Injury

The peroneal component of the sciatic nerve is most susceptible to stretch by the internally rotated, dislocated hip.

1. Its oblique course makes the peroneal nerve less mobile than the tibial nerve.

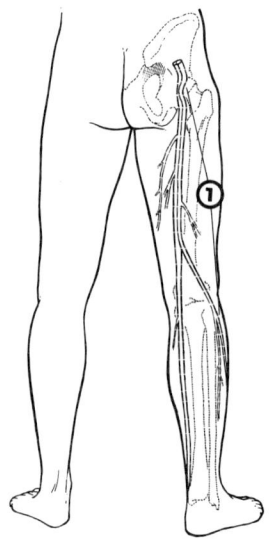

2. The peroneal nerve has a greater number of axons in cross-section and less intraneural fat for protection against trauma than does

3. The tibial nerve.

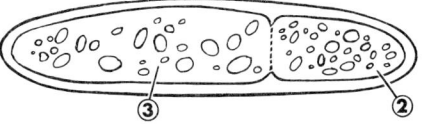

Note: Stretch injury to the nerve, as indicated by involvement of only the muscles supplied by the peroneal nerve, need not be explored, since the recovery is usually spontaneous. Surgery cannot speed recovery of a stretch injury. Operative exploration, however, may still be indicated if the type of fracture-dislocation warrants it (see page 1285).

Nerve Compression Injuries

Occasionally the nerve will be compressed by a displaced acetabular fragment or by callus formation. This may be recognized by:

1. Callus buildup producing a delayed palsy after reduction.

2. Involvement of both the tibial and the peroneal components of the nerve.

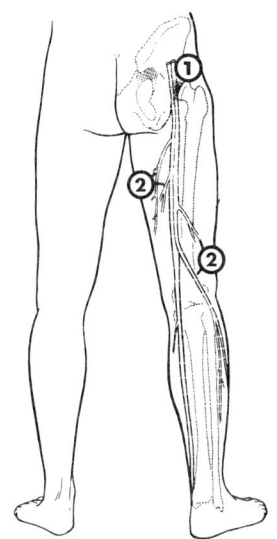

Note: Careful assessment of the patient's neurologic deficit will determine if both the tibial and peroneal nerves are injured.

These findings of nerve compression indicate the need for operative decompression. Usually this is done in conjunction with primary reduction of the hip fracture-dislocation.

Lumbosacral Nerve Root Avulsion

Rarely the posterior dislocation can avulse the fifth lumbar and first sacral nerve roots. This can be diagnosed by the patient's loss of strength in hip abductor, extensor, and external rotator muscles.

1. Myelography shows outpouching and pseudomeningocele of L5 and S1 nerve roots.

Operative treatment is not warranted for this type of injury.

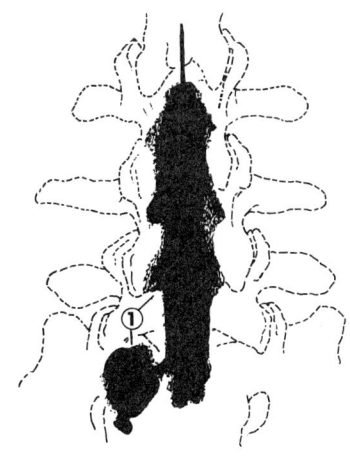

Management of Type V Dislocation With Fracture of the Femoral Head

REMARKS

Dislocations of the hip with femoral head fractures frequently require open reduction because attempts at closed reduction of the fracture fragment are usually unsatisfactory.

Most often the fracture fragment involves the inferior, non-weight-bearing third of the femoral head. This fragment can be removed surgically.

If more than one third of the femoral head is fractured, the fragment usually retains its ligamentum teres attachment. In this rare circumstance, the weight bearing fragment may be reattached after sacrificing the ligamentum teres so as to permit accurate reduction and fixation to the main femoral head surface.

The mechanical contribution of large medial head fragments to the articulation is of more significance than is the circulation from the ligamentum teres vessel. Even simple dislocations without fractures ordinarily deprive the head of this vessel's minor contribution.

In the process of fixing a large medial head fragment or removing a smaller one, the hip joint must be thoroughly explored and irrigated to remove all small osteocartilaginous fragments that are likely to become abrasive agents.

The prognosis is guarded after this major injury to the femoral head, since traumatic arthritis is highly likely. However, excision of the head fragment or accurate reduction where indicated can give the patient many years of useful and pain-free hip function.

WHEN THE FRAGMENT IS LESS THAN ONE THIRD OF THE FEMORAL HEAD

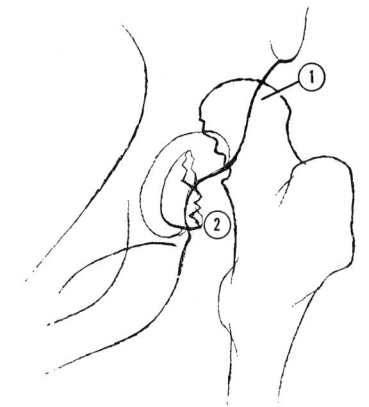

Prereduction X-Ray

1. Posterior dislocation of the femoral head.
2. Marginal fragment detached from the inferior aspect of the femoral head.

Note: Primary open reduction of the fracture-dislocation with removal of the fragment is the only accurate way to prevent femoral head abrasion and wear on the joint.

The posterior approach is preferred to avoid further vascular disruption and permit complete joint inspection.

In unusual circumstances closed reduction may be successful. Dowd and Johnson have reported successful reduction of the head fragment by full internal rotation of the hip and spica cast immobilization.

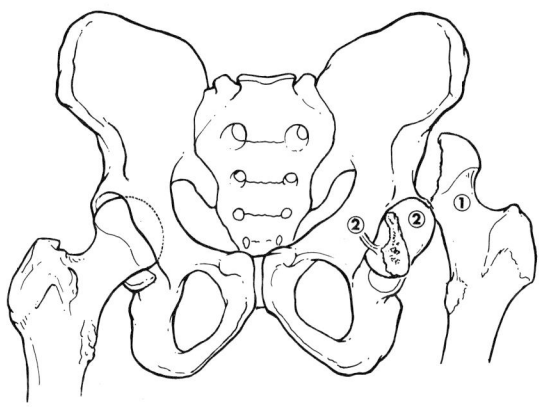

Prereduction X-Ray: Less Common Injury

1. Posterior dislocation of the femoral head.
2. The marginal fragment involves a larger weight-bearing portion of the femoral head and has retained its ligamentum teres attachment.

Note: A fragment of this size should be reattached to the femoral head to restore the normal mechanics of the articulation.

Operative Procedure: Primary Open Reduction with Removal of Loose Femoral Head Fragment

1. With the patient positioned on the uninjured side, make an incision beginning 5 cm distal to the posterior superior iliac spine and continue it lateral and distal, paralleling the fibers of the gluteus maximus muscle, to the greater trochanter. Continue the incision distal along the posterior border of the greater trochanter for 5 cm.

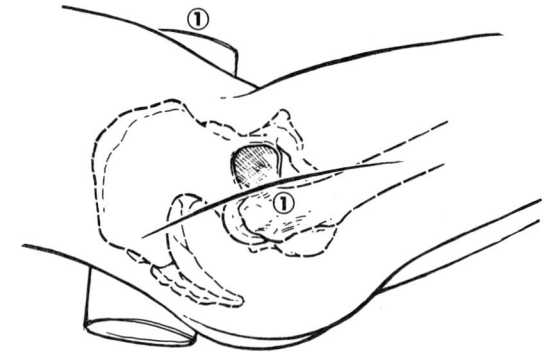

2. Deepen the incision through the deep fascia.

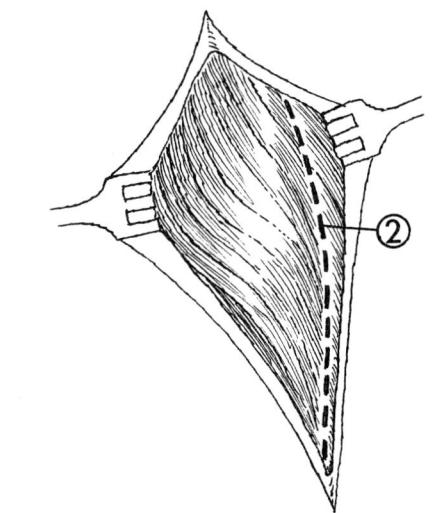

1. Split the gluteus maximus fibers and detach the muscle partially from its insertion to the fascia lata. Protect and visualize the sciatic nerve.
2. Divide the tendons of the piriformis, superior gemellus, internal obturator, and inferior gemellus muscles.

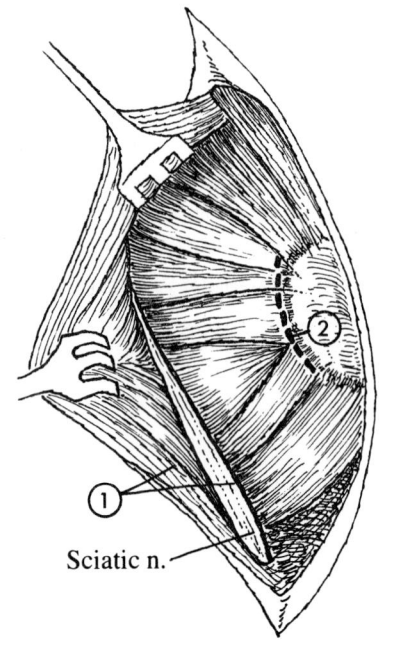

POSTERIOR DISLOCATIONS OF THE HIP

3. Retract the detached external rotators of the hip joint posteriorly.

4. By internal rotation and flexion of the dislocated hip, the marginal fragment can be located and removed.

Note: Thoroughly explore the hip joint for loose fragments. There may be quite numerous cartilaginous fragments not evident on initial x-ray.

Following thorough exploration of the joint, reduce the hip and obtain an intraoperative x-ray to assess adequacy of reduction.

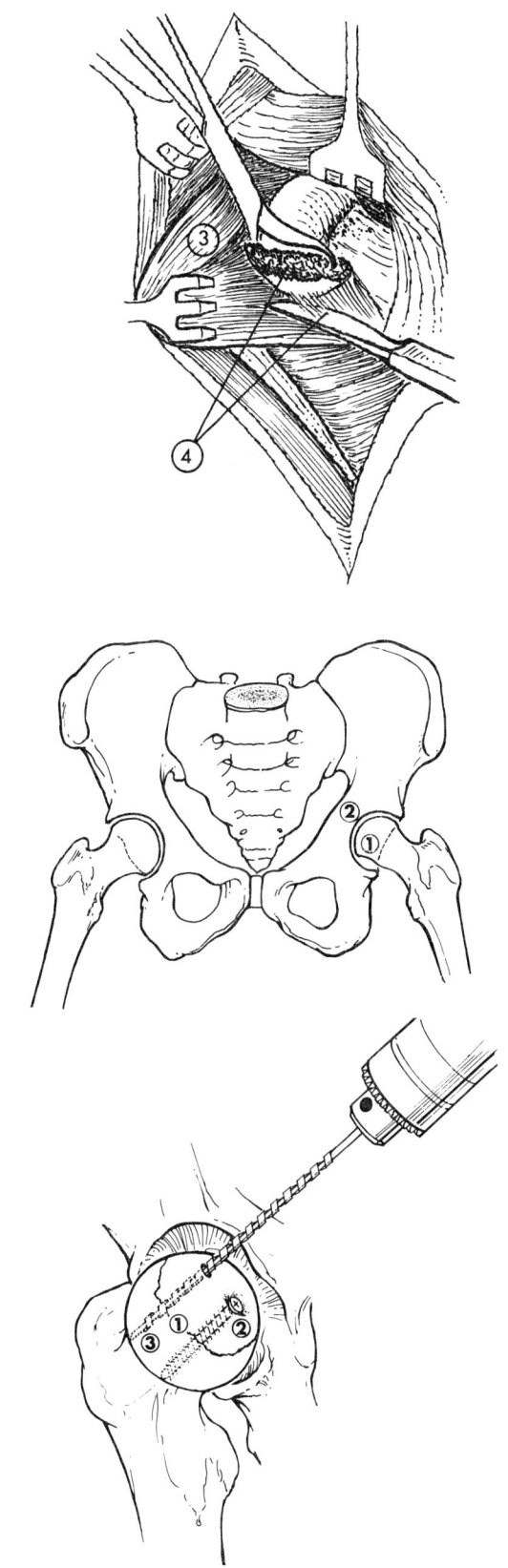

Intraoperative X-Ray after Excision of the Fracture Fragment

1. Defect is seen in the non-weight-bearing portion of the femoral head.

2. The femoral head is symmetrically reduced in the acetabulum.

Screw Fixation of the Large Medial Head Fragment (Sarmiento and Laird)

If the medial head fragment is large enough to involve the weight-bearing portion, the ligamentum teres attachment and vessel can be sacrificed to achieve reduction.

1. The freed medial head fragment is reduced and fixed to the dislocated head.

2. One screw is inserted through the soft fovea where the ligament had formerly inserted.

3. A second screw may be countersunk in the non-weight-bearing portion of the fragment, with sequentially enlarged drill holes in the head,

Screw Fixation of the Large Medial Head Fragment (Sarmiento and Laird) (Continued)

4. The fragment, and
5. The articular surface so that

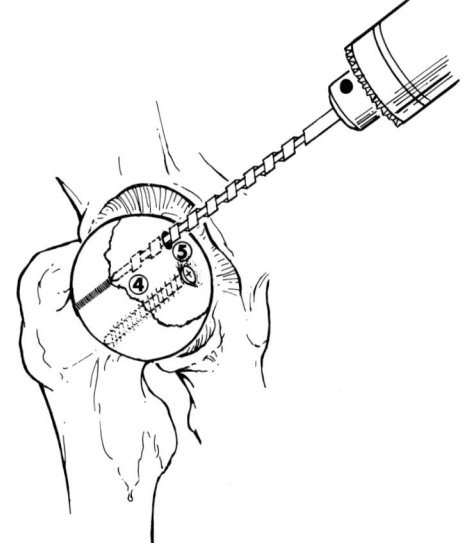

6. The screw sinks beneath the surface.

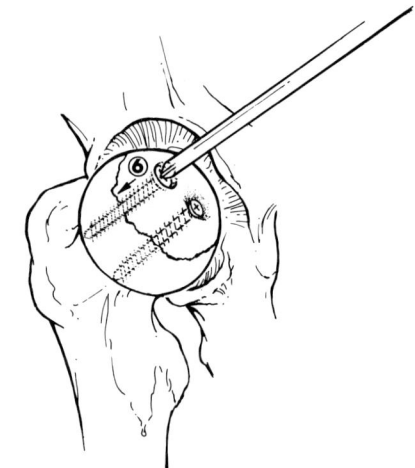

Intraoperative X-Ray After Screw Fixation of the Weight-Bearing Fragment

1. The fracture has been reduced and is held with two screws.
2. The femoral head is symmetrically reduced in the acetabulum.

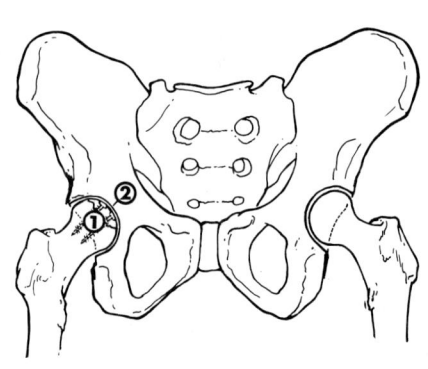

Immobilization

Apply skin traction to the lower leg. The hip is extended and the extremity is slightly abducted.

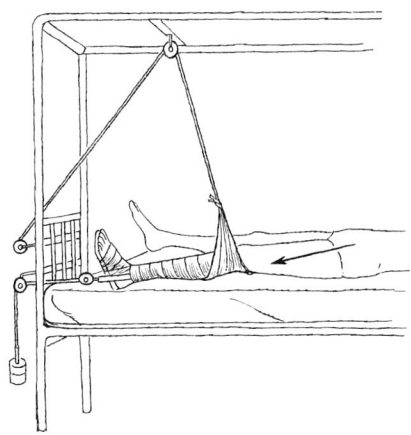

Postoperative Management

When the fracture fragment has been removed, traction should be continued for 2 to 3 weeks. During this immobilization institute active range-of-motion exercises to the hip and quadriceps exercises.

If the fracture fragment has been reduced and fixed to the femoral head, traction should be maintained for 6 to 8 weeks, depending on the stability of the reduction and radiographic evidence of union.

During the recovery phase give the patient aspirin, 3 grams daily in divided doses, since this has been shown to protect against degenerative arthritis and appears to diminish the risk of thromboembolism after hip procedures.

Progression of the patient to weight bearing with crutches should be determined by the fixation achieved at surgery as well as by the subsequent radiographic signs of union. Active range of motion should be encouraged but full weight bearing should be delayed until the fracture fragment has united.

Follow-up of patients with this type of fracture-dislocation should be a minimum of 2 years, but most significant complications will be manifested within the first year.

The patient should be warned that symptoms such as aching or stiffness in the hip or knee or occasional "giving way" will probably indicate the beginning of traumatic arthritis or avascular necrosis.

The course after injuries of this type to the orbicular cartilage is unpredictable. Clinical symptoms do not always correlate with radiographic changes.

Management of a Femoral Neck Fracture Associated with Hip Dislocation

REMARKS

The femoral neck may occasionally fracture at the time of initial dislocation, but the usual cause is overvigorous rotational manipulation at the time of attempted closed reduction.

This significant complication deprives the dislocated proximal femur of virtually all of its blood supply. It is best managed by avoiding it initially.

All closed reductions should be done with minimal violence, preferably using the Stimson maneuver, adequate anesthesia, and minimal leverage in rotating the hip (see page 1273).

Should the surgeon be faced with managing a hip dislocation combined with a femoral neck fracture, open reduction of the dislocation with rigid fixation of the surgically visualized fracture is indicated.

Primary vascular pedicle bone grafting of the fracture site should also be done if any posterior gap is evident. Even though the entire femoral head has been deprived of its blood supply, it may still provide many years of good function.

Primary prosthetic replacement of the femoral head may be indicated in the older patient with this combined injury or in the high femoral neck fracture that cannot be fixed adequately under direct visualization.

Our experience at the University of Nebraska has been that the Cathcart femoral prosthesis with an ovoid or "out-of-round" design cemented into the femoral canal has given the best long-term results for femoral neck fractures.

Should the acetabulum also be damaged, primary total hip replacement becomes the treatment of choice.

Prereduction X-Ray

1. Stump of the femoral neck is in the acetabulum.
2. Femoral head lies outside the acetabulum in a superoposterior position in relation to the acetabulum.

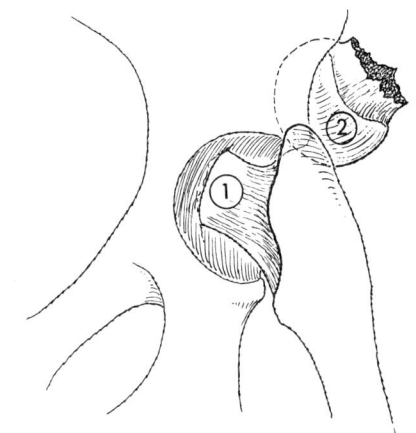

SURGICAL PROCEDURES

Either primary open reduction with internal fixation or prosthetic replacement may be chosen, depending on the indications.

Primary Open Reduction and Internal Fixation

1. With the patient positioned on the uninjured side, make an incision beginning 5 cm distal to the posterior superior iliac spine and continue it lateral and distal, paralleling the fibers of the gluteus maximus muscle, to the greater trochanter. Continue the incision distal along the posterior border of the greater trochanter for 5 cm.

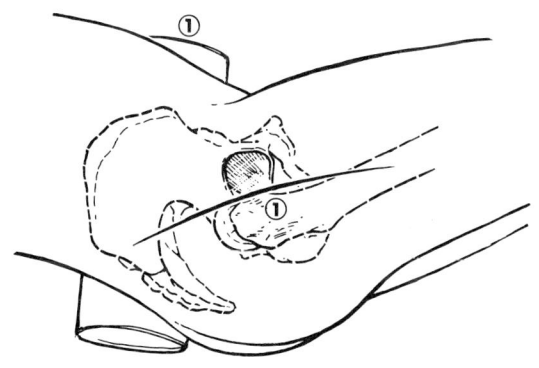

2. Deepen the incision through the deep fascia.

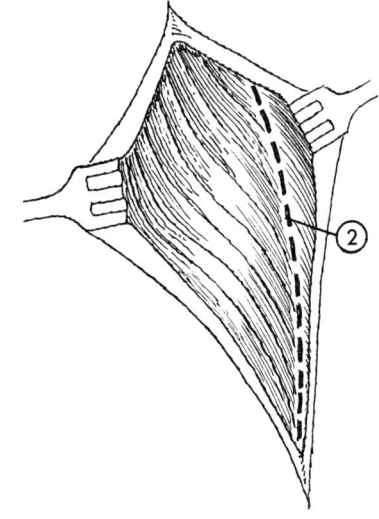

POSTERIOR DISLOCATIONS OF THE HIP

Primary Open Reduction and Internal Fixation (Continued)

1. Split the gluteus maximus parallel with its fibers and detach its insertion into the fascia lata.
2. Visualize the sciatic nerve and inspect it for any evidence of injury.
3. Divide the tendons of the piriformis, superior gemellus, internal obturator, and inferior gemellus muscles.

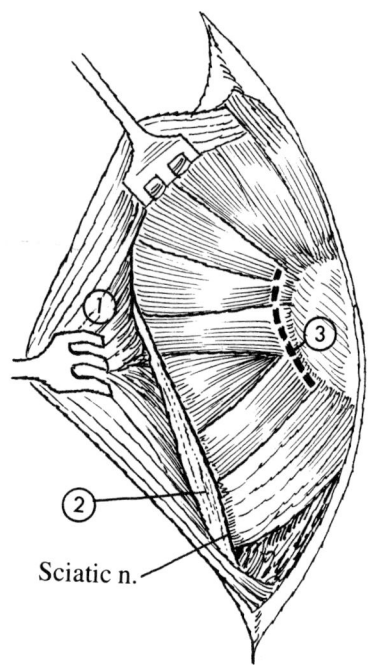

4. Retract the external rotator muscles and the sciatic nerve posteriorly.

Note: At this point the femoral head will be visualized outside of the capsule.

5. Dislocated femoral head.
6. Neck of the femur in the acetabulum.

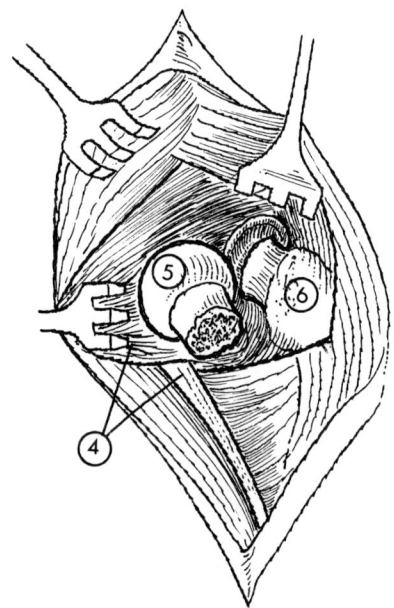

1. Under direct visualization, reduce the femoral head back onto the neck and hold the fracture compressed.
2. Fix the fracture with multiple (5 to 6) Knowles pins drilled up from the greater trochanter.
3. A pin may exit through neck provided it reenters head.
4. Pack any fracture defects with cancellous bone obtained from the trochanter or use vascularized pedicle graft from trochanter.

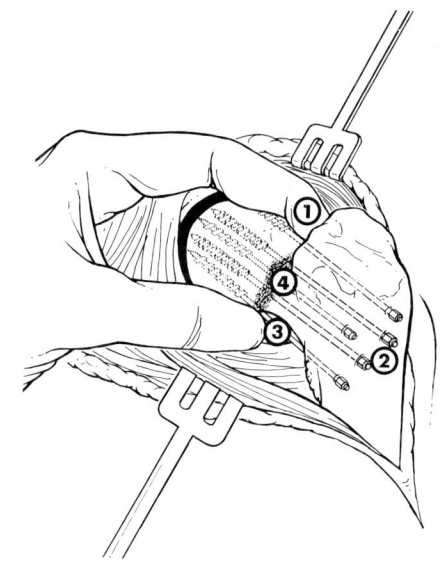

Note: After thoroughly inspecting and irrigating the hip joint for loose fragments, reduce the femoral head.

Check the rigidity of fixation by moving the hip through a full range of motion.

If the fixation is not rigid, insert additional pins or replace the femoral head with a prosthesis. Obtain intraoperative x-rays.

Intraoperative X-Ray

1. The fracture should be rigidly fixed by the pins.
2. The hip space should be symmetrically restored.

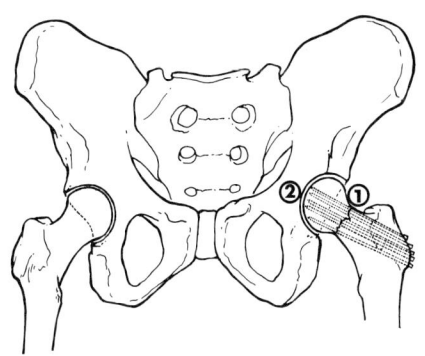

Primary Cathcart Prosthetic Replacement in Femoral Neck Fracture-Dislocation

REMARKS

For high femoral neck fracture with dislocation that cannot be held rigidly the alternative treatment is a primary cemented Cathcart prosthesis.* This prosthesis may also be used primarily for the older patient (more than 60 years) with this rare combined injury.

---

*Available from DePuy Co., Warsaw, Indiana

POSTERIOR DISLOCATIONS OF THE HIP

In the same circumstances, should the acetabular surface be damaged, total hip replacement would be the preferred primary reconstructive procedure.

The ellipsoidal or "out-of-round" design of the Cathcart prosthesis approximates that of the normal femoral head and permits synovial fluid lubrication of the acetabulum. The effect in theory and on long-term follow-up is to diminish boring of the steel prosthesis through the acetabular cartilage.

Cementing the femoral stem diminishes the tendency of the prosthesis to loosen.

OPERATIVE TECHNIQUE

1. With the patient positioned on the uninjured side, make an incision beginning 5 cm distal to the posterior superior iliac spine and continue it lateral and distal paralleling the fibers of the gluteus maximus muscle, to the greater trochanter. Continue the incision distal along the posterior border of the greater trochanter for 5 cm.

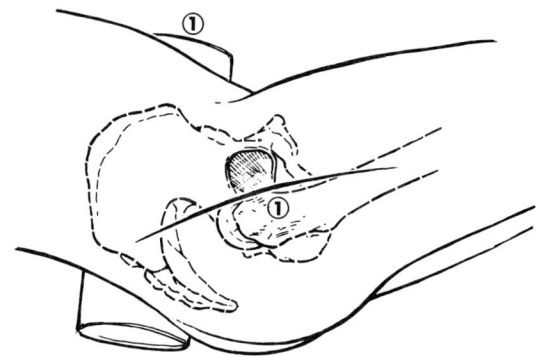

2. Deepen the incision through the deep fascia.

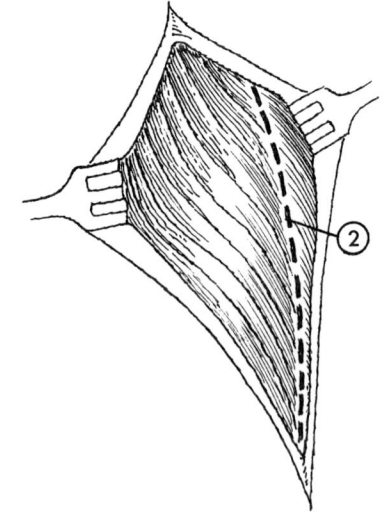

1. Split the gluteus maximus parallel with its fibers and detach its insertion into the fascia lata.
2. Displace the muscle mass posteriorly. Visualize the sciatic nerve.
3. Divide the tendons of the piriformis, superior gemellus, obturator internus, and inferior gemellus muscles.

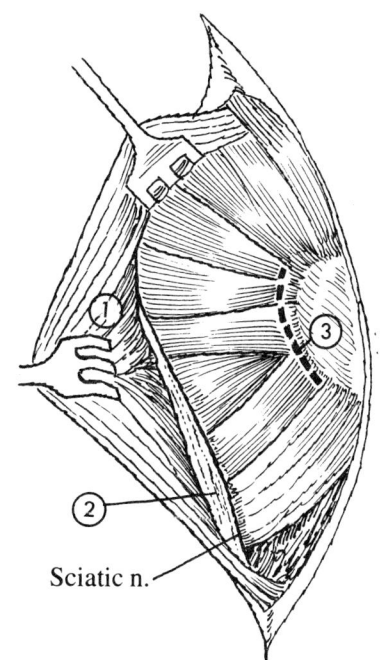

4. Retract the detached external rotators and the sciatic nerve.
5. Isolate the dislocated femoral head, which usually lies superior and posterior to the acetabulum, and remove it from the wound.
6. The neck of the femur may be in the acetabulum.

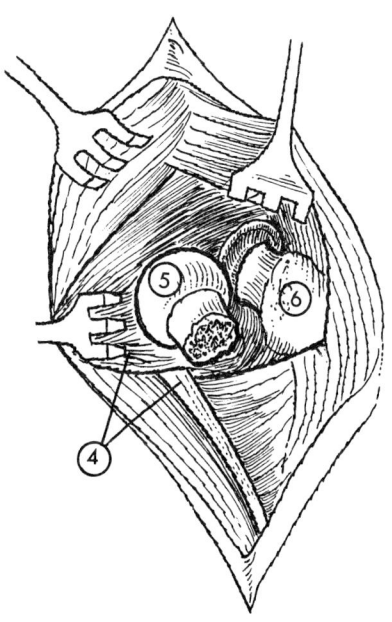

POSTERIOR DISLOCATIONS OF THE HIP

Primary Cathcart Prosthetic Replacement in Femoral Neck Fracture-Dislocation (Continued)

1. Internally rotate the extremity; this brings into full view the stump of the neck.
2. With an electric saw reshape the femoral neck to provide a seat for the Cathcart prosthesis. Enough of the calcar must remain to provide adequate support to the medial portion of the prosthesis.
3. Ream the medullary canal completely with a rasp so as to remove all cancellous bone.
4. Cut out a notch in the greater trochanter with a "starter," which permits easy insertion of the prosthesis.

Note: Choose a prosthesis that is of the same size as the femoral head removed. Also check the size of the prosthesis by placing it directly into the acetabulum before insertion of the stem into the medullary canal.

1. After the proper size prosthesis has been selected, fill the thoroughly reamed medullary canal with a batch of methyl methacrylate cement. Drive the Cathcart prosthesis into the cemented canal, and
2. Seat the neck of the prosthesis on the calcar.
3. The shape of the femoral prosthesis is designed to allow synovial fluid to perfuse the acetabulum.

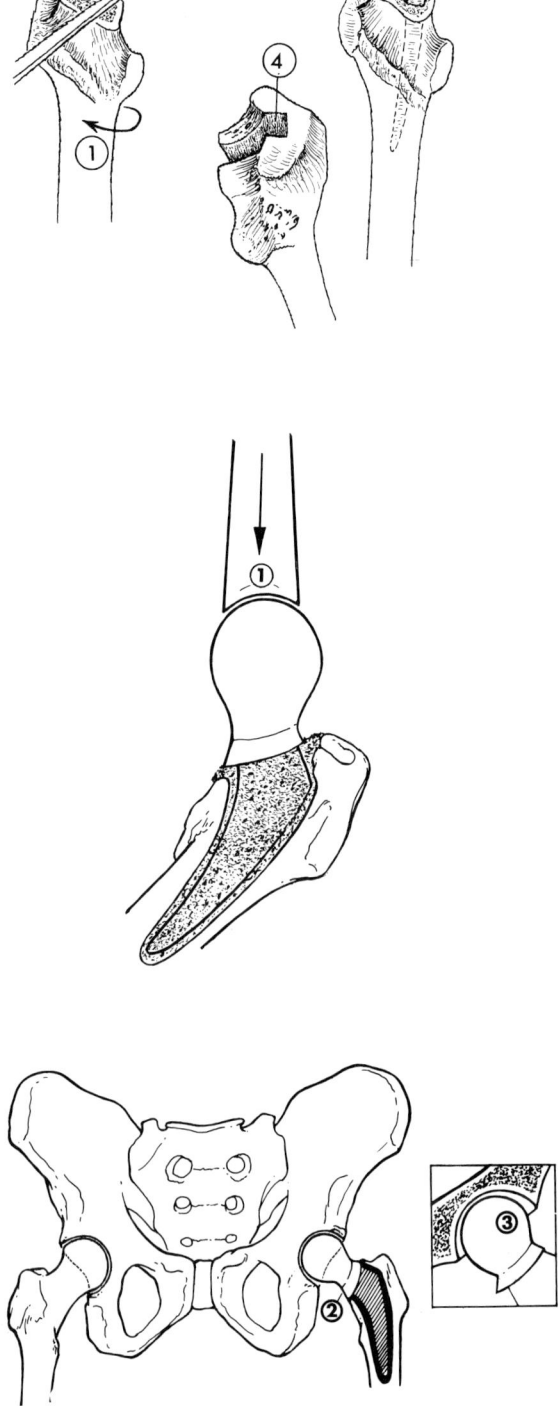

POSTOPERATIVE MANAGEMENT FOR FEMORAL NECK FRACTURE-DISLOCATION

Postoperative protection for the hip depends on the procedure employed and the degree of stability evident at the time of operation.

If the Cathcart or total hip prosthesis was chosen to replace the fractured femoral neck, the operated leg need only be supported with an abduction device to protect against flexion and external rotation.

The patient may be allowed to bear weight with a walker or crutches by the third postoperative day.

Crutch walking should be continued for 6 to 8 weeks, after which time the patient may advance to a cane.

If the fracture-dislocation was fixed internally, the hip should be immobilized in traction for 3 to 4 weeks.

The patient may then gradually begin active range-of-motion exercises to the hip and may start crutch walking.

Crutch walking must be continued for a minimum of 4 to 6 months to protect the healing of the femoral neck fracture.

The patient should be cautioned that progressive pain or stiffness of the hip or knee or "giving way" of the hip may indicate the onset of traumatic arthritis or avascular necrosis.

While the patient is immobilized in traction, start aspirin, 3 grams a day in divided doses, since this has been shown to protect against traumatic arthritis and also appears to minimize the incidence of thromboembolism after hip procedures.

A postoperative abduction splint may be useful for 3 to 5 days after prosthetic replacement to prevent the patient from flexing and adducting the hip and thereby risking re-dislocation.

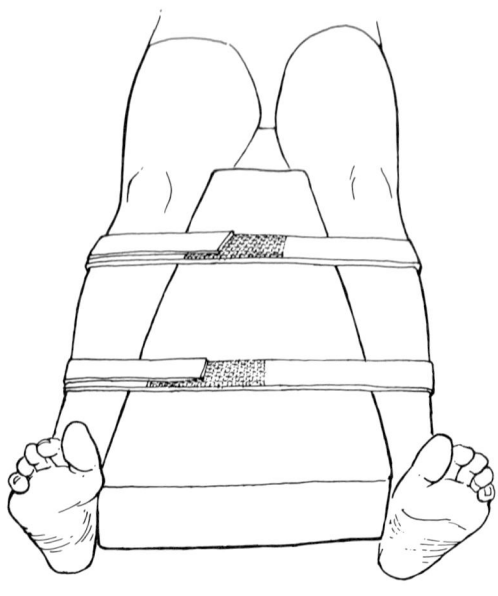

Dislocation of the Hip Joint with Fracture of the Shaft of the Femur

REMARKS

Fracture of the femoral shaft combined with dislocation of the hip frequently results from two separate mechanisms. The first dislocates the hip and throws the victim around or out of the car. The second injury is incurred as the patient lands on the dislocated side and fractures the femur.

This combined injury is treacherous because in 50 to 60 per cent of reported cases the fractured shaft masks the dislocation of the hip.

All x-rays of long bone fractures must include the joints proximal and distal to the fracture. In addition, routine x-ray of the pelvis in any seriously injured patient, particularly with lower limb fractures, will avoid this diagnostic lapse.

Management of the fracture-dislocation generally requires intramedullary nailing of the shaft fracture in order to reduce the hip.

Occasionally with distal femoral fractures, closed reduction of the hip is possible without fracture fixation, but in the vast majority of injuries the surgeon should prepare for open reduction of the fracture and frequently of the dislocation as well.

Should the proximal injury be unrecognized, the hip dislocation frequently causes nonunion of the femoral shaft fracture. This requires intramedullary nailing and bone grafting. An open reduction of the dislocated hip may be done at the time of nailing, but the preferred reconstructive procedure for a hip that has been chronically dislocated for more than three months is total hip replacement (see page 1312).

POSTERIOR DISLOCATIONS OF THE HIP

Prereduction X-Rays

UNRECOGNIZED HIP DISLOCATION WITH FEMORAL SHAFT FRACTURE

Note: This diagnostic lapse could be avoided by insisting that the x-ray always include the joint above and the joint below the fracture.

1. The femoral shaft fracture is angulated medially.
2. The proximal fragment is in adduction rather than the usual position of abduction.
3. The lesser trochanter is internally rotated and is not visible.
4. The hip joint has been omitted from the x-ray.

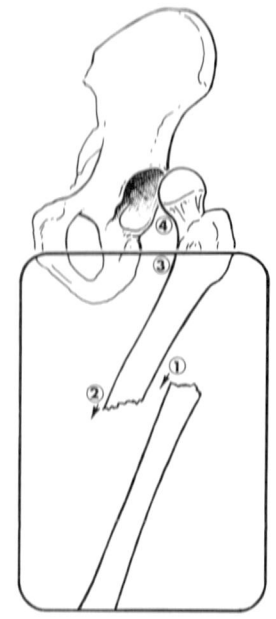

TYPE III FRACTURE-DISLOCATION OF THE HIP

1. The femoral head is dislocated posteriorly.
2. The acetabular rim is comminuted in multiple fragments.
3. The femoral shaft has sustained a high fracture.

Note: This type of fracture-dislocation of the hip requires open reduction. The femoral shaft fracture can be fixed by closed intramedullary nailing at the same time.

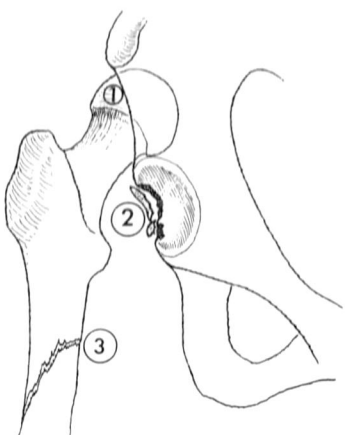

Manipulative Reduction

For acute, relatively undisplaced shaft fracture with hip dislocation, one or two attempts at closed reduction are worthwhile.

In most instances the shaft fracture prevents the surgeon from applying any traction on the hip.

Fixation of the shaft by either closed or open intramedullary nailing permits reduction of the hip dislocation.

Note: Closed reduction of the dislocation may be possible if the femoral shaft fracture is in the distal third or the hip is subluxated rather than completely dislocated.

Manipulative Reduction
(Continued)

1. The patient is placed in the supine position on the floor.
2. An assistant makes downward pressure on the anterosuperior spines of the ilium.
3. The operator makes upward traction on the leg with the hip flexed 90 degrees.
4. Another assistant applies direct pressure on the dislocated femoral head in an upward and inward direction.

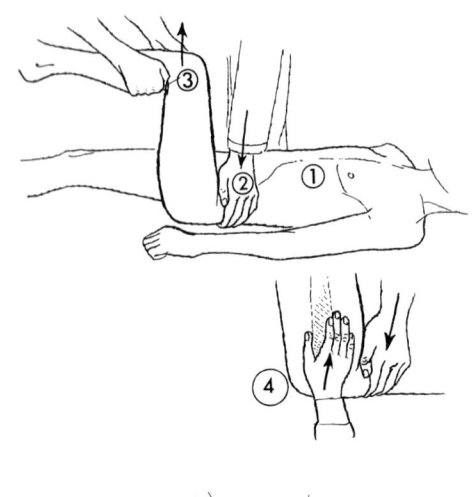

After the head enters the acetabulum,
1. While upward traction is maintained,
2. Lower the thigh to the floor to the extended position.

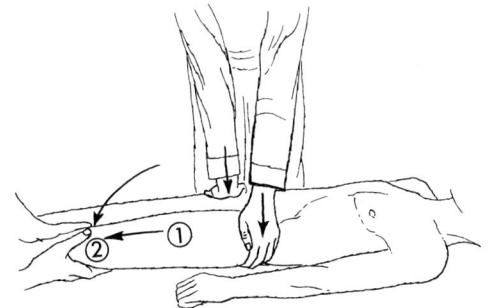

Operative Management of Hip Dislocation Associated with Femoral Shaft Fracture.

In most instances, stabilization of the femoral shaft fracture is necessary to provide sufficient leverage to reduce the hip dislocation. This is particularly true if the fracture is in the proximal or middle third or if the dislocation is old.

1. The femur is reduced and stabilized by either open or closed intramedullary nailing.
2. Following stabilization of the femur shaft, the fracture-dislocation of the hip is opened, the joint is cleared of all loose fragments, and the dislocation is reduced under direct visualization.

Note: Occasionally for Type I dislocation with femoral shaft fractures, the hip may be reduced by a closed method following stabilization of the shaft.

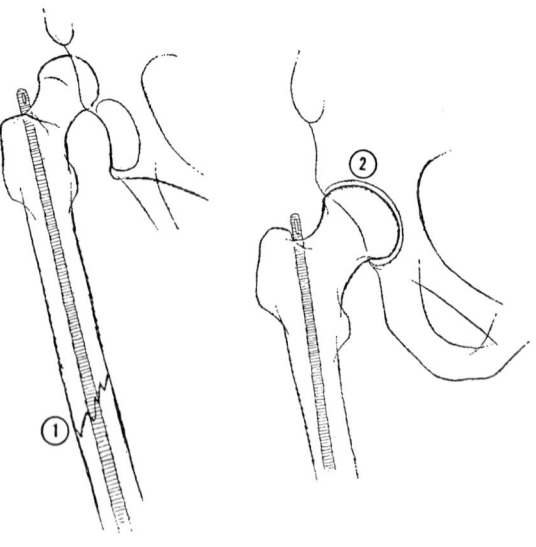

Postreduction Management

Immobilize the injured limb postoperatively in 2.3 to 3.2 kg (5 to 7 lb) of skin traction until soft tissue swelling subsides.

If the hip was stable after reduction and the fracture was rigidly fixed by the intramedullary nail, prolonged immobilization is not necessary.

There is no evidence to indicate that early weight bearing increases avascular necrosis or traumatic arthritis, provided that joint reduction has been anatomic and no loose bodies persist in the joint.

If the hip was unstable at the time of reduction or if fixation of acetabular fragments was necessary, continue traction for 2 to 3 weeks as necessary to permit healing of the acetabular rim.

During the period of prolonged immobilization, give the patient aspirin, 3 grams daily in divided doses, which has been shown to protect against degenerative arthritis and appears to diminish the risk of thromboembolism.

Follow-up of patients with serious dislocations and fracture-dislocations of this nature should be a minimum of 2 years. Most significant complications will be manifested within the first year. Warn the patient that symptoms such as aching or stiffness in the knees or an occasional "giving way" may indicate the beginning of traumatic arthritis or avascular necrosis.

Old Unreduced Dislocations of the Hip

REMARKS

Old unreduced traumatic posterior dislocation of the hip is usually the result of an accident in which the patient's comatose condition, a fracture of the ipsilateral femur or tibia, or dislocation or injury to the opposite hip masks the dislocation.

Leaving the hip dislocated leads to consistently poor results.

In many instances a primary reconstructive procedure gives results superior to attempt at open or closed reduction. This is particularly true if the fracture-dislocation is a Type IV or Type V.

In a young patient with a Type I dislocation of less than three months' duration, closed reduction should be attempted with the consideration that avascular necrosis may occur. Preliminary heavy skeletal traction is necessary to overcome soft tissue contractures if closed reduction is to succeed.

Open reduction and removal of bone fragments with internal fixation of the fractured acetabular lip may yield good results in a young patient with a Type II or Type III fracture-dislocation of less than three months' duration.

For Type IV or Type V fracture-dislocation or a dislocation that has been out for more than three months, primary reconstructive procedures, particularly total hip joint replacement, offer the best results.

Unrecognized Type I Dislocation of Less than Three Months' Duration

1. AP x-ray shows isolated posterior dislocation of the hip one month after injury.

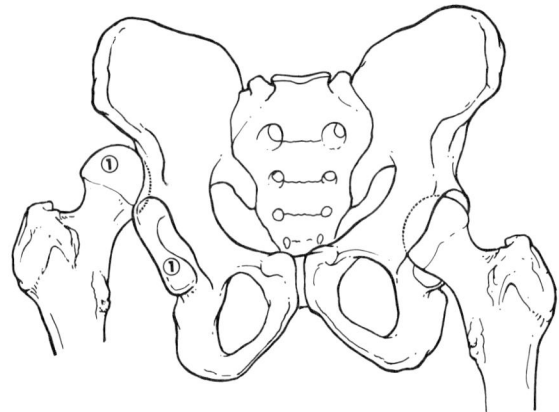

2. Oblique view shows no damage to the acetabular rim or femoral head.

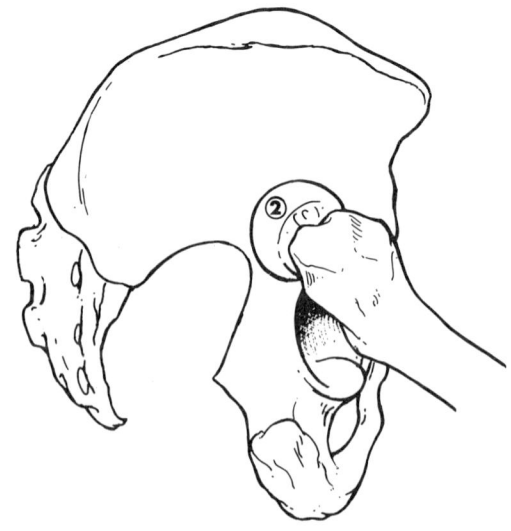

Technique of Closed Reduction: Heavy Skeletal Traction (after Gupta and Shravat)

1. To stretch the soft tissues contracted around the dislocated hip use heavy—up to 18 kg (40 lb)—traction applied to a skeletal pin in the distal femur. Use sedation and muscle relaxation as necessary.
2. After 5 to 7 days of traction, the x-ray should show that the femoral head has been pulled to or below the level of the acetabulum.
3. Gradually abduct the limb while slowly decreasing the amount of traction.
4. The femoral head should seat gradually and atraumatically into the acetabulum.

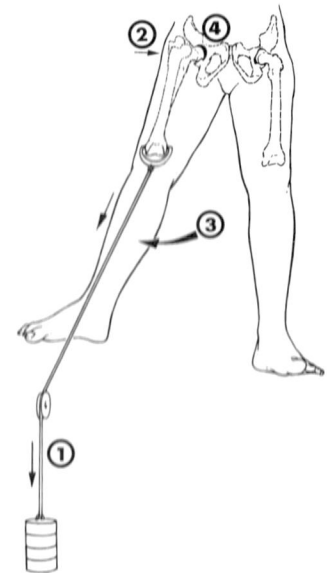

Postreduction Management

Decrease the skeletal traction weight to 5 kg (11 lb) and continue traction for 2 to 3 weeks.

After 2 to 3 weeks of traction, begin crutch walking.

Encourage active non-weight-bearing exercises for another month while the patient walks on crutches, and then permit progressive weight bearing.

The patient should be followed with periodic x-rays for at least 2 years to detect changes of avascular necrosis or traumatic arthritis.

Late Open Reduction for Type II or Type III Fracture-Dislocation

PREREDUCTION X-RAY

1. X-ray of the hip 11 weeks after injury shows a posterior Type II fracture-dislocation with comminution of the acetabular rim.
2. The femoral head shows no evidence of traumatic arthritis.

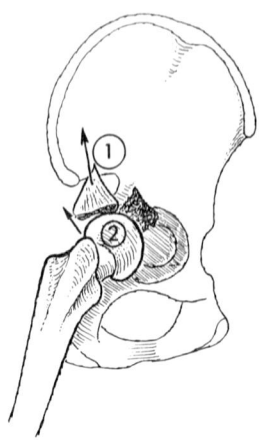

Open reduction and fixation of the acetabular rim should be performed as described on page 1286.

Late Open Reduction for Type II or Type III Fracture-Dislocation (Continued)

Follow-up x-ray

Eight years after open reduction and acetabular fixation, the patient has almost normal hip function:
1. The joint space is maintained.
2. There is increased sclerosis on x-ray of the acetabular injury.
3. There are no signs of traumatic arthritis or avascular necrosis in the femoral head.

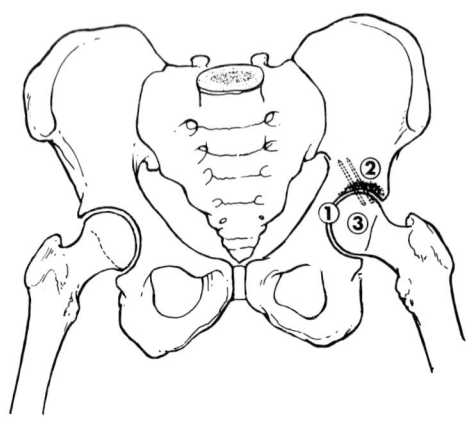

Primary Reconstructive Arthroplasty for Unreduced Type V Fracture-Dislocation

1. Type V dislocation with fracture of the femoral head was discovered in a 35-year-old victim of multiple injuries 8 weeks after initial injury.

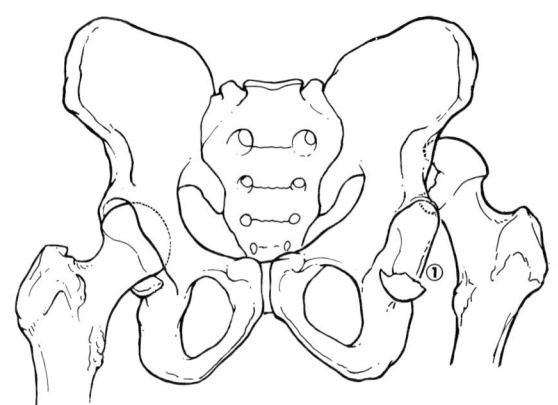

2. Total hip replacement offers the best chance for satisfactory restoration of function after this type of unrecognized injury.

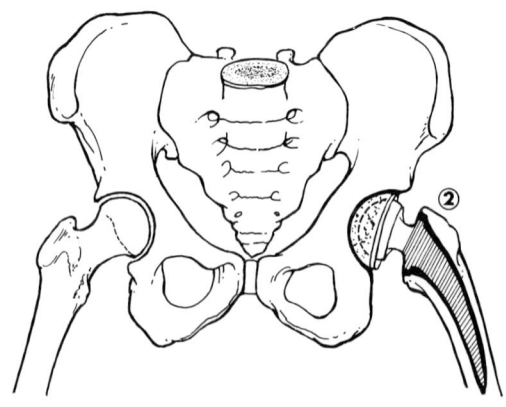

Chronic Dislocation with Acetabular Fracture

1. For chronic dislocation with fracture of the acetabulum, reconstruction of the posterior acetabular support may be necessary using a bone graft from the femoral head in addition to total hip replacement.

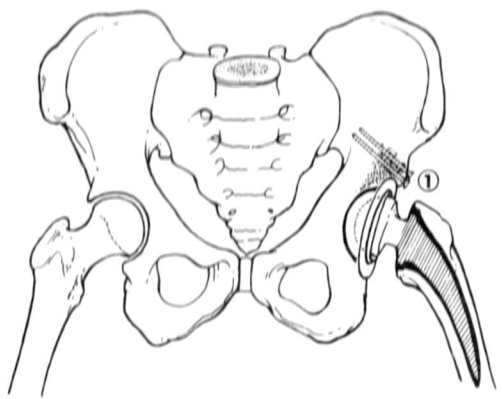

Recurrent Traumatic Posterior Dislocation of the Hip

REMARKS

Recurrent traumatic dislocation of a previously normal hip joint is relatively rare, although it does occur.

Recurrent posterior dislocation is more frequent in children than in adults. Approximately 6 per cent of childhood dislocations can recur, while at most only 1 to 2 per cent of adult dislocations are subject to recurrence.

If a dislocation recurs more than 2 to 3 times, trauma to the femoral head or sciatic nerve is possible, and operative repair should be recommended.

The major cause of recurrent dislocation is a large defect in the posterior capsule with large synovial outpouching or a false joint.

Treatment is by operative excision of the posterior pouch and repair of the capsular defect.

Although the exact cause for this abnormality to develop after dislocation is not certain, the most common factor is immobilization of only a few days following closed reduction of the posterior dislocation.

POSTERIOR DISLOCATIONS OF THE HIP

Appearance on Arthrogram

1. An arthrogram in a hip with recurrent dislocation demonstrates that there is a defect in the posterior capsule that forms an outpouching permitting recurrence.

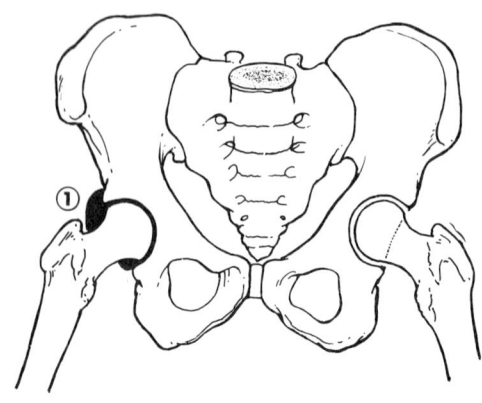

Operative Repair

The hip is approached posteriorly and
1. The synovial outpouching is excised, exposing the hip joint.

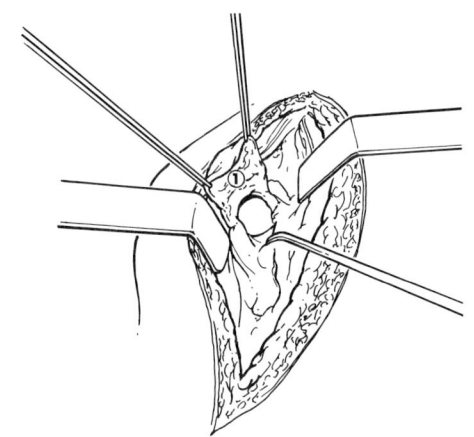

2. The defect is repaired by "double breasting" the lower part of the capsule over the upper part with sutures.

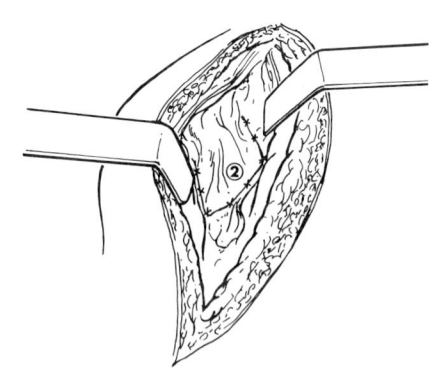

Postoperative Management

The hip should be immobilized in a light walking hip spica cast for 6 weeks postoperatively to insure satisfactory healing and to prevent flexion of the hip.

When soft tissue is completely healed, after 6 weeks, remove the cast and begin active range-of-motion exercises, protecting the hip with crutches for an additional 4 to 6 weeks.

ANTERIOR DISLOCATIONS OF THE HIP

REMARKS

Anterior dislocation of the hip is not common, occurring in 10 to 12 per cent of all traumatic dislocations.

The femoral head may dislocate anteromedially toward the obturator foramen or anterolaterally toward the pubis.

Obturator dislocation most often results from forceful abduction and external rotation and extension that causes the neck of the femur to impinge against the acetabulum and the trochanter to lever against the ilium. The femoral head is then forced out through a tear in the lower, anterior aspect of the joint capsule.

The mechanism for the less frequent and more difficult pubic dislocation appears to be a forceful hyperextension and external rotation of the hip. This thrusts the head directly anteriorly or anterolaterally out of the acetabulum and through the capsule above the iliofemoral ligament. Usually this results from a sudden twist on the weight-bearing side while the hip is hyperextended.

As a rule, reduction of an obturator dislocation is readily achieved by closed methods, but closed reduction of a pubic dislocation can be quite difficult.

The usual first step in reducing the obturator dislocation is by traction and gradual flexion of the hip. This maneuver, however, is inappropriate for a pubic dislocation because it serves to tighten the already tight posterior capsular structures and thereby prevents reduction.

The first step in reducing a pubic dislocation is to place the femoral head back into the position in which it dislocated so as to retrace its path back into the acetabulum. The initial maneuver for a pubic dislocation should be hyperextension and external rotation to accomplish an atraumatic reduction.

If the mechanism of the anterior dislocation is not considered, closed reduction, particularly of a pubic dislocation, may be futile, and open reduction becomes necessary.

Closed reduction should not be attempted repeatedly because an irreducible anterior dislocation does in fact require open reduction.

Always evaluate the femoral arterial pulse before and after reduction of the dislocation. The close proximity of the femoral vessels to the hip put them at risk from anterior dislocation.

Mechanism of Obturator Dislocation

The possible mechanisms include the following:

1. The limb is abducted, externally rotated, and flexed so as to impinge the neck against the acetabulum and the trochanter against the ilium.
2. Force is applied to the back of the thigh.
3. The head of the femur is forced out of the joint.

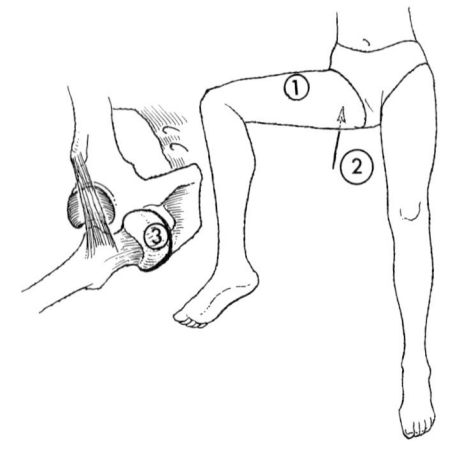

1. The limb is abducted, externally rotated, and flexed so as to impinge the neck against the acetabulum and the trochanter against the ilium.
2. Force applied to the knee passes through the femur.
3. The head of the femur is forced out of the joint through a rent in the capsule.

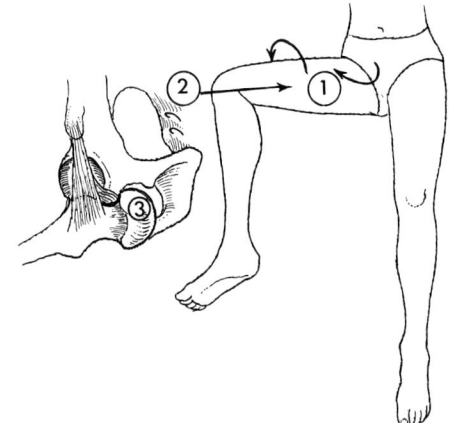

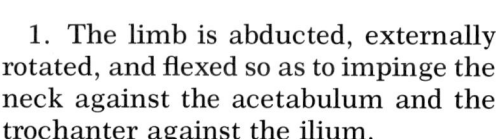

Mechanism of Pubic Dislocation

Note: Although pubic dislocation occurs less frequently than obturator dislocation, it is very difficult to reduce. The technique of reduction should be to reproduce the mechanism and retrace the path of the dislocated hip back into the acetabulum by hyperextension.

1. The patient hyperextends his hip while running.
2. A sudden twist of the hyperextended hip causes forceful external rotation.
3. The hyperextended, externally rotated femoral head dislocates through the capsule superior to the iliofemoral Y ligament.

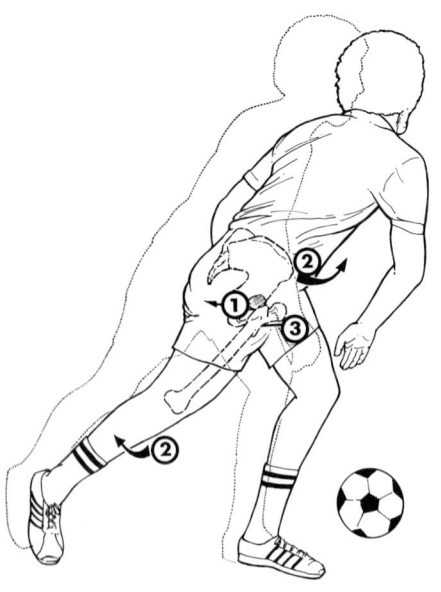

ANTERIOR DISLOCATIONS OF THE HIP

4. The posterior capsule muscles and external rotator muscles become tight and prevent reduction in flexion.

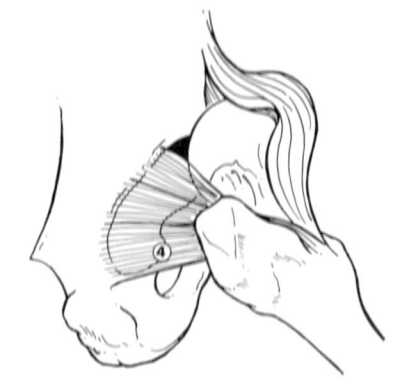

Typical Deformity

Obturator dislocation

1. The hip is slightly flexed.
2. The limb is externally rotated.
3. The thigh is abducted.

Note: In pubic dislocation, there is little or no abduction, the hip is extended, and the limb is externally rotated.

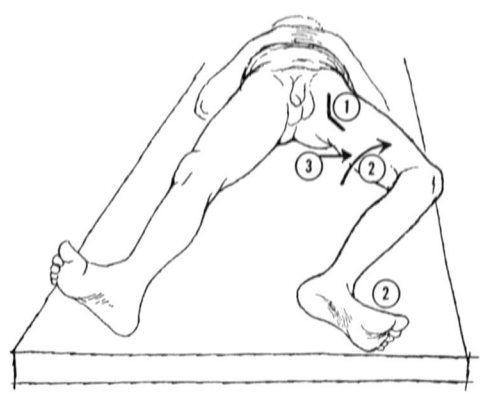

Pubic dislocation

1. The extremity is in severe external rotation (90 degrees).
2. The extremity is abducted only slightly (15 to 20 degrees) and it is slightly flexed.
3. The femoral head can readily be palpated in the inguinal region.

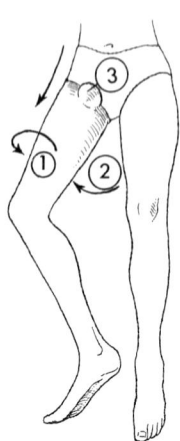

ANTERIOR DISLOCATIONS OF THE HIP

Prereduction X-Ray

Obturator dislocation

1. The femoral head rests on the obturator foramen.
2. The femur is widely abducted and
3. Flexed and
4. Externally rotated.

Pubic dislocation

1. Anteroposterior x-ray shows the cephalad displacement of the femoral head to a pubic or subspinous position.
2. The femur is externally rotated, as indicated by the position of the lesser trochanter, and is in slight abduction.

3. Lateral x-ray shows the head is anterior to the acetabulum.

CAUTION:

1. The close proximity of the femoral vessels puts them at risk from an anterior pubic dislocation. Always check circulation before and after reduction.

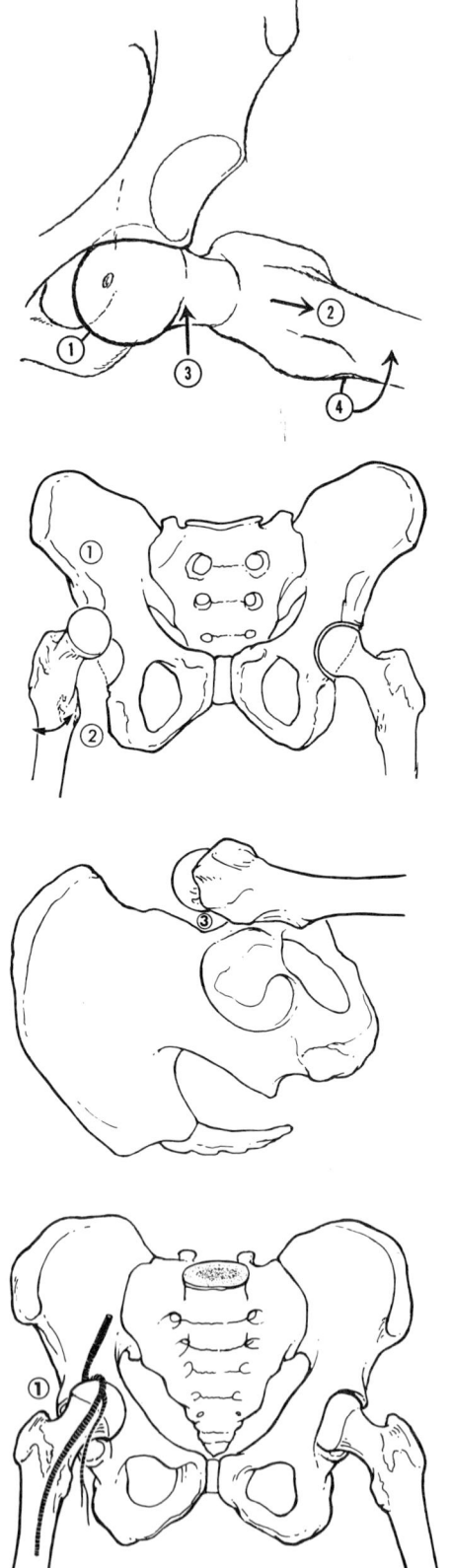

ANTERIOR DISLOCATIONS OF THE HIP

Reduction of Obturator Dislocation

This should be done under general anesthesia and with adequate muscle relaxation, although occasionally simply positioning the hip for x-ray will reduce the dislocation.

1. The patient is placed on the floor in the supine position.
2. An assistant makes downward pressure on the anterosuperior iliac spines.

3. Grasp the affected limb and flex the hip and knee to a right angle.
4. Rotate the limb to a neutral position. (This position converts an anterior to a posterior dislocation.)

5. Make steady traction on the leg directly upward, lifting the head of the femur into the acetabulum.

Note: Do not adduct the hip until it is reduced in the acetabulum; otherwise a fracture of the femoral head or neck may occur.

1. While upward traction is maintained,
2. Lower the thigh to the floor to the extended position.

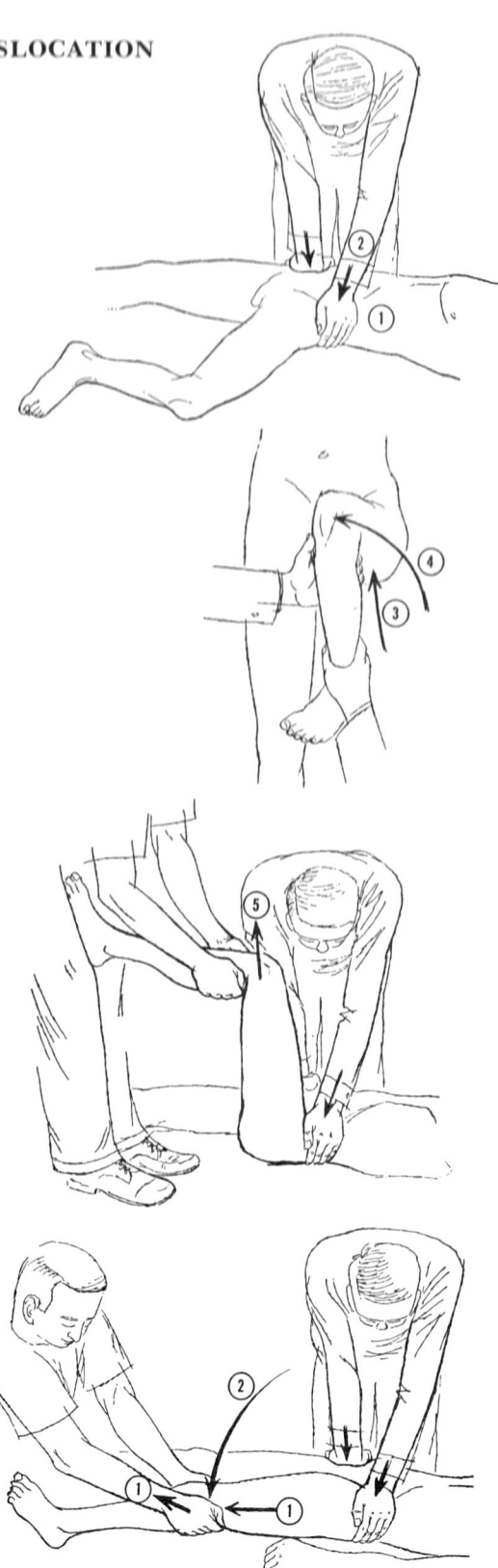

1319

Alternate Method of Reduction

If reduction is not achieved by the maneuvers just described,

1. Apply traction to the limb in the position of deformity, which is that of flexion and abduction.

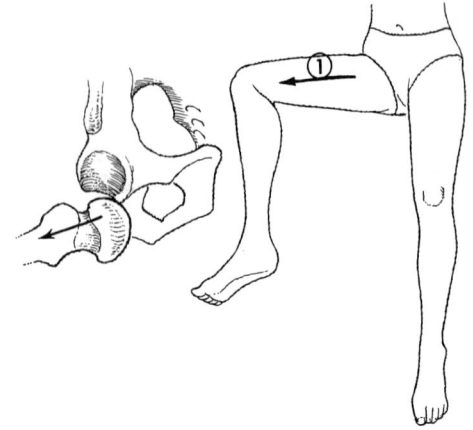

2. While traction is maintained gently bring the limb to a vertical position. This lifts the femoral head onto the anterior rim of the acetabulum.

Direct pressure over the head of the femur helps push the dislocated bone over the rim.

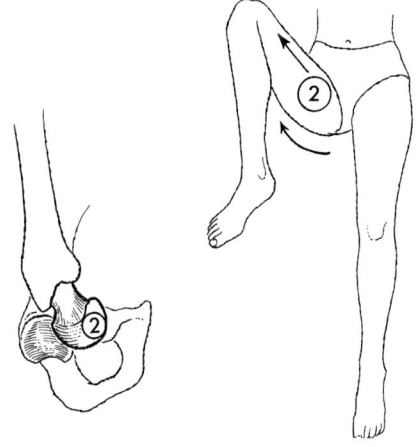

3. While traction and direct pressure are maintained, internally rotate the limb and lower the thigh to the extended position.

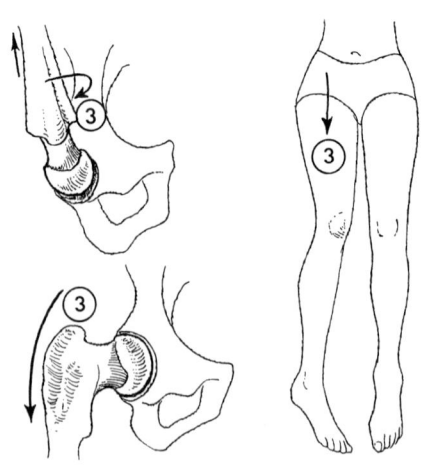

Postreduction X-Ray

1. The head of the femur is seated in the acetabulum.
2. The shaft of the femur is in the neutral position.
3. Shenton's line is intact.
4. The lesser trochanter is well visualized.

Note: Check carefully for the presence of any bony fragments within the joint. Anterior dislocation with large fracture fragments should be treated by operative reduction, as in posterior dislocation.

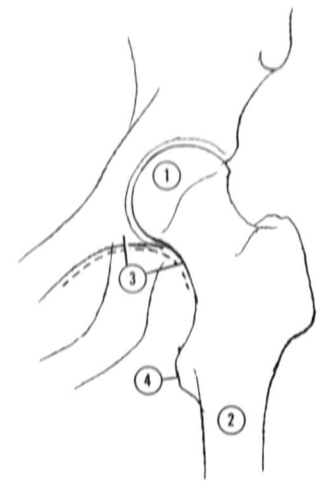

Immobilization

Apply skin traction to the lower leg.
The hip is extended and the leg is slightly abducted.

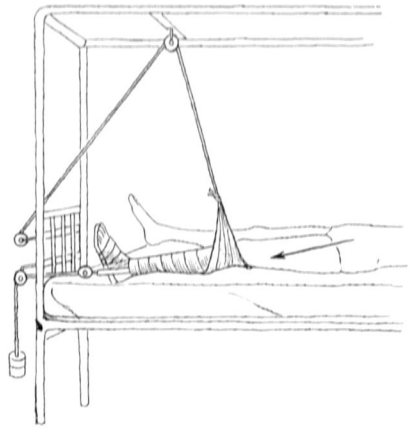

Postreduction Management

Maintain skin traction for 3 weeks.
Within a few days the patient may begin range-of-motion exercises to the hip, but hip flexion should be avoided.
During the recovery period give the patient aspirin, 3 grams daily in divided doses, which has been shown to protect against degenerative arthritis and appears to diminish the incidence of thromboembolism after hip procedures.
Continue the aspirin for 2 to 3 months, until the patient is walking independently.
The patient may begin weight bearing with crutches and may gradually increase the amount of weight borne until he can eliminate crutches. There is no evidence to indicate that early weight bearing increases the incidence of avascular necrosis or traumatic arthritis, provided that the joint reduction has been anatomic and there are no loose bodies persisting in the joint.

Follow-up of the patient with a dislocated hip should be a minimum of 2 years, but most significant complications will be manifested within the first year. Patients should be warned that symptoms such as aching or stiffness in the hip or knee or occasional "giving way" may indicate the beginning of traumatic arthritis or avascular necrosis.

REDUCTION OF A PUBIC DISLOCATION (AFTER DINGLEY AND DENHAM)

REMARKS

The less common pubic dislocation cannot be reduced by the maneuver that usually reduces an obturator dislocation of the hip.

In these instances the head is forced out of the anterior aspect of the capsule by severe hyperextension and external rotation of the hip joint, and any attempt to flex the hip is met by the firm resistance offered by the posterior capsule, which binds the head firmly on the pubis.

This dislocation is readily reduced by first hyperextending the hip, then internally rotating the limb.

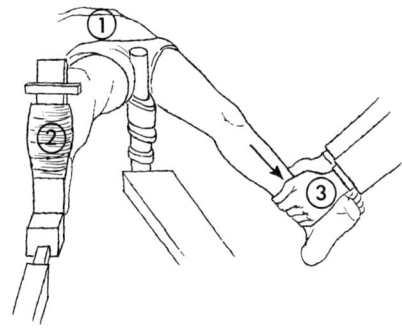

1. Place the patient on a fracture table.
2. Fasten the unaffected limb to the foot plate.
3. Make longitudinal traction in the line of the deformity.

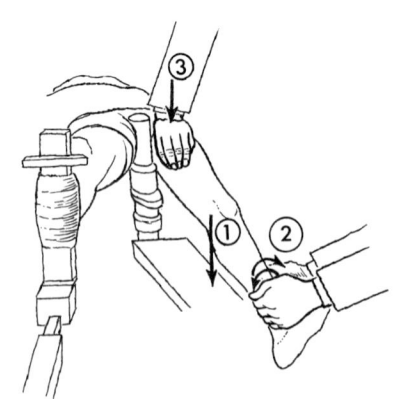

While traction is maintained:
1. Hyperextend the hip and
2. Gently rotate the femur internally and externally to disengage the femoral head; at the same time,
3. An assistant makes direct downward pressure on the femoral head.

Postreduction Management

This is the same as for uncomplicated obturator dislocation.

Unreducible Anterior Dislocation of the Hip (Fresh Dislocation)

REMARKS

An anterior dislocation usually reduces more readily than a posterior dislocation, but in rare instances the usual manipulative maneuvers fail.

This is most commonly due to inappropriate flexion manipulation for pubic dislocation. It also may be due to a penetration of the femoral head into the iliopsoas muscle or buttonholing of the femoral head through the tight iliofemoral ligament.

If after two attempts by appropriate maneuvers the surgeon cannot reduce the anterior dislocation, open reduction should be carried out.

Open reduction should also be employed for any fracture or anterior dislocation of the hip with fragments likely to be entrapped in the joint.

Operative Reduction

1. Begin the incision over the iliac crest 8 cm superior to the anterosuperior iliac spine and continue the incision straight downward on the thigh for 10 cm.
2. Divide the deep fascia over the iliac crest and develop the interval between the tensor fasciae latae and the sartorius muscles.
3. Deepen the incision on the crest to the bone.
4. Reflect by subperiosteal dissection the tensor fasciae latae, gluteus medius, and gluteus minimus muscles from the outer surface of the ilium.
5. Identify and ligate the lateral circumflex artery in the interval between the sartorius and the rectus femoris muscles.
6. Identify and divide the two heads of the origin of the rectus femoris muscle and displace the muscle downward.

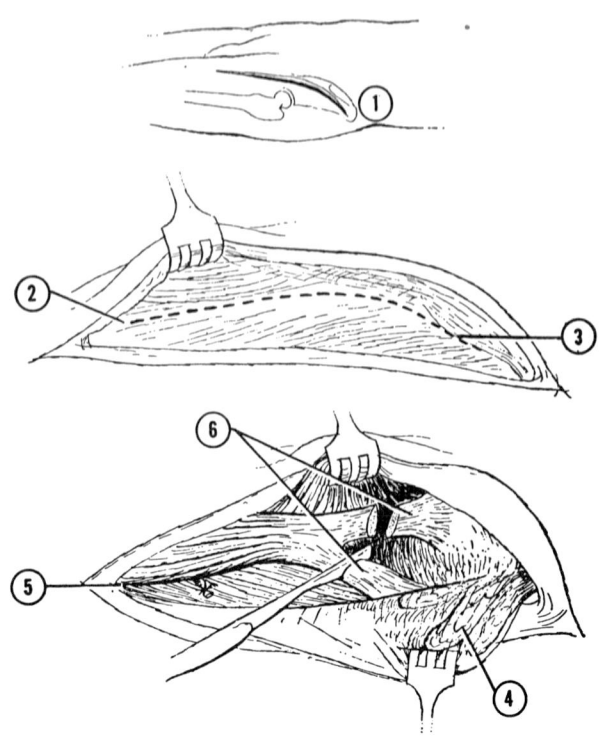

Operative Reduction (Continued)

When the femoral head has pierced the iliopsoas muscle:

1. Divide one limb of the iliopsoas muscle surrounding the neck of the femur; if necessary enlarge the hole in the capsule surrounding the femoral neck.
2. Apply straight longitudinal traction on the limb.

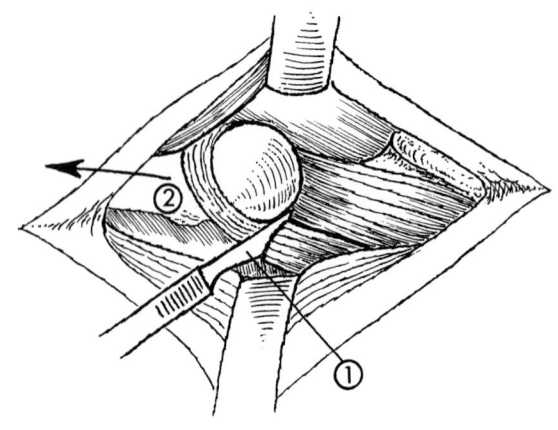

3. While traction is maintained, internally rotate the limb and
4. Apply direct pressure on the head to effect a reduction.

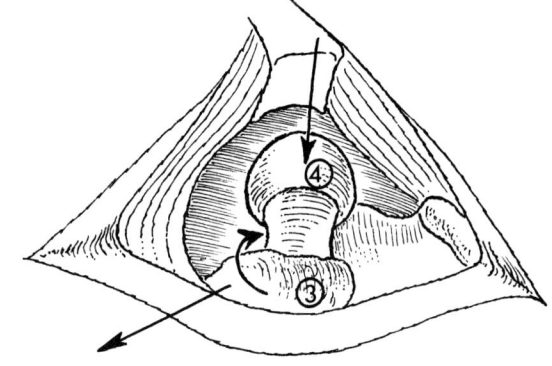

When the head has buttonholed the anterior portion of the capsule:

1. Extend the opening in the capsule proximally and distally.
2. Apply straight longitudinal traction on the limb.

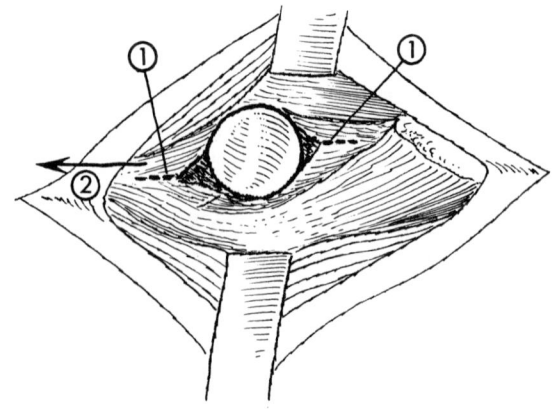

3. While traction is maintained, internally rotate the limb and
4. Apply direct pressure on the head to effect a reduction.

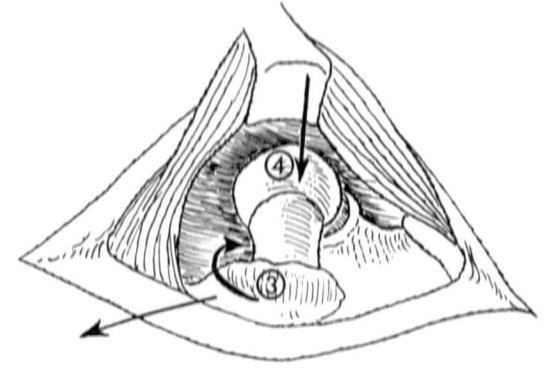

Postoperative Management

This is the same as for uncomplicated anterior dislocation reduced by the closed method.

Old Unreduced Anterior Dislocations of the Hip

REMARKS

Like posterior dislocation, anterior dislocation of the hip may go unrecognized and unreduced.

Occasionally an anterior dislocation may also recur.

In most instances, the chronic unreduced dislocation requires open reduction.

In rare circumstances, as with chronic unreduced posterior dislocation (see page 1309), particularly with fracture of the acetabulum or femoral head, a primary total hip replacement is the reconstructive procedure of choice.

Because of the close proximity of the femoral neurovascular structures, closed reduction by heavy traction is not prudent for a chronic anterior hip dislocation.

ANTERIOR DISLOCATIONS OF THE HIP

Typical Deformity

This patient exhibits a severe deformity of the extremity and trunk.

1. The lumbar lordosis is exaggerated, with scoliosis toward the affected side.
2. Pelvis on the affected side is lower and rolled anteriorly.
3. Limb is abducted and laterally rotated.
4. Hip and knee are flexed.
5. There is apparent lengthening of the limb. (There is actually also some true lengthening.)

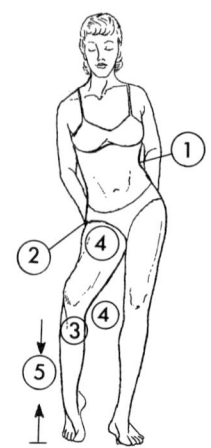

Preoperative X-Ray

1. Acetabulum is empty.
2. Head of the femur is dislocated anteriorly in the obturator position.

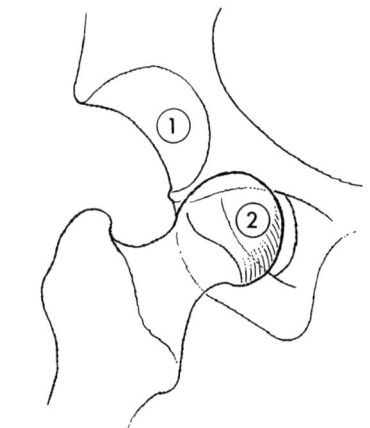

Operative Reduction

The patient is in the supine position with a pack under the affected hip. The leg is draped separately with stockinette.

1. Begin the incision over the iliac crest 2 cm posterior to the anterosuperior spine.
2. Continue the incision over the iliac crest and then downward on the leg in the interval between the tensor fasciae latae and the rectus femoris.

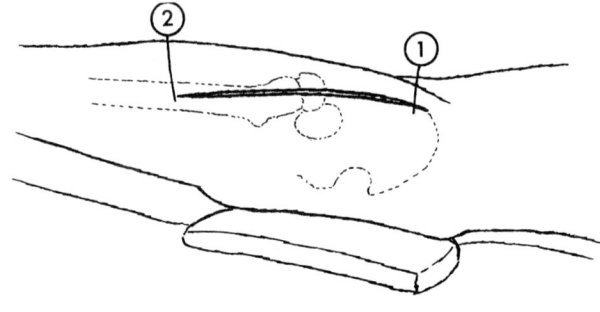

ANTERIOR DISLOCATIONS OF THE HIP

3. Ligate the ascending branch of the lateral femoral circumflex artery and accompanying vein found crossing the wound.

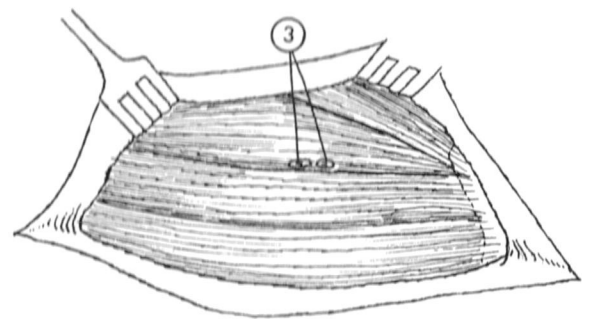

1. Deepen the incision on the iliac crest to the bone, and by subperiosteal dissection reflect the tensor fasciae latae and the gluteus medius and gluteus minimus from the side of the ilium.
2. Isolate and detach the reflected head and the straight head of the rectus femoris.
3. Detach the tendon of the sartorius and the iliopsoas.

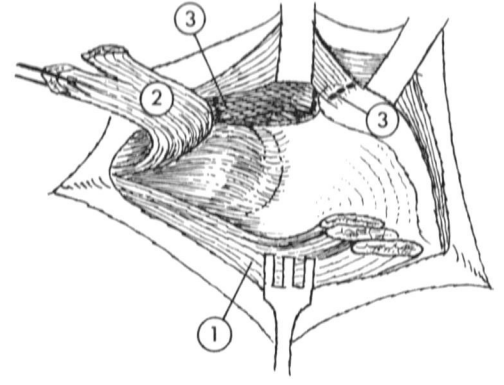

4. Displace all these muscles medially.

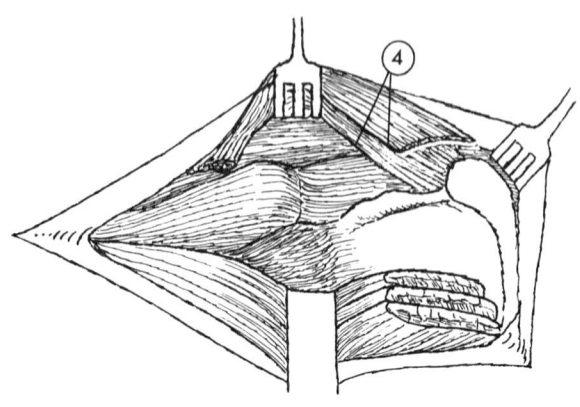

1327

Operative Reduction (Continued)

1. Palpate the femoral head under the pectineus and adductor longus muscles.
2. With a sharp curette excise all fibrous tissue and adherent capsule from the acetabulum.

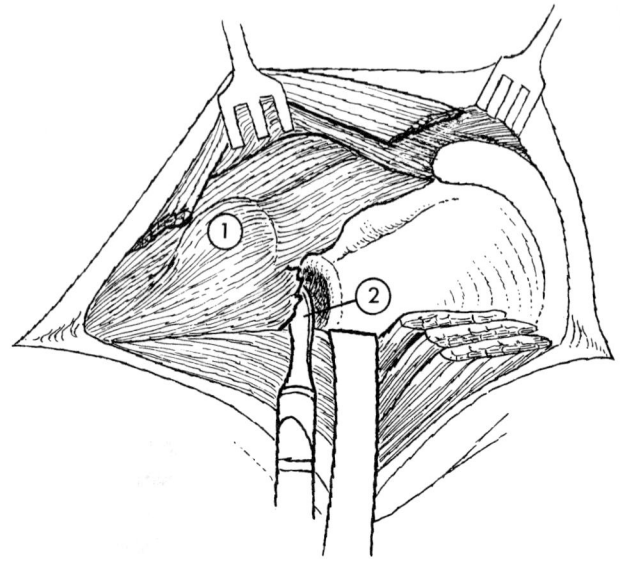

1. Retract medially the pectineus together with the femoral vessels and nerve.
2. Excise all fibrous tissue surrounding and binding the femoral head until the head is freely mobilized.

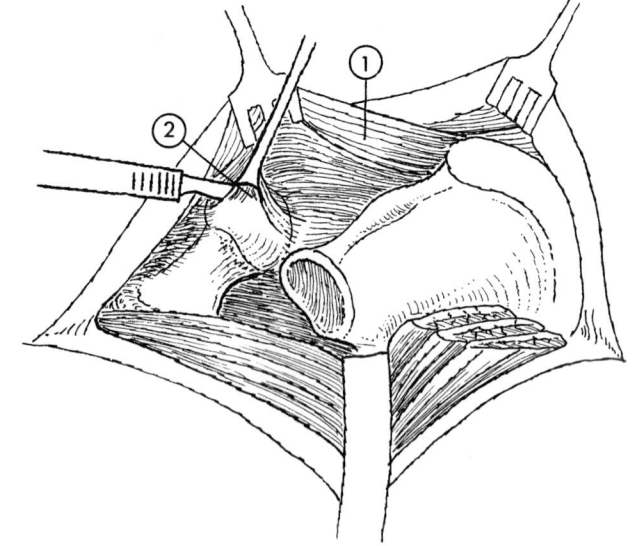

ANTERIOR DISLOCATIONS OF THE HIP

Mobilize the femur further by:
1. Flexing the hip to 90 degrees.
2. Apply traction with the extremity slightly adducted.
3. Internally and externally rotate the femur.

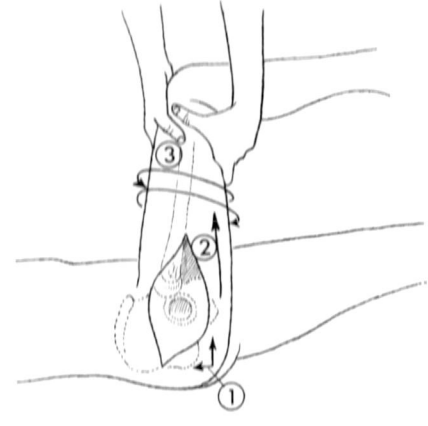

Reduce the dislocation by:
1. Flexing the hip to 90 degrees.
2. Apply traction to the adducted extremity.
3. While traction is maintained, internally rotate the extremity.

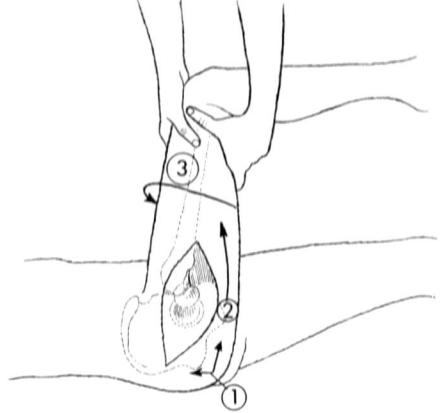

Postreduction X-Ray

1. Head of the femur is seated in the acetabulum.
2. The shaft of the femur is in neutral position.
3. Shenton's line is intact.
4. The lesser trochanter is well visualized.

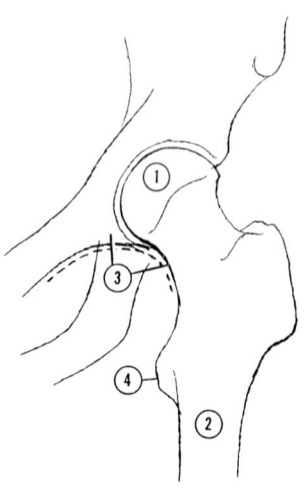

Primary Total Hip Replacement for Chronic Anterior Dislocation

Open reduction of the chronic anterior dislocation is indicated if it is less than three months old.

For chronic dislocations of longer than three months' duration and for dislocations associated with significant fractures of the acetabulum or femoral head, primary total hip replacement becomes the reconstructive procedure of choice (see page 1312).

TRAUMATIC DISLOCATION OF THE HIP IN CHILDREN

REMARKS

Traumatic dislocation of the hip is considerably less common in children than in adults.

In a child younger than 6 years of age, the hip may dislocate with minimal trauma, such as a blow on the back while the child is stooping. Dislocations in this age group are usually reduced without difficulty and without subsequent complications.

In older children, hip dislocation follows more significant trauma, most frequently resulting from athletic injuries, falls from a significant height, or motor vehicle accidents.

Only 15 to 20 per cent of childhood dislocations are associated with fractures of the acetabulum or of the femoral head, indicating the usually less severe mechanism. This is in contrast to adult dislocations, 50 per cent or more of which have some associated fracture.

The outcome of a dislocated hip in a child can be correlated with the severity of the initial injury, particularly as indicated by an associated fracture of the acetabulum or femoral head.

Delay of more than 24 hours prior to reduction also increases the chance of avascular necrosis, particularly if severe trauma produced the injury.

The incidence of avascular necrosis and traumatic arthritis after dislocation in a child is considerably less than after the same injury in the adult.

Prompt, atraumatic closed reduction and selective use of primary open reduction for a dislocation with significant associated fracture or an irreducible dislocation are as important in the treatment in the child as in the adult.

Subsequent to reduction, it is wise to immobilize the active child and to prevent weight bearing. There is some evidence that weight bearing less than two months after reduction may adversely affect the outcome.

TRAUMATIC DISLOCATION OF THE HIP IN CHILDREN

TECHNIQUE OF REDUCTION

Reduction should be atraumatic, and general anesthesia with good muscle relaxation is important.

Rarely, for simple dislocations in the child younger than 6 years, reduction can be accomplished without anesthesia using Stimson's gravity method.

Indications for open reduction in the child are the same as in the adult, namely, significant acetabular or femoral head fracture (see page 1286).

Gravity Method (Stimson's Maneuver)

1. The patient is positioned prone with lower limbs hanging from the end of the table.
2. The pelvis is immobilized by the assistant.
3. The surgeon holds the ankle and flexes the knee of the dislocated limb to 90 degrees while pulling downward several minutes on the dislocated limb.
4. Gentle rocking or rotatory motion of the limb directs the head toward the acetabulum.
5. The assistant pushes the trochanter into the acetabulum to complete the reduction.

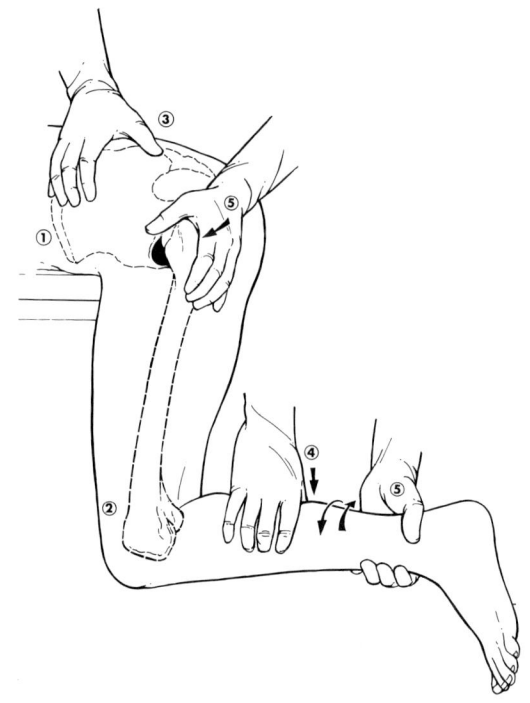

Alternate Method

The child is under general anesthesia.

1. While an assistant presses downward on the anterosuperior spine of the pelvis,
2. Flex the hip to 90 degrees.
3. Make gentle traction upward and inward.

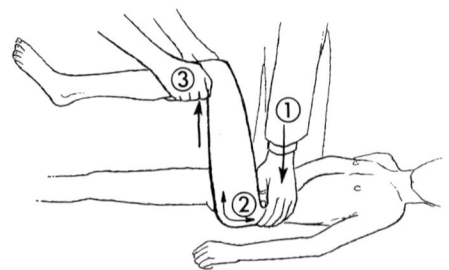

Postreduction X-Ray

1. Femoral head is seated in the acetabulum.

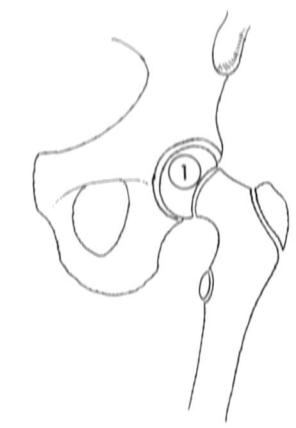

Postreduction Management

Apply a plaster spica.
1. The hip is extended.
2. The extremity is slightly abducted.

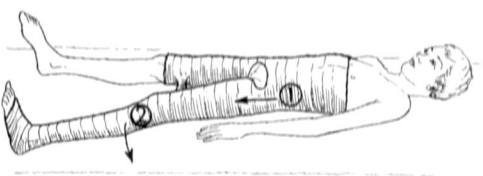

Maintain the plaster spica for 4 to 6 weeks.
After 4 to 6 weeks allow full weight bearing and normal activity; these children need no physical therapy.

or

Apply skin traction to the leg.
1. The hip is extended.
2. Use 1.7 to 4.5 kg (4 to 10 lb) of traction depending on the size of the child.
After 6 weeks permit ambulation on crutches with no weight bearing on the affected extremity.

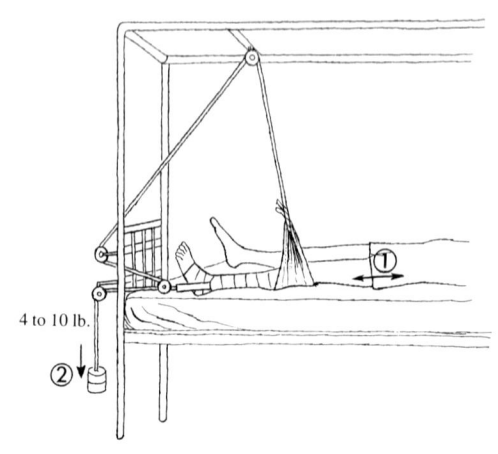

Protect the hip from weight bearing for 2 months from the time of injury.

After 2 months permit partial weight bearing on crutches and then full weight bearing.

Crutches are discarded as soon as the patient feels he has no further need of them.

CAUTION

Follow the child for at least 2 years with periodic x-rays to determine the status of the hip.

Caution the parents that if the child starts complaining of aching in the hip or knee, occasional "giving way," or stiffness, traumatic arthritis or avascular necrosis may be developing.

Avascular necrosis and traumatic arthritis are both less common after hip dislocation in a child than after the same injury in an adult.

FRACTURES OF THE ACETABULUM

REMARKS

The regions of the acetabulum that are most often fractured are three:

1. The superior dome or weight-bearing portion is the most important area. Fractures in this region have the poorest results.
2. The posterior portion or rim of the acetabulum. This area maintains joint stability. Fractures should be sufficiently reduced to prevent redislocation.
3. The inner wall. This is the thinnest portion and the most frequently fractured area of the acetabulum. Disruption of this area has little effect on hip function.

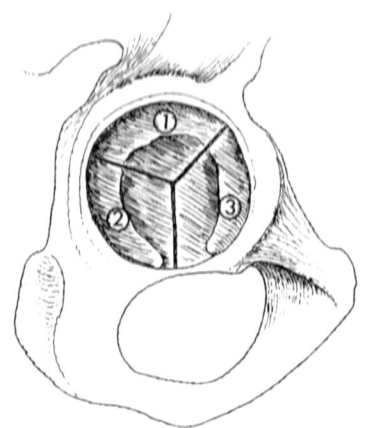

These three areas correspond roughly to the original divisions formed by the triradiate cartilage as the acetabulum develops.

Development of the Acetabulum with Growth

1. Ilium.
2. Ischium.
3. Pubis.
4. Triradiate synchrondrosis.

Note: The three bones meet at the triradiate cartilage in the acetabulum. These three parts roughly correspond to the superior, posterior, and anterior segments of the acetabulum that are involved in fractures of the acetabulum.

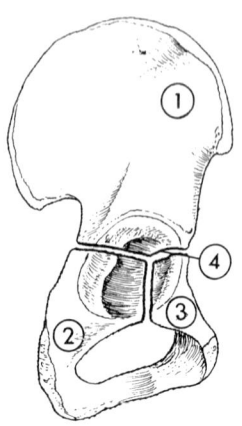

FRACTURES OF THE ACETABULUM

Mechanisms of Injury

The mechanism of injury generally determines the nature of the fracture.

1. A fall on the greater trochanter produces
2. A linear fracture of the acetabulum or
3. A complete fracture of the inner wall with varying degrees of intrapelvic protrusion.

Note: This is the most common mechanism and type of acetabular fracture.

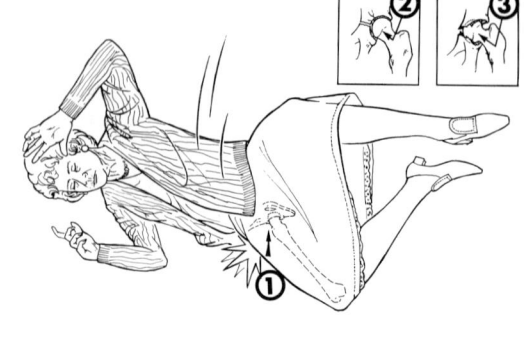

1. A force applied to the long axis of the femur with the knee and hip flexed produces
2. A posterior acetabular fracture or fracture-dislocation as the hip is adducting and flexing or

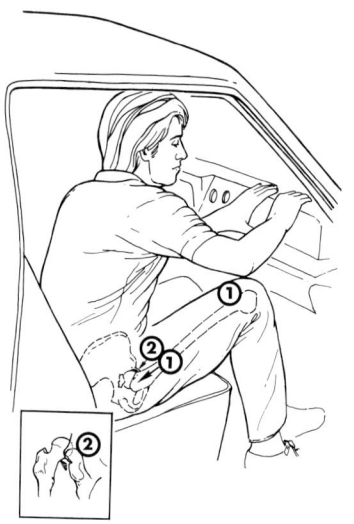

3. A fracture of the superior dome or bursting fracture as the hip is abducting and extending.

These are the most serious acetabular fractures and are likely to cause the poorest results.

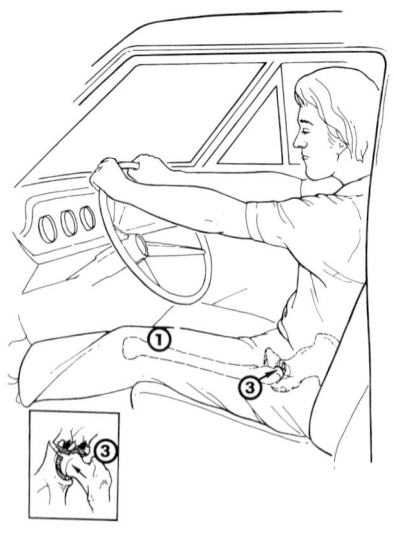

X-Ray Technique

Complete radiographic assessment is essential to determine the extent of the acetabular fracture.
1. The injured patient lies supine.
2. A right oblique view and
3. A left oblique view help to visualize all the acetabular fractures.

Note: Tomography of the acetabulum is also necessary prior to embarking on any operative intervention in these comminuted fractures.

Computerized tomography, if available, may be very helpful for ascertaining the extent of the fracture.

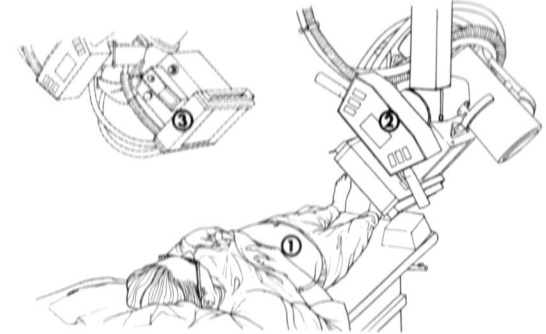

Linear Fractures of the Acetabulum

Remarks

This lesion is usually the result of a blow of minimal intensity on the lateral aspect of the greater trochanter.

In general the prognosis is good; complications such as aseptic necrosis, traumatic arthritis, and myositis ossificans are rarely encountered.

Mechanism of Injury

1. Blow on the lateral aspect of the trochanter.
2. Linear undisplaced fractures of the acetabulum.

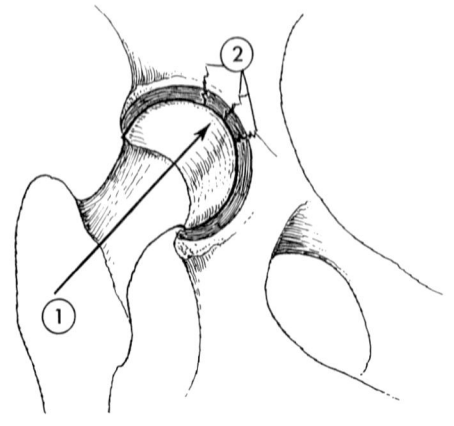

FRACTURES OF THE ACETABULUM

Appearance on X-Ray

1. The fracture is readily demonstrable by anteroposterior x-ray.

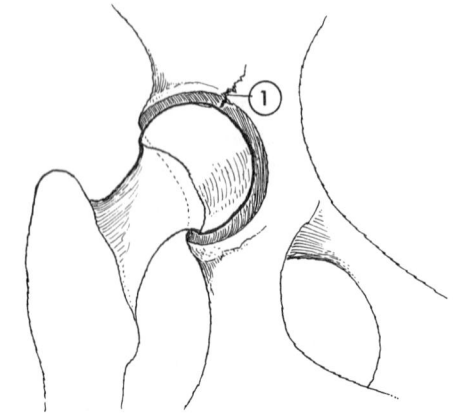

Immobilization

Apply skin traction.
The hip is extended.
Apply 2 to 3 kg (4.5 to 6.5 lb) of weight.

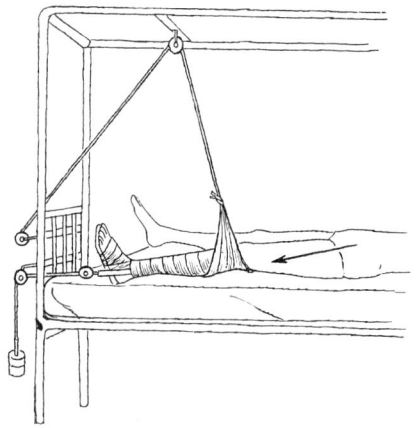

Management

Maintain traction for 1 to 2 weeks.
Start skateboard abduction exercises during the first or second week to maintain motion in the hip joint.

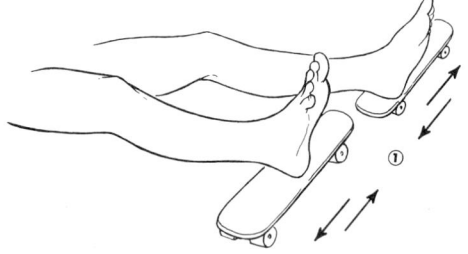

Pain usually disappears within 3 to 6 weeks.
Most patients may be out of bed and using crutches by the third week.
Crutches and external support can usually be discarded by the tenth week.
Recheck the patient with x-rays approximately every 4 to 6 months for 2 years following the injury.
Most of these injuries heal without residual complications.

Fracture of the Posterior Acetabulum

REMARKS

Fractures of the posterior acetabulum are usually associated with posterior dislocation. They may be merely small fractures of the rim or sizable fractures of a larger portion of the posterior wall, which cause instability.

These fractures most often result from a severe blow to the anterior aspect of the knee with the knee and hip flexing. This is the same mechanism that produces a Type II or Type III posterior fracture-dislocation.

It is important to recognize the true nature of this problem. Frequently a standard anteroposterior x-ray will not demonstrate the size of the acetabular fracture or any significant posterior instability of the hip.

Oblique views are always needed to visualize the area of disruption adequately.

The major factors likely to cause a poor result after a posterior acetabular fracture are:
1. Persistent instability of the hip.
2. A delay in reduction of an associated hip dislocation.
3. Femoral head damage.

Primary open reduction of the injury is indicated when there is a Type II or Type III posterior dislocation. Exploration of the hip is necessary in these injuries to remove abrasive, loose osteocartilaginous fragments, as described on page 1286.

Open reduction is also indicated when the posterior fragment must be reduced and fixed to restore joint stability.

Because of its close proximity to the posterior acetabulum, the sciatic nerve is involved in about 35 per cent of these fractures. Most often, the injury stretches the peroneal branch. Spontaneous recovery may be anticipated.

When both the tibial and peroneal components are involved or when the palsy is delayed for several days, operative exploration is indicated for neurolysis because the nerve is likely to be entrapped at the fracture site (see page 1290).

Types of Posterior Acetabular Fractures

1. An acetabular rim fracture was not adequately visualized on a standard anteroposterior x-ray owing to position of femoral head.

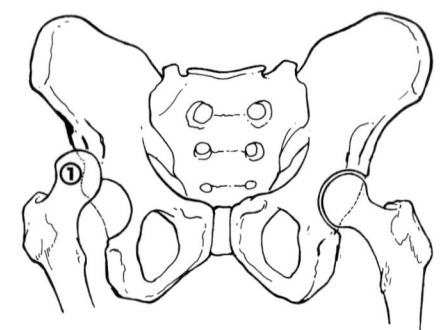

2. An oblique x-ray showed a large displaced fragment, which required operative reduction and fixation for hip stability.

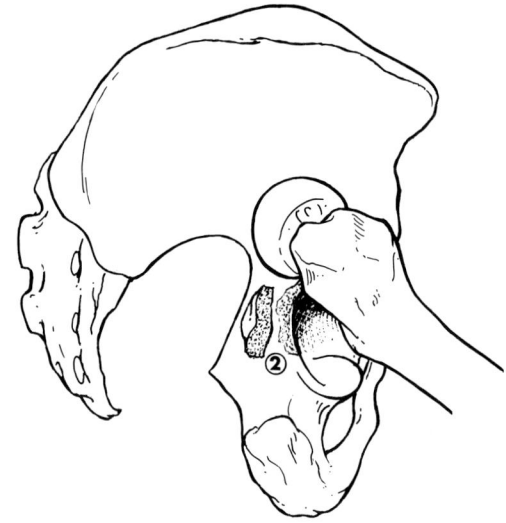

1. A Type III dislocation with comminuted fracture of the posterior acetabulum should be treated by operative reduction, as described on page 1286.
2. Outcome depends on minimizing damage to the femoral head, by removing intra-articular loose fragments, and stabilizing the posterior rim.

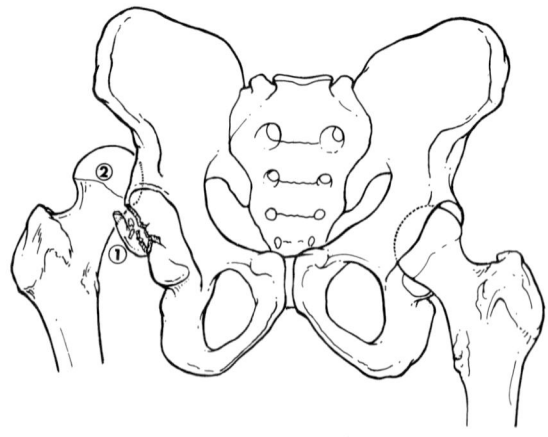

Immobilization

Apply skin traction.
The hip is extended.
Apply 2 to 3 kg (4.5 to 6.5 lb) of weight.

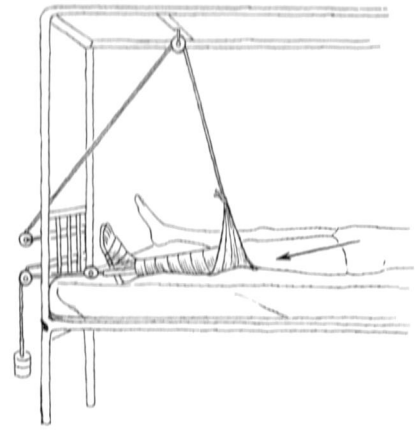

Subsequent Management

Maintain traction for 2 to 3 weeks.
Start skateboard abduction exercises during the first or second week to maintain motion in the hip joint.

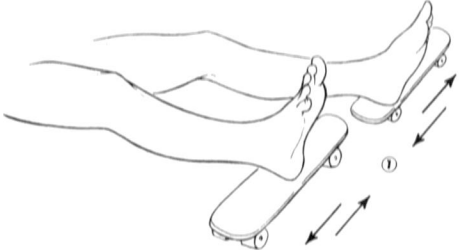

Pain usually disappears within 3 to 6 weeks.
Most patients may be out of bed and using crutches by the third week.
Crutches and external support can usually be discarded by the third week.
Recheck the patient with x-rays approximately every 4 to 6 months for two years following the injury.
Most of these injuries heal without residual complications.

POSTERIOR ACETABULAR FRACTURE WITH LARGE FRAGMENT OR POSTERIORLY UNSTABLE HIP

Prereduction X-Ray

1. X-ray of the hip in flexion shows instability posteriorly.
2. The lesser trochanter is not visualized owing to internal rotation from the dislocation.
3. The posterior fragment requires prompt stabilization, and the joint should be explored as described on page 1286.

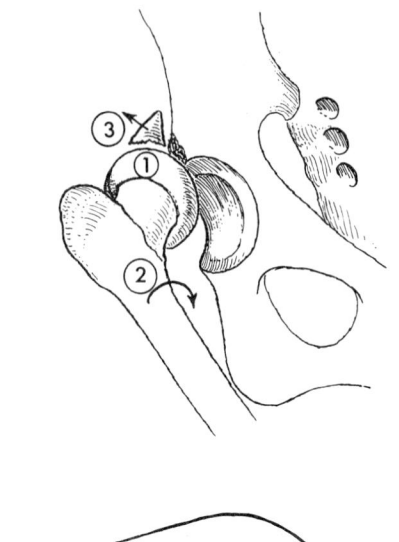

Postreduction X-Ray

1. The posterior acetabular fragment has been stabilized with two screws.
2. Flexion of the hip no longer produces posterior subluxation.

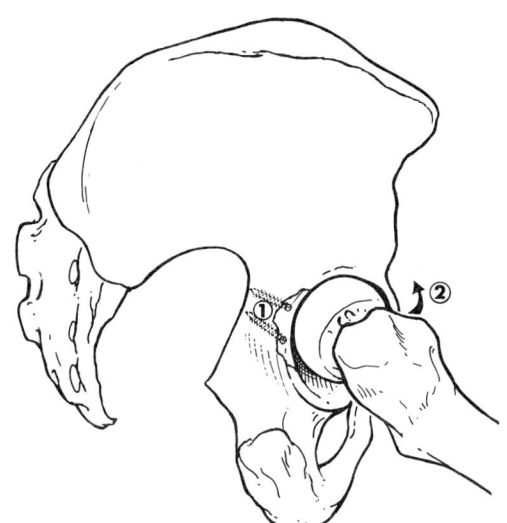

Subsequent Management

Immobilize the patient in traction for 4 weeks to permit healing of the disrupted soft tissues.

During immobilization, start aspirin, 3 grams daily in divided doses, since this has been demonstrated to protect against traumatic arthritis and appears to diminish the incidence of thromboembolism.

The patient may start active abduction exercises while in traction to regain full hip motion.

After 4 weeks discontinue traction and start progressive weight bearing on crutches. There is no evidence that early weight bearing increases the incidence of traumatic arthritis or avascular necrosis, provided that the reduction has restored normal articular surfaces and there are no abrasive fragments within the joint.

Follow-up after repair of an unstable hip should be at least two years, although most complications will be manifested within the first year.

Advise the patient that signs of aching or stiffness in the hip or knee or occasional "giving way" may be the first indications of traumatic arthritis or avascular necrosis.

The outcome should be good if the hip was stabilized promptly and there was no damage to the femoral head.

Fracture of the Inner Acetabular Wall

REMARKS

This is the most common type of acetabular fracture because of the thinness of the inner wall, particularly in the elderly.

Most often the mechanism is a direct blow to the greater trochanter.

The intrapelvic protrusion of the femoral head may range from minor to severe.

The vast majority of the injuries, even with severe protrusion, can be treated by closed methods with good to excellent results.

It is not necessary to reduce the displaced acetabular wall provided that the femoral head is restored to its proper position and is held under a stable superior acetabular dome.

Open reduction of these injuries is not only difficult but usually without benefit.

For any protrusion, primary manipulation should be done under anesthesia. The head can be reduced by adducting the lower limb so as to pull the protruding head out from the acetabulum.

Skeletal traction can then be used to maintain the reduction until redisplacement does not occur.

If the acetabular fracture is comminuted and, particularly, if any of the weight-bearing dome surface is involved, traction should be prolonged for 12 weeks.

Sciatic nerve palsy may occur with this injury, but it is less common than with posterior acetabular fractures and usually does not require operative exploration of the nerve. Stretch injury of the nerve usually recovers spontaneously.

FRACTURES OF THE ACETABULUM

Initial X-Ray

1. Inner wall fracture of the acetabulum without protrusion.
2. Superior dome of the acetabulum is intact.
3. Femoral head and dome are in normal relationship.

Note: This fracture needs no manipulative reduction.

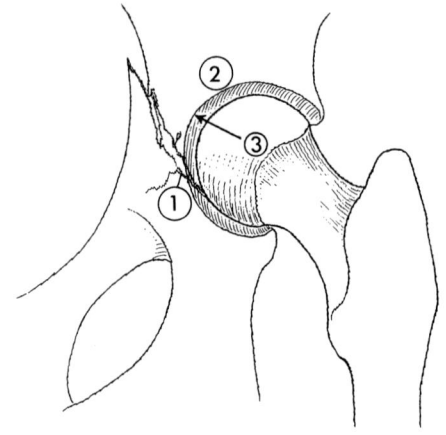

Immobilization

Apply skin traction.
The hip is extended and the leg is slightly abducted.

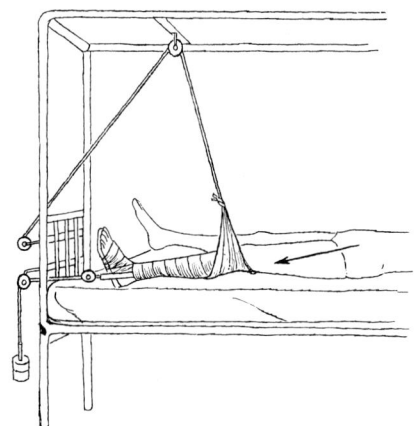

Subsequent Management

Maintain traction for 2 to 3 weeks.
Start skateboard abduction exercises during the first or second week to maintain motion in the hip joint.

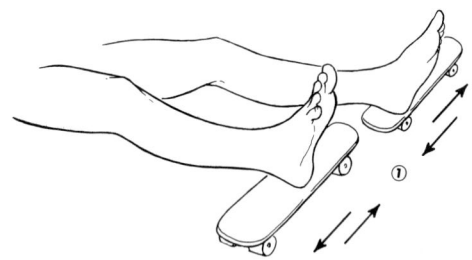

Pain usually disappears within 3 to 6 weeks.
Most patients may be out of bed and using crutches by the third week.
Crutches and external support can usually be discarded by the tenth week.
Recheck the patient with x-rays approximately every 4 to 6 months for 2 years following the injury.
Most of these injuries heal without residual complications.

FRACTURE OF INNER ACETABULAR WALL WITH INTRAPELVIC PROTRUSION OF THE FEMORAL HEAD

Prereduction X-ray

MODERATE PROTRUSION

1. Fracture of the inner wall with inward displacement.
2. Fracture of the pubic rami.
3. Femoral head is displaced inward.
4. Acetabular dome is intact.

Note: This fracture must be reduced so that the femoral head and the acetabular dome are in normal relationship.

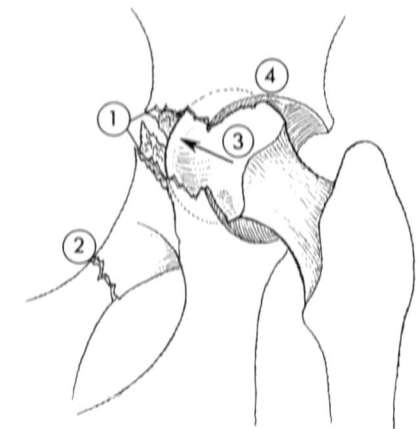

MARKED PROTRUSION

1. Fracture of the inner wall with severe inward displacement.
2. Fracture of both pubic rami.
3. Severe intrapelvic protrusion of the femoral head.
4. The acetabular dome is intact.

Note: This unstable fracture must be reduced and reduction then maintained by longitudinal and lateral traction.

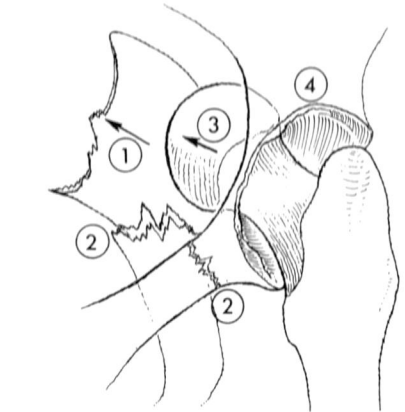

Closed Reduction: Lipscomb Technique

Under general anesthesia,
1. The patient is turned on the uninjured side.
2. Side traction is applied using triangulated pins that penetrate both cortices of the femur in the subtrochanteric region.
3. A folded pillow bolster is placed between the thighs.
4. The injured hip is adducted to pull the femoral head out of the acetabulum while traction is applied to the trochanter.

Note: The pins for lateral traction should not enter the synovial space of the hip. It is the scissoring effect of the pins, which are crossed and wired or tied snugly together, that prevents them from pulling out.

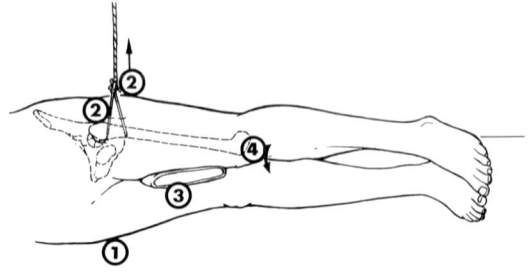

Maintenance of Reduction

1. Heavy traction of up to 13 kg (27 lb) is applied to the triangulated pins. The position of the pins prevents them from falling out.
2. Traction of 9 to 13 kg (20 to 27 lb) is applied to the distal femoral pin.

Note: The amount of traction depends on the size of the patient and the degree of displacement.

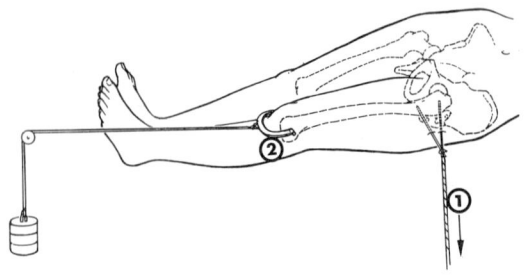

Postreduction X-Ray

1. Some persistent displacement of the inner acetabular wall will not affect hip function.
2. The femoral head is seated under the dome in normal position.

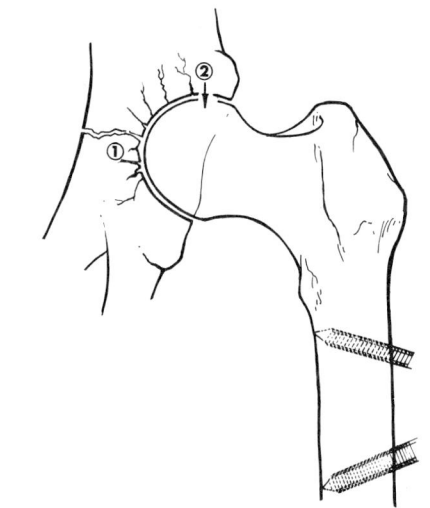

Subsequent Management

1. Gradually decrease the traction to 3 kg (6.5 lb) of lateral pull and
2. 6 to 7 kg (13 to 15 lb) of distal femoral pull by four weeks.
3. Permit active range of motion, particularly abduction exercises to the hip and flexion exercises to the knee.
4. A splint such as the Fry exercise splint* is useful for permitting abduction exercises while maintaining traction.

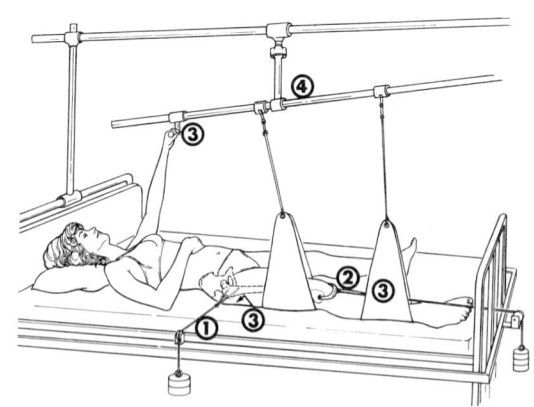

---

*Available from Orthopaedic Equipment Corporation, Bourbon, Indiana 46504.

Continue the traction for twelve weeks to permit complete healing of the inner wall.

Shorter periods of traction are associated with poorer results.

During immobilization, give the patient aspirin, 3 grams a day in divided doses, since this has been shown to protect against traumatic arthritis and appears to diminish the incidence of thromboembolism.

After 12 weeks, traction may be discontinued and the patient may be allowed up on crutches with partial weight bearing.

Full weight bearing is generally possible by 4 to 6 months.

Fractures of the Superior Acetabular Dome

REMARKS

Fractures of the superior dome may range from types that leave the relationship between the dome and femoral head undisturbed to those that completely disrupt the entire acetabulum.

Because of the usually strong superior acetabular structure, these injuries must be caused by major trauma.

The overall results of these fractures are the poorest of all acetabular injuries; however, long-term clinical results frequently are considerably better than indicated by radiographic appearance.

Among the prime determinants of end result is the amount of damage inflicted on the femoral articular surface. This cannot be changed by even the most anatomic operative fixation of the acetabular fracture.

Treatment should be directed at preventing further damage to the femoral articular surface. This can usually be accomplished by heavy femoral traction to decrease surface contact and by early non-weight-bearing motion to remold the articular fibrocartilage.

The fractured articular surface should be treated as an autoarthroplasty. Non-weight-bearing abduction motion can remodel the polymerizing scar tissue of the damaged articular surface and encourage fibrocartilage formation.

Closed reduction and heavy skeletal traction can usually restore the congruity of the acetabular dome sufficiently to prevent abrasive wear on the femoral surface.

Even if closed reduction is incomplete, open reduction should be attempted only if the fragments are sufficiently large to be manipulated and fixed as necessary to restore congruity.

In general, the results from operative treatment are no better than with skeletal traction and early abduction exercise. The risk of a bad result from operation is high, particularly when the fracture is managed by a surgeon who rarely operates on this severe fracture. Postoperative infection has been as high as 26 per cent in some series.

Prior to the development of total hip replacement, the surgical risk might have been worthwhile. It is now imperative to avoid infection so that total hip replacement may still be offered to the symptomatic patient.

Mechanism of Injury

For fracture of the dome of the acetabulum (as an isolated lesion):
1. The femur is almost completely extended.
2. Force is transmitted directly upward onto the dome of the acetabulum.
3. A large fragment of the dome is sheared off and is displaced upward and slightly backward.
4. The femoral head is dislocated upward.

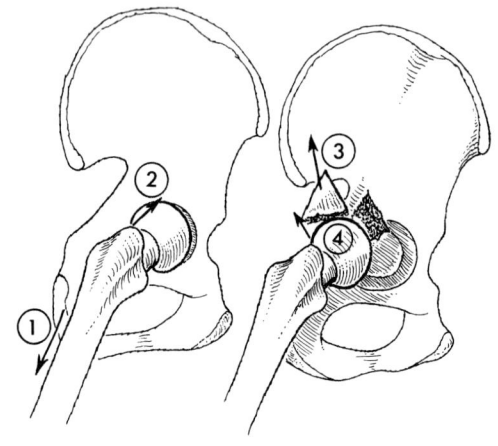

For superior and bursting fractures of the acetabulum (the dome is preserved):
1. Femur is almost completely extended and slightly abducted.
2. Force is transmitted upward and inward onto the acetabulum.
3. The superior dome is intact.
4. Fracture of the posterior portion of the acetabulum.
5. Fracture of the inner wall.

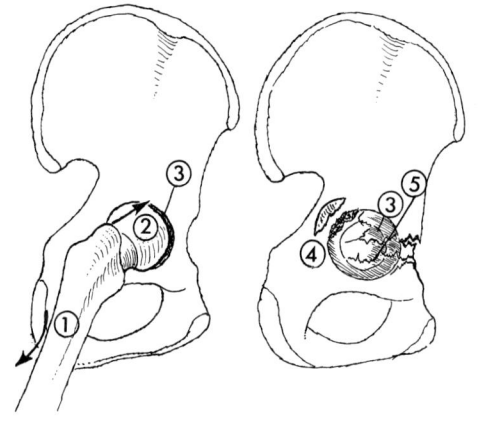

or
1. The dome is comminuted.
2. The inner wall is disrupted.
3. The femoral head is displaced inward.

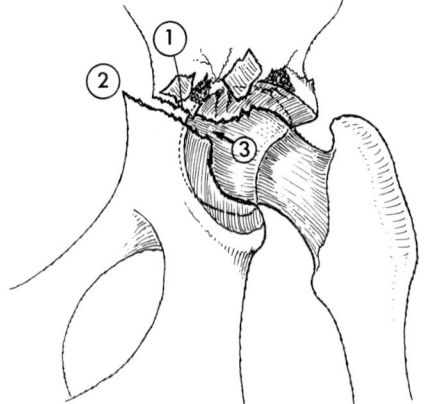

or
1. The dome is comminuted.
2. The inner wall is markedly disrupted.
3. The femoral head is displaced inward.
4. Fracture of the superior and inferior pubic rami.

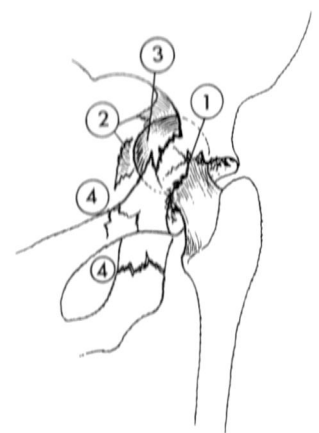

MANAGEMENT OF SUPERIOR DOME FRACTURE OR BURSTING FRACTURE WITHOUT DISPLACEMENT

The superior dome and the femoral head are in normal relationship.

Appearance on X-Ray

1. Fracture of the superior dome without displacement.
2. Femoral head is in normal relationship with articular surface of the dome.
3. Fracture of the inner wall.

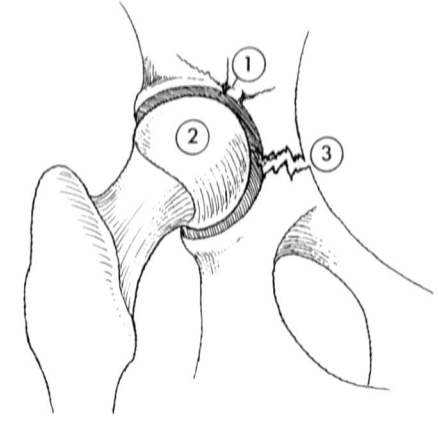

or
1. Fracture of the superior dome without displacement.
2. Fracture of posterior rim in acceptable position.
3. Fracture of inner wall.

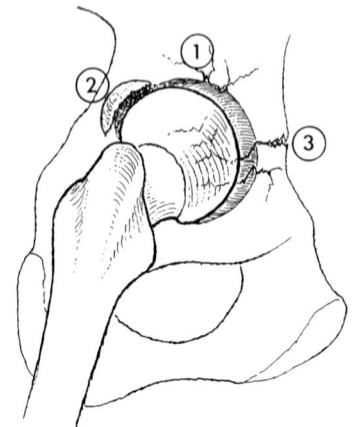

Reduction

These fractures need no reduction.

Immobilization

Apply skin traction.
The hip is extended.
Apply 2 to 3 kg (4.5 to 6.5 lb) of weight.

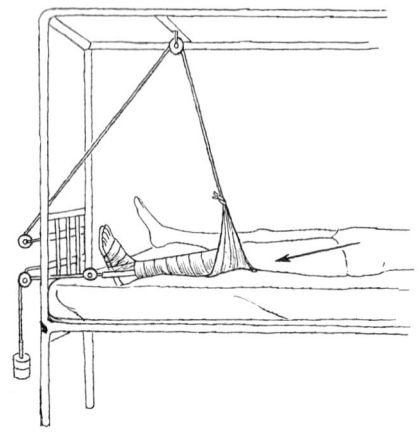

Subsequent Management

While the patient is in traction, start aspirin, 3 grams daily in divided doses. Aspirin has been shown to protect against degenerative arthritis and appears to diminish the risk of thromboembolism after hip procedures.

Maintain traction for 6 weeks. This is longer than with undisplaced linear acetabular fractures because the weight-bearing surface is involved.

During this period start skateboard abduction exercises and active exercises for the quadriceps.

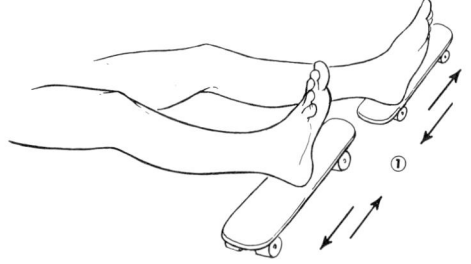

After 6 weeks, permit crutch walking without bearing weight on the affected limb.

After 12 to 16 weeks, depending on the severity of the particular surface injury, permit progressive weight bearing on the affected limb.

Normally the patient may return to full weight bearing by 6 months.

The majority of these patients regain normal hip function without any residual osteoarthritis or avascular necrosis; however they should be followed for at least 2 years after injury.

The major determinant of outcome is the amount of damage to the femoral head rather than the acetabular fracture.

MANAGEMENT OF SUPERIOR DOME FRACTURE OR BURSTING FRACTURES WITH DISPLACEMENT OR COMMINUTION OF THE SUPERIOR DOME

REMARKS

Closed manipulative reduction with a 12-week period of traction can be effective management of these difficult injuries.

Accurate anatomic reduction is not the primary determinant of a satisfactory result. Frequently the clinical result after these injuries is considerably better than expected on the basis of radiographic evidence.

Closed reduction can achieve close to normal acetabular-femoral head relationships. Only rarely, if closed reduction leaves large displaced acetabular fragments that abrade the femoral head, open reduction can be of some value.

Prereduction X-Ray

1. The acetabular dome is comminuted.
2. The inner wall is disrupted.
3. The femoral head is protruding.
4. The superior and inferior pubic rami are fractured.

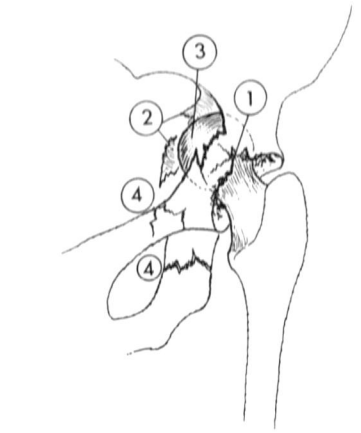

Technique of Closed Reduction (After Lipscomb)

Under general anesthesia,
1. The patient is turned on the uninjured side.
2. Side traction is applied using triangulated pins that penetrate both cortices of the femur in the subtrochanteric region.
3. A folded pillow bolster is placed between the thighs.
4. The injured hip is adducted to pull the femoral head out of the acetabulum while traction is applied to the trochanter.

Note: The pins for lateral traction should not enter the synovial space of the hip. It is the scissoring effect of the pins, which are crossed and wired or tied snugly together, that prevents them from pulling out.

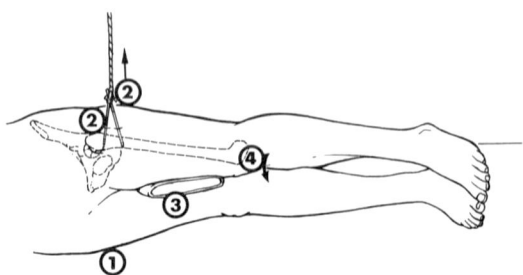

Maintenance of Reduction

1. Heavy traction of up to 13 kg (29 lb) is applied to the triangulated pins. The position of the pins prevents them from falling out.
2. 9 to 13 kg (20 to 29 lb) of traction is applied to the distal femoral pin.

Note: The amount of traction depends on the size of the patient and the degree of displacement.

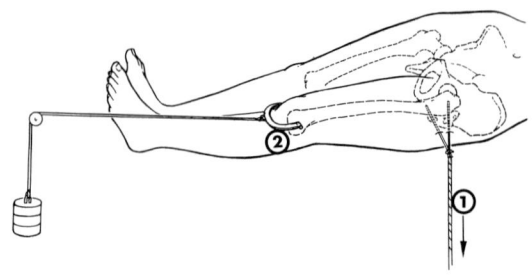

Postreduction X-Ray

1. The acetabular dome remains comminuted but
2. There is a fairly normal relationship between the dome and the femoral head.
3. The femoral head has been pulled back under the dome.
4. The inner wall remains disrupted.

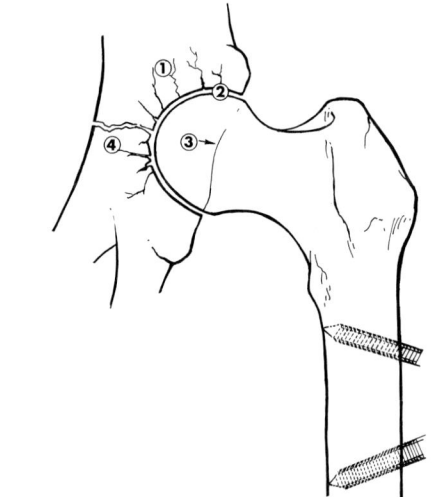

Postreduction Management

1. Gradually decrease the traction to 3 kg (6.6 lb) of lateral pull and
2. 6 to 7 kg (13 to 15.5 lb) of distal femoral pull by 4 weeks.
3. Permit active range of motion, particularly abduction exercises of the hip and flexion exercises to the knee.
4. The Fry exercise splint* is useful for permitting abduction exercise while maintaining traction.

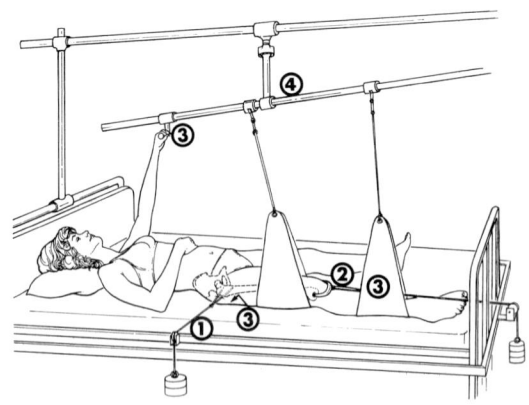

---

*Available from Orthopaedic Equipment Corporation, Bourbon, Indiana 46504.

FRACTURES OF THE ACETABULUM

Continue the traction for 12 weeks to permit complete healing of the inner wall.

Shorter periods of traction are associated with poorer results.

During immobilization, give the patient aspirin, 3 grams a day in divided doses, which has been shown to protect against traumatic arthritis and appears to diminish the incidence of thromboembolism.

After 12 weeks, traction may be discontinued and the patient may be allowed up on crutches with partial weight bearing.

Full weight bearing is generally possible by 4 to 6 months.

OPERATIVE FIXATION OF SUPERIOR DOME FRACTURES

REMARKS

Operative intervention should only be utilized if it is likely to improve results significantly over closed reduction with adequate skeletal traction.

Surgical fixation is usually necessary when the dome fracture consists of a few loose, large fragments that cause hip instability or are displaced sufficiently to abrade the femoral articular surface.

Internal fixation is not needed to stabilize an inner wall fracture associated with the dome fracture. The inner wall injury has minimal effect on hip function.

Comminuted dome fractures are not candiates for internal fixation.

If a femoral head deteriorates after the injury, total hip replacement should be offered the patient when fracture of the subchondral bone consolidates. The need for total hip replacement should be determined only on the basis of the patient's pain not radiographic changes.

Indications and Limitations of Operative Fixation

POSTREDUCTION X-RAY

1. A large fragment of the dome is displaced superiorly and posteriorly.
2. The femoral head is unstable.

Note: Fixation of this dome fracture will help to stabilize the hip joint.

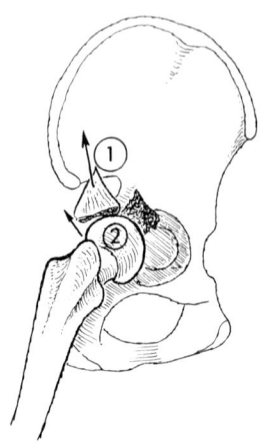

Indications and Limitations of Operative Fixation (Continued)

Preoperative x-ray (after attempted closed reduction)

1. A triangular fragment has been turned 180 degrees.
2. Incongruity of the articular surface persists despite skeletal traction, and the displaced fragment abrades the femoral head.

Note: Operative fixation is indicated here to prevent further damage to the femoral articular surface.

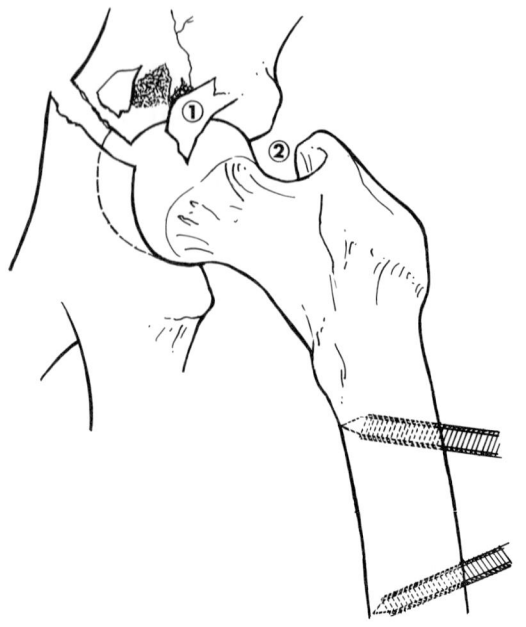

Prereduction x-ray

1. The dome is comminuted sufficiently to prevent adequate internal fixation.
2. The inner wall is disrupted, but this should not impair hip function.
3. The femoral head is protruding inward.

Note: Because of the comminuted acetabular dome, internal fixation is unlikely to improve the result. Closed reduction and heavy skeletal traction are preferred.

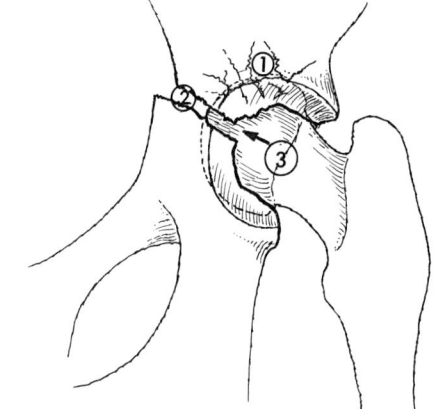

Operative Procedure

1. The patient is in the lateral position. Begin the skin incision 5 cm distal and lateral to the posterior superior iliac spine and extend it distally, paralleling the fibers of the gluteus maximus muscle, to the posterior superior aspect of the greater trochanter. Continue the incision distally for 8 cm in line with the posterior border of the trochanter.

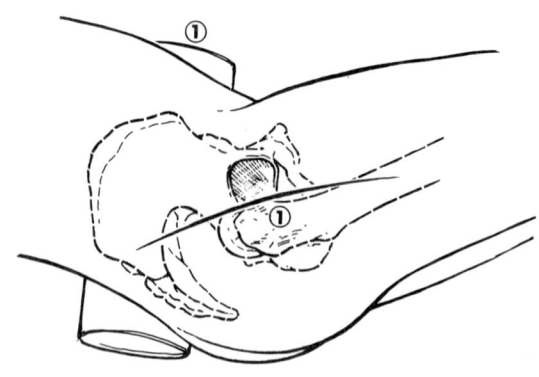

2. Deepen the incision through the gluteus maximus muscle by separating its fibers parallel to the skin incision.

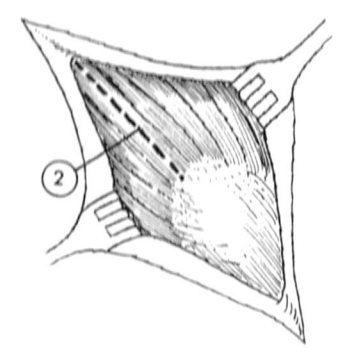

3. Divide the insertion of the gluteus maximus into the fascia lata for 5 cm in line with the vertical limb of the skin incision.

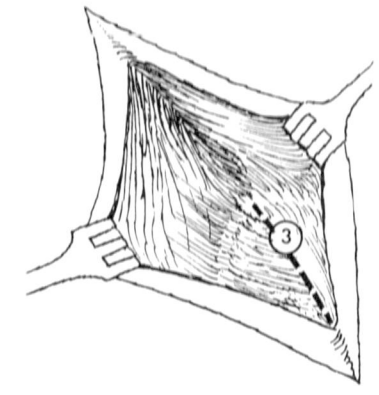

1. Visualize the sciatic nerve.
2. Sever the tendons of the piriformis, gemelli, and obturator internus muscles at their sites of insertion into the greater trochanter.

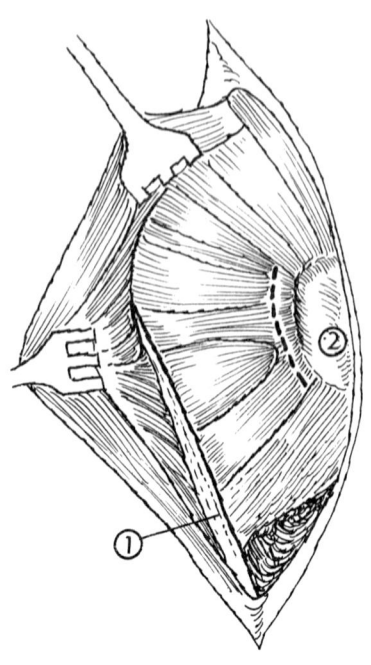

Operative Procedure (Continued)

3. Retract the rotator muscles posteriorly together with the sciatic nerve. This brings into view:
4. The femoral head.
5. Disrupted capsule.
6. Detached fragment of the dome.
7. Raw surface of the superior portion of the acetabulum.

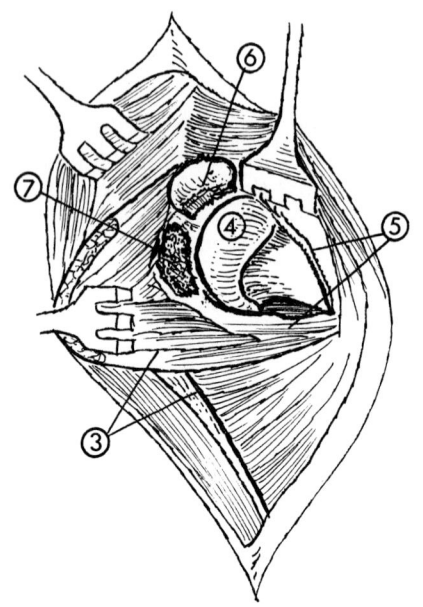

1. Insert a flat blade retractor into the pelvis opposite the acetabulum between the greater sciatic notch and the ischial spine.
2. By subperiosteal dissection reflect the gluteus minimum muscle superiorly. This brings into view:
3. Superior and posterior portions of the acetabulum.

Note: Beyond this stage of the operation, the technique depends upon the pathologic condition found.

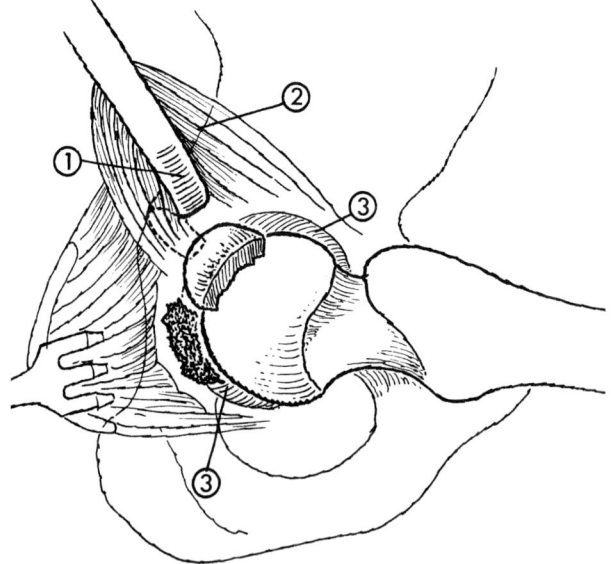

For single bony fragment

When the lesion comprises a large single bony fragment, clean the raw surfaces of the detached fragment and the acetabulum of any debris.

1. Replace the fragment in its anatomic position.
2. Fix it to the ilium with one or two screws.
3. Direct the screws obliquely upward to engage the thick portion of the ilium.

Note: If the hip was dislocated or subluxated superiorly, explore the joint thoroughly and irrigate thoroughly for loose bodies. Evaluate range of motion and joint stability on the table and obtain an intraoperative x-ray to assess the position of the screws.

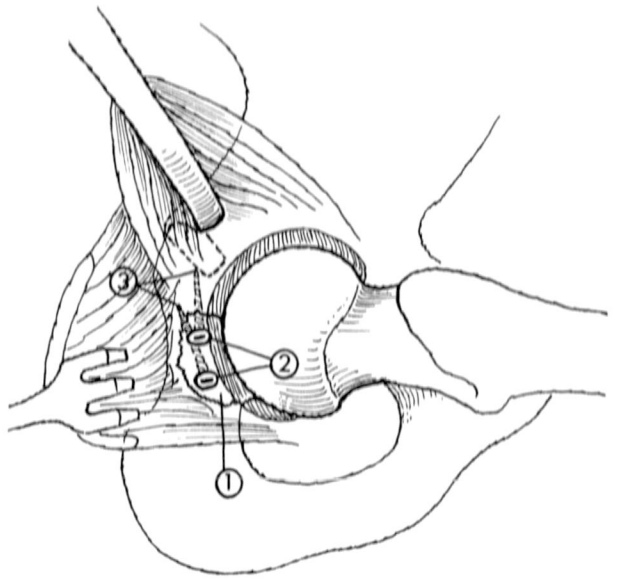

Intraoperative x-ray

1. The large acetabular fragment is reduced and fixed with two screws.
2. The head and roof of the acetabulum are congruous.

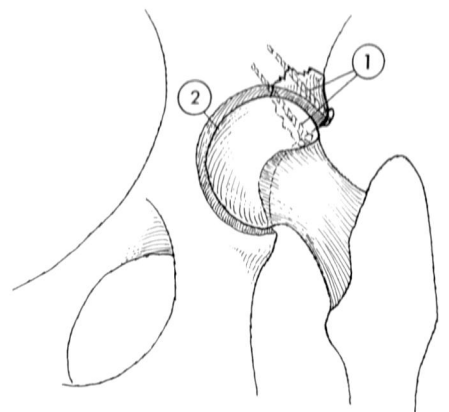

Operative Procedure (Continued)

For several fragments

When the displaced dome comprises several fragments,
1. If there is some inward displacement of the head, make traction on the femur downward and laterally. (The head must be concentrically reduced).
2. Reassemble the large fragments. (Small loose fragments can be discarded; large fragments must be replaced).
3. Fix them in the anatomic position to the ilium with screws. (Inspect the femoral head. Remove all small fragments of bone and cartilage that lie in the joint and might interfere with accurate reduction.)

Note: Assess range of motion of the hip on the operating table and obtain intraoperative x-rays to evaluate the position of the screws.

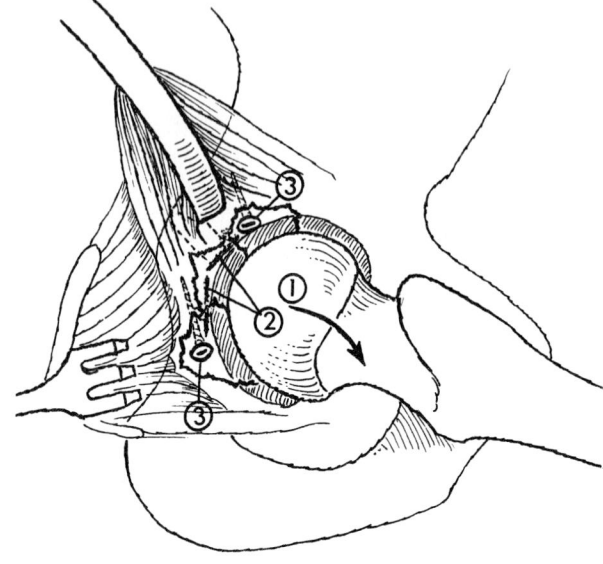

Intraoperative x-ray

1. The acetabular fragments are reassembled and fixed to the ilium with screws.
2. The femoral head and roof of the acetabulum are in normal relationship.
3. The fracture of the inner wall is not completely reduced; this is of no significance.

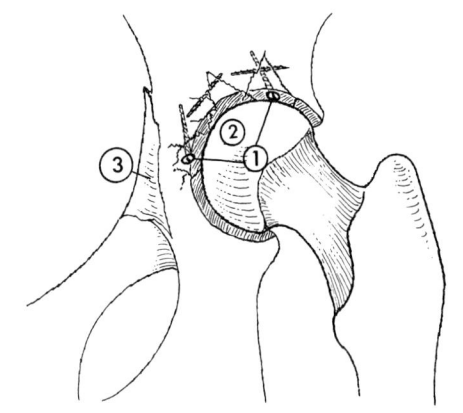

Immobilization

Apply skeletal traction.
1. Insert a threaded pin in the distal femur.
2. Place the limb in a thigh splint or a similar device that allows abduction exercises.
3. The hip and knee are extended.
4. Apply 10 to 12 kg (22 to 26 lb) to maintain the joint space.

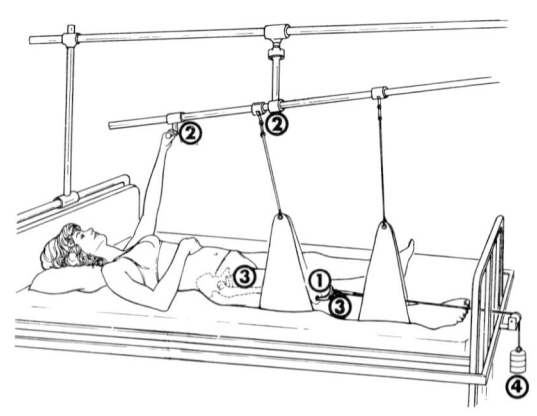

Subsequent Management

Maintain traction for 6 to 12 weeks, depending on the degree of fracture disruption.

If the femoral head has protruded centrally, 12 weeks of traction is generally necessary to insure adequate healing and prevent redislocation.

While the patient is in traction, start active abduction exercises to promote remodeling of the articular surface.

Traction may gradually be discontinued by the end of 12 weeks and crutch walking may be started.

Full weight bearing is usually possible by 6 months.

Follow the patient closely for two years for radiographic evidence of traumatic arthritis or avascular necrosis. The majority of these complications will be evident within the first year.

Fracture with Chronic Disruption of the Acetabulum and Displacement of the Femoral Head

REMARKS

Acetabular fractures that do poorly are usually evident from the onset.

A decision can usually be made within the first year regarding the need for reconstructive total hip replacement. This should be based on the patient's pain symptoms and functional limitations rather than radiographic changes. Frequently the clinical result is far superior to the radiographic picture.

For chronic acetabular deficiency after these fractures, bone grafting from the excised femoral head, as described by Dunn and Hess, can be effective to reconstruct the acetabulum for support of the prosthesis.

Preoperative X-Ray

1. One year after acetabular fracture, the dome remains comminuted and the joint space has been destroyed.
2. The inner wall has been disrupted.
3. There is chronic medial and posterior displacement of the femoral head.

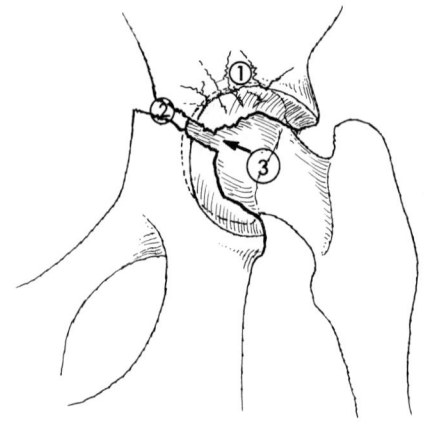

X-Ray After Reconstruction by Total Hip Replacement (After Dunn and Hess)

1. The disrupted dome has been grafted with bone from the excised femoral head.
2. The inner wall has been filled with bone graft.
3. A protrusio ring is used to prevent central migration of the prosthesis.

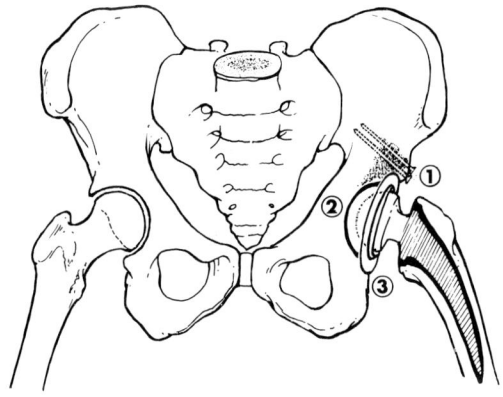

SUMMARY: COMPLICATIONS AND PITFALLS IN MANAGING HIP DISLOCATIONS AND FRACTURE OF THE ACETABULUM

REMARKS

This section has emphasized the acute complications of hip dislocations and acetabular fractures, which are many. Acute complications include commonly associated injury to the knee, either bony or ligamentous; injury to the sciatic nerve, from either stretch or compression; chronic dislocation, unrecognized either because the patient is comatose or because fracture of the ipsilateral femoral shaft has masked it; and fracture of the femoral neck associated with the dislocation or overvigorous attempts at closed reduction.

Awareness of these potential acute complications and complete clinical and radiographic assessment of the patient's injury can prevent or significantly diminish long-term complications.

The major long-term complication of hip injury is traumatic arthritis. Avascular necrosis, or what is interpreted as such on x-ray, occurs at about half the frequency of traumatic arthritis.

Primary open reduction of fracture-dislocation of the hip as advocated by Epstein can be expected to lower the rates of traumatic arthritis to about 17 per cent and of avascular necrosis to about 5 per cent.

Open reduction of acetabular dome fractures without dislocation has never been shown to decrease the frequency of traumatic arthritis or avascular necrosis. Operative intervention for the acetabular injuries without dislocation must be extremely selective.

The major determinants of outcome are the degree of initial injury inflicted on the femoral head, the absence of abrasive osteocartilaginous intra-articular fragments, and the promptness with which a dislocation is reduced. (Central protrusion is the only type of hip dislocation in which promptness of reduction is not critical for the end result.)

Ninety to 95 per cent of the bad results from dislocations and fractures of the acetabulum will be evident within the first year. The majority are manifest from the outset.

Total hip replacement with or without bone graft reconstruction of the acetabulum offers significant relief for the majority of patients disabled by these injuries.

RADIOGRAPHIC APPEARANCE OF CHRONIC COMPLICATIONS

Often, the radiographic changes of traumatic arthritis and avascular necrosis are impossible to differentiate.

Microscopic study of excised portions of the femoral head most often show that the bone is viable but that the articular cartilage has been involved by traumatic arthritis.

Myositis ossificans may also occur.

Traumatic Arthritis

Traumatic arthritis has occurred after posterior dislocation of the hip joint.
1. Narrowed joint space.
2. Marginal osteophytes of the acetabulum and femoral head.
3. Cystic areas in the femoral head.
4. Flattening of the femoral head.

Avascular Necrosis of the Femoral Head

1. Triangular area of increased density.
2. Collapse and flattening of the subchondral bone.
3. The joint space is preserved in the early phase, but it is lost when secondary traumatic arthritis occurs.

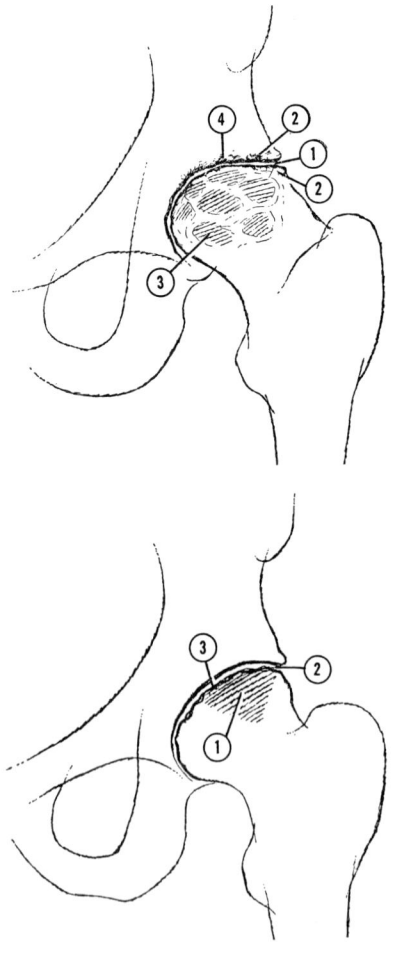

SUMMARY: COMPLICATIONS AND PITFALLS IN MANAGEMENT

Myositis Ossificans

Myositis ossificans appears to be due to hematoma and muscle trauma as a result of the injury.

It is not necessarily the result of primary operative treatment of a fracture-dislocation or early weight bearing or active exercises.

This represents calcification of the capsule rather than the muscle and may develop promptly after initial injury.

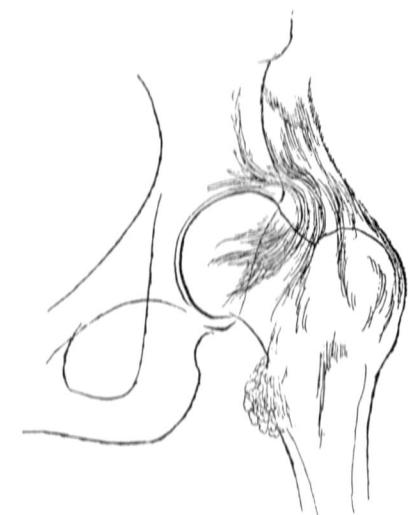

The calcification is likely to recur even following a total hip replacement, and the surgeon should be alert to this possibility.

These chronic complications can be minimized but not entirely avoided by anticipating the pitfalls during the initial management of these serious injuries.

REFERENCES

Canale, S. T., and Manugian, A. H.: Irreducible traumatic dislocations of the hip. J. Bone and Joint Surg. 61-A:7, 1979.

Carnesale, P. G., Stewart, M. J., and Barnes, S. N.: Acebatular disruption and central fracture-dislocation of the hip. J. Bone and Joint Surg. 57-A:1054, 1975.

Cathcart, R. F.: New ideas in the design and function of the Austin Moore prosthesis. Orthop. Review, Vol. II, 3:15, 1973.

Chrisman, O. D., and Snook, G. A.: Studies on the protective effect of aspirin against degeneration of human articular cartilage. Clin. Orthop. 56:77, 1968.

Connolly, J. F.: Acetabular labrum entrapment associated with a femoral-head fracture-dislocation. J. Bone and Joint Surg., 56-A:1735, 1974.

Dehne, E., and Immermann, E. W.: Dislocation of the hip combined with fracture of the shaft of the femur on the same side. J. Bone and Joint Surg., 33-A:731, 1951.

Dingley, A. F., and Denham, R. H.: Pubic dislocation of the hip. J. Bone and Joint Surg., 46-A:865, 1961.

Dowd, G. S. E., and Johnson, R.: Successful conservative treatment of a fracture-dislocation of the femoral head. J. Bone and Joint Surg. 61-A:1244, 1979.

Dunn, H. K., and Hess, W. E.: Total hip reconstruction in chronically dislocated hips. J. Bone and Joint Surg., 58-A:838, 1976.

Ehtisham, S. M.A.: Traumatic dislocation of hip joint with fracture of shaft of femur on the same side. J. Trauma, 16:96, 1976.

REFERENCES

Eisenberg, K. S., Sheft, D. J., and Murray, W. R.: Posterior dislocation of the hip producing lumbosacral nerve-root avulsion. J. Bone and Joint Surg., 54-A:1083, 1972.

Epstein, H. C.: Posterior fracture-dislocations of the hip. J. Bone and Joint Surg., 56-A:1103, 1974.

Epstein, H. C.: Traumatic dislocations of the hip. Clin. Orthop., 92:116, 1973.

Funk, F.: Traumatic dislocation of the hip in children. J. Bone and Joint Surg., 44-A:1135, 1962.

Garrett, J. C., Epstein, H. C., Harris, W. H., et al.: Treatment of unreduced traumatic posterior dislocations of the hip. J. Bone and Joint Surg., 61-A:2, 1979.

Gillespie, W. J.: The incidence and pattern of knee injury associated with dislocation of the hip. J. Bone and Joint Surg., 57-A:376, 1975.

Gupta, R. C., and Shravat, B. P.: Reduction of neglected traumatic dislocation of the hip by heavy traction. J. Bone and Joint Surg., 59-A:249, 1977.

Harris, W. H., Bourne, R. B., and Oh, I.: Intra-articular acetabular labrum: A possible etiological factor in certain cases of osteoarthritis of the hip. J. Bone and Joint Surg., 61-A:510, 1979.

Hirasawa, Y., Oda, R., and Nakatani, K.: Sciatic nerve paralysis in posterior dislocation of the hip. Clin. Orthop., 126:172, 1977.

Jennings, J. J., Harris, W. H., and Sarmiento, A.: A clinical evaluation of aspirin prophylaxis of thromboembolic disease after total hip arthroplasty. J. Bone and Joint Surg., 58-A:926, 1976.

Kleiman, S. G., Stevens, J., Kolb, L., et al.: Late sciatic-nerve palsy following posterior fracture-dislocation of the hip. J. Bone and Joint Surg., 53-A:781, 1971.

Liebenberg, F., and Dommisse, G. F.: Recurrent post-traumatic dislocation of the hip. J. Bone and Joint Surg., 51-A:632, 1969.

Lipscomb, P. R.: Fracture-dislocation of the hip. In Instructional Course Lectures, American Academy of Orthopaedic Surgeons, 18:102, 1961.

Nerubay, J.: Traumatic anterior dislocation of hip joint with vascular damage. Clin. Orthop., 116:129, 1976.

Nixon, J. R.:. Late open reduction of traumatic dislocation of the hip. J. Bone and Joint Surg., 58-B:41, 1976.

Ogden, J. A.: Changing patterns of proximal femoral vascularity. J. Bone and Joint Surg., 56-A:941, 1974.

Pennsylvania Orthopaedic Society: Traumatic dislocation of the hip in children. Final report by the Scientific Research Committee, J. Bone and Joint Surg., 50-A:79, 1968.

Rowe, C. R., and Lowell, J. D.: Prognosis of fractures of the acetabulum. J. Bone and Joint Surg., 43-A:1961.

Sarmiento, A., and Laird, C. A.: Posterior fracture-dislocation of the femoral head. Clin. Orthop. 92:143, 1973.

Scott, J. E., and Thomas, F. B.: Delayed presentation of post-traumatic posterior dislocation of the hip with acetabular rim fracture. Injury; the British Journal of Accident Surg., 5:325, 1973.

Simmons, R. L., and Elder, J. D.: Recurrent post-traumatic dislocation of the hip in children. S. Med. J. 65:1463, 1972.

Stimson, L. A.: An easy method of reducing dislocations of the shoulder and hip. M. Rec., 57:356, 1900.

Sunderland, S.: Nerves and Nerve Injuries. Edinburgh, E. & S. Livingstone, Ltd., 1968, pp. 1015–1095.

Thompson, V. P., and Epstein, H. C.: Traumatic dislocation of the hip. J. Bone and Joint Surg., 33-A:746, 1951.

Tipton, W. W., D'Ambrosia, R. D., and Ryle, G. P.: Non-operative management of central fracture-dislocations of the hip. J. Bone and Joint Surg., 57-A:888, 1975.

FRACTURES OF THE FEMUR

FRACTURES OF THE UPPER END OF THE FEMUR

Fracture of the Greater Trochanter

REMARKS

Fractures of the upper end of the femur include:
- Fractures of the greater trochanter.
- Fractures of the lesser trochanter.
- Intertrochanteric fractures (extracapsular fractures).
- Fractures of the neck of the femur (intracapsular fractures).

REMARKS

This may be considered an incomplete intertrochanteric fracture resulting from a direct blow on the bony prominence.

Displacement of the trochanteric fragment is rare, since most of the soft tissues remain attached to the femur.

UNDISPLACED FRACTURE

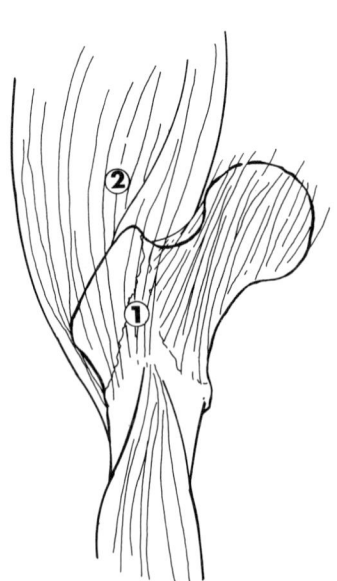

Prereduction X-Ray

1. Linear fracture through the greater trochanter.
2. Surrounding soft tissue attachments prevent displacement.

Management

The patient should be treated symptomatically.
Permit protected weight bearing with crutches.
Apply ice to the injured area to relieve pain.
Continue protected crutch walking for four to six weeks until the patient is free of pain.

SLIGHTLY DISPLACED FRACTURE

Prereduction X-Ray

1. Fracture of the greater trochanter is comminuted.
2. Fragments are displaced slightly and should be reduced.

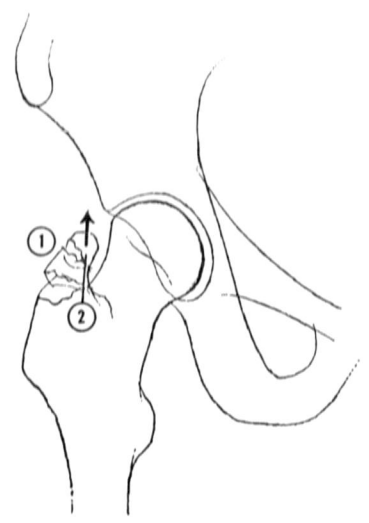

Reduction and Immobilization by Pantaloon Spica

1. A light pantaloon spica is applied to the abducted hip.
2. The knees are free and the patient is allowed protected weight bearing with crutches.

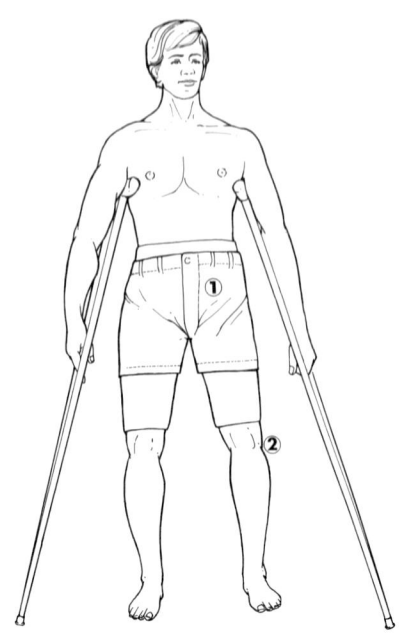

Postreduction X-Ray

The upper end of the shaft of the femur is in apposition with the avulsed greater trochanter.

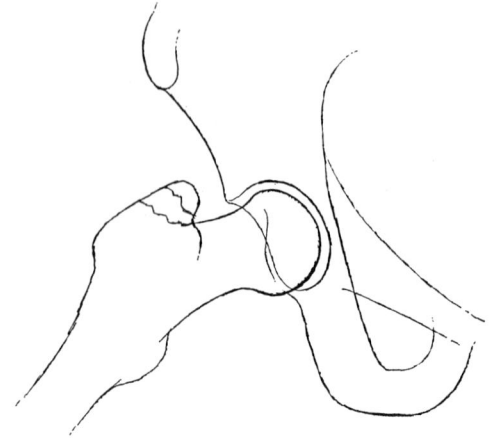

Postreduction Management

Remove the plaster cast at the end of six weeks.
Have the patient continue walking with crutches or cane until the hip is pain free.

Fracture of the Lesser Trochanter

REMARKS

This fracture, a commonly associated lesion in comminuted intertrochanteric fractures of the femur, may be ignored because it in no way materially affects the ultimate result.
In some instances the epiphysis of the lesser trochanter is avulsed by the iliopsoas muscle; the same mechanism may pull off the lesser trochanter in adults.

Prereduction X-Ray

Avulsion of the lesser trochanter.
1. The fragment is displaced upward by the iliopsoas muscle.

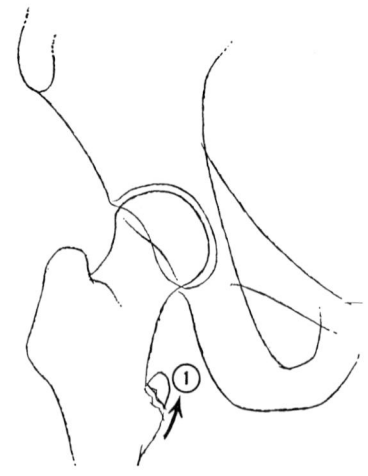

Initial Management

1. The patient is made comfortable by positioning in bed with the hip flexed.
2. The position can be maintained temporarily with the limb on pillows.

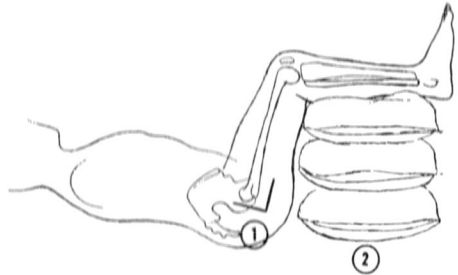

Subsequent Management

Maintain the hip in a flexed position for two to three days while the initial pain and swelling subside.

Treat the patient symptomatically with analgesics and application of ice to the area of the injury.

Permit protected walking with crutches for three to four weeks.

The patient may discard the crutches when the hip is pain free and he can walk without a limp.

Intertrochanteric Fractures

REMARKS

Intertrochanteric fractures include all extracapsular fractures from the greater trochanteric region of the femur to a point 5 cm below the lesser trochanter.

These fractures, which are most often produced by minor trauma or a fall, are injuries of old age. The annual incidence in people more than 70 years old is 5 per 1000, and in people more than 80 years old the incidence is 19 per 1000.

About 70 per cent of patients are women because trochanteric fractures, like Colles' fractures and proximal humeral fractures, are failures of osteoporotic bone.

Hip fractures have always been associated with a high mortality rate, which continues to hover today around 30 per cent, depending on the patient's age and preoperative physical and mental status. The results when these fractures are sustained by elderly, institutionalized patients are even worse, in terms of survival and ability to walk again.

Surgical management does little to alter the significant mortality rate of hip fracture, but effective operative fixation can relieve the patient's discomfort and disability.

Since not all hip fractures require internal stabilization, the first thing the physician should consider, after assessing the general health and mental status of the patient, is the stability of the fracture.

A small percentage of intertrochanteric fractures will be intrinsically stable, as indicated by the patient's ability to control and lift the injured leg with minimal discomfort. These will heal well with protected weight bearing and support of the limb against external rotation deformity.

The majority of patients, however, will present with shortened, externally rotated limbs requiring internal stabilization to give a reasonable chance for independent walking and living.

Intertrochanteric fractures may occasionally occur in young adults or children, most often as a result of significant direct violence to the hip. These fractures generally require internal fixation to prevent malunion and coxa vara deformity.

The optimum treatment demands a realistic appraisal, first of the needs of the patient and second of the technical requirements of the fracture itself.

NEEDS OF THE PATIENT

As Miller has reported in his study from Charlottesville, the average age of patients with hip fractures is 73 years.

More than 70 per cent of these patients are women, 30 per cent manifest cerebral dysfunction, 18 per cent have symptoms from arthritis, 16 per cent have congestive heart failure, 14 per cent have diabetes, and 8 per cent are subject to pulmonary disease.

Thirty per cent of these patients die within one year after hip fracture. In many the cause of death is judged to be pulmonary embolism, myocardial infarction, or pneumonia, but the majority succumb to the inanition of old age.

The older the patient, the less likely will be her survival or ability to walk subsequent to the fracture. Fewer than one third of the patients more than 80 years of age are alive and walking one year later. This percentage diminishes even further in patients suffering from cerebral dysfunction.

In the elderly patient with osteoporotic bone, intramedullary pin fixation via techniques such as Ender's closed method (see page 1379) appears most satisfactory because it is technically simple and is least likely to add to the patient's multiplicity of problems.

The likelihood that the patient less than 60 years old will survive a hip fracture exceeds 80 per cent. In this younger patient with less osteoporotic bone, firm mechanical fixation is important to prevent deformity and to restore the ability to walk independently. The most effective mechanical support for these fractures can be provided by open reduction and fixation using compression screw techniques (see page 1382).

Careful assessment of the patient and the type of fracture permits the physician to maximize his contribution to the patient's well-being and to minimize his role as part of the patient's disease.

FRACTURES OF THE UPPER END OF THE FEMUR

TYPES OF FRACTURES AND TECHNICAL CONSIDERATIONS

Many varieties of fractures occur in the trochanteric region.

Their stability can be estimated both by the degree of initial clinical deformity and by adequate radiographic visualization of the fracture. Comminution of the strong medial cortex frequently indicates significant instability.

TYPE I: STABLE, UNDISPLACED FRACTURE

This type is characterized by a fracture line traversing the intertrochanteric region. The fracture is extracapsular and, as a rule, the greater and lesser trochanters are not implicated.

Usually this is an incomplete fracture and is stabilized by the surrounding soft tissues (capsule and muscle), which remain attached at the fracture site. This fracture is especially likely in a young male patient less than 65 years of age and without advanced osteoporosis.

In this undisplaced fracture, the major deforming force is the weight of the leg, which causes external rotation and varus tilt of the fracture unless the limb is supported.

If one prevents the tendency toward external rotation, this fracture may be effectively treated nonoperatively.

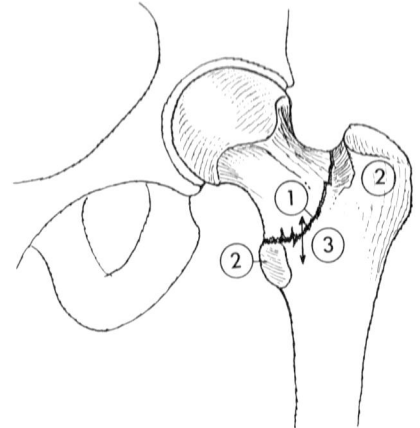

Appearance on X-Ray

1. Fracture line extends along the intertrochanteric line.
2. The trochanters are not involved.
3. The proximal and distal fragments are in normal anatomical alignment.

TYPE II: DISPLACED FRACTURE WITHOUT COMMINUTION OF THE MEDIAL CORTEX

In this lesion, the main fracture line extends completely along the intertrochanteric region and the proximal fragment tilts into varus deformity. Both trochanters may be implicated, and in some instances the greater trochanter is split and pulled posteriorly.

Since the medial cortex remains relatively intact, the fracture will be stable once it is reduced and fixed adequately.

This is the most common type of intertrochanteric fracture and may be stabilized either by intramedullary Ender's rods or by compression screw technique.

Appearance on X-Ray

1. Fracture through the intertrochanteric line.
2. Varus deformity of the proximal fragment.
3. Comminution of the greater trochanter.
4. Fracture of the lesser trochanter without involvement of the medial cortex.
5. External rotation of the distal fragment.

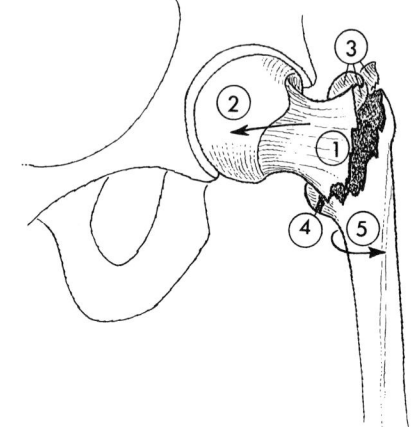

1. Fracture through the intertrochanteric line and into the greater trochanter.
2. Varus deformity of the proximal fragment.
3. Comminution of the greater trochanter.
4. Vertical split of the greater trochanter.
5. Avulsion and medial displacement of the lesser trochanter.

Note: Since the medial cortex remains intact, varus displacement is minimized.

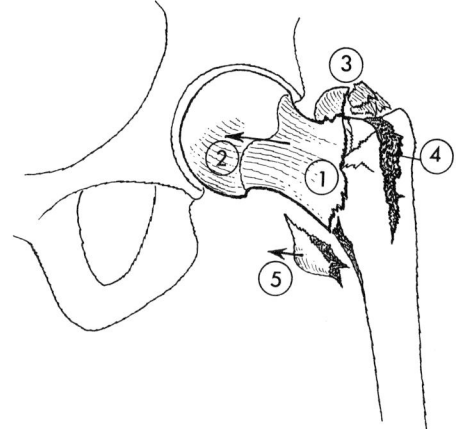

Type III: Vertically Displaced Fracture With Comminution of the Medial Cortex

This fracture is unstable owing to comminution of the medial cortex, which permits vertical displacement of the proximal fragment into a pronounced varus position.

Quite frequently, these fractures can be stabilized, not by trying to restore normal anatomical relationships but by fixing the distal fragment in its medially displaced position.

Appearance on X-Ray

1. Split fracture of the greater trochanter.
2. Comminuted fracture of the medial cortex and medial displacement of the distal fragment.
3. Pronounced varus deformity of the proximal fragment due to the loss of medial support.
4. Comminution of the posterior cortex, which also contributes to fracture instability.

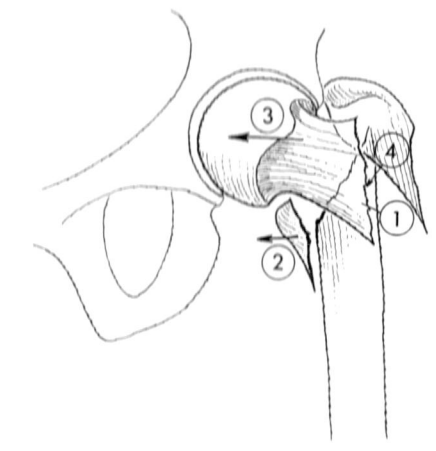

Type IV: Intertrochanteric Fracture With Subtrochanteric Component

This uncommon fracture is extremely unstable owing to the loss of subtrochanteric support, which ordinarily carries the most concentrated load of any area of the femur. The fracture is the most difficult to reduce and stabilize adequately and is fraught with complications. If one uses a nail and plate, plate failure and varus deformity of the fracture are common. Supplemental fixation is usually necessary.

Appearance on X-Ray

1. Fracture through the intertrochanteric region.
2. Comminution of the greater trochanter.
3. Fracture of the medial cortex.
4. Spiral fracture involving the subtrochanteric region of the femur.

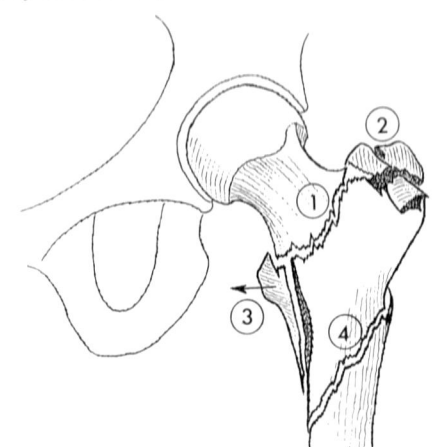

MANAGEMENT OF INTERTROCHANTERIC FRACTURES

Nonoperative Management of Type I (Undisplaced) Fracture

REMARKS

Occasionally a patient, particularly a younger patient, who presents with a stable, undisplaced fracture may be treated with bed rest.

Should this fracture heal in a slight varus position, it is not detrimental to hip function.

During the recovery period, the limb should be supported to prevent external rotation deformity while the patient lies in bed.

Initial X-Ray

1. Fracture line extends along the intertrochanteric region.
2. The greater and lesser trochanters are not involved.
3. The proximal and distal fragments are in normal anatomic alignment.

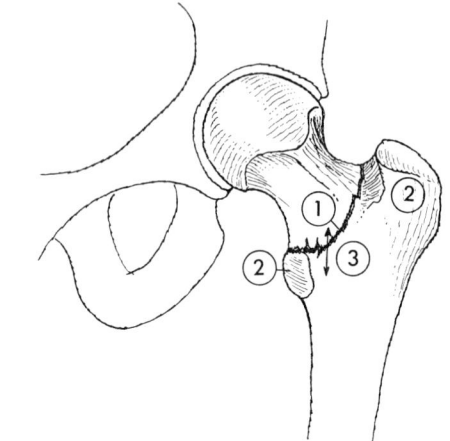

Initial Management: Buck's Traction

1. Apply a removable prepadded traction splint.
2. The medial and lateral straps prevent rotational deformity.
3. The foot piece prevents foot drop.
4. Minimum (3 to 4 kg) traction is necessary.

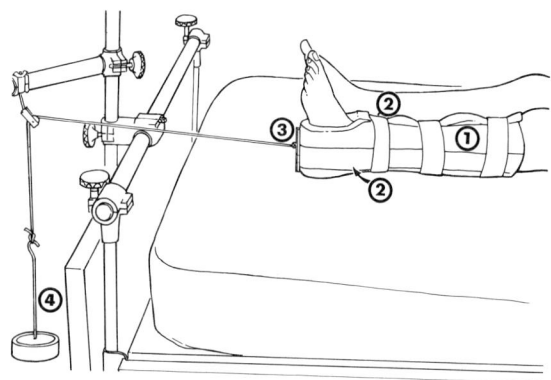

Subsequent Management

As the patient's pain subsides over the first week or two after injury, traction may be removed and active exercises to the hip and thigh muscles may be started.

Begin crutch walking when the patient has regained muscle control of the limb.

The patient should support the weight of the limb by toe touching rather than by trying to hold the fractured limb completely off the ground.

Reapply the splint without traction when the patient is in bed so as to support the fractured leg against external rotation deformity.

Continue crutch or cane walking for 12 to 16 weeks until the fracture is healed clinically and radiographically.

X-Ray 12 Weeks After Injury

1. The fracture has settled into slight varus position, which does not impair hip function.
2. Intramedullary callus has filled in the fracture line.

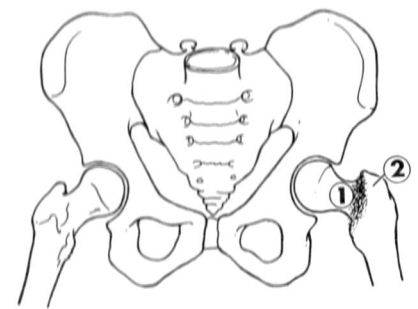

OPERATIVE MANAGEMENT FOR TYPE II, TYPE III, AND TYPE IV FRACTURES

Initial Evaluation of the Patient

1. The majority of patients with intertrochanteric fractures are elderly and present with an obviously shortened, externally rotated limb from an unstable extracapsular fracture.

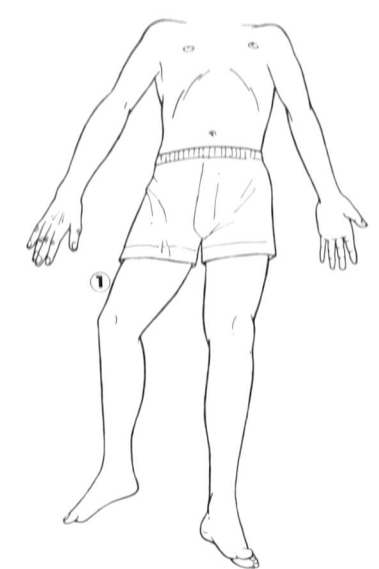

2. Obtain anteroposterior and lateral x-rays to confirm the clinical diagnosis.
At the same time, obtain a chest x-ray to evaluate for cardiopulmonary problems such as heart failure and pneumonia.

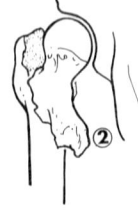
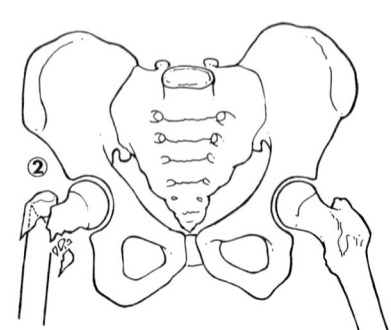

Initial Treatment

1. Many patients are dehydrated and have depleted blood volume. Evaluate levels of electrolytes, glucose, and blood urea nitrogen and begin necessary replacements.
2. Intermittent or indwelling catheterization is necessary to evaluate urine output and prevent urination in bed.
3. Apply light (3-kg) Buck's traction to support the hip preoperatively.

Note: These patients tolerate the supine position poorly, and they should undergo operative fixation of the fracture within 24 to 48 hours if their general medical condition allows.

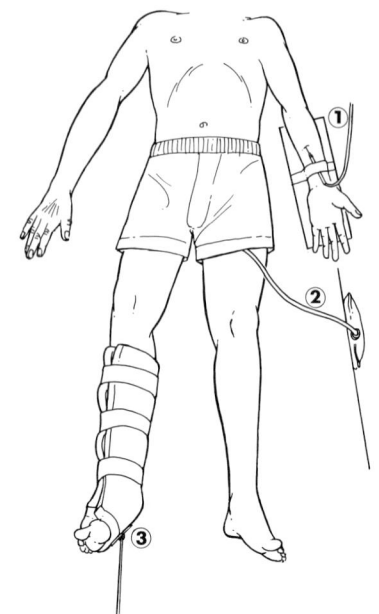

SURGICAL CONSIDERATIONS

REMARKS

Well-controlled general anesthesia is safer in the elderly and less likely than spinal anesthesia to result in complications, particularly cerebral dysfunction.

The operation should be done on a fracture table with image-intensified fluoroscopy.

Evaluate the preoperative x-rays to choose the type of fixation necessary, but be prepared to change your plans during the procedure.

The primary objective is to reduce the fracture to a stable position and to hold that position with the appropriate internal fixation devices.

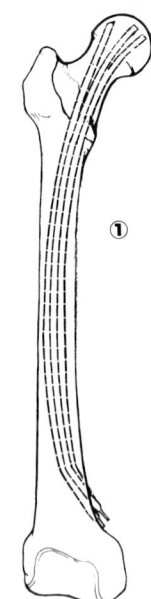

1. The simplest, least disruptive method of supporting these fractures in the elderly patient with osteoporotic bone is multiple intramedullary pins inserted by Ender's method from the distal femur.

The major complication in this method is loss of fracture stability, particularly rotational stability. A number of these patients also have pain at the point of insertion of the pin (in the distal femur).

2. For unstable fractures in the younger patient (less than 65 years), compression screw fixation with the sliding nail technique is a consistently effective method. Compression screws are designed to impact while reduction is maintained. A high-angle 150-degree nail is preferable because it most closely parallels the weight-bearing force across the fracture line and most readily permits fracture impaction. The sliding components of the nail prevent penetration through the femoral head, which has been the most common complication with non-sliding nails.

The major disadvantage of open reduction with compression screw fixation is the risk of subsequent wound infection.

3. Occasionally with intertrochanteric fractures that have a comminuted medial cortex (Type III), the fracture must be stabilized by permitting medial displacement of the distal fragment and holding the fracture in the medially displaced position.

4. The uncommon but difficult to treat intertrochanteric fracture with a subtrochanteric component (Type IV) requires supplemental fixation in addition to the usual nail-and-plate devices or intramedullary nails.

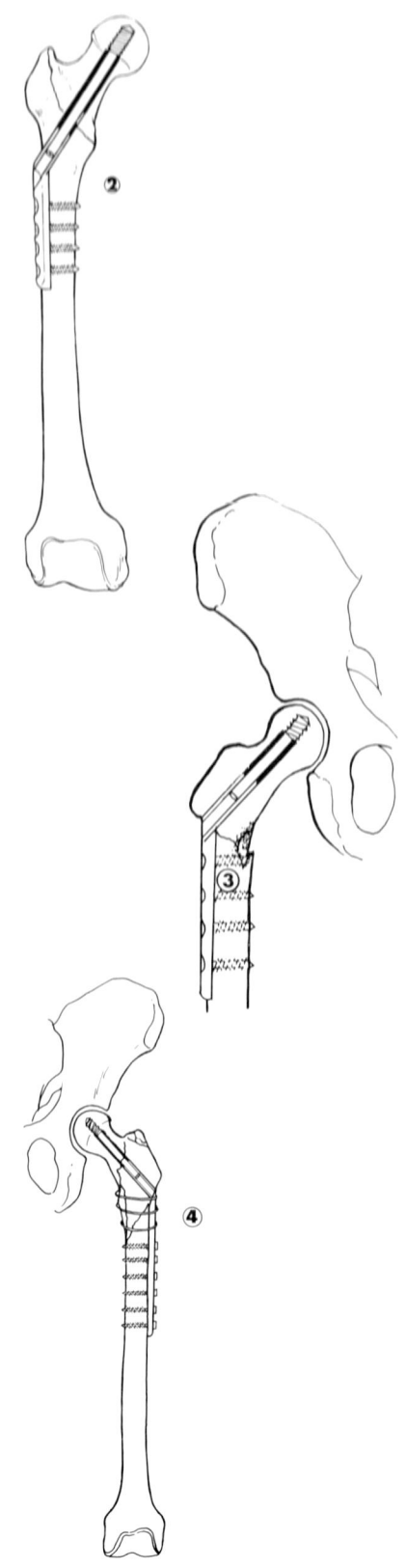

FRACTURES OF THE UPPER END OF THE FEMUR

TECHNIQUE OF FRACTURE REDUCTION

Prereduction X-Rays

ANTEROPOSTERIOR VIEW

1. Fracture occurs through the intertrochanteric line.
2. The proximal fragment is in varus.
3. There is comminution of the greater trochanter.
4. There is a fracture of the lesser trochanter without involvement of the medial cortex.
5. The distal fragment is rotated externally.

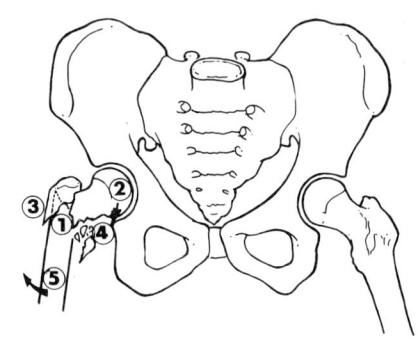

LATERAL VIEW

1. Because of external rotation of the distal fragment, the fracture has opened anteriorly.
2. The posterior cortex is also fractured.

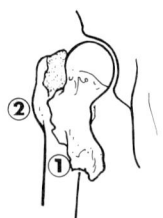

Position of the Patient

The patient is anesthetized in bed and is then transferred to the fracture table. General anesthesia is safest and is least likely to cause cerebrovascular or cardiopulmonary complications.

1. The unfractured limb is abducted widely to make room for the fluoroscopic tube and to tilt the pelvis upward on the uninjured side. *Do not abduct the fracture.*
2. The fractured limb is fixed to the table in neutral position.
3. Pull on the fractured limb sufficiently to tighten the knee ligaments.
4. Internally rotate the fractured limb slightly to reduce or close the anteromedial cortex.

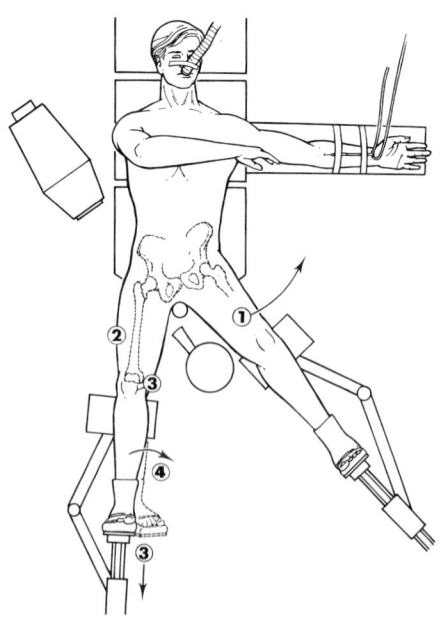

Postreduction X-Rays

Anteroposterior view

1. Tilting the pelvis by abducting the opposite leg rotates the proximal fragment into valgus.
2. The intertrochanteric fracture is aligned but is not distracted by excess traction.
3. The trochanteric fragments are not critical for stability.
4. The medial cortex is in contact apposition.

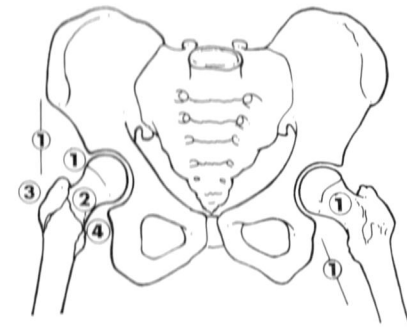

Lateral view

1. Internal rotation has closed the anteromedial gap.
2. The posterior cortex remains open slightly.

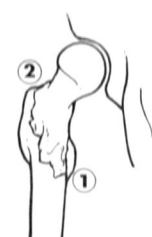

FIXATION BY ENDER'S NAIL METHOD

Note: This procedure is particularly indicated for relatively stable fractures in elderly patients with osteoporotic bone. It requires image-intensified fluoroscopy and complete familiarity with the instrumentation.

1. Make an 8-cm skin incision from the adductor tubercle and carry it proximally.
2. Dissect between the adductor magnus and the vastus medialis to reach the medial surface of the femur.
3. About 3 cm proximal to the adductor tubercle, a transverse branch of the medial superior geniculate artery is seen on the periosteum.
4. Perforate the bone at this point with a Steinmann pin and then widen the hole with 1.5-cm drill.

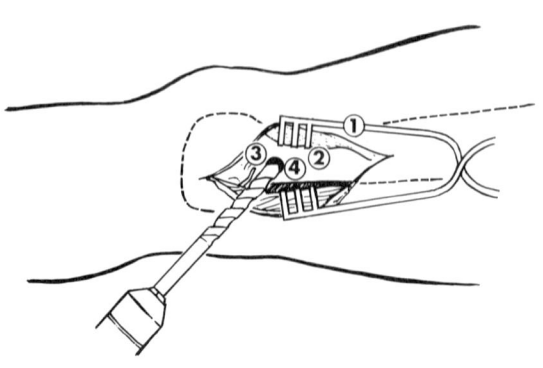

1. Determine the necessary length of the first nail by placing it on the limb over the drapes and checking the position with the fluoroscope. The nail should project well up over the head.
2. Insert three to five Ender's nails and drive them across the fracture to within 5 mm of the hip joint as seen on fluoroscopy. The first nail should be hammered in medially along the calcar.
3. The other nails are bent so as to fan out into the head. Nail position can be adjusted by rotating the nail during insertion. The nails should reach close to the hip joint and should diverge in the femoral head.
4. The flat ends of the nails should be smoothly seated on the femoral cortex.

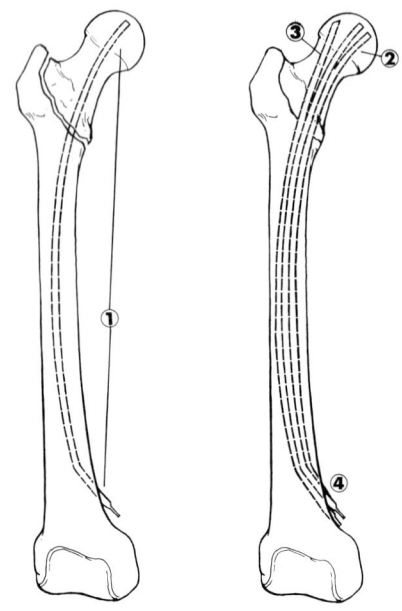

For Unstable Fractures Not Reduced by Preoperative Traction

Note: This procedure can be technically difficult and requires experience.

1. Lift the thigh up and rotate the fractured limb externally 90 degrees.
2. Apply sufficient traction to bring the distal fragment down, but avoid excess traction.

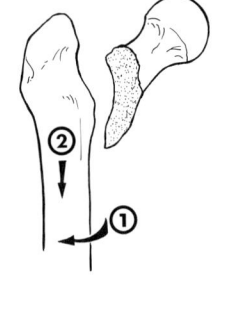

3. Insert the first nail and hitch the proximal fragment with the nail tip.

4. Then, by internal rotation of the aligned fracture, further reduction can be accomplished and the other nails can be inserted.

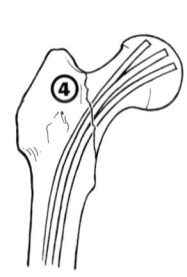

For Unstable Intertrochanteric Fractures With a Subtrochanteric Component (Type IV)

1. Insert two pins from the medial condyle into the femoral head.
2. Insert two pins from the lateral condyle into the greater trochanter.

Note: Fixation of this type of fracture with Ender's nails may not be mechanically stable. Postoperative traction or external cast support is recommended.

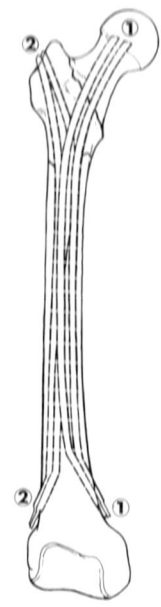

Subsequent Management

Following the operation the patient can begin bearing weight with a walker or crutches.

Some degree of backing out of the nails occurs in most cases, but usually this does not cause symptoms.

Occasionally, if the insertion site is too distal on the femur and too close to the medial condyle, the nails cause knee pain and require re-insertion or removal.

Protect the leg against a tendency to externally rotate at the fracture. This can be done by supporting the limb with a removable splint while the patient is in bed.

1. Avoid external rotation deformity, which can occur when the patient lies in bed.

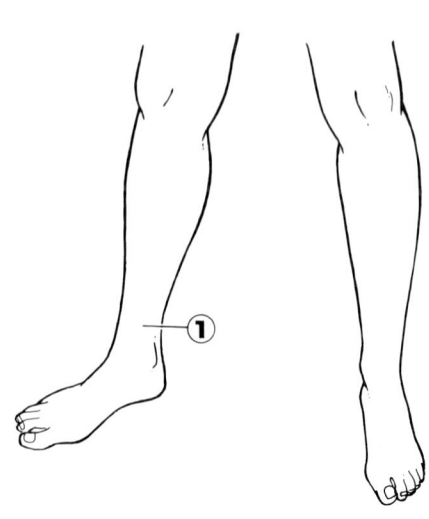

Subsequent Management
(*Continued*)

2. Support the limb for four to six weeks with a padded splint using an outrigger to prevent rotation.

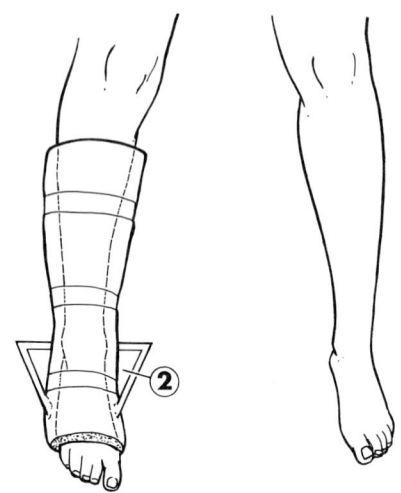

FIXATION BY HIGH-ANGLE COMPRESSION HIP SCREW (AFTER SOUTHWICK)*

This technique is particularly indicated for unstable fractures or fractures in young patients with hard cortical bone, in contrast to the indication for Ender's pinning, which is primarily for a relatively undisplaced fracture in an elderly patient with osteoporotic bone.

Closed reduction is accomplished on the fracture table as previously described (see page 1378).

Appearance on X-Rays

ANTEROPOSTERIOR VIEW

1. Tilting of the pelvis by abducting the opposite leg rotates the proximal fragment into valgus.
2. The intertrochanteric fracture is aligned but is not distracted by excess traction.
3. The trochanteric fragments are not critical for stability.
4. The medial cortex is in contact apposition.

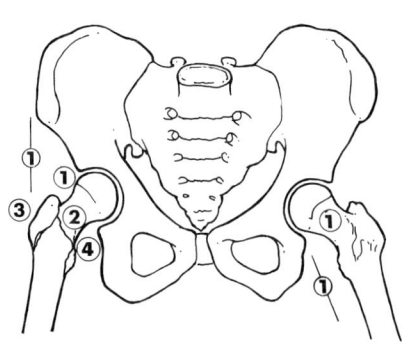

LATERAL VIEW

1. Internal rotation has closed the anteromedial gap.
2. The posterior cortex remains open slightly.

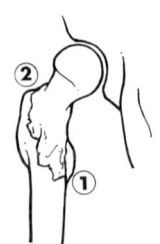

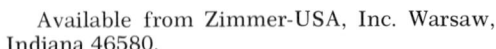

*Available from Zimmer-USA, Inc. Warsaw, Indiana 46580.

Operative Procedure

1. Begin the skin incision from 2 cm above the greater trochanter and extend it distally 15 cm.

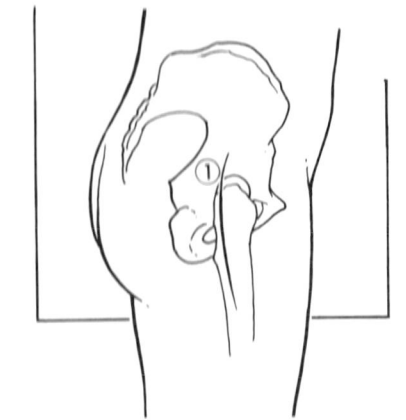

2. Cut the fascia lata at the posterior edge of the vastus lateralis.
3. Cut the posterior aspect of the vastus lateralis and elevate it anteriorly with a Bennett retractor.

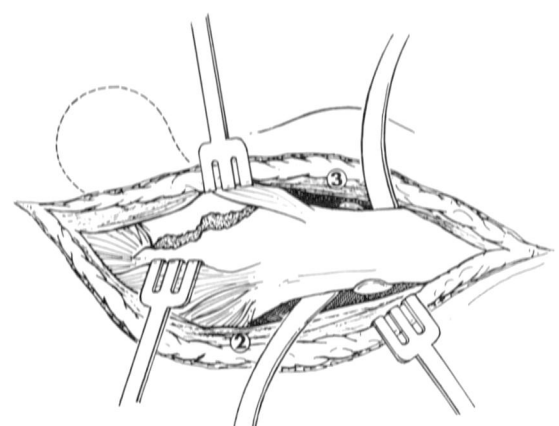

1. Using a 6-mm drill, start the hole for the guide pin 5 cm below the lower ridge of the greater trochanter, or 2 cm below the lesser trochatner.
2. Use a fixed, 150-degree angle guide to insert a heavy 3-mm guide pin and direct it into the head using image-intensified fluoroscopy.
3. The pin should be inserted almost centrally or slightly toward the medial calcar of the neck and well into the subchondral bone of the head.
4. Measure the length of the guide pin and subtract 1.2 cm to determine the proper length of the lag screw.

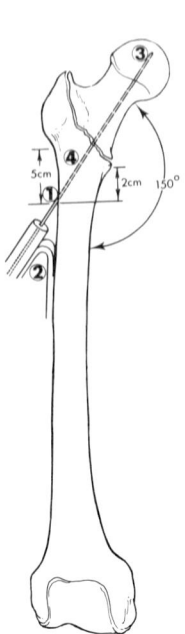

FRACTURES OF THE UPPER END OF THE FEMUR

Operative Procedure
(Continued)

1. Prepare the lateral cortex by drilling with a cortical step drill and take care to avoid bending the guide pin during the drilling.

2. Advance the drill into the bone until the lower portion of the second notch reaches the lateral cortex.

Note: Should the guide pin be pulled out during this drilling, it must be re-inserted prior to the next step.

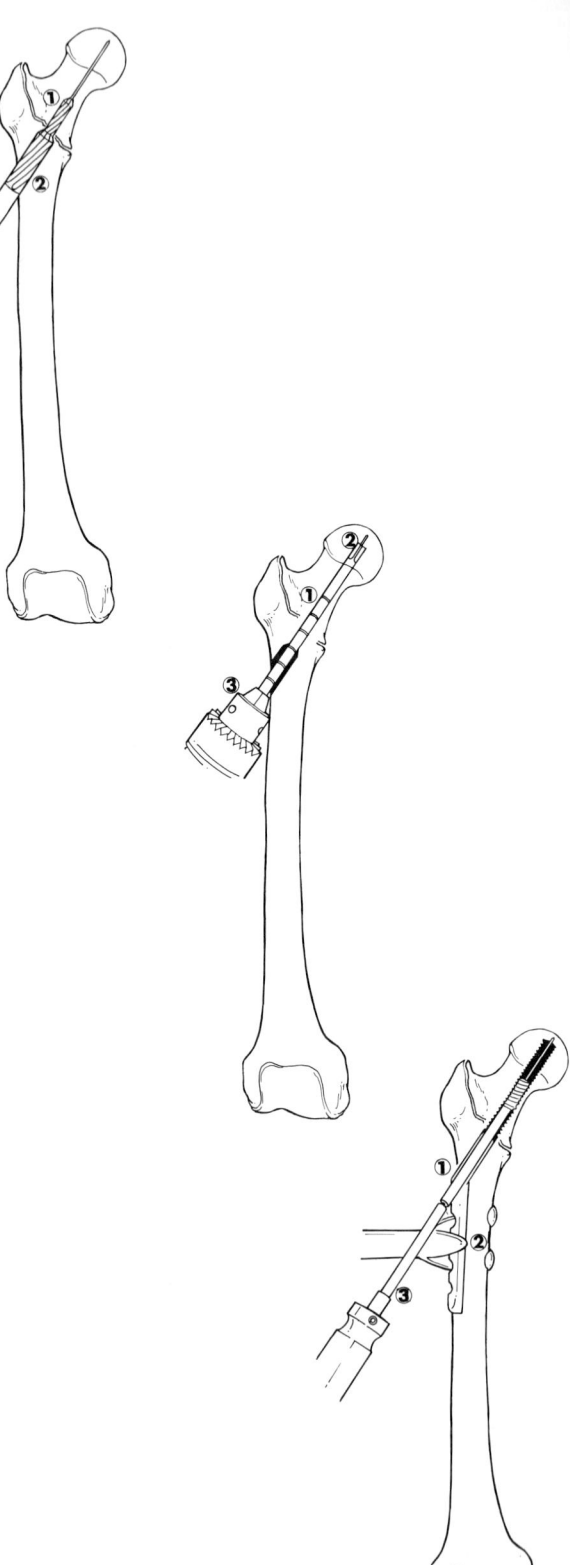

1. The lag screw reamer is then used to drill the femoral neck to the appropriate length determined from the guide pin.

2. The reamer is advanced to within 1 cm of the head.

3. The inferior portion of the ring which indicates the appropriate length should reach the lateral cortex.

Note: For hard bone, a bone tap should first be used to prepare the channel for the lag screw.

1. The lag screw and the side plate combination are then inserted in collapsed position over the guide pin.

2. The plate is held against the shaft with a Lowman clamp.

3. A special, hollow-milled screwdriver fits over the guide pin and engages a slot on the base of the screw. The lag screw is then advanced appropriately into the head.

1. The lag screw penetrates to within 1 cm of the articular surface.
2. The screw must be overlapped by at least 1.8 cm with the compression tube.
3. Buttress screws then fix the plate to the cortex. They should extend through both cortices of the distal fragment.
4. When adequate position is confirmed by fluoroscopy, release traction on the limb and compress the fracture with an impactor.

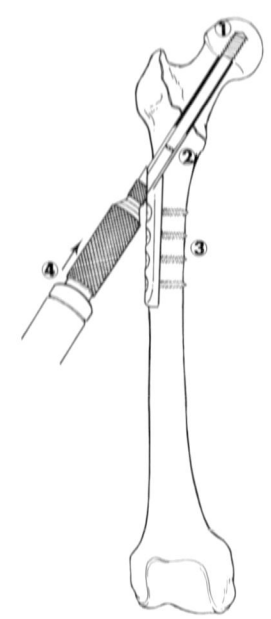

X-Ray After Impaction

1. Fracture line is closed.
2. The lag screw has started to slide through the compression tube to permit further fracture impaction.

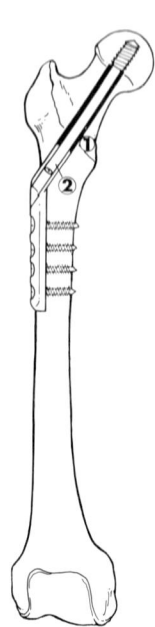

FRACTURES OF THE UPPER END OF THE FEMUR

Management of Unstable Fracture by Compression Screw

PREOPERATIVE X-RAY

1. A pronounced varus deformity is evident.
2. There is comminution of the medial cortex with loss of calcar support to the fracture.

Note: Medial support of the fracture may be regained by using the compression screw to displace the distal fragment medially.

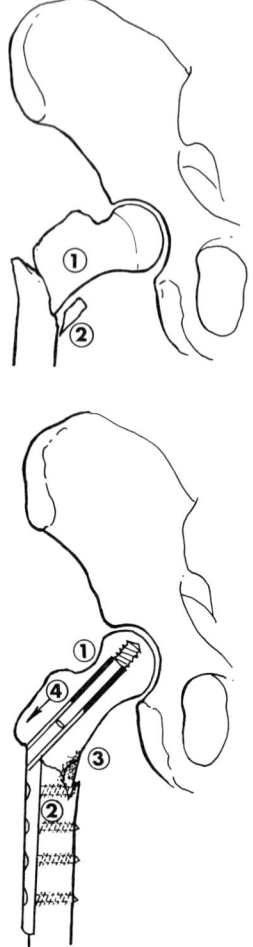

POSTOPERATIVE X-RAY

1. The compression screw is seated well in the head.
2. The distal fragment has been allowed to displace medially by the compression device.
3. The comminuted medial cortex has been stabilized by the position of the fragment.
4. There is impaction of the fracture, as indicated by retraction of the screw.

Management of an Intertrochanteric Fracture with a Subtrochanteric Component (Type IV)

REMARKS

Intertrochanteric fracture with subtrochanteric component presents the greatest difficulty of all intertrochanteric fractures. The tendency to varus and torsional deformities is great.

Mechanical failure is common unless the fracture is firmly held.

When the displaced, unstable component is in the intertrochanteric region, the fracture is best stabilized by compression screw technique using supplemental cerclage wire fixation on the subtrochanteric component. It is important that the plate be fixed to the distal fragment by at least six buttress screws passing through both cortices.

When the major instability is in the subtrochanteric region, the fracture may be fixed by Zickel nail technique (see page 1395) or, rarely, by Ender nail technique (see page 1381).

FRACTURES OF THE UPPER END OF THE FEMUR

PREOPERATIVE X-RAY

1. There is a fracture through the intertrochanteric region.
2. The greater trochanter is comminuted.
3. The medial cortex has been fractured and medial stability is lost.
4. There is continuation of the fracture into the subtrochanteric region.

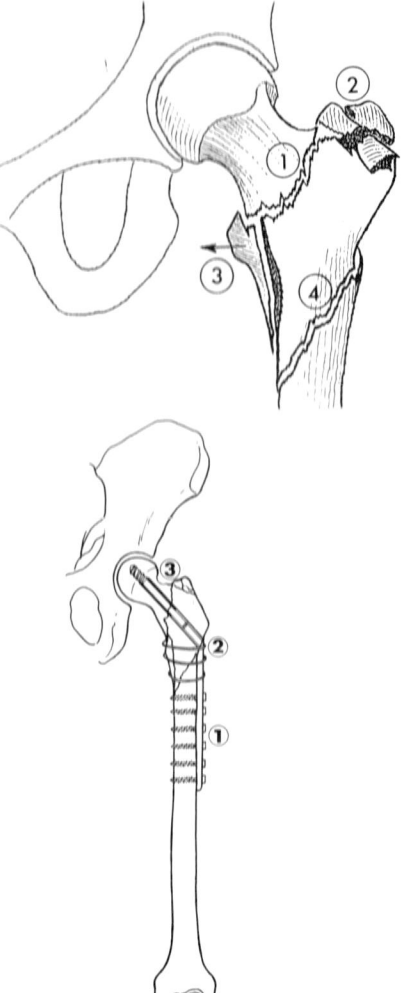

POSTOPERATIVE X-RAY

1. Circumferential wire fixation gives additional support to the fracture and the plate to prevent varus deformity of the subtrochanteric region.
2. The subtrochanteric component is stabilized by the long plate with six screws through both cortices of the distal fragment.
3. The intertrochanteric component of the fracture is stabilized by the sliding compression screw.

POSTOPERATIVE MANAGEMENT

Avoid prolonged use of intravenous solutions in these elderly patients. Start oral administration of fluids promptly.

Strong analgesics should be avoided because they frequently produce an adverse affect and cause the elderly patient to become agitated and confused. Aspirin is preferable for pain relief following operative fixation of the elderly patient's hip fracture.

Allow the patient to get out of bed or to stand using a tilt table on the second postoperative day.

With stable reduction of the fracture, the patient may progress to walking with the assistance of a walker. Partial weight bearing on the fractured side may be permitted.

The patient can usually advance to a cane by 12 to 16 weeks, at which time there is generally radiographic evidence of healing.

The patient should continue using the cane indefinitely after the fracture to assist and protect the injured side.

Check the progress of the fracture healing at intervals of approximately 6 weeks until union is evident.

Complications of Intertrochanteric Fractures

REMARKS

The major complication of intertrochanteric fractures is death. Perioperative (three-month) mortality averages 15 per cent and one-year mortality is 25 to 30 per cent.

There is some correlation between immediate operation and the mortality rate. Cain found the highest surgical mortality in patients operated on within the first day after injury. An intertrochanteric fracture need not be treated as a surgical emergency in an elderly patient; only after complete evaluation of the patient's underlying problems should surgery be performed.

Rehydration and restoration of blood volume are particularly critical preoperative precautions.

Approximately 80 per cent of surviving patients may be expected to return to an ambulatory status after hip fracture. Technical complications, including nail failure, nail penetration into the joint, infection, and occasionally even arterial injury, account for a number of failures.

Nail Penetration from Malreduction

1. A fixed-angle nail inserted at a low angle and
2. Without reduction and impaction of the medial cortex results in
3. Anterior protrusion of the nail with loss of fracture reduction.

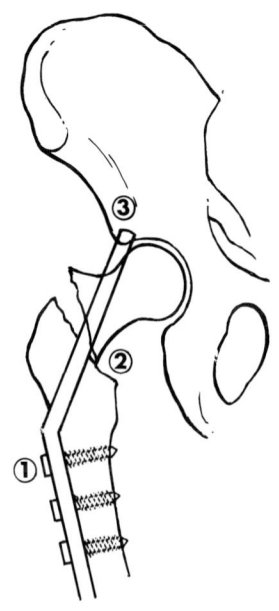

Prevention

1. A sliding nail inserted at an 150-degree angle permits fracture impaction without nail penetration.

Note: The barrel of the sliding nail should be inserted, if at all possible, only through the distal fragment and not across the fracture.

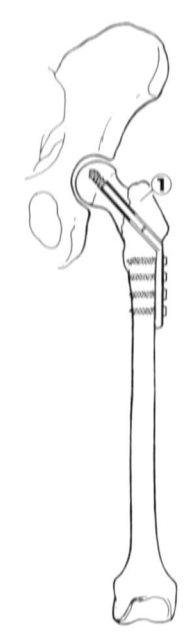

Complications from a Short Nail

A short nail for an intertrochanteric fracture may cause
1. Complete loss of fracture reduction or
2. A fatigue fracture of the femoral neck.

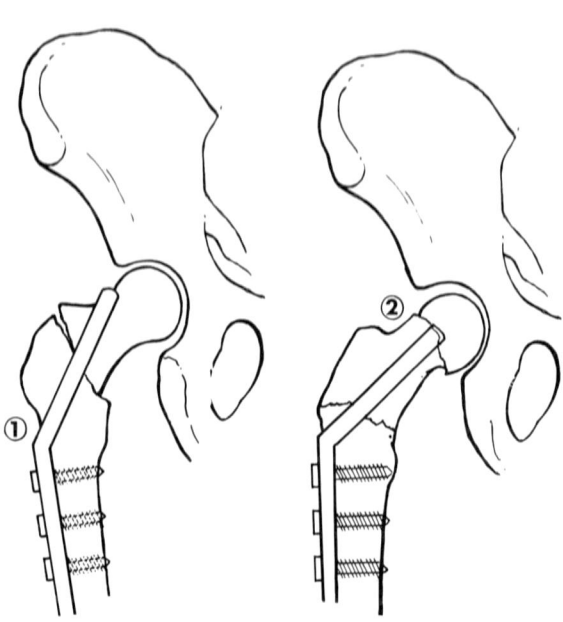

Infection

Superficial and deep infection occurs in approximately 5 per cent of fractures treated by open reduction and internal fixation. Prophylactic antibiotics begun immediately prior to operation and continued for the first postoperative day may diminish the incidence of wound infection from operative fixation.

Infection (Continued)

1. Intramedullary rods where indicated can eliminate the risk of wound infection but
2. May slightly increase the risk of technical failure and loss of fracture reduction.

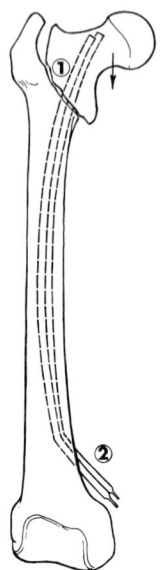

Intertrochanteric Fractures in Infants and Children

Intertrochanteric fractures are uncommon in children and usually are produced by significant trauma. Frequently the child has been run over by a car or has fallen on the hip from a height.

Most often the fracture extends up into the base of the neck and is displaced.

The major and common complications include coxa vara, avascular necrosis of the femoral epiphysis, and premature closure of the physeal line. The frequency of these complications is directly related to the degree of initial fracture displacement.

Fractures that are not displaced may be treated by a spica cast applied with the opposite leg in abduction to tilt the pelvis and maintain the proximal fracture fragment in slight valgus position.

Intertrochanteric and cervicotrochanteric fractures with initial displacement are best treated by closed reduction and internal fixation with 2 to 3 Knowles pins to prevent coxa vara deformity and nonunion.

To avoid premature physeal closure, the fixation pins should not cross the physeal lines. Premature closure may still occur, however, because of the nature of the injury. Following pin fixation of these fractures, it is well to immobilize the young child in a spica cast for 4 to 6 weeks to insure and protect fracture healing.

Avascular necrosis occurs fairly frequently (in approximately 25 per cent of cases). It is especially likely to follow displaced cervicotrochanteric fracture.

The type of primary treatment does not appear to influence or alter the complication of avascular necrosis. Changes of avascular necrosis are usually noted 9 to 18 months after the injury. Involvement may vary from injury of the entire capitofemoral epiphysis to increased sclerosis of the femoral neck above the fracture line.

The prognosis, should avascular necrosis develop, is better if the child was younger than 10 years of age at the time of fracture.

The severity of radiographic changes of avascular necrosis does not correlate with the clinical symptoms. Many young patients with avascular necrosis after fracture may enjoy 20 or more years of useful function before painful symptoms develop.

UNDISPLACED INTERTROCHANTERIC FRACTURE

Prereduction X-Ray

1. Intertrochanteric fracture is complete but not displaced.
2. There is minimal decrease in the neck-shaft angle.

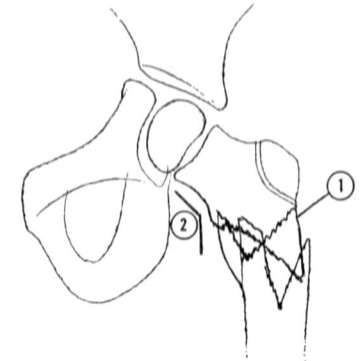

Reduction and Immobilization

1. The child is placed in a bilateral spica cast with the opposite limb abducted to tilt the pelvis upward.
2. The fractured limb is in neutral position and
3. Slight valgus position.

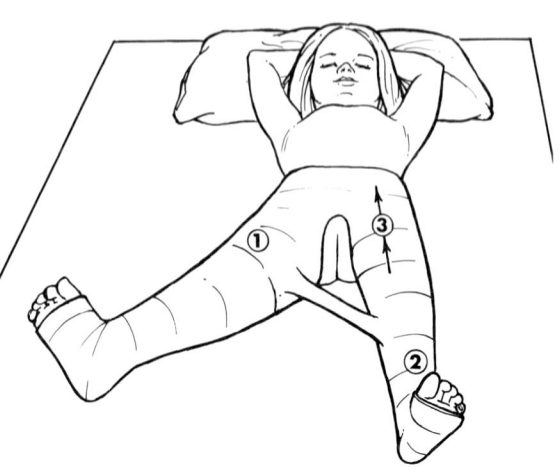

Management

Fractures of this nature usually heal within 8 weeks, after which the spica may be removed. Following removal of the cast, no special therapy is necessary in young children, since they usually regain motion and ability to walk quite readily.

DISPLACED INTERTROCHANTERIC FRACTURE

Prereduction X-Ray

An intertrochanteric fracture has occurred and has displaced into coxa vara deformity. Increased fracture angulation is likely unless this injury is reduced and fixed internally.

X-Ray After Closed Reduction and Knowles Pin Fixation

Note: The fracture is reduced on a fracture table as described for intertrochanteric fractures in adults (see page 1378).

1. The femoral neck angle has been restored to normal or close to normal.
2. The intertrochanteric fracture is fixed with three Knowles pins. Care is taken that the pins do not cross the physeal lines.

Note: In small children two Knowles pins will be adequate to hold this fracture.

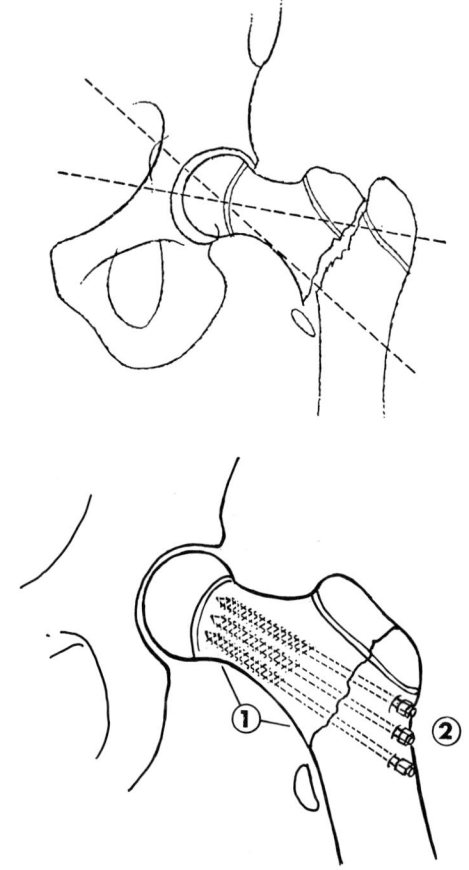

Postreduction Management

Following the operative fixation of the fracture the child is immobilized in a bilateral spica cast (see page 1391), which protects the fracture from too-vigorous activities.

The cast may be removed at four to six weeks, depending on radiographic signs of healing.

Allow the child to walk with crutches for two to three months longer.

Advise the parents that the injury needs to be followed closely over the subsequent year for development of avascular necrosis, since this may be still possible even though the fracture is well healed.

The Knowles pins usually become buried in bone quite rapidly and need not be removed unless they cause symptoms.

Should avascular necrosis become evident on follow-up, the child should be treated with continued protected crutch walking in the same manner as he would be treated for Legg-Perthes disease.

The prognosis, should posttraumatic avascular necrosis develop, is better if the child was less than ten years of age at the time of fracture.

Subtrochanteric Fractures

SUBTROCHANTERIC FRACTURES WITHOUT INTERTROCHANTERIC COMPONENT

REMARKS

The mechanical problems of stabilizing fractures in the subtrochanteric region are formidable, and these fractures are notoriously the most difficult to treat. They are associated with varying degrees of comminution and are more difficult than other fractures of the trochanteric region to reduce and fix.

The greatest compression stress on the femur during weight bearing is concentrated in the medial subtrochanteric region. This means that fixation devices must be particularly well designed to withstand the stress of weight bearing.

Typically, a nail-plate fixation without supplemental fixation is inadequate to hold a subtrochanteric fracture, and mechanical failure of the device with nonunion of the fracture is the result.

Mechanism of Nail-Plate Fixation Failure

1. Comminuted subtrochanteric fracture with loss of the medial cortical buttress shifts all the forces of weight bearing onto the plate fixation.
2. The force of weight bearing produces a bending moment (F × d) on the nail-plate fixation.
3. Failure of the nail plate can occur.

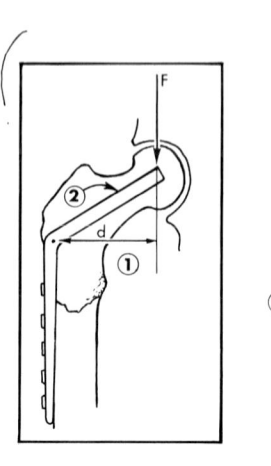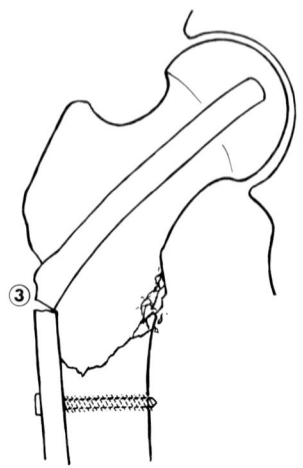

Mechanism of Nail-Plate Fixation Failure (Continued)

1. Torsional forces also contribute to the varus tendency of these fractures.
2. Rotation of the long distal fragment can cause the screw to pull loose and fixation to fail.

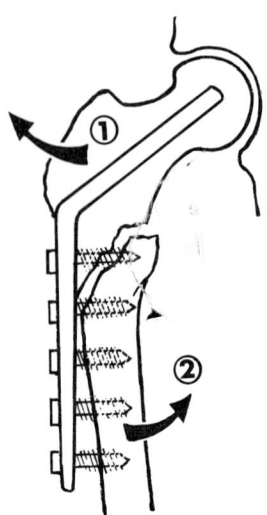

Preferable Fixation by Zickel Nail

1. Intramedullary Zickel nail provides support along the line of medial stress.
2. The proximal fragment is controlled by the triphlanged nail and by
3. The large diameter of the proximal rod.
4. The intramedullary fixation device controls the distal fragment and stabilizes the fracture until it is healed.
5. Supplemental fixation may be needed for support against the torsion.

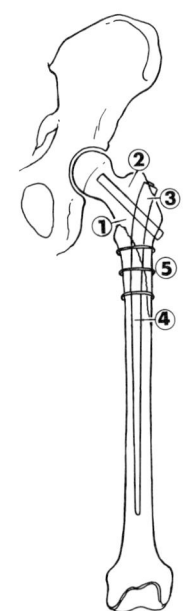

Fractures that are suitable for fixation with the Zickel nail include:
1. Short oblique fractures with and without comminution.

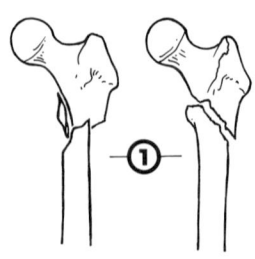

2. Long oblique fractures with and without comminution. These fractures should also be fixed with cerclage wire.

3. High transverse, subtrochanteric fracture with comminution of the medial cortex; this fracture also requires bone grafting to replace the medial cortical buttress.

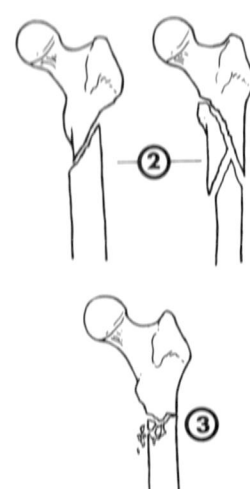

Because of the biomechanical principle involved, intramedullary nail fixation is most effective in decreasing the bending moment (F × d) at the fracture. External nail-plate fixation, no matter how strongly constructed, will always be less satisfactory because it is inserted at a mechanically greater disadvantage. Nail-plate fixation is most suitable for intertrochanteric fractures with subtrochanteric component.

INTERTROCHANTERIC FRACTURE WITH SUBTROCHANTERIC COMPONENT

1. The intertrochanteric fracture is stabilized best by sliding compression screw technique.
2. A long side plate with supplemental fixation by cerclage wire and bone grafting are necessary to stabilize the subtrochanteric fracture.

Note: A Zickel nail is not suitable here because it is liable to comminute the intertrochanteric fracture, thereby providing inadequate fixation.

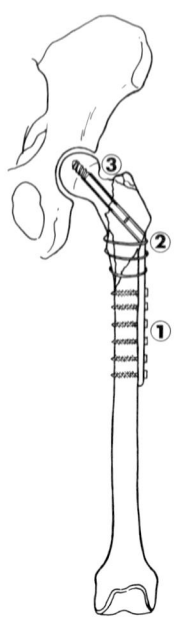

REDUCTION AND ZICKEL NAIL FIXATION FOR SUBTROCHANTERIC FRACTURE WITHOUT INTERTROCHANTERIC COMPONENT

1. The patient is placed on the operating table in a supine position with the pelvis slightly elevated on a bolster.
2. Begin a curved posterolateral incision 8 cm proximal to the greater trochanter and continue it distal to the fracture. Divide the fascia lata along the line of the skin incision.

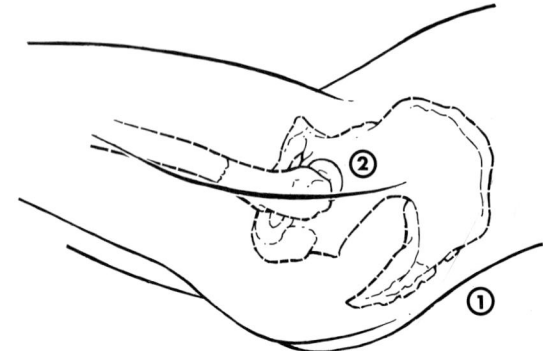

1. Develop the interval between the tensor fasciae latae and gluteus muscles and reflect the former medially, exposing the tip of the trochanter and the insertion of the gluteus medius.
2. Displace the vastus lateralis anteriorly, and by sharp dissection divide it longitudinally 1.5 to 2.5 cm anterior to the linea aspera; in the subtrochanteric region, continue the incision forward into the tendinous origin of the muscle.

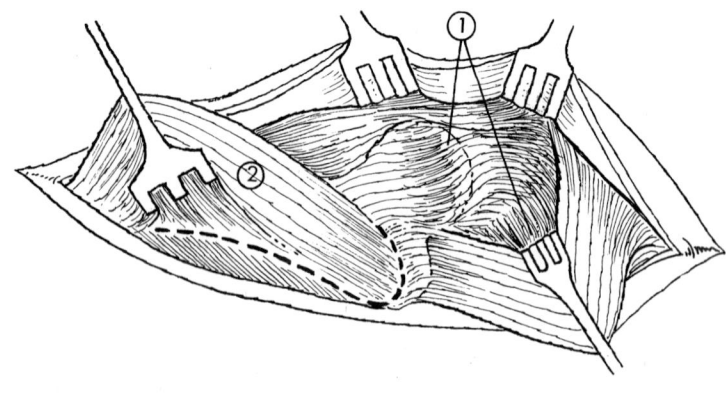

3. By subperiosteal dissection, elevate the muscle from the femur and retract it anteriorly and toward the midline. This exposes the entire upper end of the femur.

4. Maintain the exposure by hooking the edges of two Bennett retractors around the shaft of the distal fragment of the femur.

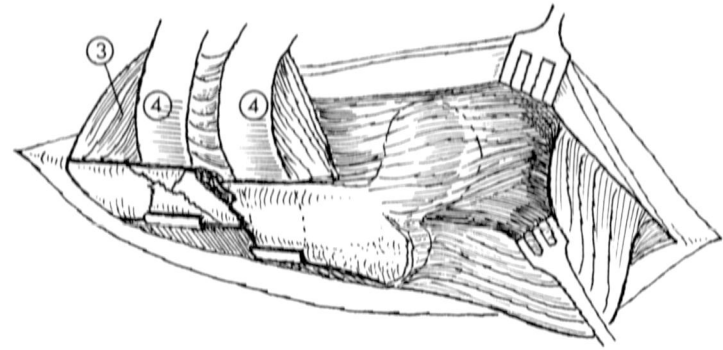

1. Elevate the distal fragment into the wound.

2. Determine the exact diameter of the medullary canal by passing long-handled drills of varying sizes into the distal fragment until the one having the correct diameter is found; it should fit snugly in the canal but not tightly.

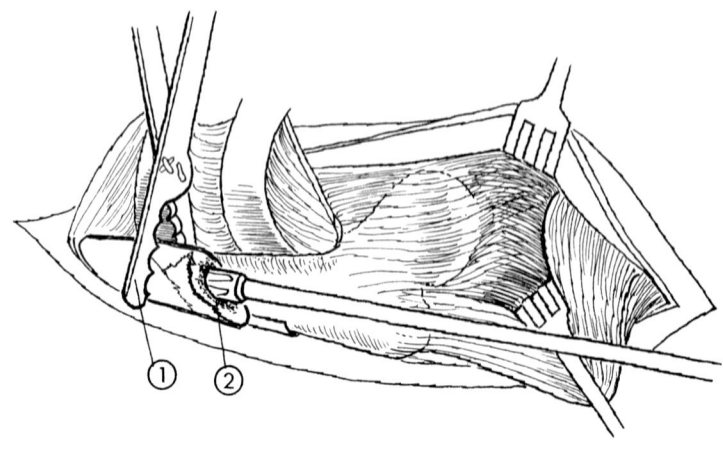

3. Test for the appropriate size of intramedullary rod to insure proper fit down the canal. This is important because the danger of later extension of the fracture down the femoral shaft is avoided.

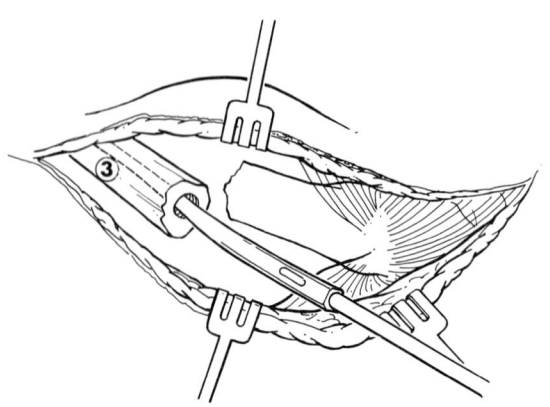

1. Ream the trochanteric fragment, beginning with a small reamer and advancing to a larger one.

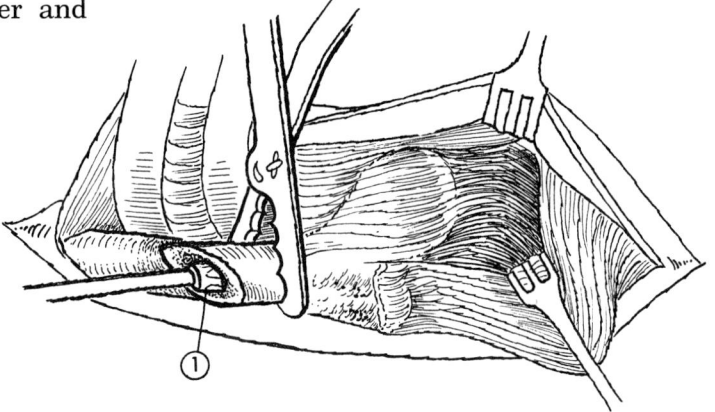

2. Osteotomizing the proximal cortical tip of the greater trochanter through a split in the gluteus medius helps orient the reamer.

3. The trochanteric canal should be reamed to a large diameter (17 mm) to allow insertion of the wide proximal end of the rod.

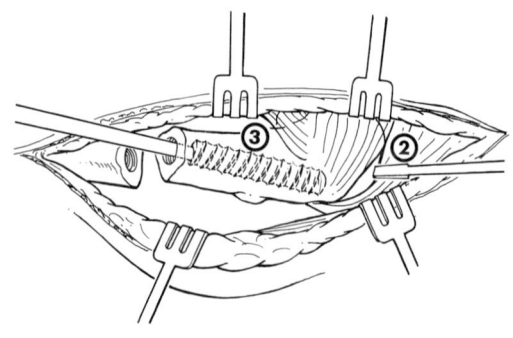

1. The fracture is reduced and is held with clamps.
2. The rod is assembled with a tunnel locater attached and driven through the prepared channel with the hip adducted.

Note: The rods are manufactured for left or right side; make sure to use the correct rod and to orient it properly.

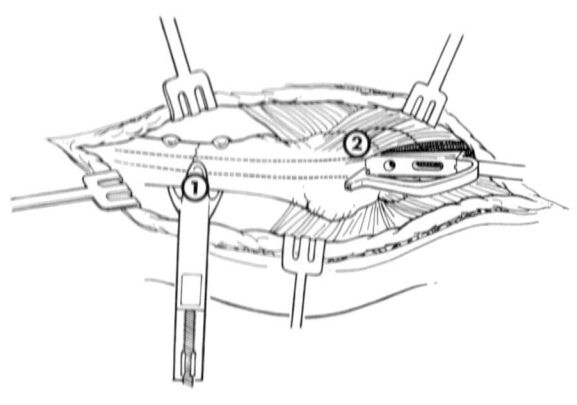

1. The position of the rod's tunnel in the trochanter is indicated by the tunnel locator.
2. The degree of anteversion of the femoral neck is determined by palpating the neck. Usually there is a 15 degree anteversion with reference to the operating table.
3. When the rod is fully seated, a guide-wire is drilled through the tunnel locater and the position is ascertained by x-rays taken in two planes.
4. The guide-wire should be near the medial cortex on the anteroposterior view and in the center of the neck on the lateral view.

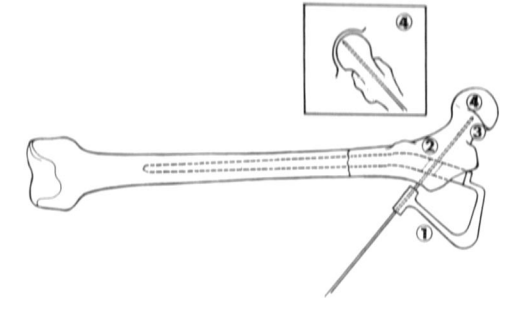

1. If the position of the guide-wire is satisfactory, the tunnel locater is removed and a 1.3-cm cannulated reamer is used to drill the cortical hole over the wire. A triphlanged nail is then inserted.

Note: X-rays taken at this time should show accurate placement of the nail.

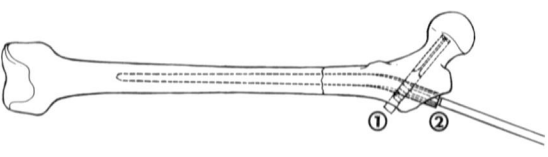

2. The nail is locked into the rod with a set screw.
3. Circumferential 18-gauge wire should now be applied around the fracture if there is fracture comminution or instability from a long oblique fracture.
4. Apply bone grafts taken from the pelvis to any persistent defects in the medial weight-bearing cortex.

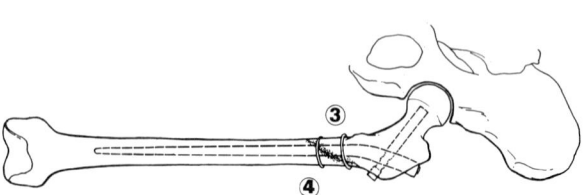

FRACTURES OF THE UPPER END OF THE FEMUR

Postoperative Management

Support the limb in Buck's traction for 3 to 5 days until the acute swelling and pain subside.

The patient may begin standing with crutches within the first week.

Support the limb against external rotation deformity by reapplying the Buck's traction until the patient has full control of the muscles.

The patient should continue with protected walking using crutches or a walker until fracture union is evident. Union, on the average, takes about 17 weeks.

The most common problem after Zickel nail fixation is external rotational deformity of the fracture. This may be prevented by proper placement of the nail during surgery and by postoperative support to prevent the weight of the limb from externally rotating the distal fragment.

If there is any question about fracture stability, add the external support of a cast-brace with a pelvic band or a mini-spica (see page 1404).

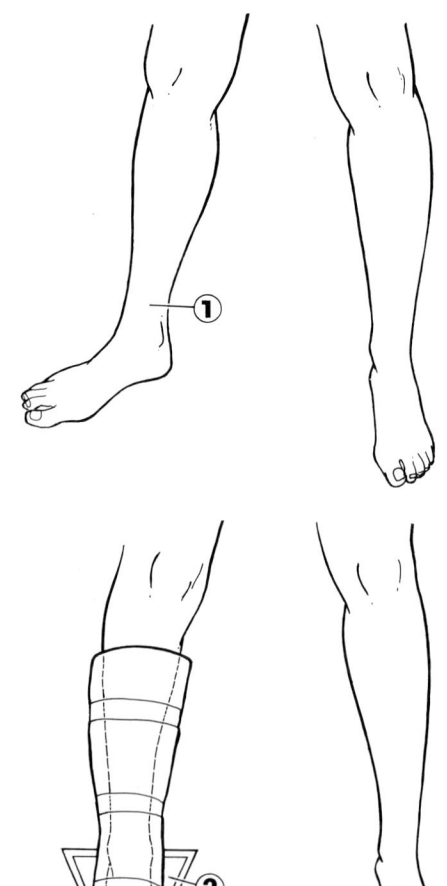

1. If the patient turns the fractured leg externally while lying in bed postoperatively,

2. Support the limb for 4 to 6 weeks using a padded splint with an outrigger.

NONOPERATIVE TREATMENT OF SUBTROCHANTERIC FRACTURE

REMARKS

Subtrochanteric fractures may occur in infants and young children as well as adults.

In contrast to displaced intertrochanteric fractures in children, which require operative fixation, subtrochanteric fractures may be treated by closed techniques.

The basic deformity to be corrected is flexion and external rotation of the proximal fracture fragment. Reduction is accomplished by aligning the distal fragment with the proximal fragment by flexion and external rotation.

For infants younger than 2 years of age who weigh less than 15 kg, Bryant's traction may occasionally be needed to correct flexion deformity of the proximal fragment. Often, subtrochanteric fractures in children less than 10 years of age may be treated by immediate spica application (see page 1501).

For older children as well as adults with subtrochanteric fractures, use 90–90-degree traction to align the distal fragment with the proximal fragment.

As the fracture solidifies, the limb may be slowly extended, and by 3 to 4 weeks a walking mini-spica or a cast-brace with a pelvic band can be applied.

The external support must maintain the rotational alignment of the fracture and must protect the fracture against varus tilting. The cast or cast-brace must be applied with the fractured limb abducted 30 to 40 degrees and externally rotated 15 to 20 degrees so as to hold reduction.

Using closed reduction with 90–90-degree traction and appropriately applying cast or cast-brace in the early phases of fracture healing, the physician can encourage rapid fracture union and permit the child or adult to return promptly to preinjury functional level.

Typical Deformity

1. Consistently the upper fragment displaces into flexion abduction and external rotation.
2. The distal fragment lies posterior and medial to the proximal fragment.

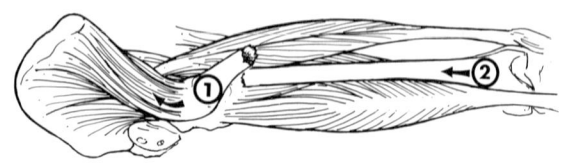

Appearance on X-Ray

1. Flexion and external rotation of the proximal fragment and
2. Internal rotation of the distal fragment
3. Appears on x-ray as a varus deformity.

Note: This is primarily a three-dimensional torsional alignment rather than strictly a varus deformity in the frontal plane.

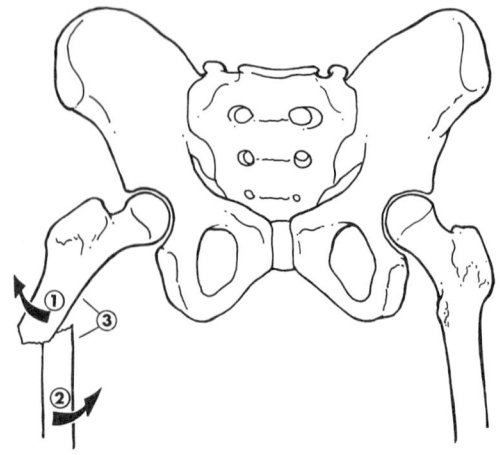

Technique of Reduction and Immobilization in Children Younger Than 2 Years (Bryant's Traction)

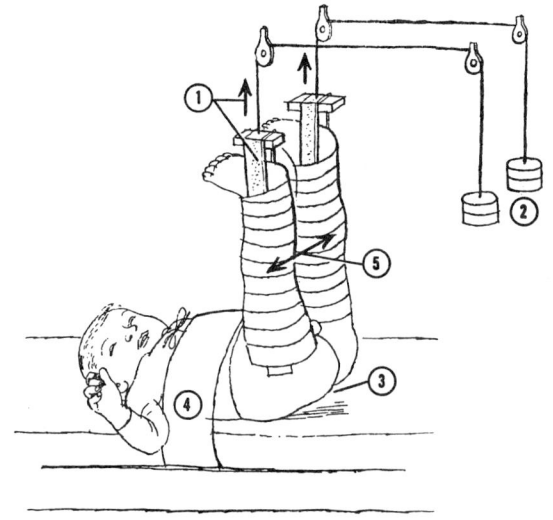

1. Apply overhead traction to both limbs. Use a strip of foam rubber instead of adhesive plaster.
2. Use pulleys and weights but not fixed traction.
3. Weight should be sufficient to elevate the sacrum from the bed.
4. Always use a restraint.
5. Keep the legs well abducted.

CAUTION

Bryant's traction should not be used in children heavier than 15 kg or older than 2 years of age because of the risk of limb ischemia.

Be careful not to hyperextend the child's knees in Bryant's traction, because this also may affect popliteal circulation.

The traction need not be heavy but it should be sufficient (1 kg) to lift the child's buttocks off the bed and to permit changing of diapers.

Check the child's toes for circulation and motor function daily, and remove traction if there is suspicion of circulatory or neurologic impairment. Both limbs must be checked, as the unfractured leg also may be subject to ischemic muscle necrosis.

Subsequent Management

Bryant's traction is maintained either in the hospital or at home for 3 weeks.

At the end of 3 weeks the fracture is usually solidifying and not tender, and traction may be discontinued.

A spica cast may be applied for 3 weeks longer.

Six weeks after injury the fracture should be well healed in a child this age, and external support may be discarded.

The child may then be allowed gradually to resume standing or weight bearing, depending on age and on ability to ambulate prior to injury.

90–90 Traction in Older Children and Adults

With the patient under general anesthesia or adequate local anesthesia:

1. A 3-mm threaded Steinmann pin is inserted medially, 2 cm proximal to the adductor tubercle on the fractured side.
2. Sterile gauze dressings are placed over the pin site and a traction bow of the correct size is applied to the Steinmann pin.
3. A light, well-padded below-knee cast is applied to keep the ankle in neutral position.

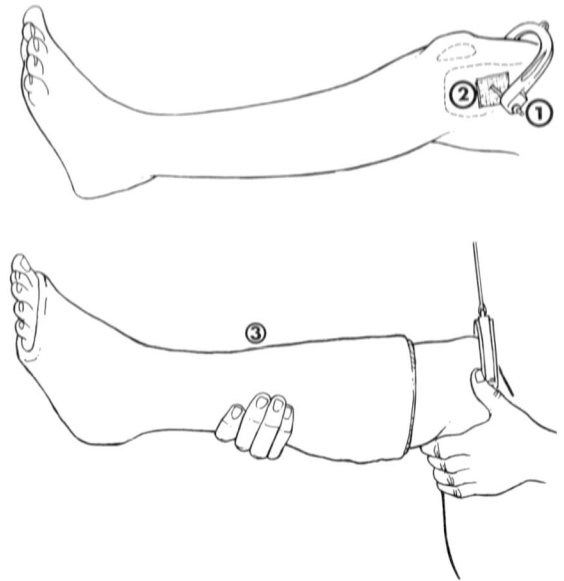

1. The fractured thigh is suspended in a position of 90 degrees of hip flexion and slight external rotation.
2. The knee is flexed 90 degrees and
3. The leg is supported in a sling or from plaster loops in the cast.

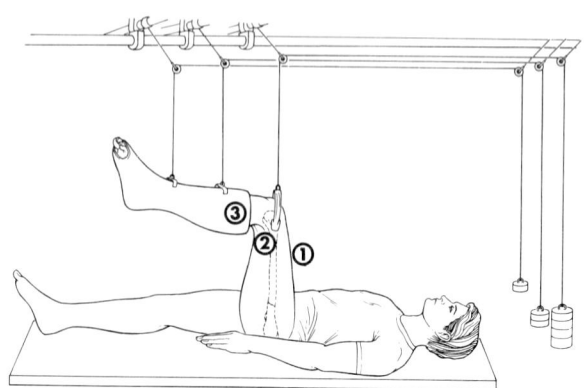

FRACTURES OF THE UPPER END OF THE FEMUR

Subsequent Management

Avoid over-distracting the fracture; the pull of traction on the distal fragment is aided by the pull of gravity on the proximal fragment. Usually, 5 kg of traction is sufficient in children and 10 kg in adults.

Confirm reduction by anteroposterior and lateral x-rays with the patient in traction. By the third to fourth week the knee and hip may be gradually extended while traction is maintained.

When the fractured limb has been extended, apply a mini-spica or cast-brace.

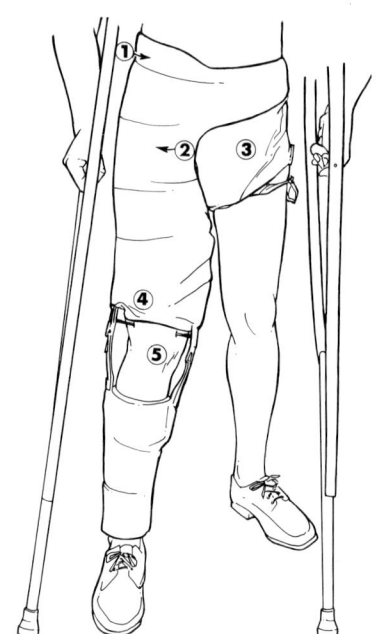

Application of a Mini-Spica

1. The mini-spica is wrapped snugly around the pelvis.
2. The hip on the fractured side is abducted and externally rotated.
3. The unfractured hip is left free of the cast.
4. The knee is allowed to move on the fractured side using brace hinges.
5. The traction pin is left in the distal femur until the stability of the fracture can be determined during weight bearing.

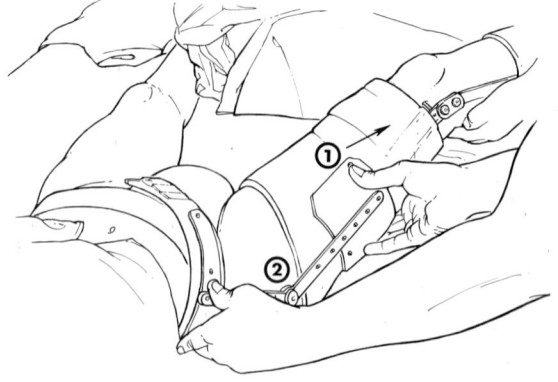

Application of Cast-Brace

1. A cast-brace is applied with the limb in the abducted, externally rotated position.
2. The pelvic band with hip joint attached to the cast-brace holds the fractured limb in continued abduction and external rotation.

3. The patient walks on the fractured limb in the abducted position, maintaining a valgus reduction of the subtrochanteric fracture.

4. The traction pin is left in the distal femur until the stability of the fracture can be ascertained during weight bearing.

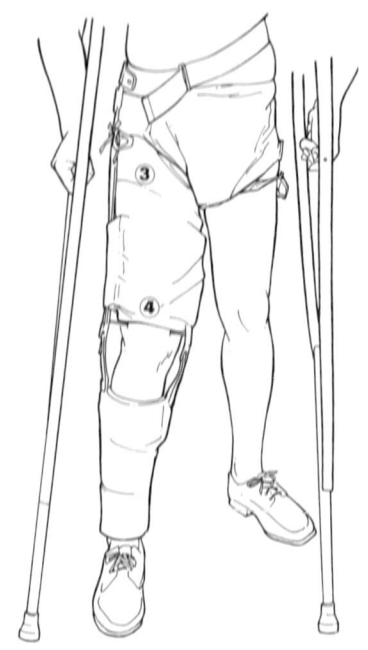

Appearance on X-Ray

Prior to mini-spica or cast-brace application,

1. Torsional deformity is evident at the fracture site. This apparent varus angulation is a combination of external rotation of the proximal fragment and internal rotation of the distal fragment.

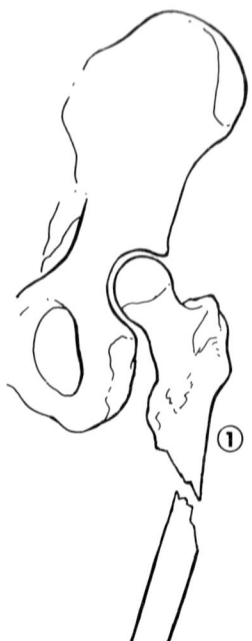

Appearance on X-ray (Continued)

After application of cast-brace with pelvic band,

2. The pelvic band attachment is maintaining the fractured limb in abduction and external rotation and

3. Torsional deformity at the fracture site has been corrected.

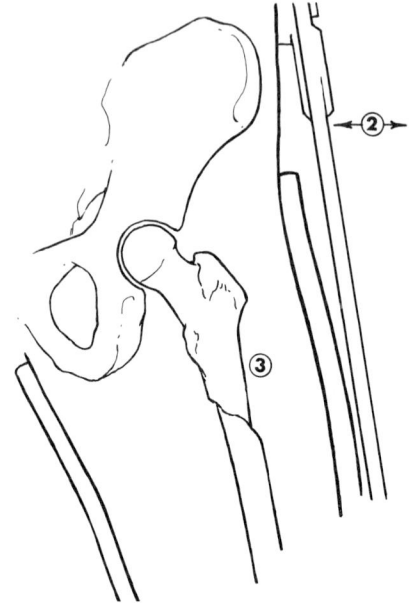

Subsequent Management

If the fracture proves unstable, intermittent traction may be used, employing the pin that is still in the distal femur.

In most instances the alignment of the fracture can be maintained with either the mini-spica or the cast-brace and the patient is discharged from the hospital.

Follow the position of the fracture with periodic x-rays for 2 months after discharge. The mini-spica or cast-brace can be removed by 12 to 14 weeks, the average time for fracture healing in adults with subtrochanteric fractures.

In children, the fracture may heal twice as rapidly as in adults, and the mini-spica or cast-brace can be removed by 6 to 8 weeks.

FRACTURES OF THE NECK OF THE FEMUR

REMARKS

Since this fracture is a common affliction of the aged, increasing life expectancy has made the medical and sociologic problems of management quite significant.

Femoral neck fractures occur 4 to 5 times more frequently in women than in men, because of the relatively greater degree of osteoporosis in women. The average age for a patient sustaining this fracture is 73.

The 5-year survival rate in this age group is consistently around 50 per cent. Of those who survive, only half treated by internal fixation will have acceptable clinical results. The other half will suffer either of two major complications, nonunion or segmental collapse of the femoral head.

The likelihood of complications depends primarily on the degree of initial displacement of the fracture, but even initially undisplaced fractures are subject to segmental collapse.

Undisplaced or impacted fractures generally do well with either nonoperative or operative treatment. Nonoperative management carries approximately an 80 per cent chance of good to excellent results, whereas 90 per cent of impacted femoral neck fractures are likely to have good to excellent results if fixed internally.

Currently, most undisplaced fractures are treated with multiple Knowles pins to prevent displacement.

The frequency of complications with the displaced femoral neck fracture has earned it the designation "unsolved fracture."

Recent attempts at surgical solution have included multiple pins, pins and screws, compression screws, and cross screws, all of which in the surviving patient still result in a nonunion rate of approximately 30 per cent. Late segmental collapse in healed fracture also occurs in about 30 per cent.

Open reduction and primary bone grafting has been reported to lower the complication rate, but the applicability of this method must be studied further.

The insolubility of the displaced femoral neck fracture in the elderly has led to the use of primary femoral prosthetic replacement. This appears especially applicable in patients older than 70 years whose life expectancy is 5 years or less.

With a cemented femoral prosthesis, the majority of patients with femoral neck fracture, rather than experiencing the prolonged and frustrating complications of nonunion or segmental collapse, can be restored to early, pain-free ambulation for their remaining years.

Attempted closed reduction and internal fixation, described in the literature, have little to recommend them for the elderly patient. The femoral neck fracture should not be considered primarily a challenge to the orthopedic surgeon's ego to the detriment of the elderly patient who needs and desires to get back on her feet as quickly as possible.

Still, the fracture occurs sufficiently often in younger patients that we must continue to attempt solutions other than primary prosthetic replacement for the combined problems of fracture instability and circulatory damage to the femoral head.

One factor that does not appear to contribute as significantly to complications as was previously thought is the delay prior to operation. In a large prospective study of 1500 femoral neck fractures, Barnes and co-workers found no essential effect on the rate of union or segmental collapse when operative fixation was delayed up to 1 week.

Before choosing the alternative modes of treating a femoral neck fracture, the surgeon must consider the mechanics and classification of the fracture as well as the effect of the injury on circulation to the femoral head.

MECHANISM OF FEMORAL NECK FRACTURE

REMARKS

The difficulties in fixing this fracture stem directly from the mechanism of injury.

Kocher pointed out in 1896 that the fracture results from firm fixation of the head by the anterior capsule and iliofemoral ligaments while the neck rotates externally.

Clinically, this frequently results from sudden twisting of the elderly patient's osteoporotic femoral neck with simultaneous vertical loading of the extended hip.

The patient often does not sustain the fracture because of a fall; she fractures the hip first and then falls.

With an undisplaced fracture, the patient may be able to continue to walk but with an antalgic limp.

In most instances the patient presents with a painful, shortened limb, an external rotation deformity, and inability to put weight on the leg.

CAUTION

Any elderly patient with hip pain after a rotatory injury must be treated and protected for a femoral neck fracture despite equivocal or contrary radiographic evidence. Frequently radiographic changes are not evident for 1 to 2 weeks after the injury. Fatigue fractures may also occur in young people, e.g. military recruits, and these often require bone scanning for initial detection (see page 1423).

Femoral neck fractures show a consistent pattern produced by indirect external torsional mechanisms. The fracture line runs obliquely from the distal medial cortex or calcar to the proximal lateral cortex or region of the epiphyseal scar (see also page 1464).

The epiphyseal scar and the strong ascending trabeculae act as stress concentrators and insure the constancy of the fracture.

The only variation is the point of failure of the calcar, which may be at varying distances from the head.

These fractures then must be considered subcapital since by far the majority begin just beneath the head.

The diagnosis "transverse cervical fracture," implying a lower fracture, should be abandoned because it generally stems from misinterpretation of the radiographic appearance of the fracture, which varies depending on the degree of internal rotation of the limb.

Obliquity of the Fracture Line in Subcapital Fractures

1. Fracture line begins at the superior cervicocapital junction.
2. Fracture line extends obliquely through the neck to the inferior cortex.
3. Beak of the neck is attached to the proximal fragment.

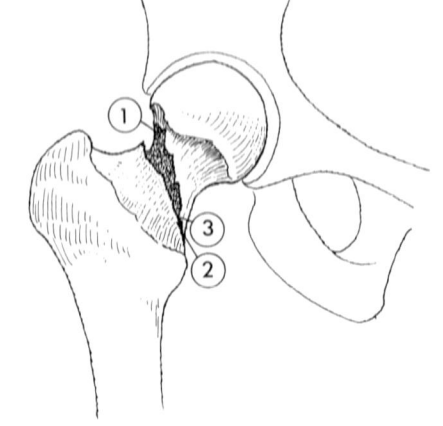

1. An oblique subcapital fracture may be misinterpreted as a transcervical fracture, depending on the degree of rotation of the fractured limb at the time of x-ray.
2. Rotation of this subcapital fracture causes it to appear lower in the neck and to be misinterpreted as a "transcervical fracture."

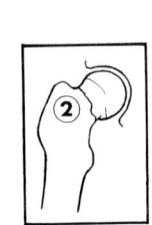
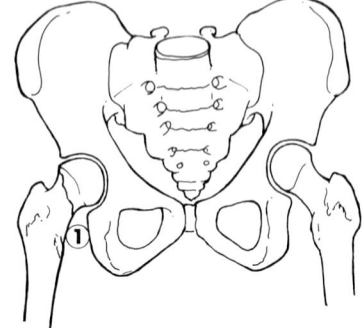

CLASSIFICATION OF SUBCAPITAL FRACTURES ACCORDING TO DEGREE OF ROTATIONAL INSTABILITY (AFTER GARDEN)

Garden's classification or staging of femoral neck fractures according to the degree of rotational instability and displacement is useful in selecting treatment and determining prognosis.

When results from these fractures are discussed, it must be made clear at what stage the fracture was at presentation, because results vary considerably according to the degree of fracture instability.

The Role of Lateral Rotation of the Limb in the Mechanism of Subcapital Fracture of the Neck of the Femur

1. The extremity rotates laterally.
2. The pelvis rotates in the opposite direction.
3. Tension force is applied at the anterior aspect of the neck as
4. Compression force is applied at the posterior aspect of the neck.
5. Incomplete fracture occurs perpendicular to the long axis of the neck.
6. The capital fragment is in slight valgus.

Note: This is equivalent to a Stage I fracture, or incomplete fracture. Prognosis is good.

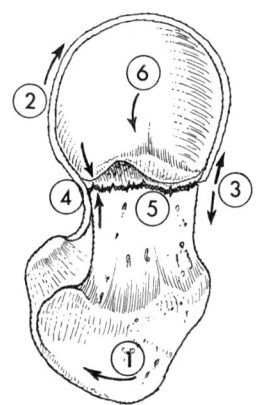

As the forces continue:
1. The fracture is completed and
2. The capital fragment is in normal position with the distal fragment.
3. The posterior neck is not comminuted.
4. The posterior retinaculum is intact.

Note: This is equivalent to a Stage II fracture, or complete fracture without displacement. Prognosis is good, provided that the fracture is not allowed to displace.

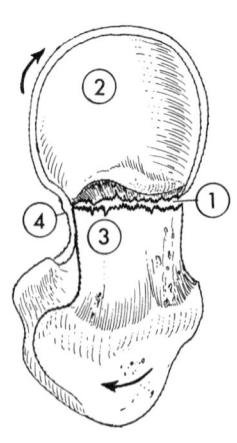

With further external rotation of the limb:
1. The femoral head rotates internally.
2. The limb rotates externally.
3. The fracture line opens anteriorly.
4. The posterior cortex is compressed at the fracture line but not collapsed.
5. The posterior retinaculum is still intact and the fragments are not detached.

Note: This is equivalent to a Stage III fracture, or complete fracture with partial displacement. Prognosis is guarded, but if rigid fixation is achieved, fracture union is likely.

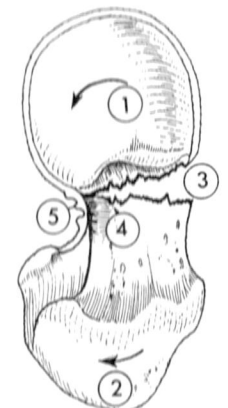

With further external rotation of the limb and complete displacement and detachment of the fragments:
1. The limb rolls out to full external rotation.
2. The distal fragment displaces superiorly.
3. The head rotates back into its normal position in the acetabulum.
4. The neck fragment rotates anterior to the head.
5. Complete collapse of the posterior cortex occurs with separation of a large triangular fragment from the posteroinferior cortex adjacent to the head.
6. The posterior retinaculum is disrupted, permitting complete detachment of the fragments.

Note: This is equivalent to a Stage IV fracture, with complete fracture and full displacement. Prognosis is poor. Open reduction with posterior bone grafting or prosthetic replacement is indicated, depending on the age of the patient.

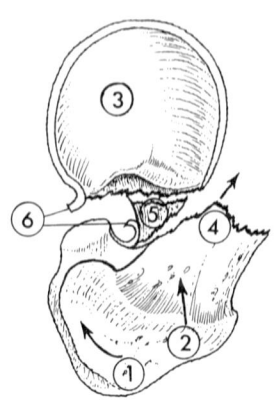

GARDEN'S STAGING OF SUBCAPITAL FRACTURES — ANTEROPOSTERIOR APPEARANCE

Stage I: Incomplete Subcapital Fracture

1. Incomplete fracture of the neck.
2. External rotation of the distal fragment.
3. The proximal fragment is in valgus.
4. The medial trabeculae of the head and the trabeculae of the neck form an angle greater than 180 degrees.

Note: This is a stable fracture with a good prognosis, provided that it does not become complete and does not displace.

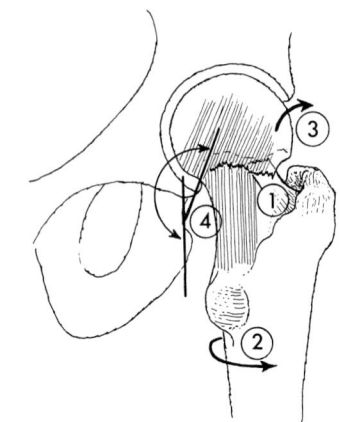

Stage II: Complete Subcapital Fracture Without Displacement

1. There is a complete oblique fracture through the neck.
2. The capital fragment is not displaced.
3. The distal fragment is in normal alignment with the proximal fragment.
4. The medial trabeculae of the head make an angle of approximately 160 degrees with those of the femoral cortex.

Note: Lateral rotation of the distal fragment may cause displacement of the fragments, thus producing a fracture of Stage III or IV.

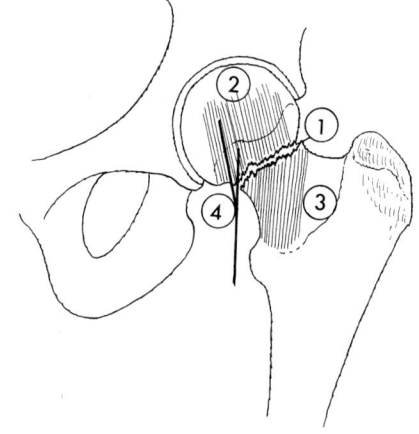

The posterior cortex of the femur is still not collapsed and the posterior retinaculum is intact.
This is a stable fracture with a good prognosis, provided that it is not allowed to displace.

Stage III: Complete Subcapital Fracture with Partial Displacement

1. The distal fragment is rotated laterally.
2. The proximal fragment is tilted into varus and rotated medially.
3. The medial trabeculae of the head are not in alignment with those of the pelvis.

Note: The posterior cortex of the neck is not collapsed; the posterior retinaculum is still intact holding the fragments together, but this may be injured.

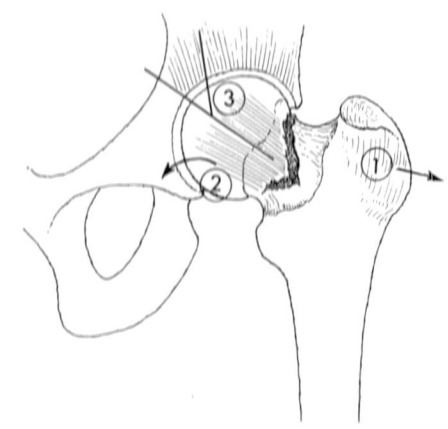

Further lateral rotation of the distal fragment will convert this lesion to a Stage IV fracture.

This fracture, if properly reduced, can be converted to a stable fracture with a good prognosis.

Stage IV: Complete Subcapital Fracture with Full Displacement

1. The capital fragment is completely detached from the distal fragment and has returned to its normal position in the acetabulum; its medial trabeculae now are in alignment with those of the pelvis.
2. The distal fragment is rotated laterally.
3. The distal fragment is displaced upward and anterior to the proximal fragment.

Note: The posterior cortex of the neck has collapsed and the posterior retinaculum is stripped or torn from the posterior aspect of the neck.

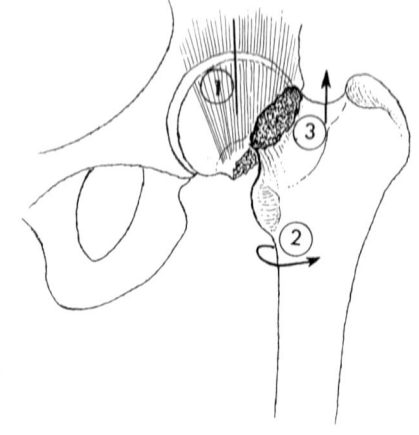

This fracture is difficult to reduce perfectly; even if the reduction is achieved, the defect in the posterior cortex renders it unstable. The prognosis is poor.

Primary prosthetic replacement or open reduction with posterior bone grafting is indicated, depending on the patient's age.

MEASUREMENT OF THE HEAD-NECK RELATIONSHIPS

The weight-bearing trabeculae of the head, neck, and pelvis lie in line with the pathways of stress.

In subcapital fractures a change in the relationship of the weight-bearing trabeculae in the pelvis, head, and neck indicates fairly accurately the relationship of the proximal fragment to the distal fragment.

In the anteroposterior view the medial trabeculae of the head make an angle of approximately 160 degrees with those of the femoral cortex.

In the lateral view the medial and lateral trabeculae of the head converge and intersect on a straight line running through the center of the neck. Hence, the normal anteroposterior-lateral arrangement of the weight-bearing trabeculae of the head and neck can be expressed as 160/180 (Garden).

Garden and other investigators have found that to achieve satisfactory results, alignment of the fracture must be within the range of 155 to 180 degrees on the AP view and 180 to 155 degrees on the lateral view.

Other useful determinants of malreduction include wedging of the hip joint space, extreme tilting of the capital fragment in any direction, widening of the joint space, and disturbance of Shenton's line.

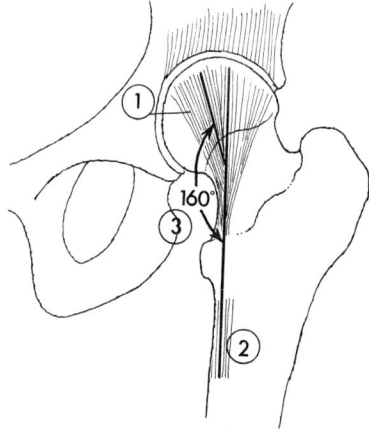

Anteroposterior X-Ray — Normal Anteroposterior Alignment

1. Medial trabeculae of the head.
2. Medial cortex of the femur.
3. These make an angle of approximately 160 degrees.

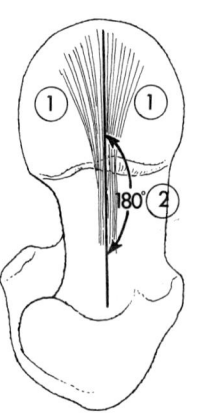

Lateral X-Ray — Normal Lateral Alignment

1. Medial and lateral trabeculae intersect on
2. A straight line running through the center of the neck — 180 degrees.

FRACTURES OF THE NECK OF THE FEMUR

Capital Fragment in Valgus

1. Medial trabeculae of the head.
2. Medial cortex of the femur.
3. These make an angle of 180 degrees.

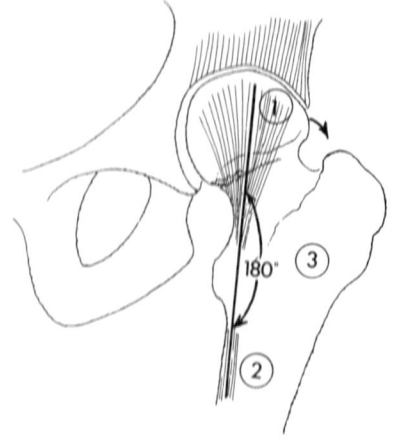

Capital Fragment in Varus

1. Medial trabeculae of the head.
2. Medial cortex of the femur.
3. These make an angle of 135 degrees.

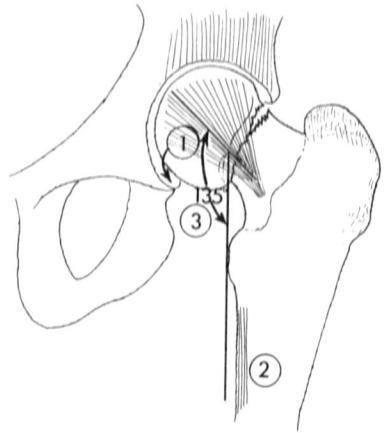

OTHER DETERMINANTS OF MALREDUCTION

1. Wedging of the joint space.

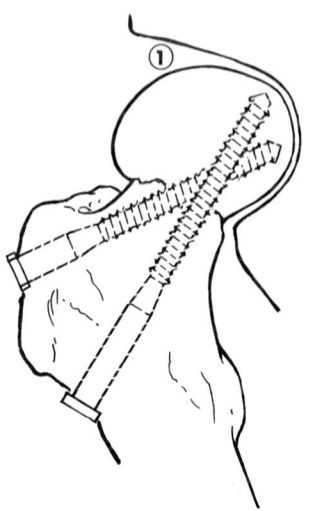

2. Extreme tilting of the capital fragment.

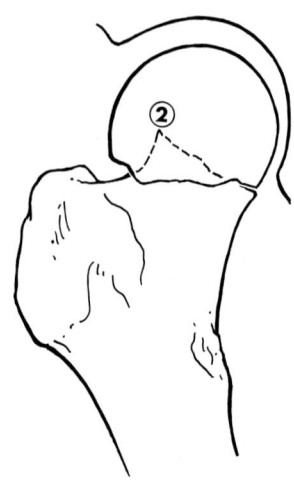

3. Widening or narrowing of the joint space.

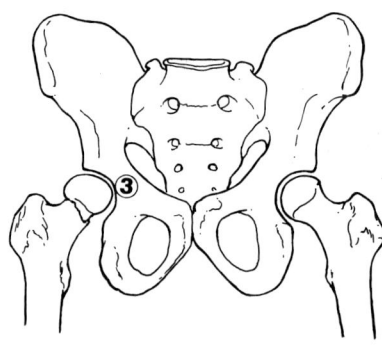

4. Interruption of Shenton's line.

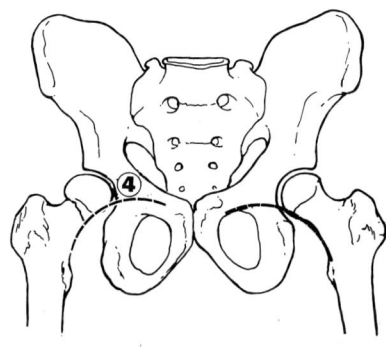

SIGNIFICANCE OF POSTERIOR COMMINUTION FOR FEMORAL NECK FRACTURE STABILITY

REMARKS

The anterior surface of the femoral neck is convex and the head of the femur overhangs the posteroinferior portion of the neck.

In elderly people the flared posteroinferior juncture of the head and neck is thin and friable. When subjected to compression forces it readily crumbles. However, the type of lesion produced is fairly constant: a triangular piece of bone separates from the posteroinferior surface of the neck at its point of union with the head, producing a collapse of the posterior cortex.

This defect in the posterior and inferior cortices is responsible for the instability of subcapital fractures in the Stage IV category. This fracture is difficult to reduce, and even if anatomic reduction is achieved, the defect in the posterior cortex still persists, rendering the reduced fracture unstable.

The loss of the posterior support prevents adequate stability with the usual internal fixation techniques. To overcome instability, open reduction and posterior bone grafting may be necessary.

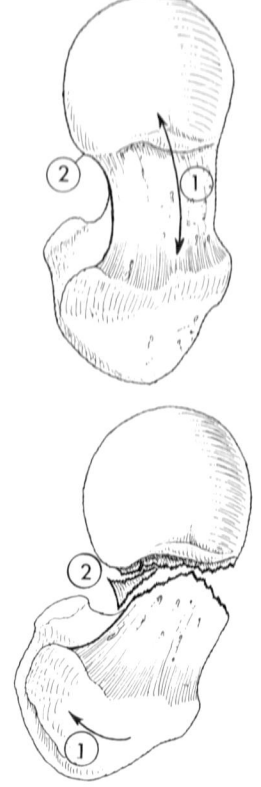

Lateral View of the Upper End of the Femur

1. Anterior convexity of the neck of the femur.
2. Overhang of the femoral head over the posteroinferior cortex of the neck.

Collapse of the Posteroinferior Cortex of the Neck in Stage IV Fracture

1. The distal fragment is in full lateral rotation
2. Compression of the posterior cortex results in comminution of the cortex with separation of a triangular piece of bone.

Note: This type of fracture in a young person is a prime indication for open reduction and posterior bone grafting.

CIRCULATORY CHANGES ASSOCIATED WITH FEMORAL NECK FRACTURE

REMARKS

Most of the blood supply to the femoral head is derived from three sources:
The posterior superior retinacular vessels.
The posterior inferior retinacular vessels.

The artery of the ligamentum teres.

The retinacular vessels are derived from the medial femoral circumflex, as previously described on page 1264. They supply the growing femoral epiphysis in childhood and the femoral head in adulthood. These vessels enter through the capsule along its intertrochanteric insertion and then course along the femoral neck, enveloped in retinacular folds of the capsule, to enter the bony foramina just distal to the articular surface. These vessels, because of their long course, are quite vulnerable to injury. The superior retinacular vessels are particularly liable to disruption by a displaced femoral neck fracture.

The artery of the ligamentum teres is usually a branch of the obturator artery. It penetrates the head at the fovea capitis but supplies a very small volume of the head (10 per cent). This vessel may become a source of revascularization after a completely displaced femoral head loses its superior and inferior retinacular supply.

Blood Supply of the Femoral Head

1. Posterior superior retinacular vessels.
2. Posterior inferior retinacular vessels.
3. The artery of the ligamentum teres.

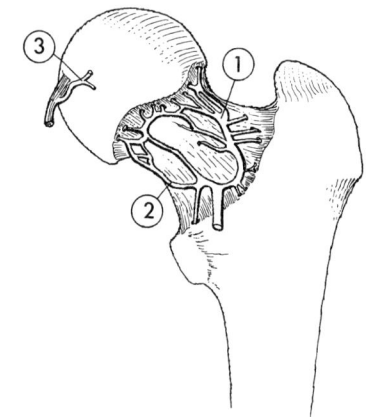

PATHOLOGY OF THE FRACTURE'S CONTRIBUTION TO NONUNION

REMARKS

Because of the unique elongated position of the femoral neck within the joint capsule, the femoral neck fracture must heal without the benefit of external callus from either periosteum or surrounding soft tissues.

Fracture healing comes almost entirely from the intramedullary callus, which in the undisplaced fracture is usually quite adequate.

With complete displacement of the fracture, however, the proximal fragment loses its circulation quite promptly, as evidenced by death of the blood-forming and fat-forming cells in the marrow. Fracture healing then must depend on callus formation from the viable distal medullary canal across the proximal fragment.

Fracture healing from a viable distal fragment to a "dead" proximal fragment is quite possible provided that fixation is adequate, but frequently stabilization is inadequate owing to posterior cortical comminution. Fracture union consequently is mostly by dense fibrous tissue.

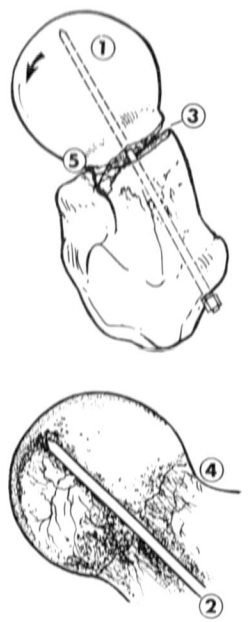

1. Complete displacement has disrupted the retinacular vessels and has caused necrosis of the proximal fragment.
2. Pins stabilize the fracture.
3. The fracture gap is filling with some new bone formed by appositional growth but also by fibrous tissue.
4. There is no external callus evident.
5. The posterior cortical buttress is lost allowing motion at the fracture site, particularly with external rotation of the limb.

Note: The lack of external callus, the loss of circulation to the proximal fragment, and the external rotational instability all contribute to the high rate of nonunion in a displaced femoral neck fracture.

PATHOLOGY OF THE FRACTURE'S CONTRIBUTION TO SEGMENTAL COLLAPSE OF THE FEMORAL HEAD

Segmental collapse results from the failure of subchondral bone weakened by the response to the injury. This has been called "avascular necrosis," which implies that the bone having lost its circulation, dies and crumbles away. Actually, dead bone retains its structural properties, and it is only the vascular response to the dead bone that weakens the structure and causes the collapse.

Circulation to the femoral head is inevitably damaged by the displaced fracture, which runs from the epiphyseal scar obliquely downward.

The superior retinacular vessels are torn consistently with any fracture displacement, and the inferior vessels may or may not remain intact.

The superior segment of the head is most often rendered ischemic, but in a large percentage of displaced fractures the entire head may lose its blood supply.

The extent of the dead bone cannot be determined by changes in radiographic density. Increased radiographic density is usually the result of new bone depositing on dead bone and consequently is a sign of viability.

Bone scanning with technetium-99m sulfur-colloid, which is taken up by the marrow cells in viable femoral heads, is the most reliable indicator of avascular necrosis currently available (see page 1452).

Segmental collapse occurs consistently in the region of the dead bone just beyond the border of the revascularization front. Failure in this region of healing causes the subchondral bone to fatigue and to pull away its support for the articular cartilage. Traumatic arthritis then results.

Segmental collapse occurs much more readily when biomechanical loading across the hip joint is altered by abnormal reduction of the femoral head fragment. The weakened subchondral bone will fatigue quite readily when the intra-articular stresses are concentrated by malreduction, particularly in a valgus position.

1. Revascularization into the area of dead bone weakens the trabeculae.
2. The failure occurs through the dead bone just beyond the border of revascularization.
3. Collapse of subchondral bone produces a crescent defect beneath the articular cartilage.
4. Lack of support for the articular cartilage results in traumatic arthritis of the joint surface.

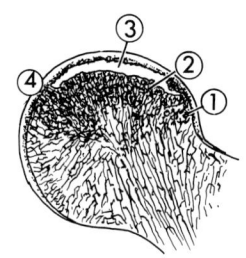

Note: The diagnosis of avascular necrosis can be made prior to segmental collapse by bone scan using technetium-99m sulfur-colloid, which is taken up by viable marrow cells in the femoral head (see page 1452).

Flattening of Head (Forerunner of Segmental Collapse)

1. Fracture line.
2. Flattening of weight-bearing area of the head (seen as early as six months after injury).

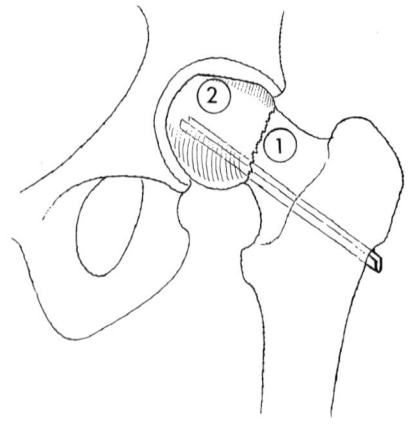

Segmental Collapse

1. Fracture line almost obliterated.
2. Segmental collapse (may occur as late as three years after injury).

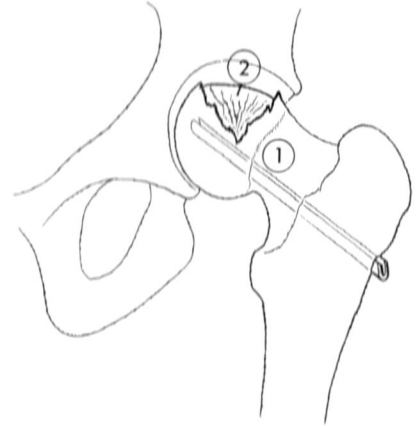

BIOMECHANICS OF THE HIP JOINT AND THE EFFECT OF FRACTURE REDUCTION ON SEGMENTAL COLLAPSE

REMARKS

According to Rydell, the hip is not a ball-and-socket joint. The head pivots in the acetabulum, which is constructed like a gimbal.

The normal "out-of-round" design of the femoral head in the acetabulum causes the joint to pivot about the superior weight-bearing portion of the femoral head.

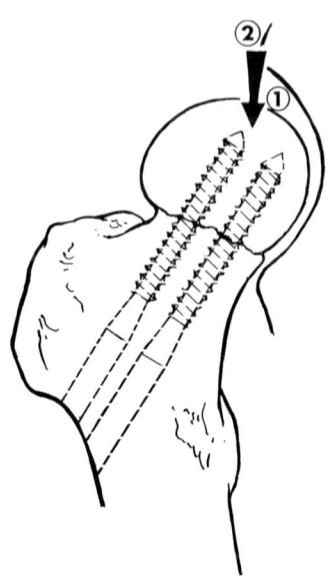

1. Reduction of the subcapital fracture in excessive valgus position causes the joint space to become wedge-shaped and concentrates weight bearing on a narrow point of the head.
2. The articular surface of the head is pushed outside the joint.

Note: The injury to the femoral head circulation produced by the fracture and the altered biomechanics of the joint produced by reduction in excessive valgus position are the chief factors leading to segmental collapse.

Evaluation of Patients for Femoral Neck Fractures

REMARKS

Suspect that any patient who complains of hip pain after a fall or after repetitive strain has sustained an undisplaced femoral neck fracture. The sole physical finding may be hip pain produced with gentle internal rotation of the femur.

A patient complaining of hip pain, particularly an elderly patient, should have adequate anteroposterior and lateral x-rays to rule out this common injury.

Femoral neck fractures may also result from fatigue of the relatively weak femoral neck in young persons, particularly military recruits in basic training.

If a femoral neck fracture is suspected but is not detected on standard x-rays, bone scans should be obtained about 5 to 7 days after onset of symptoms.

Undisplaced and unrecognized fractures of the femoral neck have the potential for serious complications whether they are impacted fractures in the elderly or stress fractures in the young.

X-Ray Evaluation Techniques

FOR ANTEROPOSTERIOR VIEW

1. Always obtain an anteroposterior view of the pelvis rather than of the hip. This permits comparison with the opposite side.

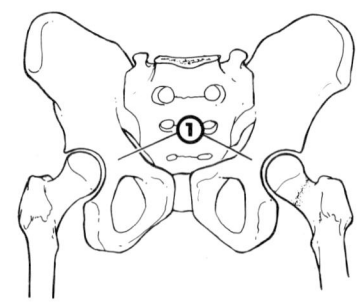

FRACTURES OF THE NECK OF THE FEMUR

For lateral view

1. A true lateral x-ray is obtained without moving the injured limb excessively. The tube is placed under the involved limb at a 30 degree-angle from the shaft and is directed toward a point midway between the greater trochanter and the crest of the ileum.

2. The x-ray cassette is held against the patient's flank above the iliac crest.

Note: If the radiographic evidence is negative despite clinical suspicion of a femoral neck fracture, protect the patient's hip with crutches and obtain a bone scan 5 to 7 days later.

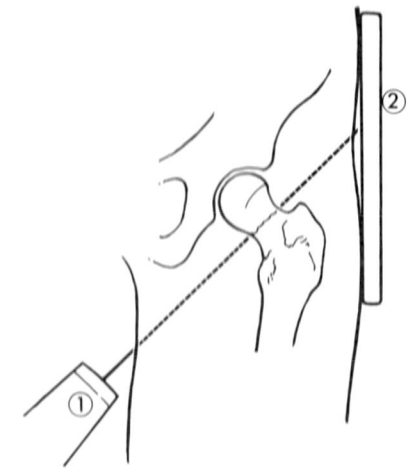

Bone Scan for Occult Fractures

1. The bone scan shows increased activity in the left femoral neck of a 28-year-old man with hip pain of 10 days' duration after beginning basic military training. The original x-ray of this lesion showed no abnormalities.

2. X-ray after the bone scan shows a fatigue fracture, as indicated by increased sclerosis of the femoral neck.

Note: Prompt diagnosis of fatigue fractures in this area requires a high index of suspicion and early use of bone scanning, if necessary. Fatigue fractures and impacted femoral neck fractures can be treated much more effectively before they displace than after.

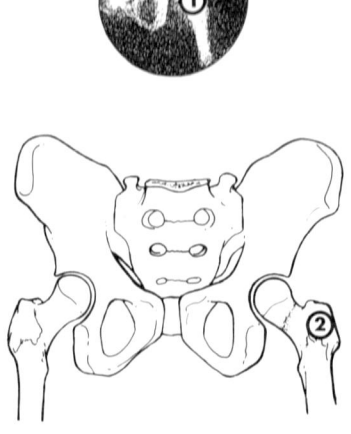

Management of Femoral Neck Fractures

REMARKS

Management of the femoral neck fracture must be chosen primarily according to the degree of initial fracture displacement and the age of the patient. The most common fracture is displaced and occurs in a patient who is chronologically and physiologically more than 70 years of age. For this patient the most effective treatment is primary femoral prosthetic replacement.

For the next most common fracture, the impacted Stage I or Stage II fracture, multiple Knowles pins offer the best opportunity for healing without complications.

There is evidence from the work of Crawford that the patient with a truly impacted or Stage I femoral neck fracture may be treated by protected crutch walking without internal fixation. If Crawford's criteria are truly present and the patient wishes to accept a 10 to 15 per cent chance of displacement, nonoperative treatment may be employed.

Stage III fractures are displaced and require closed reduction. Rigid fixation using a compression screw protects against external rotational loading across the fracture.

Completely displaced Stage IV fractures, particularly in younger patients who are not candidates for primary prosthesis, require open reduction and fixation with bone grafting of the comminuted posterior cortex. This offers the patient statistically the best chance for accurate reduction of the fracture and diminished incidence of segmental collapse of the femoral head.

MANAGEMENT OF STAGE III AND STAGE IV FEMORAL NECK FRACTURES IN THE ELDERLY PATIENT

REMARKS

Studies comparing results of primary internal fixation and primary prosthetic replacement in these fractures done by the same surgeons indicate that these fractures are best treated in the elderly by primary femoral prosthetic replacement. A femoral prosthesis is also indicated for a fracture in a patient with a seizure disorder or spasmodic Parkinsonian condition who cannot protect the hip adequately after internal fixation.

The major objection to femoral prosthetic replacement has been a fairly high incidence of loosening in the femoral canal or erosion of the steel prosthesis through the acetabular cartilage.

Newer femoral prostheses, such as the Cathcart type, are designed to be cemented in the femoral canal and are ellipsoidal in order to more closely approximate the natural shape of the femoral head. These features diminish loosening and also permit synovial fluid to flow between the steel prosthesis and the acetabular cartilage to diminish the chance of erosion.

We have found at the University of Nebraska that the Cathcart cemented prosthesis provides a good to excellent method of restoring the elderly patient to her preinjury ambulatory status with minimal long-term symptoms from either acetabular erosion or stem loosening.

Technique of Inserting a Cemented Cathcart Prosthesis

1. The patient is in the lateral position.
2. Approach the hip through a posterior incision, which begins 5 cm distal to the posterior superior iliac spine and parallels the fibers of the gluteus maximus. It runs distally one fingerbreadth posterior to the trochanter for approximately 5 cm.

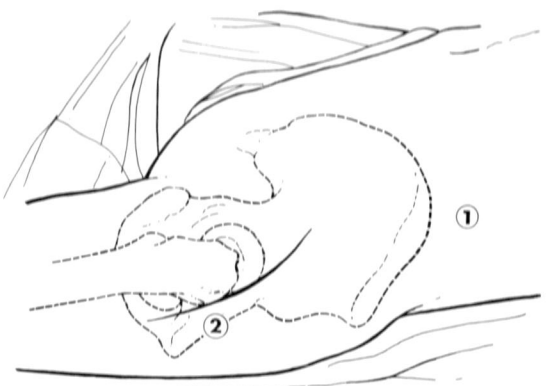

1. Split the gluteus maximus along the line of the incision and release its insertion partially into the fascia lata.
2. Visualize and protect the sciatic nerve.
3. Divide the tendons of the piriformis, the superior gemellus, the obturator internus, and the inferior gemellus to expose the hip capsule.

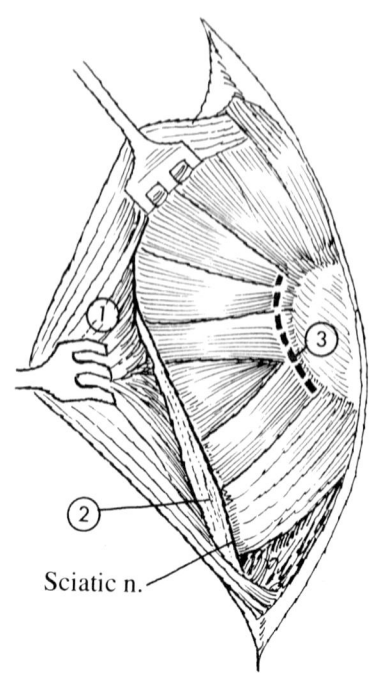

Technique of Inserting a Cemented Cathcart Prosthesis (*Continued*)

4. Open the hip capsule with a T-shaped incision to expose the fracture.
5. Cut the femoral neck at an angle to parallel the neck of the prosthesis and to seat the prosthesis on the calcar 1.5 cm above the lesser trochanter.
6. Ream the medullary canal completely with a rasp so as to remove all cancellous bone.

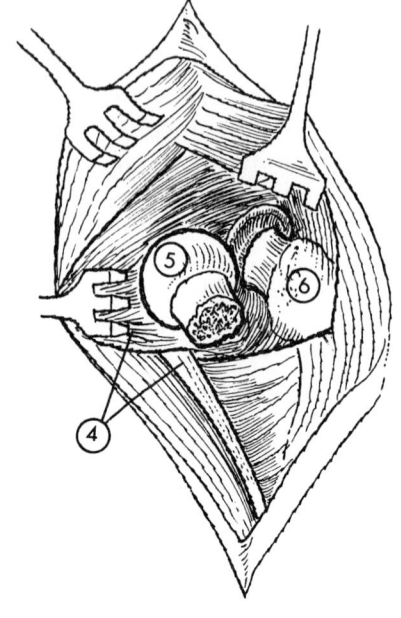

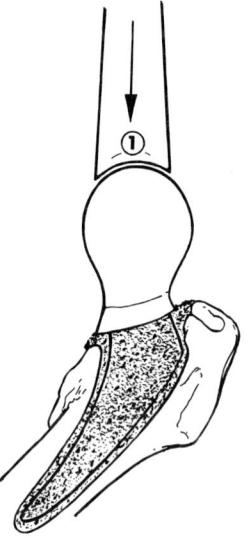

1. After the proper size prosthesis has been selected, fill the thoroughly reamed medullary canal with a batch of methyl methacrylate cement and introduce the prosthesis.

2. Drive the Cathcart prosthesis into the cemented canal and seat the neck of the prosthesis on the calcar.
3. The "out-of-round" shape of the femoral prosthesis is designed to allow perfusion of the acetabulum by synovial fluid and to diminish the likelihood of acetabular erosion.

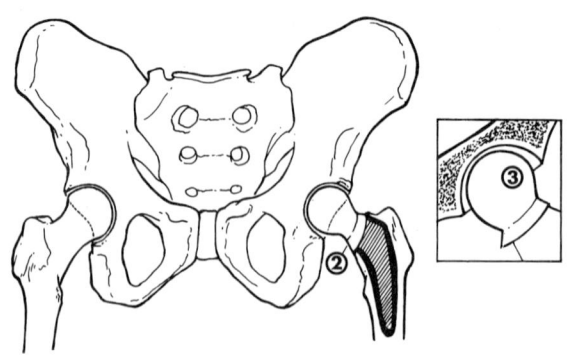

Postoperative Management

Protect the hip by supporting it in an abduction device to prevent flexion and external rotation.

The patient may be allowed to bear weight with a walker or crutches by the third postoperative day.

Crutch walking or use of the walker should be continued for 6 to 8 weeks, after which the patient may advance to a cane.

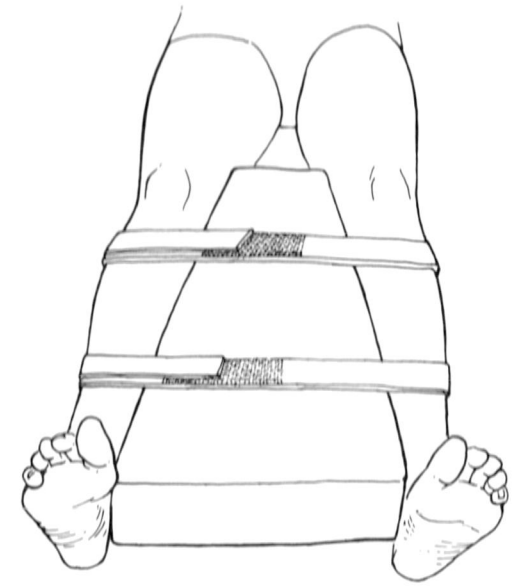

MANAGEMENT OF STAGE I AND STAGE II IMPACTED SUBCAPITAL FRACTURES

REMARKS

For the second most frequent type of fracture, fixation by multiple Knowles pins offers the best opportunity of healing without complication. If the patient is willing to accept a roughly 10 per cent chance that the fracture will "slip" and meets the criteria established by Crawford, nonoperative treatment may be acceptable.

Crawford's criteria for diagnosis of a stable impacted fracture include:
1. No shortening or external rotation of the limb.
2. Very little discomfort in the hip joint on active or passive motion.
3. Ability of the patient to perform active internal rotation of the limb.
4. Impaction should be evident on both anteroposterior and true lateral x-ray views.

Impacted Fracture Suitable for Crawford's Nonoperative Management

1. Both the anteroposterior and
2. True lateral views show the fracture impacted in the valgus position.

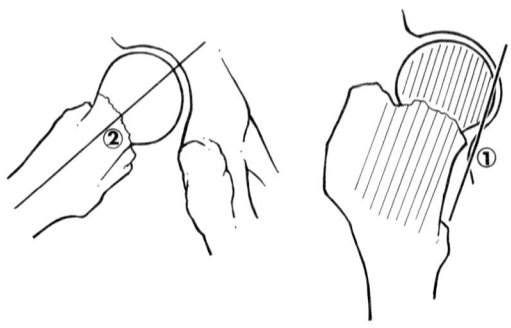

Impacted Fracture Unsuitable for Nonoperative Management

1. Anteroposterior x-ray shows what appears to be a valgus impacted fracture.
2. A true lateral x-ray indicates displacement of the fracture to a degree that would prohibit the fracture from healing adequately and that is therefore unacceptable.

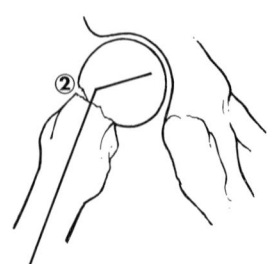
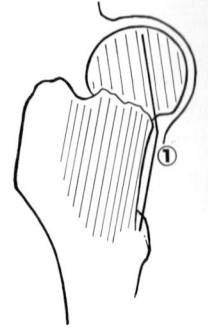

Nonoperative Management

During recovery, the patient may use a walker or crutches with toe-touch weight bearing as tolerated. Insistence that the patient refrain completely from weight bearing only accentuates the problem. The muscle activity required to maintain the limb off the ground produces loading across the hip that is greater than loading from simple weight bearing.

The patient should avoid rotating the affected limb and should continue using external assistive devices for at least four months, until the fracture shows radiographic evidence of union.

KNOWLES PIN FIXATION FOR STAGE I AND STAGE II FRACTURES

REMARKS

These undisplaced fractures in the elderly patient, who cannot adequately protect the hip against torsional injury, should be treated by fixation with multiple Knowles pins.

This procedure is generally safe and effectively protects the fracture against torsional injury and displacement.

Knowles pin fixation is recommended in most impacted and undisplaced Stage I and II fractures.

Preoperative X-Ray

IMPACTED VALGUS FRACTURE

1. Fracture line.
2. Head is in slight valgus. (The angle that the medial trabeculae of the head makes with the lateral cortex of the femur must not exceed 180 degrees.)
3. Head sits squarely on the neck in the lateral view.

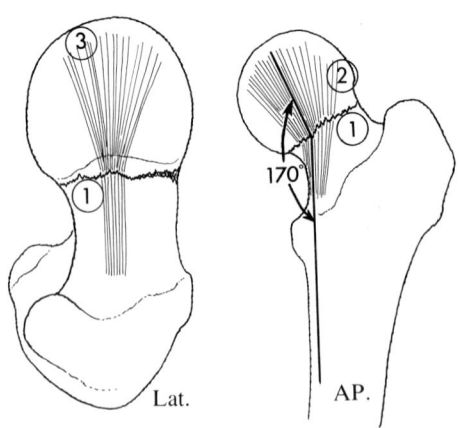

FRACTURES OF THE NECK OF THE FEMUR

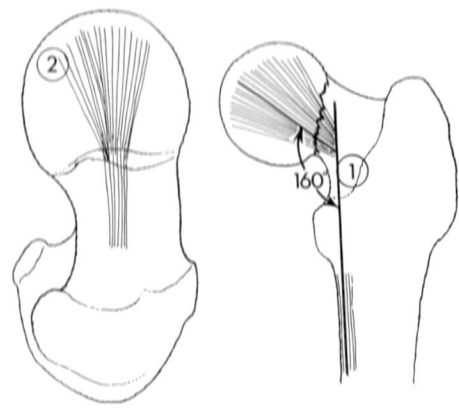

UNDISPLACED FRACTURE

1. On the anteroposterior view, the medial trabeculae of the head make an angle of 160 degrees with the lateral cortex of the femur.
2. Head sits squarely on the neck in the lateral view.

Operative Procedure

This procedure is best done on a fracture table with image-intensified fluoroscopy.

Be sure that adequate anteroposterior and lateral views can be obtained with the x-ray equipment.

The patient is anesthetized in bed and then is transferred to the table carefully to avoid disimpacting the fracture.

General anesthesia is safest and the least likely to cause cerebrovascular or cardiopulmonary complications in the elderly patient.

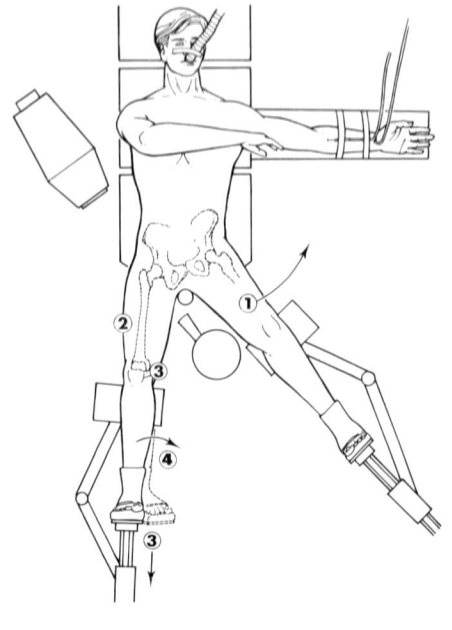

POSITION OF PATIENT

1. The unfractured limb is abducted to make room for the fluoroscopic tube.
2. The fractured limb is fixed to the table in neutral position.
3. Avoid applying any traction to the fractured limb other than that necessary to support the knee.
4. Internally rotate the fractured limb slightly.

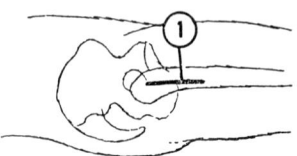

INSERTION OF GUIDE PINS

1. Make an 8-cm incision on the lateral aspect of the thigh just below the greater trochanter and centered on the shaft of the femur.

Operative Procedure (Continued)

2. Deepen the incision to the bone and by subperiosteal dissection expose the base of the trochanter and the upper end of the femur for approximately 7 cm.

3. Two to three centimeters below the lower margin of the greater trochanter and directly opposite the lesser trochanter, drill a hole 3 mm in diameter and direct it at an angle of approximately 45 degrees with the lateral cortex.

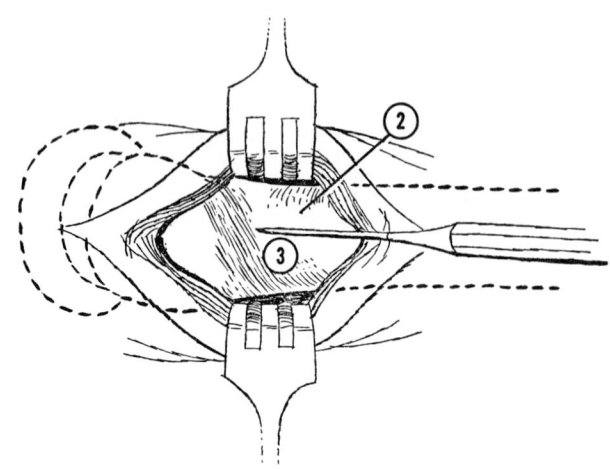

4. Pass a guide pin 3 mm in diameter into the neck and head. Pin position, as determined on the fluoroscope, should be in the subchondral bone.

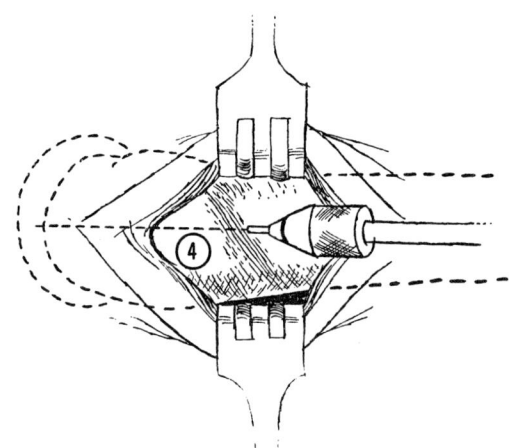

INTRAOPERATIVE X-RAYS

Take both anteroposterior and lateral views.

1. Pin lies in the center of the neck and head.
2. Pin makes an angle of 45 degrees with the shaft. This is the desired angle.

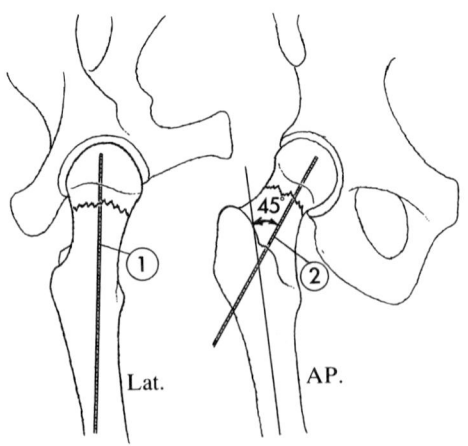

Insertion of Knowles Pins

The proper length for the Knowles pins is determined by the exact length of the guide pin. Leave the guide pin in place while the first two Knowles pins are inserted.

1. The first Knowles pin is inserted anterior and superior to the guide pin.

2. The second Knowles pin is inserted posterior and inferior to the guide pin. The guide pin may now be removed.

3. Two additional pins are inserted paralleling the first two.

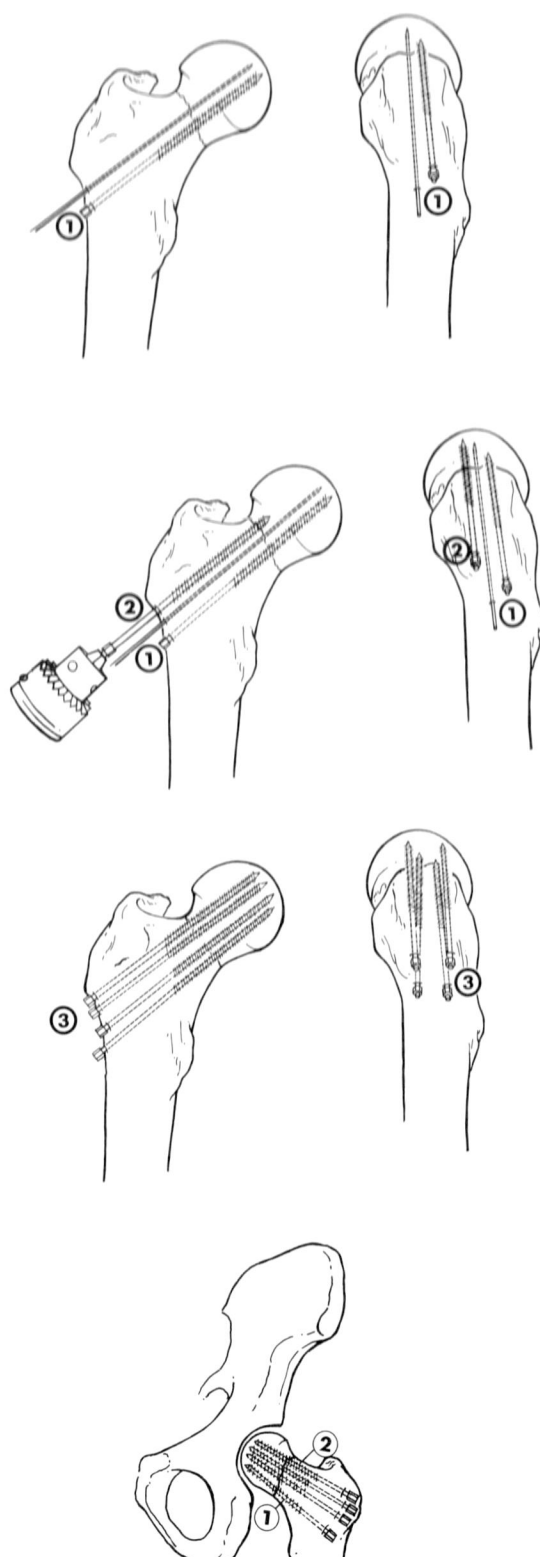

Postoperative X-Rays

Anteroposterior view

1. The two lower pins lie close to the calcar at an angle of approximately 150 degrees.
2. The upper pins lie close to the superior neck and head.

Note: If the pin exits partially through the neck and reenters the head, fixation is quite satisfactory.

1431

Postoperative X-Rays (Continued)

LATERAL VIEW

3. The anterior pins are close to the anterior cortex of the neck.
4. The posterior pins are close to the posterior cortex of the neck.

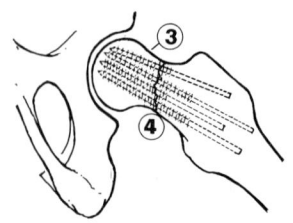

Postreduction Management

Encourage active exercises of the hip and knee as soon as the postoperative pain subsides.

The patient should be out of bed and standing in parallel bars by the second day, and she should progress to walking with a walker or crutches as soon as she regains her balance.

Toe-touch weight bearing may be allowed for balance.

After any hip injury, prolonged sitting in a chair should be avoided because it increases the likelihood of pelvic vein thrombosis.

The patient should continue with crutches or a walker for four months until the fracture is healed clinically and radiographically.

She should continue using a cane indefinitely after a hip fracture.

PARTIALLY DISPLACED (STAGE III) AND FULLY DISPLACED (STAGE IV) FEMORAL NECK FRACTURES

REMARKS

Management of these difficult femoral neck fractures with significant rotational displacement must be based primarily on the patient's physiological and emotional needs.

The patient who is older than 70, with 5 years or less life expectancy, is best treated by primary femoral prosthesis. The cemented femoral prosthesis as described on page 1426 is most likely to give prompt and satisfactory results.

Johnson and Crothers have shown that the differences in results of treatments for displaced fractures are clear-cut and indicate a higher failure rate after nailing than for prosthetic replacement. In studies with adequate follow-up of displaced fractures, the failure rate from nailing remains between 30 and 50 per cent despite numerous refinements of technique.

In a younger patient who is willing to accept the 40 per cent chance of complications and who can tolerate a secondary procedure, nailing seems indicated. At present the use of a high-angle compression hip screw offers very effective support provided that the posterior cortex is not comminuted.

For completely displaced fractures, particularly in young patients, open reduction and posterior bone grafting are indicated. This is the only way to insure accurate reduction and to correct the loss of posterior cortical support, which is responsible for many of the technical failures from nail fixation.

Prior to internal fixation, scanning of the femoral head with technetium-99m sulfur-colloid may detect significant areas of avascular necrosis and confirm the need for posterior bone grafting to minimize the likelihood of segmental collapse.

Preoperative X-Rays

PARTIALLY DISPLACED FRACTURE

1. The capital fragment is in varus position.
2. The distal fragment is rotated laterally.
3. The medial trabeculae of the head make an angle of 135 degrees with the medial cortex of the femur.

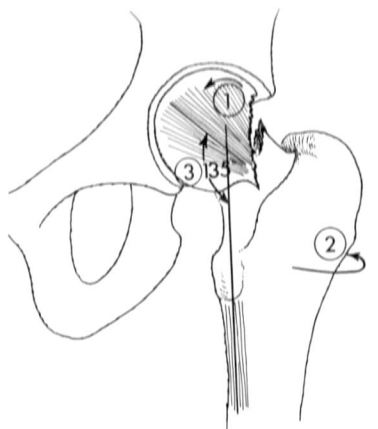

FULLY DISPLACED FRACTURE

1. The capital fragment is in its normal position in the acetabulum.
2. The distal fragment is fully rotated laterally.
3. The medial trabeculae of the head make an angle of 160 degrees with the medial cortex of the femur.

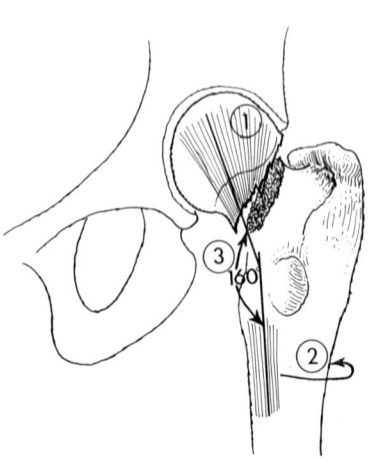

Operative Procedure: High-Angle Compression Hip-Screw Technique for Femoral Neck Fractures (After Southwick)

POSITION OF PATIENT

The patient is anesthetized in bed and then is transferred to the fracture table. General anesthesia is safest and least likely to cause cerebrovascular or cardiopulmonary complications.

Image-intensified fluoroscopy is required for this procedure. Prior to starting the operation be sure that the x-ray equipment is functioning satisfactorily and adequate anteroposterior and lateral views can be obtained.

1. The unfractured limb is abducted widely to make room for the fluoroscopic tube and to tilt the pelvis upward on the uninjured side.
2. The fractured limb is fixed to the table in neutral position.
3. Light traction is applied to the fractured limb sufficiently to tighten the knee ligament.
4. The fractured limb is internally rotated 45 degrees to correct the external rotation of the distal fragment.

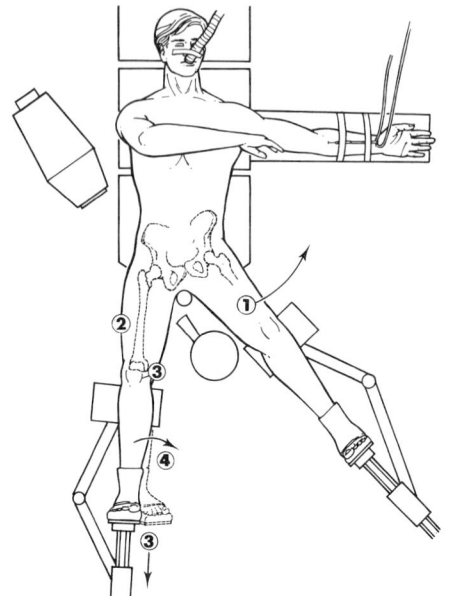

AVOID ABDUCTION OF THE FRACTURED LEG

1. Abduction of the fractured leg only serves to open up the fracture site medially.
2. By abducting the opposite leg while tilting the pelvis, the proximal head fragment can be brought over the distal neck fragment into the valgus position.

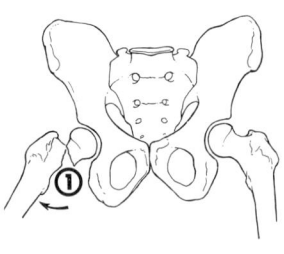

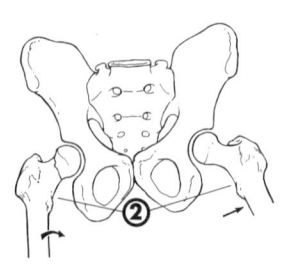

Postreduction X-Ray

Reduction must be satisfactory on both the anteroposterior and lateral view.

1. The anteroposterior view shows the fracture is in 170 degrees of valgus.
2. The lateral view shows the fracture aligned in the correct 180 degree position.

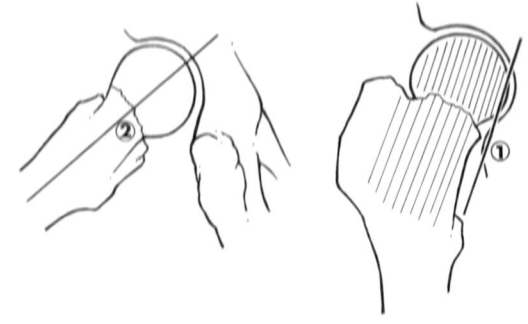

Operative Technique (After Southwick)

1. Begin the skin incision 2 cm above the greater trochanter and extend it distally for 10 cm.

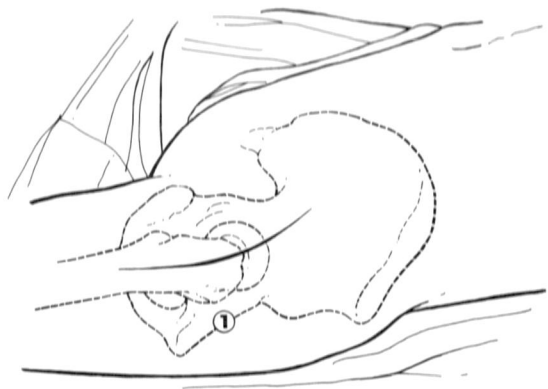

2. Cut the fascia lata at the posterior edge of the vastus lateralis.
3. Cut the posterior aspect of the vastus lateralis and elevate it anteriorly with the Bennett retractor.

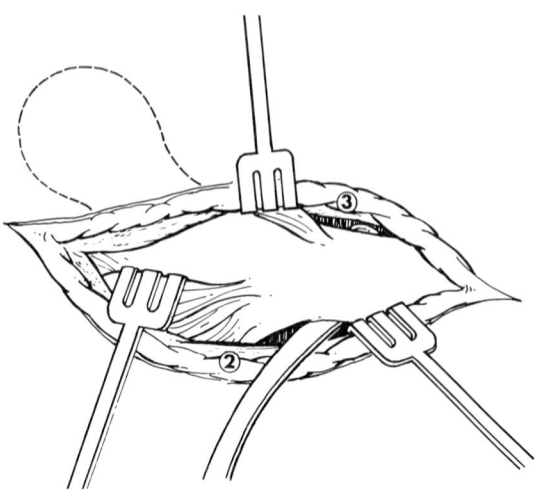

Operative Procedure: High-Angle Compression Hip-Screw Technique for Femoral Neck Fractures (After Southwick) (*Continued*)

1. Using a 6-mm drill, start the hole for the guide pin 5 cm below the lower ridge of the greater trochanter.
2. Use a fixed, 150-degree angle guide to insert a heavy 3-mm guide pin and direct it into the head under image-intensified fluoroscopy.
3. The pin should be inserted almost centrally or slightly toward the medial calcar of the neck and well into the subchondral bone of the head.
4. Measure the length of the guide pin and subtract 1.2 cm to determine the proper length of the lag screw.
5. Drive the pin into the acetabular cortex about 1 cm, making sure it is well seated.
6. Insert another guide pin superiorly to help stabilize the fracture.

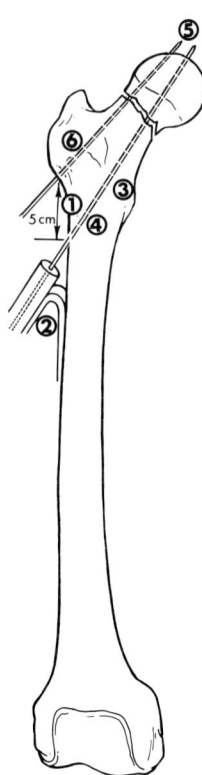

1. Prepare the lateral cortex by drilling with a cortical stop drill and take care to avoid bending the guide pin during the drilling.
2. Advance the drill into the bone until the lower portion of the second notch reaches the lateral cortex.

Note: Should the guide pin be pulled out during this drilling, it must be re-inserted prior to the next step.

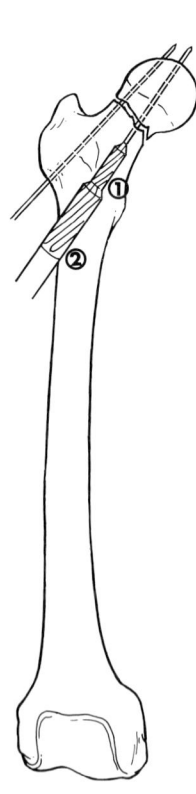

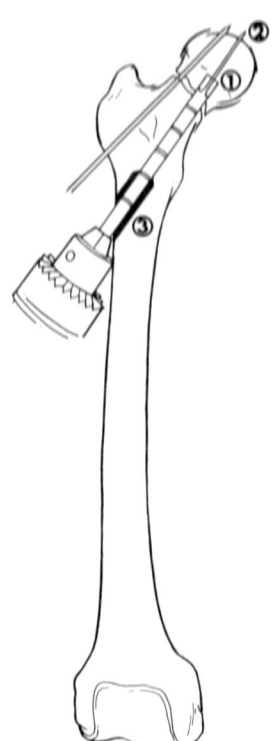

1. The lag screw reamer is then used to drill the femoral neck to the appropriate length, which is determined from the guide pin.
2. The reamer is advanced to within 1 cm of the head.
3. The inferior portion of the ring, which indicates the appropriate length, should reach the lateral cortex.

Note: After the reaming, tap a channel for the lag screw threads with a bone tap.

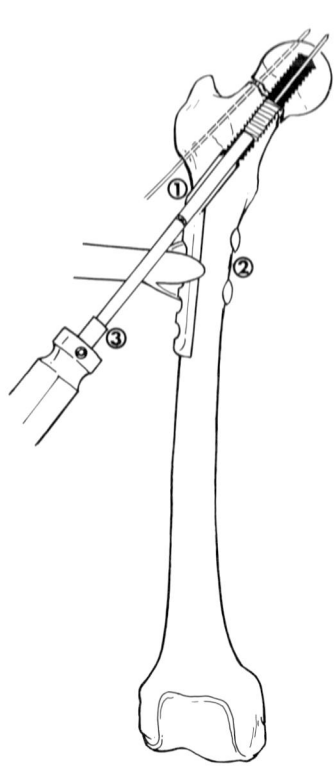

1. The lag screw and the side plate combination is then inserted in the collapsed position over the guide pin.
2. The plate is held against the shaft with a Lowman clamp.
3. A special, hollow-milled screwdriver fits over the guide pin and engages a slot on the base of the screw. The lag screw is then advanced appropriately into the head.

Operative Procedure: High-Angle Compression Hip-Screw Technique for Femoral Neck Fractures (After Southwick) (Continued)

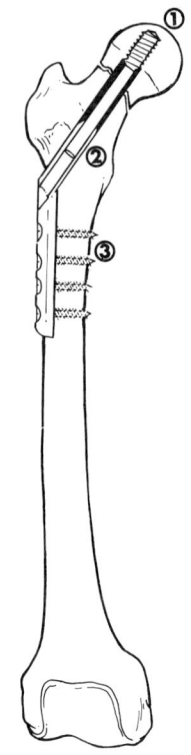

1. The lag screw penetrates to within 1 cm of the articular surface.
2. The screw must be overlapped by at least 1.8 cm with the compression tube.
3. Buttress screws then fix the plate to the cortex. They should extend through both cortices of the distal fragment.

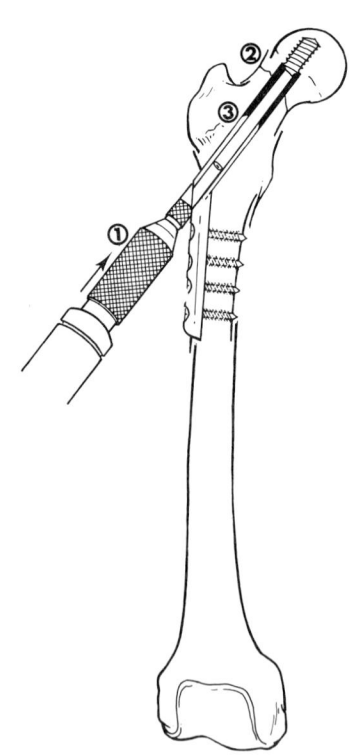

1. When adequate position is confirmed by fluoroscopy, remove the supporting guide pin, release traction on the limb, and impact the fracture.
2. Impaction closes the fracture line.
3. The lag screw slides through the compression tube to permit fracture impaction.

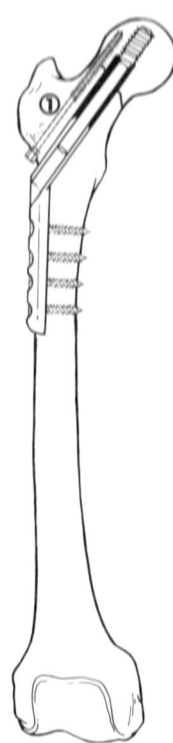

1. After impaction over the lag screw, insert a Knowles pin superiorly to add rotational stability.

Postoperative Care

Prophylactic administration of antibiotics during surgery and for two days following surgery is indicated in these patients.

The patient may be allowed out of bed on the second day following surgery.

The patient is encouraged to walk in parallel bars or with a walker as soon as she regains her balance.

Protective crutch walking or use of a walker must be continued for 12 to 16 weeks, until the fracture has healed clinically and radiographically.

Take x-rays periodically for the next year to evaluate for segmental collapse of the femoral head.

OPEN REDUCTION AND POSTERIOR BONE GRAFTING OF DISPLACED FEMORAL NECK FRACTURES (AFTER MEYERS, MOORE, AND HARVEY)

REMARKS

This method is particularly indicated in young adult patients, for whom the prognosis with displaced femoral neck fractures has been quite poor.

By direct visualization the comminuted posterior femoral neck cortex, which is the chief cause of rotational fracture instability, can be reinforced using cancellous bone and a vascular pedicle bone graft.

FRACTURES OF THE NECK OF THE FEMUR

Position of Patient

1. After administration of general anesthesia and endotracheal intubation, the patient is placed in the prone position on the fracture table.

2. The involved limb is secured to the footplate and placed in light traction with slight abduction and as much internal rotation as possible.

Note: Image-intensified fluoroscopy or equipment for adequate x-rays must be available for anteroposterior and lateral views. The reduction of the fracture is checked on preliminary x-rays.

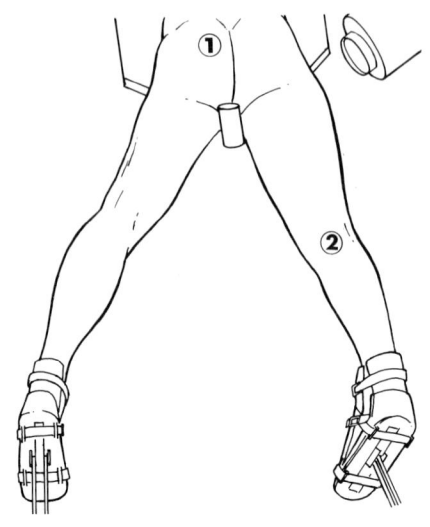

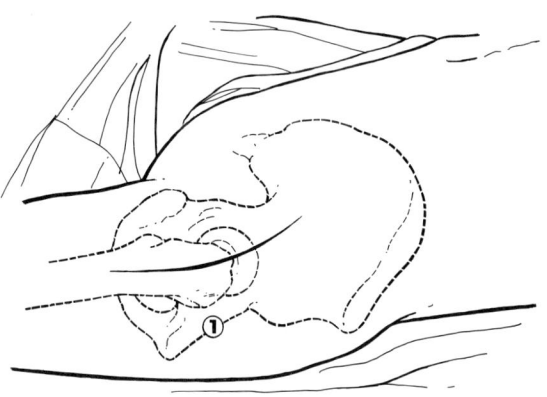

Surgical Approach

1. The incision starts 8 cm cephalad and posterior to the superior margin of the greater trochanter. It continues to the tip of the greater trochanter and then along the lateral aspect for a distance of 15 to 20 cm.

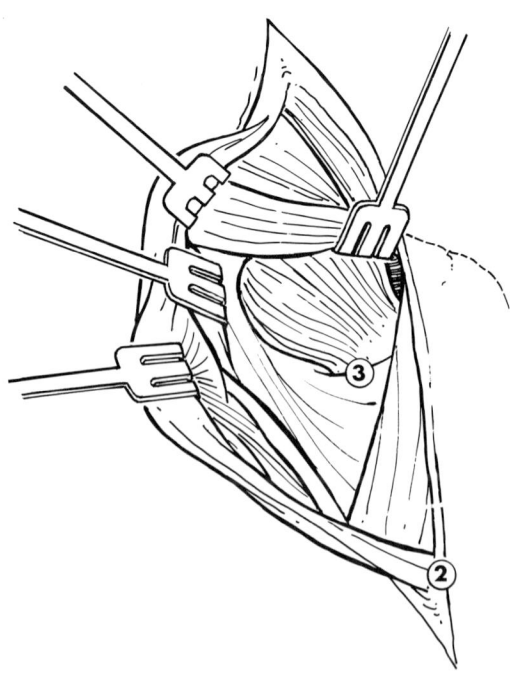

2. The deep fascia is cut and the subgluteal bursa is removed to expose
3. The borders of the quadratus femoris muscle insertion.

1440

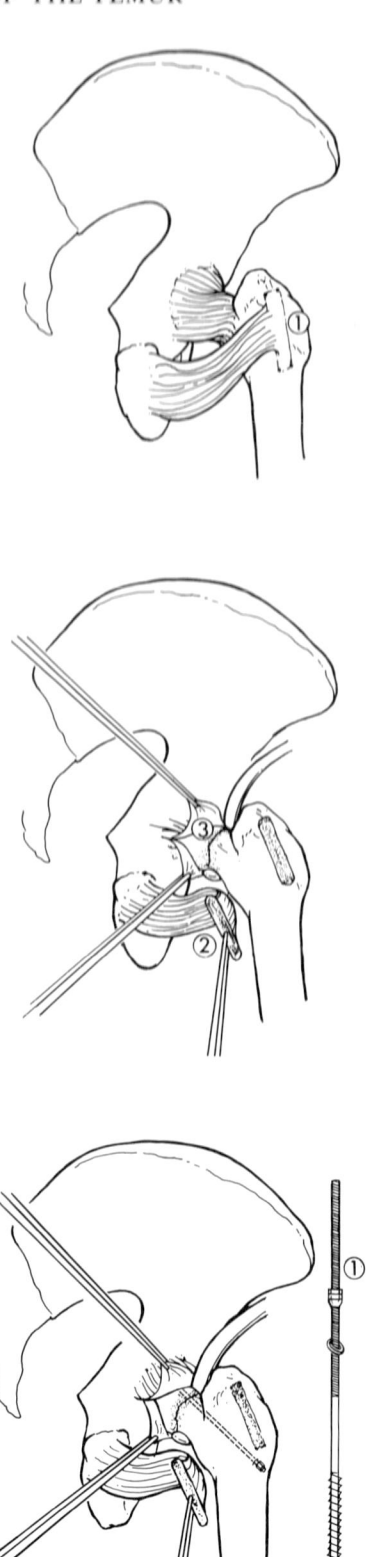

1. A muscle pedicle graft is outlined with drill holes around the insertion of the quadratus and a pedicle graft is taken.

Caution: This is the most difficult part of the procedure. Take graft carefully to avoid fracturing it.

2. The graft and its muscle attachment are bluntly dissected from the posterior capsule and

3. The capsule is opened with a T-shaped incision to expose the fracture. Small retractors bring the fracture site into full view and demonstrate the comminution of the posterior cortex. Final reduction is completed under direct visualization.

1. A Hagie pin or Knowles pin is then inserted through a hole, 4.5 mm in diameter, previously drilled from the lateral femoral cortex. This is located approximately 2 cm distal to the base of the greater trochanter and 0.5 cm anterior to the linea aspera.

1441

Surgical Approach (Continued)

2. When the first pin is in a satisfactory posteroinferior position and up into the subchondral bone, as demonstrated on x-ray, the remaining Knowles or Hagie pins are inserted.

3. Prior to insertion of all the pins, any defect in the posterior cortex of the neck is packed with cancellous bone chips.

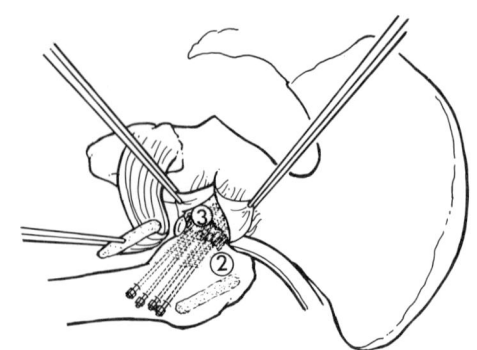

1. A mortising chisel is placed along the posterior aspect of the femoral neck and is driven up into the femoral head for 1 to 2 cm.

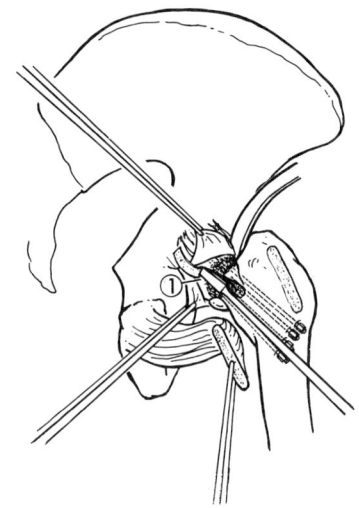

2. The proximal end of the pedicle graft is then driven into the prepared slot in the head and is impacted.

3. One or two screws are placed through the distal portion of the pedicle graft into the trochanteric region.

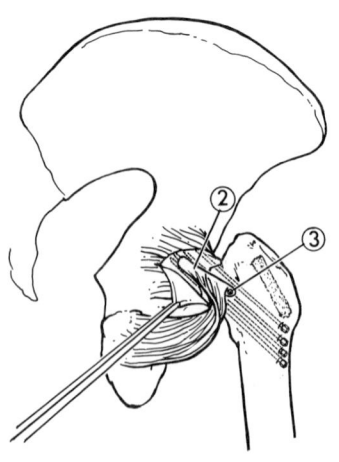

Postoperative Management

The patient is permitted out of bed as soon after operation as his condition permits.

He is started on toe-touch walking in parallel bars by the third or fourth day.

He may advance to a walker or crutches depending on his strength and agility.

Protected walking is continued for 12 to 16 weeks, until union can be recognized on x-ray.

The patient should return periodically for x-rays for at least two years to evaluate for segmental collapse of the femoral head.

Use technetium-99m sulfur-colloid scans to evaluate the circulatory status of the femoral head (see page 1452).

Basilar Fracture of the Neck of the Femur

REMARKS

This lesion is encountered less commonly than subcapital fractures.

Internal fixation by means of a high-angle compression hip screw offers the most effective means of management (see page 1434).

Prereduction X-Ray

Low cervical fracture with displacement.

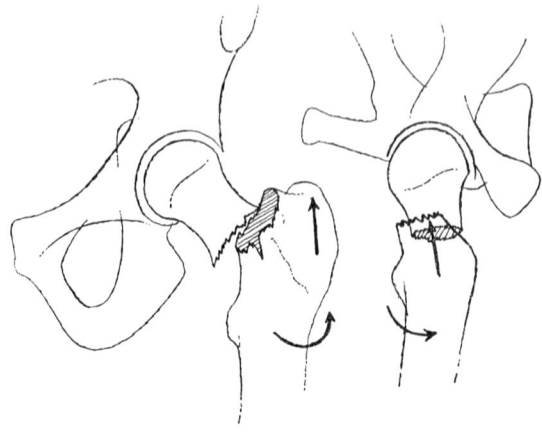

Postreduction X-Ray

The fragments are in normal alignment and are held by the compression hip screw.

1. The x-rays on the first postoperative day with initial weight bearing show impaction of the trabeculae.
2. Compression of the fracture is indicated by slight protrusion of the lag screw through the tube.

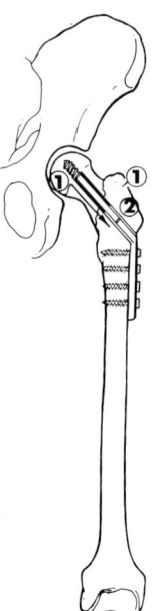

Fractures of the Femoral Neck in Children

REMARKS

Fractures of the femoral neck are rare injuries in children, occurring at less than 1 per cent of the frequency in adults.

In contrast to the indirect torsional mechanism that produces the adult hip fracture, the usual mechanism in children is direct violence to the hip. The child commonly is run over by a motor vehicle or falls on the hip from a height.

Approximately one third of these children will sustain other serious injuries, such as a fractured pelvis or a head injury, that may cause delay in treatment of the hip fracture or even failure to recognize it promptly.

The majority of femoral neck fractures in children are transverse or midcervical fractures.

The entire group of hip fractures can be classified according to Delbet and Colonna into four types:

Type I: physeal fracture or traumatic separation of the epiphysis.
Type II: a transcervical fracture.

FRACTURES OF THE NECK OF THE FEMUR

Type III: a cervicotrochanteric fracture.
Type IV: intertrochanteric fracture.

TYPE I: TRAUMATIC EPIPHYSEAL SEPARATION

The Type I fracture should be distinguished from the slipped upper capital femoral epiphysis by its occurrence in children less than nine years of age and its sudden onset following significant injury.

Because this is an epiphyseal injury, it should be treated with closed methods. Rarely in a young child the epiphysis is completely dislocated and requires open reduction.

In all reported cases of open reduction of these injuries, there has been significant subsequent avascular necrosis.

Closed treatment of acute fractures of the physis permits the remaining growth potential in young children to remodel the deformity.

Gentle closed reduction and external immobilization using traction and/or a spica cast is the safest and surest way of managing traumatic separation of the proximal femoral epiphysis in a child younger than nine years. This is in contrast with an acute slip in the adolescent, for which internal fixation with multiple pins is necessary (see pages 201 and 208).

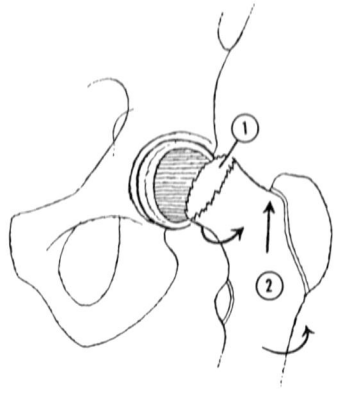

Prereduction X-Ray

1. Complete traumatic separation of the proximal femoral epiphysis.
2. The femoral shaft is externally rotated and is displaced upward.

Note: Unless the epiphyseal injury is recognized, it may be mistaken for a dislocation because of the displacement of the femoral neck.

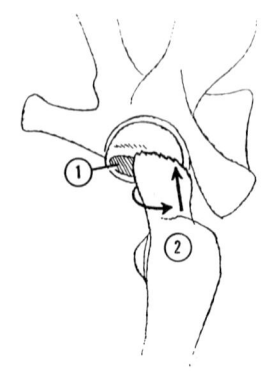

Management

1. The patient is placed in light Buck's traction (3 to 4 kg, depending on body weight).
2. Internal rotation straps are applied to the distal femur and leg to bring the distal fragment into line with the femoral epiphysis.

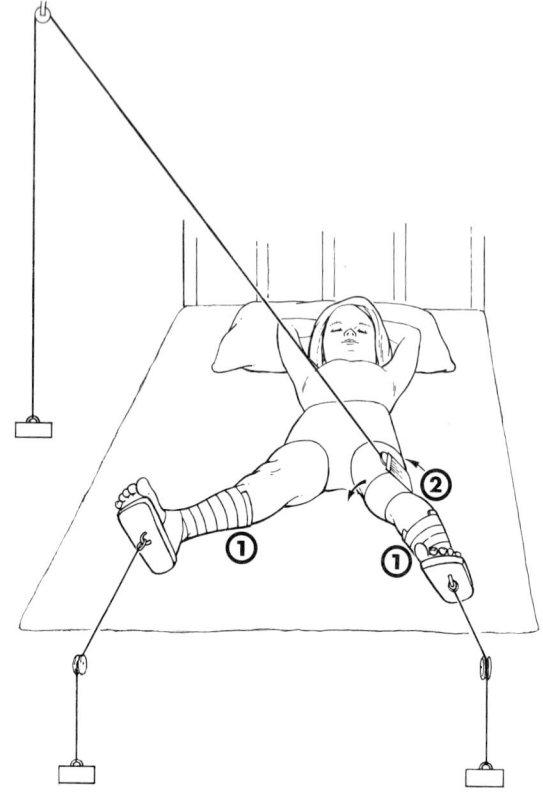

Postreduction X-Ray

1. Usually satisfactory reduction can be achieved by slight traction and internal rotation.
2. Some persistent displacement and widening of the physis is acceptable.

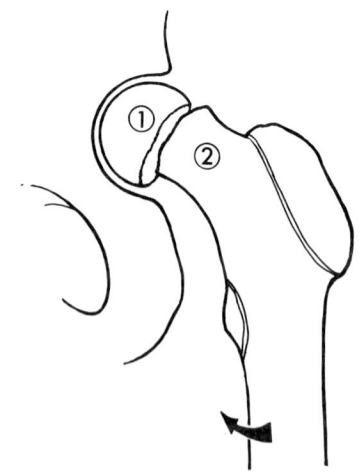

X-Ray Two and One-Half Years Later

1. There are some increased radiographic densities in the femoral head but the head remains viable.
2. There is shortening of the femoral neck and slight coxa vara.
3. The physis remains open and contributes to growth of the proximal femur.

Note: The physis would have closed if pins had been used to support the displaced femoral epiphysis and the end result would have been much less satisfactory.

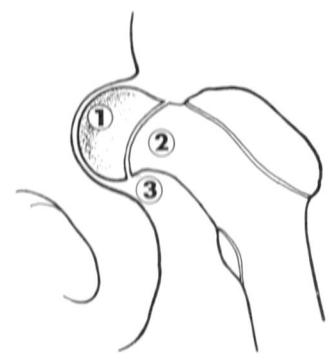

TYPE II (TRANSCERVICAL) AND TYPE III (CERVICOTROCHANTERIC) FRACTURES

REMARKS

These are the most common types of femoral neck fractures in children and are associated with a high incidence of complications, particularly avascular necrosis, coxa vara, nonunion, and premature epiphyseal arrest.

Avascular necrosis of the epiphysis causes most of the poor results. It occurs in about 50 per cent of these injuries.

The likelihood of complications is directly related to the initial degree of fracture displacement.

The severity of avascular necrosis is dependent on the age of the child at the time of fracture. A patient younger than ten years reconstitutes avascular bone much as in Legg-Perthes disease, but an older child usually is left with a destroyed hip.

The tendencies to coxa vara and nonunion can be diminished by closed reduction and fixation with two to three Knowles pins. The pins should be inserted to avoid penetrating either the femoral capital or the trochanteric epiphysis and causing premature epiphyseal arrest.

Following reduction and pin fixation, external support in a spica cast insures additional protection to the hip and is usually wise in a young child with this injury.

Prereduction X-Rays

Transcervical fracture

1. Transcervical fracture with
2. Coxa vara deformity.

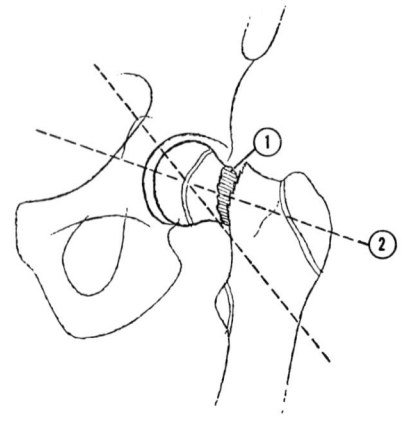

Cervicotrochanteric fracture

1. Fracture through cervicotrochanteric area.
2. Severe diminution of the femoral neck angle.

Note: These fractures are both fixed as previously described with Knowles pins using image-intensified fluoroscopy to position the pins exactly (see page 1429).

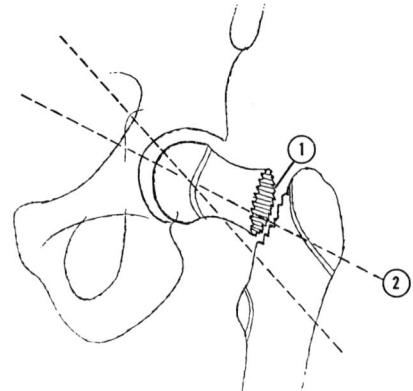

Postreduction X-Rays

1. Three Knowles pins have been inserted to hold the cervical fracture without involving the proximal femoral epiphyseal line or the trochanteric apophysis.
2. The coxa vara deformity has been corrected.

Note: For younger children with less bone, two Knowles pins may be satisfactory.

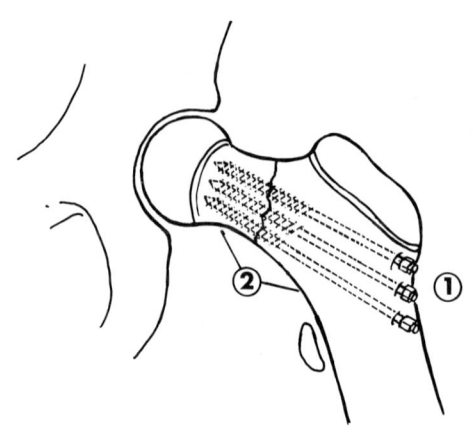

Postoperative Management

The child is immobilized in a bilateral spica cast for 6 weeks after reduction and fixation of the fracture.

The cast is removed after 6 weeks, and if the fracture is healing clinically and radiographically, the child may start crutch walking. Continue crutch walking for at least six months to protect the femoral head during revascularization.

Follow these patients carefully and caution them that if pain develops in the hip they should resume using crutches.

On the average, avascular necrosis becomes radiographically evident within 9 months following injury with a range of 1.5 to 18 months.

The Knowles pins need not be removed routinely unless they are producing symptoms.

TYPE IV (INTERTROCHANTERIC) FRACTURE IN CHILDREN

This is discussed under intertrochanteric fractures in adults and is managed in a similar manner (see page 1382).

Complications of Femoral Neck Fractures

REMARKS

The high mortality rate in femoral neck fractures, which is at least 15 per cent within three months of injury, should always be kept in mind in selecting treatment.

The most common complications resulting from the fracture itself include avascular necrosis of the femoral head, nonunion, and segmental collapse.

Avascular necrosis may be minimal or severe. The treatment required may vary from protection with a Legg-Perthes brace in a young child to total hip replacement in the elderly patient who becomes symptomatic after pin fixation.

Nonunion and malunion after a femoral neck fracture can be treated in the young patient by corrective osteotomy. This is designed to change the femoral neck alignment and salvage a useful hip.

Bone scanning using technetium-99m sulfur-colloid should be done prior to operative correction in order to determine the viability of the femoral head.

Meyers and co-workers have shown that posterior pedicle grafting may salvage these hips despite evidence of avascular necrosis provided that segmental collapse has not occurred. The posterior pedicle graft promotes prompt fracture union and revascularization of the head.

If the femoral head shows loss of sphericity, indicating segmental collapse from avascular necrosis, a femoral prosthesis or total hip arthroplasty becomes necessary.

Occasionally, the patient will present with previously unrecognized displaced femoral neck fracture. In the young individual with greater than ten years' life expectancy, provided that there is no segmental collapse, open reduction and posterior pedicle bone grafting are indicated.

In the older patient with previously unrecognized femoral neck fracture, prosthetic replacement is statistically most likely to provide satisfactory functional results.

MANAGEMENT OF UNTREATED FRACTURE OF THE FEMORAL NECK FOUR TO SIX WEEKS OLD

REMARKS

The viability of the femoral head can be determined with 95 per cent accuracy by a technetium-99m sulfur-colloid bone scan, as described by Meyers and co-workers.

Treat this fracture in the younger patient with open reduction and posterior pedicle bone grafting.

In the older patient with bone scan evidence of avascular necrosis or segmental collapse, prosthetic replacement is the wisest choice.

Prereduction X-Ray of Unrecognized Hip Fracture in a Patient Less than 60 Years of Age

1. The anteroposterior view shows varus displacement of the femoral neck.
2. The distal fragment is rotated externally, as evidenced by the appearance of the lesser trochanter.
3. The distal shaft is displaced superiorly.

This fracture should be treated by open reduction and posterior pedicle bone grafting (see page 1439).

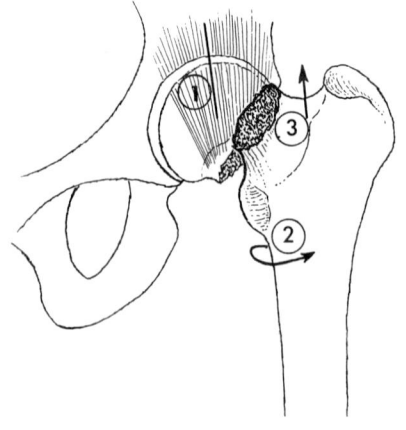

Postoperative X-Ray

1. The head is reduced in slight valgus position.
2. The neck is impacted into the head.
3. The posterior pedicle bone graft is evident.
4. Fracture fixation has been achieved by four Haggie pins.

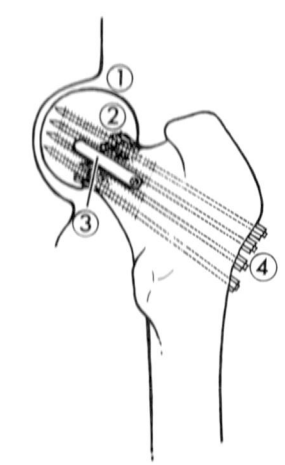

NONUNION OF THE FEMORAL NECK WITH A VIABLE HEAD

REMARKS

The viability of the head can best be determined by a preoperative bone scan using technetium-99m sulfur-colloid, as described by Meyer and co-workers.

In the patient older than 70 years, nonunion may be managed by total hip replacement to allow prompt functional rehabilitation.

The preferable procedure in most nonunions without extensive femoral head damage or resorption of the neck is open reduction and posterior pedicle bone grafting (see page 1439).

Prereduction X-Ray

1. Only minimal absorption of the femoral neck exists.
2. The plane of fracture is almost vertical.
3. The femoral head is adducted but there is no evidence of segmental collapse.

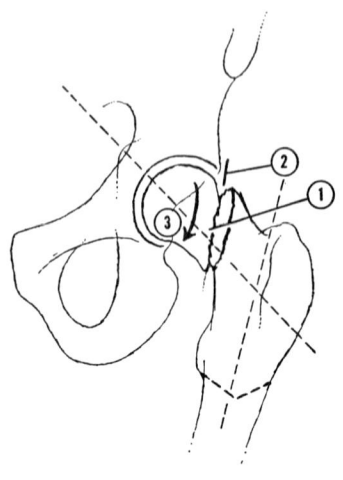

Preoperative Evaluation of the Vascularity of the Femoral Head with Technetium-99m Sulfur-Colloid (After Meyer and Co-workers)

REMARKS

In contrast to bone-seeking radioisotopes, which are picked up whenever there is bone production, technetium-99m sulfur-colloid is specific for deficient or severely impaired circulation in any tissue, including bone.

The method provides a qualitative rather than a quantitative evaluation of the circulatory status of the femoral head.

It must be done with the lower limbs completely internally rotated to achieve the best image of the hip joint circulation and eliminate the image of the greater trochanter.

1. Normal technetium-99m sulfur-colloid scan shows equal flow to both hips.

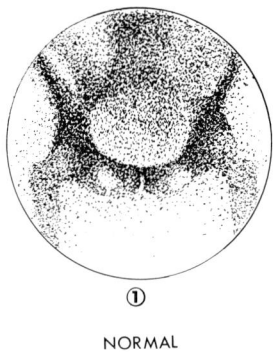

NORMAL

2. A scan in an ununited displaced fracture indicates impaired circulation to the injured hip and normal circulation to the opposite hip.

Note: A muscle pedicle graft is designed to speed revascularization of the injured femoral head and prevent segmental collapse.

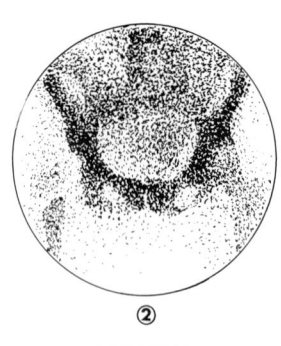

ABNORMAL

1. Five years after internal fixation and posterior muscle pedicle graft, the fracture is healed and there is no evidence of late segmental collapse.

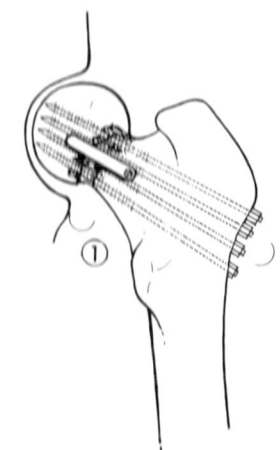

2. Nonunion in a patient older than 65 years is best treated by total hip joint arthroplasty.

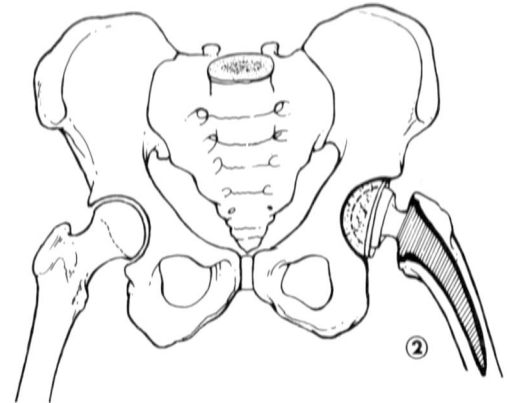

NONUNION WITH NONVIABLE FEMORAL HEAD AND SEGMENTAL COLLAPSE

REMARKS

With this particular injury the chances of achieving satisfactory union and an asymptomatic hip joint are so low that a primary prosthetic replacement is generally the treatment of choice, particularly in the patient older than 65.

Before offering the younger patient a total hip arthroplasty, always use the pseudarthrosis test: The patient's present disability and pain must be sufficient that it would be improved even if the total hip arthroplasty were complicated and required conversion to a pseudarthrosis.

Indications for Prosthetic Arthroplasty

On the preoperative x-ray of this 32-year-old patient,

1. There is complete absorption of the femoral neck.
2. The femoral head is dense and nonviable, as indicated by technetium-99m sulfur-colloid bone scan.
3. There is segmental collapse of the subchondral bone.

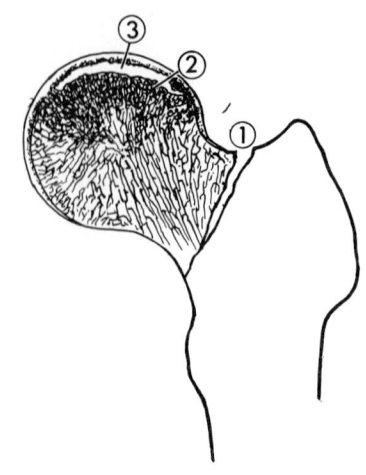

1. The femoral head has been replaced with total joint arthroplasty.

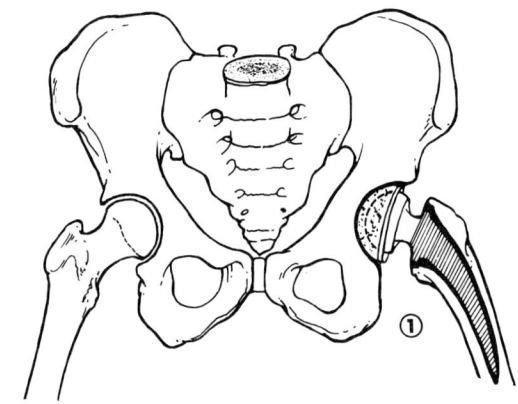

Pseudarthrosis Test Prior to Total Hip Arthroplasty

Prior to performing total hip replacement, always consider whether the patient's present symptoms could still be relieved by a resectional or Colonna arthroplasty of the joint if the total hip replacement were to fail.

1. A Colonna arthroplasty is preferable because placing of the greater trochanter into the acetabulum gives stability.
2. The hip abductors are transferred down to the lower level of the shaft of the femur.

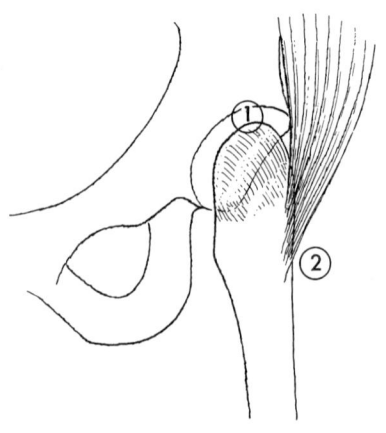

COXA VARA DEFORMITY AFTER FEMORAL NECK FRACTURE IN A CHILD

REMARKS

Coxa vara deformity may cause a painful limp and require operative fixation.

The deformity is particularly likely to follow closed treatment of a child's femoral neck fracture by abduction spica cast. For this reason multiple Knowles pins are the treatment of choice for femoral neck fractures in children (see page 1444).

Prereduction X-Ray

1. A femoral neck fracture in a 14-year-old boy has healed with pronounced coxa vara deformity.

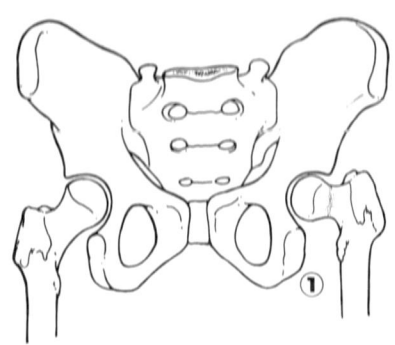

X-Ray After Valgus Angulation Osteotomy

1. A blade plate is angled to achieve the desired correction of the femoral neck and is inserted into the trochanteric region.
2. An osteotomy is made parallel to the blade in the trochanteric region. An appropriate size wedge is removed to achieve a valgus angulation of the femoral neck.

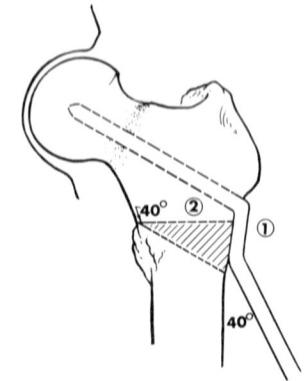

3. The osteotomy is closed and the plate is fixed to the shaft with screws.

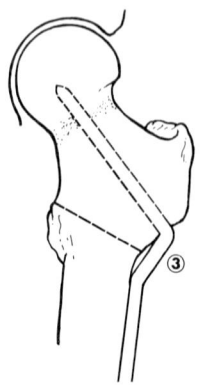

FRACTURES OF THE FEMORAL SHAFT

REMARKS

In contrast to fractures of the hip, which usually result from minimal and indirect injury, fractures of the femoral shaft are generally produced by high-impact mechanisms.

Femoral shaft fractures occur most often from motor vehicle accidents, falls from significant heights or gunshot injuries. Also, the average age for femoral shaft fracture is 33 years, whereas that for hip fracture is 73 years.

The most common locations and types of femoral shaft fracture, in order of occurrence, are:
1. Supracondylar-intracondylar region or distal third.
2. Transverse fracture in middle third.
3. Proximal third, just above the isthmus where the femur narrows.
4. Comminuted fracture in middle third.

Each fracture type carries different liabilities and different biomechanical considerations that influence choices of management.

Twenty to 25 per cent of patients with femoral shaft fractures sustain other major injuries that affect treatment.

Head injuries occur in 15 per cent of patients and ipsilateral tibial fractures occur in 10 to 15 per cent.

Because of often extensive hemorrhage in these fractures, fat emboli and other shock-like states can be expected in 6 to 10 per cent of patients. Prompt restoration of blood volume and close monitoring of mental status are important components of treatment.

In 3 per cent of femoral shaft fractures, the adjacent superficial femoral or popliteal artery is injured. Prompt recognition and repair of these vascular injuries are essential for limb survival.

Twenty per cent of femoral shaft fractures are open injuries and require immediate wound cleansing and treatment to prevent infection (see page 125).

Initial Immobilization

The fracture deformity should be corrected and held by
 1. A Hare splint

2. Military antishock trousers (MAST).

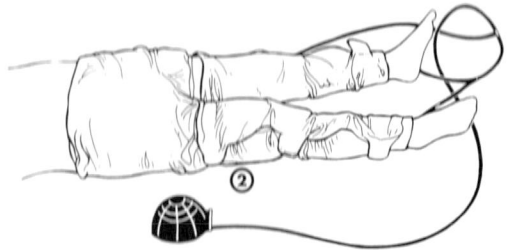

Note: The antishock trousers may be useful for immediate treatment of hypovolemic shock. They should not be inflated for more than 2 to 3 hours about the fracture because swelling and the rigid external compression may cause muscle ischemia. They should be deflated slowly and with careful blood pressure monitoring to avoid reproducing hypovolemic shock (see Appendix).

The physician should always check the distal CNS (circulation, neurologic function, and sensation), and inspect the skin over the splinted fracture to be sure that the fracture is not open.

EMERGENCY MANAGEMENT

REMARKS

Most patients lose from 2 to 4 units of blood with these injuries. Prompt blood volume replacement is essential to prevent hypovolemic shock and delayed shock syndromes such as fat embolism (see pages 77 and 83).

As the patient's blood volume is being restored and the airway is insured assess the patient for all possible injuries.

X-rays should be taken with a portable x-ray machine in the emergency room rather than in the x-ray department, for which the patient would have to be transported. The x-ray department tends to be the most dangerous place in the hospital for acutely injured patients.

X-rays of the long bone fracture must always include the joints proximal and distal to the injury. Any patient injured seriously enough to sustain a femoral shaft fracture must also have an x-ray of the pelvis. Two to 3 per cent of these fractures will have associated fracture or dislocation of the proximal femur.

Open fractures must be treated expeditiously. Associated head injuries are not contraindications to prompt fracture cleansing and debridement, provided that the patient shows no signs of increased intracranial pressure.

Associated chest and abdominal injuries should be assessed and treated promptly. Delaying treatment of an open fracture to "observe" the victim for possible intra-abdominal or head injury too often causes a septic fracture to become the life-threatening problem.

General anesthesia is usually the safest technique to permit adequate wound cleansing of the open fracture while still monitoring the patient's central nervous system and cardiovascular function.

Gunshot and shotgun fractures are managed either by local excision of the wound or complete exploration of the fracture, depending on whether the injury is high-velocity or low-velocity (see page 132).

Thorough initial assessment and management of the fracture makes definitive treatment much less complicated.

SKELETAL TRACTION

When the patient's initial evaluation (or emergency treatment for an open femoral fracture) is completed, the fracture can be immobilized by skeletal traction.

Distal femoral traction is the most effective way of controlling fracture alignment whether closed or open treatment is eventually instituted.

1. Insert a 3-mm threaded Steinmann pin into the medial aspect of the distal femur at the level of the superior patellar pole.

Note. Do not use a power drill to insert the pin because it might burn the hard cortical bone and cause a ring sequestrum.

2. Be sure that the pin runs perpendicular to the long axis of the femur to permit fracture reduction.

3. The pin should be inserted with the knee flexed to avoid damage to the popliteal vessels in Hunter's canal.

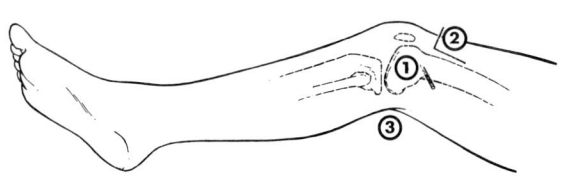

1. Support the fracture in balanced traction with a Harris splint.

2. Apply 10 kg of traction initially. The fracture should be distracted slightly during the first few days. If necessary, increase the traction to 20 kg.

3. The hip and knee are flexed 15 degrees.

4. The apparatus is supported by weights to maintain balance of the limb.

Note: The patient is allowed to move in bed with the aid of a trapeze bar.

5. A foot support holds the foot at right angles.

6. The foot of the bed is elevated 30 degrees for counter traction.

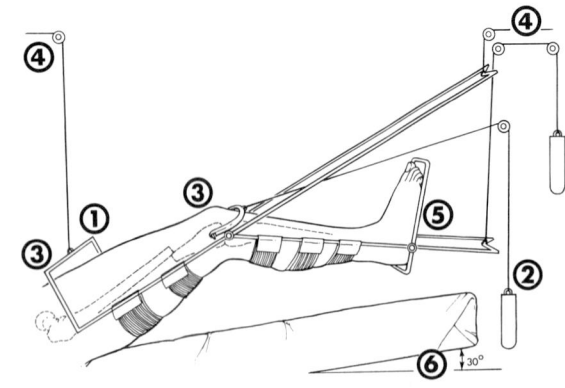

FRACTURES OF THE FEMORAL SHAFT

CAUTION

The patient should not have the head of the bed elevated because it completely alters the mechanics of traction.

In addition, the patient should not sit in bed while in traction because sitting would encourage pelvic vein thrombosis and pulmonary embolism.

Postreduction X-Ray

Always obtain *true* anteroposterior and lateral views. Too often the x-rays "lie" about the reduction because the view is oblique rather than parallel to the fracture.

1. Anteroposterior view, which commonly is not centered over the fracture, appears to show that the fracture is slightly distracted.
2. A true lateral view centered over the fracture shows incomplete reduction.

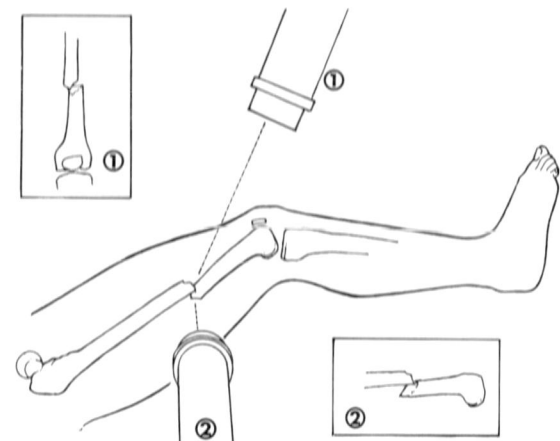

Definitive Treatment

REMARKS

Selection of the definitive treatment should be based on the physician's appreciation of the biology of fracture healing as well as the mechanics.

The most effective methods include closed intramedullary nailing by the Küntschner technique, open reduction and fixation by diamond or fluted-nail technique, and closed reduction and cast-brace immobilization.

Closed nailing of the femoral fractures is a highly complex technique requiring a skilled operating team and a complete and diverse set of special equipment, including an appropriate operating table and C-arm image-intensified fluoroscopy. The method should be limited to regional centers and should not be employed by the individual surgeon in the community hospital with only occasional experience. Technical complications may be considerable if the procedure is not followed exactly.

In most instances in which internal fixation is required, because of either fracture instability or failure to reduce the fracture initially by closed methods, open reduction and fixation by a Schneider nail is most effective. Use of the Küntschner nail should be reserved for the closed intramedullary method for which it was designed. It is not as satisfactory either biologically or biomechanically in the open technique as the Schneider nail.

Plate fixation has been used for femoral shaft fractures but is associated with an extremely high rate of complications, which include failure of fixation, nonunion, and refracture through the end screw hole. Secondary fracture is always possible through the end screw hole, where the stress from the relatively elastic bone is transmitted to the rigid plate. Because of the risk of refracture and the unfavorable distribution of stress, the plate should always be removed in a secondary operation. Plate fixation is the least satisfactory of all the techniques employed for femoral fracture union.

Closed reduction of the femoral shaft fracture with cast-brace application by two to six weeks after fracture proves to be the least complicated and most effective method of management for most femoral fractures. It does not provide the immediately spectacular results of closed nailing, but healing time and restoration of function are essentially the same.

The cast-brace method does not require complex or expensive equipment but does demand the basic necessity of the physician's good judgment. The technique is particularly suited for fractures in the distal half of the femur and comminuted shaft fractures, i.e., the types of fracture least suited for intramedullary nailing.

Transverse midshaft fractures and fractures in the proximal half can be managed effectively by the cast-brace method if the physician anticipates and prevents problems of shortening and angulation.

Early cast-brace treatment allows the physician to maximize the biologic healing processes but demands that he understand the biomechanics of femoral fracture deformities.

TECHNIQUE OF CLOSED REDUCTION AND EARLY CAST-BRACE IMMOBILIZATION

REMARKS

The traditional nonoperative methods of femoral shaft fracture treatment, which include prolonged skeletal traction and spica cast immobilization, yield consistently poor results. Nonunion or malunion requiring eventual operative treatment has been reported in 11 to 29 per cent of cases, shortening of more than 2 cm in 14 to 30 per cent, and refracture in 4 to 17 per cent.

The most commonly reported disability after nonoperative treatment of femoral fracture has been knee stiffness and weakness, which have occurred in at least 30 per cent of cases treated by prolonged nonoperative immobilization.

The cast-brace technique introduced by Mooney and co-workers permits closed reduction of the fracture and mobilization of the patient and the knee. The method encourages controlled fracture motion and stimulates healing by abundant external callus formation. Fractures of the femoral shaft, which like the humeral shaft has richly vascularized surrounding soft tissue envelopes, are particularly suited to this method of treatment.

Closed reduction and cast-brace technique maximizes the natural healing processes, particularly when employed within the first 6 weeks after injury. It also eliminates fracture disease or disuse atrophy of joints and muscles, which have commonly followed the usual nonoperative methods of management.

Closed reduction and cast-brace immobilization require judgment regarding fracture mechanics. It is essential to understand that the three-dimensional appearance and function of the patient's limb, rather than a two-dimensional radiograph, is the ultimate determinant of successful treatment.

Three-Dimensional Biomechanics of Fracture Deformities

Treatment by closed reduction and cast-brace application requires a three-dimensional conceptualization of the fracture deformity rather than the two-dimensional approach encouraged by strict reliance on radiographs.

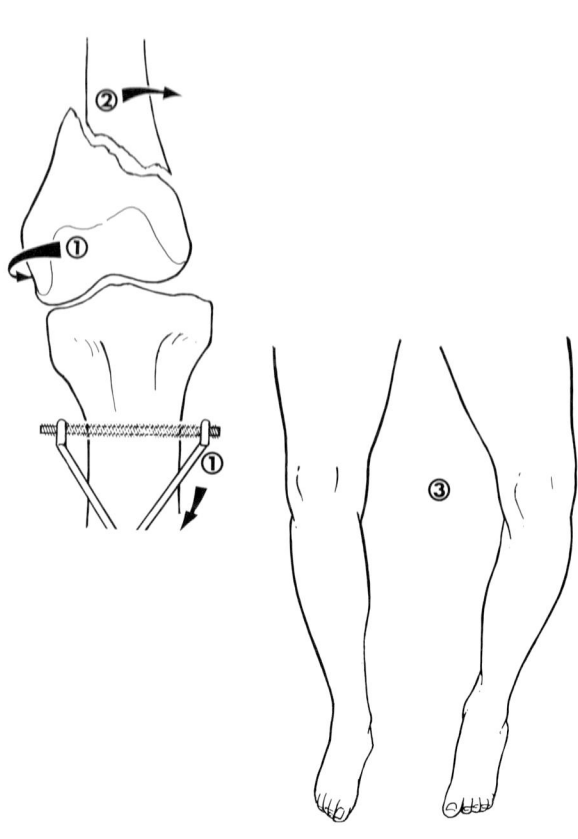

Supracondylar and Distal Femoral Fractures

A common deformity after supracondylar fracture of the femur is genu varum. This is produced by:

1. Traction rotating the distal fragment internally.
2. The proximal fragment rotates externally while the patient lies in bed. The flexed position of the knee in skeletal traction disguises the torsional malalignment.
3. The malalignment is interpreted radiographically as genu varum, but the torsional component is evident clinically.

Supracondylar and Distal Femoral Fractures (Continued)

Valgus deformity from supracondylar fracture can be produced by:

1. A loose long-leg cast, which when combined with the weight of the distal limb causes:

2. External torsion of the distal fragment.

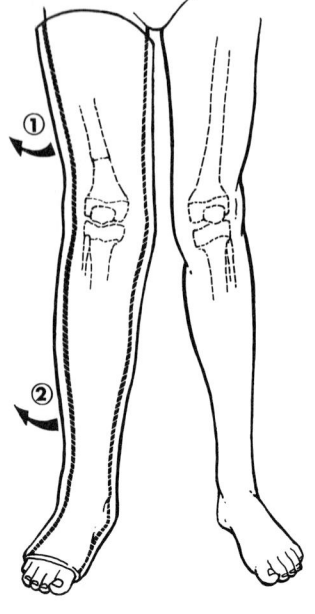

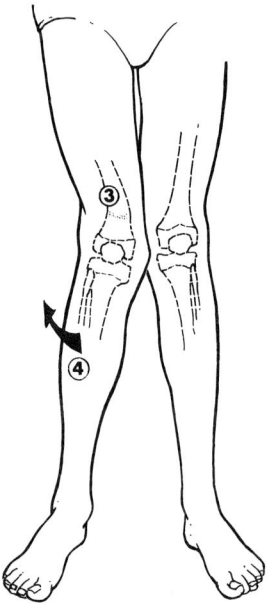

3. The result is interpreted radiographically as a valgus angulation but actually is due to

4. Torsional external rotation deformity, as seen clinically.

Varus and valgus deformity are prevented by early application of cast-brace with
 1. The knee extended and
 2. In slight valgus.

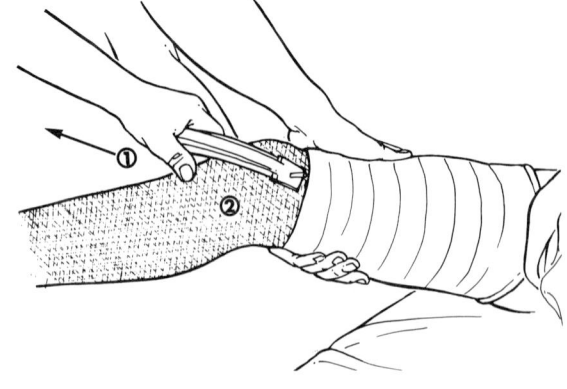

3. Motion at the knee joint permitted by the cast-brace eliminates the torsion on the fracture site that would be produced by a long-leg cast with the knee in extension.

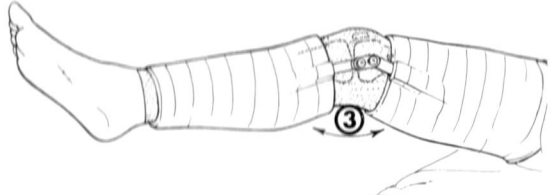

Distal femoral fracture fragments consistently displace:
1. Posteriorly owing to the mechanism of injury, which is a direct blow to the distal femur.
2. Tibial traction or flexion of the knee does not correct the deformity caused by the original mechanism of injury.

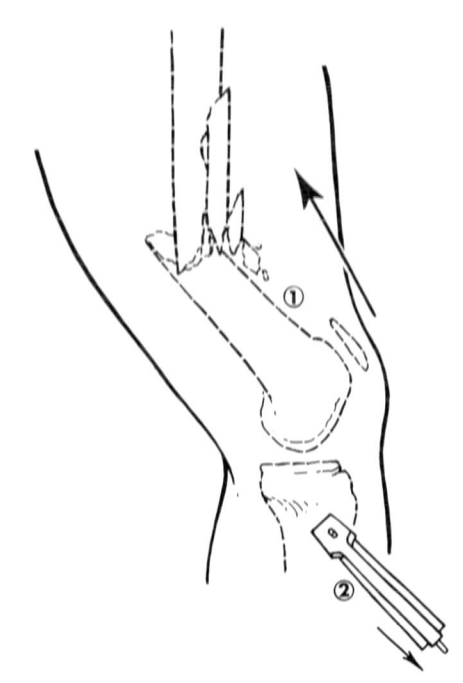

3. The deformity is corrected by direct pull on the distal fragment using a skeletal traction pin in the femoral condylar area.

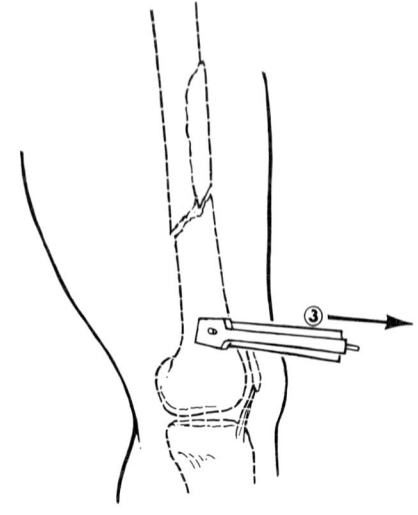

Torsional Fractures of the Middle and Proximal Shaft

Yamada has shown that the direction of torsional loading consistently determines the obliquity of the fracture. For example:

1. Internal twisting of a bone specimen produces a fracture line running from distal lateral to proximal medial.

2. A femoral shaft fracture produced by internal torsion or pronation runs from the distal lateral to the proximal medial cortex.

3. External torsion of a bone specimen produces a fracture line running from distal medial to proximal lateral.

4. A femoral shaft fracture, which is produced by external torsion or supination, runs from the distal medial to the proximal lateral cortex.

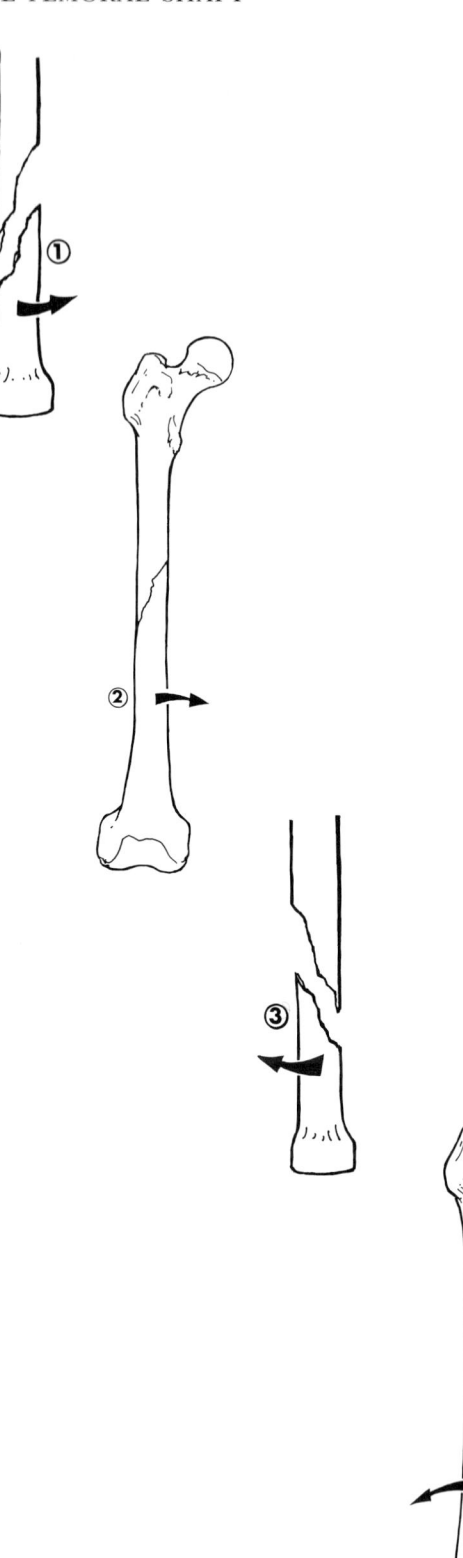

FRACTURES OF THE FEMORAL SHAFT

Analyzing the torsional components of the fracture helps to anticipate deformities and to choose appropriate methods for fracture reduction.

1. Midshaft oblique fractures produced by external torsion may lock in a displaced position.
2. They are reduced by internal torsion of the distal fragment on the proximal fragment.

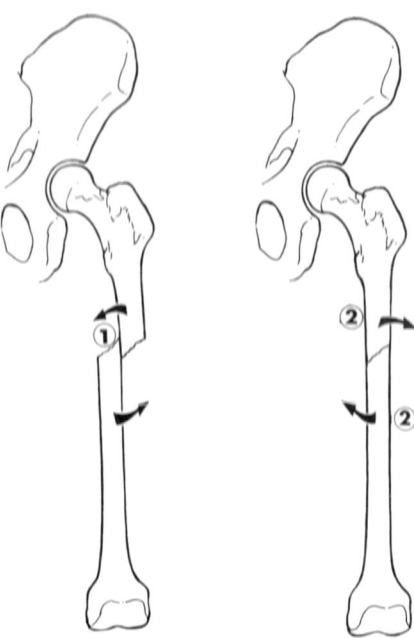

Torsional deformities should be anticipated with proximal femoral fractures.
1. A proximal femoral fracture is frequently produced by internal torsion

OR

2. A long oblique fracture of the proximal femur can result from external torsion.

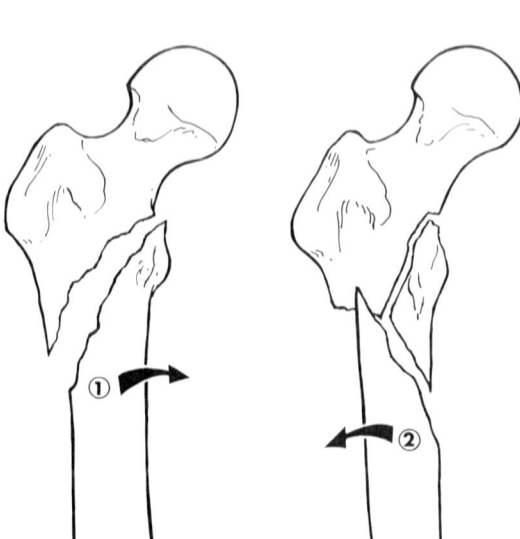

Note: Since the weight of the limb tends to rotate these proximal femur fractures, there is a high incidence of plate failure associated with them. This can frequently be prevented by using 90–90-degree traction or a cast-brace applied with a pelvic band or a mini-spica to hold proper rotation reduction (see page 1401).

1465

Transverse Fractures of the Midshaft

These are produced by direct loading or bending and cause translational deformities. Because of the tendency to shorten, these fractures are best treated by intermittent traction or open reduction and internal fixation.

1. Initial alignment of the transverse midshaft fracture is satisfactory in the cast-brace.
2. Shortening occurs with weight bearing, but this can be prevented by intermittent skeletal traction in the cast-brace or by open reduction and internal fixation.

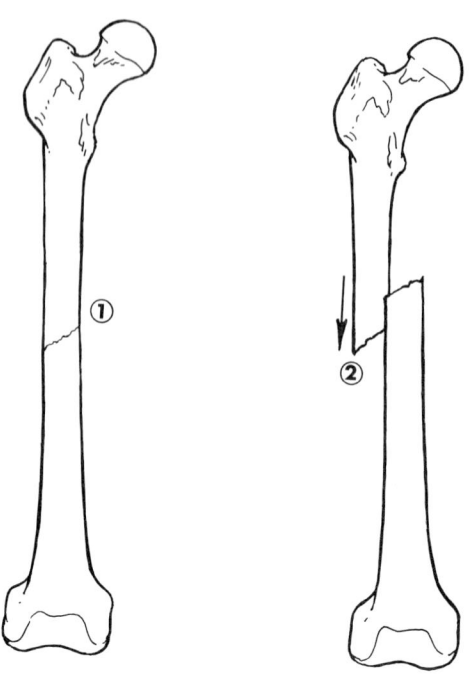

COMMINUTED SHAFT FRACTURES

These fractures are stable in the cast-brace because of internal "stiction" of the fragments.

The bone tends to shorten 1 to 2 cm whether closed or open treatment is employed.

Persistent attempts to maintain length with a comminuted fracture may produce distraction and nonunion.

1. Comminuted midshaft fracture prior to cast-brace application.
2. Comminuted fracture heals in a slightly shortened position accepted at the cast-brace application.
3. Callus is external periosteal type encouraged by early muscle function in the cast-brace.

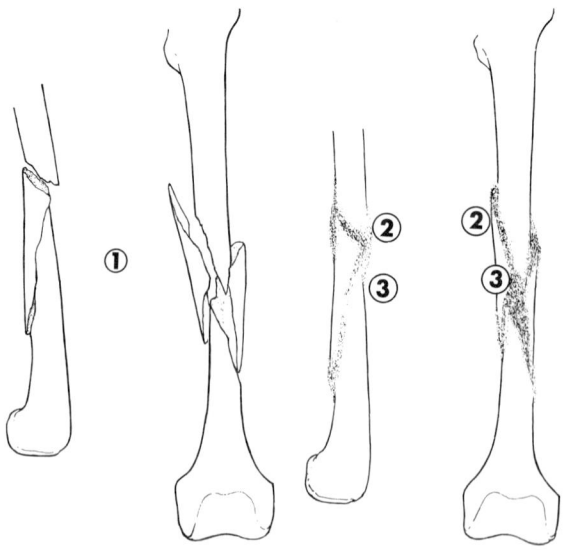

Iatrogenic Fracture Comminution

1. This fracture with a long proximal extension is unsuitable for intramedullary nailing.
2. Attempted intramedullary nailing causes comminution of the proximal fragment.

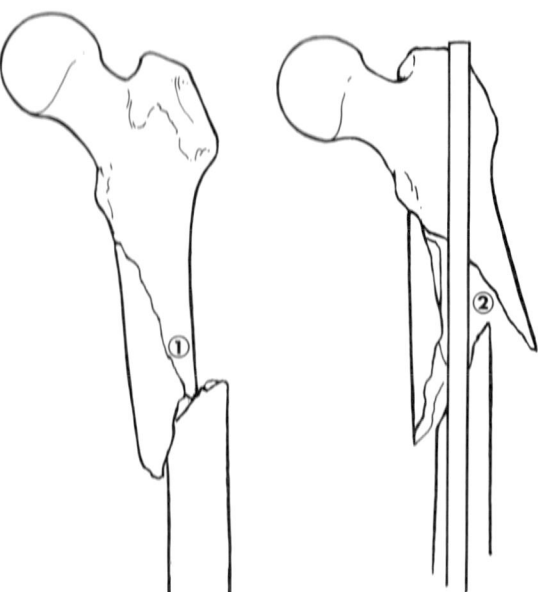

3. Supplemental external immobilization with a cast-brace provides adequate reduction of the fracture and healing in a satisfactory position of function.

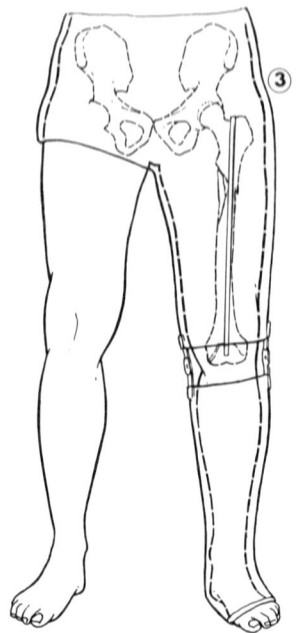

TECHNIQUE OF CLOSED REDUCTION AND CAST-BRACE APPLICATION

REMARKS

The fracture should be reduced by slight distraction prior to the cast-brace application.

FRACTURES OF THE FEMORAL SHAFT

If the reduction is unsatisfactory in skeletal traction, e.g., as in a locked oblique fracture, the patient should be given an anesthetic to permit manipulation. In most instances, the cast-brace can be applied with the patient in bed and lightly sedated.

The duration of skeletal traction varies from a few days to three or four weeks, depending on the initial stability of the fracture.

Fractures in the distal shaft that are relatively undisplaced at the time of presentation, and oblique fractures produced by indirect torsional loading can be treated by cast-brace application within the first few days.

Fractures in the midshaft or proximal shaft are best immobilized for several weeks to permit the edema to subside and some initial fracture stability to develop.

With the patient in bed, the traction is released and:

1. An assistant maintains steady traction.
2. A Spandex*stocking is rolled over the leg and across the pin.
3. An assistant continues to support the leg with traction while a 12.5-cm roll of plaster is applied snugly to the thigh.

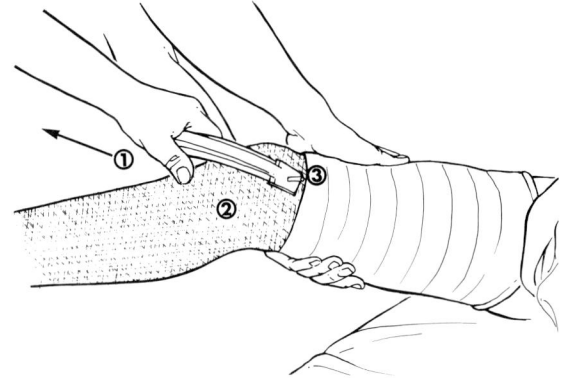

1. Fractures in the distal third are reduced by holding the knee in extension and external rotation.

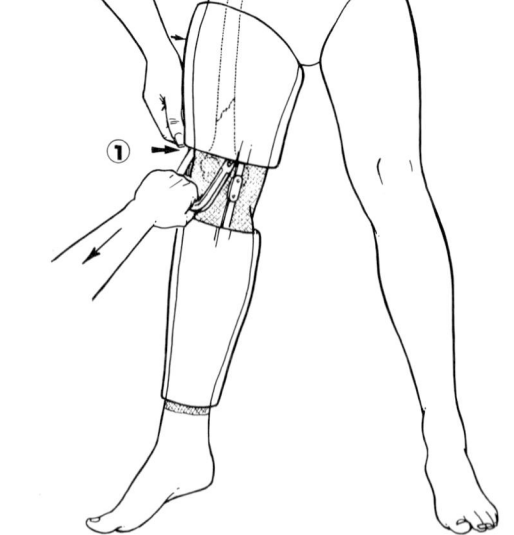

---

*Available from United States Manufacturing, 623 Central Avenue, Glendale, California 91209.

FRACTURES OF THE FEMORAL SHAFT

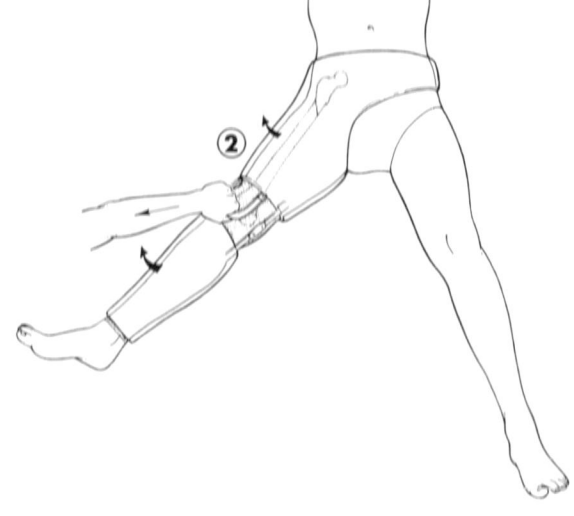

2. Fractures in the proximal third, which are produced by internal torsion, are held in external rotation and abduction.

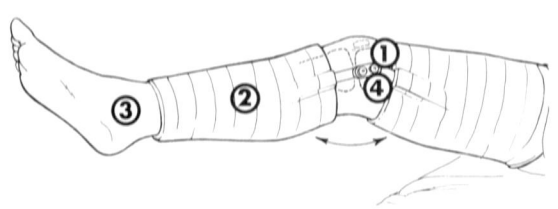

1. The pin is not incorporated in the plaster cast, but the cast ends just above the pin. This permits intermittent skeletal traction if necessary.

2. The lower leg cast is applied over 1 to 2 layers of cast padding.

3. The foot is left out of the cast because the traction pin supports the weight of the cast.

Note: The pin must be a heavy, 3-mm to 5-mm threaded pin to permit this technique. It is removed at 6 weeks when it is no longer needed for skeletal traction.

4. The knee joint is centered over the adductor tubercle.

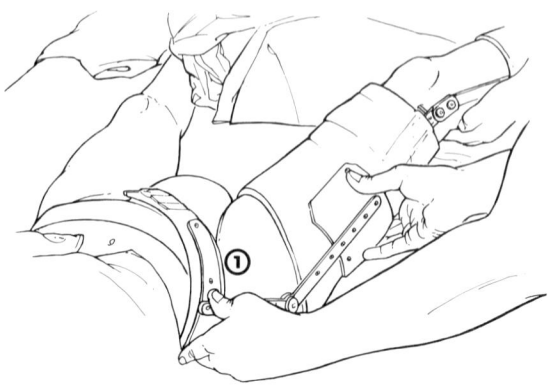

1. Fractures in the middle and proximal femoral shaft frequently require a pelvic band or

1469

2. A mini spica to maintain the hip in abduction and external rotation.

Note: A pelvic band or mini spica is critical for immobilizing the more proximal fractures. Hardy has shown that the fixed abduction provided by these devices maintains the soft tissue pressures within the thigh necessary to prevent fracture displacement and to dissipate fracture translation.

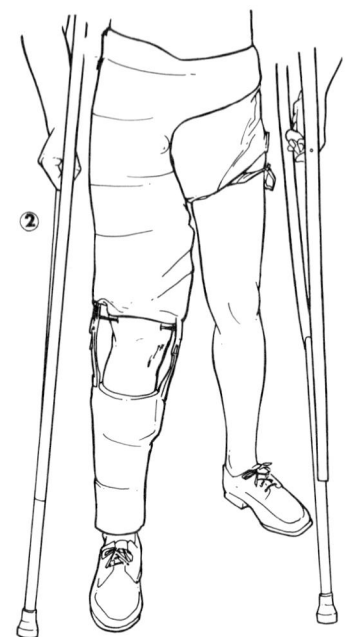

Postreduction Management

The patient is usually comfortable in the device and after several days is allowed to start crutch walking and weight bearing as tolerated.

1. When not walking the patient is kept in skeletal traction.

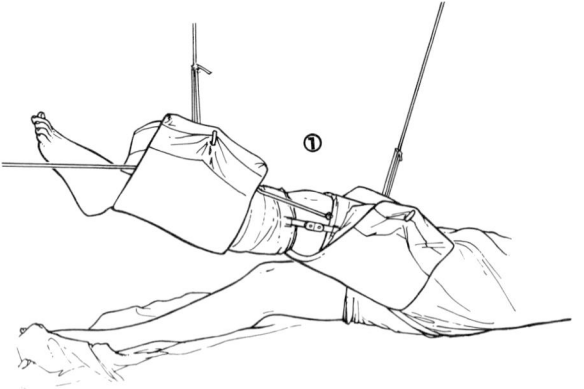

2. The traction may be readily removed to allow ambulation.

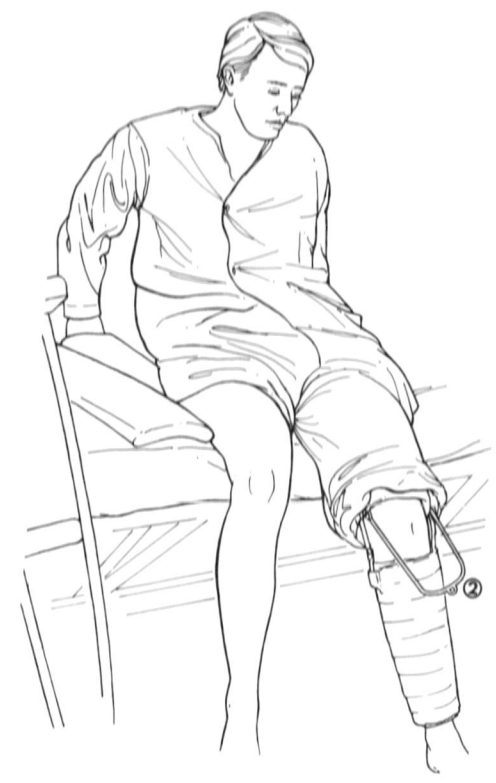

The position of the fracture is observed by frequent x-rays during the week or two after reduction.

Be certain that the x-ray technique is consistent because an oblique x-ray will alter the appearance and interpretation.

1. A true lateral view shows satisfactory reduction after cast bracing.

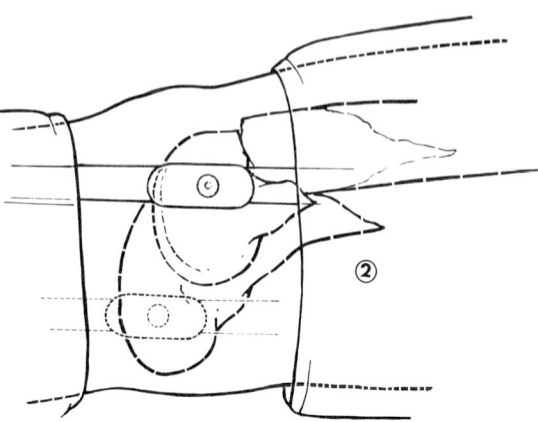

2. This "lateral" x-ray is actually an oblique view, as indicated by the 45 degree offset of the knee hinges. An x-ray like this causes concern that the fracture reduction has become unacceptable, whereas it is the x-ray technique that is the problem.

Subsequent Management

If the position is stable in the cast-brace after 1 to 2 weeks of observation in the hospital, the patient may be discharged.

He should return for outpatient evaluation on a biweekly basis. The skeletal traction pin may be removed approximately 6 weeks after injury and the foot incorporated in the cast.

By 12 to 16 weeks, the majority of these fractures are healed sufficiently and the cast-brace can be removed.

The fracture is considered healed when the patient can bear full weight on the limb without external support and has no limp or pain.

Characteristically, the fracture heals with abundant external callus and the patient regains full range of knee motion.

Occasionally with fractures in the supracondylar region that involve the quadriceps apparatus there is persistent limitation of knee flexion.

INTERNAL FIXATION FOR FRACTURES OF THE SHAFT OF THE FEMUR

REMARKS

Ideally, intramedullary nail fixation is done by the closed method as first described by Küntschner. The many technical considerations and the array of equipment necessary for this are best described by Hansen and Winquist, who suggest that optimal results can be achieved only in regional centers.

The majority of femoral fractures can be treated by closed reduction and cast-brace immobilization with results equal to or better than those of internal fixation, provided that the physician appreciates the potential complications and utilizes the method appropriately.

Ten to 15 per cent of shaft fractures are best treated by open reduction and intramedullary fixation, either because adequate reduction cannot be achieved by closed means or because the patient sustains associated injuries to the hip or knee.

Open reduction and internal fixation should be avoided in patients younger than 16 and in open fractures because of inordinate complication rates.

Where indicated, however, open reduction and internal fixation are best accomplished by the Schneider nail method, which has proven to be the biomechanically and biologically most sound technique for this application.

1. Schneider's four-flanged nail utilizes the double I beam principle to give maximum strength to the solid nail.
2. The flanged edges that engage the intramedullary surfaces minimize fracture rotation.
3. The grooves between the flanges allow intramedullary revascularization promptly across the fracture site.
4. The graduated sawtooth ends cut a trough for the four flanges of the nail as it is driven down the medullary canal. This keeps the nail from being "hung up."

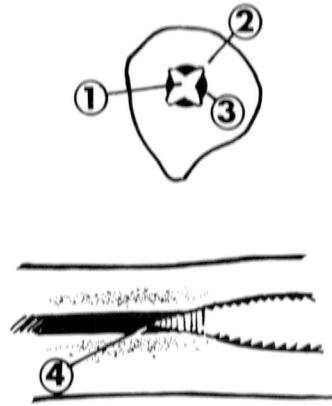

Special instrumentation is minimal with the technique and includes one drive-extractor with an extra one on hand, a 9-mm drill, a set of 10 mm to 13 mm nails with lengths ranging from 30 to 48 cm, and standard orthopedic instruments including bone clamps, bone hooks, and retractors for fracture reduction.

Fixation may have to be supplemented by cerclage wires, transcortical screws placed tangential to the nail, and/or external immobilization with the cast-brace.

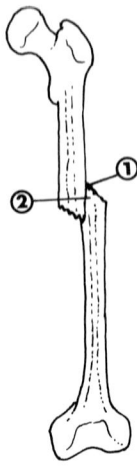

Preoperative X-Ray

1. Short oblique fracture of the upper third that has been unstable in the cast-brace.
2. There is overriding and unacceptable shortening of the fragments.

Preoperative X-Ray (Continued)

3. The length of the nail is determined preoperatively via a scanogram centered over the top of the trochanter and the knee of the other leg.

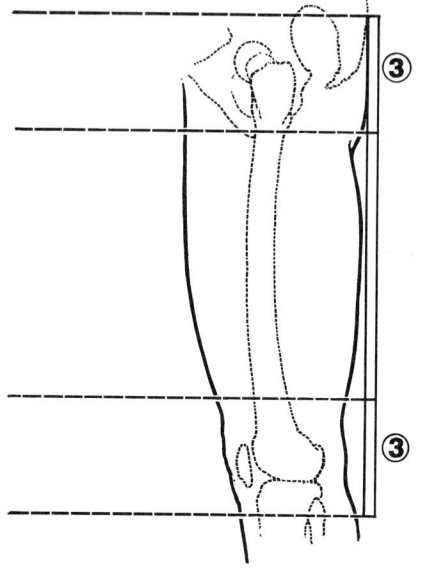

Operative Technique (Under General Anesthesia)

1. The patient is in the complete lateral position lying on the unaffected side. The hip and knee on the affected side are flexed.

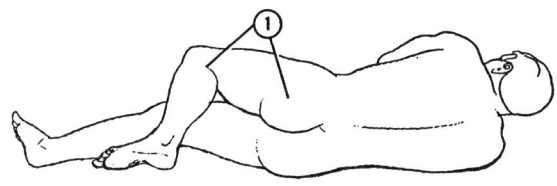

1. Make an incision on the posterolateral aspect of the thigh beginning 7 cm above the fracture and terminating 7 cm below it.

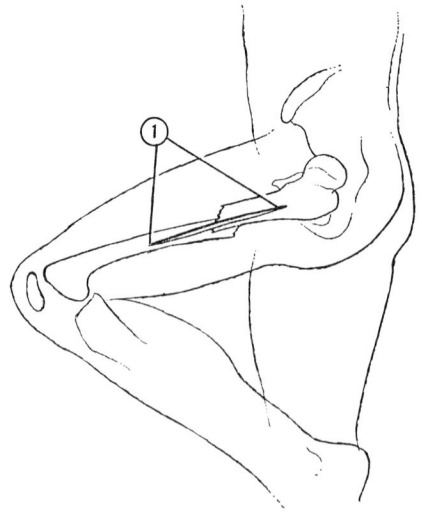

1. Divide the fascia lata in the line of the skin incision, exposing the posterior portion of the vastus lateralis.
2. Retract the vastus lateralis anteriorly.
3. This exposes the lateral intermuscular septum.
4. Make an incision along the anterior margin of the intermuscular septum down to the bone.
5. Expose the posterolateral aspect of the femur and fracture site by subperiosteal dissection.

Note: In the middle third the second perforating branches of the profunda artery and vein are encountered crossing the wound; these must be ligated.

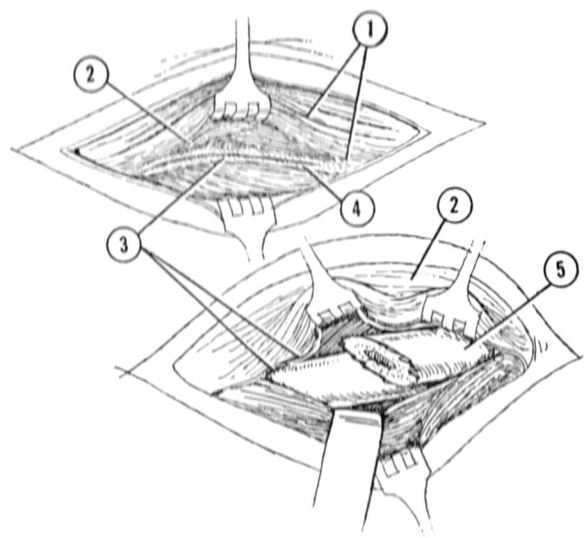

1. Deliver the proximal fragment out of the wound, keeping the distal fragment adducted out of the way. The 9-mm drill is then placed up the proximal medullary canal.

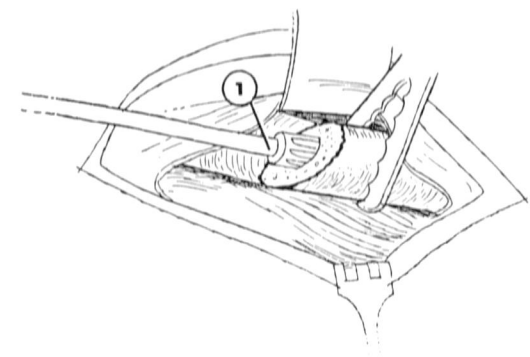

2. Drill upwards to make a pilot hole to avoid comminuting the greater trochanter or neck.

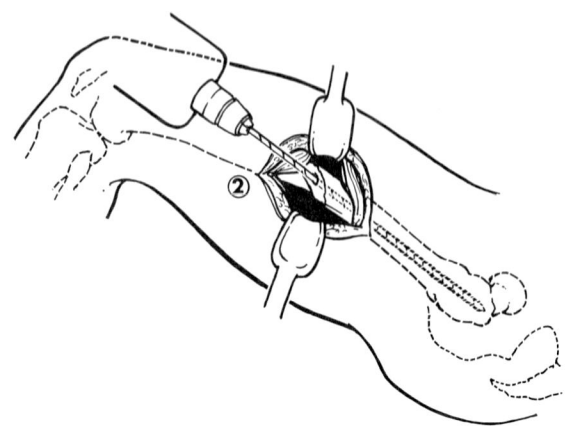

Operative Technique (Under General Anesthesia) (Continued)

3. The width of the femoral nail is determined by passing nails of likely sizes up the proximal medullary canal and selecting the one that is snug and a little tight. This nail is then driven up the canal and out the top of the trochanter.

Note: The leg should be placed in adduction as the nail is driven proximally.

4. Make a small incision over the protruding nail and drive the lower end of the nail to the end of the fracture.

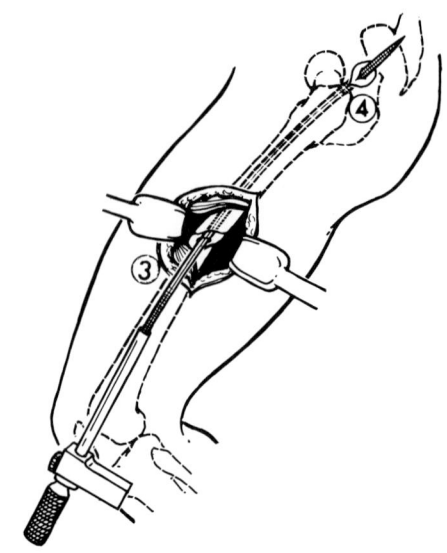

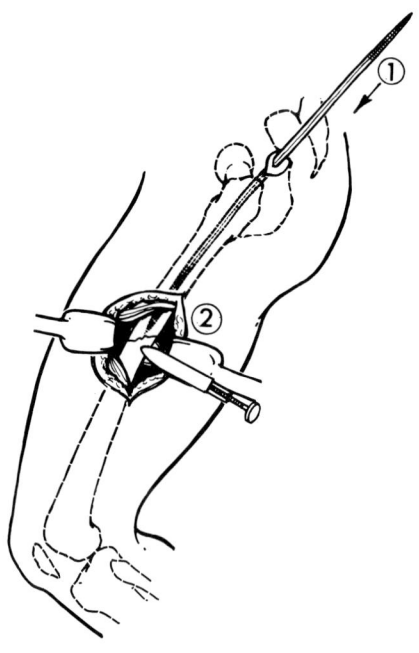

1. The patient is given rapid-acting curare and the fracture is reduced using traction and rotation of the fracture fragments.

2. The nail is then passed through the distal medullary canal. The distal canal is not reamed because it is larger than the proximal shaft canal.

Note: The nail must be of proper length as determined by preoperative scanogram to permit adequate fracture fixation. Obtain an intraoperative x-ray to insure that the nail length is adequate.

3. While intraoperative x-ray is being obtained, "fish-scale" the fractur site to lay slivers of bone close to the fracture region.

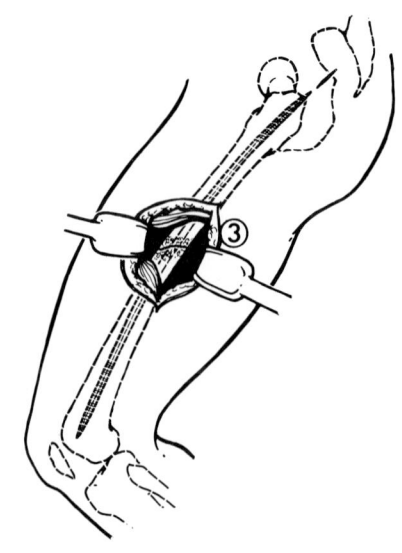

Intraoperative X-Ray

1. The nail must be drive distally to engage in the heavy cancellous bone in the supracondylar region.
2. The nail should be left about 1 cm above the neck of the femur.

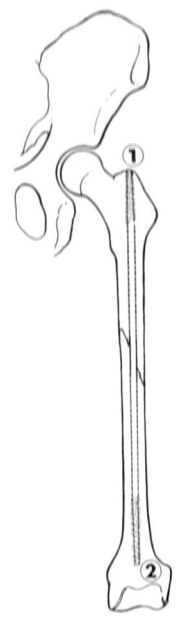

Supplemental Fixation Techniques

1. For long oblique fractures that still have some rotation despite the nail, apply multiple cerclage 18-gauge stainless steel wires.
2. For less than satisfactory fixation of the distal fragment apply cortical screws inserted tangentially to the nail.
3. When there is any question about the degree of fracture stability or the reliability of the patient use external support by means of a cast-brace.

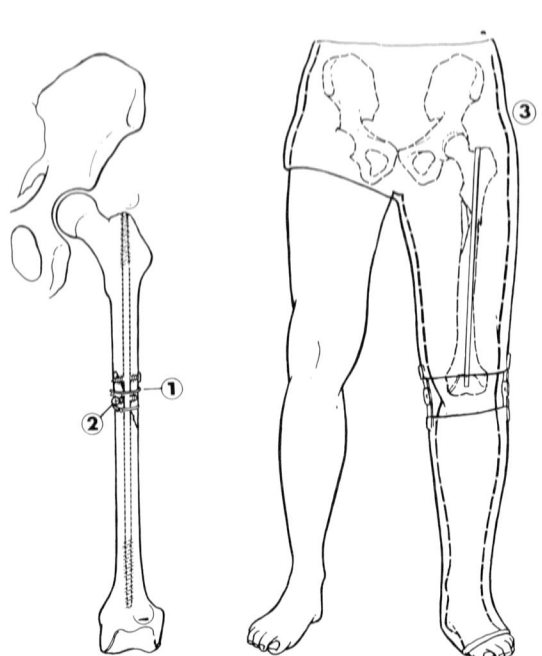

POSTOPERATIVE CARE

Apply a compression dressing for the first few days while the patient is immobilized in balanced suspension.

Gradually mobilize the patient in bed and encourage range-of-motion exercises to the knee and hip joints.

When the patient regains control of thigh muscles, he may be allowed to walk with crutches; this is usually about the third or fourth postoperative day, depending on the degree of fixation and the patient's motivation.

The patient may employ partial weight bearing with stable fixation of the fracture.

Full weight bearing should not be permitted until the x-ray shows evidence of solid fracture union, usually by 10 to 12 weeks.

The nail generally should be removed when there is complete obliteration of the fracture site, especially in young patients. This should be done only after an interval of at least one year.

Complications of Femoral Shaft Fractures

REMARKS

Complications from femoral shaft fractures may be life-threatening or limb-threatening. The immediately potential complications include death from hypovolemic shock, delayed shock (fat embolism syndrome), and sepsis.

Death in the later stages of fracture healing most commonly results from pneumonia in the elderly patient or pulmonary embolism in any patient subjected to prolonged immobilization.

A femoral shaft fracture may frequently cause blood loss of 1500 to 2000 ml, but continued shock after adequate blood volume replacement indicates either major arterial laceration or bleeding from other sites.

Three per cent of femoral fractures are associated with major arterial injury that requires immediate repair.

Arterial repair and fasciotomy of the muscle compartments of the leg, if necessary, should take priority over internal fracture fixation. Keep in mind that the major cause for disruption of a peripheral artery is infection, not fracture instability.

Fracture Management After Arterial Repair

In most instances the fracture may be immobilized externally using:
1. Skeletal traction allowing a slight shortening of the fracture

OR

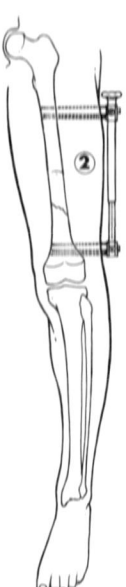

2. A Wagner-type external fixation device.

Note: Internal fracture fixation may be necessary for extremely unstable fractures likely to damage the arterial repair. In most instances external support is the most expeditious method of management.

DELAYED SHOCK: FAT EMBOLISM SYNDROME

Patients who sustain significant trauma that produces femoral fractures must be monitored closely for delayed shock, or fat embolism syndrome.

Any sudden alteration in the patient's mental status indicates the need to evaluate blood gases and treat promptly (see page 82).

SEPSIS

REMARKS

Overwhelming sepsis may occur with open femoral fractures, particularly when the wounds involve the buttock region.

Thorough cleansing of the wound and open treatment of the fracture as an abscess are essential. Prophylactic broad-spectrum antibiotics may be used only if combined with complete wound cleansing and open treatment.

Always scrutinize the postoperative x-ray for evidence of retained foreign material; with contaminated wounds, plan a second wound exploration and debridement in the operating room 3 to 5 days after initial wound treatment.

Anaerobic infections (tetanus and gangrene) after an open femoral fracture are extremely lethal and should be prevented by the methods described on pages 125 to 129.

Do not worry about secondary closure of the wounds in the thigh. These invariably heal spontaneously by intussusception of the wound edges, provided that infection is eliminated and soft tissue immobilization is adequate (preferably a cast-brace).

Many open femoral fractures result from gunshot or shotgun wounds (see page 132).

Fractures produced by low-velocity, low-caliber gunshot wounds do not require surgical exploration but may be treated by local wound excision.

Close-range, high-velocity shotgun fractures demand surgical exploration and debridement, since foreign material and wadding are frequently retained at the fracture site.

Close-Range Shotgun Fracture of the Femur

1. The wound of entrance is left open after debridement.
2. The fracture site is thoroughly explored in the operating room.
3. Two shotgun wads are removed from the medial side of the thigh.
4. The femoral artery is visualized and found intact.

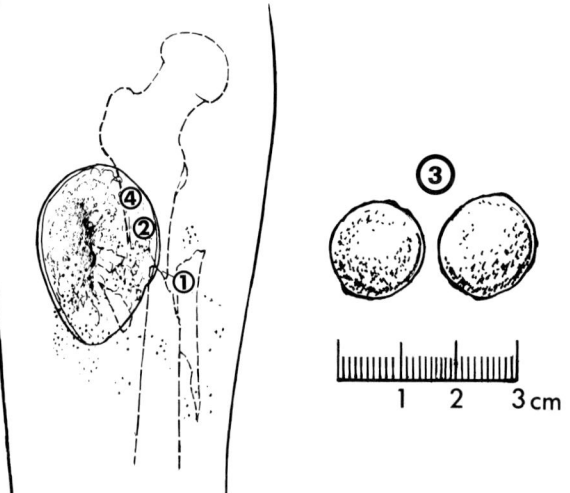

The fracture is treated in skeletal traction and then by external cast immobilization.

Six months after injury:
1. The comminuted fracture is healed.
2. The soft tissue wound has closed by intussusception without skin graft.

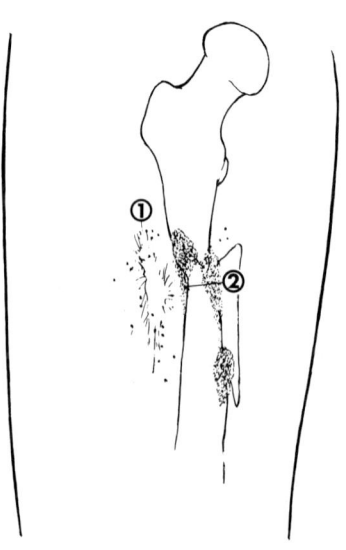

.22-Caliber Gunshot Fracture of the Femur

1. The wound is treated by superficial debridement without exploring the fracture.
2. The fracture is treated with traction and a cast-brace.
3. Healing is evident at 16 weeks.
4. The bullet has not been removed.

Note: Surgical exploration is indicated with low-velocity gunshot wounds only if the bullet is likely to have penetrated a joint, such as the hip or knee.

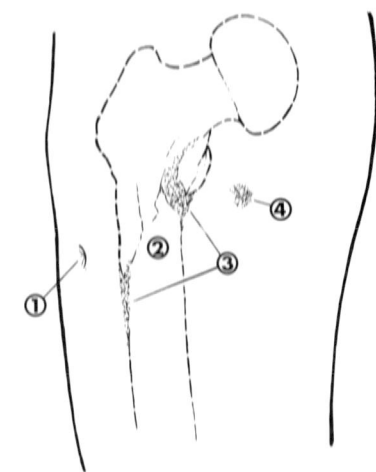

DISLOCATION OR FRACTURE OF THE HIP COMPLICATING FEMORAL SHAFT FRACTURES

REMARKS

Three per cent of femoral shaft fractures have an associated hip dislocation or femoral neck fracture. Half the time this injury is missed because of inadequate x-ray technique.

X-rays of the pelvis and hip region are therefore essential in any patient with a femoral shaft fracture.

Internal fixation is usually necessary to manage these combined injuries adequately.

In most instances, stabilization of the femoral shaft fracture is necessary to provide sufficient leverage to reduce the hip dislocation. This is particularly true if the fracture is in the proximal or the middle third or the dislocation is old.

Prereduction X-Ray of Unrecognized Dislocation with Femoral Shaft Fracture

1. The femoral shaft fracture is angulated medially.
2. The proximal fragment is adducted rather than in the usual abducted position.
3. The lesser trochanter is internally rotated and not visible.
4. The hip joint had been omitted from the initial x-ray.

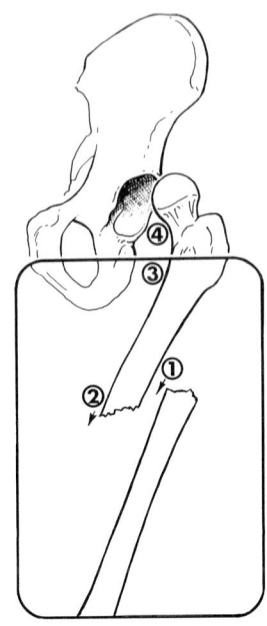

FRACTURES OF THE FEMORAL SHAFT

Reduction Technique

1. The femur is reduced and stabilized by intramedullary nailing.
2. Following stabilization of the femoral shaft the dislocation of the hip is reduced.

Note: This may require open reduction, particularly if there are loose fragments within the joint (see page 1306).

Prereduction X-Ray of Femoral Neck Fracture with Femoral Shaft Fracture

1. The shaft fracture is completely displaced.
2. Femoral neck fracture is relatively undisplaced.

Note: Intramedullary nail fixation of the shaft by a Schneider or Küntscher technique is likely to comminute and displace the neck fracture. Ender's rod fixation is preferable and may be supplemented by Knowles pin fixation of the femoral neck fracture.

Postreduction X-Ray

1. Femoral shaft fracture has been stabilized by Ender's rods.
2. Knowles pins have been used to supplement fixation of the femoral neck.

Note: External support with a cast-brace is usually necessary to protect the shaft fracture after Ender's rod fixation.

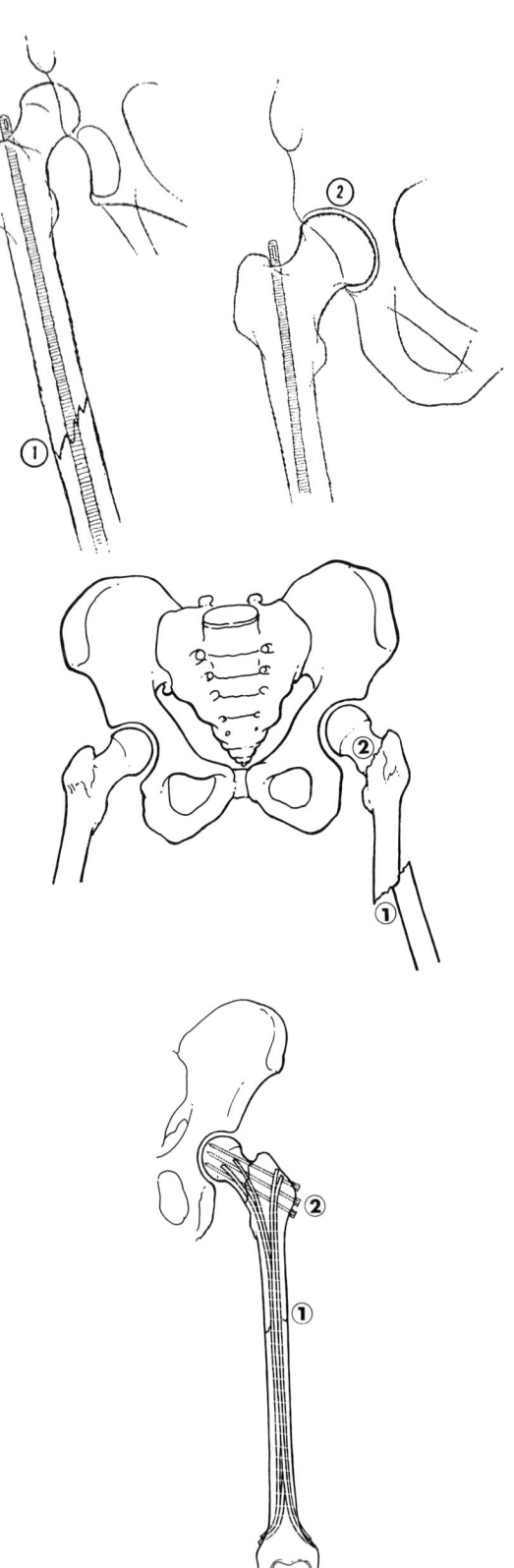

KNEE INJURIES ASSOCIATED WITH FEMORAL SHAFT FRACTURES

REMARKS

In addition to hip injuries, watch for the occasional ligamentous injury of the knee or fracture of the patella that may be associated with the femoral shaft fracture.

These usually require operative repair of the knee injury and internal fixation of the shaft fracture to permit rehabilitation of the patient's limb.

Closed treatment becomes extremely difficult for this fracture because of the knee injury. In addition, early rehabilitation and restoration of knee motion is inadequate if skeletal traction is used to immobilize the femoral shaft fracture.

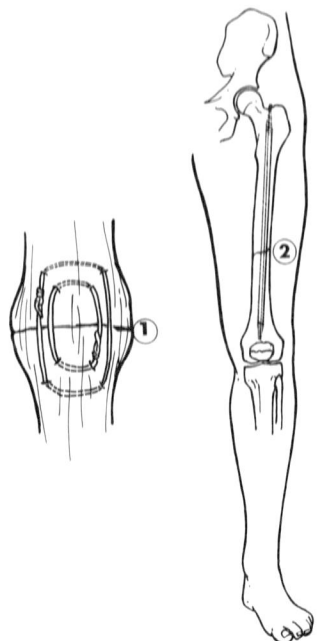

The treatment of choice for a patellar fracture with femoral shaft fracture is:
1. Repair the patella by cerclage wire.
2. Fix the femoral shaft fracture with an intermedullary Schneider nail.

TIBIAL FRACTURE ASSOCIATED WITH FEMORAL SHAFT FRACTURE: "THE FLOATING KNEE"

REMARKS

An ipsilateral tibial fracture associated with the femoral shaft fracture has been called "the floating knee" owing to the loss of proximal and distal support about the joint.

In the series reported by Connolly, Dehne, and LaFollette, 14 per cent of femoral shaft fractures were associated with tibial fractures. In

19 of 20 patients with these combined injuries treated by closed reduction and cast-brace method, both fractures healed. Satisfactory knee motion was evident in all except two fractures, in which there was comminution of the tibial articular surface.

Closed reduction and cast-brace immobilization are quite effective for managing the significant "floating knee" problem. Internal fixation is rarely needed if the physician appreciates the mechanics of fracture reduction and the requirements of knee joint alignment.

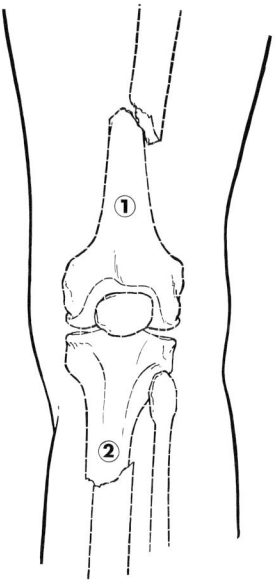

Prereduction X-Ray

1. A displaced fracture of the distal femur.
2. A relatively undisplaced ipsilateral tibial fracture.

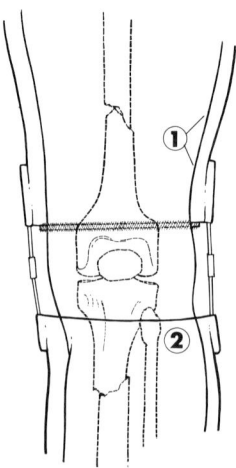

Postreduction X-Ray

1. The femoral fracture is reduced by femoral traction and is immobilized in the cast-brace.
2. The tibial fracture is adequately immobilized in the lower portion of the cast-brace.

Note: The femoral fracture usually heals faster than the tibial fracture. The cast-brace is removed at 12 to 14 weeks and the tibial fracture is then protected with a short-leg walking cast.

COMPLICATIONS OF CLOSED TREATMENT

REMARKS

The objectives of treatment are (1) to achieve fracture union and (2) to restore length and alignment of the limb to as close to normal as possible.

Closed cast-brace management is quite successful at achieving the first objective of fracture union. Its main complications result from failure to maintain satisfactory length and alignment.

Anatomic reduction of the fracture should always be a goal, but less than anatomic end-to-end apposition may frequently be quite satisfactory and even necessary. Comminuted shaft fractures often must impact 1 to 2 cm in order to permit healing.

Transverse fractures heal quite promptly in bayonet rather than end-to-end apposition. External callus formation and remodeling restore bone architecture close to normal quite effectively.

Choosing treatment on the basis of radiographic evidence rather than the clinical appearance of the limb may lead to inappropriate or unnecessary surgical treatment. However, ignoring a fracture's progressive angulation or shortening during the critical first 6 to 8 weeks of healing will also lead to unsatisfactory results.

Mechanically, the reduction should restore the normal gait relationships of the hip and knee joints. Slight angulation or overriding of the fracture fragments that maintains joint alignment is acceptable.

Varus or torsional malalignment, which throws the knee joint out of its normal relationship to the hip, should be avoided. Quite frequently the only reliable indicator of torsional malalignment is visual inspection, not radiographic appearance.

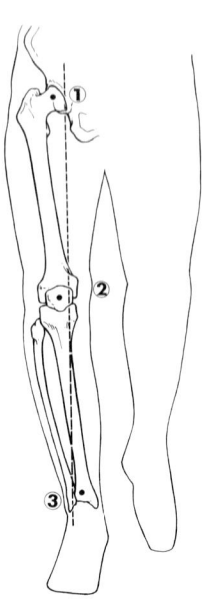

The weight-bearing line from the center of gravity falls:
1. Medial to the hip.
2. Medial to the knee.
3. Lateral to the ankle.

Bayonet apposition in either:
1. The lateral plane or
2. The anteroposterior plane may be accepted provided that the axis of the hip and motion of the knee joint are not altered.

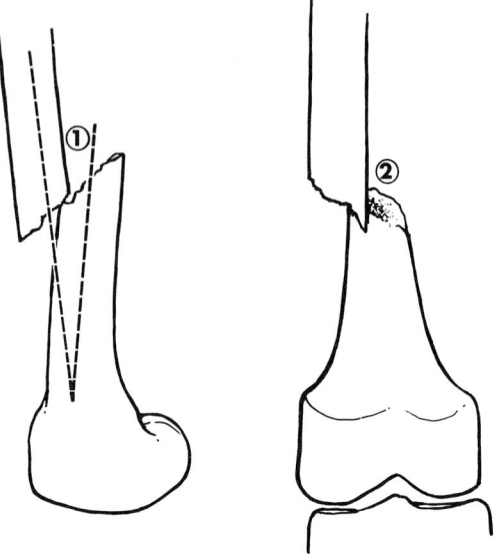

1. Bayonet apposition that maintains normal joint relationships permits fracture healing with normal clinical appearance and functional restoration.

End-to-end fracture apposition with torsional angulation is unacceptable.

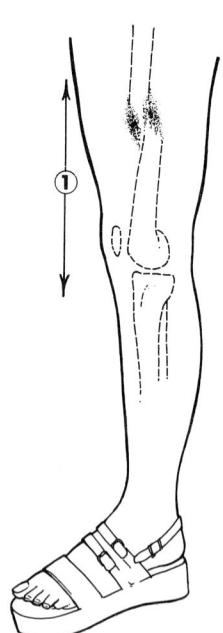

1. External torsion of the proximal fragment.
2. Internal torsion of the distal fragment.
3. Appears on x-rays as a varus angulation.
4. Torsional malalignment of the hip and knee joint centers of motion will affect both cosmetic appearance and function of the limb and must be prevented.

Note: A five-degree to ten-degree increase in varus or torsional malalignment noted after the patient starts weight bearing in a cast-brace should not be accepted, since it is likely to increase as the fracture heals. Apply a pelvic band or mini-spica to prevent torsional malalignment.

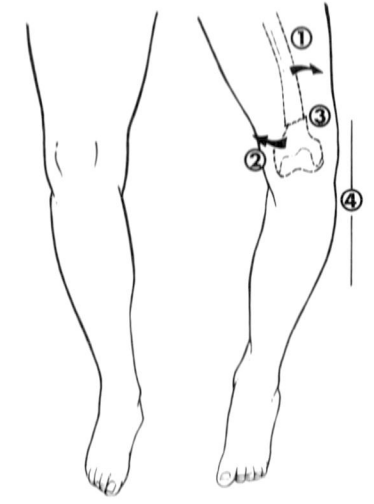

Potential Complications with Closed Treatment

1. A transverse fracture may shorten excessively.
2. A proximal femoral fracture may displace into a flexion deformity.

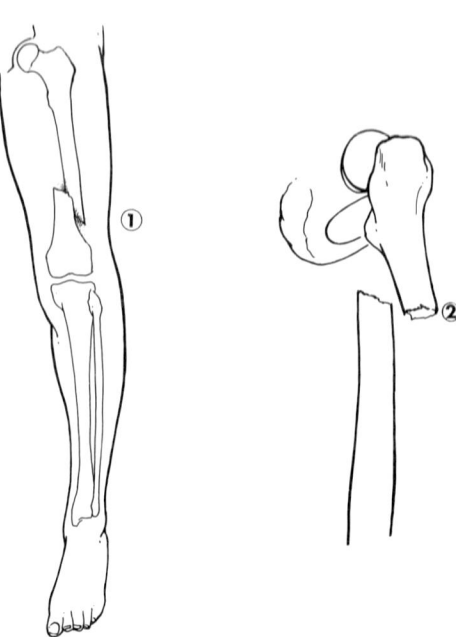

Potential Complications with Closed Treatment (Continued)

3. Internal fixation may still be used promptly if the fracture proves unstable after early cast-brace application.

Note: The surgeon who utilizes early closed reduction and cast-brace technique should be alert for these potential complications of unsatisfactory alignment during the first 4 to 6 weeks and should be prepared to correct them by either operative or nonoperative methods.

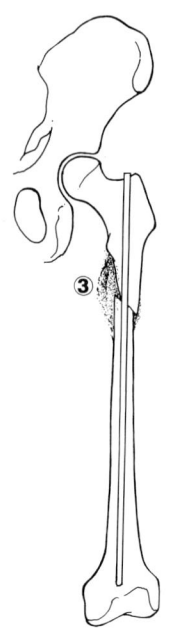

REFRACTURE

REMARKS

Refracture may occasionally occur after apparently satisfactory union with closed cast-brace treatment.

Patients who have learned to walk during the healing stages may be overconfident when the cast-brace is removed and may discard the external support too quickly.

Protected crutch walking is advisable for at least six weeks after removal of the cast-brace.

Refracture of this type is generally undisplaced and usually requires reapplication of either a cast-brace or an adjustable thigh support.*

1. Refracture of an incompletely healed segmental fracture two weeks after removal of the cast-brace.

---

*Available from Orthomedics Incorporated, 8332 Iowa Street, Downey, California 90241, and from United States Manufacturing, 623 Central Avenue, Glendale, California 91209.

FRACTURES OF THE FEMORAL SHAFT

2. The femur was stabilized and protected by an adjustable thigh support.

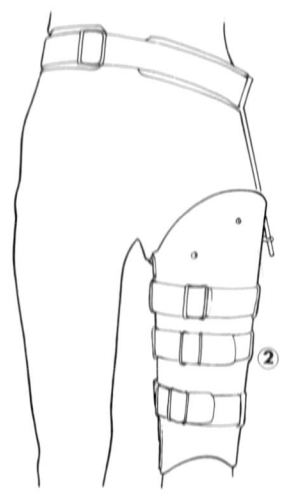

3. Refracture healed in 12 weeks.

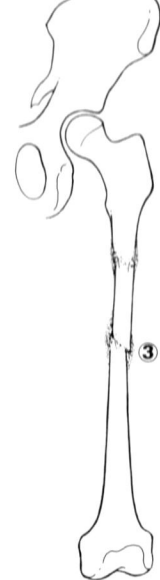

OCCULT INFECTED CLOSED FRACTURE

REMARKS

Although secondary infection of a closed long bone fracture is unusual, it does occur, particularly in patients with multiple injuries.

Fever, increasing pain, and an enlarging thigh mass should cause one to suspect the diagnosis, particularly in a patient who has been unconscious for a time.

Underlying systemic disease, diabetes mellitus, or a source of infection such as an intravenous or urinary catheter may lead to secondary seeding of the fracture hematoma.

1. Suspect the diagnosis if the x-ray shows gas shadows developing about the closed fracture.

Note: Prompt surgical drainage is mandatory. The fracture may then be immobilized with a cast-brace.

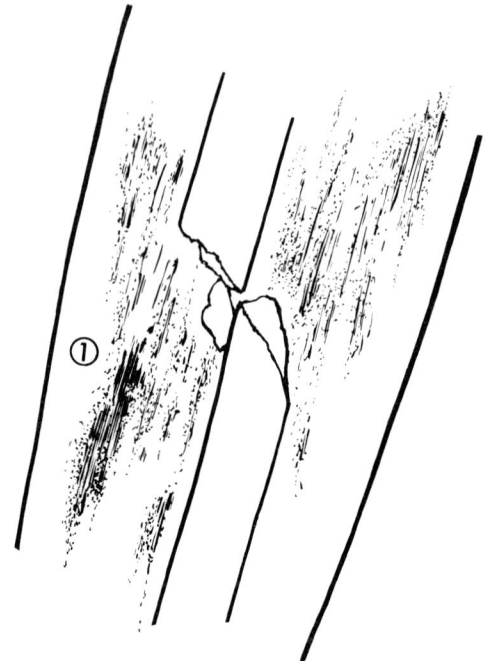

COMPLICATIONS OF INTERNAL FIXATION

REMARKS

The technical complications from internal fixation are potentially many.

Planning the operation carefully in order to be prepared for these common complications is among the surgeon's primary responsibilities.

Among the most common complications are:

1. Impaction of a nail that is too wide and shatters the femur.

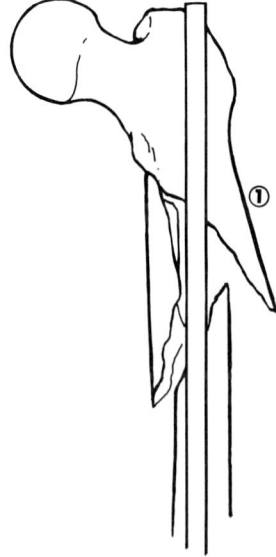

2. Use of a nail that is too short.
3. Use of a nail that is too small and allows fracture rotation.

Note: All of these complications can be salvaged by the use of supplemental internal or external fixation (see page 1467).

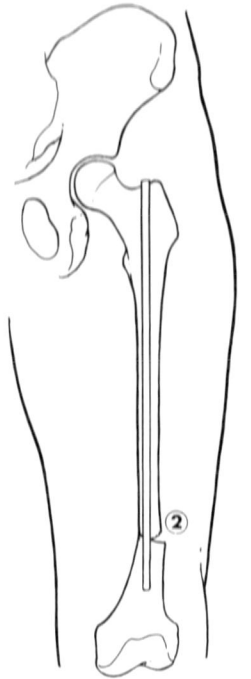
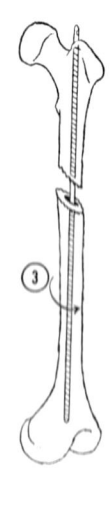

The use of plate fixation for the femur is particularly prone to complication and should be limited to selected cases.

1. The torsion on the screws fixing the fracture commonly causes loosening or breakage and failure of fixation.
2. The junction between the elastic bone and the inelastic plate creates stress concentration even after the fracture is healed and subjects the patient to the risk of refracture.

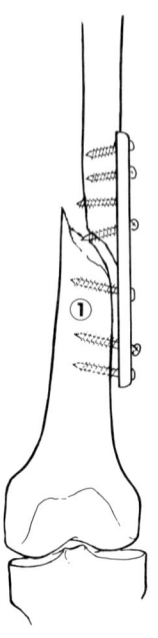
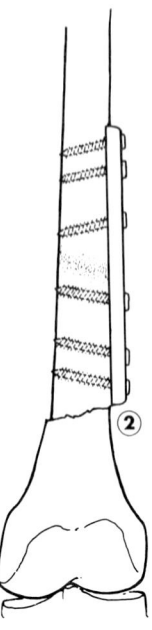

Infection

REMARKS

Infection occurs in 3 to 6 per cent of reported series of patients treated by open reduction and internal fixation.

The major signs of infection are sudden pain in the fracture or wound area, swelling, and increased temperature.

In order to detect these significant indicators early, prophylactic antibiotics should be continued for no more than 36 hours postoperatively. Prolonged use of antibiotics only masks the abscess that has developed and now requires surgical drainage.

Delaying prompt surgical treatment of the infected wound while procrastinating with antibiotic treatment makes the ultimate outcome much worse.

Management of the Infection After Intramedullary Nailing

1. Leave the nail in place. This permits treatment of the infection without having to deal with an unstable fracture.

2. Open the wound widely and drain completely. Treat this as a soft tissue abscess and do not attempt wound closure.

Note: Once adequate surgical drainage has been accomplished and wound cultures are obtained, start appropriate intravenous antibiotics. However, the primary treatment is surgical drainage.

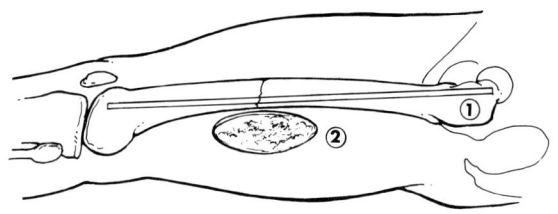

1. Use external support of the bone and soft tissue with a cast-brace when the infection is under control.

2. External support of the soft tissue by the rigid cast dressing permits spontaneous healing of the soft tissue wounds while the fracture heals.

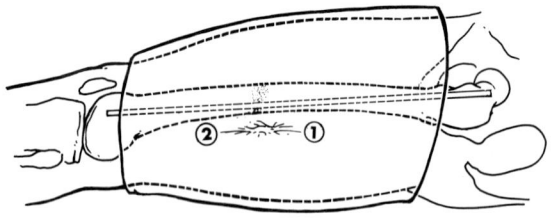

Nonunion

REMARKS

Nonunion is gratifyingly uncommon after femoral shaft fractures treated by functional methods including either the cast-brace or internal fixation. This is in contrast with former results from "conservative treatment" and with results from plate fixation of the femur.

A femoral shaft fracture that remains locally tender and does not support weight six months after injury should be considered nonunited.

The true status of the slowly healing shaft fracture may be difficult to ascertain, particularly after intramedullary nailing. Before categorizing the fracture as nonunited, obtain stress x-rays under fluoroscopy to be sure that the fracture moves or rotates. If no motion is evident, continue protected weight bearing with crutches to permit further consolidation of the fracture.

Effective methods of treating nonunion include bone grafting, use of more rigid fixation devices or a larger intramedullary nail, and electrical osteogenesis.

Electrical osteogenesis is a new method that stimulates intramedullary callus formation by low-voltage electrical signals. It causes considerably less morbidity than bone grafting or internal fixation of a nonunited fracture and is the current treatment of choice for this problem.

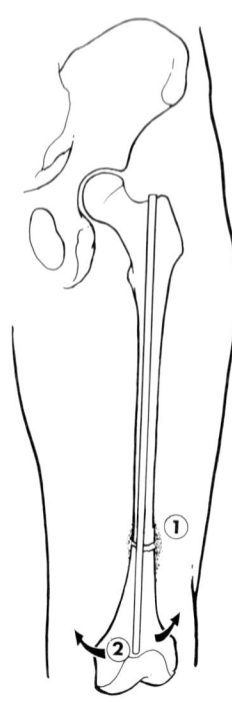

Preoperative Condition and X-Ray of Nonunited Femoral Shaft Fracture

1. The fracture is still painful with weight bearing and a defect is evident six months after intramedullary nailing. Joint alignment is satisfactory.

2. Stress testing under fluoroscopy demonstrates 5 to 10 degrees of motion of the distal fragment.

Technique of Electrical Osteogenesis — Semi-Invasive Technique (After Brighton and Co-Workers)

These electrodes should be inserted under sterile conditions with good radiographic control, preferably by image-intensified fluoroscopy. A common cause of nonunion after operative fixation or open fracture is chronic infection. This may come to light as electrical stimulation is begun, and the patient should be advised of this possibility.

In most patients, local anesthesia is satisfactory to insert the electrodes.

1. Four insulated electrodes are inserted percutaneously directly into medullary canal of the fracture.

Note: The electrodes do not contact each other or the intramedullary nail. For this reason image-intensified fluoroscopy is quite helpful during insertion.

2. The insulation is scraped from the ends of the electrodes and four leads are attached from the battery pack.

3. The anode pad is attached to the skin and the unit is activated.

4. The monitor is checked to make sure that the current level is satisfactory.

5. An external support is applied to protect the electrodes.

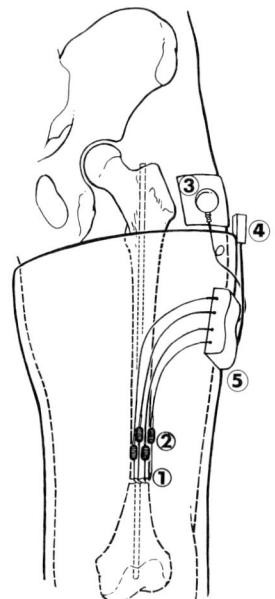

Subsequent Management

The patient may be up on crutches but should avoid weight bearing that might pull out the electrodes.

Most patients can be discharged from the hospital on the day of or the day after electrode insertion.

The anode pad should be changed every 2 to 3 days and the patient should be seen monthly to monitor the battery pack and the position of the electrodes by x-ray.

The electrodes are left in place for twelve weeks and are then removed.

X-Ray after Twelve Weeks of Electrical Stimulation

1. The electrodes have been removed and the fracture line is seen to be filling in with intra-medullary callus. Tenderness and motion are no longer evident at the fracture.

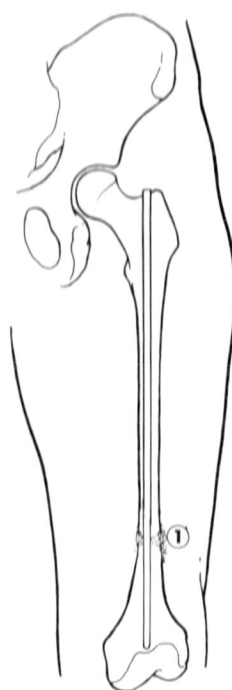

CAUTION

Continue to protect the fracture with crutches and/or external support for 2 to 3 months after electrical stimulation until consolidation is advanced.

MALUNION

REMARKS

If a nonunited or healed fracture has developed a position detrimental to joint function or has shortened excessively, surgical correction is necessary.

The major indication for correction of malunion is disability from joint malposition because resultant strain on the knee will cause pain and walking difficulty.

Moderate degrees of angulation of the shaft may be tolerated and can be remodeled provided that torsional malalignment has not occurred at the knee joint.

In each instance the physician must determine what is true impairment of function and what is merely a radiographic "malunion" of little functional significance. Many apparent malunions are within the range of biomechanical tolerance for normal gait.

A limp that persists after treatment may frequently be the result of poor gait habits learned during crutch walking. Many such limps can be unlearned and do not require surgical correction.

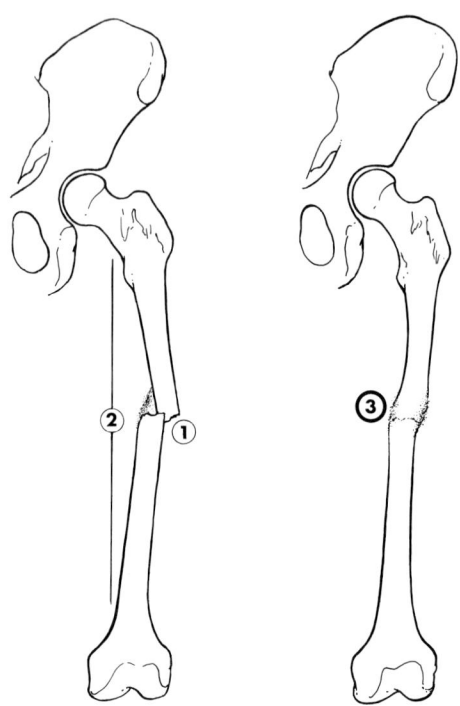

Angulated Fracture that Remodels

1. A varus angulation has developed in a fracture of the proximal half while the patient was in traction for six weeks.

2. The alignment of the hip and knee were satisfactory because internal torsion was prevented.

3. One year after fracture, remodeling has decreased the angulation by laying down bone on the medial side of the fracture and resorbing bone on the lateral side.

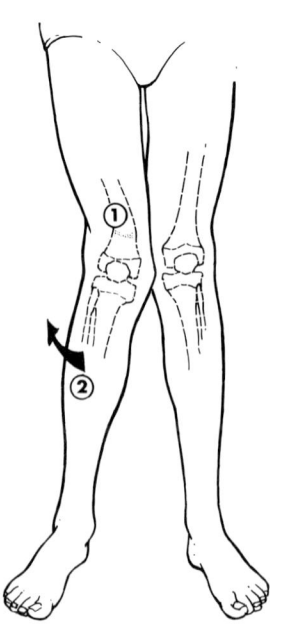

Example of Malunion

1. External torsional deformity has occurred after treatment of distal femoral fracture by a long leg cast. The weight of the cast has caused the distal fragment to turn outward.

2. The torsion of the knee joint has shifted the axis of the knee motion out of proper weight-bearing alignment with the hip.

1. The knee joint was realigned by derotational osteotomy.

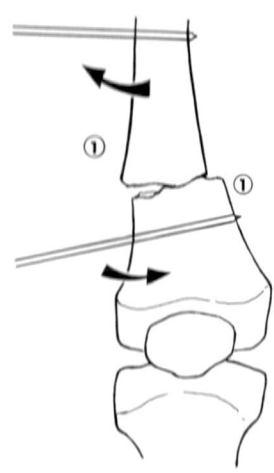

2. The proximal and distal pin transfixion maintained correct position.

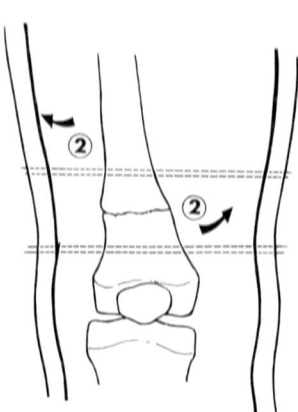

Appearance 14 Weeks after Derotational Osteotomy

1. The osteotomy has healed and corrected the torsional malalignment of the knee as seen on x-ray and
2. On clinical examination.

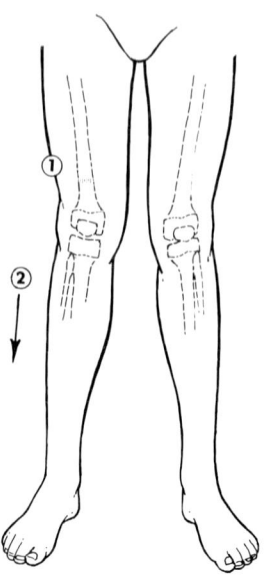

Malunion after Internal Fixation

1. The nail, which was too small to keep the fracture aligned, has broken.
2. Fracture gap and nonunion are evident.
3. Torsional deformity has occurred at the knee joint.

X-ray taken after operative reduction shows:

4. The fracture site has been explored and filled with cancellous bone.
5. The broken nail is replaced with a heavier nail that fills the canal.
6. The torsional deformity of the knee joint has been corrected.
7. Additional cancellous bone is inserted external to the fracture.

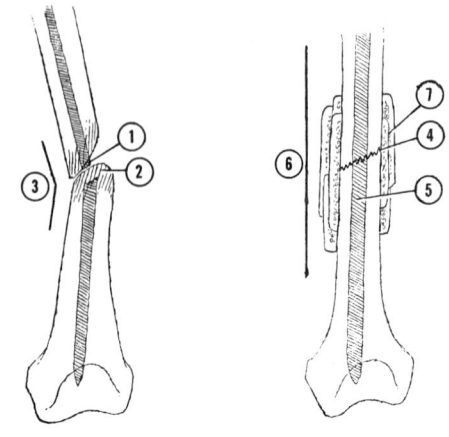

MALUNION FROM EXCESSIVE SHORTENING

Most often, shortening of 2 to 3 cm can be accommodated by simple methods such as a shoe lift.

If shortening is excessive (5 cm or more) operative intervention may be necessary.

The lengthening should be accomplished gradually using external fixation devices such as the Wagner apparatus.*

PREOPERATIVE X-RAY

1. A neglected shaft fracture has healed with 6 cm of overriding producing significant disability.

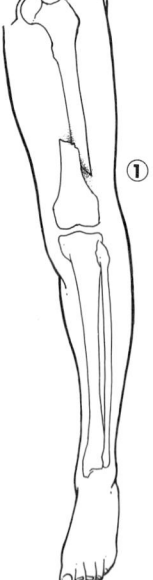

*Available from Synthes LTD, P.O. Box 529, Wayne, Pennsylvania 19807.

POSTOPERATIVE X-RAY

1. The Wagner apparatus* is attached to the proximal and distal fragments by Schanz screws.
2. The fracture site has been explored and the callus has been osteotomized.
3. The desired length is achieved slowly by daily extension of the apparatus. The limb is restored almost to its anatomic length.

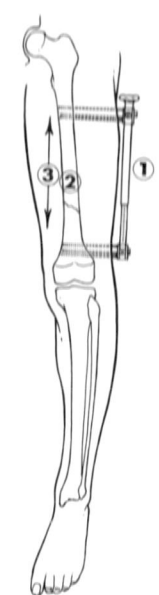

SUBSEQUENT MANAGEMENT

The external fixation is continued for 12 to 14 weeks, until new callus is evident on x-ray.

The fixation may be removed but the fracture should be protected by a cast-brace or external support with crutches until it is completely solidified.

Bone graft or electrical osteogenesis may be necessary to stimulate union after lengthening of fracture.

KNEE STIFFNESS

REMARKS

When prolonged spica cast immobilization was standard treatment for femoral shaft fractures, knee stiffness was a common residual complication.

Since treatment has incorporated the concepts of early functional range of motion using either cast-brace support or intramedullary rod fixation, knee stiffness is uncommon.

Occasionally when the fracture involves the distal femur or is associated with injuries to the knee such as a patellar fracture, knee stiffness may persist despite a functional exercise program as previously described (see page 138).

If knee flexion is less than 90 degrees four months or more after the fracture has been well-healed, knee manipulation can be quite useful. The method is an effective way of releasing the usual cause of the knee stiffness, which is intra-articular and quadriceps adhesions.

Manipulation should be done cautiously; extreme leverage should never be applied to the knee.

---

*Available from Synthes LTD, P.O. Box 529, Wayne, Pennsylvania 19807.

FRACTURES OF THE FEMORAL SHAFT

Technique of Knee Manipulation

The patient should be given a general or spinal anesthetic and the muscles should be completely relaxed. The table is lowered completely.

PREMANIPULATION POSITION

1. The patient's hip is flexed to 90 degrees and
2. The patient's thigh is supported by an assistant.
3. The knee flexion is seen to be limited to 60 degrees.

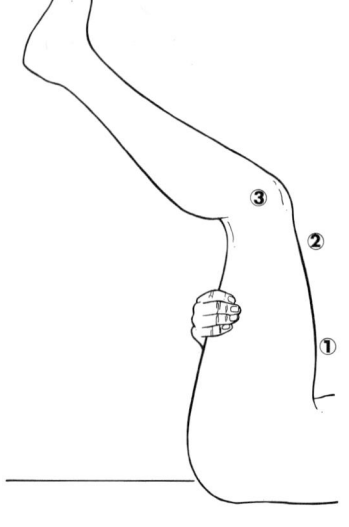

MANIPULATION

1. The surgeon grasps the proximal tibia.

Caution: Do not use the distal tibia for grasp, since this would apply extreme leverage to the knee.

2. The knee is repeatedly and firmly flexed and pushed to the point where stiff resistance is met.
3. After 10 to 15 flexion strokes, the intra-articular and subpatellar adhesions release and the knee flexes beyond 90 degrees.

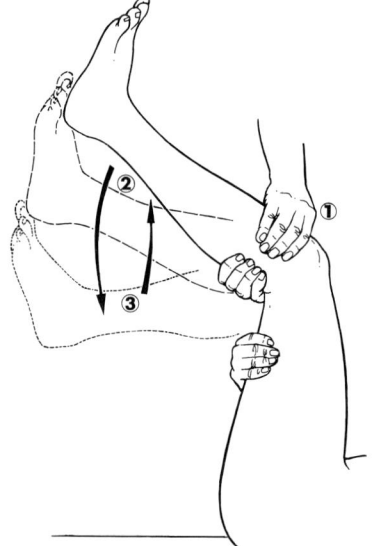

SUBSEQUENT MANAGEMENT

Obtain intraoperative x-rays to be certain that no fracture has occurred during the manipulation.

Aspirate the knee joint and inject long-acting anesthetic (Bupivacaine) to permit postoperative exercise.

Immobilize the knee with a dorsal splint, maintaining the flexed position for 1 to 2 days after the manipulation.

The patient should begin active exercises and passive stretching exercises (see page 138). The splint may be discarded as soon as active flexion reaches or exceeds 90 degrees.

Femoral Shaft Fractures in Children

REMARKS

Femoral shaft fractures in young children, as in adults, are frequently associated with severe trauma. Forty per cent or more will sustain significant associated injuries, including head injuries, multiple associated fractures, and severe abrasions.

In the young child or infant with a femoral shaft fracture, always look for fractures elsewhere, which might be indicative of child abuse.

Traditionally, shaft fracture in an infant has been treated by Bryant's traction whereas Russell's traction has been used in the older child. Serious complications such as skin slough or Volkmann's ischemic contracture have accompanied skin traction techniques.

Irani and co-workers have shown that young children may be safely and effectively treated by immediate spica cast immobilization. If no other injuries have occurred, the fracture can be aligned in the emergency room without anesthesia. The initial shock and pain from the fracture can be minimized and the patient can be returned promptly to a familiar home environment. This technique when used appropriately is the treatment of choice for children younger than 10 years of age.

Nonunion is almost unheard of in a child's femoral fracture. Consequently, open reduction and internal fixation should be avoided. Rarely, failure to reduce the fracture due to entrapment of the adjacent sciatic nerve or soft tissues may indicate open reduction and internal fixation.

The major complication has been considered to be overgrowth on the side of the fracture; however, with the technique of immediate spica cast application, the growth response after the fracture heals in children younger than 10 years consistently balances the leg lengths.

Shortening may persist in children older than 10 years of age with transverse fractures that heal with more than 2 cm of overriding. Fractures of the transverse type in children older than 10 are best treated by either Russell's or skeletal traction to maintain length.

TECHNIQUE OF IMMEDIATE SPICA IMMOBILIZATION FOR CHILDREN YOUNGER THAN TEN YEARS (IRANI AND CO-WORKERS)

REMARKS

The physician using this technique must first carefully evaluate the child for injuries elsewhere.

FRACTURES OF THE FEMORAL SHAFT

Immediate reduction is carried out in the emergency room without anesthesia as soon as the clinical diagnosis of femoral shaft fracture is made.

This technique reduces the danger of shock and makes the child more comfortable and less fearful during transportation.

1. The heel of the fractured limb is grasped in one hand and the calf in the other to apply traction and stabilize the fracture.

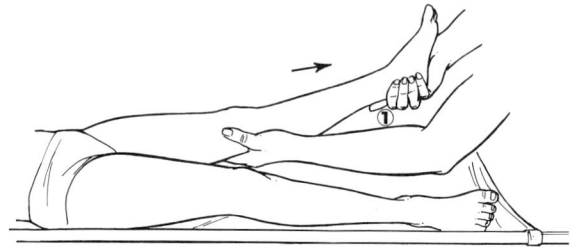

2. The knee is flexed to 40 to 60 degrees and the child is slid distally toward one side of the stretcher.

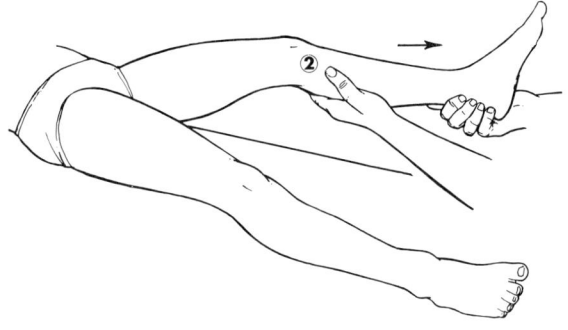

3. An assistant applies a long leg cast to the fractured limb.

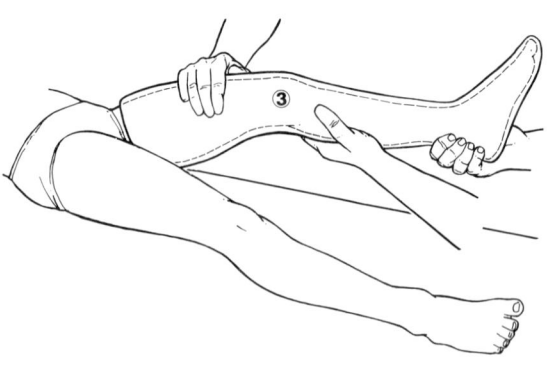

1. After the leg cast is applied, the child is placed on a spica table.
2. The hip is slightly flexed.
3. A 1½ hip spica is then applied.

Note: In children younger than 5 years, apply a double hip spica to permit handling of the small patient.

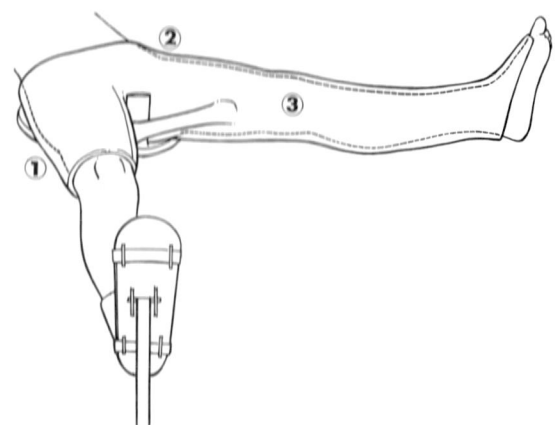

Only after the spica cast is complete are x-rays taken to verify the type and position of the fracture.
1. In children of all ages the sole of the cast is removed beneath the foot.
2. This prevents the child from pushing forcefully against the cast, which tends to cause overriding of the fracture fragments, and
3. It diminishes pressure necrosis on the back of the heel.

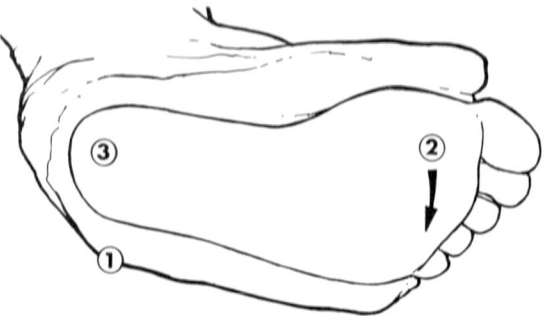

X-Rays Following Immediate Spica Application

Initial radiographic evaluation is secondary to the immediate alignment of the limb and immobilization of the fracture.

Any angulation of the fracture site can be corrected subsequently, within the first week after cast application. This is frequently necessary.

FRACTURES OF THE FEMORAL SHAFT

Transverse Fracture

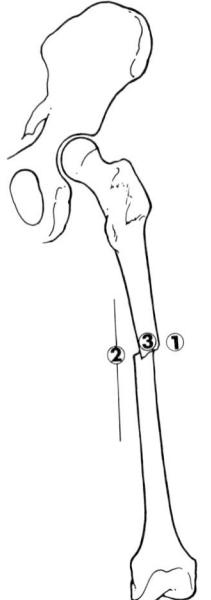

1. A transverse fracture of the junction of the upper and middle thirds.
2. Medial angulation of up to 15 degrees may be accepted.
3. One to 2 cm of overriding can be accepted.

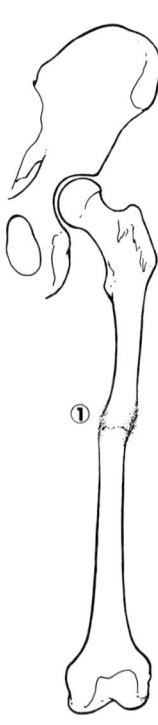

1. X-ray of healing fracture at three months shows remodeling in process.

1. Posterior angulation should be corrected to avoid recurvatum of the knee.
2. X-ray after cast wedging shows satisfactory correction of the angulation.

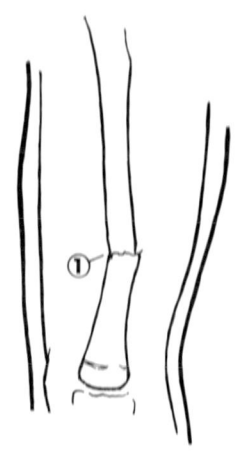 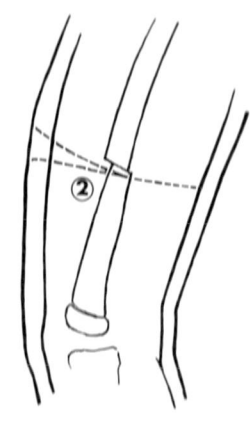

1. The lateral x-ray of a subtrochanteric fracture in a 7-year-old child shows 20 degrees of anterior angulation and overriding, which can be accepted in a child this age.
2. X-ray 2 years after treatment shows remodeling of the subtrochanteric fracture.

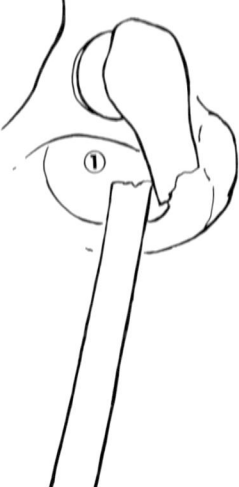 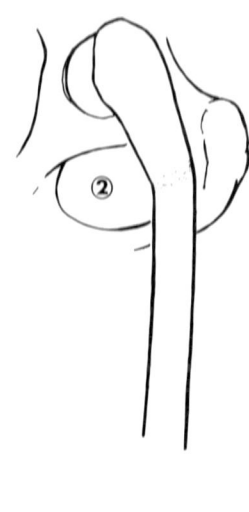

1. Transverse fractures in a child older than 10 years and
2. Shortening of more than 2 cm will not correct with growth.

Note: This much shortening in a child this age should not be accepted. The fracture should be treated in traction.

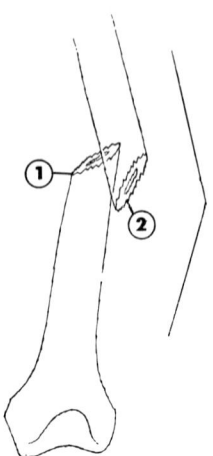

FRACTURES OF THE FEMORAL SHAFT

SUBSEQUENT MANAGEMENT

If a child is suspected of having other injuries such as a cerebral concussion, he should be admitted to the hospital for observation. The average length of stay in the hospital for this patient is 4 days.

The child should be examined daily for the first few days after spica cast application and then at weekly intervals on an outpatient basis.

The spica cast may be removed after 6 weeks in children younger than 2 years.

For children between 3 and 6 years, the cast can be removed from 8 to 10 weeks after injury.

For children 7 to 10 years old, immobilization is continued for 12 weeks.

Check union of the fracture by x-ray after removal of the spica.

The child may be permitted progressive ambulation at home after removal of the cast. Physical therapy is not required.

Although there may be evidence of either slight shortening or slight overgrowth for the first year after injury, with maturity the leg lengths generally become equal.

OTHER METHODS OF MANAGEMENT

REMARKS

Immediate spica cast immobilization is preferable for most fractures in children younger than 10 years. Other methods have been used such as Bryant's traction, particularly for young children who need to be followed for other potential problems.

In general, Bryant's traction should be avoided owing to inordinate complications from skin slough or muscle necrosis.

The technique is illustrated here mainly to warn of its hazards.

Technique of Bryant's Traction

1. Apply overhead traction to both legs; use strips of foam rubber secured by elastic cotton bandage.
2. Use pulleys and weights, not fixed traction.
3. The weight should just lift the buttocks off the mattress.
4. Use a restraint.

Note: In high femoral shaft fractures the legs should be widely abducted.

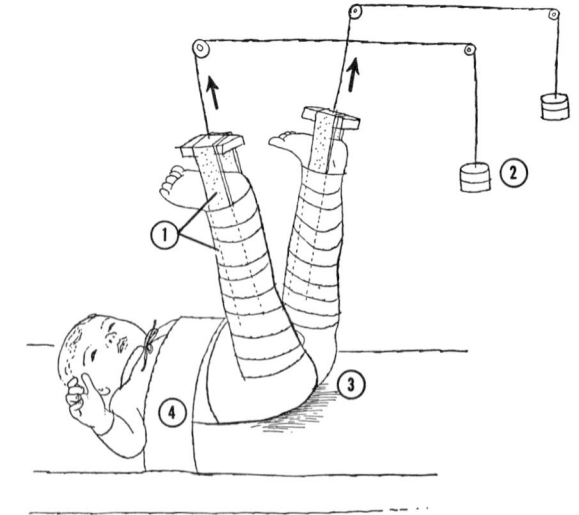

Postreduction X-Ray

1. Alignment is restored.
2. Slight overriding is acceptable.
3. Callus is evident.

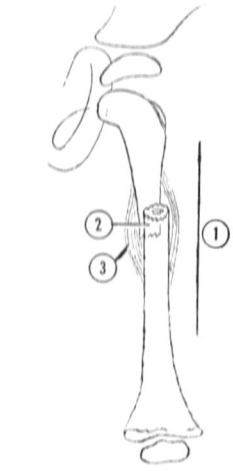

CAUTION

1. Ischemic muscle necrosis or
2. Severe skin slough may result from this technique in children older than 2 years or heavier than 15 kg (see page 68).

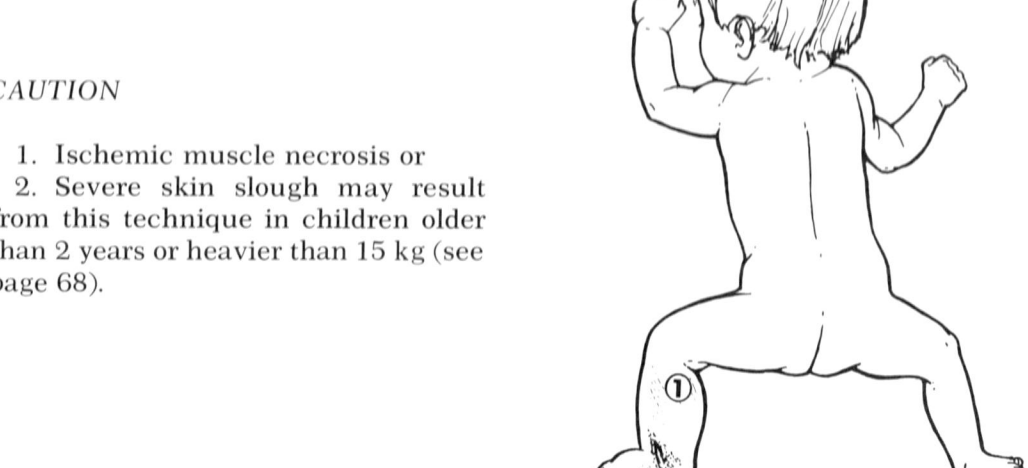

TRANSVERSE FRACTURES IN CHILDREN MORE THAN 10 YEARS OLD

REMARKS

Transverse fractures in children older than 10 years tend to shorten if treated by immediate spica immobilization.

Overriding of more than 2 cm is unacceptable in these patients because it is likely to persist and not be corrected by growth.

Management of this type of fracture should be by traction. Most often this can be done using Russell's traction to keep the leg length and prevent overriding.

Prereduction X-Ray

1. Fracture of the middle third of the shaft.
2. Marked overriding.
3. Adduction of the upper fragment and abduction of the lower fragment.

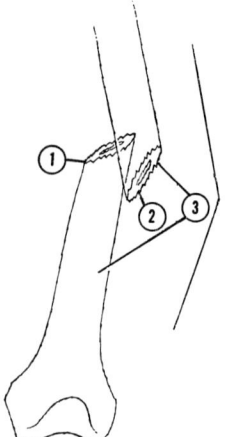

Reduction and Immobilization (Russell's Traction)

1. Make skin traction on the lower leg. (Use foam rubber strips instead of adhesive plaster.)
2. The knee is supported in a canvas sling lined with a sheet of foam rubber and supported from an overhead beam.
3. Pulley systems A and B maintain the limb in the desired position.
4. The leg rests on one or two pillows with the knee flexed slightly.
5. Two to 3 kg (3–6 lb) usually suffice to restore alignment and reduce excessive overriding.
6. Abduct the leg 45 to 60 degrees.
7. Elevated foot of bed for counter traction.
8. Foot plate prevents rotation.

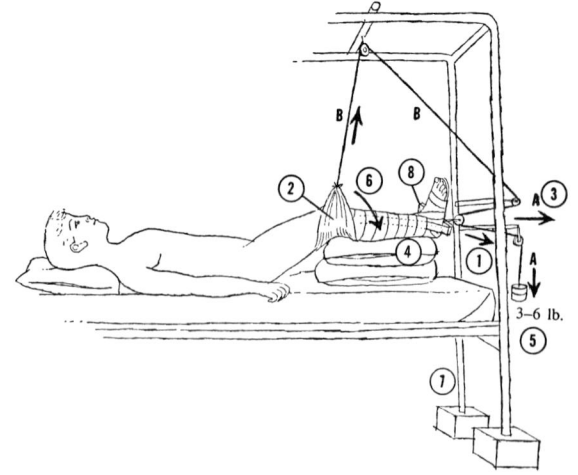

Postreduction X-ray (After Russell's Traction)

1. The fracture is aligned correctly without angulation.
2. There is less than 1 cm of overriding.

Note: If the overriding does not correct with 3 kg of skin traction, use skeletal traction. Skin traction of more than 3 kg will cause the child's skin to slough.

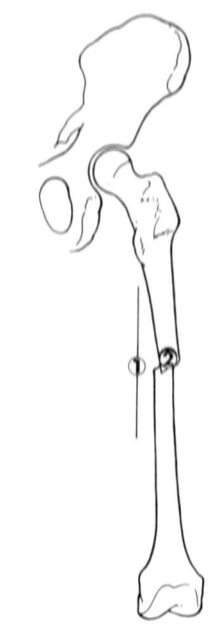

For Excessive External Torsion in Traction

1. Apply traction to both legs.
2. Use internal rotator moleskin traction to correct external rotation.

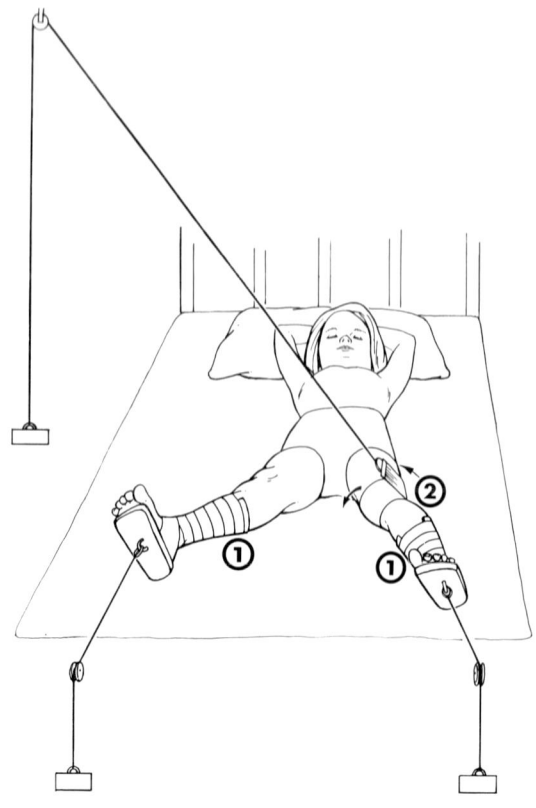

For Excessive Valgus Angulation

In the event that angulation is not corrected by single leg traction, apply skin traction to the opposite leg.

1. Reduce weight on the affected limb.
2. Increase the weight on the unaffected limb. This tilts the pelvis distally on the unaffected side and corrects the angulation of the fracture on the affected side.

Note: This is especially applicable to fractures of the upper and middle thirds with adduction of the proximal fragment.

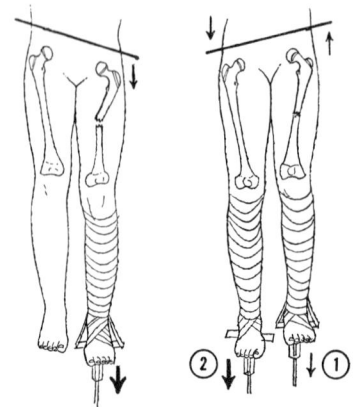

Subsequent Management for Fractures in Children Older than Ten Years

The Russell's traction should be checked several times daily and adjusted as necessary. These children tend to be quite mobile in bed and need to be followed closely.

Check the patient's feet regularly for evidence of circulatory embarrassment or neurologic impairment.

Keep the limb in traction until callus is no longer tender. This generally requires 2 to 3 weeks.

A cast-brace may then be applied as described for adult fractures at this level (see page 1467).

The patient may be allowed up on crutches following cast-brace application. The alignment of the fracture must be followed carefully, since these patients are very active once the cast-brace is applied and the fracture may angulate in the plaster.

By 10 weeks the fracture is usually united and the cast-brace may be discarded.

Continue protected crutch walking for an additional month until complete fracture union is evident on x-ray.

FRACTURES OF THE LOWER END OF THE FEMUR

Supracondylar Fractures and Fractures of the Distal Third

REMARKS

Among the most common of all femur fractures are those in the lower third and supracondylar region.

Forty-five per cent are sustained by minor injuries to osteoporotic bone. Most commonly this occurs when the elderly person falls on the flexed knee. These heal uneventfully with minimal complications, provided that unnecessarily prolonged immobilization is avoided.

Twenty per cent are open fractures and require prompt surgical cleansing and debridement of the wound. The temptation to discard loose bone fragments should be resisted during surgical debridement because iatrogenic bone defects are a common cause of nonunion.

Supracondylar fractures rarely injure major peripheral vessels but fractures in the distal third just above the supracondylar region carry a high risk of vascular disruption.

Monitor distal circulatory status carefully.

Despite numerous internal fixation devices, overall results are far superior with closed methods. The flared distal femur with its wide medullary canal and thin cortex present serious biomechanical challenges to internal fixation.

Standard intramedullary nails provide poor fixation in the widened canal of this region. If internal fixation is necessitated either because of a pathological fracture or because of the patient's extreme debility, the Zickel distal femoral nail provides reasonably satisfactory fixation. It must often be supplemented by external support.

Attempted operative fixation is particularly likely to be disastrous in a comminuted supracondylar fracture extending up into the shaft.

Compared with operative fixation, closed reduction and early cast-brace management can be relatively simple, particularly if one considers the mechanics of the injury.

Consistently, the direct blow to the distal femur with the knee flexed causes posterior displacement of the distal fragment and anterior displacement of the proximal fragment.

The objective of reduction is to pull the distal fragment distal and forward into alignment with the proximal shaft. This cannot generally be accomplished by tibial traction across the joint no matter how much the knee is flexed.

Direct upward pull by means of skeletal traction on the distal fragment is essential to reverse the mechanisms of injury.

TYPES OF SUPRACONDYLAR FRACTURES (AFTER NEER AND CO-WORKERS)

REMARKS

These fractures may vary depending on the mechanism of injury and the degree of displacement.

Most can be effectively treated with closed reduction techniques and early mobilization of the knee.

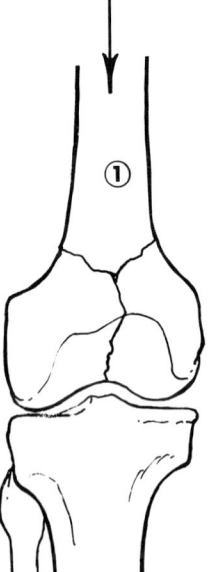

1. Type I has minimal displacement.

2. Type II may have medial or lateral displacement of the condyles.

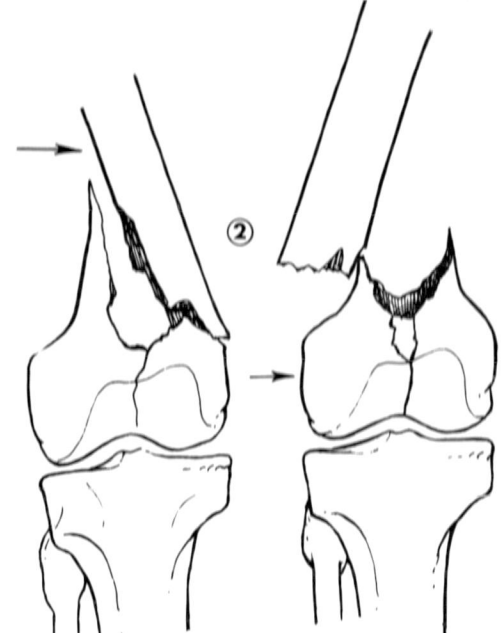

3. Type III is a combination of supracondylar fracture and fragmented shaft.

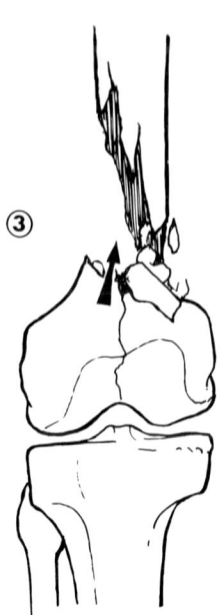

FRACTURES OF THE LOWER END OF THE FEMUR

TYPE I: FRACTURES WITH MINIMAL DISPLACEMENT

REMARKS

In minimally displaced fractures the fracture line may or may not extend into the intercondylar region.

They can be readily reduced and immobilized with the knee in a posterior extension splint until acute swelling subsides.

Subsequently, patients can be put in cast-brace and allowed to start weight bearing and range-of-motion exercises.

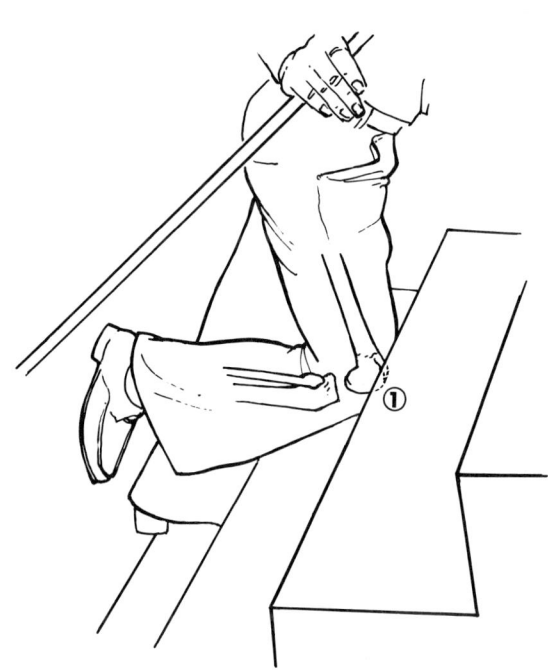

Mechanism

1. These usually occur in elderly patients from a fall on the flexed knee.

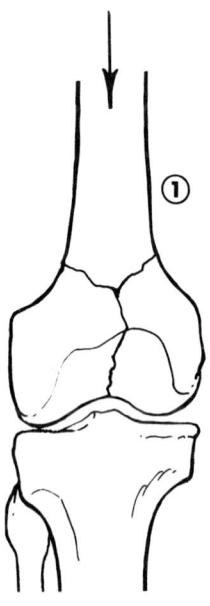

Appearance on X-Ray

1. X-rays show a typical impaction fracture of an osteoporotic bone.

Note: Intercondylar extension of the fracture line does not alter treatment.

Cast-Brace Management

With swelling of the knee joint it is wise to aspirate the joint and immobilize the fracture in a posterior splint with the knee extended for three to five days.

When swelling subsides, apply a cast-brace.

1. The knee is extended and in slight valgus.
2. The cast-brace is molded firmly over the condyles and
3. In the popliteal region to prevent displacement on flexion.

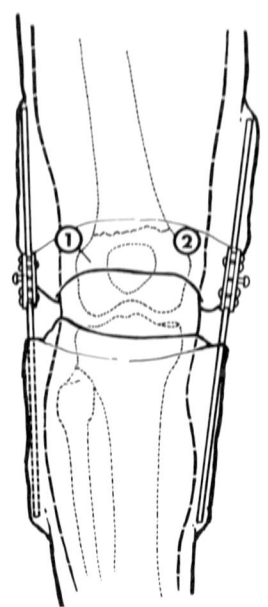
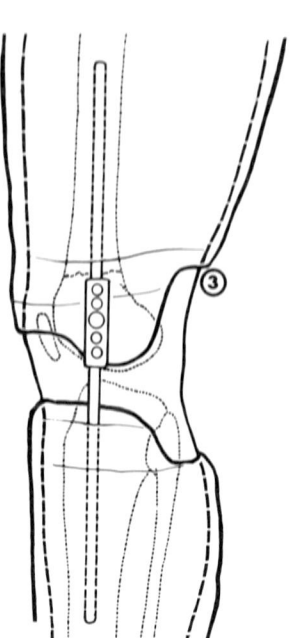

Subsequent Management

Forty-five degrees of knee flexion and full extension should be possible in a cast-brace.

The patient is allowed to walk with crutches and bear weight as tolerated on the fractured side.

Healing is usually prompt in the cancellous bone, and the cast-brace may be removed at six weeks.

Have the patient continue crutch walking for six to eight weeks, until fracture union is complete and knee flexion and extension are close to normal.

FRACTURES OF THE LOWER END OF THE FEMUR

TYPE II: SUPRACONDYLAR FRACTURE WITH MEDIAL OR LATERAL DISPLACEMENT OF THE CONDYLES

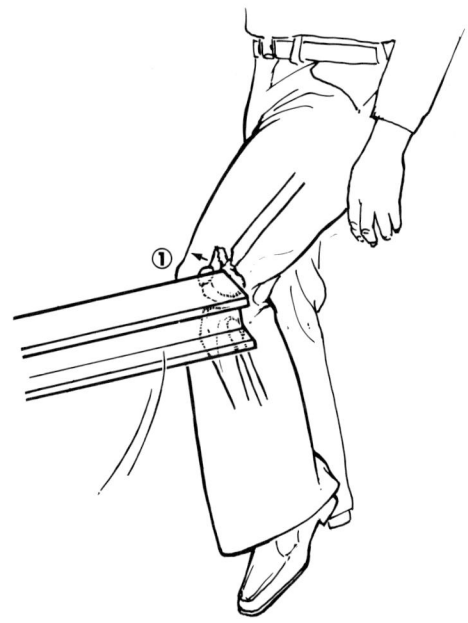

Mechanism

1. A severe blow to the anterolateral side of the flexed knee causes the condyles to displace medially and rotate internally.

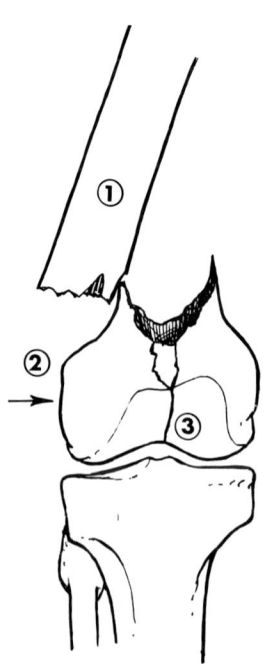

2. The shaft thrusts anteriorly and laterally and may be driven out through the lateral portion of the extensor apparatus and through the skin. Condyles displace medially and rotate internally.

3. Intercondylar or T fractures may be present in more than half of these fractures, but the separation is usually minimal.

Alternate Mechanism

1. Severe blow to the lateral side of the extended limb displaces the shaft medially and

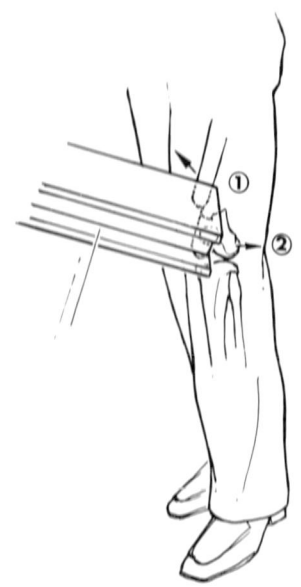

2. The condylar fragment displaces laterally.

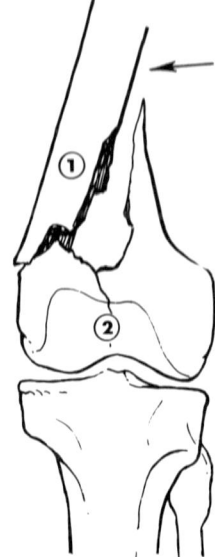

Management

These fractures may be open owing to penetration of the proximal fragment through the skin. Disruption of the quadriceps apparatus is usually not severe.

Injury to the adjacent popliteal vessels is always possible in this area and the distal circulation must be carefully monitored.

The displaced condylar fracture must be reduced by direct traction using a heavy threaded Steinmann pin inserted in the distal femur.

Management (Continued)

1. Because the mechanism of fracture consistently produces posterior angulation,
2. Tibial traction is usually ineffective for reduction.

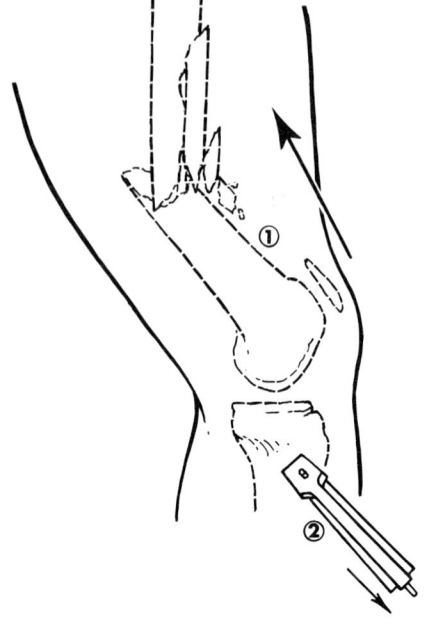

1. The pin should be inserted in the distal femur even though there may be intercondylar fractures.

Note: If the condyles are split widely, they may fixed with Knowles pins but this is more often necessary with Type III fractures (see page 1525).

2. The traction should be directed upward to pull the condylar fragment, which has displaced posteromedially or posterolaterally, back into line with the proximal fragment.

Note: Do not try to reduce a posterior displacement by knee flexion. It is due to the initial mechanism of the injury and is not produced by gastrocnemius pull.

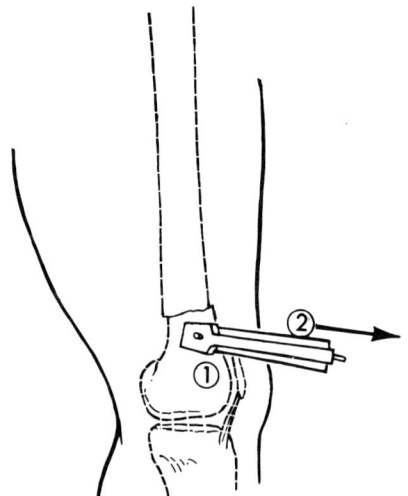

TORSIONAL DEFORMITY WITH A SUPRACONDYLAR FRACTURE

Significant internal torsional deformity is usually associated with this fracture.

The most common complication of the injury is a varus deformity of the knee produced commonly by traction rotating the condylar fragment inward.

1. Initial anteroposterior x-ray shows external rotation of the proximal fragment, indicated by the position of the lesser trochanter.

2. There is internal rotation and medial displacement of the condylar fragment.

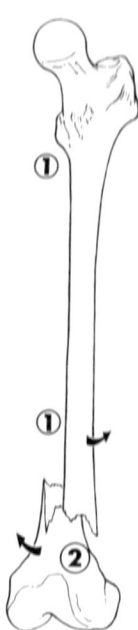

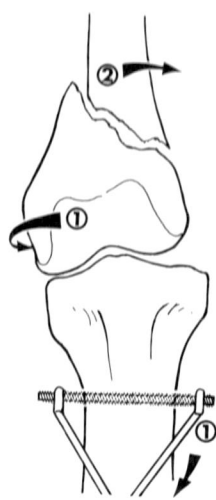

1. Prolonged skeletal traction may rotate the distal fragment internally while

2. The proximal fragment remains externally rotated.

3. The result is a "varus" deformity of the knee from the torsional malalignment.

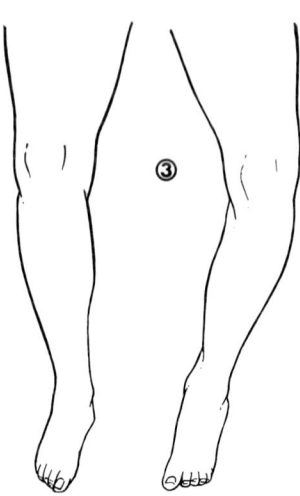

Correction of Torsional Alignment by Cast-Brace Application

1. A cast-brace is applied with the knee extended using distal femoral traction to reduce the fracture.
2. By visual estimation the knee is placed in slight valgus position and
3. Slight external rotation.

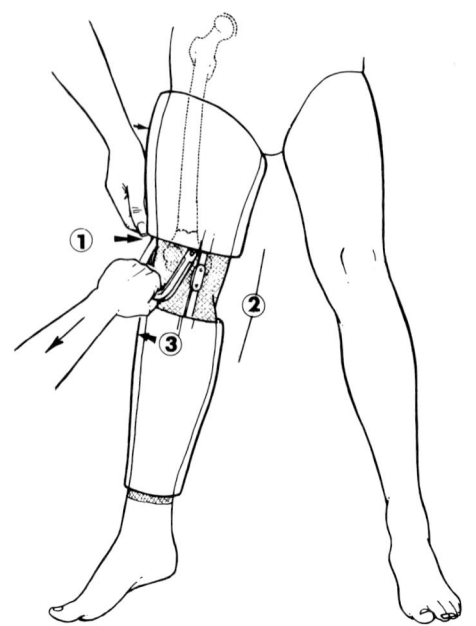

1. The cast is molded firmly about the femoral condyles down to the pin.
2. The pin is left in the distal femur to be used for 1 to 2 weeks of intermittent traction if necessary to maintain stability.

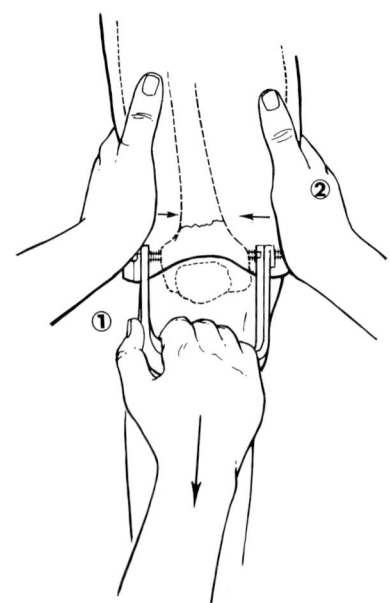

CAUTION

Avoid ending the cast too far above the knee joint.

1. A cast that is too high or ends too near the fracture site will allow varus and valgus loading of the fracture.

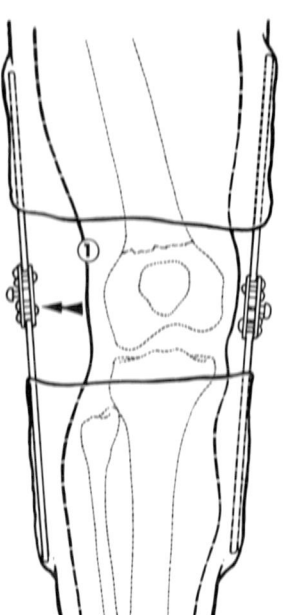

2. The cast should be molded well down over the condyles and

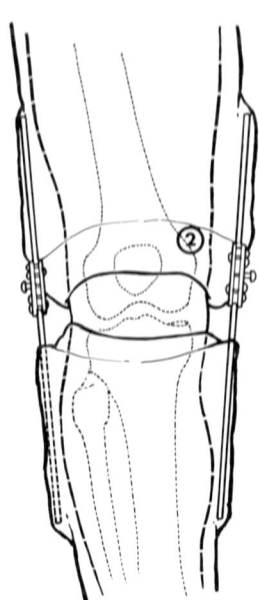

3. The clearance in the popliteal area should be sufficient to allow 45 degrees of knee flexion.

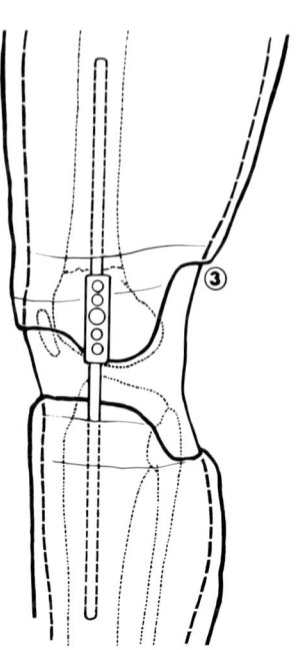

Subsequent Management

The patient is allowed to bear weight on the fractured limb as tolerated. If the fracture proves to be unstable, the traction may be applied to maintain alignment during the early healing phases.

Thirty to 60 degrees of knee motion is usually possible in the cast brace, and full active extension should be emphasized.

The fracture is usually sufficiently healed by 8 to 10 weeks to allow removal of the cast-brace.

Continue external protection with crutches or a cane for 2 months while the fracture continues to heal.

Therapy should emphasize active range of motion of the knee to regain full extension and at least 90 degrees of flexion.

Full flexion may not be obtainable if the quadriceps mechanism has been severely damaged at the time of fracture.

TYPE III: SUPRACONDYLAR FRACTURE WITH INVOLVEMENT OF DISTAL FEMUR

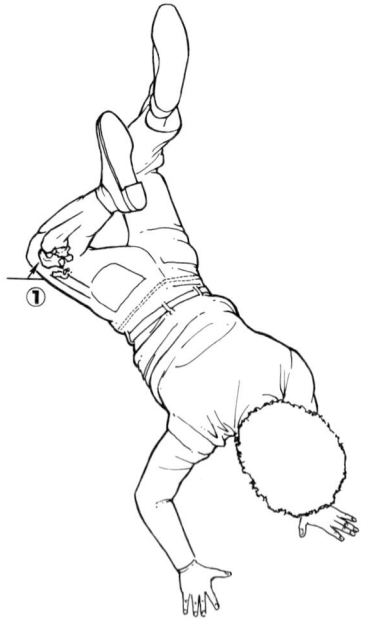

Mechanism

1. This fracture is produced by extreme violence to the anterior aspect of the flexed knee as occurs in a fall from a height or in a motorcycle accident.

2. The shaft penetrates the quadriceps mechanism and injures it severely. Frequently the end of the fragment protrudes through the skin.
3. The shaft fragments in multiple pieces.
4. Protruding bone fragments may impinge on the patella tract or
5. Threaten the popliteal artery posteriorly.

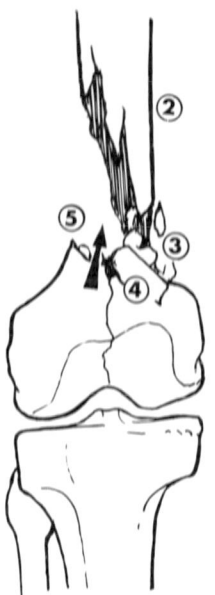

Initial Management

Surgical debridement is frequently necessary because these fractures are often open. During the surgical procedure do not remove any of the multiple small pieces of bone; this could produce a fracture gap that osteoblastic healing could not bridge.

Associated tibial fractures occur in about a third of cases but may be treated by closed cast-brace methods.

The condylar fragments may be split widely in these fractures.

Patients with Type III fractures are most prone to develop internal rotational or varus knee deformities owing to prolonged maintenance in traction. Healing time is significantly longer than in Type I or Type II fractures.

Closed reduction with skeletal traction of the distal femur and early cast-brace application, as described for Type II fracture, is the treatment of choice for this injury. It permits prompt fracture healing and early functional return of knee motion.

An alternate, effective method is Zickel nail fixation.

Technique of Closed Treatment of Type III Fractures

1. A comminuted Type III fracture with fragmentation of bone is evident.

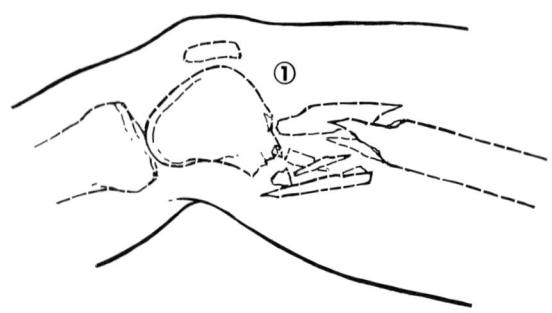

2. The fracture is aligned by distal femoral traction and a cast-brace is applied and is molded firmly over the femoral condyles.

Note: The cast-brace must come down well over the condyles to provide adequate support (see page 1521).

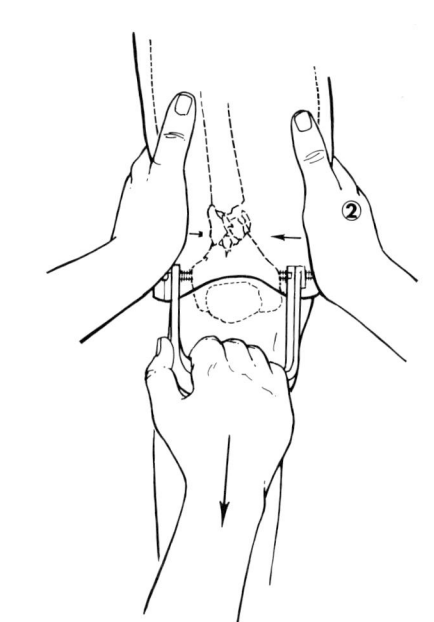

3. Healing is evident at 16 weeks. One to 2 cm of shortening is acceptable to permit fracture impaction and bony union.

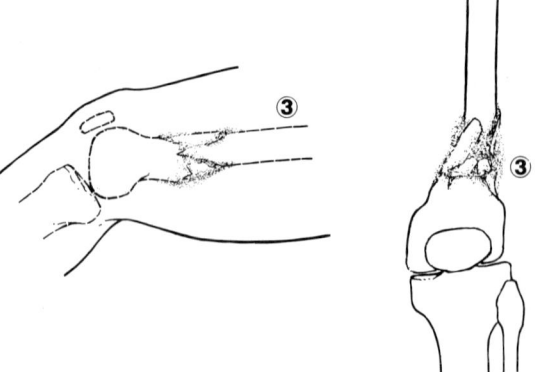

Technique of Knowles Pin Fixation

1. A widely displaced condylar fragment may be reduced and held with percutaneous Knowles pins. The comminuted shaft and condylar fracture may then be immobilized with the cast-brace method.

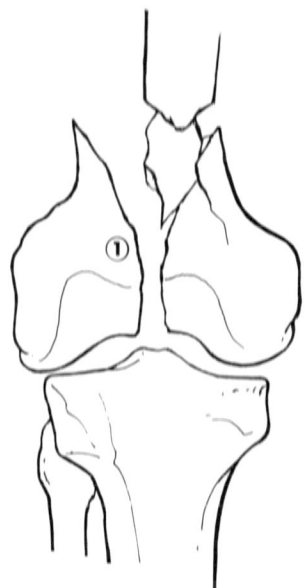

2. Healing is evident at 16 weeks. One to 2 cm of shortening is acceptable to permit fracture impaction and bony union.

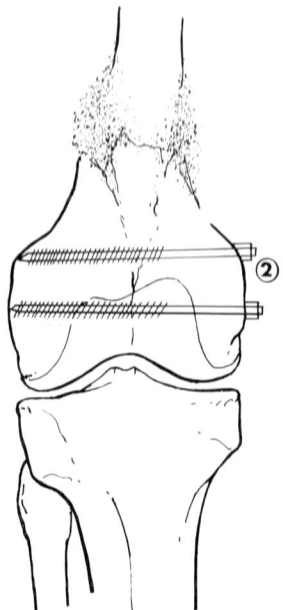

Postreduction Management

The patient should be allowed to bear weight on the fractured limb as tolerated.

Range of motion to full extension and approximately 40 degrees of flexion should be possible with the cast-brace.

A condylar fracture with comminuted femur fracture is generally healed by 12 to 16 weeks, at which time the cast-brace may be removed.

Protected weight bearing with crutches should be continued for two months longer until complete healing is evident on x-ray and the patient has regained maximum knee motion.

OPERATIVE REDUCTION AND INTERNAL FIXATION

REMARKS

The wide flared medullary canal and thin cortex of the distal femur make fractures in this region serious challenges for either intramedullary nail or plate fixation.

The majority of fractures in this area can be most effectively treated by closed reduction. Knee joint function can be restored by cast-brace technique, as previously described.

Pathologic fractures, fractures with arterial injury, nonunion, and, rarely, displaced supracondylar fractures in victims of multiple trauma require fixation, which can be achieved effectively with Zickel nailing of the distal femur. The method allows intramedullary support and does not have the mechanical deficiencies of plate fixation.

Operative Procedure

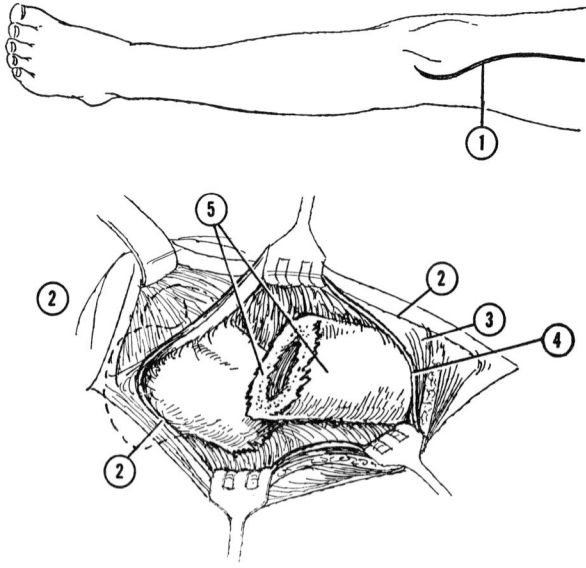

Note: The patient is positioned supine and the leg is draped so that the knee may be flexed and extended.

1. Make a 12-cm to 15-cm incision on the anterolateral aspect of the distal end of the thigh between the rectus femoris and the vastus lateralis. At the upper end of the patella the incision curves laterally to the level of the joint line, then gently anteriorly.

2. The iliotibial band is preserved and retracted posteriorly.

3. Develop the interval between the rectus femoris and the vastus lateralis, exposing the vastus intermedius.

4. Incise longitudinally the vastus intermedius and the periosteum.

5. By subperiosteal dissection expose the ends of the bone fragments.

After washing all clots and loose fragments from the wound,

1. Make downward traction on the leg.
2. Reduce the fracture with a bone clamp or elevator.

Note: In T condylar fractures the knee joint must be entered to insure anatomic reduction of the condyles.

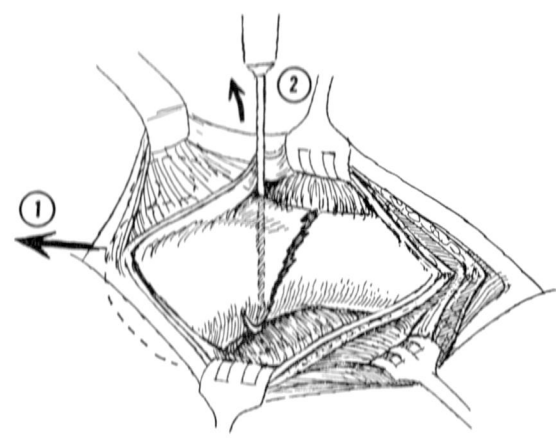

1. A short medial incision is made vertically at the adductor tubercle anterior to the medial collateral ligament.

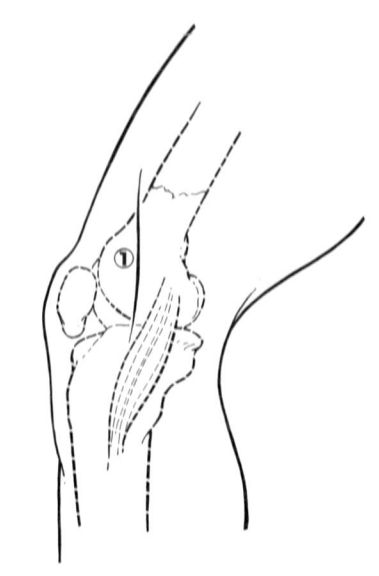

2. Marker wires are drilled into the medial and lateral condyles and an x-ray is taken to determine the level for insertion of the appliance.

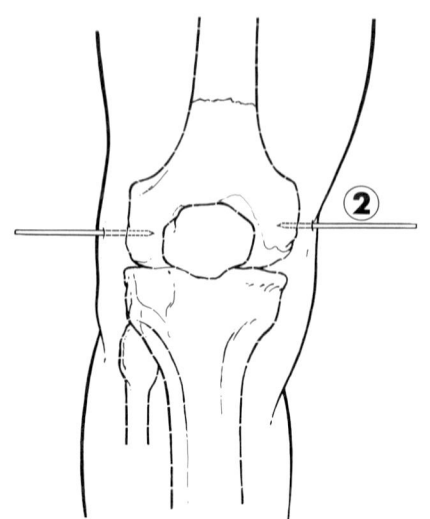

FRACTURES OF THE LOWER END OF THE FEMUR

Operative Procedure (Continued)

1. Condyle holes are made with drills and curettes.
2. A reamer is directed obliquely toward the opposite cortex of the shaft proximal to the fracture.

Note: In osteoporotic bone, minimal reaming should be done. The medial and lateral rods are inserted simultaneously.

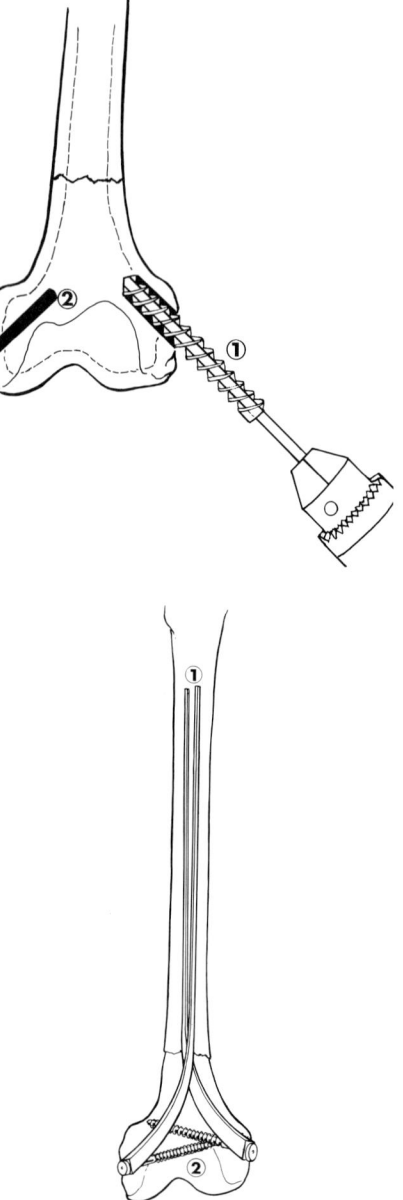

1. After x-rays in two planes are taken to determine proper placement of the rods,
2. The distal tunnel of the rod is drilled with a 4-mm drill and cancellous screws are inserted through the tunnel.

More x-rays should be taken to insure satisfactory position.

Subsequent Management

Frequently bone grafting, supplemental internal cerclage wiring, or external cast-brace immobilization may be necessary.

The patient should be allowed to bear weight with crutches and begin active range-of-motion exercises to the knee joint postoperatively as soon as swelling subsides.

With proper selection of patients and application of the device, complications are few and healing is usually prompt. Knee motion, however, is frequently limited after operative fixation in this region.

Unicondylar Femoral Fractures

REMARKS

Unicondylar femoral fractures are rare injuries that frequently are associated with injuries elsewhere and quite often go unrecognized.

When they are recognized their significance may not be appreciated and they may be treated by inappropriate closed methods.

By altering the condylar profile, unicondylar fractures seriously impair the mechanics of knee motion, even if displacement is minimal. Most require open reduction and internal fixation.

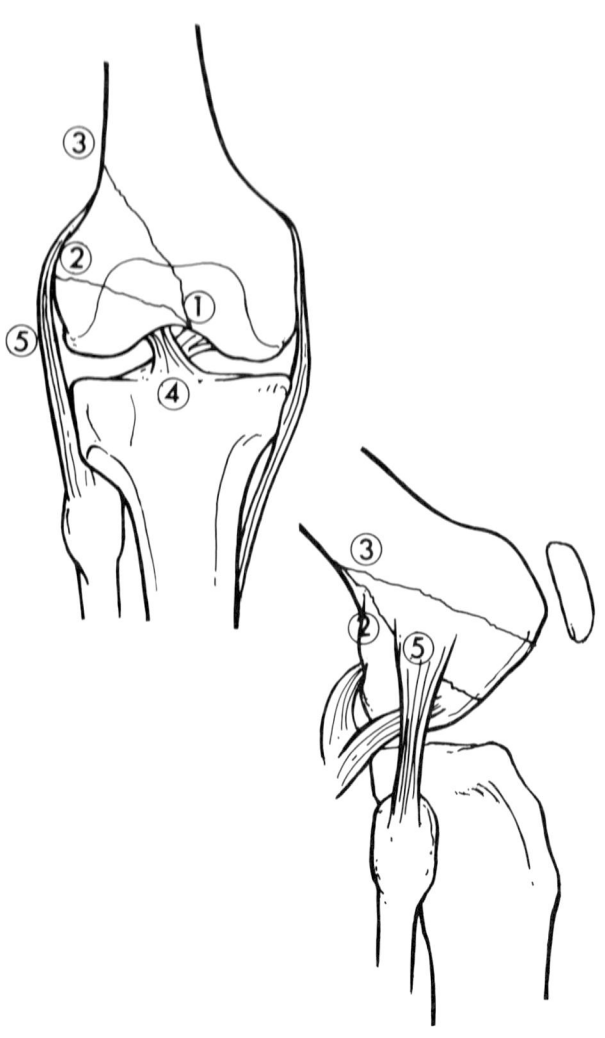

Fractures of the Lateral Condyle

About two thirds of the unicondylar fractures involve the lateral condyle.

Typically, the fracture line

1. Begins in the intercondylar region and runs either
2. Transversely

OR

3. Obliquely and laterally.
4. The anterior cruciate and
5. Part or all of the lateral collateral ligament remain attached to the fragment.

1529

Fractures of the Medial Femoral Condyle

Fractures of the medial condyle are less common than those of the lateral condyle. These usually run:
1. In a sagittal direction to include
2. The medial collateral ligament but usually not the posterior cruciate ligament.

Note: In fractures of the medial condyle, besides disrupting the articular surface, there is significant risk of avascular necrosis owing to the impaired circulation in this area.

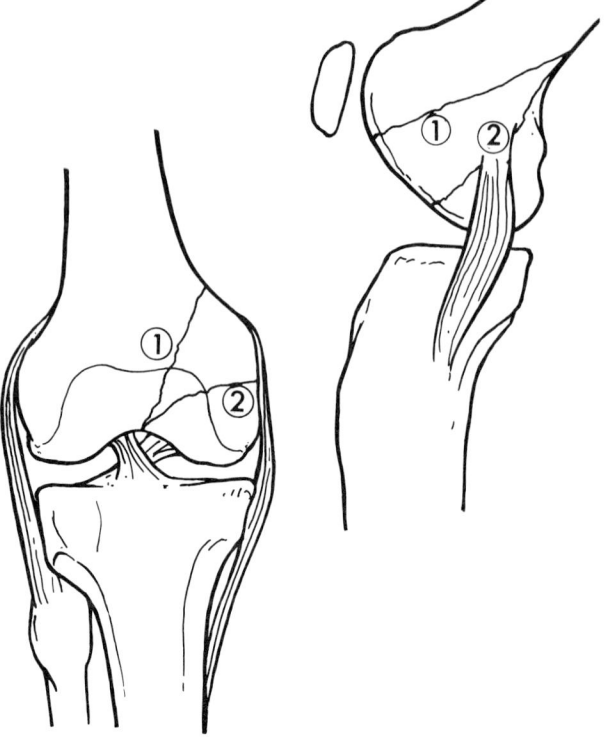

MANAGEMENT OF UNICONDYLAR FRACTURES

Prereduction X-Rays

LATERAL CONDYLAR FRACTURE

Displacement is identical in all types of lateral condylar fracture.
1. With a lateral femoral condylar fracture, the fragment displaces
2. Superiorly and
3. Posteriorly and externally.

Note: The displacement creates a "step-off" that may be masked on standard anteroposterior x-rays of the condyles. Always obtain complete axial patellar views and tomograms to ascertain the degree of displacement.

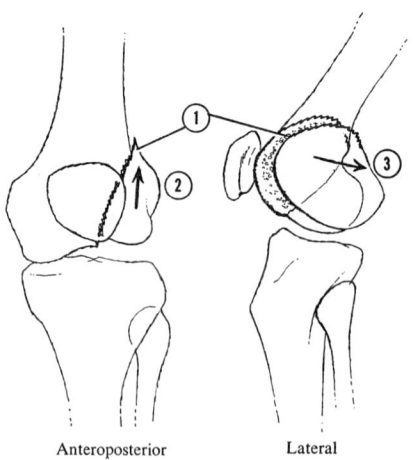

Anteroposterior   Lateral

FRACTURES OF THE LOWER END OF THE FEMUR

Medial condylar fracture

Note: Because of the disruption of the blood supply to this area, avascular necrosis is common following this type of fracture.

1. Fracture of the medial femoral condyle.
2. The condylar fragment is displaced upward.
3. The condylar fragment is displaced and tilted backward.

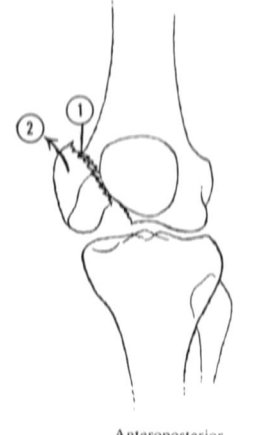
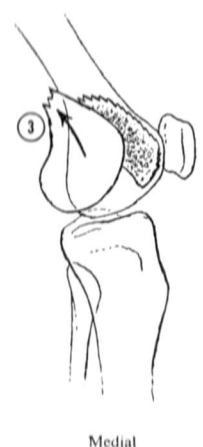

Anteroposterior   Medial

Apparently undisplaced fracture of the lateral condyle

Note: Quite frequently these fractures are more displaced than is evident on the initial x-ray.

1. Fracture of the lateral femoral condyle appears to be undisplaced on anteroposterior and standard lateral x-rays.
2. An axial view of the patellofemoral joint shows significant displacement, indicating the need for operative fixation.

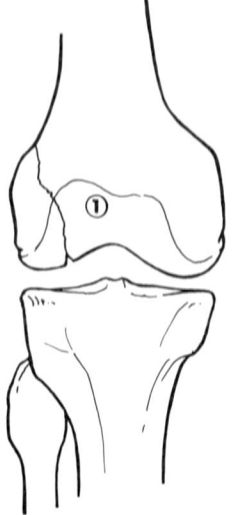
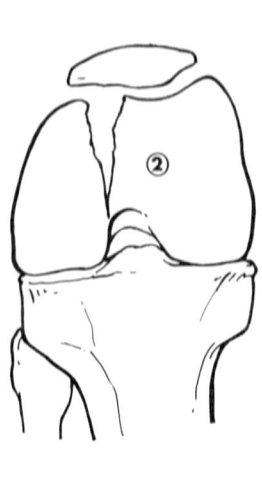

Because of the likelihood of displacement even with cast application, open reduction and internal fixation are the treatment of choice for femoral condylar fractures.

Fixation of the fragment is best accomplished with screws inserted perpendicular to the fracture line, usually in an anterior-to-posterior direction.

Preoperative radiographic assessment should be accurate to determine the true direction of the fracture.

Operative Reduction and Internal Fixation

1. Make a 12-cm to 15-cm incision on the anteromedial aspect of the thigh in the interval between the rectus femoris tendon and the vastus medialis muscle. Continue the incision downward around the patella.

Note: For lateral condylar fractures a similar approach is made on the lateral side of the joint between the rectus femoris and the vastus lateralis.

2. Divide the fascia lata, the medial aponeurotic expansion, and the joint capsule in the line of the incision.
3. Proximally develop the interval between the tendon of the rectus femoris and the vastus medialis muscle.
4. Split the vastus intermedius longitudinally and expose the distal end of the femur and condyle by subperiosteal dissection.
5. Divide the synovial membrane, exposing the knee joint.

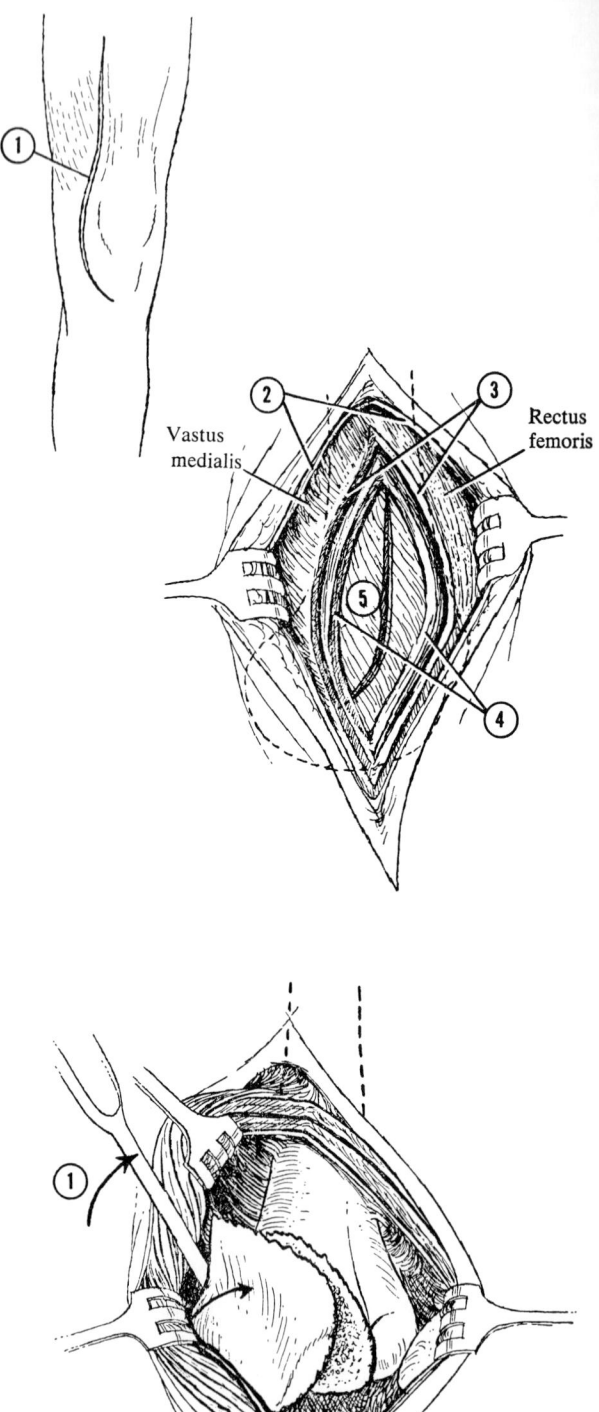

1. Under direct vision lever the medial condyle into its normal position.

2. Fix the fragment with one or two screws inserted perpendicular to the fracture and in an anterior-to-posterior direction.

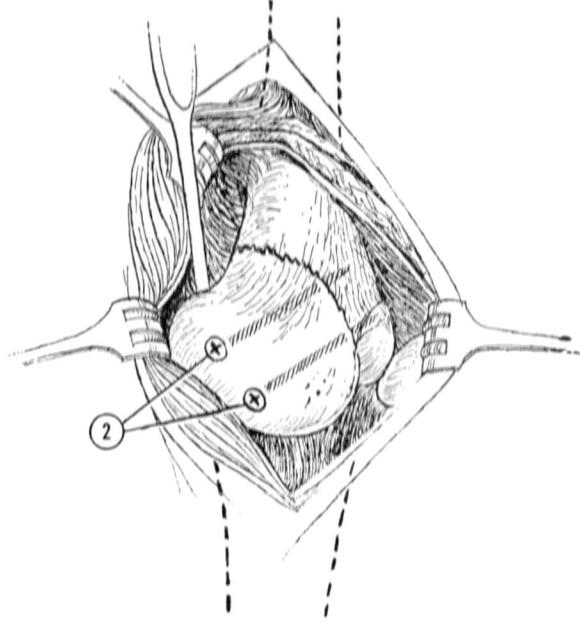

Postreduction X-Ray

The condylar fragment is in its normal position and is secured with two screws.

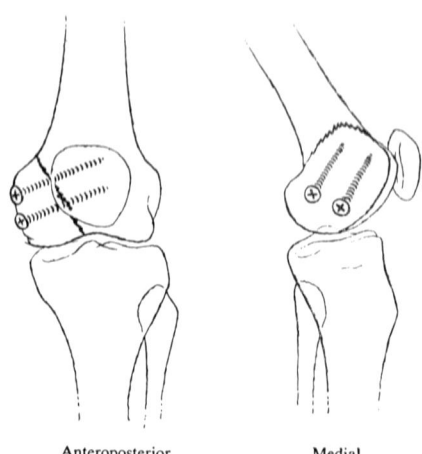

Anteroposterior   Medial

Immobilization

1. Apply a plaster cast from the groin to the toes.
2. The knee is slightly flexed.
3. The foot is at a right angle.

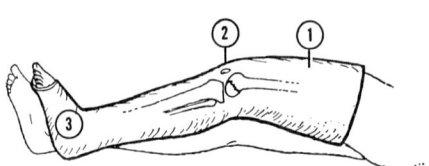

Postoperative Management

Encourage the patient in active quadriceps contraction while in the cast.

Remove the cast at the end of three weeks.

Begin a program of active range-of-motion exercises to the knee.

The patient should protect the knee with crutch walking for six to eight weeks longer, until the fracture site has completely filled in.

For fractures of the medial condyle, crutch walking should be continued for at least four months owing to the risk of vascular injury to the condylar fragment. Caution the patient that the complications of avascular necrosis and traumatic arthritis may occur and that the knee should be radiographed periodically for at least two years after this injury.

UNICONDYLAR FRACTURE IN THE FRONTAL PLANE

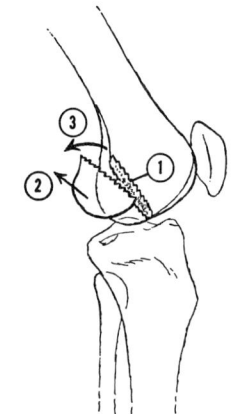

Prereduction X-Ray

1. Fracture of the posterior portion of the medial femoral condyle.
2. The fragment is displaced backward and
3. Rotated.

Operative Reduction and Internal Fixation

1. The incision begins just posterior to the biceps tendon; it extends downward to the level of the horizontal flexion crease; it continues horizontally across the popliteal space in the flexion crease and continues distally for 2 inches between the tendon of the semitendinosus and the medial head of the gastrocnemius.
2. Divide the deep fascia in the line of the incision.
3. Develop the interval between the tendon of the semitendinosus and the medial head of the gastrocnemius, exposing the posterior joint capsule.

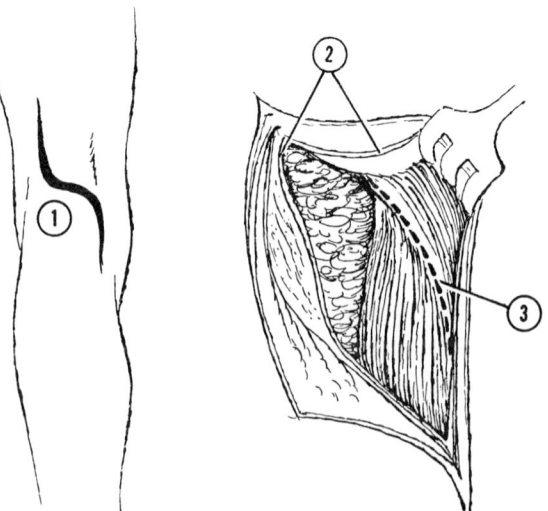

FRACTURES OF THE LOWER END OF THE FEMUR

1. Divide the joint capsule longitudinally, exposing the posterior aspect of the medial femoral condyle.
2. Lever the condylar fragment into its normal position.
3. Secure the fragment with two screws.

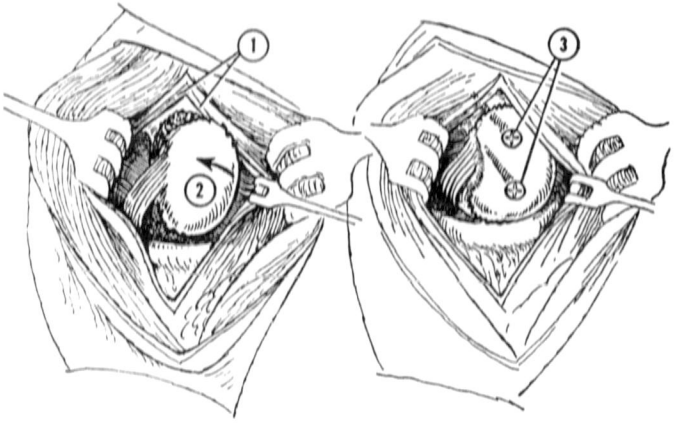

Postreduction X-Ray

The condylar fragment is in its normal position and is fixed by two screws.

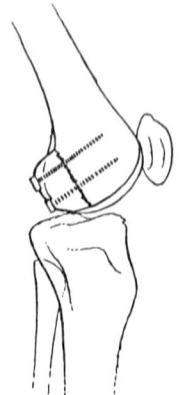

Immobilization

1. Apply a long leg plaster cast from the groin to the toes.
2. The knee is slightly flexed.
3. The foot is at a right angle.

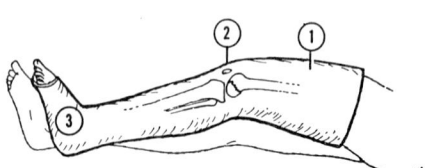

Postoperative Management

Encourage the patient in active quadriceps contraction while in the cast.

Remove the cast at the end of three weeks.

Begin a program of active range-of-motion exercises to the knee.

The patient should protect the knee with crutch walking for six to eight weeks until the fracture site has completely filled in.

For fractures of the medial condyle, crutch walking should be continued for at least four months owing to the risk of vascular injury to the condylar fragment. Caution the patient that the complications of avascular necrosis and traumatic arthritis may occur and that the knee should be radiographed periodically for at least two years after this injury.

Other Fractures of the Distal Femur

REMARKS

Other fractures in the distal femoral area include epiphyseal injuries, which are discussed in Chapter 2, and osteochondral fractures, which are discussed with knee injuries in Chapter 16. These discussions should be considered in managing these fairly common and frequently difficult fractures of the femur.

SUMMARY: PITFALLS OF MANAGING FEMORAL FRACTURES

The major technical pitfalls in treatment of intertrochanteric fractures have been wound infection and mechanical failure of fixation. By selecting intramedullary Ender rods in older patients with osteoporotic bone and sliding compression screw techniques for unstable fractures, the surgeon can minimize these technical pitfalls. Use of image-intensified fluoroscopy has aided significantly in preventing technical problems.

Femoral neck fractures present dual problems of nonunion due to poorly vascularized cortical bone and segmental collapse of an avascular femoral head. In the average elderly patient (older than 70), these complications are so common that primary prosthetic replacement is most satisfactory for displaced femoral neck fracture. Displaced femoral neck fractures in young adults often result in disastrous problems of nonunion or segmental collapse; open reduction and posterior pedicle grafting currently offer the best chance to avoid them.

Subtrochanteric fractures offer serious challenges to fixation by either open or closed methods. The torsional and bending loads on the femur in this region are extreme. Deformity and nonunion are likely to follow if fixation by either internal or external methods is inadequate. Intramedullary fixation with a Zickel nail protects against bending loads in this area but it allows torsional external rotational deformity. Long oblique fractures and fractures in which the medial cortex is comminuted may defeat the best surgical fixation devices. The surgeon managing subtrochanteric fractures must be prepared to use both internal and external immobilization techniques.

In managing transverse midshaft fractures by closed methods, the physician must anticipate the most common complication, shortening due to translational displacement. Schneider rod fixation or cast-brace treatment with intermittent distal femoral traction provides the most direct way of avoiding this pitfall.

Comminuted shaft fractures are poor candidates for open reduction and internal fixation because the resultant fixation is usually inadequate. Closed reduction and cast-brace treatment of these fractures is biologically and biomechanically most effective. Physicians using cast-brace technique must be alert to the potential complications of shortening and angulation and must be prepared to correct them early in the course of treatment.

Fractures of the supracondylar region and distal femur present characteristic deformities due to the consistent posterior displacement and internal rotation of the distal fragment. The deformity is produced by the mechanism of the original injury and not by muscle pull. It is combated by direct upward traction using a skeletal pin inserted in the distal fragment. Attempts to correct it by tibial traction across the knee are frequently ineffective. Once the distal fragment is realigned, external immobilization with a cast-brace holds the reduction, aided by intermittent traction as necessary.

Femoral shaft fractures in children less than 10 years of age are relatively simple to manage by immediate spica cast application. The tragic pitfall of ischemic muscle necrosis, produced by skin traction that elevates the limbs excessively, can be completely eliminated by immediate application of the spica cast.

Unicondylar fractures of the distal femoral articular surfaces, although rare, frequently present more than their share of complications. The displacement of the condylar fracture is often not recognized on x-ray or is treated by ineffective closed methods. Accurate operative reduction and internal fixation are necessary to avoid the frequent pitfalls of this relatively uncommon injury.

REFERENCES

Baker, D. M.: Fractures of the femoral neck after healed intertrochanteric fractures. J. Trauma, 15:73, 1975.

Barnes, R., Brown, J. T., and Garden, R. S., et al.: Subcapital fractures of the femur. J. Bone and Joint Surg., 58-B:2, 1976.

Brighton, C. T., Friedenberg, Z. B., Zemsky, L. M., et al.: Direct-current stimulation of non-union and congenital pseudarthrosis. J. Bone and Joint Surg., 57-A:368, 1975.

Cain, J.: Intertrochanteric fractures of the hip. A review of 200 cases. Resident Thesis. Vanderbilt U. Med. Center, 1973.

Canale, S. T., and Bouland, W. L.: Fracture of the neck and intertrochanteric region of the femur in children. J. Bone and Joint Surg., 59-A:431, 1977.

Casey, M. J., and Chapman, M. W.: Ipsilateral concomitant fractures of the hip and femoral shaft. J. Bone and Joint Surg., 61-A:503, 1979.

Cathcart, R. F.: New ideas in the design and function of the Austin Moore prosthesis. Orthop. Review, 2:15, 1973.

Connolly, J. F., Dehne, E., and LaFollette, B.: Closed reduction and early cast-brace ambulation in the treatment of femoral fractures. J. Bone and Joint Surg., 55-A:1581, 1973.

Connolly, J. F., and King, P.: Closed reduction and early cast-brace ambulation in the treatment of femoral fractures. J. Bone and Joint Surg., 55-A:1559, 1973.

Crawford, H. B.: Conservative treatment of impacted fractures of the femoral neck. J. Bone and Joint Surg., 42-A:471, 1960.

Dencker, H.: Technical problems of medullary nailing. Acta Chir. Scand., 130:185, 1965.

Funk, F. J., Wells, R. E., and Street, D. M.: Supplementary fixation of femoral fractures. Clin. Orthop. and Related Research, 60:41, 1968.

Garden, R. S.: Malreduction and avascular necrosis in subcapital fractures of the femur. J. Bone and Joint Surg., 53-B:183, 1971.

REFERENCES

Hansen, B. A., and Sogardis, J.: Impacted fractures of the femoral neck treated by early immobilization and weight-bearing. Acta Orthop. Scand., 49:180, 1978.

Hansen, S. T., and Winquist, R. A.: Closed intramedullary nailing of fractures of the femoral shaft. Part II: Technical considerations. In Instructional Course Lectures, The American Academy of Orthopaedic Surgeons, 27:90, 1978.

Hardy, A. E.: Pressure recordings in patients with femoral fractures in cast-braces and suggestions for treatment. J. Bone and Joint Surg., 61-A:365, 1979.

Irani, R. N., Nicholson, J. T., and Chung, S. M. K.: Long-term results in the treatment of femoral-shaft fractures in young children by immediate spica immobilization. J. Bone and Joint Surg., 58-A:945, 1976.

Johnson, J. T. H., and Crothers, O.: Nailing versus prosthesis for femoral neck fractures. J. Bone and Joint Surg., 57-A:686, 1975.

Jones, C. W., Morris, J., Shea, J., et al.: A comparison of the treatment of trochanteric fractures of the femur by internal fixation with a nail plate and the Ender technique. Injury, 9:35, 1977.

Kavanaugh, J.: Occult infected fracture of the femur. J. Trauma, 18:813, 1978.

Klenerman, L., and Marcuson, R. W.: Intracapsular fractures of the neck of the femur. J. Bone and Joint Surg., 52-B:514, 1970.

Kuderna, H., Boyler, N., and Collon, D. J.: Treatment of intertrochanteric and subtrochanteric fractures of the hip by the Ender method. J. Bone and Joint Surg., 58-A:604, 1976.

Lesin, B. E., Mooney, V., and Ashby, M. E.: Cast-bracing for fractures of the femur. J. Bone and Joint Surg., 59-A:917, 1977.

Lombardo, S. J., and Harvey, J. P.: Fractures of the distal femoral epiphysis. J. Bone and Joint Surg., 59-A:742, 1977.

Meyers, M. H., Harvey, J. P., and Moore, T. M.: Treatment of displaced subcapital and transcervical fractures of the femoral neck by muscle-pedicle-bone graft and internal fixation. J. Bone and Joint Surg., 55-A:257, 1973.

Meyers, M. H., Moore, T. M., and Harvey, J. P.: Follow-up notes on articles previously published in the Journal. Displaced fracture of the femoral neck treated with a muscle-pedicle graft. J. Bone and Joint Surg., 57-A:718, 1975.

Meyers, M. H., Telfer, N., and Moore, T. M.: Determination of the vascularity of the femoral head with technetium 99m-sulphur-colloid. J. Bone and Joint Surg., 59-A:658, 1977.

Miller, C. W.: Survival and ambulation following hip fracture. J. Bone and Joint Surg., 60-A:930, 1978.

Neer, C. S., Grantham, S. A., Foster, R. R.: Femoral shaft fracture with sciatic nerve palsy. JAMA, Vol. 214, 13:2307, 1970.

Neer, C. S., Grantham, S. A., and Shelton, M. L.: Supracondylar fracture of the adult femur. J. Bone and Joint Surg., 49-A:591, 1967.

Niemann, K. M., and Mankin, H. J.: Fractures about the hip in an institutionalized patient population. J. Bone and Joint Surg., 50-A:1327, 1968.

Prather, J. L., Nusynowitz, M. L., Snowdy, H. A., et al.: Scintigraphic findings in stress fractures. J. Bone and Joint Surg., 59-A:869, 1977.

Protzman, R. R., and Burkhalter, W. E.: Femoral-neck fractures in young adults. J. Bone and Joint Surg., 58-A:689, 1976.

Ratliff, A. H. C.: Fractures of the neck of the femur in children. Orthop. Clinics N. Am., 51:903, 1974.

Ratliff, A. H. C.: Traumatic separation of the upper femoral epiphysis in young children. J. Bone and Joint Surg., 50-B:757, 1968.

Roberts, J. B.: Management of fractures and fracture complications of the femoral shaft using the ASIF compression plate. J. Trauma, 17:20, 1977.

Rydell, N.: Biomechanics of the hip-joint. Clin. Orthop. and Related Research, 92:6, 1973.

Schneider, H. W.: Use of the 4-flanged self-cutting intramedullary nail for

REFERENCES

fixation of femoral fractures. Clin. Orthop. and Related Research, 60:29, 1968.

Seinsheimer, F.: Subtrochanteric fractures of the femur. J. Bone and Joint Surg., 60-A:300, 1978.

Sevitt, S., and Thompson, R. G.: The distribution and anastomoses of arteries supplying the head and neck of the femur. J. Bone and Joint Surg., 47-B:560, 1965.

Smith, L. D.: Hip fractures. J. Bone and Joint Surg., 35-A:367, 1953.

Southwick, W. O., et al.: Hip fixation using a high angle key-free compression hip screw. A technical description. Zimmer USA, Inc., 1978.

Stevens, J., and Ray, R. D.: An experimental comparison of living and dead bone in rats. J. Bone and Joint Surg., 44-B:412, 1962.

Trillat, A., Dejour, H., and Bost, J.: Unicondylar fractures of the femur. Rev. Chir. Orthop. 61:611, 1975.

Trueta, J., and Harrison, M. H. M.: The normal vascular anatomy of the femoral head in adult man. J. Bone and Joint Surg., 35-B:442, 1953.

Turner, B., Cochran, R., and Dobry, C.: The results of cemented Cathcart endoprostheses in elderly patients with acute femoral neck fractures. Presented at American Association for Surgery of Trauma, Chicago, 1979.

Wertheimer, L. G., and Lopes, S. D. F.: Arterial supply of the femoral head. J. Bone and Joint Surg., 53-A:545, 1971.

Yamada, H.: Strength of Biological Materials. Huntington, N. Y.: Robert E. Krieger Publishing Co., 1973, pp. 1–16.

Zickel, R. E.: An intramedullary fixation device for the proximal part of the femur. J. Bone and Joint Surg., 58-A:866, 1976.

Zickel, R. E., Fietti, V. G., Lawsing, J. F., et al.: A new intramedullary fixation device for the distal third of the femur. Clin. Orthop. and Related Research, 125:185, 1977.

INJURIES OF THE SOFT TISSUES AND BONY ELEMENTS OF THE KNEE JOINT

ANATOMIC FEATURES

STATIC MEDIAL SUPPORT STRUCTURES

The medial support structures may be considered as five components.

1. The anterior third of the medial capsule or capsular ligament extends from the medial edge of the patella tendon and patella to the leading edge of the tibial collateral ligament. This portion of the capsule is reinforced by the extensor retinaculum.

2. The midportion includes the deep capsular ligament, which lies deep to the tibial collateral ligament.

3. The posterior third of the capsule sweeps around the posterior corner as a thickening known as the posterior oblique ligament.

4. The tibial collateral ligament is the strongest medial stabilizer and runs from the femoral condyle to approximately 8 cm below the joint line.

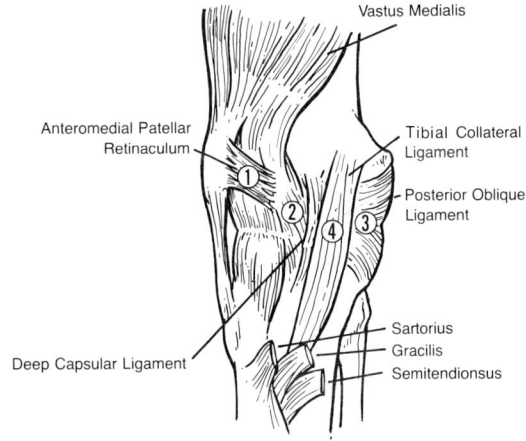

5. The semimembranosus provides some static support to the medial knee. It is primarily a dynamic stabilizer inserting into the posterior capsule to form an oblique popliteal ligament and

6. Attaching to the rim of the meniscus to retract the meniscus posteriorly.

7. The semimembranosus also attaches to the medial tibial surface deep to the tibial collateral ligament.

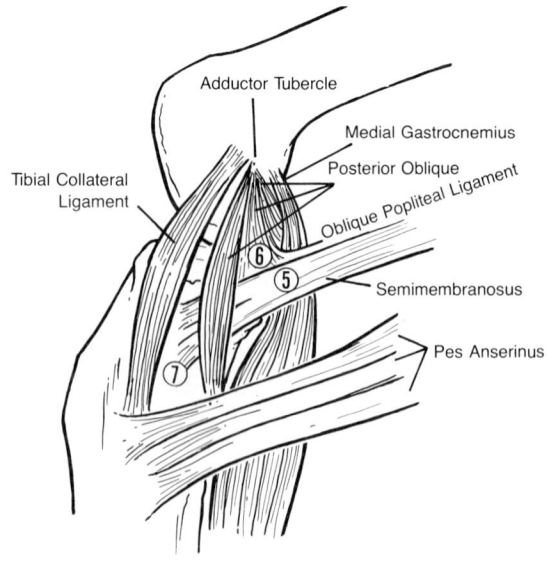

ANATOMIC FEATURES

Other static support structures in addition to the medial knee joint ligaments are:
1. The cruciate ligament.
2. The medial meniscus.
3. The bony contour of the femoral condyles locked in the tibial plateau.

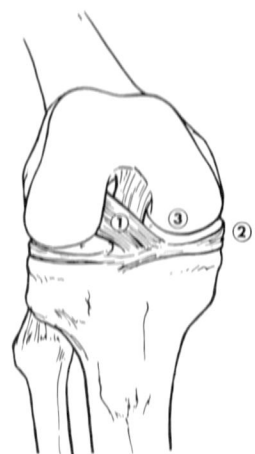

DYNAMIC MEDIAL SUPPORT STRUCTURES

The dynamic medial support structures are:
1. The vastus medialis obliquus (see page 1545),
2. The pes anserinus muscles (sartorius, gracilis, and semitendinosus),
3. The semimembranosus muscle, which is the primary dynamic stabilizer on the posteromedial aspect, and
4. The medial gastrocnemius.

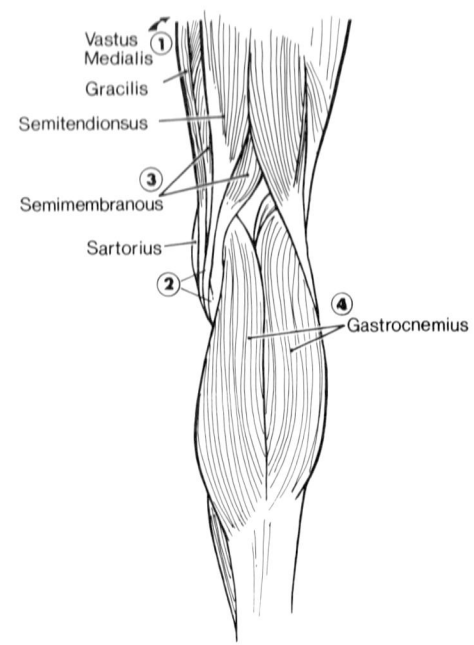

ANATOMIC FEATURES

STATIC LATERAL SUPPORT STRUCTURES

The static lateral support structures of the knee can be divided into anterior, medial, and posterior components.

1. The anterior third includes the capsular ligament reinforced by the patellar retinaculum. This extends back to the anterior border of the iliotibial band and attaches to the articular margin of the proximal tibia but has no attachment to the femur.

2. The middle third of the lateral support is composed of the deep capsular ligament beneath the iliotibial band. The deep capsular ligament extends as far posteriorly as

3. The fibular collateral ligament. This ligament is a relatively small, tendon-like structure weaker than the tibial collateral ligament.

4. The posterior third includes capsular and noncapsular ligaments forming the arcuate complex, which comprises the fibular collateral ligament, the arcuate ligament, and the tendo-aponeurotic portion of the popliteus muscle.

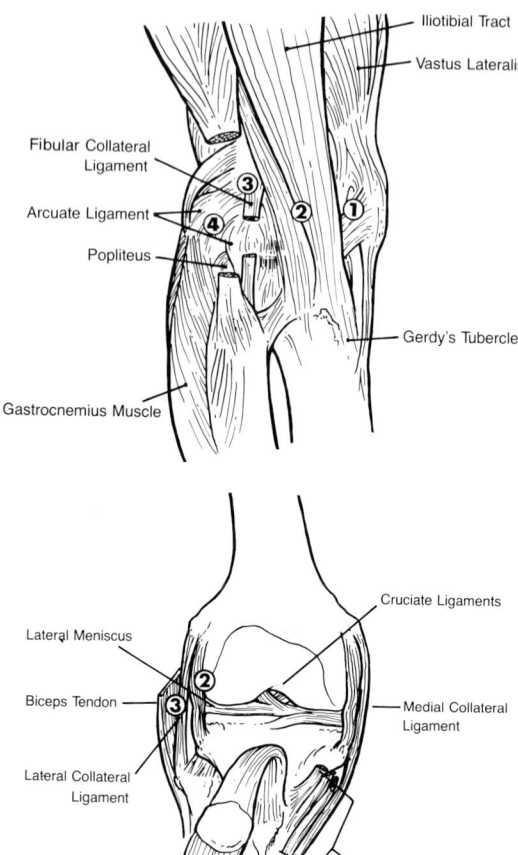

DYNAMIC LATERAL SUPPORT STRUCTURES

The dynamic lateral support structures are:

1. The vastus lateralis.
2. The popliteus running deep to the fibular collateral and serving as both a dynamic and static support. The aponeurosis of the popliteus inserts into the posterior horn of the lateral meniscus and serves to retract the horn posteriorly.
3. The biceps tendon, which is the main dynamic lateral stabilizer. The portion that invests the fibular collateral ligament is dynamically most important.
4. The lateral gastrocnemius.

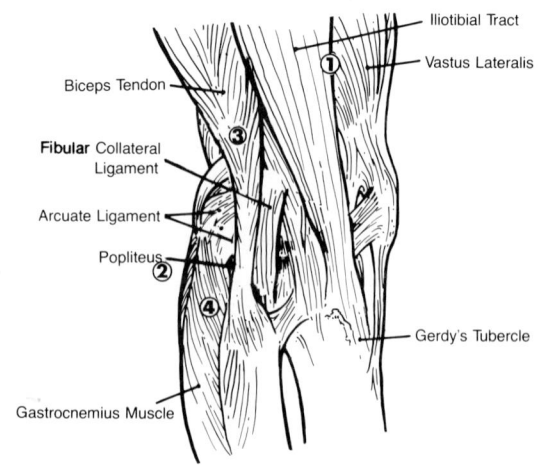

ANATOMIC FEATURES

POSTERIOR SUPPORT STRUCTURES

The major posterior support structures include:
1. The posterior capsule, which stabilizes the knee in full extension.
2. An oblique popliteal ligament or capsular ligament. This runs from the semimembranosus tendon obliquely across the posterior aspect of the joint.
3. The arcuate ligament, formed where the capsule arches over
4. The popliteus tendon inserting onto the oblique popliteal ligament as well as the posterior horn of the lateral meniscus.
5. The medial and lateral heads of the gastrocnemius both have tendinous insertions, particularly through the medial femoral condyle and blend in with the posterior capsule.

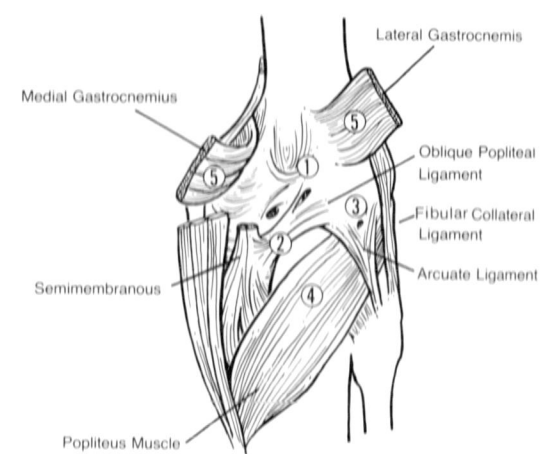

QUADRICEPS FUNCTION

All the long components of the quadriceps including the vastus lateralis, the vastus intermedius, the vastus medialis longus (VML), and the rectus femoris are able to extend the knee fully.

These systems also serve to decelerate the forward gliding of the femur on the tibia during the stance phase of gait. There is great synergy between the quadriceps apparatus and the posterior cruciate ligament to accomplish this deceleration (see page 1546).

In addition, the oblique fibers of both the vastus medialis and the vastus lateralis stabilize the patella in a mediolateral direction.

The vastus medialis has two divisions:
1. The vastus medialis longus (VML) and
2. The vastus medialis obliquus (VMO).

Note: These structures are always anatomically distinct and may have different innervation.

3. The vastus lateralis also has obliquely oriented fibers in the distal portion that are not as distinct as the VMO.

Note: The orientation of these fibers indicates that they function particularly to stabilize the patella in the mediolateral direction.

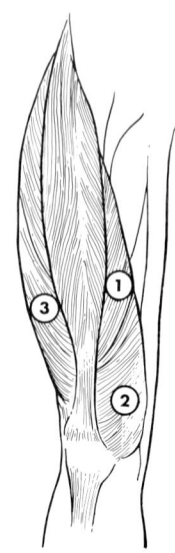

1545

The quadriceps muscles may effectively support the knee against instability in one plane.

Rotatory instability is most often prevented by the hamstring muscles posteriorly.

The efficiency of the quadriceps muscles is enhanced by the patella, which provides greater leverage as the knee is going into full extension. The patella is especially useful in functions such as stair climbing and should not be removed when there is another choice.

The patella is not merely a sesamoid bone because the patellofemoral joint is a true synovial joint and subject to osteoarthritis.

Insufficiency of the medial quadriceps mechanism may permit patellar subluxation or dislocation, which can easily be confused with ligamentous disruption.

CRUCIATE LIGAMENTS

The cruciate ligaments are fan-shaped and each spirals on itself. This ingenious arrangement serves as a means of insuring that some portion of the ligament is taut throughout the entire range of knee motion.

Marshall and coworkers have shown that the anterior cruciate is the first line of defense against anterior displacement of the tibia on the femur and also against hyperextension of the knee. It contributes stability against internal rotation of the tibia in extension as well as against valgus stress on the knee.

Hughston and coworkers have shown that the posterior cruciate is responsible for the basic stability of the knee. It provides a central axis about which normal and abnormal internal and external rotation occurs. If the posterior cruciate is intact, any instability is rotational about its axis. When the posterior cruciate is torn, all instabilities are straight, i.e., the knee opens like a door on a hinge when a valgus or varus stress is applied.

The posterior cruciate combines with the extensor apparatus (the quadriceps muscles and tendons, the patella and patellar tendon, and the extensor retinaculum) to prevent anterior displacement of the femur on the fixed tibia during stance phase of walking and running.

Anterior Cruciate Ligament (ACL)

1. The anteromedial portion of the ACL tightens as the knee flexes and checks anterior displacement of the tibia.

2. In full extension, the posterolateral portion is tightest and prevents hyperextension as well as varus and valgus instability.

Note: An anterior cruciate ligament that is partially intact at surgery may still allow anterior tibial displacement.

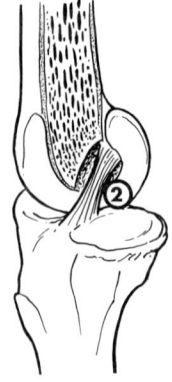
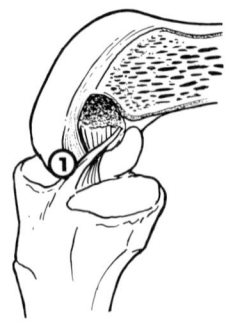

Posterior Cruciate Ligament

1. The posterior cruciate ligament has an anterolateral band that tightens as the knee flexes.

2. The short, thick posteromedial band tightens with the knee extended. This also tightens during internal rotation of the tibia with the knee in either flexion or full extension.

Note: In full extension, the posterior cruciate allows minimal abduction or adduction opening of the knee, even after the capsular ligaments and collateral ligaments as well as the posterior capsule have been removed.

If the posterior cruciate is intact, forced internal rotation of the tibia causes the femur and tibial surface to coapt and thereby prevents drawing of the tibia forward even though the anterior cruciate is torn.

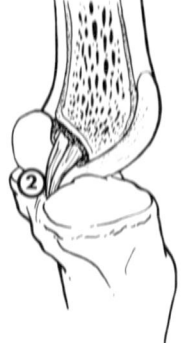
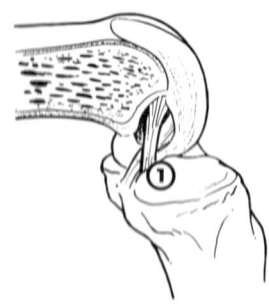

INJURIES TO THE LIGAMENTS OF THE KNEE JOINT

REMARKS

The knee is among the most exposed and vulnerable to injury of all the body's articulations. It is particularly subject to injury among young athletes, who require extremely high performance from their knees.

Systematic evaluation of the injury will help determine which instability the injury is likely to produce.

Mechanisms of Injury

The knee is susceptible to a variety of injuries. Among the most common are those produced by:
1. Valgus external rotation mechanisms.
2. Varus internal rotation mechanisms.
3. Hyperextension mechanisms.
4. Injury to the flexed knee.

VALGUS EXTERNAL ROTATION MECHANISMS

Characteristically, an individual such as a football player sustains a blow to the posterolateral aspect of the knee, which forces it into valgus and rotates the femur inward on the fixed, externally rotated tibia.

In this mechanism, the first structures to fail are the medial collateral ligaments; first usually the deep layer firmly attached to the medial meniscus and then the superficial layer.

If the force continues, the cruciate ligament absorbs the stress and gives way partially or completely.

Ordinarily the meniscus is not directly injured by this mechanism but usually is detached from the meniscofemoral or meniscotibial portions of the medial capsular structures.

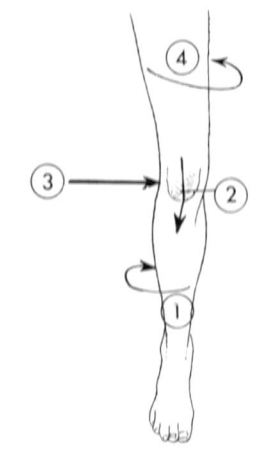

1. The foot is fixed; the leg rotates outward.
2. The knee is flexed.
3. The direct stress posteriorly forces the knee medially and rotates the femur internally.
4. The femur is forcefully rotated internally relative to the fixed tibia.

Pathologic Results of Valgus-External Rotation Injury

1. Tears of the superficial and deep portions of the medial ligaments may extend into the posterior capsule.
2. Detachment of the medial meniscus from the deep layer of the medial capsular structure.

Note: The meniscus is not torn in its substance ordinarily.

3. Partial or complete tear of the anterior or posterior cruciate ligaments.

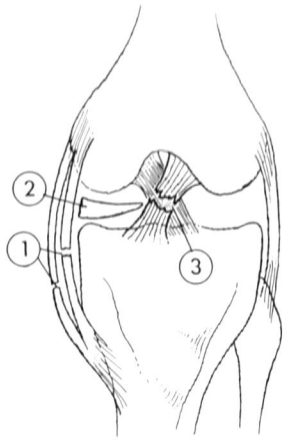

VARUS-INTERNAL TORSIONAL MECHANISMS INJURING THE LATERAL JOINT STRUCTURES

The lateral joint structures, unlike the medial support structures, are not generally injured by a direct blow to the knee. Most commonly the mechanism of injury is a fall, as when a basketball player lands after jumping, loses his balance, and falls forward with internal rotation and varus stress on the knee.

The area of injury most often is the midthird of the lateral capsule. Frequently there is an associated injury to the anterior cruciate and less frequently to the lateral meniscus and iliotibial tract.

1. Most often the victim lands on the leg while off balance.
2. He falls forward with an internal rotational stress.
3. At the same time a varus stress is applied during the fall.
4. The thigh and femur rotate externally.

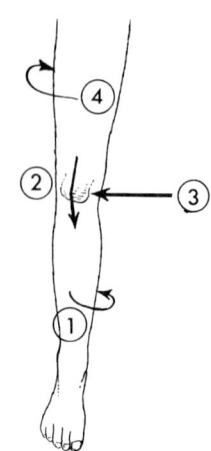

Pathologic Results of Varus-Internal Rotation Injury

1. Most often the injury is in the midthird of the lateral capsular structure.
2. Rarely, the iliotibial tract may be torn.
3. The lateral meniscus may be detached at its periphery but it is rarely torn in its substance.
4. There may be partial or complete tears of the anterior or posterior cruciate ligaments.

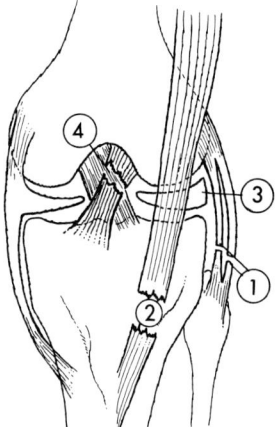

HYPEREXTENSION INJURY TO THE KNEE

REMARKS

The anterior cruciate ligament is the main ligamentous protection against hyperextension of the knee. An isolated injury to the anterior cruciate ligament may occur, with forced hyperextension and internal tibial rotation.

Characteristically, the patient feels or hears a "pop" in the knee and the knee swells as a result of hemorrhage from the vascular supply to the cruciate.

INJURIES TO THE LIGAMENTS OF THE KNEE JOINT

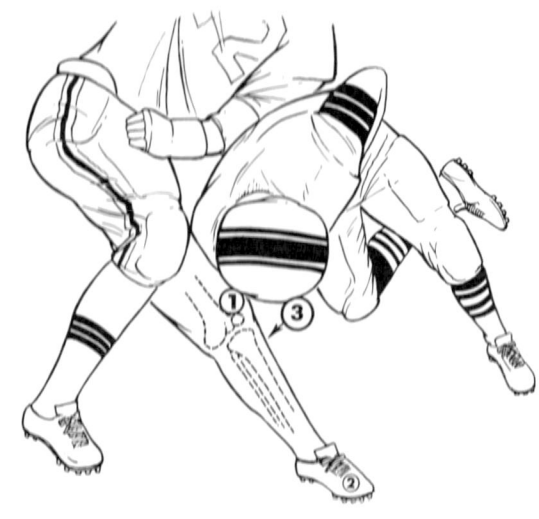

1. The victim is hit as he brings all his weight down on the extended knee.
2. The foot is slightly internally rotated.
3. The direction of the load is anterolateral, causing hyperextension and further internal rotation.

Pathologic Results of Hyperextension and Internal Rotation

1. The cruciate ligament may be torn at its femoral or tibial attachment or

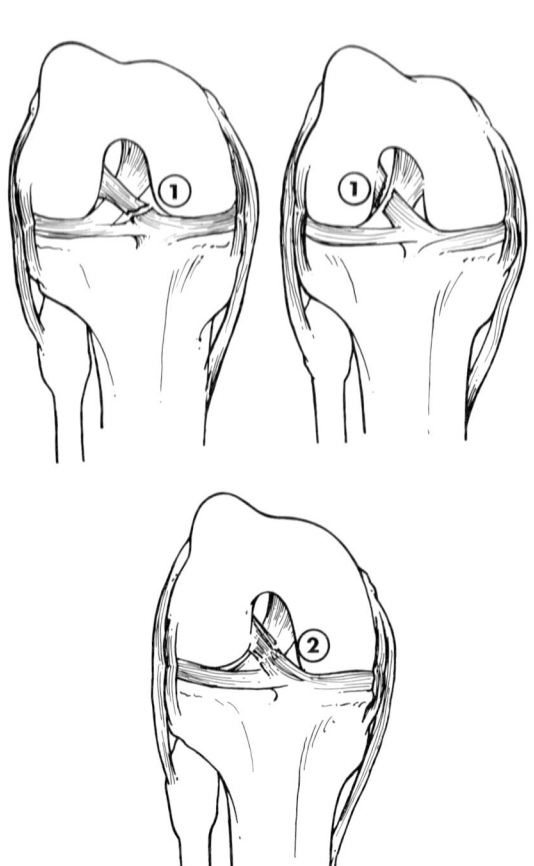

2. Within the substance itself.

Note: Frequently the cruciate is torn from hyperextension and internal tibial torsion without direct contact to the front of the leg.

Pathologic Results of Hyperextension and Internal Rotation (Continued)

3. With forceful direct contact to the anterior medial aspect of the tibia, the posterolateral capsule or arcuate complex will also be injured.

Note: The early functional disability after an anterior cruciate ligament rupture is probably not from the cruciate itself but rather from associated injury to the capsular structures.

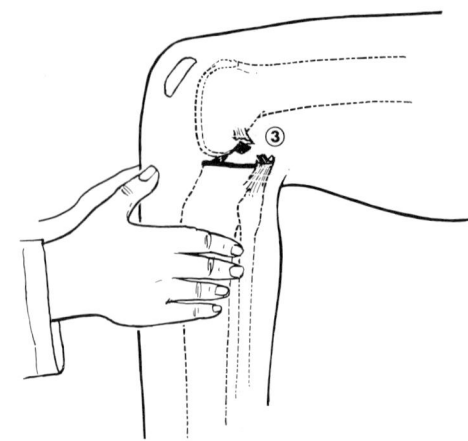

INJURY TO THE FLEXED KNEE

These injuries are less common than injuries to the extended knee but do occur in automobile accidents or in falls from heights.

1. In a fall from a height, the victim lands on the flexed knee; or, in an automobile accident, the victim sustains a direct blow from the dashboard to the proximal tibia with the knee flexed.

2. This mechanism drives the tibia posterior in relation to the fixed femur.

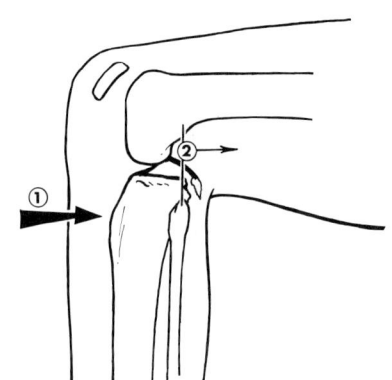

Pathologic Results of Injury to the Flexed Knee

1. The posterior cruciate ligament is torn from its tibial attachment.

2. The posterior lateral and posterior medial capsule structures, in addition to the posterior horn of the meniscus, may often be torn.

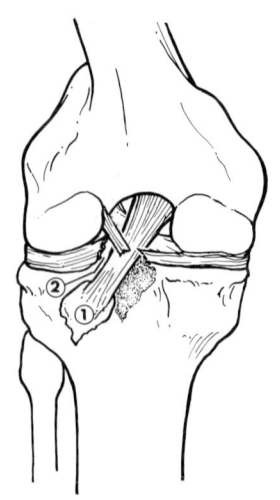

Evaluation of Ligamentous Injuries of the Knee

REMARKS

Hemarthrosis, pain, and functional limitation after a knee injury should alert the physician to a potentially disabling problem and should not be routinely dismissed as simply a knee sprain.

Physical examination of the acutely injured knee should begin with inspection for evidence of local injury, ecchymosis, swelling, and circulatory change.

Extensive periarticular swelling frequently indicates complete capsular ruptures. Complete disruption of the capsule may allow all of the fluid to leak out of the joint, causing a surprisingly benign-appearing injury.

Always palpate both knees carefully to elicit areas of tenderness or structural defects, as might be associated with acute rupture of the quadriceps tendon, dislocation of the patella, or complete ligamentous injury.

Observe the patient's ability to move the knee actively, particularly to determine if there is a locking or passive block to full extension or if there is an inability to actively extend the knee because of disruption of the extensor apparatus.

Testing for instability may be done under local anesthesia after joint aspiration and should include valgus and varus stress, posterior and anterior drawer testing, and rotatory testing.

X-rays taken while performing the stress test can document the nature of the instability. Single-contrast arthrography, including medial, lateral, and anteroposterior stress x-rays, are most effective in assessing the degree and location of the ligamentous damage.

The patellofemoral joint should not be forgotten because subluxation of the patella frequently causes hemarthrosis and pain and so can be confused with ligamentous or meniscal injuries.

Management of the injury should be based on the degree of damage revealed by complete evaluation.

Arthroscopy may also be used as an adjunct to physical examination of the injured knee with hemarthrosis (see page 1691).

TESTS TO EVALUATE LIGAMENTOUS INJURIES

Abduction and Adduction Stress Test

1. The patient lies on the table with the hip extended over the edge to relax the hamstrings.
2. The examiner places one hand on the lateral side of the thigh and one hand above the ankle.
3. The test is done with the knee in full extension and in 30 degrees of flexion.

Note: Test the uninjured leg first to assure that it will not cause pain and to compare the degrees of lateral mobility.

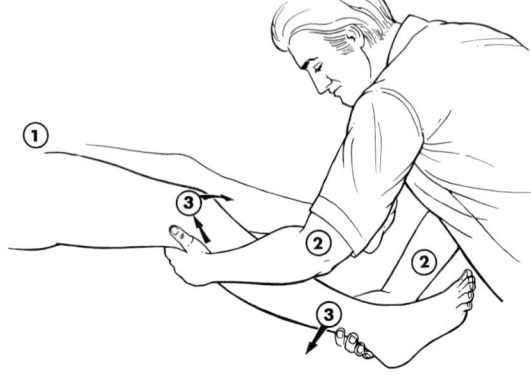

4. Adduction stress test is done with the patient in the same position and the examiner's hands reversed to apply load on the knee in the opposite direction.

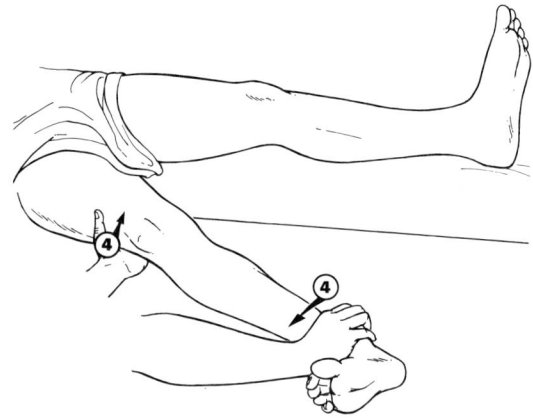

Test for Anterior Drawer Sign

1. The patient lies with the hips flexed 45 degrees and the knees flexed 90 degrees.
2. The examiner rests gently on the patient's feet and checks the uninjured knee first.
3. The tibia is drawn forward in external rotation, neutral rotation, and internal rotation.
4. Forward displacement of .5 cm. more than on the uninjured side and without a firm endpoint is a positive result.

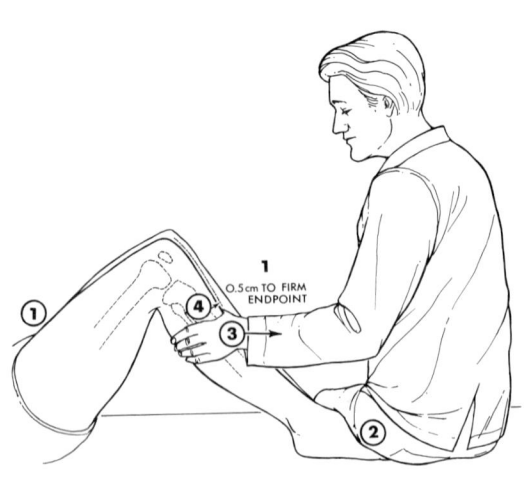

INJURIES TO THE LIGAMENTS OF THE KNEE JOINT

1. A positive anterior drawer test may indicate
2. Disruption of the anterior cruciate and
3. Frequently, disruption of the deep capsular structures, either medially, laterally, or both.

Note: Perform the anterior drawer test with the tibia rotated in various positions to evaluate for capsular and posterior cruciate damage.

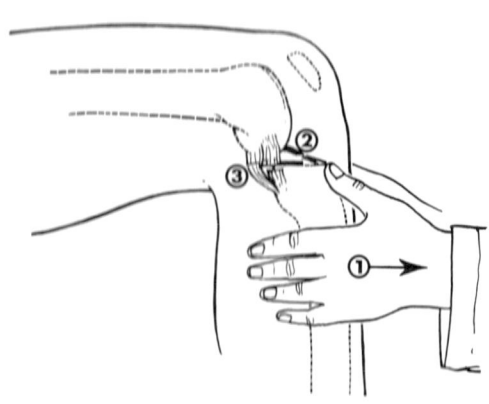

1. A positive drawer sign with the tibia externally rotated is indicative of anteromedial instability from posteromedial capsular and cruciate injury.
2. A positive drawer sign in neutral rotation indicates lateral capsular and sometimes medial capsular damage in addition to cruciate injury.

Anteromedial   Anterolateral

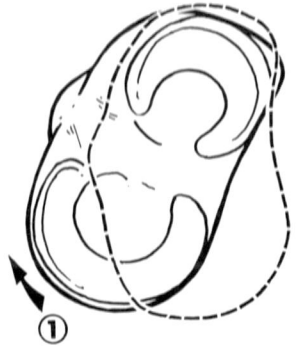 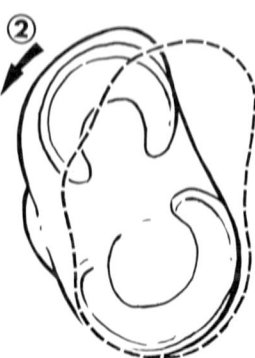

Intact Posterior Cruciate

3. Result of the anterior drawer test is negative if the tibia is internally rotated and the posterior cruciate is intact. The posterior cruciate ligament serves to coapt or lock the femoral and tibial articular surfaces in internal rotation. Persistence of a drawer sign in internal rotation is indirect evidence for posterior cruciate injury (see pages 1546 and 1557).

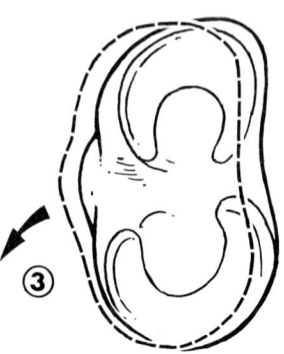

Lachman Test for Anterior Cruciate Tear

The Lachman test correlates better with an isolated anterior cruciate tear than does the anterior drawer test.

1. The patient's knee is flexed slightly, approximately 20 degrees.
2. The examiner's hands grasp the distal femur and the proximal tibia.

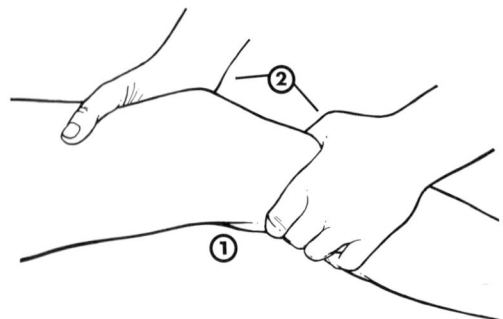

3. The tibia is drawn forcefully forward and backward on the femur. An increase of 3 to 5 mm of greater draw in comparison with the opposite, uninjured knee is a positive result.
4. Anterior translation of the tibia obliterates the infrapatellar tendon slope and is a sign of anterior cruciate damage.

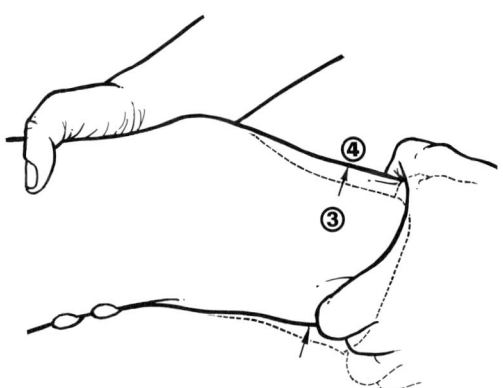

Test for Posterior Drawer Sign (Sag Test)

1. It is important to determine whether the laxity is anterior or posterior. The loss of normal anterior contour of the proximal tibia indicates that the knee is sagging posteriorly. If the posterior cruciate ligament is intact, this sag should be eliminated by internally rotating the leg.

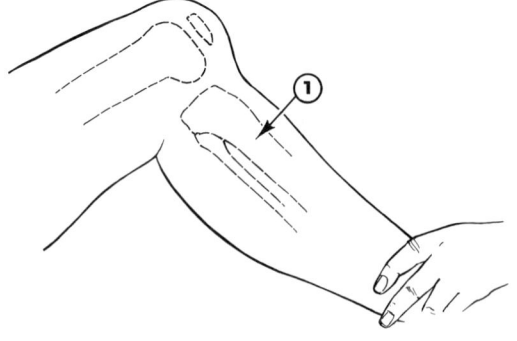

1. Internal rotation of the tibia coapts the femur on the tibial articular surface, if the posterior cruciate ligament is intact. This eliminates posterior displacement.

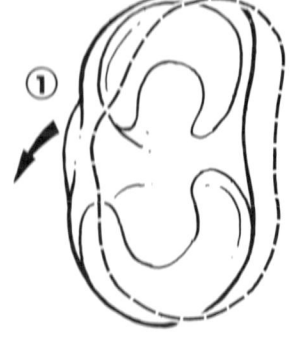

2. Posterior displacement in neutral rotation indicates, most often, posterior cruciate disruption.

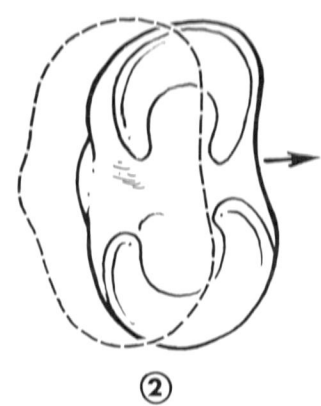

3. Posterior displacement in external rotation may be due to a posterolateral capsular damage with an intact posterior cruciate. The status of the posterior cruciate is evaluated by trying to eliminate the drawer sign with the knee in internal rotation.

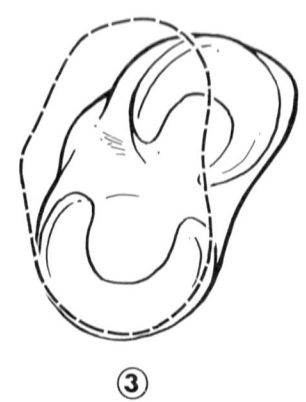

Tests for Anterolateral Instability

Injury to the anterior cruciate combined with disruption of the mid-third of the lateral capsule frequently produces anterolateral instability. In acute injuries, this may be evident from an anterior drawer test with the tibia held in neutral rotation demonstrating anterolateral instability. Hamstring tightness may frequently prevent adequate drawer testing in the acute injury. In this circumstance, a Slocum test should be employed.

Chronic anterolateral instability can be detected by the jerk test.

Slocum Test

This test is peformed with the patient in the side-lying position and is frequently the only one that can be done in an acute injury with any measure of success.

1. The patient's opposite hip and knee are flexed to get them out of the way of the knee that is being examined.
2. The torso is rotated to a point where the weight of the injured limb is borne on the heel. This exerts a valgus sag on the knee. When anterolateral subluxation of the tibia is present, a forward projection of the tibia on the femur can be palpated at the lateral side of the knee.
3. The examiner's right thumb is placed behind the head of the fibula and the index finger palpates the anterior aspect of the subluxated lateral tibial plateau.
4. The left thumb is placed behind the lateral femoral condyle.
5. With the knee in valgus and the tibia internally rotated, the knee is flexed by pushing anteriorly with both thumbs. The tibia then reduces from its anteriorly subluxed position, owing to the pull of the iliotibial band as the knee reaches between 25 and 40 degrees of flexion. This strong band luxates posteriorly, pulling or jerking the tibial condyle back into its normal position.

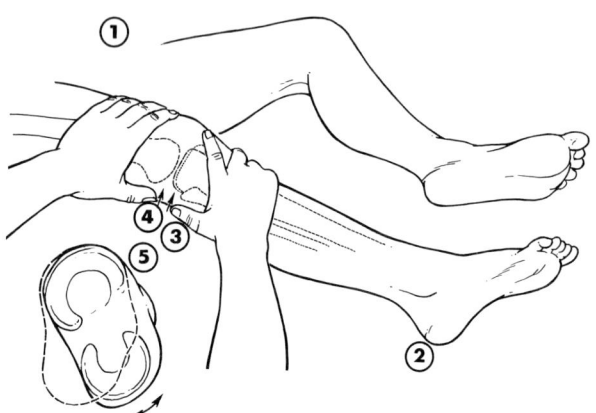

Jerk Test

1. The patient is supine with the hip flexed and the thigh adducted. The examiner's hand holds the foot internally rotated.
2. The examiner's opposite hand is lateral to and palpating behind the fibular head.
3. The patient's knee is moved from 90 degrees of flexion to full extension while valgus load is applied.

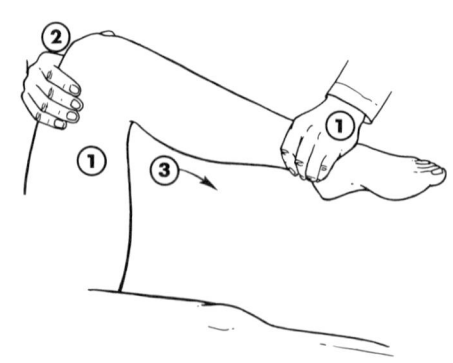

1. At 20 to 30 degrees of flexion, a sudden break in the smooth gliding is felt. This is a *jerk* in engineering terms, which is a sudden change in acceleration.

2. The jerk is due to the lateral tibial condyle subluxating anteriorly from the lateral femoral condyle at about 30 degrees of knee flexion. It then reduces at 10 to 15 degrees of flexion.

Note: In the awake patient, it is most important that the patient subjectively report this maneuver as causing the knee to go out of place.

Reversing the knee motion by going from 0 to 90 degrees of flexion produces the pivot shift test of MacIntosh, with the same abnormal motion being felt.

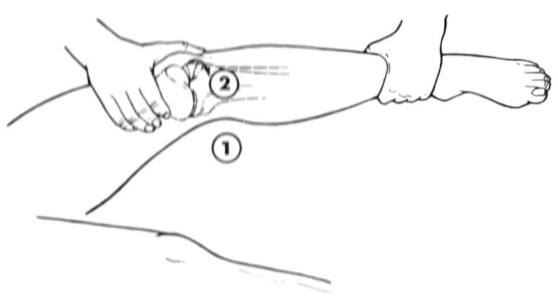

SINGLE-CONTRAST ARTHROGRAPHY TO EVALUATE ACUTE KNEE INJURIES

REMARKS

Wang and Marshall have shown the value of single-contrast arthrography in assessing injuries to the medial, lateral, and cruciate ligaments. It can be done in an emergency situation and with much less need for the technical assets usually required for arthrography technique.

After a plain film is taken to rule out the possibility of fracture, the needle is inserted under sterile technique in the superomedial third of the joint. The hematoma is aspirated from the joint.

Then, 10 ml of Renografin 60 and 5 ml of Xylocaine are injected into the knee.

1. An elastic bandage is wrapped tightly above the suprapatella bursa down to the joint line to squeeze dye into the joint space and

2. To obtain a lateral stress view for anterior drawer testing of the cruciate, the patient is positioned on his side and the knee is flexed 90 degrees.

Note: The examiner wears a lead apron and gloves. The compressive wrap keeps the dye in the intercondylar space.

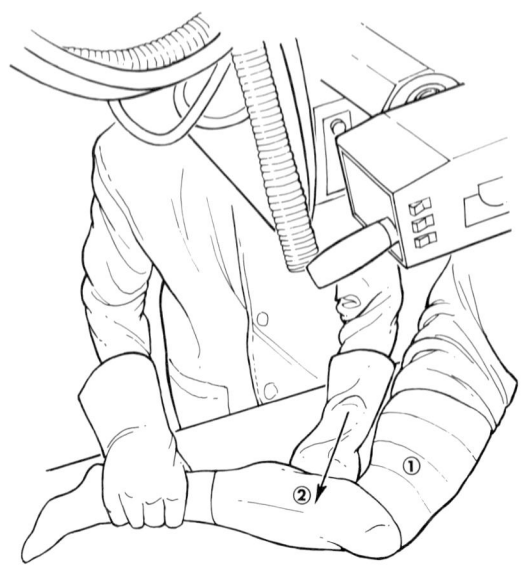

X-Ray After Arthrography

1. On the anteroposterior view, any tear in the deep medial capsular ligament will permit dye leakage.
2. When both the deep and superficial ligaments are torn, the dye extravasates beyond the smooth surface of the superficial ligament.

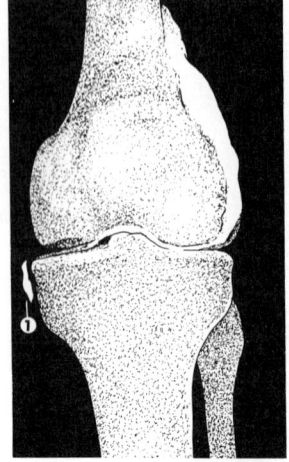
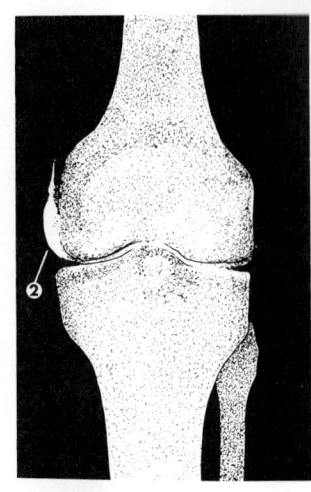

3. Dye leaking laterally or over the tubercle of Gerdy indicates lateral capsular and perhaps iliotibial band disruption.

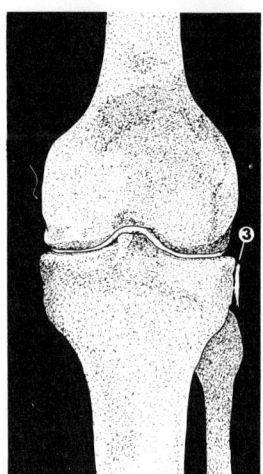

Arthrography with Lateral View

Note: To obtain adequate evaluation of the cruciate the dye must be squeezed out of the suprapatellar pouch and the film must be overexposed so that the bony condyles are quite dark.

1. When both cruciates are intact, they are seen as a sharply demarcated radiolucent band on the stress film.
2. If the anterior cruciate ligament is ruptured, it is not seen throughout its length.

Note: This simple method is not adequate to evaluate completely for a torn cartilage. However, it is of practical value to assess for the location and severity of ligamentous damage and to determine the grade of ligamentous injury.

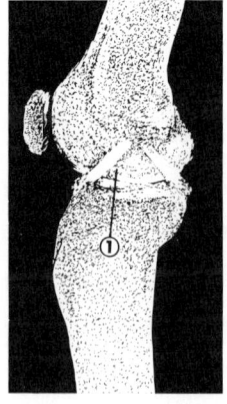
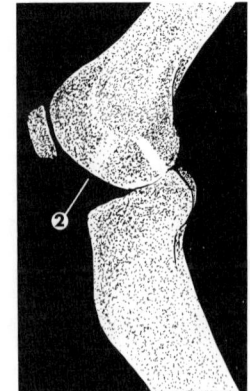

Grading of Medial Ligamentous Injuries

REMARKS

Disruption of the medial support structures generally can be graded as one of three types. This grading is based on:

The mechanism of the injury and the functional stability or instability after the injury.

Symptoms of pain, tenderness, and swelling.

Abduction stress testing in 0 and 30 degrees of flexion and drawer testing.

Stress x-rays and arthrograms of the injured knee.

The differing symptoms and findings as well as prognosis for functional recovery dictate different treatments depending on the grade of the injury. Grades I and II are usually best treated by nonoperative, early functional rehabilitation. Grade III injuries usually result in sufficient disruption of the support structures that prompt operative repair is indicated.

Care must be taken in evaluating the medial capsular injury to evaluate for combined injury to the cruciates or lateral capsular structures as well.

GRADE I MEDIAL LIGAMENT INJURY (FIRST-DEGREE SPRAIN)

This injury results from incomplete injuries to a few fibers of the medial ligaments.

There is no history of functional instability or "giving way" of the knee with weight bearing after injury. Swelling and tenderness about the knee are minimal.

Abduction stress testing at 0 and 30 degrees of flexion is normal, and the anterior drawer test is negative.

X-rays show no evidence of fracture about the joint or the medial joint opening and an arthrogram, if performed, shows no extravasation of dye.

GRADE II MEDIAL LIGAMENT INJURIES (SECOND-DEGREE SPRAIN)

These injuries result from more significant or greater tears of fibers with preservation of the gross structural integrity of the medial ligament.

The patient does not experience significant functional instability or "giving way" after the injury. This incomplete injury does cause more pain and significantly more swelling and tenderness than a Grade I or Grade III injury.

Abduction stress testing at 30 degrees of flexion may demonstrate slight (less than 5 mm) opening. Abduction stress is normal at 0 degrees.

The anterior drawer test is negative.

X-rays may occasionally show small avulsion fractures at the ligamentous insertion on the femur, but the joint does not open on application of medial stress. There may be slight extravasation evident on arthrography, particularly in the immediate periarticular region.

GRADE III MEDIAL LIGAMENT INJURY (THIRD-DEGREE SPRAIN)

This injury results from complete rupture of the ligament, either within its substance or at its point of bony attachment.

There is usually gross functional instability immediately after the injury but pain is less severe than with Grade II injury. This may be confusing and lead to underestimation of the injury, since an athlete with unstable but relatively pain-free Grade III injuries may be able to bear weight by locking the knee using the quadriceps.

There is instability of 5 mm. or more on application of valgus stress at 30 degrees but the knee is stable in full extension.

Note: Instability of the knee in full extension indicates a posterior cruciate ligament disruption superimposed on the Grade III medial ligamentous tear (see page 1599).

Stress x-rays show pronounced opening, and arthrography, if performed, demonstrates extravasation of the dye into the soft tissues at a distance from the joint.

Pathologic Results of Grade I and Grade II Medial Ligament Injuries

1. These most often involve the superficial portion of the ligament. Both injuries are incomplete tears of the ligament or occasionally small avulsion fractures from the ligamentous insertion of the bone.
2. The deep capsular ligaments and
3. The posterior cruciate ligaments are intact. The anterior cruciate may be torn.

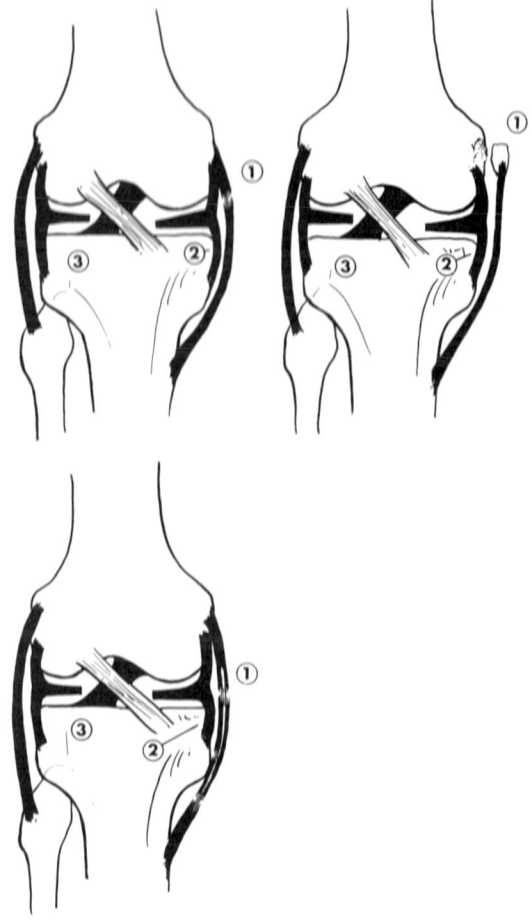

Pathologic Results of Grade III Medial Ligament Injuries

1. The ligament is disrupted in its important deep and superficial layers in most instances.
2. The anterior cruciate ligament is frequently torn.
3. The posterior cruciate ligament is intact unless there is instability in extension.

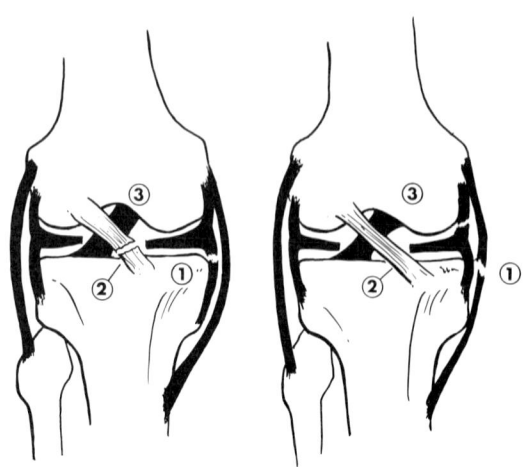

Pathology with Grade III Injuries and Instability in Full Extension

If the knee opens with mediolateral stress in full extension:
1. The posterior cruciate ligament, the key stabilizer of the knee, must be torn.
2. The superficial and deep medial ligaments are torn.
3. The meniscus is detached from its capsular ligament but is not usually torn in its substance with an acute injury.

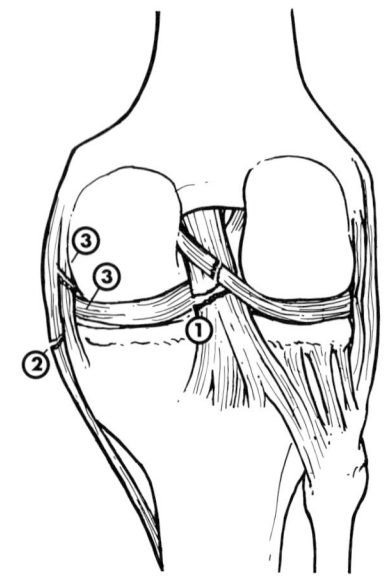

Examples of Grade I and Grade II Injuries (Limited to Medial Support Structures)

Note: Both the superficial and deep portions of the ligament may be avulsed from the femoral or tibial insertions, torn in their substance or detached from the meniscus.

The intact posterior cruciate prevents instability in full extension. Injuries to the collateral ligament will heal without surgery but deep capsular ligamentous injuries are best treated operatively.

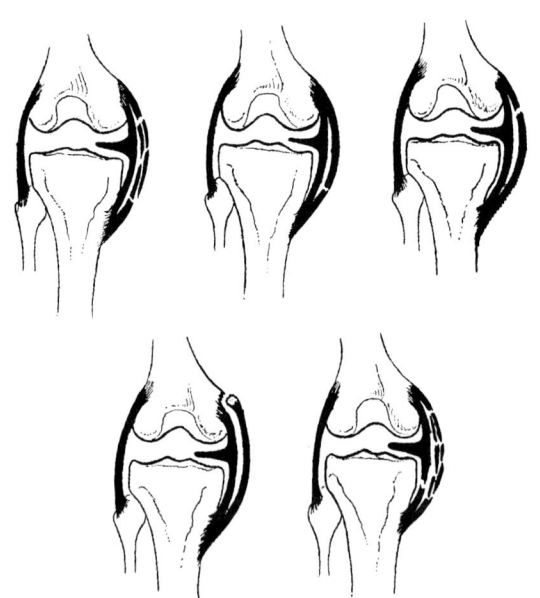

Examples of Type III Injuries (Combining Medial Capsular and Posterior Cruciate Tears)

Note: Most often the acute injury produces a detachment of the meniscus from the meniscofemoral or meniscotibial ligament rather than a complete tear. Chronic instability of the meniscus eventually will cause it to tear in its substance.

Instability of the knee in full extension indicates that the primary stabilizer of the knee, the posterior cruciate, has been disrupted.

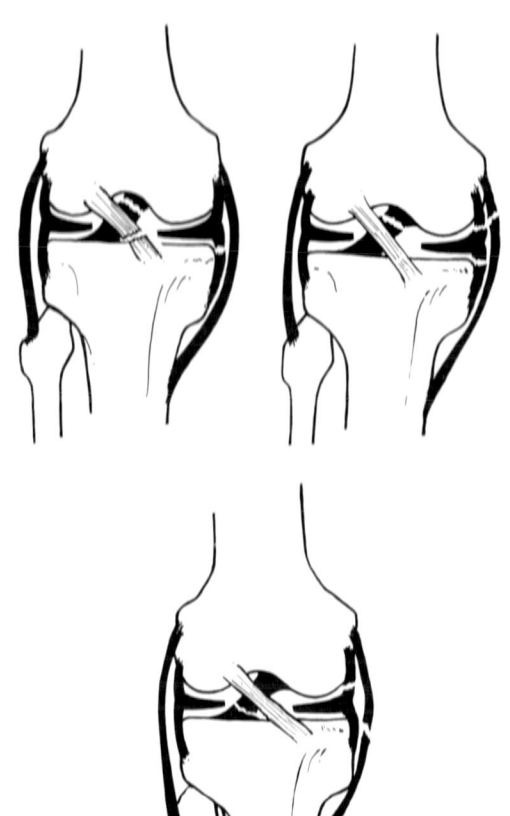

X-RAYS OF GRADE III INJURY

1. There may be widening of the medial joint space.
2. Bone fragments may be evident from avulsion of the capsular structures from the condyle of the femur.

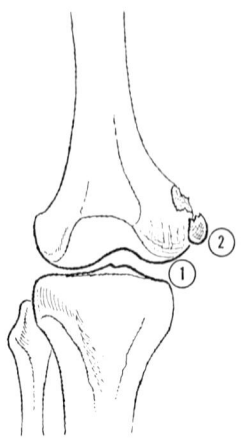

Stress X-Rays

1. Wide separation of the medial joint space is evident.
2. The subluxation of the joint is reproduced.

Note: Such wide separation is indicative of posterior cruciate ligament damage associated with medial and posteromedial capsular injury.

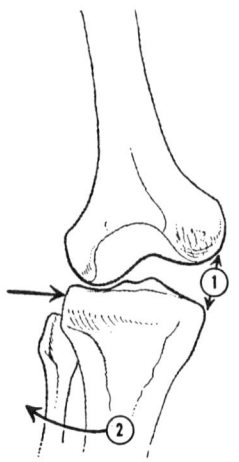

KNEE INJURIES IN ADOLESCENTS (EPIPHYSEAL OR LIGAMENTOUS INJURIES)

A valgus injury to the skeletally immature knee may produce an epiphyseal fracture, which can be mistaken for a ligamentous injury.

Epiphyseal injury can occur in patients as old as 17 years, in whom the physis may appear almost completely closed.

It is important to evaluate the unstable knee in an adolescent or teenager by stress x-ray (see page 233).

Stress-X-Ray after Epiphyseal Injury

1. Standard x-rays show no fracture of the epiphysis.

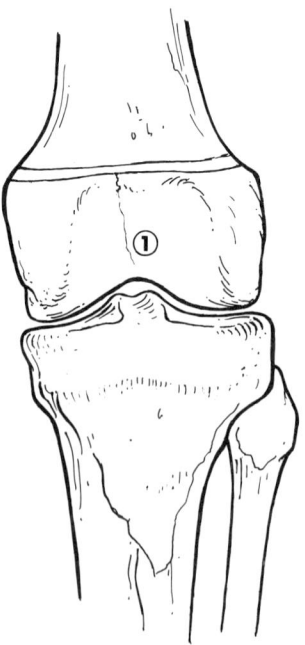

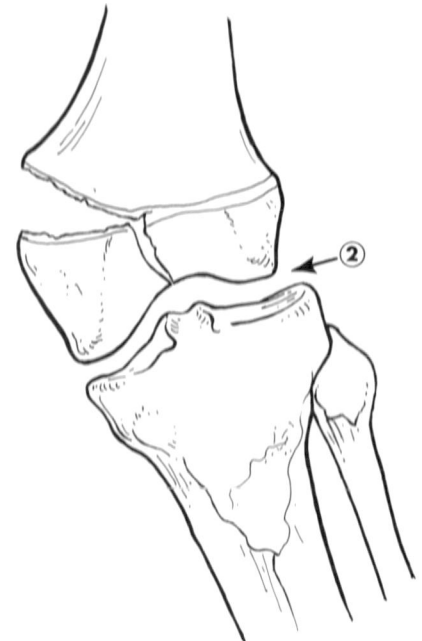

2. A stress x-ray shows the true nature of Type III epiphyseal fracture.

SINGLE-CONTRAST ARTHROGRAPHY OF GRADE III INJURIES

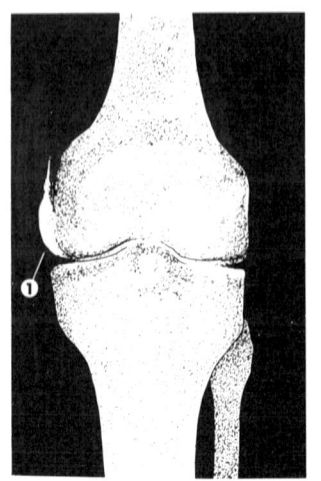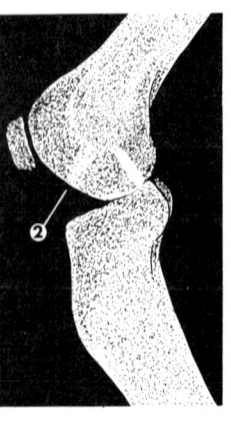

1. There is frequently complete extravasation of the dye through the superficial and deep capsular structures.

2. A lateral x-ray with anterior drawer testing shows interruption of the structure of the cruciate ligaments.

Management of Ligamentous Injuries According to Grades

REMARKS

Grade III injuries require prompt operative repair for the gross disruption of the medial joint support structures.

Grade II injuries can usually be treated nonoperatively. They should be observed and reevaluated within a week for the possibility of operative intervention.

Grade I injuries respond well to nonoperative treatment with functional reconditioning exercises.

MANAGEMENT OF GRADE I INJURIES

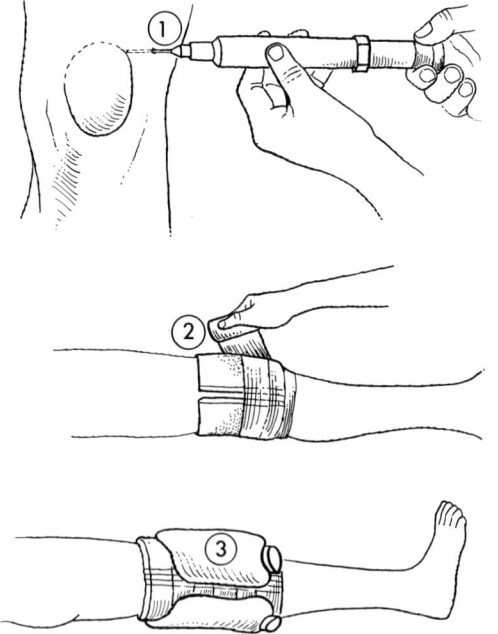

Local Treatment

1. Aspirate the knee joint of all hemarthrosis.

2. Apply a compression bandage to the knee.

3. Apply ice packs

4. After local symptoms subside protect the knee with an elastic wrapping and crutches.

INJURIES TO THE LIGAMENTS OF THE KNEE JOINT

Subsequent Management

Continue non-weight-bearing crutch-walking until the patient can ambulate pain free and without a limp.

Start immediate quadriceps muscle exercises and continue with ice packs until the swelling subsides.

Follow the patient closely. By the end of the first week the effusion should be almost resolved and full extension should be possible. Full flexion usually does not return until the second week.

By the end of two weeks there should be less tenderness in the ligamentous area, and progressive resistive quadriceps muscle exercises may be instituted.

By the end of the third week the knee should be tight and the ligaments should not be tender. At this point the patient may begin jogging exercises and may progress to normal activities.

If the patient's progress in the first week does not coincide with this anticipated course, the injury should be reevaluated for more significant disruption than Grade I.

MANAGEMENT OF GRADE II INJURIES

REMARKS

Nonoperative management is usually preferable with Grade II injuries, but the patient should be examined carefully within the first week for evidence of a more significant injury.

Keep in mind that with these Grade II injuries the mediolateral laxity with stress applied on the knee at 30 degrees of flexion should not exceed 5 mm. The anterior and posterior drawer tests should be negative. The ligamentous tenderness should become well-localized and should not remain diffusely tender. In the first week, the patient should rapidly gain motion and stability, and the tenderness should subside.

Local Treatment

1. Aspirate the knee joint, particularly if an arthrogram has been performed, so as to eliminate the dye and hematoma.
2. Apply a compression bandage and elevate the limb with ice packs for one to two days.

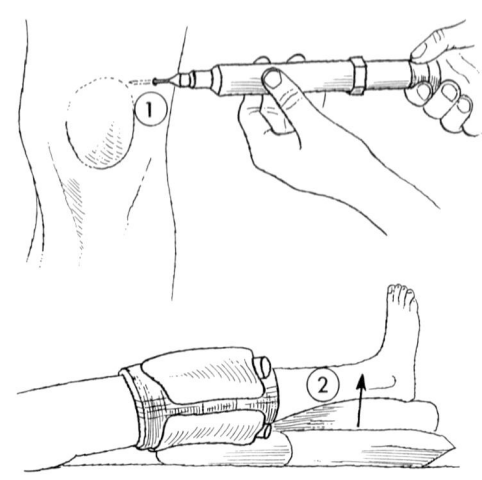

Subsequent Management

Allow the patient to walk with toe-touch weight bearing on crutches. Begin immediate quadriceps exercises and follow closely.

Full extension of the knee should return by seven to ten days, and flexion should be improving by two weeks.

The major criteria for improvement and recovery are diminishing swelling and tenderness in the knee and ligamentous area with progressive recovery of full motion.

Each patient must be managed individually. The patient who does not demonstrate expected recovery within the first seven to ten days should have the knee examined under anesthesia for evidence of more significant instability than Grade II.

SURGICAL MANAGEMENT OF GRADE III INJURIES

REMARKS

Since this injury most typically is caused by momentary subluxation of the knee joint due to a valgus stress with the tibia externally rotated, significant instability may follow.

The injury frequently includes the deep capsular ligament as well as the tibial collateral ligament. The posterior oblique ligament and medial half of the posterior capsule may also frequently be involved.

Ordinarily the capsular ligaments attaching to the meniscus are torn, but the meniscus itself usually remains intact. In addition to the medial capsular structures, the cruciates or lateral capsule structures may also be damaged and must be carefully evaluated prior to surgery.

If this injury heals without adequate surgical repair, the patient may well be bothered by "giving way" of the knee when he changes direction as in cutting, pivoting, or twisting.

Adequate surgical repair should be performed on all the potentially damaged areas, including the posteromedial corner of the knee.

Price and Allen have shown that, if at all possible, the medial ligament repair should be done with preservation of the meniscus. The menisci serve as shock absorbers and carry over half the load of weight bearing at full extension. They also transmit significant load in flexion and particularly enhance mediolateral stability. These functionally important structures should never be discarded without good reason.

Operative Repair of Disrupted Medial and Posterior Capsular Structures (Hughston Incision)

The posterior corner is the focal point of this incision, which exposes all possible tears in the medial and posterior capsular structures as well as the posterior cruciate ligament.

1. The patient is supine with the hip flexed and abducted 45 degrees and the knee flexed approximately 90 degrees.
2. The incision begins proximally over the hamstrings on the posteromedial aspect of the thigh and is carried distally along the joint line to the patellar tendon and then swung distally along the anteromedial surface of the tibia.

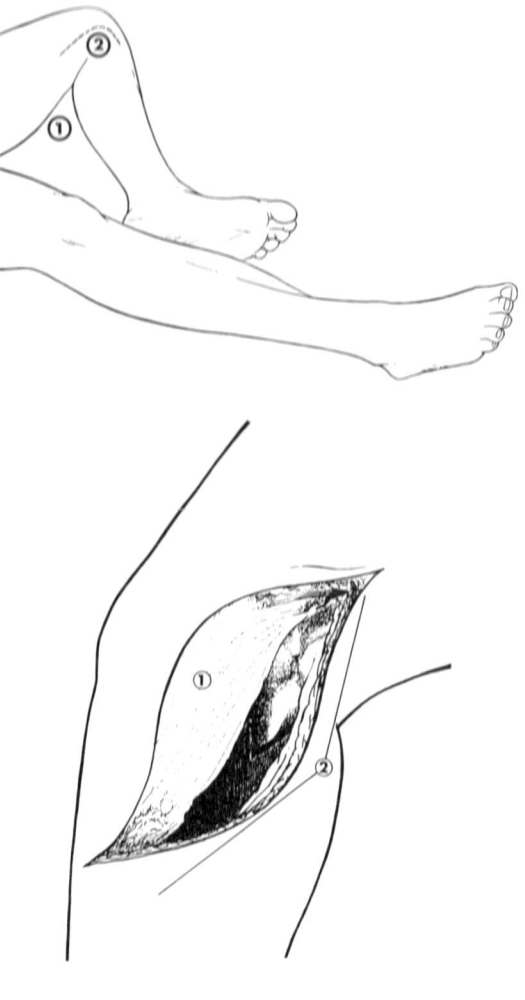

1. The skin and subcutaneous tissue are not dissected from the underlying fascia. The fascia lata is incised in line with the skin.
2. The proximal flap is reflected to reach the distal portion of the vastus medialis, and the distal flap is reflected for reaching the pes anserinus.

1. Areas of hemorrhage indicate the tear of the tibial collateral ligament.
2. Reflection of the torn tibial collateral ligament and retinaculum discloses the tears in the meniscotibial or meniscofemoral ligaments.

When there is no obvious tear initially, vertical incisions are made anterior and posterior to the tibial collateral ligament to inspect the capsular ligaments, both meniscofemoral and meniscotibial portions.

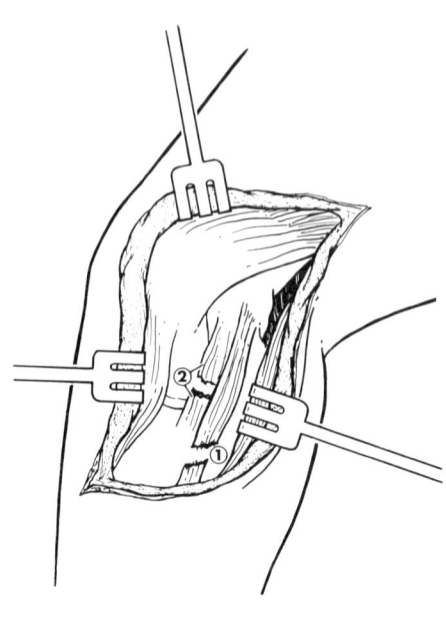

Operative Repair of Disrupted Medial and Posterior Capsular Structures (Hughston Incision) (Continued)

1. The posterior capsule must be thoroughly inspected and palpated.

2. If the posterior cruciate ligament is torn, it can be reached by retracting or releasing the medial head of the gastrocnemius (see page 1601).

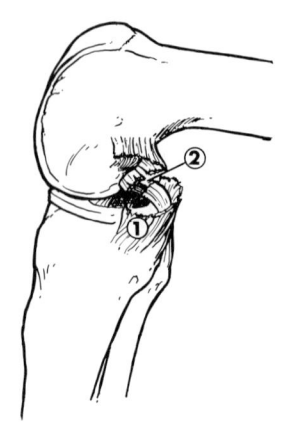

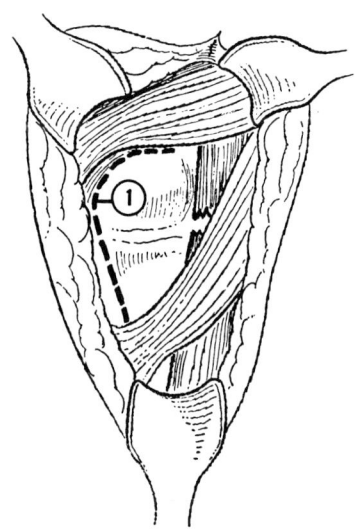

1. The joint is then exposed and explored through an anteromedial incision made through the retinaculum and capsule.

2. The entire joint should be visualized through this approach, and the cruciate ligaments and meniscus are inspected.

Note: The mere presence of a cruciate ligament does not indicate its functional capacity.

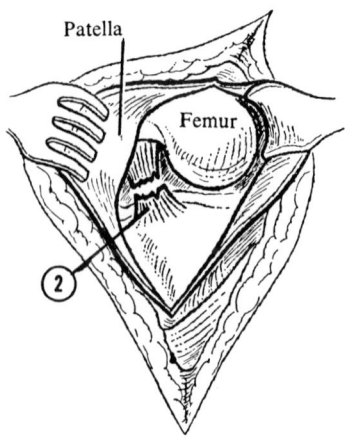

3. Perform an anterior drawer test while directly palpating the cruciates to determine their functional stability.

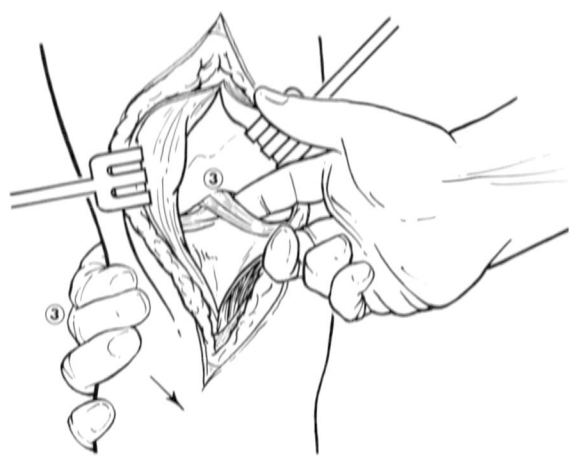

4. If the anterior cruciate ligament has a "mop end" tear in its substance, it should be resected. Otherwise the ligament should be repaired with the knee in 30 degrees of flexion.

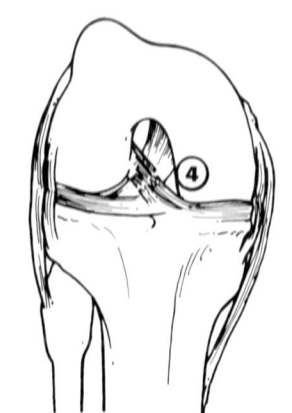

Method of Repair of Cruciate Ligaments *(see page 1594)*

When the ligament is avulsed from the tibia with or without a fragment of bone:
1. Reattach the end of the ligament by a mattress suture passing through two drill channels made in the medial tibial condyle.
2. If the bony fragment is large, anchor it to its tibial bed with a screw.

When the femoral attachment of the anterior cruciate ligament is torn:
3. Reattach the end of the ligament by a mattress suture passing through two drill channels made obliquely through the lateral femoral condyle.

After repair of the intra-articular structures, proceed with repair of the meniscal ligaments and posterior oblique ligament as necessary.

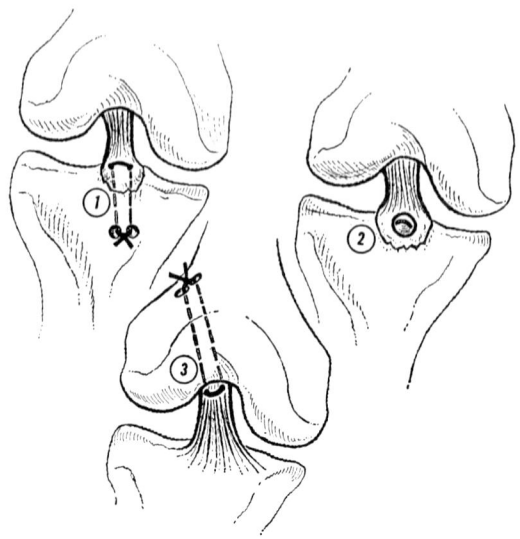

Repair of the Meniscofemoral and Meniscotibial Ligaments

REMARKS

The meniscofemoral and meniscotibial ligaments are formed by the deep fibers of the medial capsular ligament and are separate and distinct from the superficial and tibial collateral ligament. The meniscofemoral and meniscotibial ligaments quite frequently rupture at different levels in so-called tears of the tibial collateral ligament.

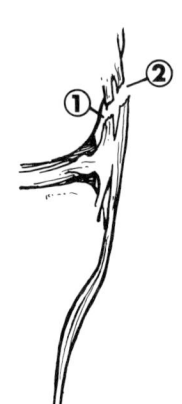

1. Proximal disruption of the meniscofemoral ligament is generally accompanied by
2. Proximal tear of the tibial collateral ligament.

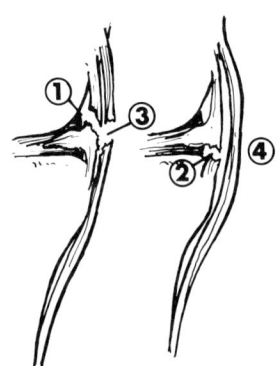

1. Central tears of the capsular or meniscofemoral ligament or
2. The meniscotibial portion of the capsular ligament may be associated with
3. Central tear of the tibial collateral ligament or
4. Attenuation of the collateral ligament.

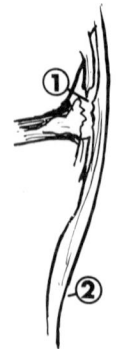

1. Central tears of the meniscofemoral or meniscotibial ligament may be associated with
2. Distal tears of the medial collateral ligament.

Technique of Repair

1. Proximal tears are resutured to bone through superficial drill holes proximal to the articular cartilage. The meniscofemoral and tibial collateral ligaments are sutured together.
2. If possible, the deep and superficial layer of ligaments should be repaired separately. Occasionally, with central tears it is necessary to repair both ligaments with one stitch sutured to the meniscus.
3. Tears of both the meniscofemoral and the meniscotibial ligaments can be repaired by suturing them into the periphery of the meniscus.

Note: The entire posteromedial aspect of the knee must also be inspected and palpated to determine whether the important posterior oblique ligament requires repair.

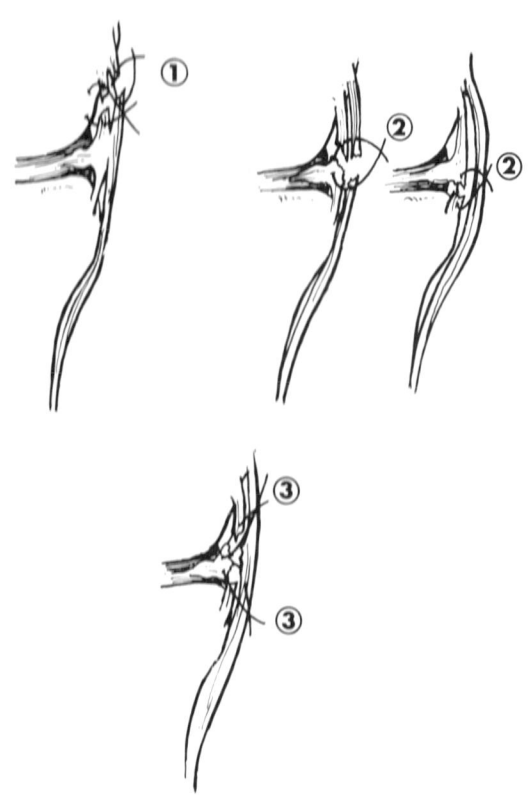

Technique of Repair of Posterior Oblique and Tibial Collateral Ligaments (After Hughston)

1. Three nonabsorbable mattress sutures are placed along the axis of the posterior oblique ligament (POL). These must be anchored distally in the ligament at the posterior corner of the tibia and
2. Proximally at the attachment of the ligament to the adductor tubercle.
3. The POL is then drawn forward as tightly as possible to the femoral epicondyle with the knee in 60 degrees of flexion.

Note: This repair advances the ligament approximately 5 mm. and gives it mechanical advantage.

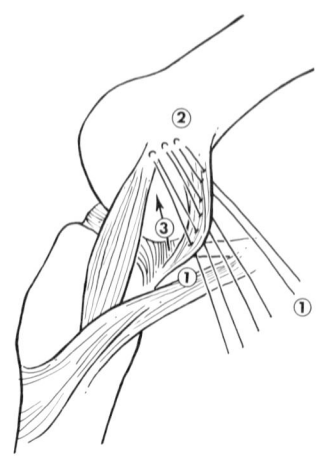

Technique of Repair of Posterior Oblique and Tibial Collateral Ligaments (After Hughston) (Continued)

1. The tibial end of the POL is advanced anteriorly and
2. Sutured to the periosteum of the tibia.

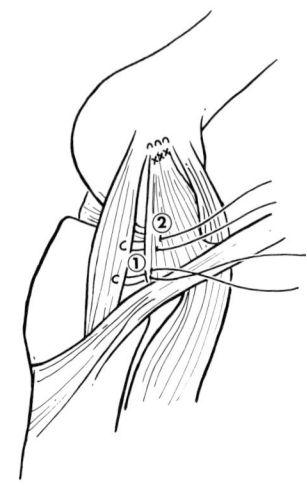

3. The third basic stitch in the midportion of the POL pulls it into the repaired tibial collateral ligament but does not go through the capsular ligament into the joint.

Note: The meniscus should be left intact and stabilized by this repair rather than being removed. The meniscus is removed only in the rare instance in which it has been torn through its substance.

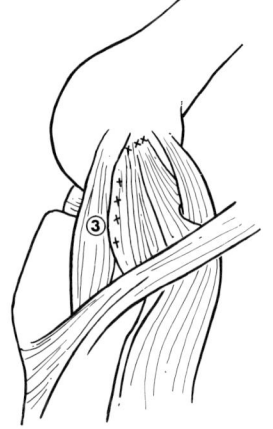

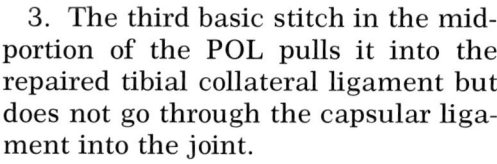

1. If the tibial arm of the posterior oblique ligament has been detached from the tibia, it can be sutured through holes drilled in bone.
2. A towel clip can be used to create a tunnel for the suture.

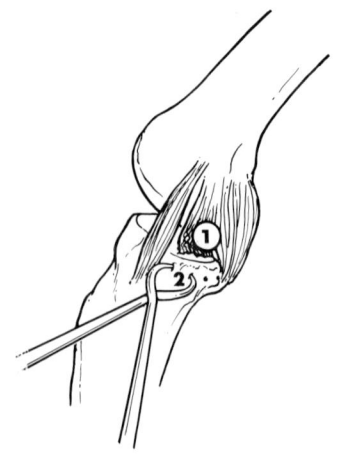

3. The sutures are tied to the bone substance for firm reattachment of the ligament to the tibia.

Note: The ligamentous repair is never tighter than at the moment it is completed. Always test for stability of the repair in 30 degrees of knee flexion. If stability is not regained the sutures should be removed at once and another attempt should be made to achieve a stable repair.

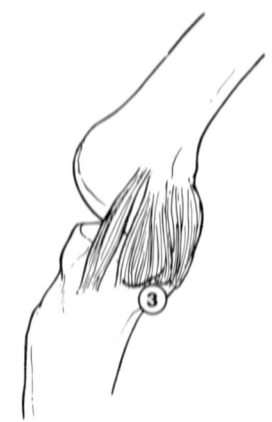

1. If the medial compartmental structures are so torn that restoration of stability proves to be impossible, reconstructive techniques such as the pes anserinus transfer, as described by Slocum and Larson, must be used.

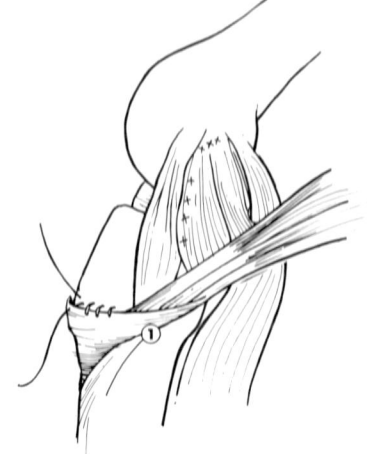

SUBSEQUENT MANAGEMENT

The knee is immobilized in a bulky Jones dressing until the immediate postoperative swelling subsides. Subsequently, a long leg cast with the knee flexed approximately 30 degrees is used for three weeks.

A cast-brace molded well down over the femoral condyles and tibial plateau is then applied and used for four to six weeks longer while the patient regains knee function.

Technique of Repair of Posterior Oblique and Tibial Collateral Ligaments (After Hughston) (Continued)

CAUTION

Avoid applying a loose cast-brace, which does not protect against varus and valgus strain.

1. The cast-brace must be carefully molded down over the condyles and patella anteriorly.

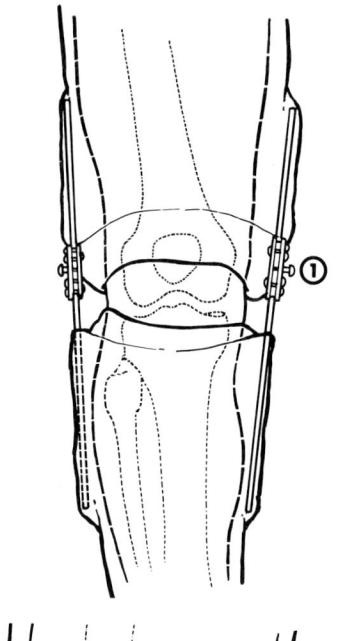

2. There should be sufficient clearance posteriorly to allow 40 to 60 degrees of knee flexion.

Note: Flexion and full extension can be controlled by stops on the hinges, if necessary, to protect cruciate ligament repairs. Avoid allowing the patient to perform full knee extension too quickly, since this will be likely to disrupt the repair of the posterior ligamentous structures.

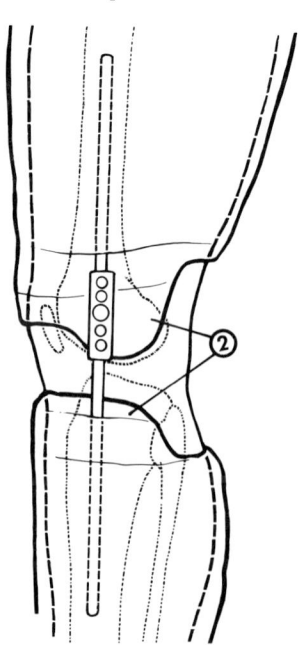

Pellegrini-Stieda Syndrome (Complication of Injury to the Tibial Collateral Ligament)

REMARKS

This disorder results from minor tears in the medial joint structure with secondary calcification of the traumatized tissue and usually requires no treatment. Occasionally the prominence on the medial femoral condyle is sufficiently large to warrant excision.

If the lesion is recognized early, the knee should be immobilized in a cylinder cast for several weeks; this treatment may effectively prevent development of soft tissue calcification.

X-Ray of Early Lesion

1. Elongated amorphous calcareous deposit in the substance of the tibial collateral ligament.

Note: This usually appears two to three weeks after the injury.

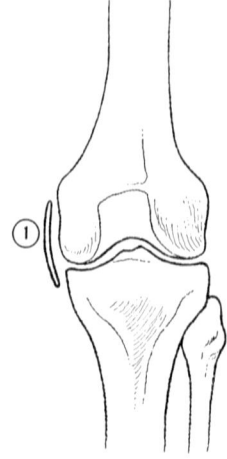

Early Management

Always anticipate and try to abort this complication in ligamentous injuries, especially of the tibial collateral ligament.

1. Apply a nonpadded plaster cylinder to the limb from the groin to just above the malleoli.
2. The knee is extended.

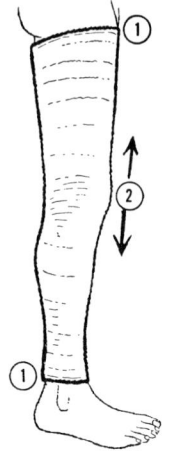

Permit weight bearing and quadriceps-setting exercises immediately.

In an early lesion, within three to four weeks after injury, the cast is left on for six weeks. At the end of this time the soft-tissue calcification may have been absorbed and gentle exercises can be allowed.

Occasionally, injection of 1 ml of hydrocortisone into the ligament will aid in absorption of the calcareous deposit or will prevent its occurrence.

Since these lesions are generally asymptomatic, operative treatment is rarely indicated.

X-Ray of Same Case after Five Weeks of Plaster Immobilization

Calcareous deposit is completely absorbed.

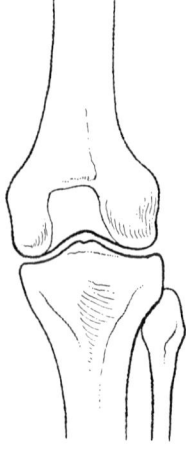

X-Ray of Late Lesion (10 to 12 Weeks after Injury)

1. Formation of discrete heterotopic bone in the region of the medial epicondyle.
2. Ossified ligament is attached to the epicondyle.

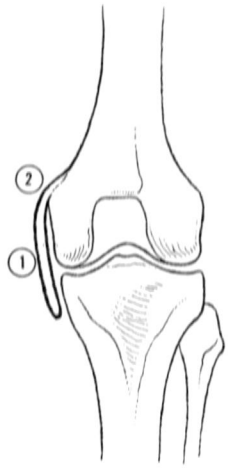

Late Management

If the bony mass becomes tender or interferes with normal knee motion, it can be excised using sharp dissection to avoid further trauma to the knee.

X-Ray of Same Case after Excision of Bony Mass

1. Heterotopic bone is excised; only a small spicule remains in the region of the femoral epicondyle.

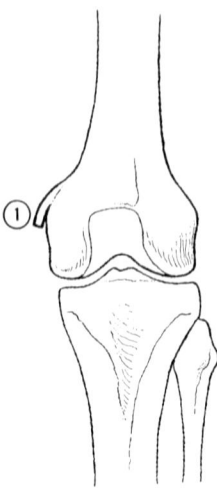

Acute Injuries Causing Anterolateral Instability

REMARKS

Injuries causing lateral instability are not as common as those causing medial instability and often go unrecognized because the clinical signs are subtle.

The mechanism most often is a forced varus strain without direct contact on the medial side of the knee. Basketball players or other athletes who land off balance after jumping are most susceptible to lateral joint injuries.

Most often the diagnosis should be suspected when the patient complains of immediate intra-articular swelling or has demonstrable lateral tenderness and puffiness or a palpable lateral defect.

The adduction or varus test of the knee in 0 and 30 degrees of flexion is frequently not helpful for lateral disruption.

Most often the diagnosis depends on the physician's awareness of the problem and prompt evaluation of knee stability within the first hour after injury, before pain, swelling, and muscle guarding mask the physical findings.

The most sensitive physical test for anterolateral instability is anterolateral displacement of the tibial surface on straight anterior drawer testing.

The pivot-shift or jerk test may be negative in the acutely injured knee, depending on how soon the examination is done after injury and how much protective hamstring tightening occurs.

X-rays of the acute injury may occasionally show an anterolateral fleck fracture from the tibial articular surface where the lateral capsule attaches.

Another radiographic finding with anterolateral subluxation is a notch in the lateral femoral condyle. Losee and coworkers pointed out that this is caused by impingement of the posterolateral margin of the subluxating tibia, much like the Hill-Sachs lesion in the proximal humerus associated with a dislocating shoulder.

Single-contrast arthrography in the acute injury that demonstrates a leak laterally or over Gerdy's tubercle offers an additional confirmation of the significant injury.

Keep in mind that acute anterolateral rotatory instability may be associated with acute anteromedial rotatory instability. Prior to repairing the medial ligaments in all acute injuries, reexamine the knee using adequate anesthesia to determine the necessity for lateral repair.

INJURIES TO THE LIGAMENTS OF THE KNEE JOINT

An additional consideration is the possibility of posterolateral instability, which is less common than anterolateral instability but still must be considered. Posterolateral rotatory instability due to a tear of the arcuate complex is demonstrated by the external rotation-recurvatum test. It should not be confused with a tear of the lateral meniscus or of the posterior cruciate ligament.

Mechanism of Injury

Carefully evaluate all patients who have had a rotatory injury to the knee with or without a direct blow to the medial aspect.

Quite often the injury results from a fall producing a varus internal rotation loading on the knee.

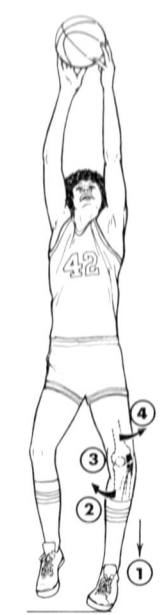

1. The individual lands on the leg while off balance.
2. He falls forward with an internal rotation and stress.
3. At the same time a varus stress is applied during the fall.
4. The thigh and femur rotate externally.

Note: The symptoms after the acute injury may be minimal or there may be mild to moderate pain over the lateral knee joint. There may also be well-localized swelling or a palpable defect over the lateral condylar region.

Diagnostic Tests for Anterolateral Instability

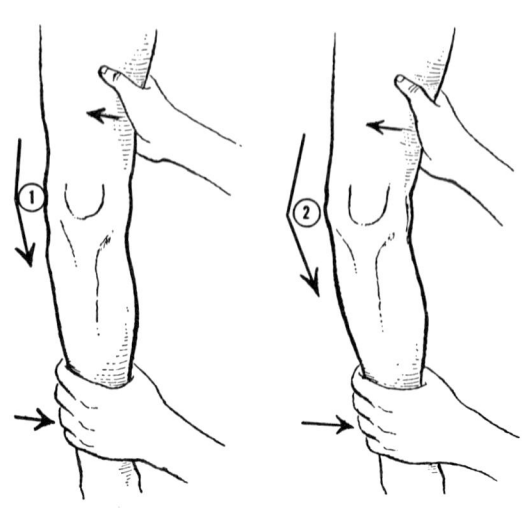

1. Varus stress of the knee after injury is usually unrevealing or at the most shows a slight increase in mobility on the injured side.
2. If there is gross instability on varus testing, usually the entire lateral capsule, the posterior cruciate ligament, and sometimes the peroneal nerve have been torn.

Note: The usual benign picture after these injuries tends to confuse the examiner unless more specific tests are employed.

1583

INJURIES TO THE LIGAMENTS OF THE KNEE JOINT

Diagnostic Tests for Anterolateral Instability (Continued)

The most specific test for acute anterolateral instability is the anterior drawer test as described by Hughston and coworkers.

It is performed using

1. Standard anterior drawer testing with the knee and tibia in neutral rotation.

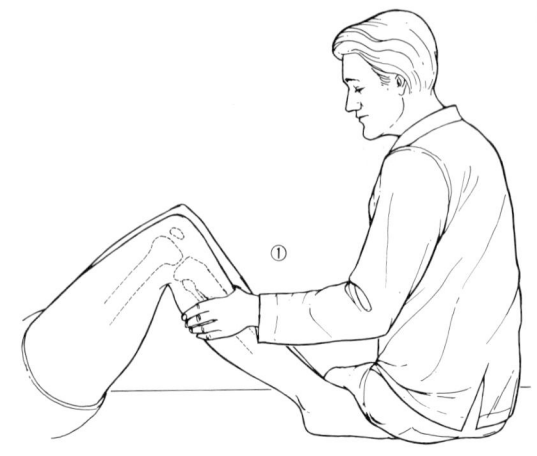

2. Anterior subluxation of the lateral plateau occurs despite drawing of the tibia straight forward, indicating anterolateral instability.

The second specific test is the jerk test, which may be negative in the acute injury owing to hamstring spasm. The maneuver should always be carried out in evaluating the knee under general anesthetic (see page 1558).

Anterolateral

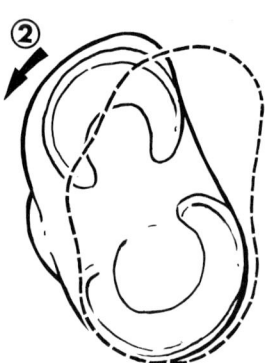

Test for Posterolateral Rotatory Instability (After Hughston)

Keep in mind that there may be a combined injury present. Anterolateral instability may be combined with anteromedial instability or with posterolateral instability.

To test for posterolateral rotatory instability:

1. Simultaneously lift each limb by the great toe, thereby causing the knee to fall into maximum recurvatum.
2. Disruption of the arcuate complex causes the injured knee to go into excessive recurvatum and
3. Causes external rotation and tibia vera.

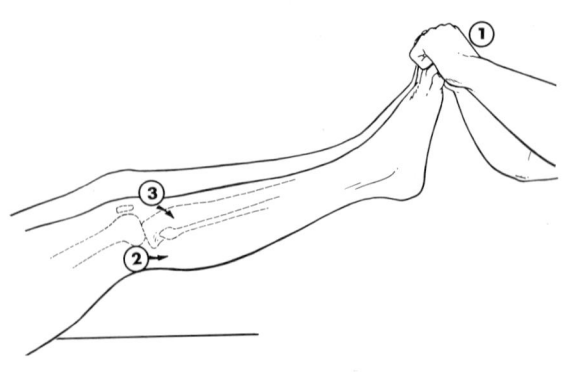

Radiographic Findings in Acute Anterolateral Instability

1. Occasionally a lateral capsular sign or avulsion of a small bone fragment from the lateral capsular attachment will be seen, indicating acute tear.

2. With chronic anterolateral instability, notching of the lateral femoral condyle can be produced by impingement of the lateral meniscus during subluxation.

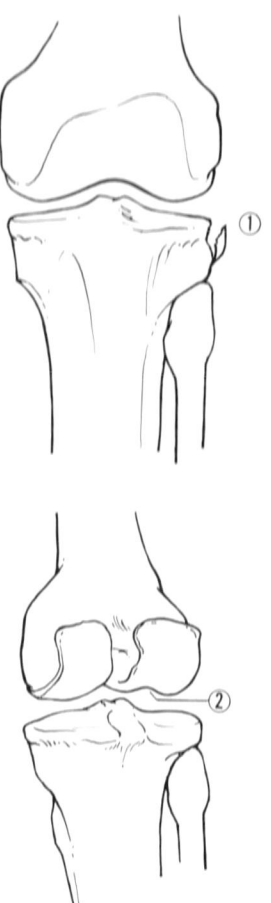

OPERATIVE TREATMENT OF ACUTE ANTEROLATERAL ROTATORY INSTABILITY (After Norwood and Coworkers)

Always repeat the examination under anesthesia immediately prior to any surgical procedure.

1. An anteromedial incision is made first to inspect the medial and lateral menisci and to inspect and palpate the cruciate ligaments during stress testing.

Note: Remove any meniscus that is torn in its substance and repair the cruciate ligament, if possible. The majority of cruciate ligament injuries are of the "mop end" type and require excision of the stump ends rather than repair (see page 1573).

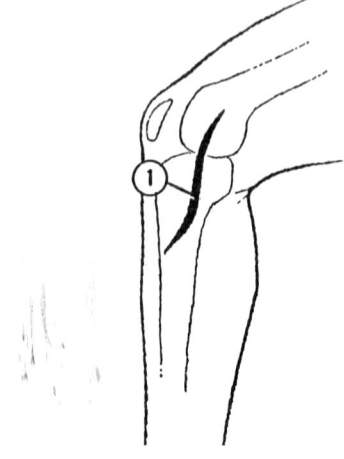

1. After any intra-articular damage is identified and treated make a lateral hockey stick incision to expose the entire lateral ligamentous structure.

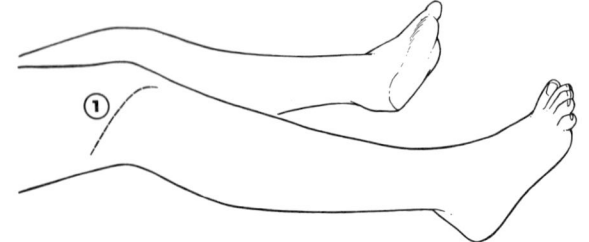

2. The majority of lateral damage has occurred in the midthird of the capsular ligament.

Note: The entire lateral aspect and posterolateral aspect of the joint should be visualized back to the arcuate complex to be sure that all areas of injury have been repaired.

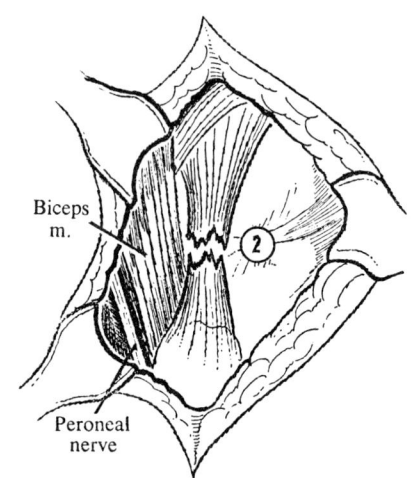

1. Repair the entire area of damage to the deep layer.
2. The superficial ligament as well as the iliotibial tract fibers should be repaired.
3. A segment is taken from the biceps tendon to reinforce the capsule and ligament repair.

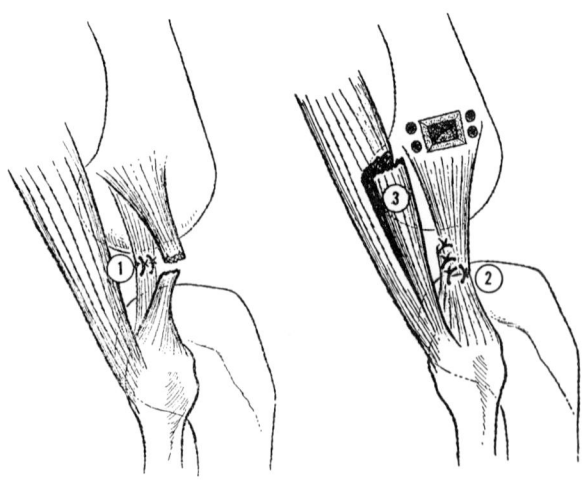

4. If the capsule and ligament repair does not result in knee stability and a negative jerk test, the repair is tightened and shortened into a trough made in the linea aspira.

5. The ligament and capsule repair is reinforced with the strip removed from the biceps tendon.

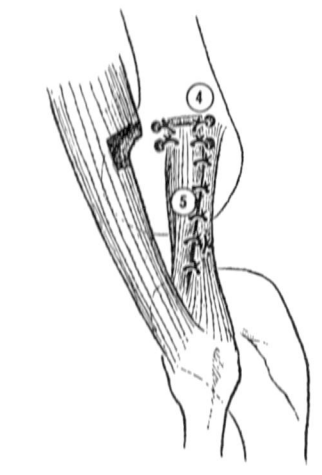

Methods of reattachment of the distal end of the fibular collateral ligament:

1. Reattachment of the ends of the ligament by interrupted sutures.
2. Anchorage of the end of the ligament in a slot made in the head of the fibula.

Note: If a fragment of bone is avulsed from the head of the fibula it may be excised or, if large, replaced in its original site.

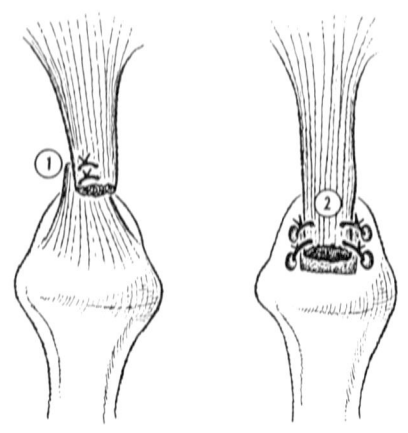

In combined lesions

When the anterior or the posterior cruciate ligaments are torn, repair is effected in the same manner as depicted on pages 1595 and 1599.

Postoperative Immobilization

The leg is immobilized in a long leg cast with the knee flexed 30 degrees for approximately three weeks.

Quadriceps-setting exercises are begun on the first postoperative day.

The patient may be up walking on crutches by the third postoperative day.

The long leg cast is removed after three weeks and a cast-brace is applied to allow the patient gradually to regain full motion. Keep the cast-brace on the knee for five to six weeks longer while continuing active quadriceps-strengthening exercises.

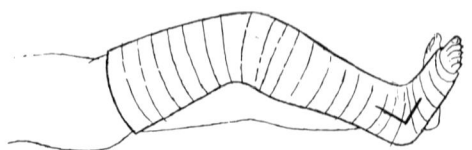

Postoperative Immobilization (Continued)

Caution

Avoid applying a loose cast-brace, which does not protect against varus and valgus strain.

1. The cast-brace must be carefully molded down over the condyles and patella anteriorly.

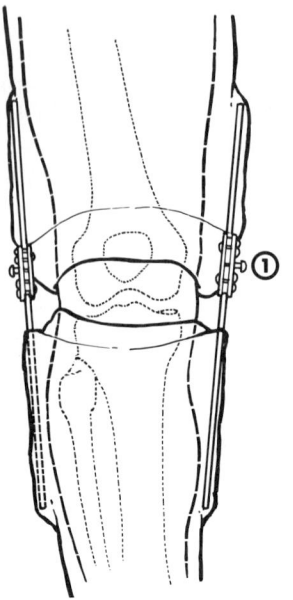

2. There should be sufficient posterior clearance to allow 40 to 60 degrees of knee flexion.

Note: Flexion and full extension can be controlled by stops on the hinges, if necessary, to protect cruciate ligament repairs.

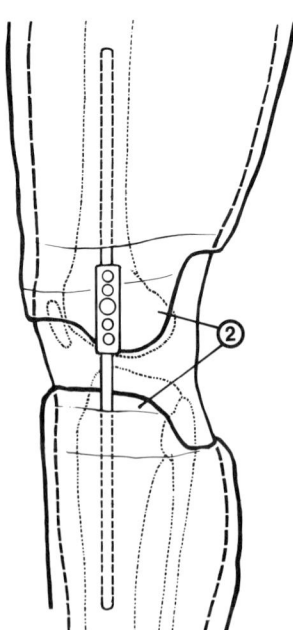

Acute Ruptures of the Anterior Cruciate Ligament and Other Injuries to the Extended Knee

REMARKS

Although rare, an isolated rupture of the anterior cruciate ligament can occur. Wang and coworkers have demonstrated that hyperextension of the knee with slight internal rotation can rupture the anterior cruciate.

Frequently, the patient will feel and hear a "pop" at the time of the injury. The knee then swells from synovial bleeding and the patient is unable to continue to actively bear weight on the leg.

Subsequently the patient may have no difficulties after the swelling subsides, although there may be episodes of the knee's "giving way" during vigorous athletic competition.

Pivoting on the extended knee is also a common cause of acute patellar dislocation, especially with a valgus strain. The associated fracture of the medial patellar border and the "fear sign" aid in differentiating this common injury from the cruciate ligament tear.

Sudden twist on the extended knee may also produce an osteochondral fracture of the lateral femoral condyle and a loose body in the knee. Usually this results from a valgus strain rather than an internal rotation loading on the knee. These patients will also hear a sudden "crack" and will develop hemarthrosis. According to Mathewson and Dandy, these fractures result from the shearing forces between the convex articular surfaces of the lateral femoral condyle and the lateral tibial plateau as they pivot under the load.

One of the most common mechanisms of cruciate ligament rupture is from a torn meniscus abutting against the ligament. Since as many as 60 per cent of young individuals undergoing meniscectomy are found to have an absent or injured anterior cruciate, the management of this problem is a common dilemma.

The diagnosis of an isolated cruciate ligament rupture has generally been based on the presence of the anterior drawer sign. Hughston has shown that the primary cause of abnormal anterior drawering of the tibia is disruption of the meniscotibial ligament rather than a tear of the cruciate. Isolated cruciate tears do not cause significant anteroposterior instability unless associated with deep capsular tears.

Isolated cruciate ligament injury does not usually require operative repair or reconstruction. Studies by Chick and Jackson, who in the course of meniscectomy found cruciate ligament disruption, indicated that 83 per cent returned to full athletic participation without repair of the cruciate. Twenty per cent of those with unrepaired cruciate injury develop some anterolateral instability as diagnosed by the jerk test, but none of these individuals required reconstructive surgery.

The majority of acute cruciate ligament tears are "mop end" disruptions through the substance. Resection of the stump is preferable to attempted repairs or uncertain reconstructive procedures. If the ligament is considered repairable, it is best done by sutures fixed through the femoral and tibial attachments. The infrapatellar fat pad and synovial membrane should be preserved to surround the repair site and permit revascularization of the ligament.

Repair of the cruciate ligament is most often done when the injury is associated with medial or lateral capsular damage. The anterolateral or anteromedial instability associated with these combined injuries is best corrected by repair of the lateral or medial capsular structures, as previously described (see pages 1574 and 1586).

Mechanism of Isolated Injury of the Cruciate Ligament

1. The victim is bearing full weight on the extended knee and is hit from the side.
2. The foot is slightly internally rotated.
3. The direction of the load causes hyperextension and further internal rotation.

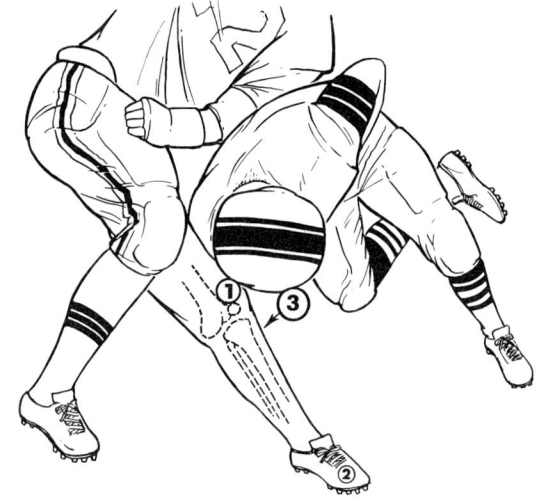

Mechanism of Cruciate Rupture from Meniscus Injury

1. A bucket-handle tear locks the knee joint and
2. The abrasion of the cruciate ligament rapidly causes disruption of the structure.

Note: Hughston has pointed out that cruciate rupture does not necessarily cause instability unless there is an associated posteromedial or lateral capsular disruption.

Cruciate tears should be distinguished from other injuries occurring to the extended knee, which include subluxated or dislocated patella, osteochondral fracture, and disruption of the posterolateral capsule.

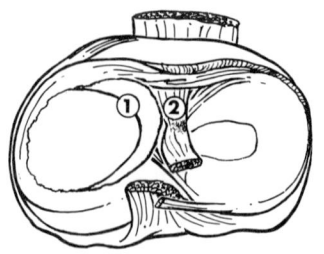

Injury to the Extended Knee Producing Patellar Dislocation

1. As the patient comes down rapidly on the knee in the hyperextended position,

2. Valgus and external rotation strains cause the patella to shift laterally.

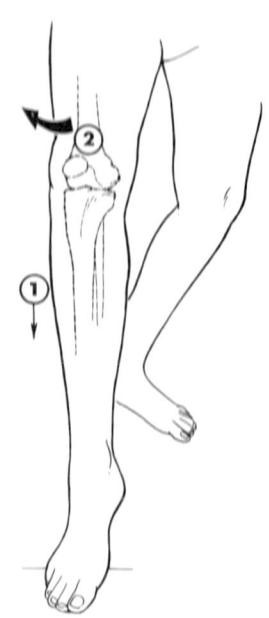

3. As the knee flexes 10 to 20 degrees, the patella dislocates or subluxates, causing the extensor mechanism to give way. The patient then suddenly falls and the patella frequently reduces spontaneously.

Note: Hemarthrosis commonly results from this injury, which should not be confused with a cruciate rupture.

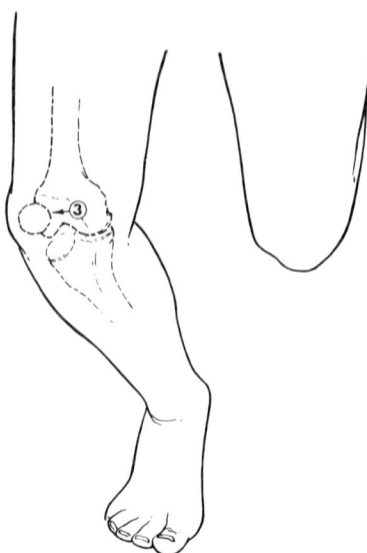

Injury to the Extended Knee Producing Patellar Dislocation (*Continued*)

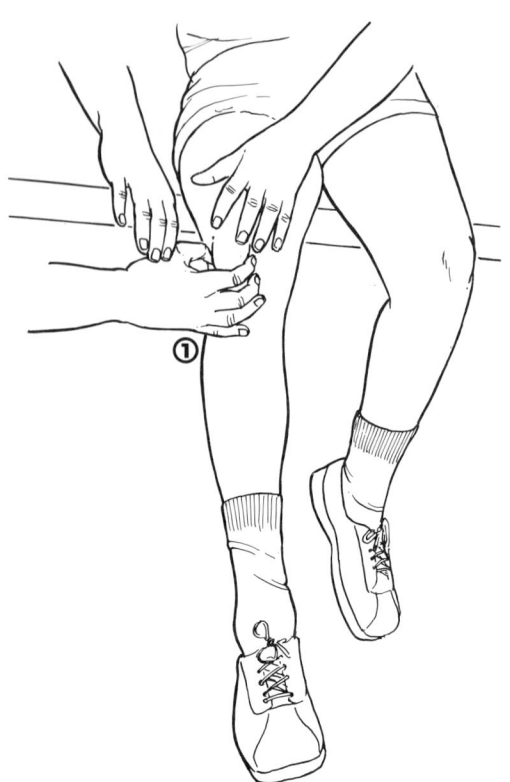

1. The diagnosis of a dislocated patella is made by elicitation of the fear sign or apprehension sign. With the knee relaxed in a flexed position, the examiner presses on the medial aspect of the patella, causing sensation of lateral instability. The patient grasps the examiner's hand in apprehension to prevent the impending dislocation.

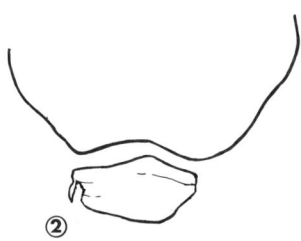

2. Oblique patellar views frequently show small medial fractures from avulsion of the retinaculum.

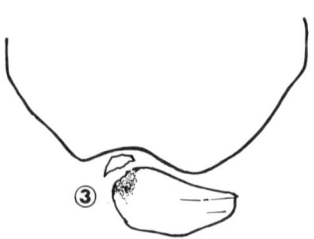

3. These fractures are to be distinguished from osteochondral fractures, which should be repaired surgically.

Osteochondral Fracture of the Lateral Femoral Condyle

Mechanism
1. A sudden hyperextension injury to the knee with valgus loading.
2. Causes impaction and shearing of the convex articular surface of the lateral femoral condyle on the lateral tibial plateau.

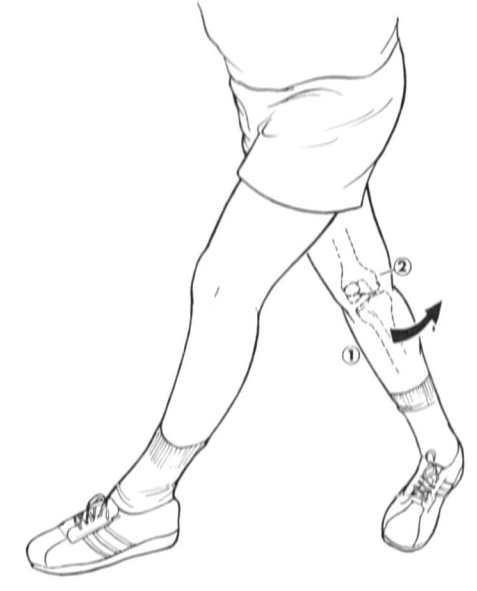

Appearance on X-Ray

Note: Unless looked for carefully, osteochondral fractures are frequently missed on x-ray.

1. There is a defect in the femoral condyle.
2. A loose fragment may be visible in the joint.

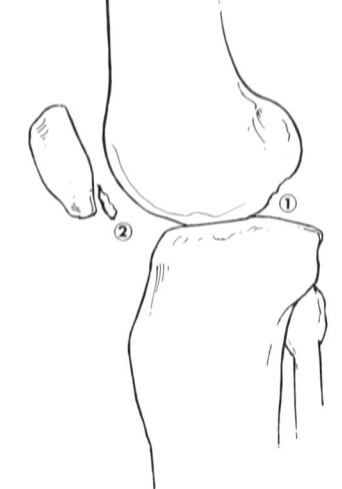

MANAGEMENT OF ACUTE ANTERIOR CRUCIATE TEARS, PATELLAR DISLOCATIONS, AND OSTEOCHONDRAL FRACTURES

Indications for Operative Repair of Cruciate Ligaments

REMARKS

Arthroscopic examinations of acutely injured knees demonstrate cruciate tear to be a common cause of hemarthrosis (see page 1691).

Arthrotomy is not usually indicated for an isolated injury to the cruciate.

Operative repair of the cruciate is usually done in conjunction with repair of the capsular ligaments (see page 1571).

Kennedy has pointed out that in at least 70 per cent of cases, the cruciate ligaments are torn in their substance rather than detached from the tibia or femur. Repair of this "mop end" type of injury is particularly ineffective and likely to result in a functionally useless structure. Resection of the "mop end" is preferable to repair.

If the ligament detaches from bone, repair can be effective. The fat pad and surrounding synovium, which supply blood for the cruciate ligament, should be preserved as much as possible in the process of repair.

Operative Repair for Detachments of the Distal and Proximal Ends of the Anterior Cruciate Ligament

(Perform the operation with a tourniquet applied around the upper third of the thigh.)

1. Expose the intercondylar region of the tibia with a medial parapatellar incision.
2. After flushing out of the joint cavity all blood clots, identify the lesion in the anterior cruciate ligament.

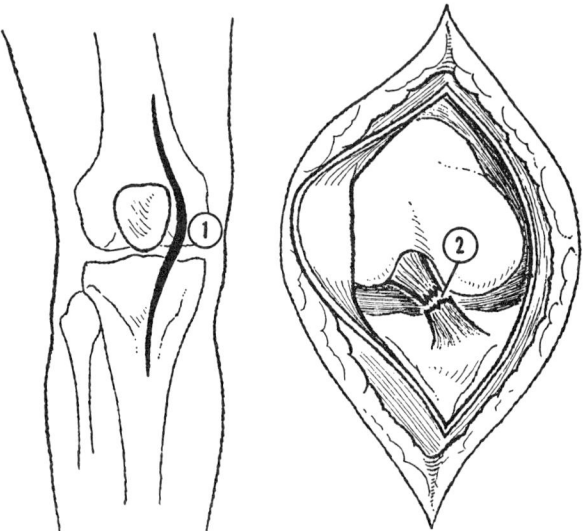

For detachment of the distal end of the anterior cruciate ligament

1. Make two parallel drill channels in the medial condyle of the tibia. They begin on the anteromedial surface of the condyle 4 cm below the tibial brim and are directed obliquely upward, backward, and inward, and issue from the superior surface of the tibia through the original site of the attachment of the ligament. (These channels may also be made from within the joint outward.)
2. Secure the ligament to its raw bed by a mattress suture tied on the anterior surface of the tibia.

Note: Do not damage the infrapatellar fat pad or surrounding synovial structures, which are important for revascularization of the repaired ligament.

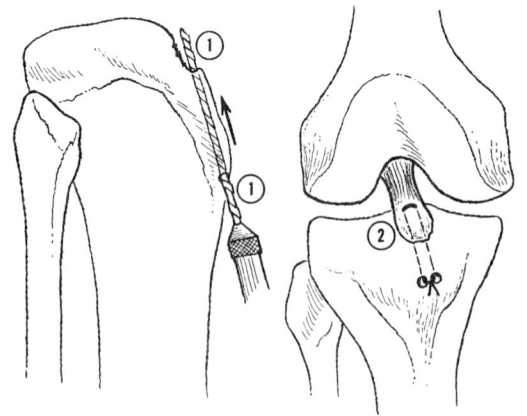

INJURIES TO THE LIGAMENTS OF THE KNEE JOINT

For detachment of the proximal end of the anterior cruciate ligament

Note: This is an exceedingly rare lesion and usually is encountered in combination with lesions of the tibial collateral ligament.

1. Pass a suture (stout silk) through the proximal end of the anterior cruciate ligament.
2. Make a 5-cm vertical incision on the lateral aspect of the thigh immediately above the lateral femoral epicondyle.
3. Make two drill holes 1 cm apart in the lateral femoral condyle and directed backward to the normal insertion of the anterior cruciate. The posterior aspect of the joint may be difficult to reach, but it is critical that the cruciate be reattached to its normal point of attachment.

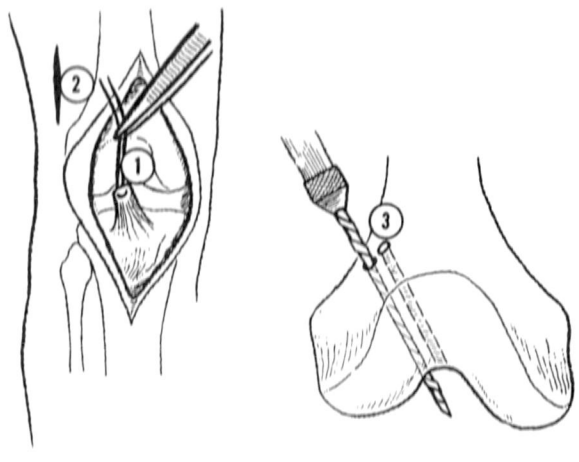

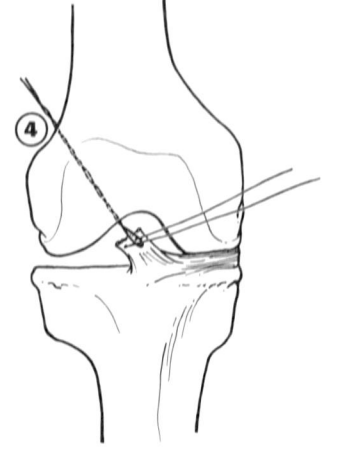

4. Pass a 20-gauge wire with a looped end through each hole and use this to direct the sutures in the ligament back up through the drill holes.

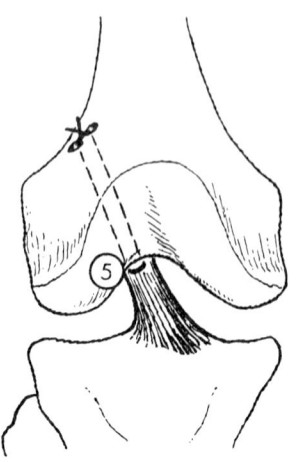

5. The suture is tied snugly over the lateral femoral condyle to maintain firm contact between the cruciate and its attachment point.

Note: After repairing the ligament, also repair its synovial sheath to promote revascularization.

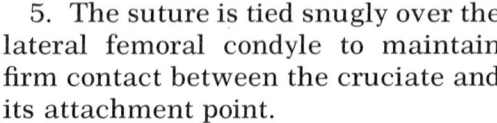

Alternate Method: Over-the-Top Repair of Anterior Cruciate Ligament Injury

An easier way of reattaching the anterior cruciate avulsed from the femoral condyle is by the over-the-top repair to its normal point of attachment, which is so very far posteriorly. This was first described by MacIntosh and with it the ligament's chance of surviving is as good as, if not better than, with repair to bone.

1. The sutures in the cruciate ligament are passed around the top of the lateral femoral condyle.
2. The suture is tied to the soft tissues behind the lateral condyle using a separate posterolateral incision.

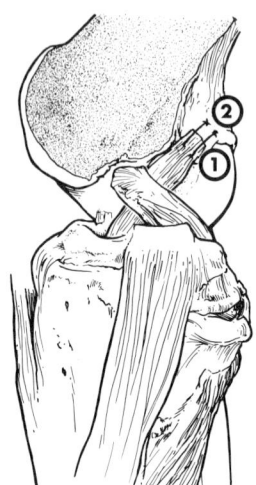

Postoperative Management

Apply a compressive dressing until immediate postoperative swelling subsides. Subsequently a long leg cast with the knee flexed approximately 30 degrees is used for three weeks.

A cast-brace molded down well over the femoral condyles and tibial plateau is then applied and used for four to six weeks longer while the patient regains knee motion.

The cast-brace, properly applied, will protect the cruciate repair against rotatory or mediolateral strain. Flexion and extension motion is not detrimental then to the repair site.

CAUTION

Avoid applying a loose cast-brace, which does not protect against varus and valgus strain.

1. The cast-brace must be carefully molded down over the condyles and patella anteriorly.
2. There should be sufficient posterior clearance to allow 40 to 60 degrees of knee flexion.

Note: Flexion and full extension can be controlled by stops on the hinges if necessary to protect cruciate ligament repairs.

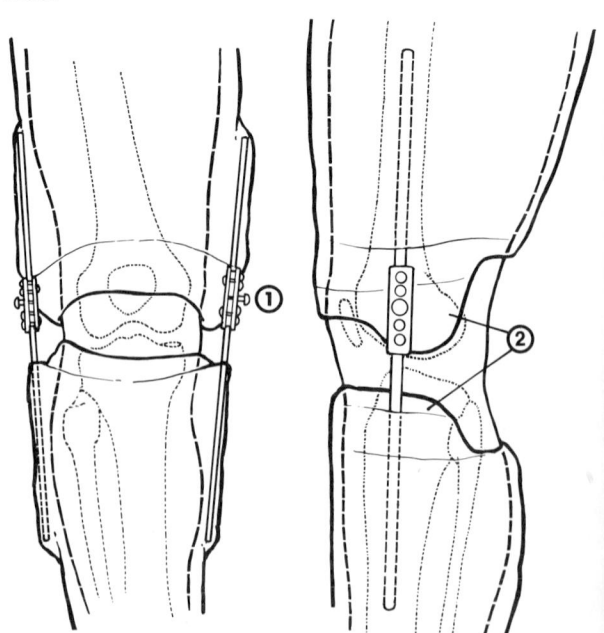

MANAGEMENT OF ACUTE PATELLAR DISLOCATION AND SUBLUXATION

Acute primary patellar subluxations and dislocations may be treated by aspiration of the knee joint followed by cast immobilization in an attempt to allow the disrupted anteromedial capsule to heal.

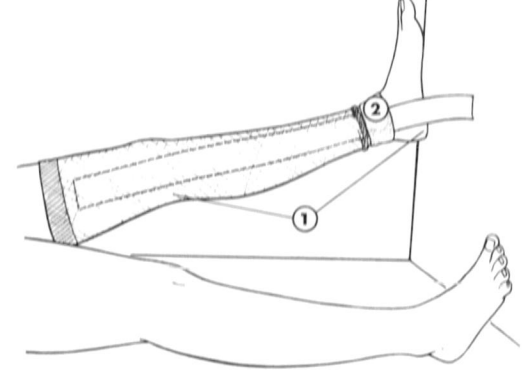

After aspirating the knee joint:
1. Apply a cylinder cast using a stockinette wrapped over 2 inch (5-cm) strips of tapes placed medially and laterally to serve as suspenders.
2. The malleoli are well padded.

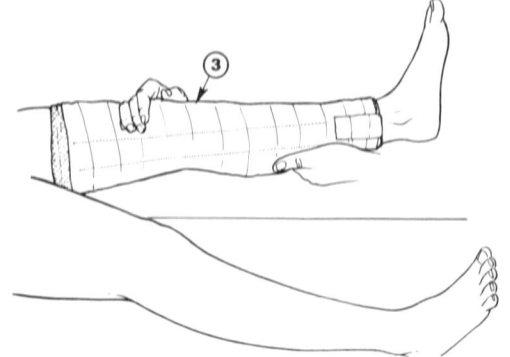

3. The plaster is molded firmly over the patella to push the patella medially and tighten the anteromedial retinaculum.

Subsequent Management

The patient is allowed to bear weight as tolerated.

During cast immobilization the patient should practice active quadriceps-setting and quadriceps-strengthening exercises.

The cast is removed after four weeks and range-of-motion exercises are started along with quadriceps and hamstring strengthening.

The patient should be advised that if recurrent subluxation or dislocation takes place, operative repair should be performed (see page 1663).

MANAGEMENT OF OSTEOCHONDRAL FRACTURES OF THE LATERAL FEMORAL CONDYLE

If the injury is detected within the first two weeks, replacement of the osteochondral fragment into the defect is possible.

Preoperative X-Ray

1. A lateral condylar fracture is evident.
2. The loose fragment is seen in the infrapatellar region.

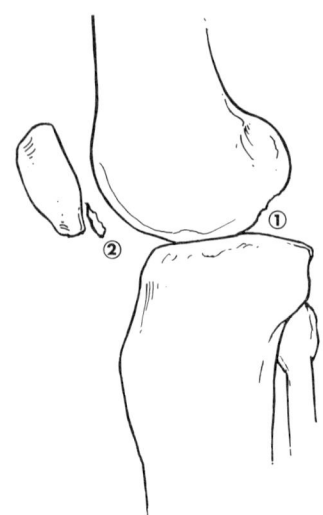

Postoperative X-Ray After Internal Fixation

1. The fragment has been replaced precisely back into its defect of origin.
2. Smillie nails are used to maintain fixation.

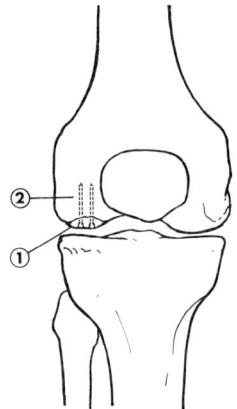

Subsequent Management

The knee is immobilized in a compressive dressing for two to three days postoperatively, until the acute swelling subsides.

Subsequently, the patient may start active range-of-motion exercises and partial weight bearing using crutches as the wound heals.

Early mobilization of the joint is essential to nourish the cartilage on the fragment and prevent it from gaining an alternative blood supply from the synovium.

Note: If the fracture is not diagnosed in the first two weeks after injury, the fragment cannot be replaced precisely and must be excised.

Acute Tears of the Posterior Cruciate Ligament

REMARKS

The posterior cruciate ligament, which runs through the central axis of the knee, is the basic stabilizer of the joint. Failure to recognize a tear or to repair it adequately usually results in a poorly functioning joint.

Anatomic dissection by Hughston and coworkers indicates that progressive tightening of the posterior cruciate ligament occurs during internal rotation of the tibia with the knee in either flexion or full extension. Also, in full extension the intact posterior cruciate allows minimal abduction or adduction opening of the joint. This is true even if the extensor retinaculum, capsular ligament, collateral ligaments, and posterior capsule have been removed. The posterior cruciate provides the basic static stability to the knee joint and the anterior cruciate and medial and lateral ligaments augment its effect.

The posterior cruciate ligament in combination with the extensor mechanism prevents anterior displacement of the femur on the fixed tibia during the stance phase of walking and running (see page 1545).

Clinical signs of an acute tear of the posterior cruciate depend on these anatomic functions. The primary signs of injury are a positive abduction or adduction stress test in extension and a positive anterior drawer test with the knee in internal rotation. The posterior drawer test may be negative in acute cases but it should also be performed (see page 1554).

With a chronic posterior cruciate tear, the posterior drawer test is positive owing to stretching of the posterior oblique and arcuate ligaments. These initially resist posterior displacement of the tibia and femur during gait despite the posterior cruciate tear. They lack the strength to withstand repetitive deceleration forces involved in normal walking, however, and eventually stretch to allow the posterior drawer test to be positive.

The posterior drawer test or sag test is also positive in acute injuries to the flexed knee such as car dashboard injuries, which displace the upper end of the tibia posteriorly. This mechanism produces acute arcuate and posterior oblique disruption as well as the cruciate tear.

If any of these signs are present, the posterior cruciate ligament must be explored thoroughly when either medial or lateral compartmental ligamentous injuries are repaired.

Mechanisms of Injury

1. Most commonly, rotational injuries are combined with varus or valgus stretch and produce
2. Tear of the posterior cruciate in association with
3. Tears of the medial or lateral ligaments.

Note: These injuries frequently disrupt the posterior cruciate ligament in its middle third or from its femoral attachment.

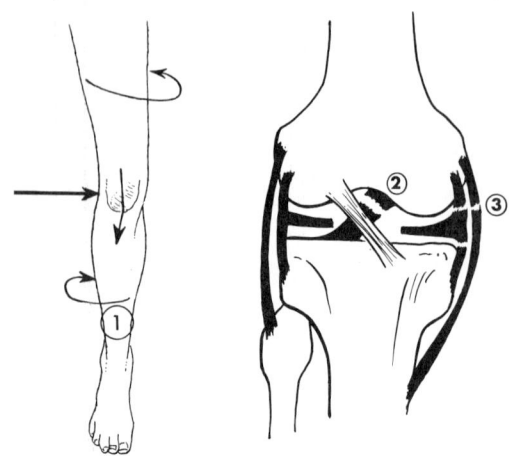

Alternate Mechanism

A less frequent but still common mechanism of posterior cruciate damage is injury to the flexed knee. For further discussion of the mechanism see page 1603.

Operative Repair of Posterior Cruciate and Medial Ligament Injuries (Hughston Approach)

1. A medial hockey stick incision is made with the patient supine, the hip abducted and externally rotated, and the knee flexed 90 degrees.
2. The incision extends along the line of the hamstrings and then along the medial joint line and curves distally at the patellar tendon.

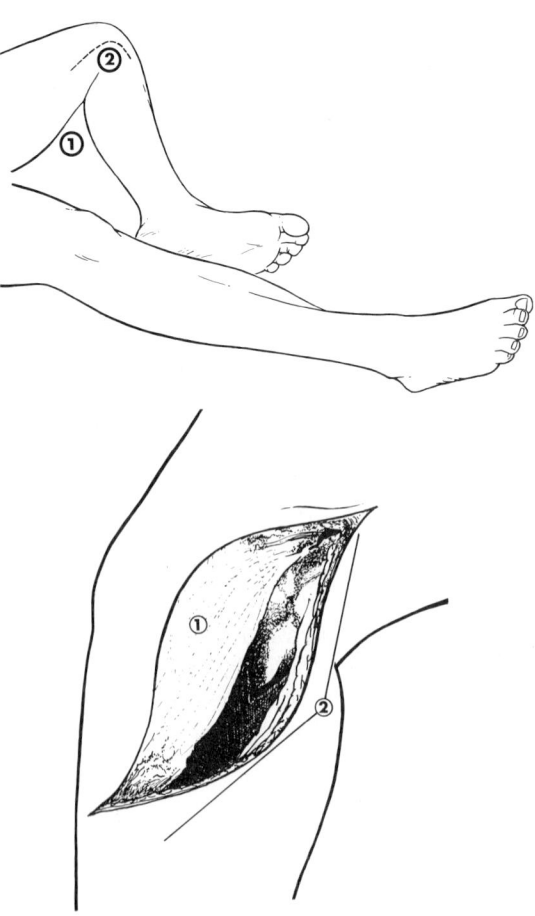

1. The skin and subcutaneous tissues are not dissected from the underlying fascia. The fascia lata is incised in line with the skin.
2. The proximal flap is reflected to reach the distal portion of the vastus medialis, and the distal flap is reflected to reach the pes anserinus.

1. In the acute injury the superficial ligaments and
2. The deep medial ligaments are irregularly and transversely disrupted, so that visualization of the entire joint is possible by abduction of the knee.

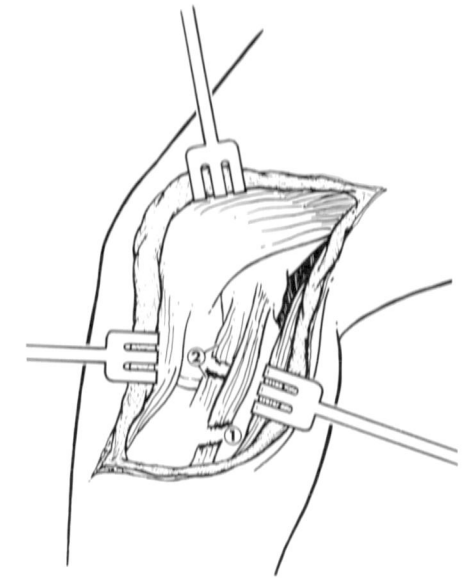

If the medial ligaments are not torn severely,
1. The knee joint is examined through a longitudinal, anteromedial retinacular incision along the medial border of the patella and the patellar tendon.
2. The posterior half of the medial meniscus and tibial attachment of the posterior cruciate are visualized through a longitudinal incision between the tibial collateral ligament and the posterior oblique ligament.
3. The posterior attachment of the posterior cruciate is exposed through an incision along the medial border of the medial gastrocnemius.

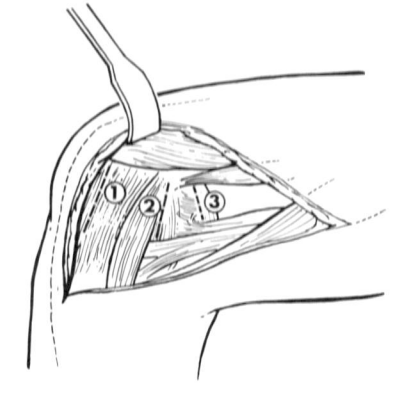

Note: For tears of the lateral ligaments associated with a posterior cruciate, a similar hockey stick incision is made on the lateral side of the knee. This must be supplemented by an anteromedial incision to examine the intra-articular structures and a posteromedial incision to expose the femoral origin of the posterior cruciate (see pages 1572, 1586, and 1594).

1. For avulsions of the ligament from the femoral attachment, the intercondylar face of the medial femoral condyle is curetted to a bleeding surface, and three parallel holes are made through the medial femoral condyle at the point of normal attachment of the posterior cruciate.
2. Heavy nonabsorbable 0 suture is passed through the three holes and is then tied to the medial femoral condyle.

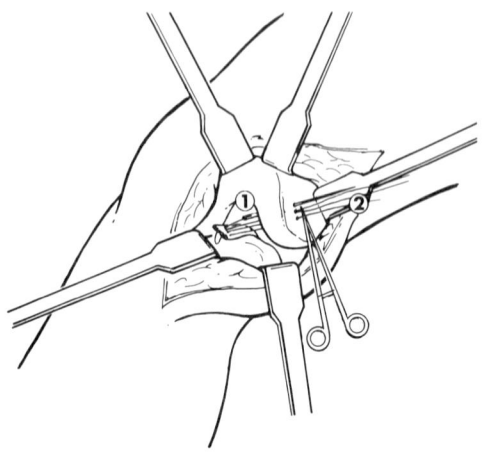

1. After tautness of the ligament is tested by light palpation and gentle abduction at 0 degrees and gentle drawer testing, the knee is flexed to 90 degrees and extended to 30 degrees while tension is maintained on the sutures. If these knee movements are associated with sliding of the sutures in and out of the hole, the site of the attachment must be repositioned because it is off-center.

Note: Before finally tying the sutures in the posterior cruciate ligament, repair the medial or lateral ligamentous injuries. Then, while the knee is flexed 45 degrees and the tibia displaced anteriorly on the femur, the sutures are tied snugly.

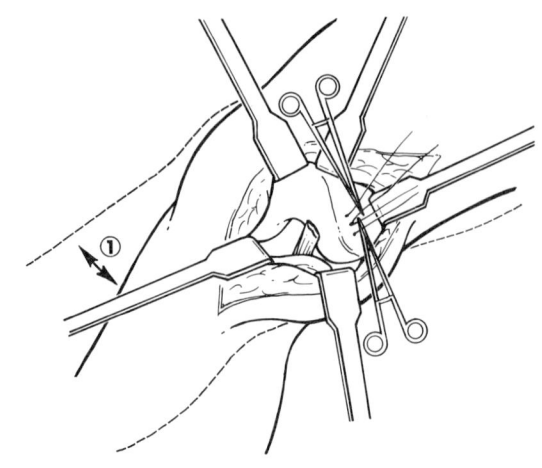

Subsequent Management

Apply a compression dressing with a thigh-to-foot plaster cast that maintains the knee in 45 degrees of flexion until the swelling subsides.

Approximately six days after operation, the postoperative dressing can be changed to a snugly fitting long leg cast.

At the end of three weeks a cast-brace may be applied, molding down well over the femoral condyles and tibial plateau. This is maintained for four to six weeks longer while the patient regains knee motion.

Avoid a too-rapid return to full extension. Flexion and extension can be controlled by stops on the hinges if necessary to protect the cruciate ligament repair.

CAUTION

Avoid applying a loose cast-brace, which does not protect against varus and valgus strain.

1. The cast-brace must be carefully molded down over the femoral condyles anteriorly.
2. There should be sufficient posterior clearance to allow 40 to 60 degrees of knee flexion.

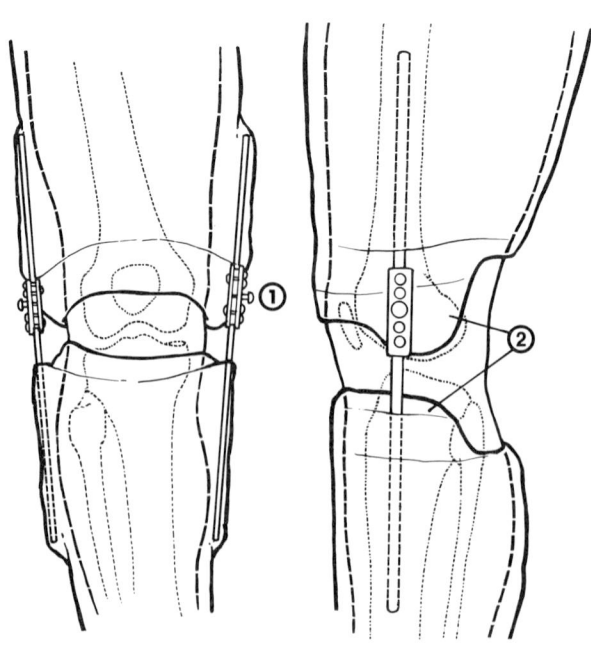

RUPTURE OF THE POSTERIOR CRUCIATE LIGAMENT FROM A DIRECT BLOW TO THE FLEXED KNEE

REMARKS

This mechanism is less common than rotatory mechanisms producing posterior cruciate ligament tears, but it does occur.

Typically, a direct blow to the anterior tibia occurs from a dashboard injury in an automobile or from a fall. The force drives the tibia posteriorly and avulses the tibial attachment of the posterior cruciate. The posterior cruciate is not attached to the posterior tibial spine but rather to the intercondylar area on the posterior aspect of the tibia.

Detachment of the posterior horn of the medial or lateral meniscus is commonly associated with posterior cruciate injury. The posterior oblique and arcuate ligaments are also likely to be ruptured.

Disruption of the posterior oblique or arcuate ligament complex results in a positive posterior drawer test. This is in contrast to posterior cruciate ligament injury from rotational mechanisms, in which there is no posterior drawer sign (see also page 1556).

Characteristically, the patient presents with a swollen knee, abrasions and lacerations on the anterior surface of the proximal tibia, and tenderness to deep palpation in the popliteal fossa.

X-rays characteristically show bone fragments of varying size and displacement from the posterior tibial surface.

For injuries with fragments of minimal size, i.e., less than 1.3 cm or minimal displacement, i.e., .3 to .5 cm, closed treatment yields satisfactory results.

For larger fragments or greater displacement, operative treatment is necessary to avoid problems with knee instability and symptomatic limitation of knee flexion.

A delayed repair of an avulsion fracture is also indicated if the fragment is large and if the patient presents with pain on walking, restricted flexion, and/or synovial effusion.

Fixation of the bone fragment may be difficult. Torisu recommends a staple rather than a screw to avoid comminution of the fragment.

The associated injury of the posterior meniscus should also be repaired. The meniscus should not be removed, if it is at all possible to keep it.

Mechanism of Injury

1. Most commonly posterior cruciate ligament injury results from a fall with the knee flexed or a direct blow to the front of the tibia, as from the dashboard in a motor vehicle accident.

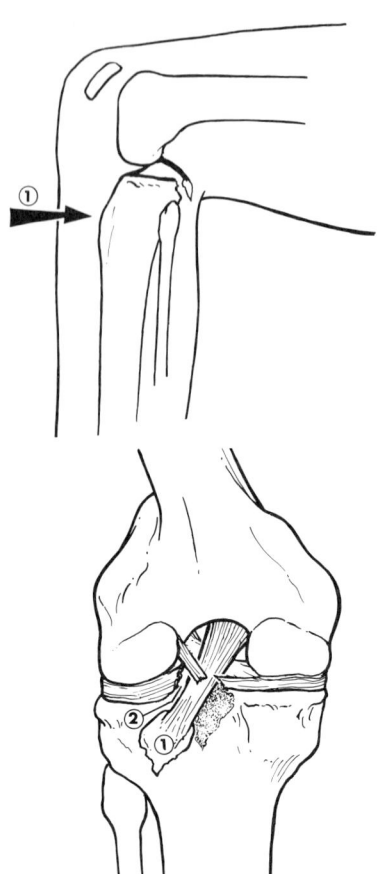

1. The posterior cruciate ligament is avulsed from its attachment to the posterior intercondylar surface of the tibia.
2. The posterior horn of the lateral meniscus may be detached.

Diagnosis

Suspect this injury in any patient who presents with abrasions or lacerations on the proximal anterior surface of the tibia, knee swelling, and popliteal pain.

Diagnostic Maneuvers: Posterior Drawer Sign

Note: This test may be limited by pain that causes the patient to guard the knee. It should be done under adequate anesthesia. Posterior cruciate disruption frequently leads to mediolateral instability with the knee in full extension when there is associated medial capsular injury (see pages 1554, 1556, 1599).

1. The knee is flexed at a right angle.
2. The femur is fixed.
3. Backward displacement of the tibia indicates a lesion of the posterior cruciate.

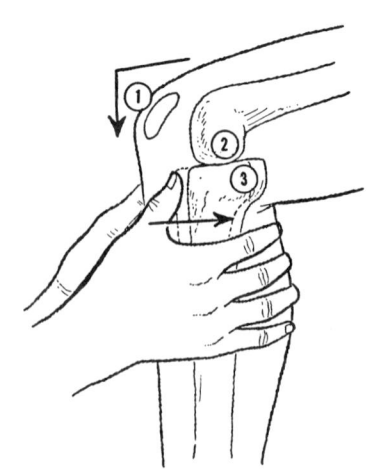

Recurvatum-Rotation Test (for Posterior Cruciate and Arcuate Complex Disruption)

1. Elevate both legs by the toes.
2. The injured leg rotates externally.
3. Hyperextension is evident on the injured side.

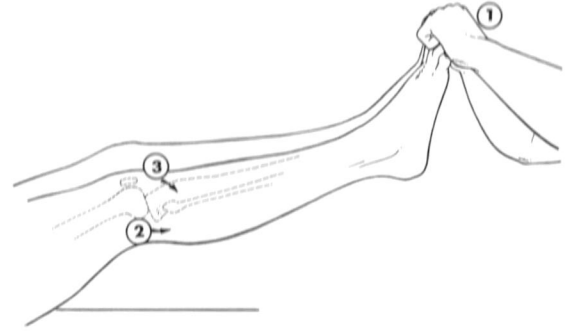

X-ray of Injury with Small Fragments Suitable for Closed Treatment

1. A fragment is less than 1 cm in size.
2. Separation is minimal, i.e., less than .3 cm.

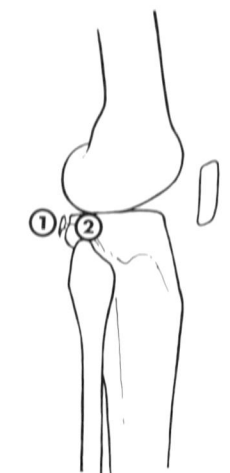

Closed Treatment

If the knee joint is swollen, it should be aspirated and:

1. A plaster cast is applied with the knee in a flexed position.
2. The tibia is pulled forward during cast application so as to relax tension on the posterior cruciate.

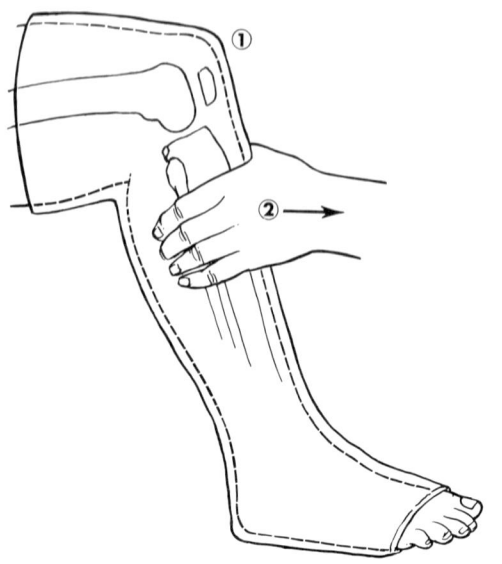

Subsequent Management

The cast immobilizes the knee in the flexed position for six weeks.

While in the cast, the patient must practice isometric quadriceps and hamstring exercises.

After the cast is removed, therapy is started to regain knee motion and quadriceps strength.

X-Ray of Injury Requiring Surgical Repair

Large fragments or fragments with more than .3 to .5 cm. of displacement should be treated operatively. Nonunion is common and causes prolonged knee trouble unless the fragments are restored anatomically.

1. Avulsion and displacement of a fragment of bone from the tibia at the site of inferior attachment of the posterior cruciate ligament.

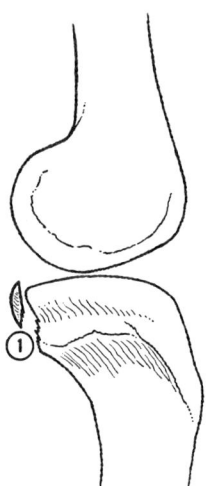

Operative Repair for Lesions of the Posterior Cruciate Ligament

1. Make a vertical S-shaped incision centered over the posterior joint line.
2. Divide the deep fascia and develop the interval between the inner head of the gastrocnemius and the tendon of the semitendinosus.

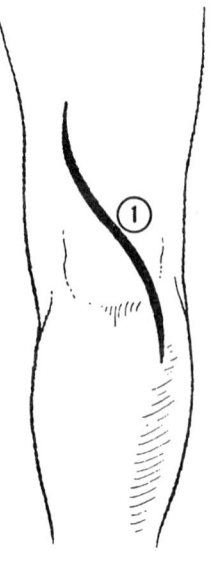
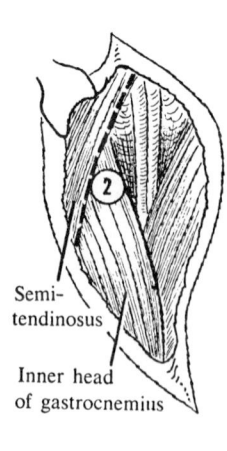

3. Cut the inner head of the gastrocnemius and displace the muscle together with the neurovascular bundle laterally, exposing the posterior capsule of the joint.

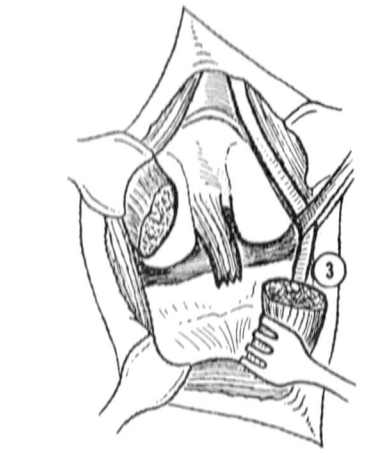

When a fragment of bone is avulsed with the ligament:
Identify the fragment of bone and the corresponding defect in the tibia.
Curette the defect free of blood clots and debris.
Secure the fragment in its normal position by one of the following methods:
1. Fasten the fragment in position by interrupted sutures passing through the surrounding capsular tissue.
2. If the fragment is large, anchor it to the tibia with a screw.
3. If the fragment is very small, anchor it to the tibia with an appropriate sized staple or with sutures passed through parallel channels, drilled 1 cm apart into the medial tibial condyle. The ends of the sutures are tied on the anterior surface of the tibia.

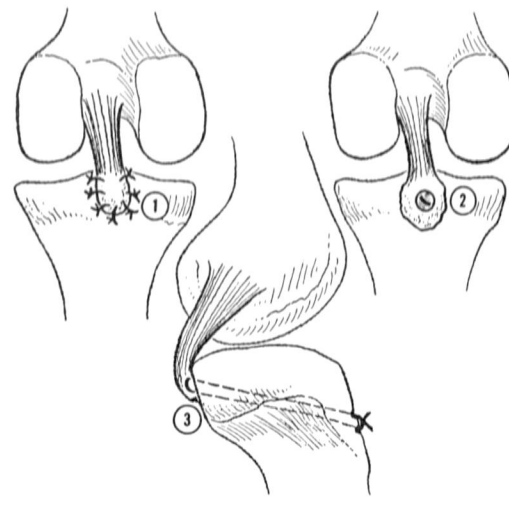

When the superior end of the ligament is detached from the femur:
1. Open the capsule and identify the posterior cruciate ligament.
2. Make two parallel drill channels in the medial femoral condyle from just above the epicondyle to the site of the attachment of the ligament. (These channels can also be made from within the joint outward.)
3. Secure the end of the ligament to the medial femoral condyle by a mattress suture passing through the distal stump of the ligament and the drill channels in the medial femoral condyle; tie the ends of the suture over the medial epicondylar area.

Note: The other torn ligaments must be sutured back firmly to their bony attachments after the cruciate is repaired.

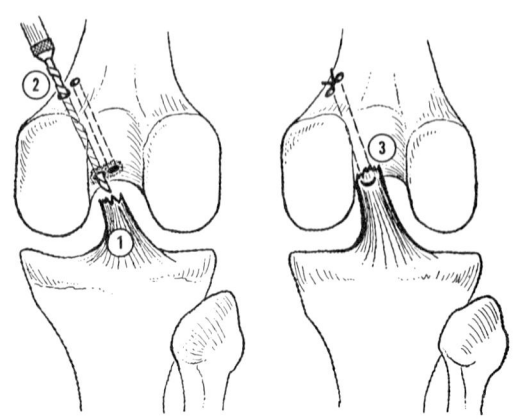

Postoperative X-Ray

1. Large bony fragment is anchored to the tibia with a screw.

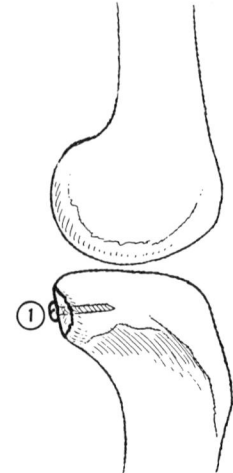

Immobilization

1. Apply a plaster-of-paris cast with
2. The knee flexed 20 degrees.
3. The toes are free.
4. The transverse and longitudinal arches are supported by molding of the cast on the foot.

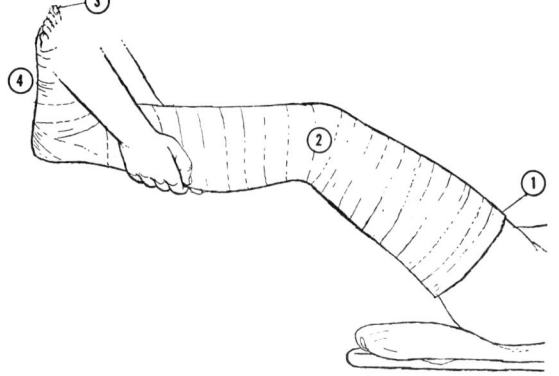

Subsequent Management

While the patient is in the cast, encourage active quadriceps and hamstring exercises.

Remove the cast at the end of four weeks and allow partial weight bearing with crutches.

At the end of six weeks, full weight bearing is usually possible.

The internal fixation need not be removed routinely.

Avulsion Fracture of the Tibial Spine

REMARKS

This lesion is comparable to detachment of the anterior cruciate ligament with a fragment of bone from its tibial attachment.

It is most commonly encountered in children from 8 to 13 years of age and is usually the result of sudden flexion and internal rotation of the knee, most characteristically in a fall from a bicycle.

The injury, when it occurs in adults, results from more violence to the knee and produces greater disruption of the joint support structures than the same injury in a child. Consequently, the prognosis for complete recovery after this injury is much better in children than in adults (see also page 234).

The degree of displacement of the bony fragments varies from none to marked. Fractures of the tibial spine in children that maintain contact with the tibial surface can be treated by aspiration of the hemarthrosis and cast immobilization with the knee in slight flexion.

Fractures that are completely dislodged or that occur in adults should be treated by open reduction and fixation of the fragment.

Open reduction and fixation should also be done for old fractures with dislodged fragments causing catching or locking of the knee joint.

Types of Fractures

A. PREREDUCTION X-RAY

1. Avulsion of the anterior tibial spine with minimal displacement.

B. PREREDUCTION X-RAY

1. Avulsion of the anterior tibial spine.
2. The fragment is moderately displaced.

C. PREREDUCTION X-RAY

1. Avulsion of the anterior tibial spine with marked displacement.
2. The fragment lies deep in the intercondylar notch of the femur.

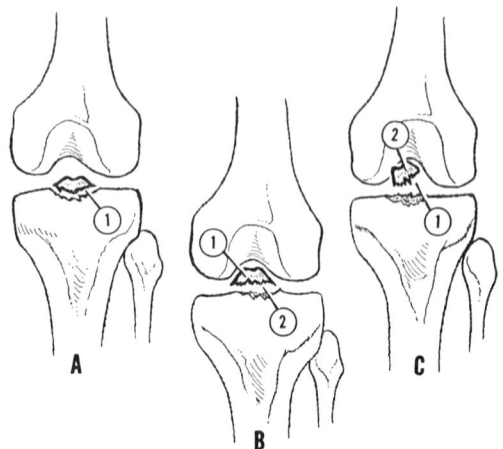

Closed Reduction by Hyperextension of the Knee

Note: Before reduction is attempted the patient is given general anesthesia and the knee is aspirated of blood and synovial fluid.

1. Force the knee gently and firmly into a position of hyperextension.
2. Then bring the knee back to the position of 180 degrees (full extension) and take check x-rays.

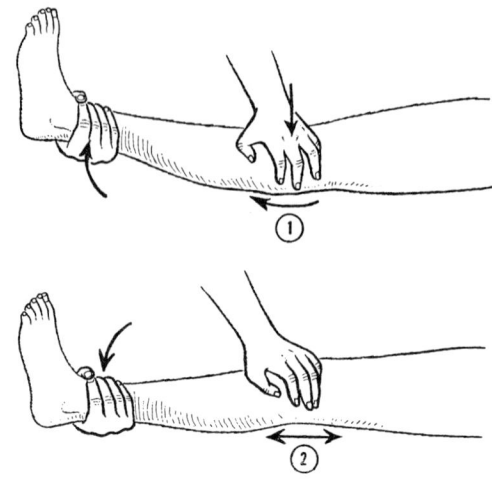

Postreduction X-ray

1. The fragment is shown in its normal anatomic position.

Immobilization

1. Apply a well-padded long leg cast.
2. The knee is in 5 degrees of flexion; it is not hyperextended.
3. The foot is dorsiflexed 90 degrees.

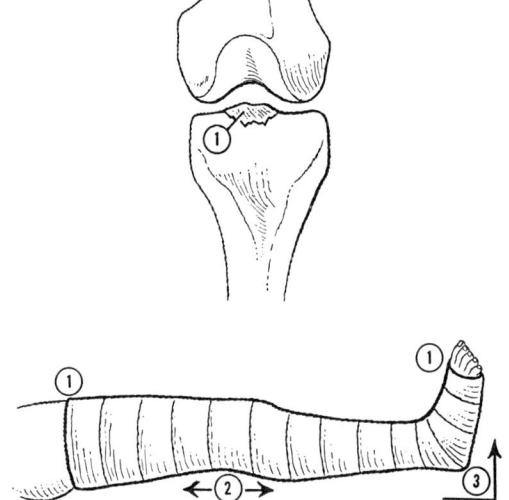

Postreduction Management

Continue cast immobilization for eight to ten weeks, until healing is evident radiographically.

During cast immobilization the patient should practice quadriceps-strengthening exercises.

When the cast is removed at eight weeks, the patient should start progressive weight bearing with crutches and should continue with active range-of-motion exercises to the knee.

By two to three weeks after cast removal the crutches may be discarded, when the strength of the quadriceps and the range of knee motion are returning to normal.

Operative Reduction

Note: This method is employed if closed methods fail to return the fragment to its normal anatomic position.

1. Expose the intercondylar region of the tibia with a medial parapatellar incision.
2. After flushing all blood clots out of the joint cavity, identify the fragment and the defect in the superior aspect of the tibia.

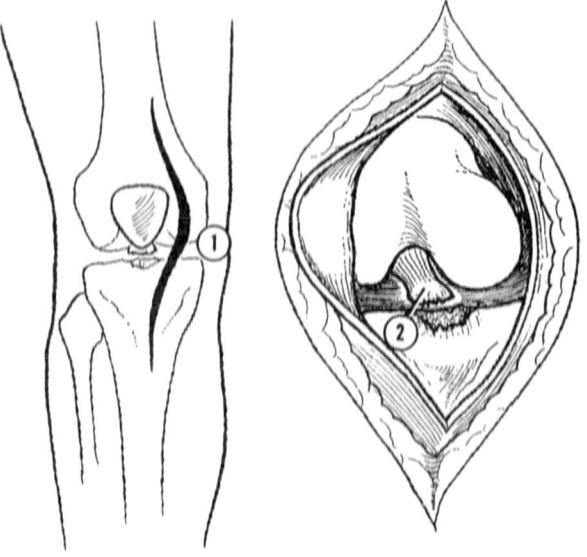

FIXATION FOR TIBIAL SPINE INJURY IN CHILDREN

1. For completely detached fragments, in order to avoid damaging the tibial epiphysis,
2. Suture the displaced fragment by simple mattress sutures to the edge of the meniscus.

MANAGEMENT IN ADULTS

1. Make two parallel drill channels in the medial condyle of the tibia. They begin on the anteromedial surface of the condyle 4 cm below the tibial brim and are directed obliquely upward, backward, and inward, and issue from the base of the defect in the intercondylar region of the tibia.
2. If the fragment is large, perforate it with two small drill holes and pass through them a stout silk suture.
3. If the fragment is small, pass the suture through the inferior end of the cruciate ligament.
4. Pass the ends of the suture through the drill holes in the tibial condyle, pull the fragment snugly in place, and tie the ends of the suture on the anterior surface of the tibia.

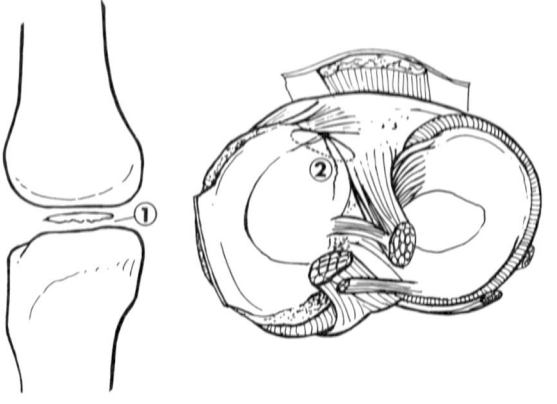

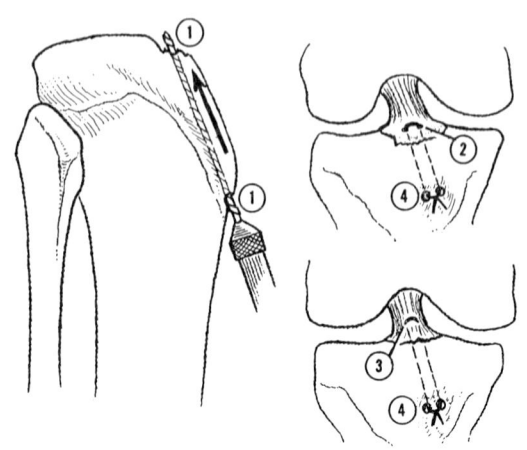

Immobilization

1. Apply a well-padded long leg cast.
2. The knee is in 5 degrees of flexion; it is not hyperextended.
3. The foot is dorsiflexed 90 degrees.

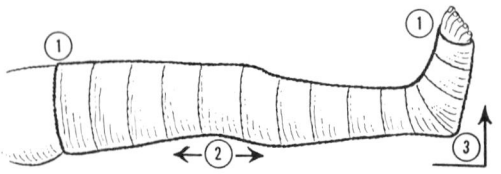

Postoperative Management

Continue cast immobilization for eight to ten weeks, until healing is evident radiographically.

During cast immobilization the patient should practice quadriceps-strengthening exercises.

When the cast is removed at eight weeks, the patient should start progressive weight bearing with crutches and should continue with active range-of-motion exercises to the knee.

By two to three weeks after cast removal the crutches may be discarded, when the strength of the quadriceps and the range of knee motion are returned to normal.

Avulsion Injuries of the Apophysis of the Tibial Tuberosity and Osgood-Schlatter's Syndrome

REMARKS

In the newborn, the tibial tuberosity is a cartilaginous projection that points downward like a tongue over the diaphysis. This cartilage projection persists until the age of 11 in girls and 13 in boys, at which time one or more centers of ossification appear that are separated from the metaphysis and epiphysis by cartilage.

Eventually the ossification centers join to the proximal tibial epiphysis and the metaphysis, and by age 18 or 19 the bony tuberosity has developed completely.

During the developmental period, an active adolescent subjects the relatively weak tibial apophysis to injury either from a direct blow or from avulsion by a sudden pull of the patellar tendon. The result is frequently a partial separation of the superior aspect of the tuberosity, which is also known as Osgood-Schlatter's syndrome. This condition is self-limited and usually responds to rest and cast immobilization in the young adolescent.

A small percentage of adolescents with Osgood-Schlatter's syndrome will have persistent pain due to nonunion of the separated bony ossicle in the superior pole of the tuberosity. This will frequently cause the teenager to limit participation in sports or vigorous activities. It will also occasionally persist and cause symptoms even in the 20-year-old military recruit. Surgical excision of the loose ossicle is indicated to relieve disabling symptoms in the older teenager or young adult.

Rarely a sudden, violent contraction of the quadriceps with the knee in a flexed position will completely avulse the tibial tuberosity. Prompt operative repair is the treatment of choice for this type of tuberosity injury.

OSGOOD-SCHLATTER'S SYNDROME

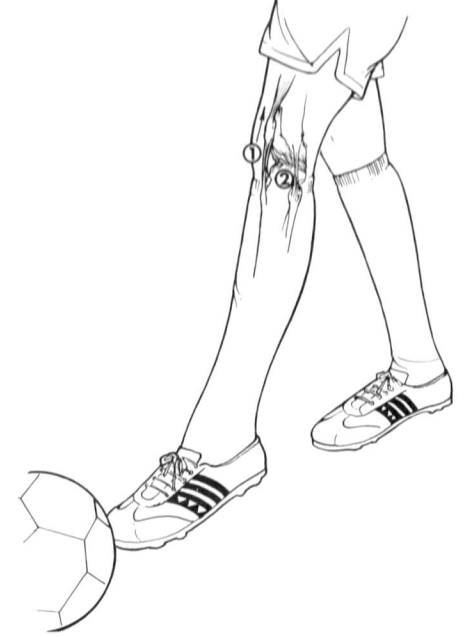

Mechanism

1. Repetitive or sudden loading of the patellar tendon produces
2. Avulsion of bone from the superior aspect of the tibial tuberosity.

Clinical Appearance

The patient is a boy or girl 11 to 15 years old who complains of painful swelling in the anterior aspect of the knee with running or going up and down stairs.

The infrapatellae bursa and peritendinous tissues are swollen.

Pain and bony motion can be reproduced by palpating the superior aspect of the tuberosity.

Appearance on X-Ray

1. An ossicle is evident in the superior aspect of the tibial tuberosity.

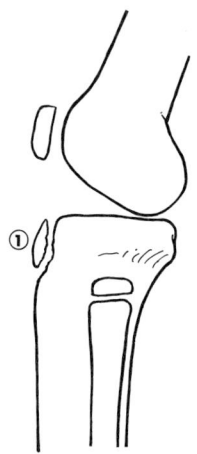

Management

1. Apply a well-padded plaster cylinder cast from the groin to above the malleoli.
2. The knee is in full extension.

Note: For persistent symptoms, it may rarely be necessary to inject a combination of local anesthetic and steroid into the infrapatellar bursa, but not into the patellar tendon, to obtain complete relief from pain.

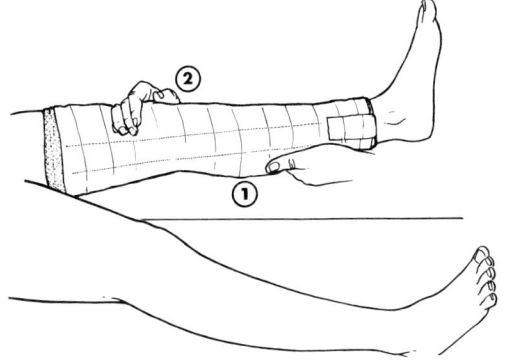

Subsequent Management

Allow the patient to bear weight with the cylinder cast and crutches. The cast is maintained for four weeks, after which it is removed.

X-Ray Three Months after Cast Immobilization

1. The tuberosity fragment is healing to the main bony portion of the tibial tuberosity.

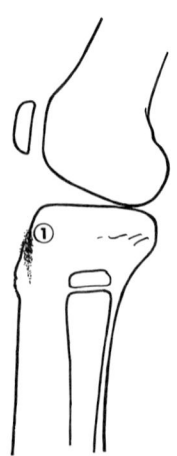

Operative Treatment of Persistent Osgood-Schlatter's Syndrome by a Patellar Tendon Transplant (Elmslie-Trillat)

In the older adolescent or young adult with recurrent intermittent symptoms from an avulsion fracture of the tibial tuberosity, operative treatment is warranted.

Removal of any loose bony ossicles and transfer of the patellar tendon medially permit the individual to resume sports and other vigorous activities that he or she has been avoiding because of recurrent knee pain.

1. A "smile" incision is made curving distally around the tibial tuberosity and up to the tibial plateaus medially and laterally. This leaves the most cosmetically satisfactory scar.
2. The infrapatella-bursa is visualized, and any loose bony ossicle is removed.
3. The tibial tubercle is osteotomized from just proximal to the insertion of the patellar tendon distally for 3 to 4 cm.

Note: The osteotomy fragment should be approximately .5 cm thick.

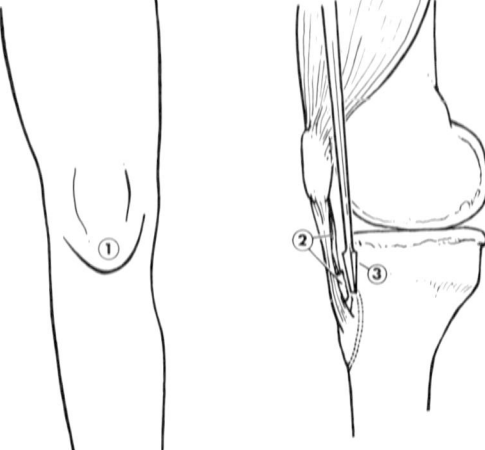

1. Periosteum medial to the tibial tuberosity is reflected medially.
2. The osteotomized tubercle with the patellar tendon and its distal periosteum intact is pivoted medially so that

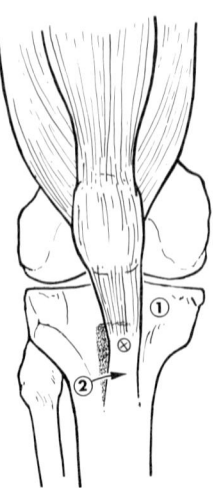

Operative Treatment of Persistent Osgood-Schlatter's Syndrome by a Patellar Tendon Transplant (Elmslie-Trillat) (Continued)

3. The patellar tendon lies in the anatomic axis of the femur with the knee flexed 45 degrees.
4. The tuberosity is fixed to the underlying bone with a cancellous screw, and the reflected periosteum is sutured to it.
5. The patella is not displaced distally.

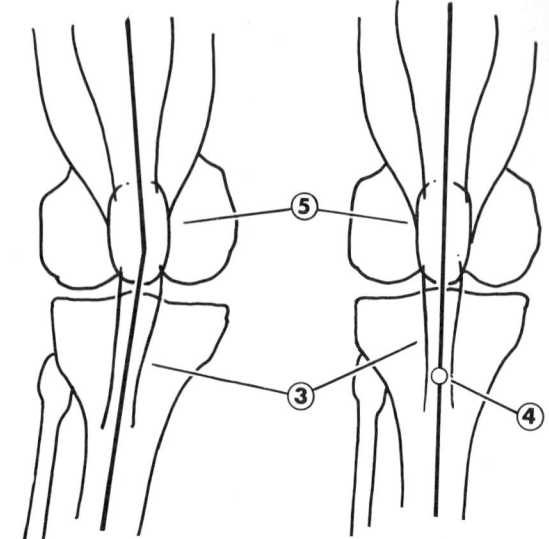

Subsequent Management

1. Apply a compression dressing around the knee.
2. Place the limb in a posterior splint from the thigh to the toes.
3. The knee is extended fully and the foot is at a right angle.

Note: Always observe the patient carefully in the immediate postoperative period for anterior compartment syndrome. This is a hazard especially after operations in this region of the leg. Severe postoperative pain and numbness in the foot are the major signs of impending ischemia as a result of swelling in the anterior compartment.

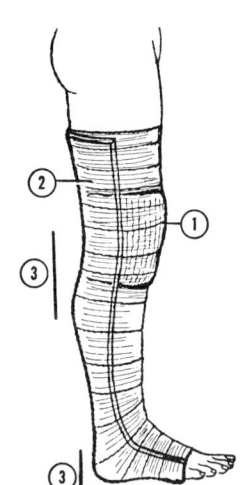

After three to five days, remove the postoperative dressing and:
1. Apply a long leg walking cast.
2. The knee is in extension.
3. The foot is dorsiflexed.

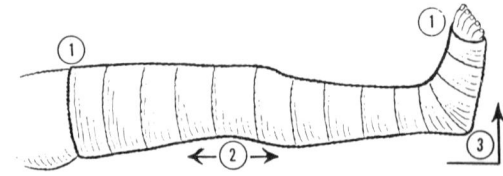

INJURIES TO THE LIGAMENTS OF THE KNEE JOINT

COMPLETE AVULSION OF THE TIBIAL TUBEROSITY

A sudden violent contraction of the quadriceps in an adolescent with immature bone may rarely completely avulse the tibial tuberosity or the proximal tibial epiphysis.

The same mechanism in the adult will cause rupture of the quadriceps tendon or the patellar tendon (see pages 1650 and 1654).

The treatment of choice in any of these injuries is prompt operative repair to restore the extensor mechanism to the knee joint.

Types of Fractures

A. PREREDUCTION X-RAY

1. The entire anterior prolongation of the tibial epiphysis is pulled away from the anterior surface of the tibia; the base of prolongation is intact.

B. PREREDUCTION X-RAY

1. The anterior prolongation is pulled away from the anterior surface of the tibia.
2. The base of the epiphyseal prolongation is fractured.

C. PREREDUCTION X-RAY

1. A small separate epiphysis of the tubercle is avulsed and pulled upward.

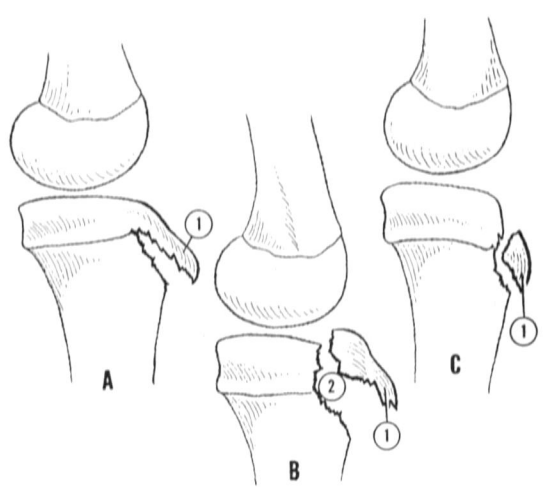

Operative Reduction

1. A "smile" incision is made curving distally around the tibial tuberosity and proximally up toward the tibial plateaus. This leaves the most cosmetically satisfactory scar.
2. Reflect the skin and the deep fascia outward, exposing the patellar tendon and the avulsed epiphysis.

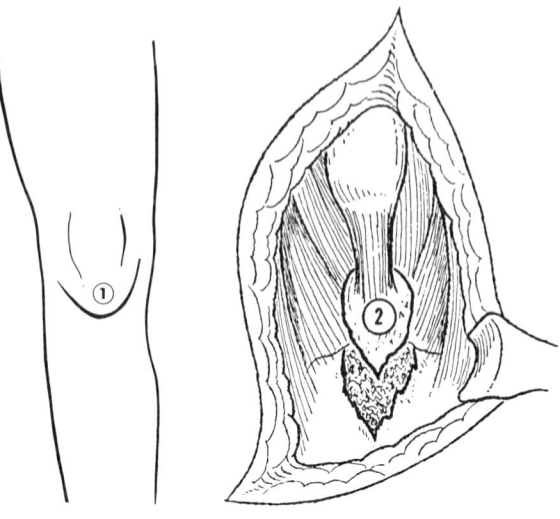

Operative Reduction (Continued)

1. Grasp the tuberosity with a towel clip and place it in its anatomic position on the anterior surface of the tibia.

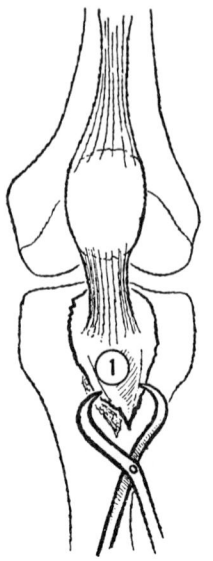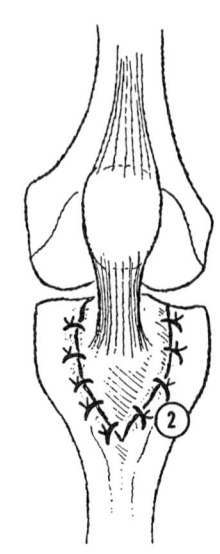

2. Fix the fracture fragment with multiple sutures or a cancellous screw drilled distally to avoid crossing the tibial epiphyseal plate if it is still open.

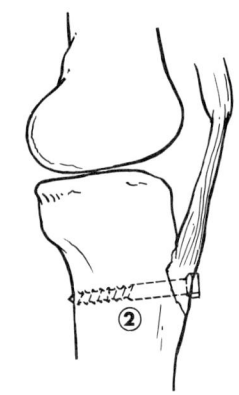

Postoperative management

1. Apply a compression bandage around the knee.
2. Place the limb on a posterior plaster splint extending from the upper third of the thigh to the toes.
3. The knee is extended fully and the foot is at a right angle.

Note: Always release the tourniquet prior to wound closure to obtain complete hemostasis and avoid periosteal vascular bleeding into the anterior compartment. Ischemic muscle necrosis is especially a hazard after operation in this region of the leg. Severe postoperative pain and numbness in the foot are the major signs of impending ischemia due to swelling in the anterior compartment.

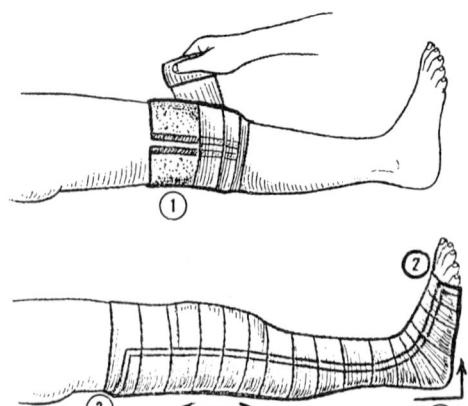

After three to five days remove the postoperative dressing and:
1. Apply a long leg walking cast.
2. The knee is in extension.
3. The foot is dorsiflexed.

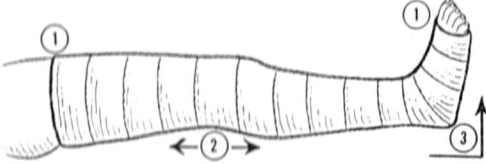

Now institute a regulated program of progressive quadriceps exercises.

Remove the cast at the end of five to six weeks and permit protected weight bearing with crutches. Now increase the intensity of the quadriceps and flexion exercises.

After the patient has regained full control of the knee joint, the crutches may be discarded. Quadriceps exercises must be continued for several months after this injury to restore full strength and function.

DISLOCATIONS AND FRACTURE-DISLOCATIONS OF THE KNEE JOINT

REMARKS

Complete dislocation of the knee, although uncommon, is a very serious injury. It carries a 30 to 40 per cent incidence of popliteal artery injury, a 35 per cent chance of peroneal nerve disruption, and a 100 per cent chance of cruciate and other ligament tears.

Common mechanisms include hyperextension forces, which produce anterior dislocation, and severe direct blows to the proximal tibia, which cause posterior, medial, or lateral dislocation.

All dislocated knees should be assumed to have limb-threatening popliteal artery injury until proven otherwise.

The dislocation should be reduced promptly under general anesthetic as a true emergency. If necessary, local injection of anesthetic into the joint space permits prompt reduction of most dislocations.

Any evidence of impaired posterior tibial or dorsalis pedis pulse after the reduction warrants prompt exploration of the popliteal artery. A warm foot in the absence of distal pulses does not indicate adequate circulation. If the popliteal circulation is not restored within 8 hours, the likelihood of amputation or ischemic muscle injury is virtually 100 per cent.

A posterior dislocation is most likely to tear the vessel. Anterior dislocation stretches it and causes extensive intimal damage; this should not be mistaken for arteriospasm but should be treated by arteriotomy to determine the extent of intimal damage. The injured segment must be resected and the artery must be repaired either by direct anastomosis or by graft. Fasciotomy is indicated in many, if not all, dislocations with arterial damage because of the markedly increased swelling following restoration of circulation (see page 67).

Peroneal nerve injury is usually extensive and the prognosis for return of function is poor. Attempted operative repair of the nerve is unwarranted. Rather, brace support and tendon transfer should be employed to restore foot control for the patient who has persistent disability from the palsy.

DISLOCATIONS AND FRACTURE-DISLOCATIONS OF THE KNEE JOINT

Once the reduction is accomplished and distal circulation is restored, the next consideration is ligamentous injury. If the knee is unstable after reduction, the chance for restoring stability is improved by operative repair, just as it would be with a combined ligamentous injury of the knee joint.

Meyers and Harvey have demonstrated the frequency of complete cruciate ligament tears with dislocation and the importance of repairing all torn ligaments, including the posterior cruciate and posterior capsular ligaments.

If there has been any impairment of circulation, ligamentous reconstruction should be delayed for at least 5 to 7 days to be sure that ischemic muscle injury will not occur. If the adequacy of distal circulation is in doubt, an arteriogram should be performed prior to any operative reconstruction of the ligaments and tourniquet ischemia should be used cautiously during operation.

Forty per cent of knee dislocations are associated with fractures including avulsions of the tibial attachment of the posterior cruciate, fractures of the tibial tuberosity, lateral or medial plateau fractures, and fractures of the femoral or tibial shaft. Fractures of the medial tibial plateau are particularly likely to produce resistant or recurrent dislocation of the knee, even during cast immobilization. Internal fixation is required to provide knee stability.

Rarely, the dislocated knee may prove resistant to reduction, particularly a posterolateral dislocation. This complication should be anticipated if there is a medial indentation due to soft tissue inclusion that becomes more pronounced with attempted reduction. Most often, open reduction may be necessary to remove structures entrapped in the joint in this rare injury.

Types of Dislocations

1. Anterior dislocation.
2. Posterior dislocation.
3. Lateral dislocation.

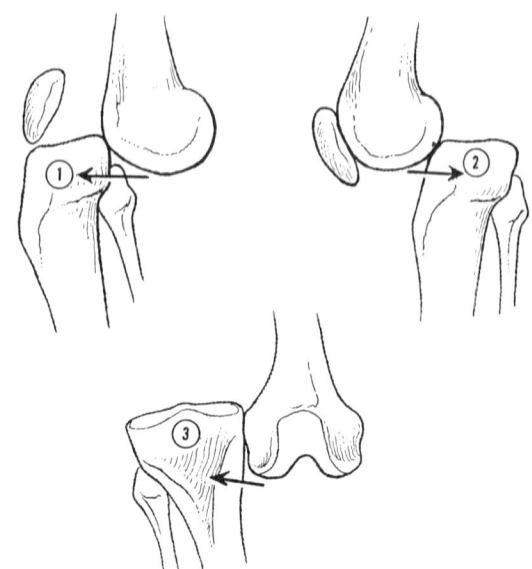

Types of Dislocations
(Continued)

1. Medial dislocation.
2 and 3. Rotatory dislocations; these are extremely rare.

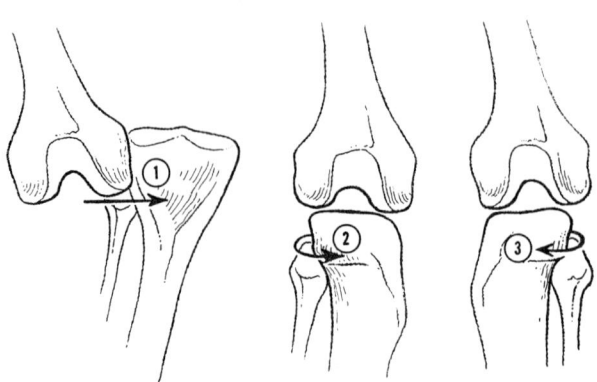

Fracture-Dislocation

1. The femoral condyle is displaced medially and posteriorly with a fracture of the medial tibial plateau.
2. The major portion of the tibial articular surface displaces anterolaterally.

Note: To achieve stability of this injury, internal fixation of the medial tibial fracture is necessary.

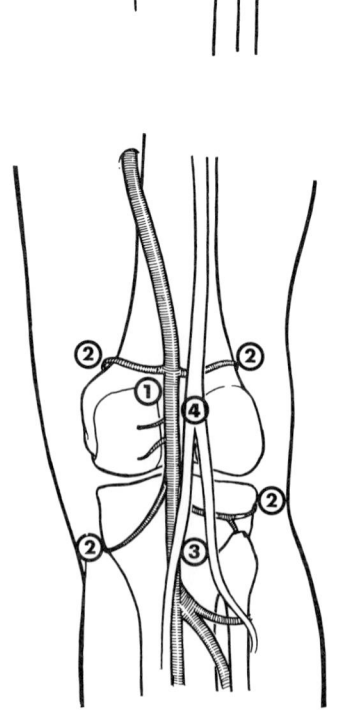

Neurovascular Anatomy

1. The exposed position of the popliteal artery and its fixation by
2. The geniculate branches and
3. The anterior and posterior branches make it susceptible to complete laceration or intimal thrombosis in 30 to 40 per cent of knee dislocations.
4. The fixed position of the common peroneal nerve makes it susceptible to severe stretch or tearing in at least 30 per cent of knee dislocations.

Note: Assume that all dislocations have significant neurovascular injury until proven otherwise by clinical and/or arteriographic examination. Arterial injury should be promptly explored and repaired. Exploration of the stretch injury of the nerve, however, is not indicated.

TECHNIQUE OF REDUCTION

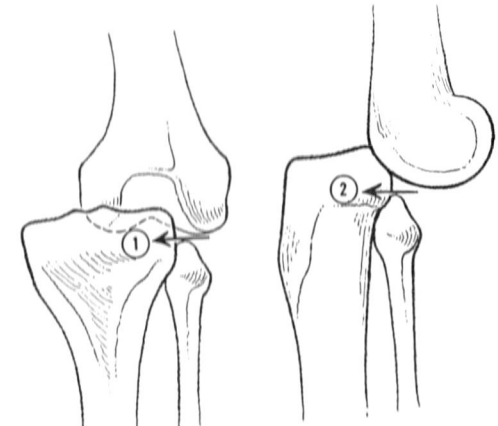

Prereduction X-Ray

1. The tibia is dislocated medially.
2. The tibia is dislocated anteriorly.

Manipulative Reduction

This should be done under either local or general anesthesia as soon as possible after the accident. The reduction technique is relatively simple and may have been accomplished by emergency rescue squad personnel, or reduction may have occurred spontaneously. Always check carefully for distal circulation if such a history is obtained.

1. An assistant fixes and makes counter traction on the thigh.
2. Another assistant makes straight traction on the leg (this usually reduces the dislocation).
3. The surgeon puts direct pressure over the displaced bones.

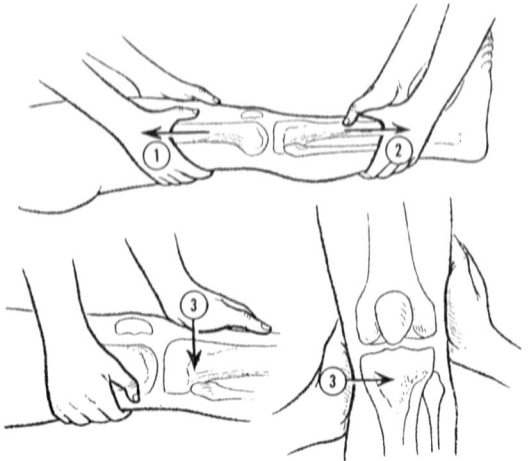

Postreduction X-Ray

1. The tibia and the femur show normal relationship to each other on the anteroposterior view.
2. There is no persistent anterior or posterior subluxation on the lateral view.

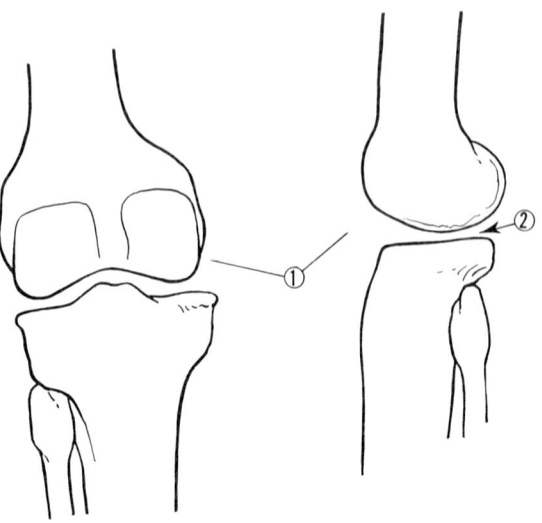

Immediate Postreduction Management

Note: Always check stability immediately after reduction to determine if there is obvious Type III instability or instability limited to one plane (see page 1554).

1. Aspirate the joint of blood and synovial fluid.
2. Apply a compression bandage extending from the groin to the midcalf.
3. Apply a posterior plaster splint from the groin to the toes.
4. The foot is dorsiflexed 90 degrees.
5. The knee is flexed 20 degrees.

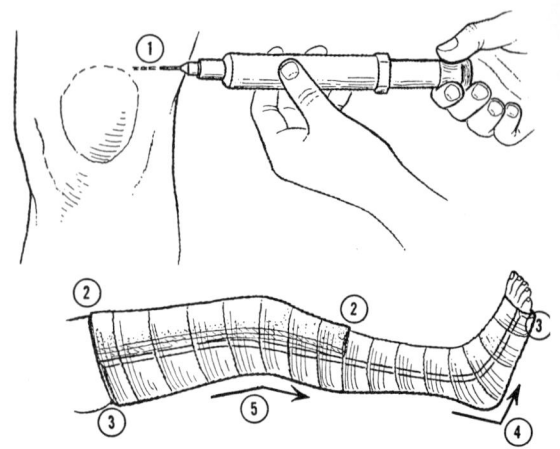

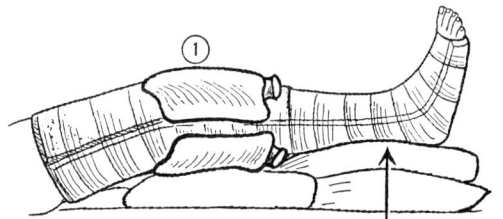

1. Elevate the limb and surround it with ice packs for 3 to 5 days while circulation is carefully evaluated.

NONOPERATIVE TREATMENT

REMARKS

Delayed operative repair is indicated for most knee dislocations owing to the usual disruption of capsular and posterior cruciate ligaments.

If the tests of the knee joint stability after reduction of the dislocation indicate that instability is of the Grade II type (see page 1562), closed treatment may be warranted. Also, if other more serious injuries or the patient's advanced age dictates, closed treatment may be necessary.

If the dislocation was posterior, immobilize the knee in flexion with the tibia pushed forward so as to encourage posterior capsular healing.

For an anterior dislocation immobilize the knee in extension.

Immobilize the knee continuously for 4 weeks and then apply a cast brace to protect the knee while motion is started.

Operative repair is indicated when there is Type III instability evident on testing after reduction (see pages 1572 and 1599).

Operative fixation is also necessary for the occasional dislocation associated with a tibial plateau fracture.

When operative treatment is employed, it is best delayed 5 to 7 days to insure adequacy of distal circulation.

Closed Treatment

1. When circulation is assured, apply a long leg cast with the knee flexed 45 degrees.
2. The tibia is pushed forward in the cast to promote tight healing of the posterior capsule in posterior dislocation.

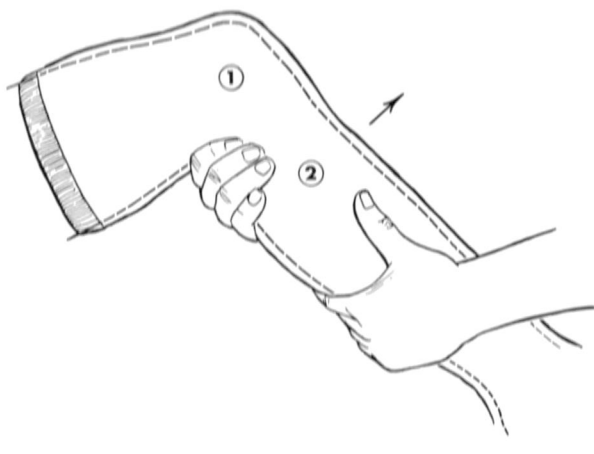

For anterior dislocation,
1. The knee is immobilized in the extended position.

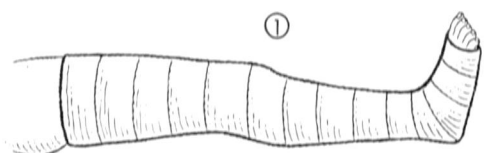

Subsequent Management

After 3 weeks remove the cast and
1. Apply a cast-brace, which protects against varus and valgus loading.
2. The plaster must be molded carefully about the femoral condyles and tibial plateaus.

Note: Continue cast-brace immobilization and active exercises of the quadriceps for 6 to 8 weeks longer. After this time remove the cast-brace and allow the patient to walk with a cane or crutches until full quadriceps strength has been regained.

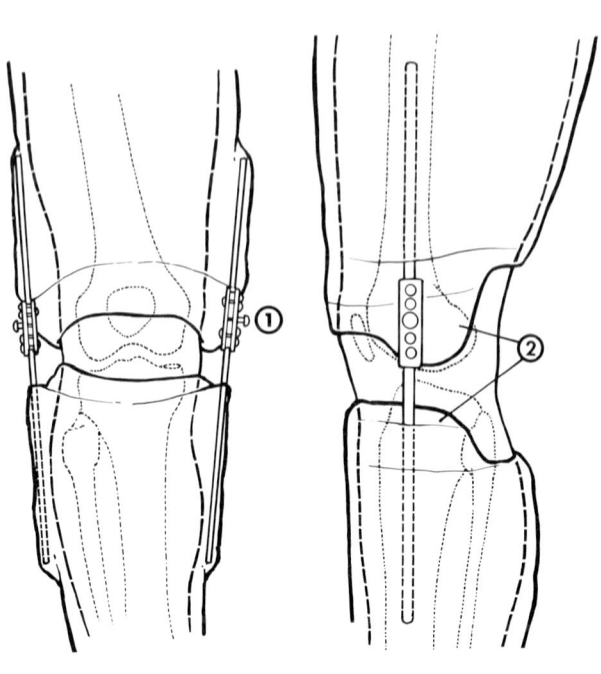

INDICATIONS FOR OPERATIVE REPAIR OF DISLOCATIONS AND FRACTURE-DISLOCATIONS OF THE KNEE

REMARKS

When there is significant Type III instability or instability in more than one plane on testing after reduction, operative repair is indicated as an elective procedure (see pages 1572 and 1599).

Surgical repair is also necessary in the presence of an open dislocation, an irreducible dislocation, or a dislocation associated with a medial plateau fracture.

Ligamentous repair should not be carried out at the time of arterial surgery unless it can be done simply without compromising the success of the vascular procedure.

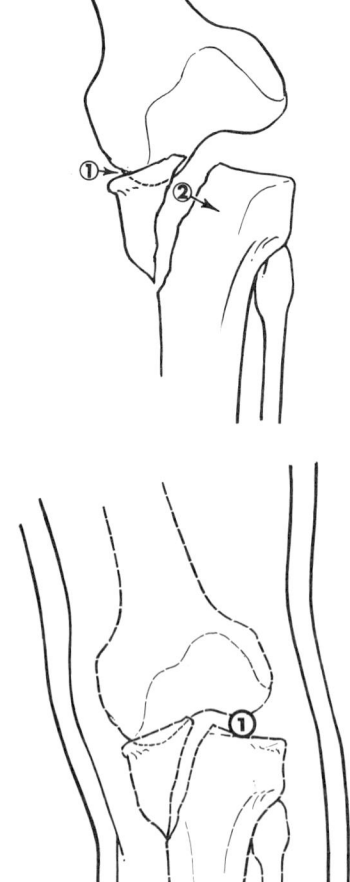

Unstable Fracture-Dislocation of the Knee

1. A fracture of the medial tibial plateau associated with medial dislocation of the femoral condyles and
2. Anterolateral dislocation of the tibial plateau.

1. The instability will recur despite cast immobilization.

2. Stabilization of the medial tibial plateau with Knowles pins is necessary to restore joint support.

3. Additional external cast support is necessary for these extremely unstable injuries.

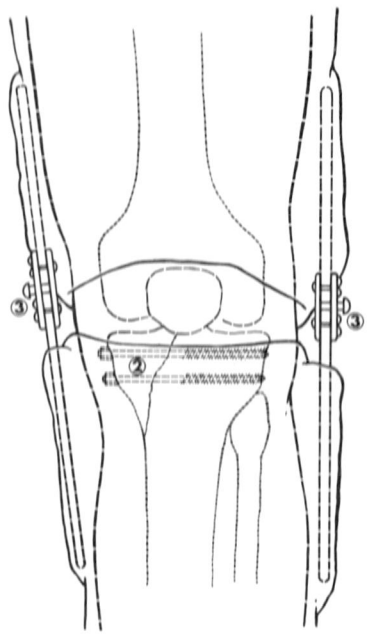

LATERAL DISLOCATION AND IRREDUCIBLE POSTEROLATERAL DISLOCATION OF THE KNEE JOINT

REMARKS

A true lateral dislocation may be difficult to reduce by closed methods when the tendons of the medial hamstrings become caught in the intercondylar notch. However, by flexing the knee beyond 90 degrees to relax the hamstrings, closed reduction may usually be accomplished.

True lateral dislocation should be distinguished from posterolateral dislocation, for which open reduction may be necessary because there is frequently an infolding of the medial ligament and capsule making closed reduction impossible.

Appearance on X-Ray: True Lateral Dislocation

1. The tibia is completely displaced lateral to the femur and
2. Pulled superiorly by the hamstrings.

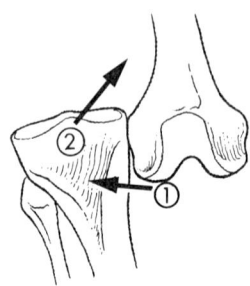

Obstruction to Reduction of True Lateral Dislocation

1. The medial hamstrings may be caught in the intercondylar notch, preventing reduction with the knee extended.

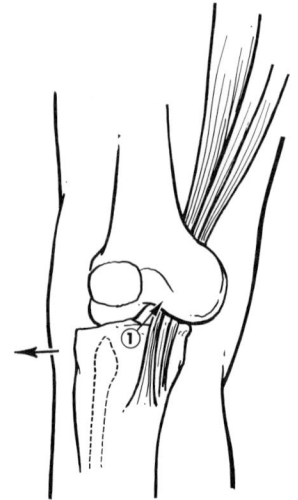

Technique of Reduction

1. The knee is flexed to 90 degrees to relax the hamstrings while the thigh is supported by an assistant.
2. The surgeon applies traction and direct pressure on the lateral tibia to reduce the dislocation.

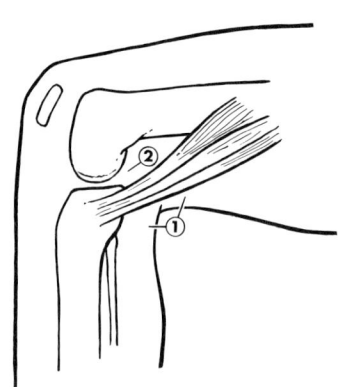

X-Ray after Closed Reduction of True Lateral Dislocation

1. The articular surface of the femur and tibia are in normal relationship to each other.
2. There is no persistent anterior or posterior subluxation after the reduction.

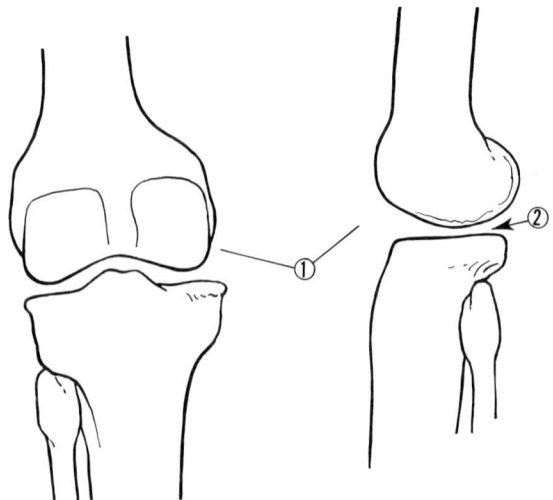

Irreducible Posterolateral Dislocation of the Knee Joint

In contrast to a true lateral dislocation the displacement of the tibia is not as marked but reduction requires operative intervention to remove the medial capsule and ligamentous structures from the joint.

Clinical Appearance

1. The knee is in slight flexion and maintained in 30 to 40 degrees of internal rotation.
2. The medial femoral condyle is prominent and palpable under the skin anteriorly.
3. Consistently there is puckering or a deep transverse groove in the skin distal to the condyle. This becomes accentuated with attempted reduction of the dislocation.

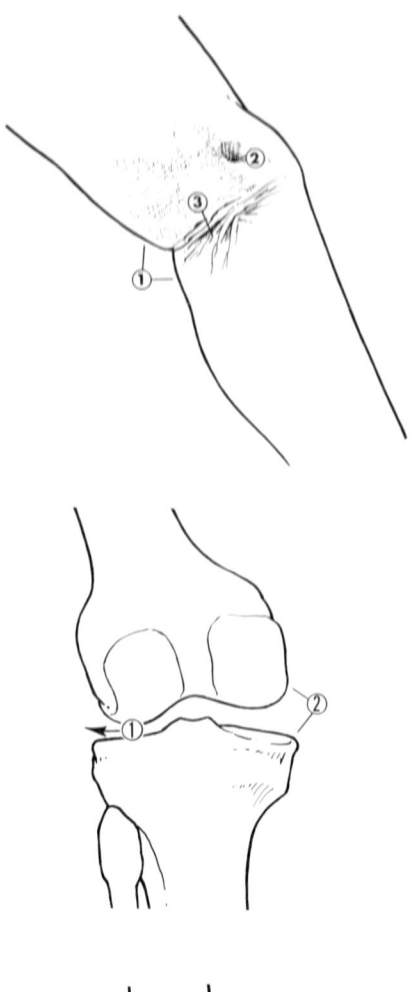

Appearance on X-Ray

Anteroposterior view

1. There is lateral displacement of the lateral condyle of the tibia relative to the femur that is never more than a quarter of the width of the condyle and nowhere near as marked as with a true lateral dislocation.
2. Because of the medial rotation of the tibia, the femoral condyle is prominent.

Lateral view

1. The medial tibial condyle is displaced or subluxated posteriorly.

Note: Closed reduction is usually unsuccessful with this rare dislocation. Open reduction is necessary to remove the infolded soft tissues and repair disrupted medial and posteromedial capsular structures.

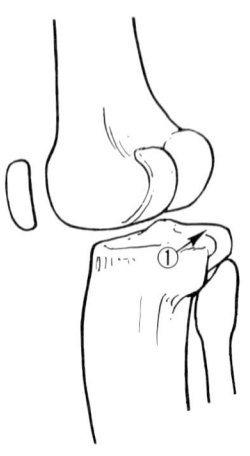

X-Ray After Open Reduction and Repair of Inverted Capsule and Ligaments

1. The articular surfaces of the femur and tibia are restored to normal relationships.
2. The posterior displacement of the tibia has been corrected on the lateral view.

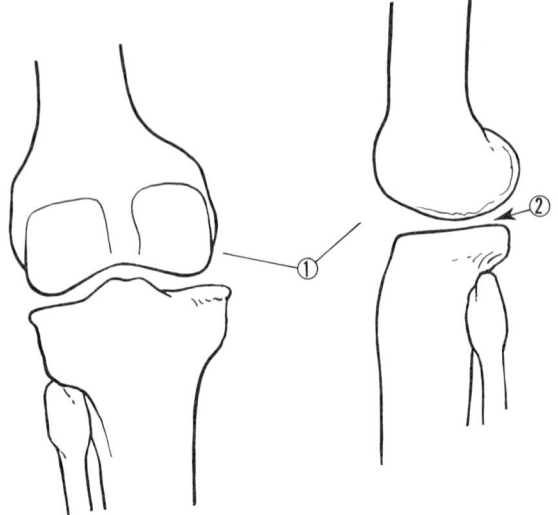

Postoperative Management

The leg is immobilized in a compressive dressing for three to five days until the swelling completely subsides, and then a long leg cast is applied.

1. The plaster cast is applied with the knee in the flexed position.
2. The tibia is pulled forward during the cast application to relax the tension on the posterior capsular structures.

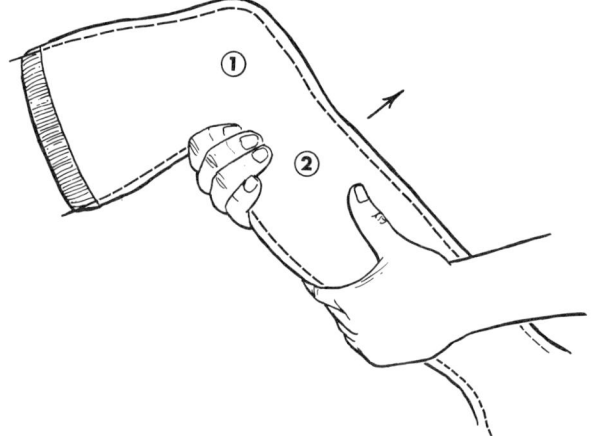

Subsequent Management

Immobilize the knee in the flexed position for four weeks.

Subsequently, remove the cast and apply a cast-brace to prevent strain of the medial capsular repair while allowing the patient to regain knee motion.

The cast-brace should be carefully applied over the condyles of the femur and tibia to provide medial and lateral stability while allowing knee flexion.

Continue with the cast-brace for four to six weeks while the patient regains full motion and control of the knee.

FRACTURES OF THE PATELLA

REMARKS

Patellar fractures are among the most common about the knee.

The patella functions to maximize the strength of the quadriceps as it shortens during full extension and to protect the articular surface of the distal femur from direct blows. Consequently, the patella is most often fractured by direct blows (e.g., dashboard injuries) to the front of the knee or indirectly by sudden, violent contractions of the quadriceps during knee flexion.

The patellar pain after fracture is usually well-localized and a defect is frequently palpable in the region of the fracture.

Characteristically, the knee swells rapidly from hemarthrosis, and aspirations should be done to relieve the joint pain. Fluid from the joint aspirate is filled with fat, which confirms the presence of a fracture.

X-rays of the injured area should include anteroposterior and lateral views as well as a patellar view, which is helpful to evaluate for osteochondral fractures from lateral patellar displacement. Care should be taken to distinguish this osteochondral fracture, which is distal and medial, from bipartite patella, which is usually superior and lateral.

The primary objective of treatment is to maintain or restore normal quadriceps function. A transpatellar fracture with 2 to 3 mm of displacement or a longitudinal fracture does not prevent full active knee extension as long as the surrounding patellar retinaculum is intact. This is particularly likely with fractures produced by direct blows to the patella. If an x-ray taken with the knee in 45 degrees of flexion demonstrates no further displacement of the fragments, the injury may be treated by protective splints or casts.

The most effective method of fixing displaced fractures of the patella is with cerclage tension-band wiring, anchoring the wire directly into bone. Weber and coworkers have demonstrated by biomechanical testing that this technique combined with repair of the retinaculum stabilizes transverse fractures sufficiently to permit knee flexion to 90 degrees without separating the fragments. Early range of knee motion is important since it significantly decreases the period of disability after fracture.

Comminuted patellar fractures may also be treated by tension-band wiring if supplemented by either parallel or oblique Kirchner wires.

Fractures of the inferior patellar pole should be fixed with cancellous screws and protected by tension-band wiring.

Rarely, the fracture may be so comminuted that patellectomy is indicated. The quadriceps and the patellar tendon must be repaired sufficiently to permit early knee motion. The patellar retinaculum should be accurately repaired as well.

Fissure and Comminuted Fractures of the Patella Without Displacement

REMARKS

These may be the result of direct or indirect force.

No displacement of the fragments or incongruity of the articular cartilage exists.

The continuity of the quadriceps apparatus is intact.

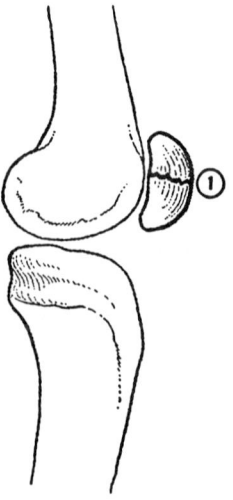

Appearance on X-Ray

1. Fissure fracture without separation of the fragments (caused by indirect force).

1. Comminuted fracture with no displacement (caused by direct force).

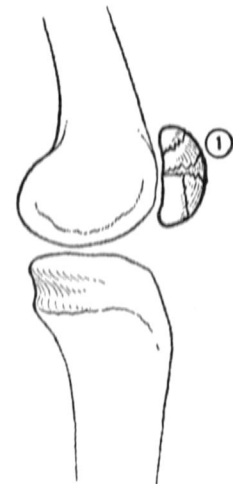

X-Ray in 45 Degrees of Knee Flexion

1. The fracture fragments remain undisplaced, indicating that the surrounding soft tissue and patellar retinaculum are uninjured.

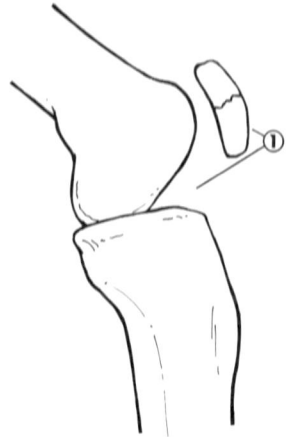

Management

Aspirate the blood from the joint cavity under aseptic conditions to relieve the pain.

Apply a compression dressing and posterior splint, elevate the leg, and place ice bags about the fracture site.

The patient may be ambulatory on crutches with bathroom privileges.

After 3 to 5 days remove the support dressing and allow active extension exercises. Knee flexion to 45 degrees may also be allowed.

The patient may progress with crutch walking but when up on crutches he should use a posterior splint to protect the knee against hyperflexion.

The protective splint is maintained for four weeks, after which it may be discarded and knee flexion exercises may be increased.

Transverse Fracture of the Patella with Separation of Fragments

REMARKS

Tension-band wiring of a patellar fracture is the treatment of choice in most instances. When done correctly, this method of fixation is sufficient to allow early, active range of motion of the knee.

This technique fixes the wires to the proximal and distal fragments using small drill holes. Two Kirschner wires may be introduced longitudinally across the fracture site to add further fixation if necessary.

Retinacular repair is also important for stability and to permit early motion after operation.

For late reconstruction of a chronic, untreated patellar fracture, see page 1657.

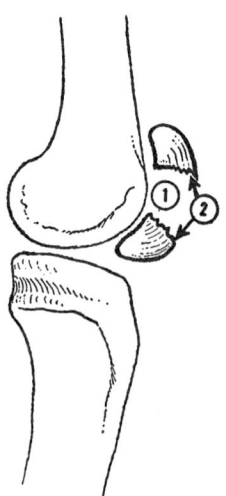

Preoperative X-Rays

1. Transverse fracture in which fragments are approximately of equal size.
2. Fragments are widely separated.

1. Transverse fracture in which the fragments are of unequal size with wide separation.

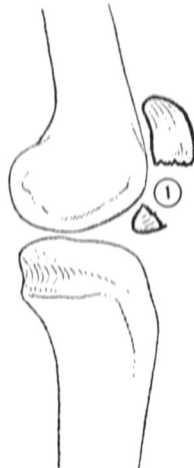

Comminuted fracture with
1. One large fragment and
2. Separation of fragments.

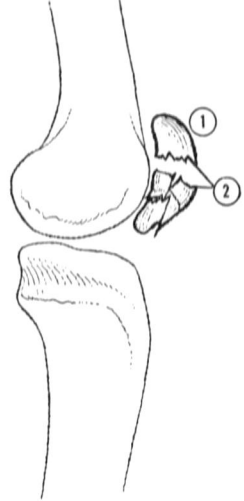

Polar fracture with
1. Comminution of smaller fragment and
2. Separation of fragments.

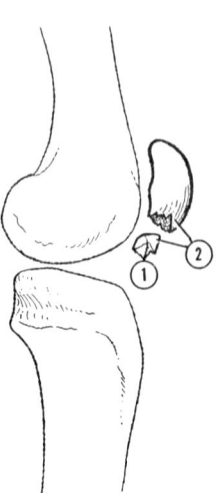

Biomechanics of Fixation

1. If the wire is placed posterior to the center of the patella, knee flexion tends to open the fracture anteriorly.
2. If the wire is placed anterior to the patella and fixed to the bone through small drill holes, the tension force is neutralized.
3. The fixation should be sufficiently stable to permit up to 90 degrees of knee flexion early after the operation.

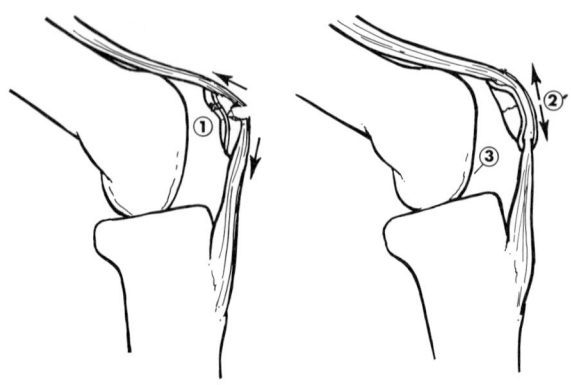

Operative Procedure

1. Make a U-shaped skin incision with its base over the distal portion of the patellar tendon.

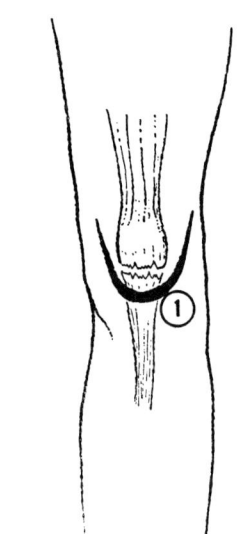

2. Reflect the skin flaps upward and downward, exposing the patella and the parapatellar regions.
3. After washing out blood clots and loose bony spicules, identify the type of fracture present.

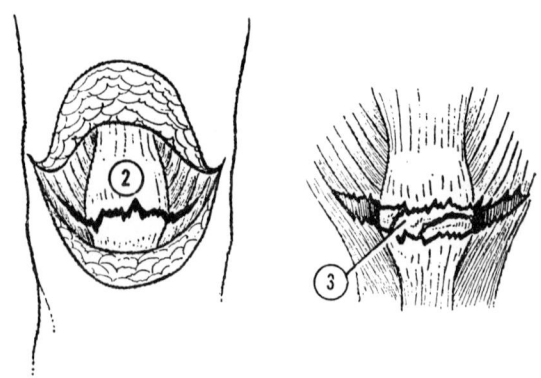

OPERATIVE PROCEDURE

For Transverse Fractures: Magnusson Wiring

1. Drill holes are made through the proximal fragment begining at the medial and lateral borders of the quadriceps tendon and then in the opposite direction through the distal fragment.
2. An 18-gauge wire (soft stainless steel) is passed through the drill holes and
3. Tightened in the suprapatellar region.

For Comminuted Fractures

1. Two Kirschner wires are passed longitudinally across the fracture.
2. An 18-gauge wire loop is passed circumferentially behind the tips of the Kirschner wires.
3. The wire loop also passes over the anterior surface of the patella.

Inferior Pole Fractures

1. For fractures of the inferior pole, stabilize the lower fragment first with a cancellous lag screw.
2. Add supplemental cerclage wire. Use an 18-gauge soft steel suture.

Note: If the fragment is too small for screw fixation, it may be removed and the patellar tendon may be fixed to the bone. However, bone-to-bone repair generally is stronger than tendon-to-bone repair.

EXCISION OF DISTAL POLAR FRAGMENTS

1. Small or comminuted distal pole fragments may be excised.

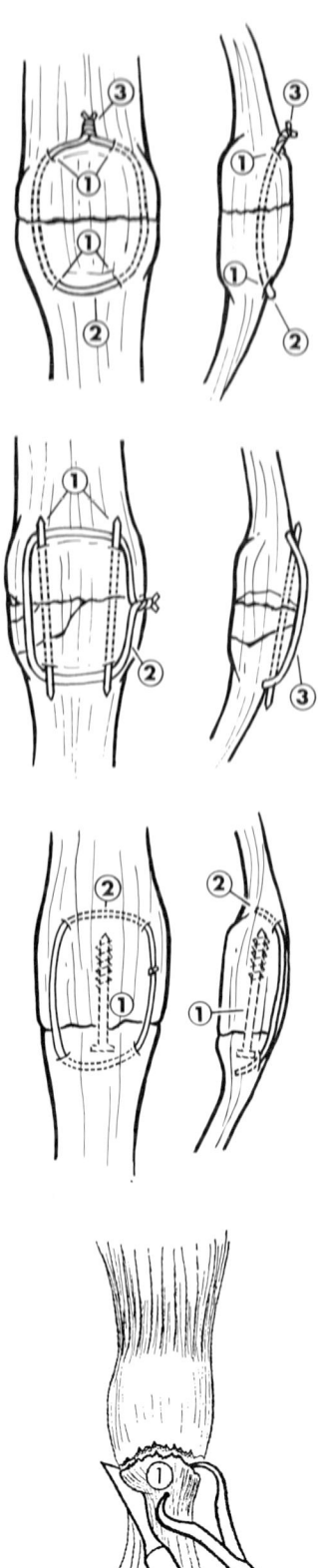

Inferior Pole Fractures
(Continued)

1. With a bone biter trim the margin of the remaining fragment to create a flat surface at right angles to the long axis of the patella.

2. Make two parallel drill channels in the fragment; they are directed downward and slightly posteriorly, opening on the fractured surface just anterior to the articular cartilage.

3. After trimming all of the devitalized tissue from the end of the tendon, pass stainless steel wire through the tendon and out through the drill holes.

4. Tighten the wire suture on the anterior surface of the fragment.

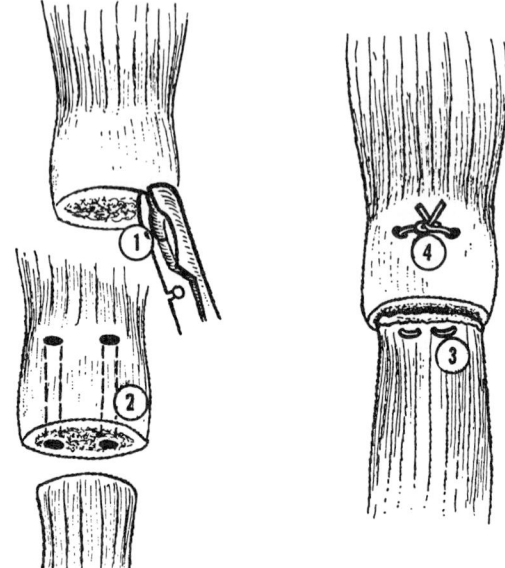

5. Approximate the edges of the rents in the retinacula with interrupted sutures.

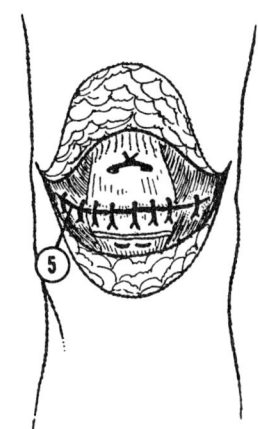

AFTER COMPLETING THE REPAIR

1. Always test the strength of the repair by flexing the knee.

2. The repair should become taut at approximately 60 degrees of knee flexion but the fixation should not loosen.

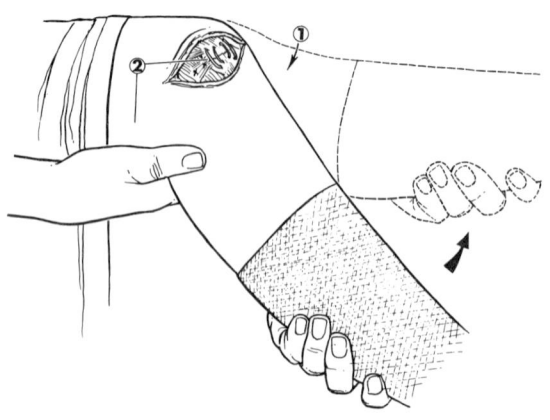

Subsequent Management

The patellar fixation should be sufficiently strong to allow the patient to begin range-of-motion exercises postoperatively without disrupting the repair site.

Immobilize the limb postoperatively in a bundle dressing for 2 to 3 days.

Subsequently begin active quadriceps-setting exercises and knee flexion to 60 degrees.

A knee exerciser can be made from a simple felt sling under the patient's thigh which allows passive knee flexion to 60 degrees.

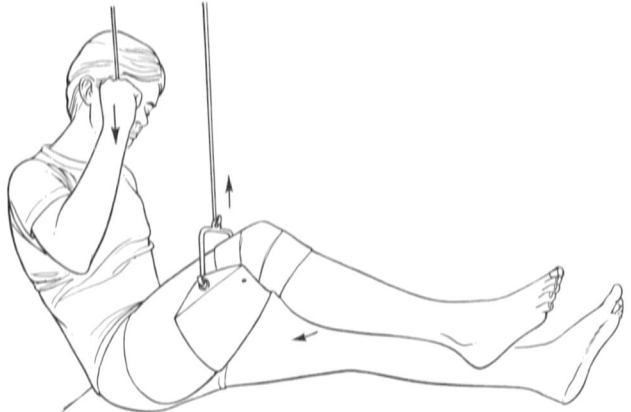

When the patient has full control of the knee, he may be up on crutches, but a posterior splint should be applied to protect the knee against sudden hyperflexion while on crutches.

Continue with the active exercises for 6 to 8 weeks after which time the patient may discard the crutches and protective splint.

Severely Comminuted Fractures of the Patella

REMARKS

Total patellectomy is justifiable in extensively comminuted fractures, which do not possess a fragment sufficiently large to provide a bony anchorage for the opposing tendon.

Preoperative X-Ray

1. Severely comminuted fracture of the patella.

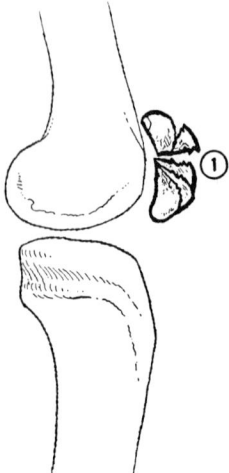

Excision of All Patellar Fragments

1. Make a U-shaped incision with its base over the distal end of the patellar tendon.

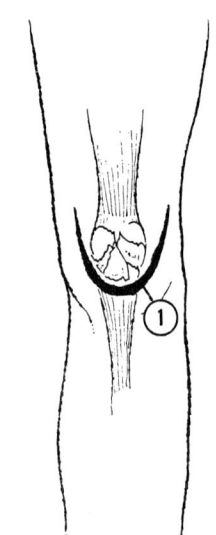

2. Reflect the skin flaps upward and downward.
3. Identify the fracture and the rents in the medial and lateral retinacula.

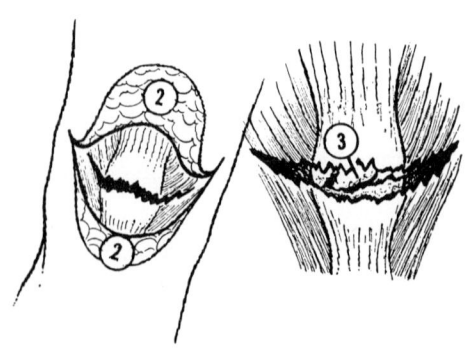

FRACTURES OF THE PATELLA

4. Grasp each fragment with a towel clip and enucleate it with sharp dissection.

5. After trimming away loose shredded fragments of the tendons and flushing the wound clear of loose fragments of bone and blood clots, overlap and plicate the edges of the tendon and the edges of the torn retinacula with mattress sutures using 0-Tevdek or a similar nonabsorbable suture.

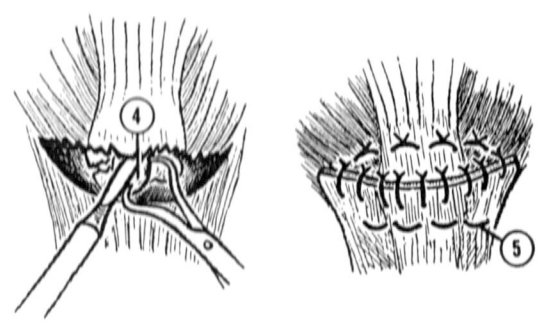

After completing the repair,
1. Always test the strength of the repair by flexing the knee.
2. The repair should become taut at approximately 60 degrees of knee flexion but sutures should not pull out.

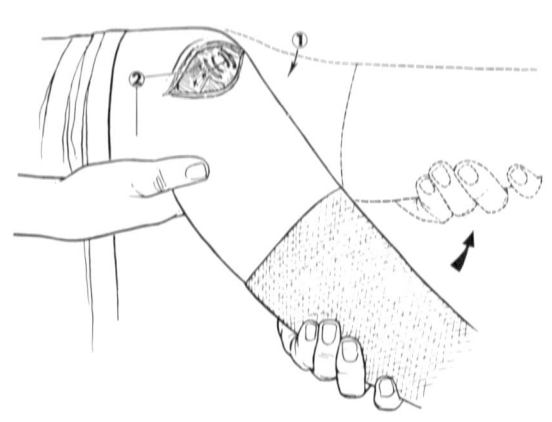

Postoperative X-Ray

1. The patella has been removed.

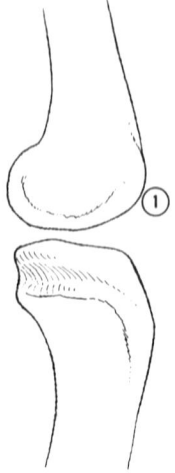

Subsequent Management

The extensor repair should be sufficiently strong to allow the patient to begin range-of-motion exercises without disrupting the repair site.

Immobilize the limb postoperatively in a bundle dressing for two to three days.

Subsequently, begin active quadriceps setting and knee flexion to 60 degrees.

Subsequent Management (Continued)

A knee exerciser can be made from a simple felt sling under the patient's thigh, which allows knee flexion passively to 60 degrees.

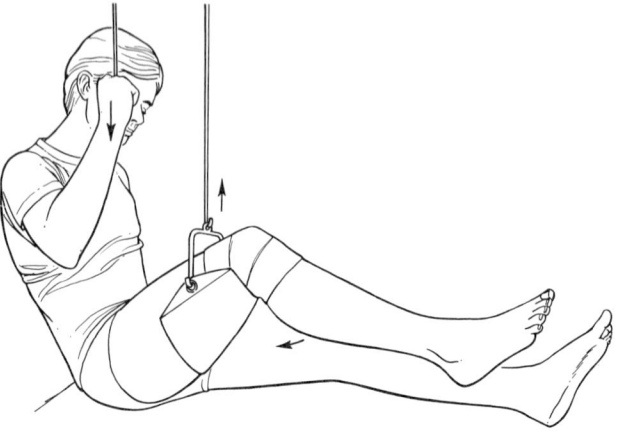

When the patient has full control of the knee, he may be up on crutches, but a posterior splint should be applied to protect the knee against sudden hyperflexion while he is on crutches.

Continue with the active exercises for six weeks, after which the patient may discard the crutches and splint protection.

Osteochondral Fractures of the Patella Associated with Dislocation

REMARKS

Small marginal fractures are frequently produced by avulsion of the medial retinaculum during lateral dislocation. These are important primarily as radiographic indicators of injury.

Approximately five per cent of acute dislocations have large intra-articular osteochondral fracture fragments. These occur when the patella slides back tangentially over the surface of the lateral femoral condyle with the knee in a flexed position. The result is a scoring of the articular surface of the medial patellar facet and lateral femoral condyles with shear fractures of the inferomedial border of the patella and the lateral femoral condyle.

Specific detailed radiographic examination of all patellar dislocations is essential and should include anteroposterior, lateral, oblique, and skyline views to assess these osteochondral fractures.

Inferomedial avulsion fracture fragments need not be replaced because they are extra-articular.

Intra-articular osteochondral fracture fragments should be removed promptly and the capsular damage should be repaired. If possible, the osteochondral fragment off the lateral femoral condyle, which may be associated with the patellar fracture, should be replaced, although usually the small amount of bone with this fragment makes reattachment impossible.

Mechanisms

AVULSION FRACTURE

1. As the patella dislocates laterally,
2. The patellar retinaculum avulses the small fragment from the medial border of the patella. This is not an intra-articular fracture and does not require open reduction.

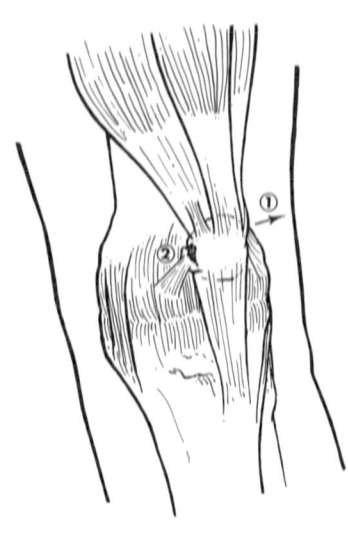

OSTEOCHONDRAL FRACTURE

1. As the patella dislocates laterally with knee flexion,
2. Shear fractures of the inferomedial patella and/or lateral femoral condyle result.

Note: Fragments in an osteochondral fracture should not be confused with bipartite patellar fragments, which are usually superior and lateral.

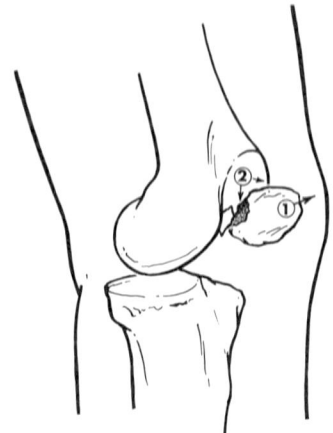

Appearance on X-Ray

AVULSION FRACTURE

1. An avulsion fracture is seen without intra-articular displacement.

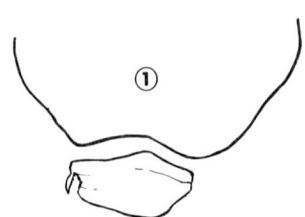

Appearance on X-Ray
(Continued)

OSTEOCHONDRAL FRACTURE

1. The inferomedial portion of the patella has been fractured and the fragment is intra-articular.

Note: If this fragment is left in its position, it frequently will enlarge owing to nourishment by synovial fluid and cause persistent and intermittent symptoms.

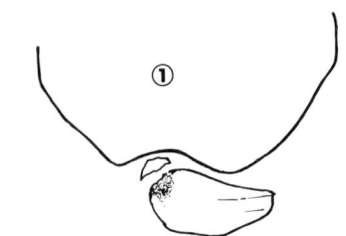

MANAGEMENT

Avulsion fracture

The injury is managed as with any acute patellar dislocation.

1. Apply a cylinder cast using a stockinette wrapped over 2 inch (5-cm) strips of tapes placed medially and laterally to serve as suspenders.

2. The malleoli are well-padded.

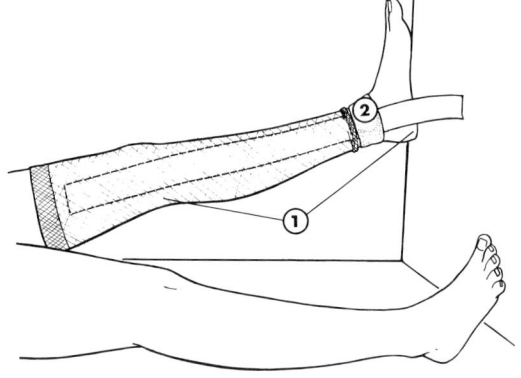

3. The plaster is molded firmly over the patella to push it medially and tighten the anteromedial retinaculum.

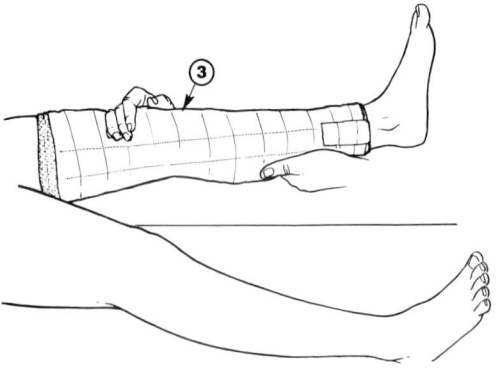

Osteochondral Fracture Associated with Patellar Dislocation

EXCISION OF FRAGMENTS

1. Make a small vertical incision directly over the fragment.
2. By sharp dissection enucleate the fragment from the fascial periosteal tissues of the patella and capsule.

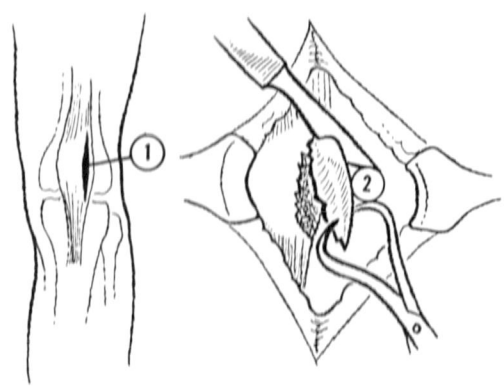

3. Trim the edges of the main fragment and make them smooth.
4. Drill holes along the edge of the patella. Do not damage the articular surface. Attach the retinaculum firmly to the bone to prevent recurrence of the dislocation.

Note: The repair must stabilize the patella to prevent recurrence of dislocations. If necessary, a reconstructive procedure such as the Elmslie-Trillot should be carried out if the patella does not track properly after retinacular repair (see page 1673).

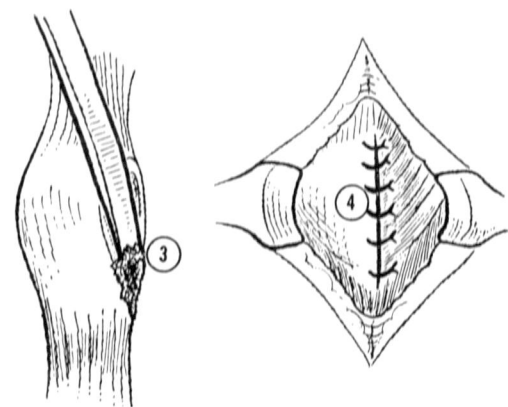

Postoperative Management

Apply a snug compression bandage around the knee.
Begin immediately quadriceps exercises and joint exercises on a regulated regimen.
After seven days allow partial weight bearing with crutches.
After one more week allow nonprotected weight bearing.

Other Osteochondral Fractures of the Patella

REMARKS

Osteochondral fracture of the patella is the most common source of loose bodies in the knee joint.

The lesion is encountered quite frequently in adolescents and young adults.

Characteristically, the fracture results from a direct blow to the patella, injuring the distal pole or one of the patellar facets.

Subsequent clinical manifestations are those of a loose body in the knee joint.

The fragment may be entirely cartilaginous and, therefore, may not be visualized on standard x-rays. Most often, there is a bony fragment attached that can be seen if adequate x-rays are made. Always take oblique as well as anteroposterior and lateral views to rule out this possibility.

The bony fragment may just appear to be a thin flake; however, this is not indicative of the true size of the loose fragment.

If these loose fragments are allowed to remain in the knee joint, quite frequently they will continue to enlarge and will form both cartilage and bone because they are nourished by synovial fluid.

Preoperative X-Ray

1. Loose body in the infrapatellar region of the knee joint.
2. Corresponding defect in the inframedial aspect of the articular surface of the patella.

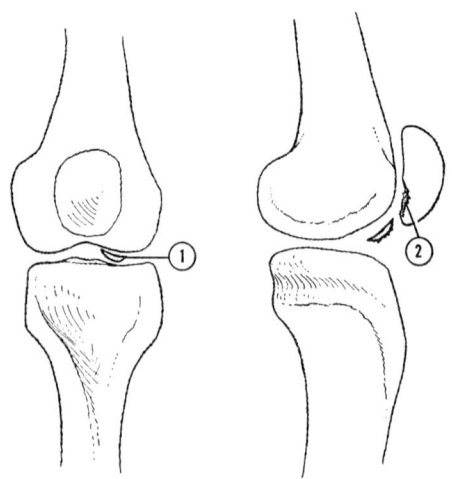

(Median Parapetellar Incision)

1. Make a skin incision on the medial aspect of the knee, beginning 2 cm proximal to the upper margin of the patella at the medial margin of the quadriceps tendon. The incision follows the medial border of the quadriceps tendon, the medial margin of the patella, and the patellar ligament, and ends just distal to the lower border of the tibial tubercle.

2. Divide the deep fascia in the line of the incision.
3. Make a vertical incision in the quadriceps tendon 1 cm lateral to its medial border and continue it distally in the capsule around the medial margin of the patella and along the medial border of the patellar tendon.

Removal of Loose Fragment

1. Divide the synovialis 1 cm from the medial border of the patella and the patellar ligament.
2. Dislocate the patella laterally and rotate it in its vertical axis so that its articular surface faces anteriorly.
3. Locate the loose body and remove it.

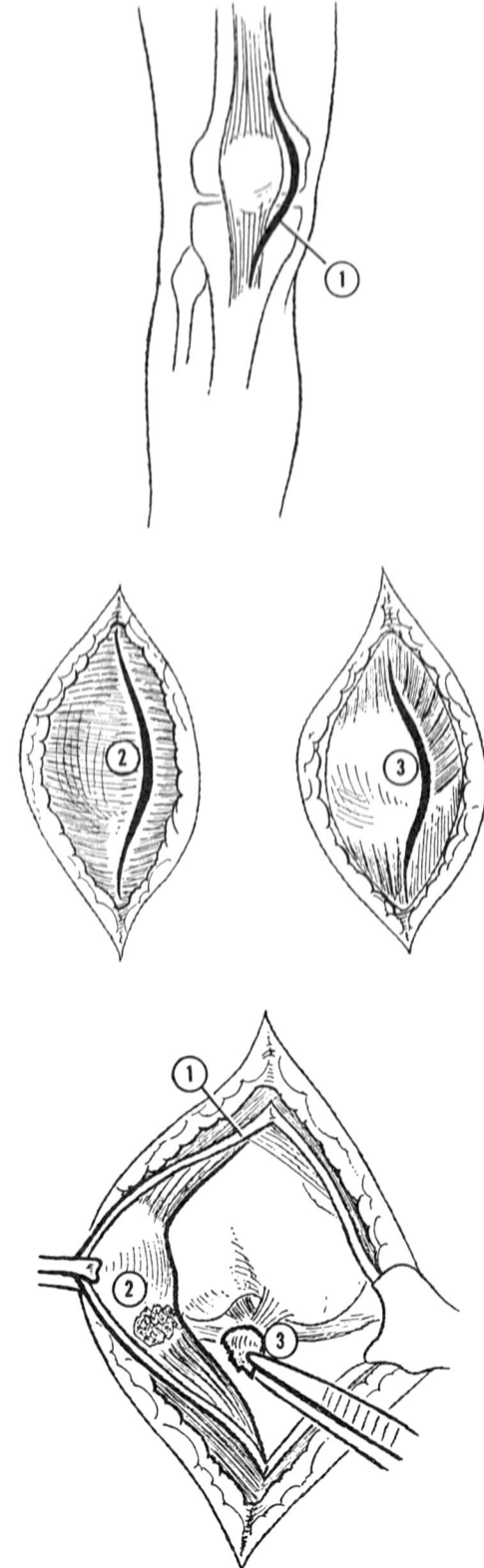

Removal of Loose Fragment (Continued)

4. Identify the defect in the articular surface of the patella and with a scalpel make smooth the irregular edges of the defect in the cartilaginous surface.

Note: Before closure flush the wound with a solution of normal saline in order to remove all blood clots and flakes of cartilage.

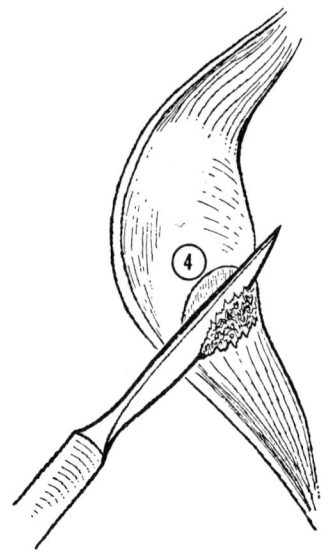

Postoperative Management

Apply a compression dressing postoperatively and elevate the leg in bed. Apply ice bags to the knee for the first 48 hours.

As soon as possible after the operation, the patient should start quadriceps-setting exercises and should actively try to extend the leg in bed.

Range-of-motion exercises, including knee flexion, can be started on the second or third postoperative day depending on the amount of swelling.

The patient may be up on crutches by the first postoperative day and should continue on crutches for at least two weeks to avoid hemarthrosis.

The crutches may be discarded by the end of the second or third week and full weight bearing may be allowed.

Active quadriceps and hamstring exercises should be continued for several months after an operation on the knee joint.

RUPTURE OF THE EXTENSOR APPARATUS OF THE KNEE JOINT

REMARKS

Rupture of the extensor mechanism of the knee joint is caused by forceful contraction of the quadriceps muscle against a force acting in the opposite direction, such as is produced when the knee is suddenly flexed by the body weight.

Rupture of the extensor apparatus may occur at one of four levels; the site is generally governed by the age of the patient.

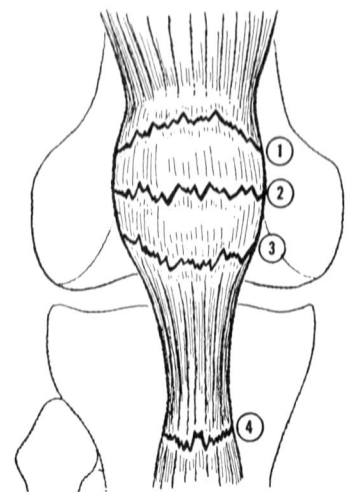

Rupture may occur:
1. At the upper pole of the patella.
2. Through the patella.
3. At the lower pole of the patella.
4. At the tibial tubercle. (The tubercle may be avulsed from the tibia.)

Immediate recognition of the lesion is imperative because repair of the apparatus in fresh lesions gives excellent results, whereas late repairs are difficult to achieve and frequently give poor results.

Do not sacrifice the patella in this lesion except as a last resort.

Rupture of the Quadriceps Mechanism

REMARKS

This injury occurs most frequently in patients older than 40 years. Characteristically, a sudden forceful contraction of the quadriceps tendon with the knee flexed overloads the extensor apparatus and causes the rupture.

Despite the patient's significant inability to extend the knee, the injury goes unrecognized with surprising frequency or is treated as "a sprained ligament."

Consistently, there is full passive extension possible in the knee but active extension may be lacking as much as 70 degrees.

A normal tendon does not rupture in its substance but tears at its insertion into bone, at the musculotendinous junction, or through the muscle belly itself. Repeated injections of cortisone weaken the tendon strength and may cause tendon rupture. Injection into weight-supporting tendons such as the quadriceps, patella, or Achilles should be avoided.

Systemic causes of rupture of the quadriceps tendon, as well as the infrapatellar tendon, include lupus erythematosus, hyperparathyroidism, and chronic acidosis or nephropathy. Secondary hyperparathyroidism with resorption of the tendo-osseous junction may also contribute to tendon rupture.

Characteristically, there is well-localized tenderness and a defect palpable above the patella. With extensive swelling, in acute injury, the gap may not be palpable. With careful examination, however, the diagnosis can be made on the basis of tenderness and loss of active extension in the absence of a patellar fracture.

Immediate operative repair is essential to permit normal knee function without external bracing.

RUPTURE OF THE EXTENSOR APPARATUS OF THE KNEE JOINT

Typical Clinical Presentation

1. There is considerable suprapatellar swelling and the distal end of the quadriceps may be palpable above the patella.

2. There is a palpable sulcus between the end of the quadriceps and the margin of the patella that is particularly evident on attempted active extension.

Note: Active extension may be lacking as much as 30 to 70 degrees.

3. There is full passive extension and no intra-articular locking or block of extension.

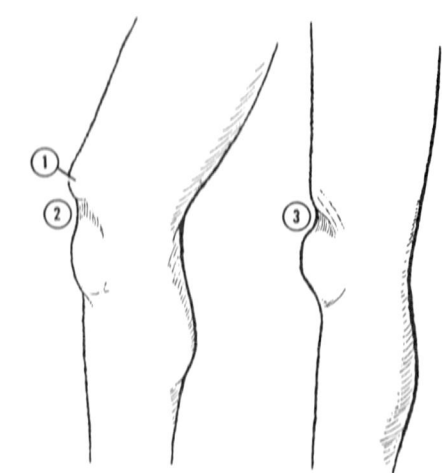

OPERATIVE PROCEDURES

Tendon-to-Tendon Repair

This method is employed when enough tissue remains on the upper margin of the patella to permit a tendon-to-tendon repair.

1. Make a U-shaped skin incision with its convexity downward; it begins over the medial femoral condyle, crosses the leg just distal to the insertion of the patellar tendon, and ends over the lateral femoral condyle.

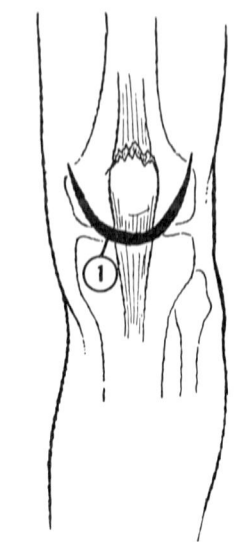

2. Reflect the skin flap and deep fascia upward, exposing the quadriceps tendon, the patella, and the patellar tendon.

3. Identify the extent of the tear in the extensor mechanism and flush out all blood clots with a solution of normal saline.

4. Trim all loose strands of tissue and devitalized tissue at the edges of the tendon.

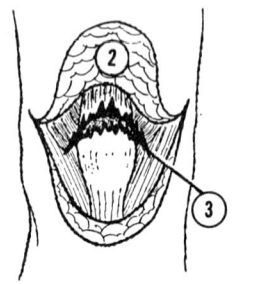
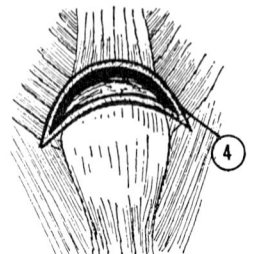

Tendon-to-Tendon Repair
(Continued)

5. Grasp the proximal end of the tendon with a towel clip and pull it down until it approximates the distal end.
6. Join both ends of the tendon with mattress sutures. Use 0-Tevdek or a similar nonabsorbable material.
7. Close the tears in the medial and lateral expansions of the tendon with interrupted sutures. (Use 0-Tevdek or a similar nonabsorbable material.)

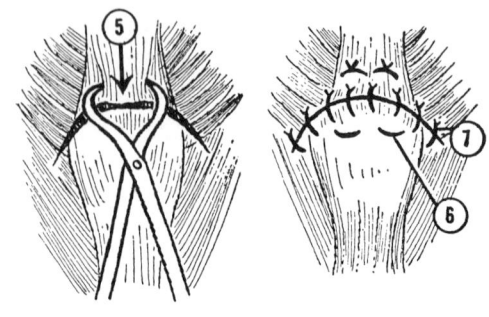

Tendon-to-Bone Repair

This method is utilized when no tendon tissue suitable for tendon-to-tendon repair remains on the upper margin of the patella.

1. Make two drill channels through the patella in its longitudinal axis.
2. Approximate the end of the tendon to the bone by a mattress suture passing through the drill channels and tied on the anterior surface of the tendon.

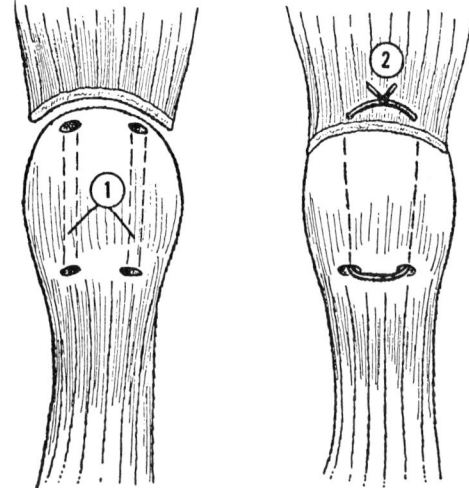

3. Repair the tears in the lateral expansions of the quadriceps apparatus by interrupted sutures.

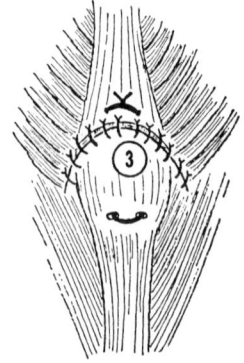

RUPTURE OF THE EXTENSOR APPARATUS OF THE KNEE JOINT

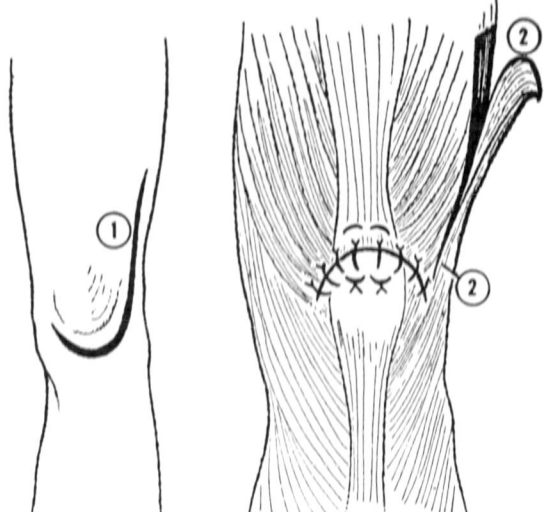

In old lesions,
1. Extend the lateral limit of the skin incision upward on the lateral aspect of the thigh 12 cm.
2. Remove a wide rectangular strip of fascia lata, leaving its base attached.

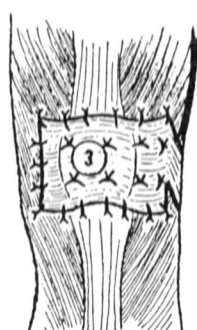

3. Reflect the strip of fascia lata over the anterior aspect of the quadriceps apparatus and secure it to the underlying tissues by interrupted sutures.

Postoperative Management

1. Apply a compression bandage around the knee.
2. Place the limb in a posterior plaster splint extending from the upper third of the thigh to the toes.
3. The knee is extended fully and the foot is at a right angle.

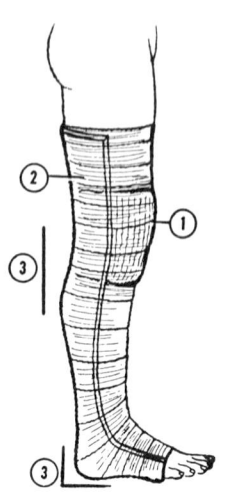

After three to five days remove the postoperative dressing and apply a long leg cast.

Now institute a regulated program of progressive quadriceps exercises.

Remove the cast at the end of five to six weeks and permit protected weight bearing with crutches; increase the intensity of the quadriceps and flexion exercises.

After eight to nine weeks permit unprotected weight bearing. Continue the exercises until maximum restoration of quadriceps power and extension and flexion of the knee are achieved.

Avulsion of the Patellar Tendon from the Patella

REMARKS

This lesion occurs commonly in young persons either from direct lacerations to the tendon or from jumping injuries.

Generally there is a complete avulsion of the tendon from the inferior margin of the patella as well as a tear in the lateral retinaculum.

A patellar tendon rupture can follow operations on the knee in which the insertion of the tendon has been disturbed.

Systemic causes of infrapatellar tendon rupture or quadriceps tendon rupture include lupus erythematosus, hyperparathyroidism, and chronic acidosis or nephropathy. Secondary hyperparathyroidism with resorption at the tendo-osseous junction can also lead to tendon rupture.

Repeated cortisone injections into the tendon weaken its strength and may cause direct rupture. Injections into weight-supporting tendons such as the patellar tendon, the quadriceps tendon, and the Achilles tendon should be avoided.

If the disruption of the patellar tendon is not recognized or if an initial repair fails, the discontinuity can be quite disabling. Late reconstruction is needed to allow the patient to walk without a brace.

Preoperative X-Rays

Fresh lesion

1. The patella is pulled upward by the quadriceps muscle.

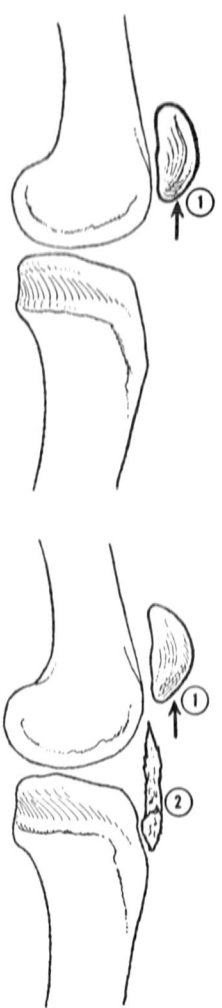

Old lesion

1. Upward displacement of the patella.
2. Heterotopic bone formation in the interval between the patella and the tibial tubercle.

Operative Repair for Early Lesion

1. Make a U-shaped skin incision with its convexity downward; it begins over the medial femoral condyle, crosses the leg just distal to the insertion of the patellar tendon and ends over the lateral femoral condyle.

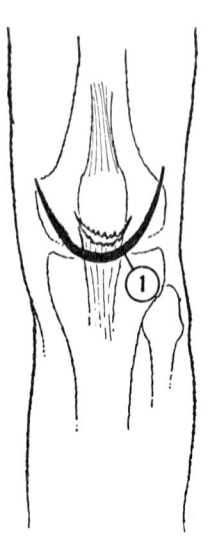

Operative Repair for Early Lesion (Continued)

2. Reflect the skin flap and deep fascia upward, exposing the quadriceps tendon, the patella, and the patellar tendon.

3. Identify the defect in the patellar tendon.

4. Remove all loose fragments of bone and trim off all devitalized strands of tissue.

5. Grasp the patella with a towel clip and pull it down until the proximal end of the tendon apposes the distal end.

6. Join both ends of the tendon with heavy mattress sutures passing close to the bone. Use 0-Tevdek or a similar nonabsorbable suture.

7. Close the tears in the lateral patellar retinaculum with interrupted sutures.

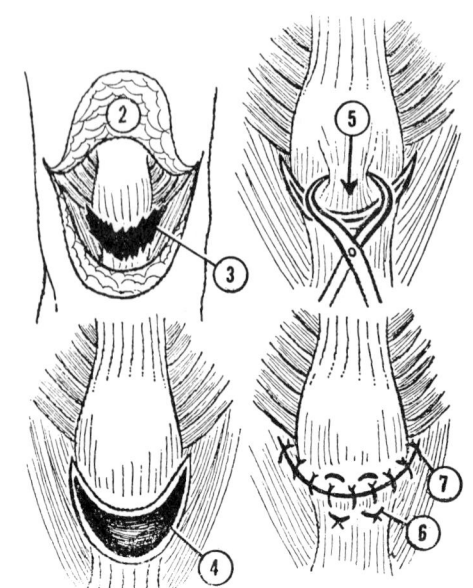

If the remainder of tendon on the patella is insufficient to effect a repair, do a bone-to-tendon repair.

1. Make two drill channels through the patella in its longitudinal axis and opening on the inferior surface of the patella.

2. Approximate the patella to the tendon by a mattress suture passing through the drill channels and tied on the anterior surface of the patella.

3. Repair tears in the lateral patellar retinaculum with interrupted sutures.

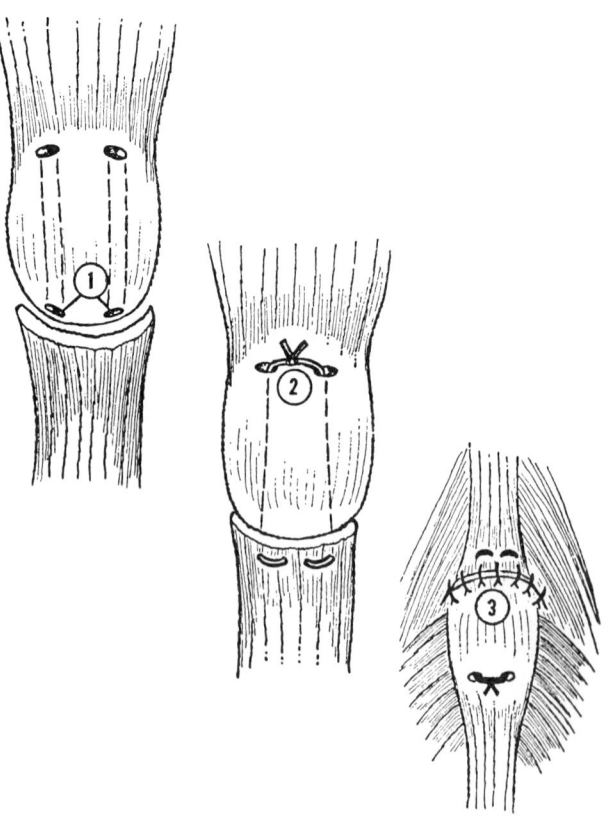

Late Reconstruction of the Patellar Tendon (After Ecker, Latke, and Glazer)

Note: This technique may also be used for chronic, untreated transverse patellar fractures.

The method used is a transfer of the gracilis and semitendinosus tendon supplemented by heavy cerclage wire. This technique is stronger than other methods such as use of fascial strips that have been previously used.

1. Begin an incision proximal and lateral to the patella and extend it distally across the midline inferior to the patella and ending at the medial flair of the tibia.
2. After dissecting flaps to expose the patella, quadriceps, and tibial tubercle, insert a Steinmann pin transversely through the proximal portion of the patella and apply distal traction.
3. Excise all scar in the remnants of the patellar tendon and mobilize the patella to lie just proximal to the joint line when the knee is in slight flexion.
4. Expose the proximal ends of the gracilis tendon and semitendinosus tendon through a separate incision. Divide them at their musculotendinous junctions and bring them out into the distal part of the first incision.

Note: The proximal ends of the tendons are sutured to the semimembranosus.

5. Two large drill holes to accommodate tendons are made transversely through the distal part of the patella and an oblique hole is made through the tibial tuberosity.

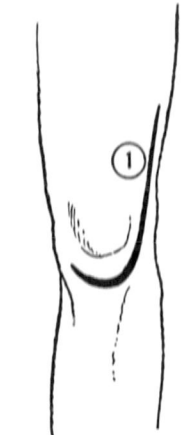

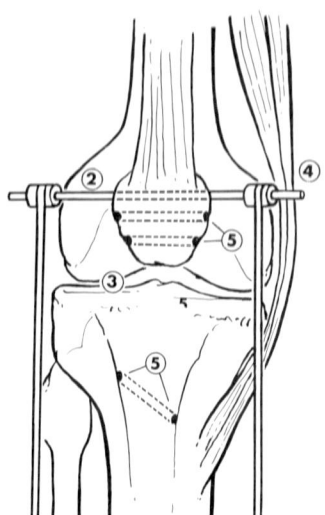

Late Reconstruction of the Patellar Tendon (After Ecker, Latke, and Glazer) (Continued)

1. Pass the semitendinosus first from medial to lateral through a hole drilled in the tibial tubercle and then from lateral to medial through a hole drilled in the patella.
2. Pass the gracilis tendon medio-laterally through a second hole in the patella.
3. Pass a heavy-gauge wire through the distal patellar hole and through the tibial tuberosity.

Note: A Dacron graft material may also be used in preference to a wire.

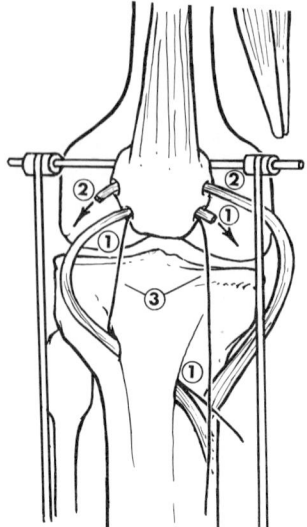

1. Maintain the patella in normal position with a traction pin and tighten the wire.
2. The tendons are then sutured to each other under tension.

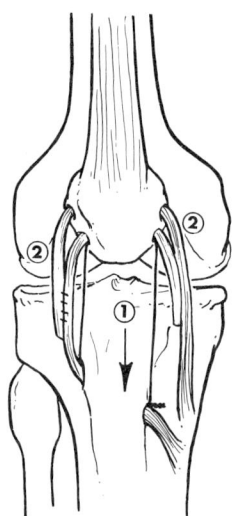

Subsequent Management

Immobilize the knee in a long leg cast in the extended position.

Six weeks postoperatively under general anesthesia remove the cast, manipulate the knee, and remove the wire.

If a Dacron graft has been used in place of a wire, it may not be necessary to remove it. However, allowing active knee motion before the wire is removed results in fragmentation of the wire.

Subsequently begin a vigorous program of straight leg raising with weights and active flexion exercises.

Avulsion Fractures of the Tibial Tuberosity in Adults

REMARKS

Avulsions of the tibial tuberosities in adults significantly impair the extensor mechanism.

This injury is analogous to fractures of the proximal tibial apophysis in children (see page 1617) and requires prompt operative reduction and repair to prevent shortening of the extensor apparatus.

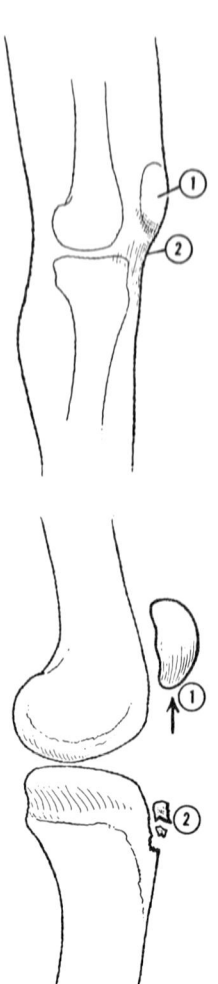

Typical Deformity

1. The patella rides high.
2. There is a sulcus immediately over the tibial tubercle. (This sulcus may be obliterated by swelling but it is always palpable.)

Preoperative X-Ray

1. The patella rides high.
2. There is fragmentation of the proximal end of the tibial tubercle.

Operative Repair

1. Make a hockey stick incision on the medial aspect of the knee; the lower limb of the incision crosses the anterior tibial crest just distal to the tibial tubercle.

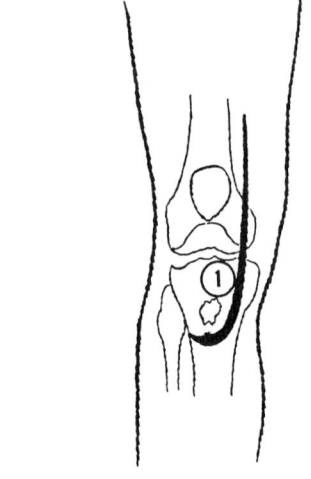

2. Reflect the skin and deep fascia outward, exposing the patella, the patellar ligament, and the tibial tubercle.
3. Identify the lesion and trim away the shredded strands of tissue and periosteum from the end of the tendon and the upper end of the tubercle.
4. Identify the extent of the tear in the medial and lateral retinacula.

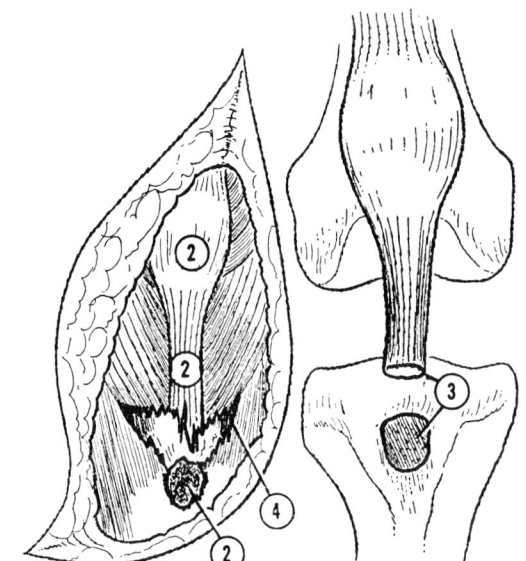

Reattach the tendon to the tibia if the tendon is torn cleanly from the tubercle or if the tendon is avulsed with a small fragment of bone after excision of the bony fragment.

1. With a sharp osteotome cut out a ledge from the tibial tubercle 1 cm deep and at right angles to the longitudinal axis of the tibia.
2. Make two drill channels through the tubercle that are directed upward and inward so that the exits are on the raw surface of the ledge.

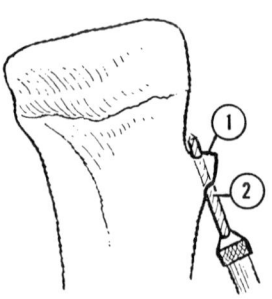

3. Grasp the patella with a towel clip and make downward traction.

4. Secure the end of the tendon to the raw surface of the ledge with a mattress suture passing through the drill channels and tied on the anterior surface of the tubercle. (Use 0-Tevdek or a similar nonabsorbable suture.)

5. Repair the tears in the medial and lateral retinacula with interrupted sutures. (Use 0-Tevdek or a similar nonabsorbable suture.)

If a large piece of bone is avulsed with the tendon use one of the two following methods.

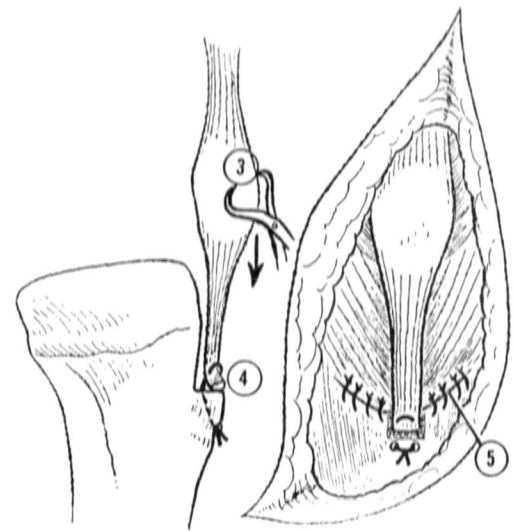

Replace the bone in its anatomic position and secure it with:

1. A mattress suture of 18-gauge wire passing through two drill channels made in the fragment and the tibial cortex or

2. A cancellous lag screw firmly fixing the fragment to the bony tuberosity.

Note: The retinaculum must also be completely repaired in addition to the patellar tendon reattachment.

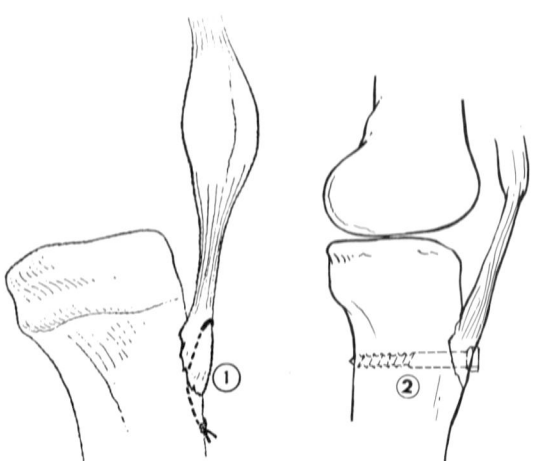

Postoperative Management

1. Apply a compression bandage around the knee.

2. Place the leg in a posterior plaster splint extending from the upper third of the thigh to the toes; the knee is extended fully and the foot is at a right angle.

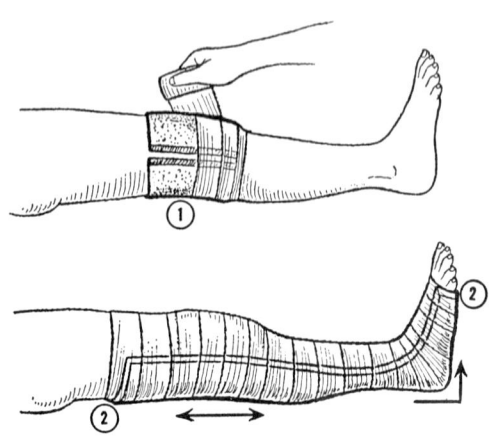

After five days, remove the postoperative splint and apply a long leg cast.

Now institute a regulated program of progressive quadriceps exercises.

Remove the cast at the end of five to six weeks and permit protected weight bearing with crutches; increase the intensity of the quadriceps and flexion exercises.

After eight to nine weeks permit unprotected weight bearing. Continue the exercises until maximum restoration of quadriceps power and extension and flexion of the knee are achieved.

DISLOCATIONS OF THE PATELLA

Acute Dislocations and Subluxations of the Patella

REMARKS

Lateral dislocation or subluxation of the patella is a common cause of knee joint instability in adolescents and young adults, particularly in teenage girls.

Medial dislocation does not occur except as a result of overvigorous surgical correction of a lateral patellar dislocation.

Most often, the patella subluxates when the extended tibia suddenly rotates externally. This causes an unstable patella to drift laterally. Subluxation over the proximal part of the lateral femoral condyle then occurs during the first 20 degrees of knee flexion.

As the patella subluxates or dislocates, the quadriceps relaxes and the knee gives away. Quite frequently the patient falls to the ground and the patella returns spontaneously to the femoral intercondylar groove. A patellar dislocation that does not reduce spontaneously is rare.

The physicians must be alert to this common cause of medial joint pain and instability and must not confuse it with a medial meniscus tear. Other injuries to the extended knee should also be included in the differential diagnosis (see page 1589).

A direct injury to the medial side of the joint or laxity from a medial capsular arthrotomy incision can also produce patellar instability.

Most often the condition occurs in individuals who are susceptible to instability because of a high-riding patella (patella alta) or the abnormality of a laterally displaced patella in a valgus knee.

Clinically the diagnosis is made apparent by palpable instability of the patella as well as by the fear sign (that is, when the surgeon attempts lateral displacement of the patella, the patient becomes so apprehensive that he grasps the examiner's hand to prevent the dislocation).

X-rays will confirm the diagnosis if patella alta is evident. This can be measured by comparing the lengths of the long axis of the patella to the long axis of the patellar tendon. Normally, this ratio is 1:1, but with patella alta it is 0.8:1.

X-rays should also be carefully scrutinized for loose osteochondral fragments. Bony fragments along the medial border of the patella are the result of avulsion of the medial patellar retinaculum. These are attached to the retinaculum and are not free fragments. Free fragments may come from the inferior patellar facet or the lateral femoral condyle and should be removed (see page 1642).

Initial treatment of an acute dislocation or subluxation can be with cast immobilization to promote healing of the disrupted medial retinaculum. Cofield and Bryan had satisfactory results without recurrences in approximately 50 per cent of patients so treated for initial patellar dislocation.

The patient with displaced intra-articular fractures or a pronounced anatomic variation likely to cause recurrent dislocation should be advised to have immediate repair of the extensor apparatus.

Of the many operations devised, the Elmslie-Trillot procedure is most effective in correcting patella alta and the lateral patellar displacement without significantly risking patella chondromalacia from overcorrection.

One should be careful in performing surgery in this area to avoid injury to the growth centers in the skeletally immature patient. Also, after any operation in this area, the surgeon should be alert to the possibility of anterior compartment syndrome in the immediate postoperative period.

Mechanism of Acute Dislocation of the Patella

1. The extended knee is subjected to sudden external rotation.
2. The patella slips superiorly over the lateral femoral condyle.

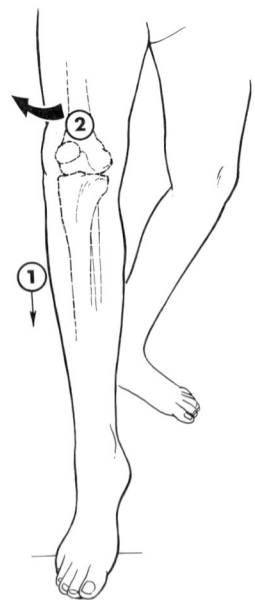

3. As the knee flexes the patella jumps over the lateral condyle and the knee collapses.

Note: Most often the knee reduces spontaneously but occasionally the patient will be brought to the physician with the patella still dislocated.

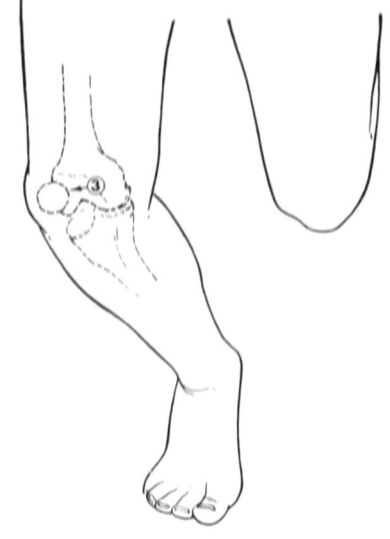

Prereduction X-Ray

1. The patella lies on the lateral aspect of the lateral femoral condyle.
2. The patella is displaced slightly downward.

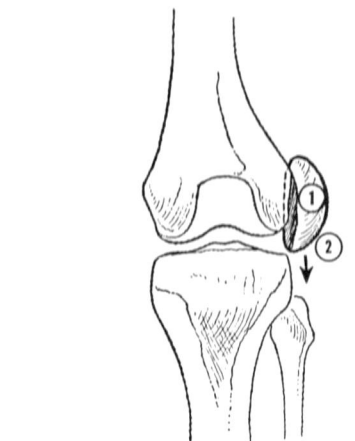

Manipulative Reduction

This can usually be done by gentle direct pressure and knee extension, but if the patient is unable to cooperate because of pain, general anesthesia may be necessary.

1. Extend the knee gradually while
2. Medialward pressure is made upon the patella, pushing it over the lateral femoral condyle.

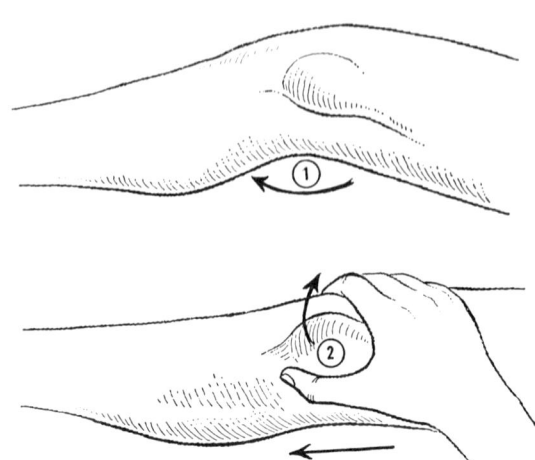

Manipulative Reduction (*Continued*)

1. The patella is in its normal position.
2. Marked swelling is usually present. Always aspirate the joint if intraarticular tension is marked.
3. Aspirate blood and synovial fluid from the joint cavity.

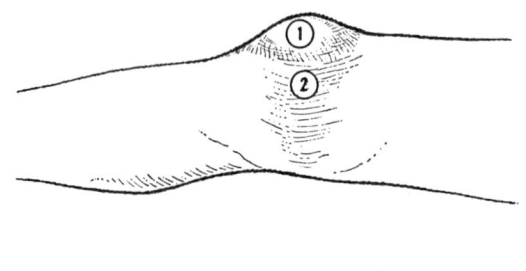
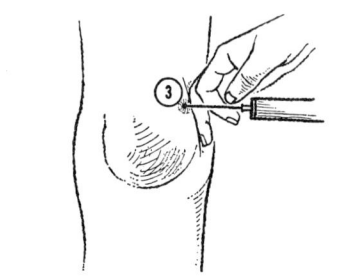

After Aspirating the Knee Joint

1. Apply a cylinder cast using a stockinette wrapped over 2-inch (5-cm) strips of tape placed medially and laterally to serve as suspenders.
2. The malleoli are well-padded.

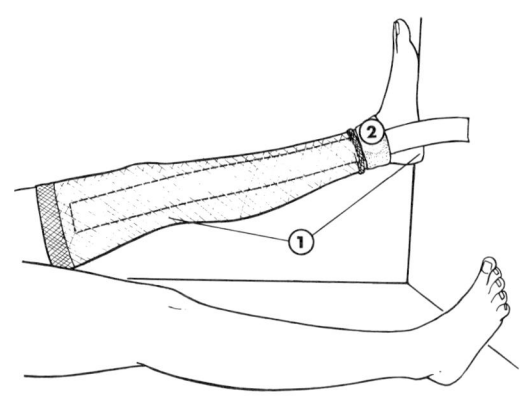

3. The plaster is molded firmly over the patella to push the patella medially and tighten the anteromedial retinaculum.

The major indications for primary operative repair after an acute dislocation are loose bodies or structural abnormalities likely to cause recurrence in active athletic individuals.

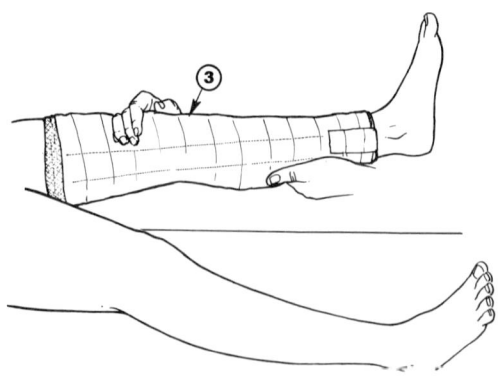

OPERATIVE REPAIR FOR LOOSE OSTEOCHONDRAL FRAGMENTS

REMARKS

Five to 10 per cent of acute patella dislocations have osteochondral fracture fragments. These should be removed because they are loose bodies in the knee joint.

Adequate patellar views are necessary to assess the size and location of these fragments.

An Elmslie-Trillot procedure is the most effective way of correcting patella alta and stabilizing the patellar mechanism without risking chondromalacia from overcorrection.

Preoperative X-Ray

1. An osteochondral fragment has been fractured off the patella in the process of dislocation.
2. This intra-articular fragment should be removed surgically and the patella should be stabilized in the process.

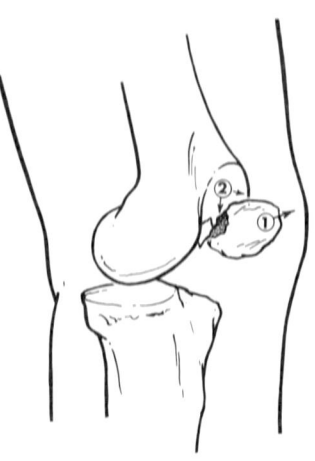

Operative Repair

1. Expose the area by a medial parapatellar incision beginning at the upper pole of the patella and 1 cm medial to it. Continue the incision around the patella and then distally medial to the patellar tendon, terminating slightly below the tibial tubercle.

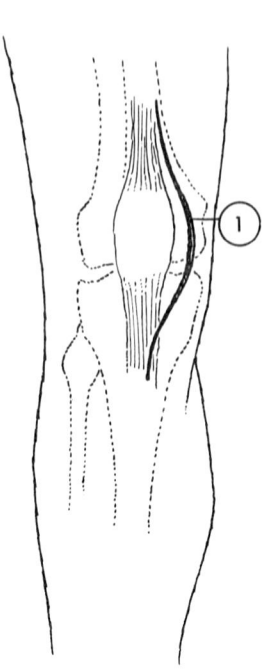

Operative Repair (Continued)

2. Retract the skin edges and divide the deep fascia to visualize the damage to the muscles, medial retinaculum, and capsule. Flush out all debris and clots with normal saline solution and carefully inspect the inside of the joint for osteochondral fragments.

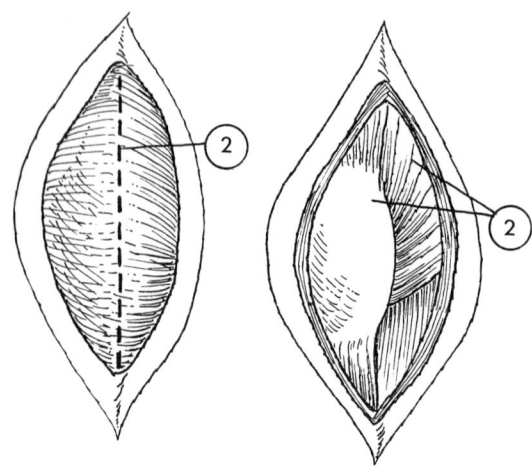

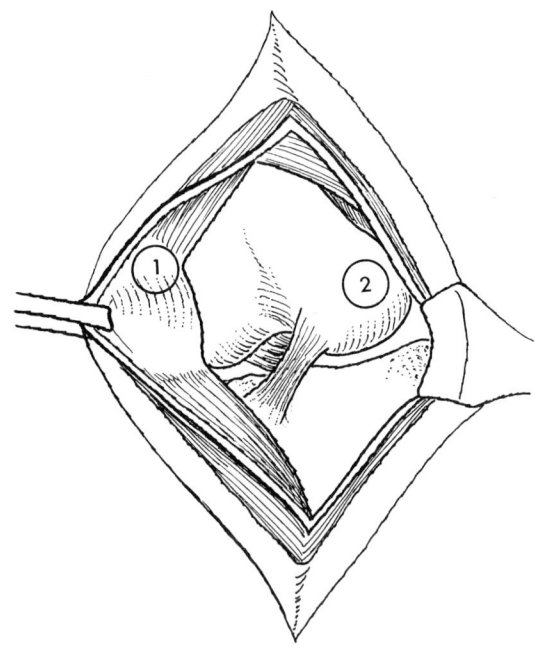

1. The articular surface of the patella is carefully inspected for the loose osteochondral fragments.
2. The articular cartilage of the lateral femoral condyle is also inspected for fracture fragments.

1. Shave off all loose fragments from the articular surface of the patella.

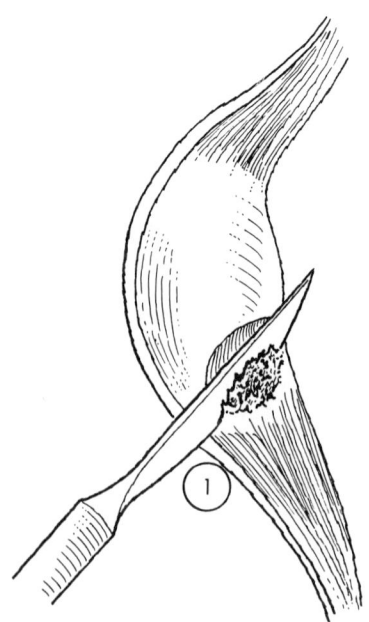

If there are no congenital alterations of the knee joint predisposing to dislocation:
1. Repair the capsule by bringing the edges together with interrupted sutures.
2. Overlap the edges of the tear in the medial retinaculum with mattress sutures.
3. Reattach the vastus medialis to the patella if it has been torn from its attachment.

If the tear is so close to the edges of the patella that closure is impossible:
4. Drill holes along the edge of the patella (do not damage the articular surface) and attach the retinaculum to bone.

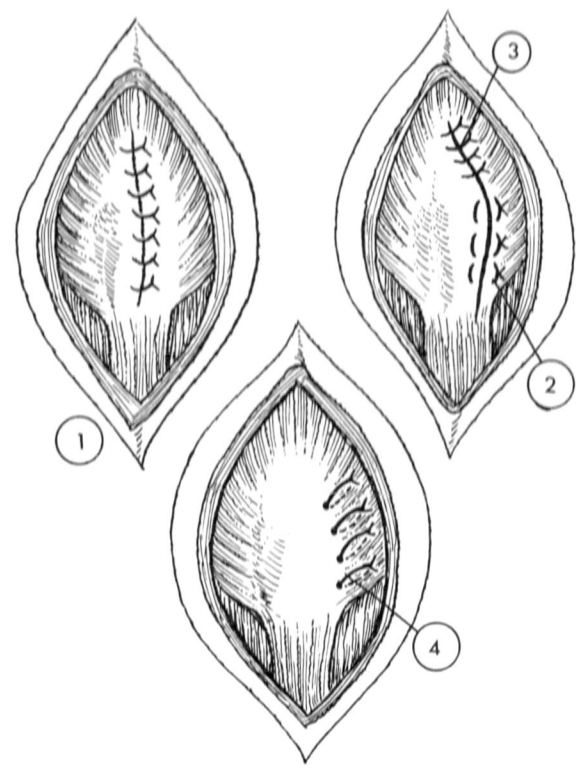

If patella alta is evident, perform an Elmslie-Trillot procedure.
5. The patellar tendon insertion is moved medially and fixed with a screw. The surgical technique is described on page 1673.

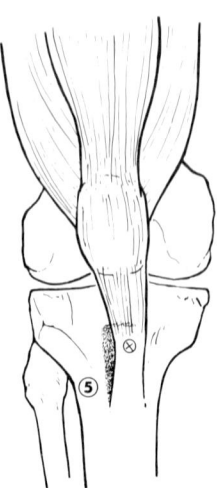

Postoperative Management

Apply a compressive dressing with the knee in extension.

After three to five days remove the compressive dressing and apply a long leg cast.

In four weeks the cast may be removed.

Active quadriceps-setting exercises are started while the patient is in the cast and are continued until full strength and range of motion have returned to the knee joint.

Recurrent Lateral Dislocation or Subluxation of the Patella

REMARKS

Approximately 50 per cent of patients who experience one patellar dislocation will have recurrence. Most often this is associated with abnormalities such as patella alta and a laterally displaced patella associated with a valgus knee.

Recurrence is most common in young adolescent girls but may be frequently seen as well in active adult men.

Frequently, the patient gives a history consistent with the patellar dislocation or subluxation that reduces spontaneously.

Clinically, the laxity of the patella can be confirmed by direct medial pressure, which elicits the fear sign (that is, when the examiner attempts lateral displacement of the patella, the patient becomes so apprehensive that he grasps the physician's hand to prevent dislocation).

X-ray is particularly helpful to confirm the clinical impression and the presence of patella alta and avulsion or osteochondral fractures.

Repeated recurrences ultimately result in symptomatic chondromalacia. Operative repair should be done to alleviate symptoms of instability and to prevent destruction of the patellofemoral articulation.

Operative repair by the Elmslie-Trillot technique effectively decreases patella alta and corrects the lateral displacement of the patella.

Clinical Evaluation: The Fear Sign

1. With the patient's knees flexed, gentle pressure made on the medial surface of the patella causes lateral displacement.
2. The patient grasps the examiner's hand because of the fear that the patella will dislocate.

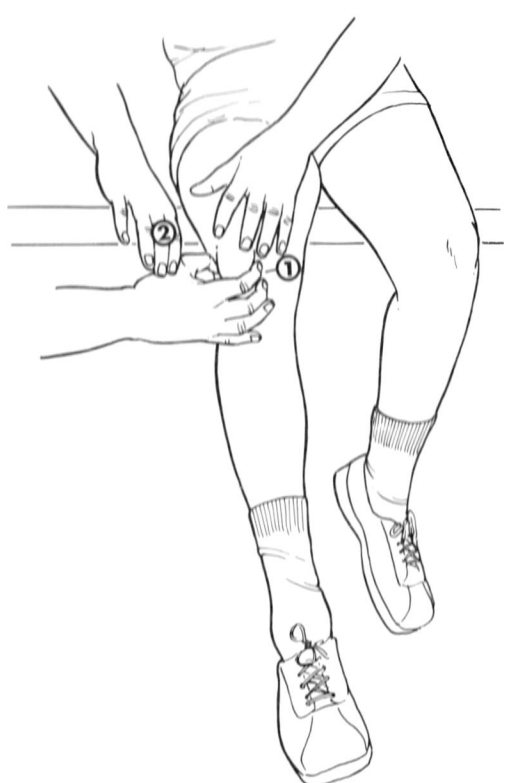

RADIOGRAPHIC EVALUATION OF RECURRENT SUBLUXATION AND DISLOCATION

Patella Alta

Insall and Salvati have shown that in a normal knee the length of the patella is approximately equal to the length of the patellar tendon.

In recurrent dislocation of the patella with patella alta, the ratio of patellar length to patellar tendon length is decreased to 0.8:1.

This high-riding patella significantly contributes to instability and lateral subluxation and eventually to chondromalacia.

Measurement of the position of the patella is based on the ratio of the greatest length of the patella to the length of the patellar tendon. The method is applicable to routine lateral x-rays with the knee in slight flexion (approximately 20 degrees).

Patella Alta (Continued)

1. In a normal knee, the length of the patella is equal to the patella tendon length — ratio is 1:1.
2. The knee with a dislocating patella has patella alta and the ratio of patellar length to patellar tendon length is 0.8:1.

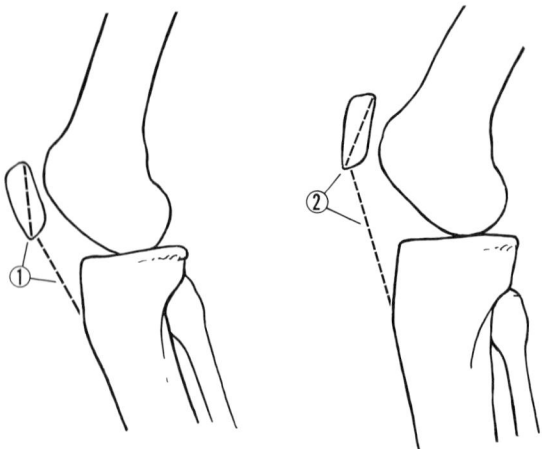

Patellofemoral Views of Recurrent Subluxation and Dislocation

NORMAL KNEE JOINT

1. The lateral condyle is well-developed.
2. The patellar groove is adequate.
3. The patella is deeply seated in the groove and its lateral articular surface is contained by the articular surface of the lateral condyle.

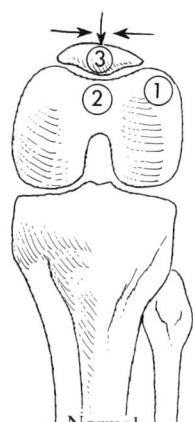

RECURRENT SUBLUXATION

1. The lateral condyle is underdeveloped.
2. The patellar groove is shallow.
3. The patella is aplastic or abnormally small and rides laterally over the condyle.
4. The articular surface of the patella is flat.

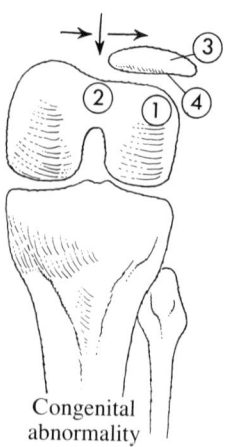

CHRONIC DISLOCATION

1. The patella lies on the lateral aspect of the femoral condyle.
2. The lateral femoral condyle is underdeveloped and flat.
3. The intercondylar groove is shallow.

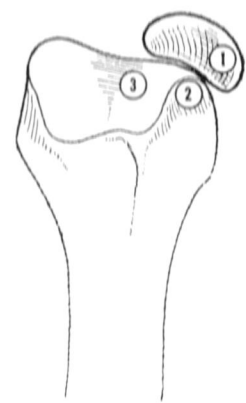

OPERATIVE REPAIR OF RECURRENT PATELLA DISLOCATION AND SUBLUXATION (ELMSLIE-TRILLOT)

This procedure should be carried out in the older adolescent or young adult patient with recurrent intermittent symptoms from patellar instability.

The Elmslie-Trillot procedure, which moves the patellar tendon medially, shortens the tendon and restores the normal one-to-one relationship between the lengths of the patella and the patella tendon.

The procedure is preferred because it achieves the necessary correction without overcorrection or increasing the risk of chondromalacia.

1. A "smile" incision is made distally curving around the tibial tuberosity and up into the medial and lateral plateaus.
2. Subcutaneous tissue is dissected free up through the prepatellar bursa so that the superior pole of the patella is exposed.
3. The medial and lateral retinacula are opened and the patellar tendon is visualized.

Note: The synovium is not opened unless there is evidence of loose osteochondral bodies within the knee.

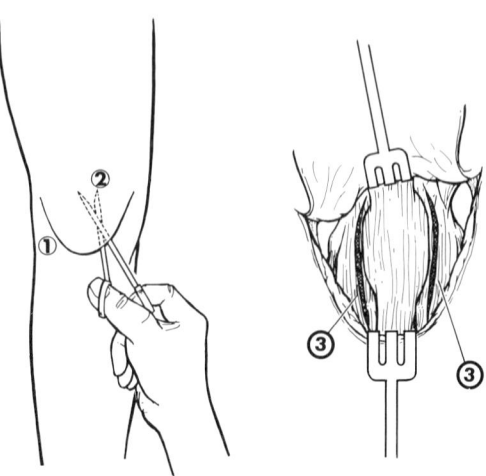

1. Periosteum medial to the tibial tuberosity is reflected medially.
2. The tibial tuberosity is osteotomized along with the patellar tendon attachment. The osteotomy fragment should be approximately 0.5 cm thick.

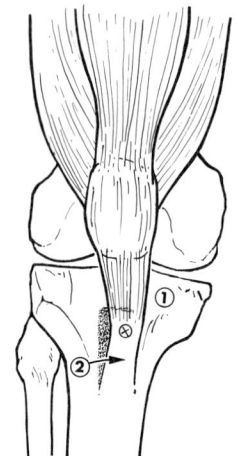

3. The tuberosity with its distal periosteum intact is pivoted medially so that the patellar tendon comes to lie on the anatomic axis of the femur with the knee flexed 45 degrees.
4. The tuberosity is fixed to the underlying bone with a cancellous screw and the reflected periosteum is sutured back to it.
5. The patella is not displaced distally by this procedure.

Note: Release the limb tourniquet to achieve hemostasis prior to closure. Do not apply a cast immediately after operation because of the risk of anterior compartment syndrome from bleeding after surgery in this region. The early sign of this catastrophe is severe pain immediately after operation followed by sensory and motor loss in the limb (see page 67).

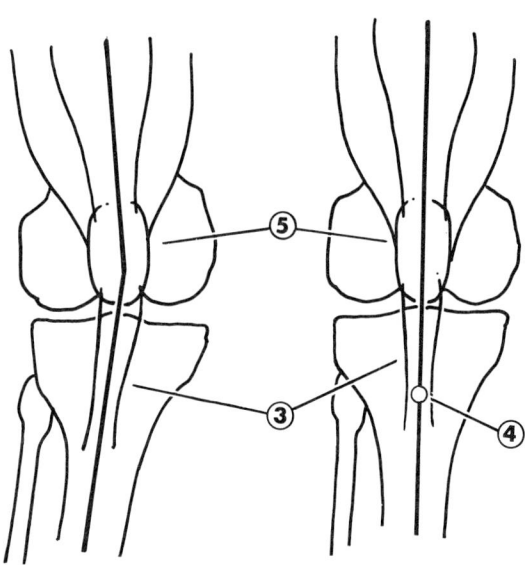

Postoperative Immobilization

1. Apply a posterior splint from the toes to the upper thigh rather than a cast. Ice applications to the operative area relieve the postoperative incisional pain.

Note: Be alert for postoperative pain in the anterior compartment.

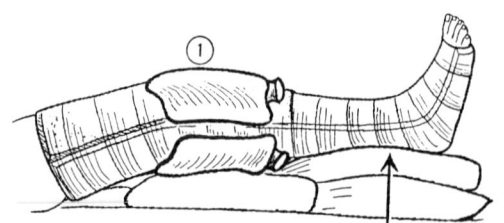

Subsequent Management

When the danger of anterior compartment syndrome has passed, usually by the third to the fifth day, apply a long leg cast with the knee in extension.

The patient may be up on crutches and should actively work on quadriceps strengthening within the first few days postoperatively.

The cast can be removed after four weeks and the patient should be started on the active extension and flexion exercise program.

When the patient has regained complete control of the knee, the crutches may be discarded.

Note: For patellar instability in younger adolescent children whose proximal epiphysis is still open, operative correction should be by soft tissue repair rather than by osteotomy, which might damage the growth center.

SOFT TISSUE REPAIR OF PATELLAR INSTABILITY IN A CHILD OR YOUNG ADOLESCENT

REMARKS

In order to avoid damaging an open proximal tibial epiphysis in a child or young adolescent, patellar stability may be achieved by releasing the lateral retinaculum, repairing the medial capsule, and advancing the vastus medialis.

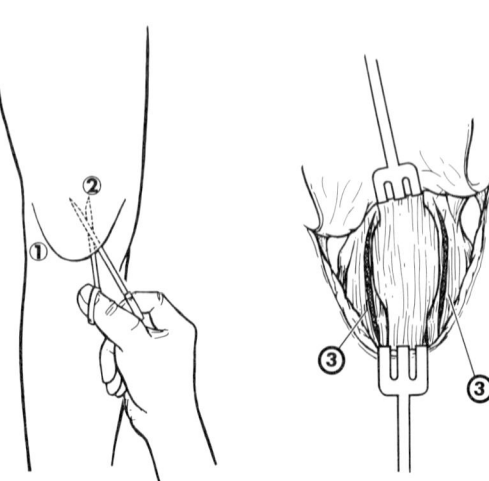

1. A smile incision is made distally curving around the tibial tuberosity and up towards the medial and lateral plateaus.

2. Subcutaneous tissue is dissected free up through the patellar bursa so that the superior pull of the patella is exposed.

3. The medial and lateral retinacula are opened and the patellar tendon is visualized.

1. The patellar tendon is mobilized distally to allow for medial repair.
2. The lateral patellar retinaculum is split from the tendon up to the superior patellar pole as far as the fascia lata. The synovium is not opened.

3. The vastus medialis and medial retinaculum are repaired and the patella and patellar tendon are overlapped as far as the midline.
4. The lateral retinaculum is not closed, but any synovium that may have been opened inadvertently should be repaired.

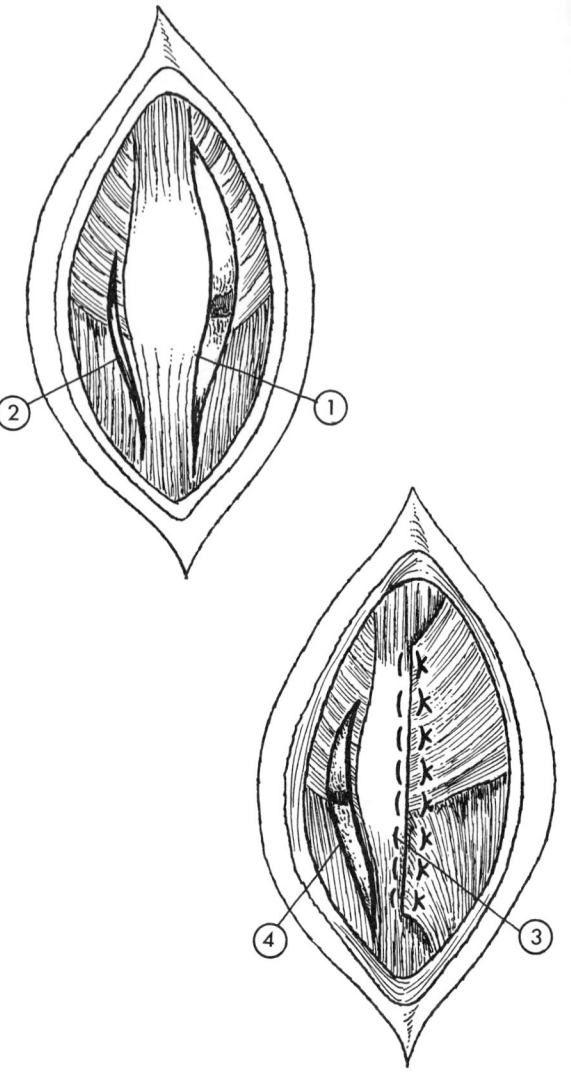

Immobilization

1. Apply a compression bandage.
2. Apply a posterior splint from the toes to the upper thigh.

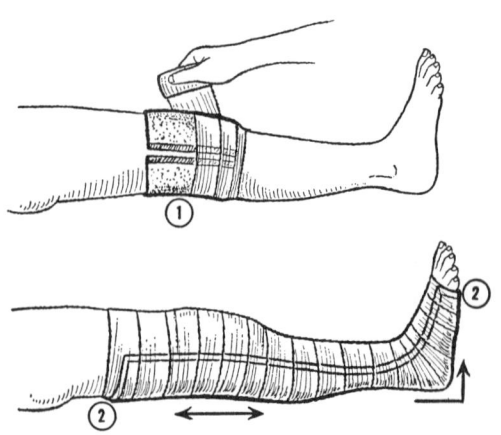

Subsequent Management

When the immediate postoperative swelling has subsided, usually by the third to the fifth day, apply a long leg cast with the knee in extension.

The patient may be up on crutches and should actively work on quadriceps strengthening within the first few days postoperatively.

The cast can be removed after four weeks, and the patient should start on an active extension and flexion exercise program.

When the patient has regained complete control of the knee, the crutches may be discarded.

OPERATIVE REPAIR FOR ADULTS WITH CHRONIC PATELLAR SUBLUXATION OR DISLOCATION AND PATELLOFEMORAL ARTHRITIS (MAQUET)

REMARKS

Chronic patellar instability in adults eventually causes patellofemoral arthritis.

The problem may be resolved with patellectomy, but it is preferable if possible to preserve the patella. Recently Maquet and others have shown that excessive patellofemoral contact stress may be relieved by anterior displacement of the tibial tuberosity.

By displacement of the tibial tuberosity forward 1.0 cm using a long osteotomy of the anterior tibial cortex, the distal aspect of the patella is raised away from its contact with the femoral surface.

The Maquet procedure can be combined with medial capsule repair, vastus medialis advancement, and lateral retinacular release to offer a satisfactory solution to the combined problem of patellar instability and patellofemoral arthritis.

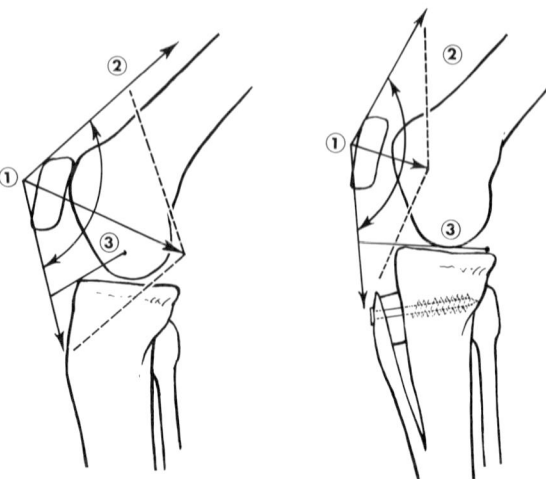

1. The Maquet principle reduces the force vector bringing the patella against the femur by
2. Opening the angle of application of the quadriceps pull through the patella to the tibia and
3. Increasing the moment of the patellar tendon.

1. The incision curves distally well down past the tibial tuberosity and then up toward the medial and lateral plateaus.

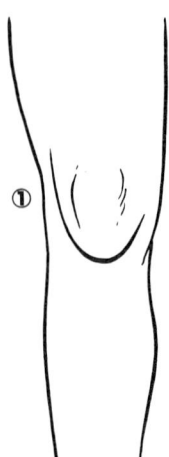

2. The subcutaneous tissue is dissected free up through the prepatellar bursa to the superior patellar pole.

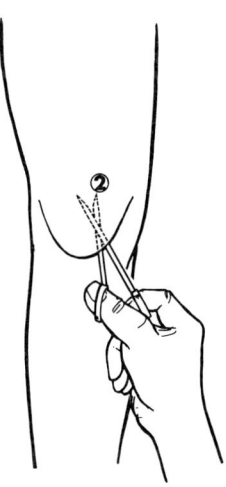

3. The medial and lateral retinacula are opened and the joint is inspected for loose bodies. The undersurface of the patella is also evaluated for the extent of patellofemoral arthritis.

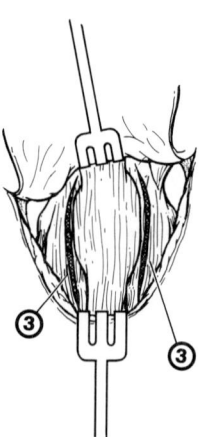

1. The tibial tuberosity is osteotomized in a long axial direction.

2. The osteotomized tibial cortex is elevated at least 1 cm and a cortical-cancellous bone graft is inserted directly beneath to maintain the elevation.

Note: Bone-bank bone serves satisfactorily for the block inserted under the cortex. If bone-bank bone is not available an autogenous graft should be taken from the proximal aspect of the patient's tibial metaphysis or from the iliac crest.

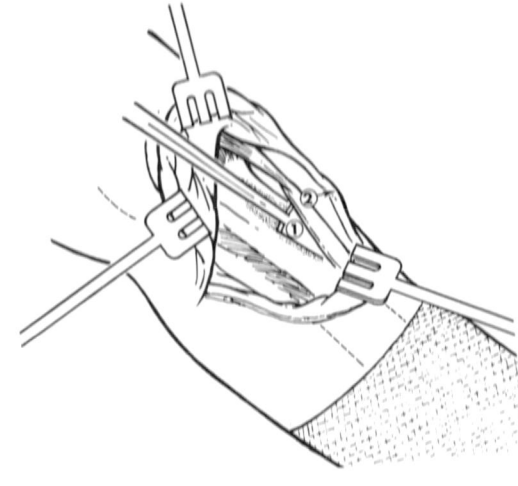

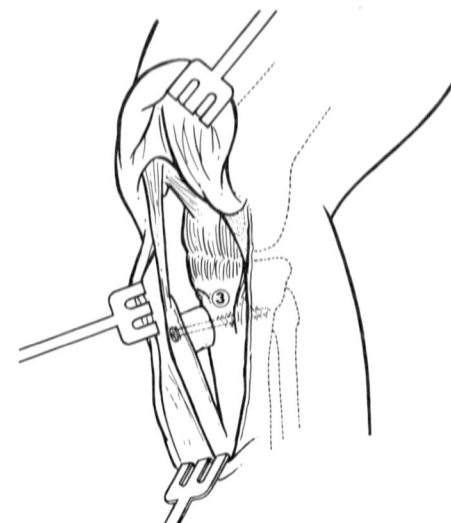

3. The cortex and bone block are fixed to the underlying metaphysis with a lag screw.

Note: The cortex elevation should be no more than 1 cm because greater elevation tends to stretch the overlying skin and cause wound necrosis.

1. After osteotomy of the tibial cortex, evaluate the patellofemoral relationship and compression with the knee flexed 45 degrees.

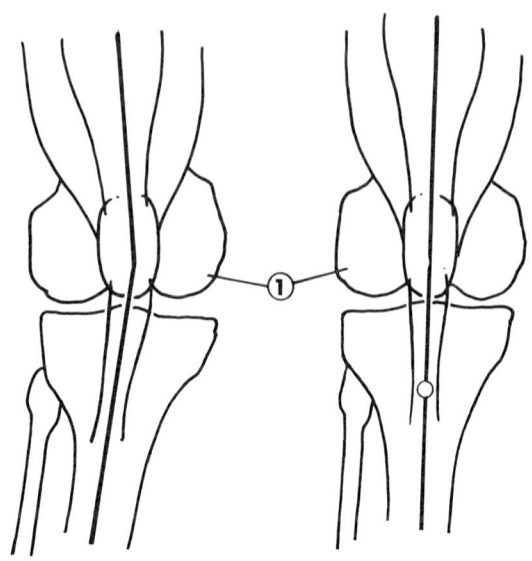

2. Release the retinacula completely to correct any tendency for lateral displacement of the patella.

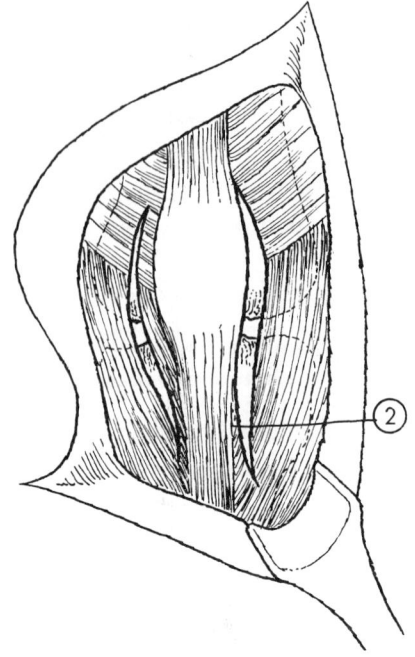

3. Advance the vastus medialis and medial retinaculum onto the quadriceps tendon and patella.
4. Leave the lateral retinaculum open but close any holes in the synovial membrane.

Note: Release the limb tourniquet prior to closure to achieve hemostasis. Do not apply a cast immediately after operation because of the risk of anterior compartment syndrome from bleeding after surgery in this region. The early sign of this catastrophe is severe pain immediately after operation followed by sensory and motor loss in the limb (see page 67).

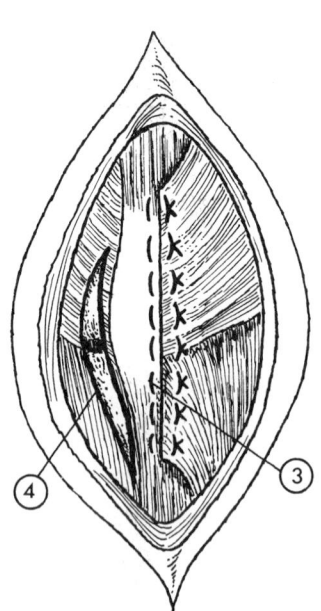

Subsequent Management

When danger of anterior compartment syndrome has passed, usually by the third to the fifth day, apply a long leg cast with the knee in extension.

The patient may be up on crutches and should actively work on quadriceps strengthening within the first few days postoperatively.

The cast can be removed after six weeks and the patient should be started on active range of motion to regain full extension and flexion in the knee joint.

Protected crutch walking is continued for at least six weeks after cast removal to insure adequate healing and protect against refracture of the cortical osteotomy.

Patellectomy

REMARKS

In the face of severe degenerative changes of both the patella and the femur, patellectomy may be indicated but it should be done only if there is no alternative. In addition a quadricepoplasty should be done to improve the tone and direction of the quadriceps mechanism.

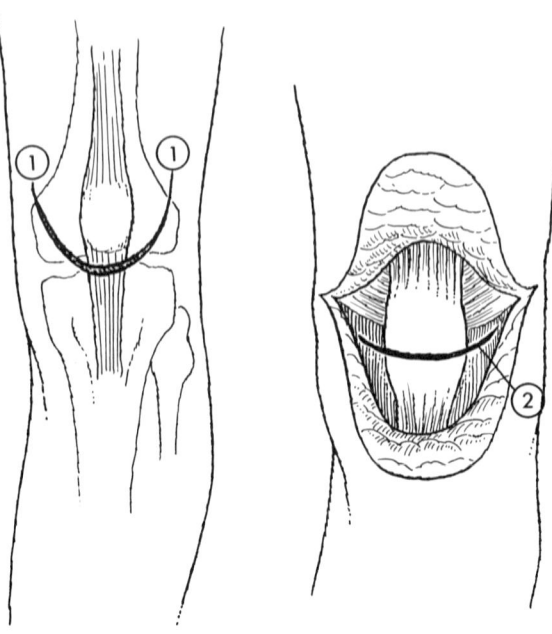

1. Over the anterior surface of the knee make a transverse U-shaped incision just distal to the patella.
2. Reflect the skin edges above and below and make a similar incision through the quadriceps expansion at the level of the distal third of the patella.

3. By sharp dissection excise the patella from the quadriceps tendon, the capsule and the quadriceps expansion, and patellar tendon. Inspect the inside of the joint for any loose bodies and shave off any degenerated loose cartilage from the femoral condyles.

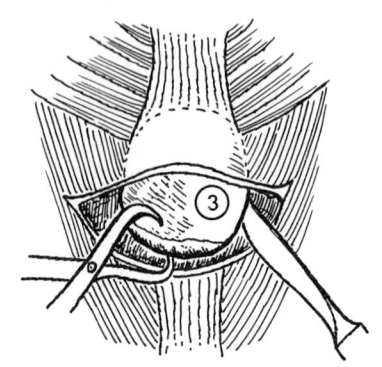

4. Pull the proximal portion of the capsule and quadriceps tendon downward and medially for 1 to 2 cm so that they overlap the distal portion of the capsule by at least 1 cm. With mattress sutures secure the edges in this position.

5. Free the insertion of the vastus medialis from the quadriceps tendon in the form of a V.

6. Pull the end of the vastus medialis downward and laterally and secure it in this position with interrupted sutures.

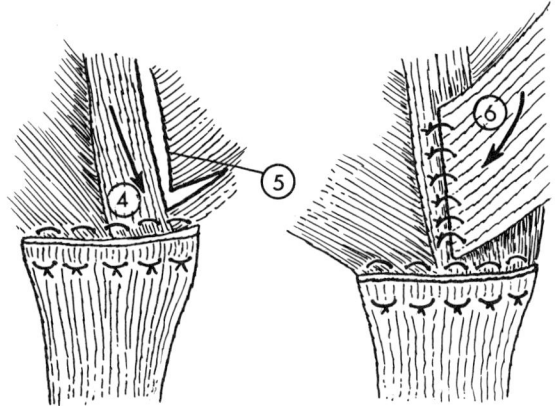

After Completing the Repair

1. Always test the strength of the repair by flexing the knee.

2. The repair should become taut at approximately 60 degrees of knee flexion but the fixation should not loosen.

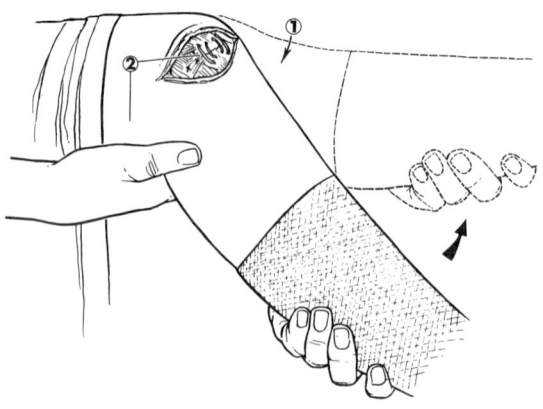

Immobilization

1. Apply a compression bandage.
2. Apply a posterior plaster splint from the toes to the upper thigh.

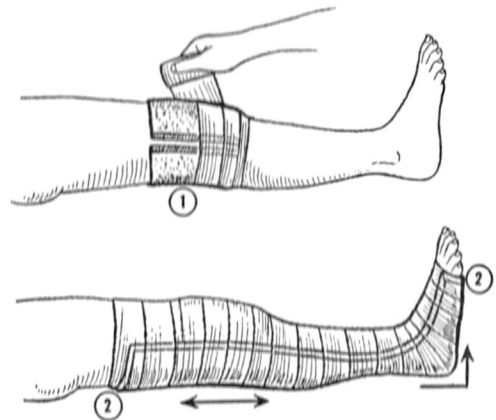

Subsequent Management

The patellar fixation should be sufficiently strong to allow the patient to begin range-of-motion exercises postoperatively without disrupting the repair site.

Immobilize the limb postoperatively in a bundle dressing for 2 to 3 days.

Subsequently begin active quadriceps sitting and knee flexion to 60 degrees.

A knee exerciser can be made from a simple felt sling under the patient's thigh which allows knee flexion passively to 60 degrees.

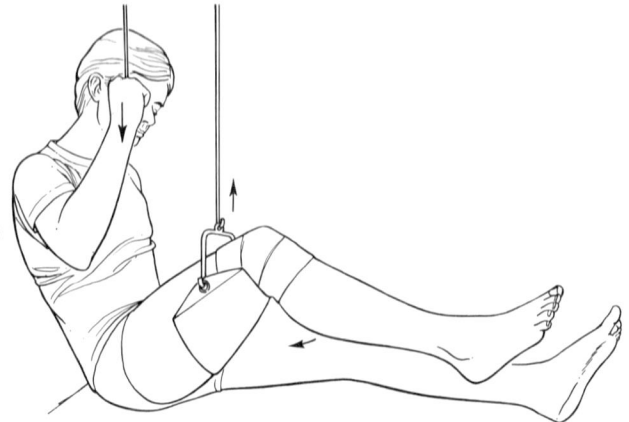

When the patient has full control of the knee he may be up on crutches, but a posterior splint should be applied to protect the knee against sudden hyperflexion while he is on crutches.

Continue with the active exercises for 6 to 8 weeks after which the patient may discard the crutches and protective splint.

Intra-articular Dislocations and Other Irreducible Rotatory Dislocations of the Patella

REMARKS

In a young child, the soft tissue attachments to the patella are lax. Direct trauma that would produce a fracture in an adult may rarely cause the patella to rotate about its longitudinal or transverse axis in a child.

Transverse rotation most often tears the superior patellar pole loose from the quadriceps, causing it to lodge under the femoral condyle with its articular surface facing the tibia.

Less frequently, the inferior patellar pole tears from the patellar tendon, and becomes wedged within the joint with its articular surface facing proximally.

Rotation of the patella about its long axis causes its articular surface to face outward.

The patient presents with a partially flexed swollen knee, and superficial abrasions about the knee joint.

Operative repair is indicated. The locked dislocation can rarely be reduced by closed methods, and the degree of soft tissue trauma to the extensor mechanism is best repaired surgically.

If the dislocation is locked within the joint, release of the remaining quadriceps attachment is usually necessary to accomplish reduction of the dislocation.

Prereduction X-Rays

ROTATORY DISLOCATION ABOUT THE TRANSVERSE AXIS

1. The quadriceps is particularly detached from the superior patellar pole.
2. The remaining retinacular attachment to the distal patella has caused rotation about its transverse axis and lodgment within the joint.
3. The articular surface of the patella faces the tibia.

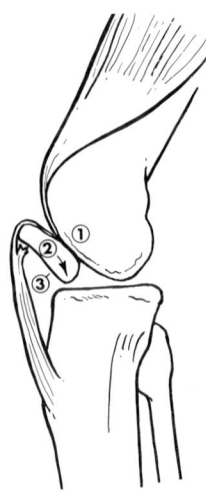

1. The inferior pole may be avulsed from the patellar tendon.
2. The patella rotates about its transverse axis to lodge in the joint.
3. The articular surface faces superiorly.

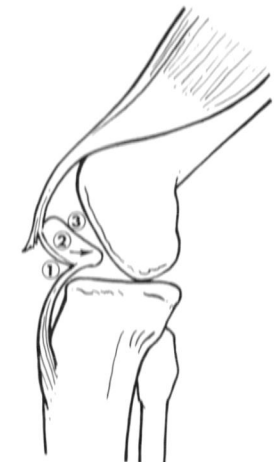

Rotatory dislocation about the longitudinal axis

1. The patella is dislocated laterally and inferiorly.
2. The articular surface faces outward and downward.
3. The medial edge of the patella is locked under the lateral border of the lateral femoral condyle.

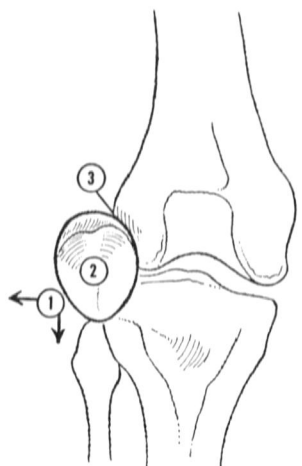

Operative Repair

Rotatory dislocation about the transverse axis

1. The joint is approached through a transverse skin incision. The remaining quadriceps attachment, which is causing the patella to rotate into the joint, is released.

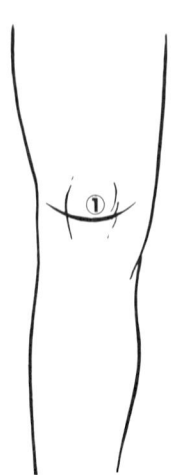

Operative Repair (Continued)

1. The entrapped patella is then removed from the joint and

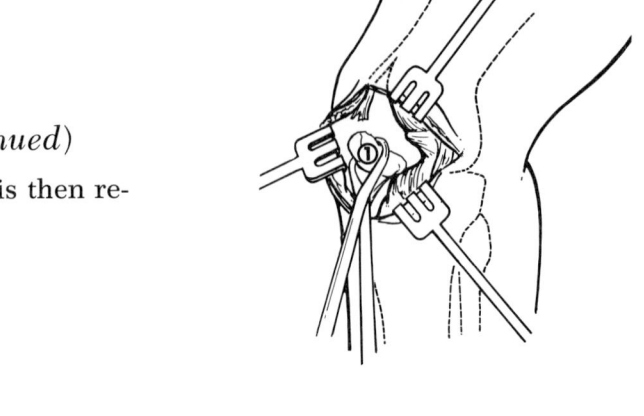

2. The quadriceps tendon is sutured back into the superior pole of the patella. The retinaculum is also repaired.

Note: If the dislocation has occurred from the less common mechanism of avulsion of the inferior patellar pole, the patellar tendon must be repaired completely.

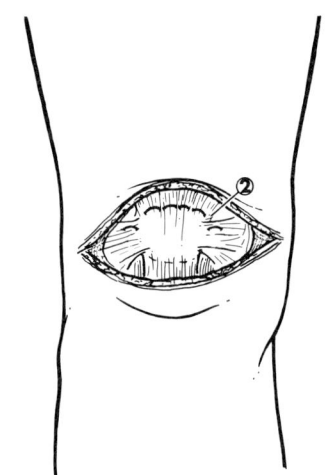

ROTATORY DISLOCATION ABOUT THE LONG AXIS

1. Make a midline skin incision over the anterior aspect of the knee joint.
2. Reflect the skin flaps and visualize the position of the patella and the soft tissue damage.

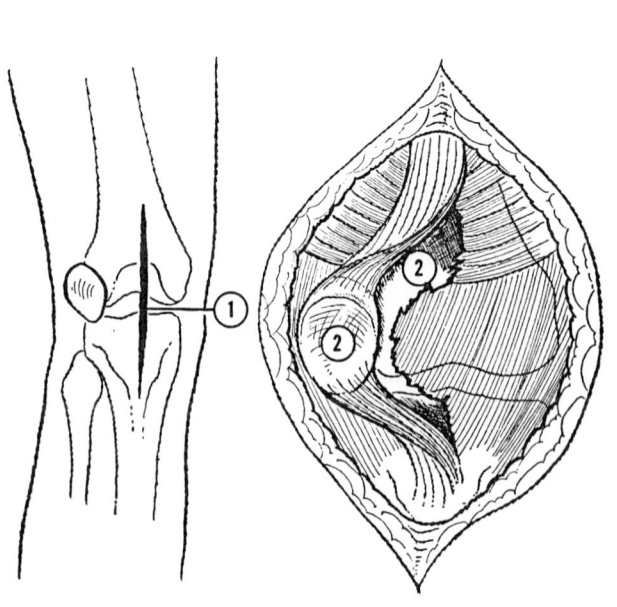

1. Grasp the patella with a towel clip; disengage its medial edge and derotate the quadriceps and patellar tendons.
2. Repair the tears in the patellar retinaculum.
3. Reattach the vastus medialis to the patella if it has been torn from its attachment.

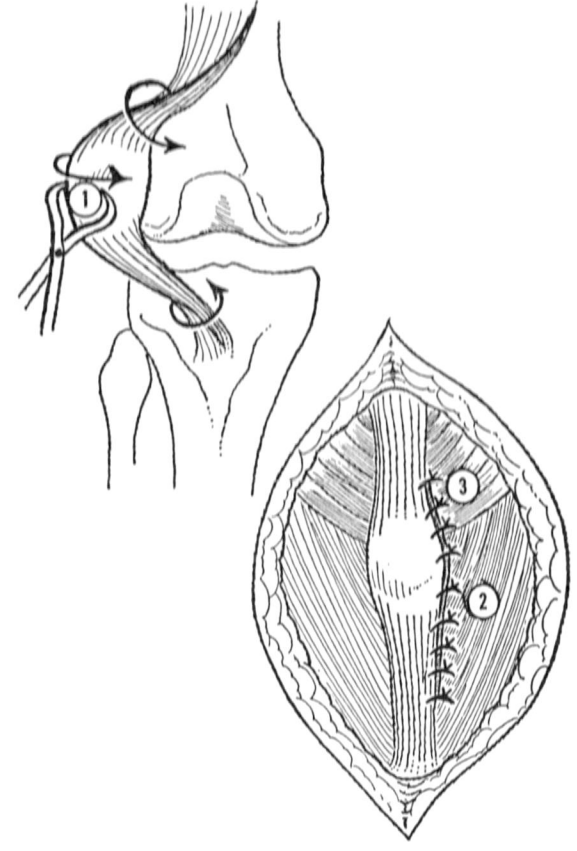

Postoperative Management

1. Immediately after completion of the operation apply a posterior plaster splint extending from the upper thigh to the toes.
2. After two weeks remove the skin sutures and apply a plaster cylinder extending from the upper thigh to just above the malleoli.

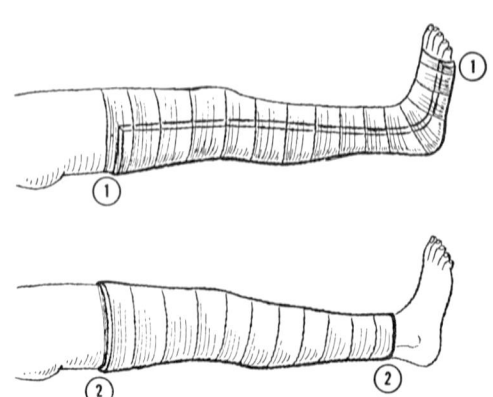

Now institute graduated quadriceps exercises and permit weight bearing.

Four weeks postoperatively remove the plaster cylinder and institute an intensive program of graduated exercises to restore normal joint motion and normal quadriceps power and volume.

SUBLUXATION AND DISLOCATION OF THE PROXIMAL TIBIOFIBULAR JOINT

REMARKS

The proximal tibiofibular joint is a rather rigid diarthrodial joint that includes a joint cavity and is surrounded by a capsule.

Acute and chronic instability and pain may result either from an isolated violent twisting injury or as an associated injury in tibial fracture.

Some individuals may rarely develop idiopathic subluxation when young and have decreasing symptoms as they reach skeletal maturity.

Most commonly, the mechanism as described by Ogden is a sudden inversion and plantar flexion of the foot causing the peroneal and toe extensor muscles to pull violently and dislocate the proximal fibula anteriorly. Simultaneously, knee flexion and external torsion of the leg springs the fibula laterally. Many individuals are anatomically susceptible to this mechanism because of unusual obliquity of the tibiofibular articulation.

Thirty to forty per cent of these patients may go unrecognized or undiagnosed. The patient usually complains of pain in the proximal fibula and frequently in the lateral popliteal fossa along the course of the stretched biceps. Occasionally these symptoms have been mistaken for meniscal injuries and the patient has undergone meniscectomy without relief.

Pain is usually accentuated by dorsiflexion and everting the foot.

Peroneal nerve symptoms may also result from acute or chronic tibiofibular dislocation.

Types of Tibiofibular Dislocation

1. The most common type is an anterolateral dislocation associated with a sudden twisting injury to the leg.

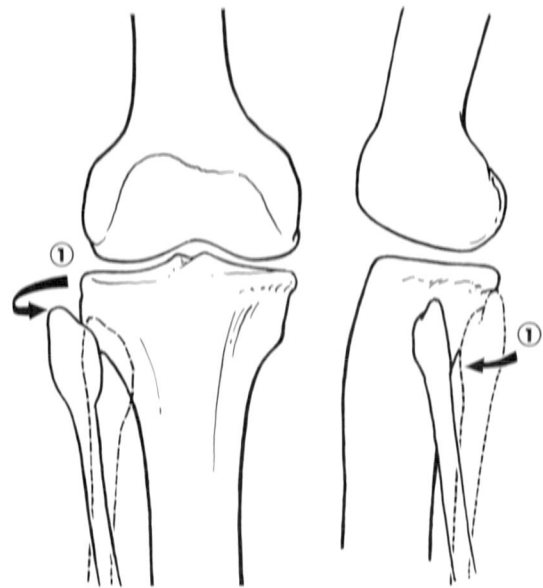

2. A posteromedial dislocation may rarely occur from direct violence to the knee, as when the knee is caught between two car bumpers or hit while on horseback.

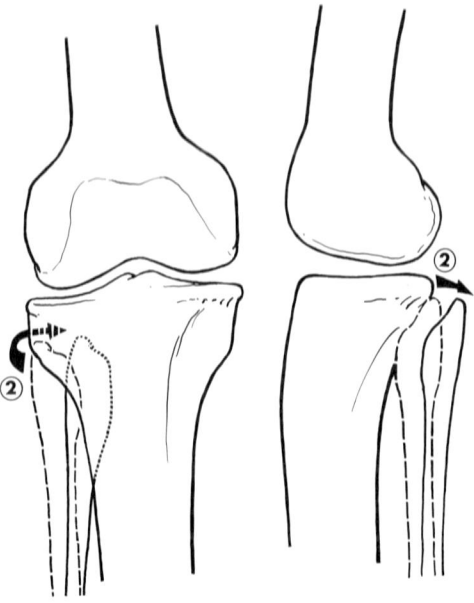

Types of Tibiofibular Dislocation (Continued)

3. Superior dislocation may be associated with congenital joint laxity or may result from shortening of the tibia after a childhood fracture.

Note: Idiopathic subluxation may be found in children with general joint laxity.

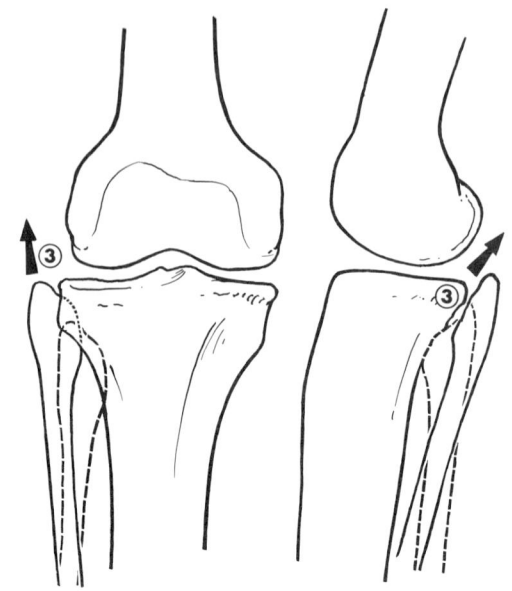

Management

For acute traumatic dislocation, reduction can usually be accomplished by:
1. Everting and dorsiflexing the foot.
2. Flexing the knee at least 90 degrees to relax the biceps and fibular collateral ligament.
3. Snapping the fibular head back into its articulation using direct pressure.

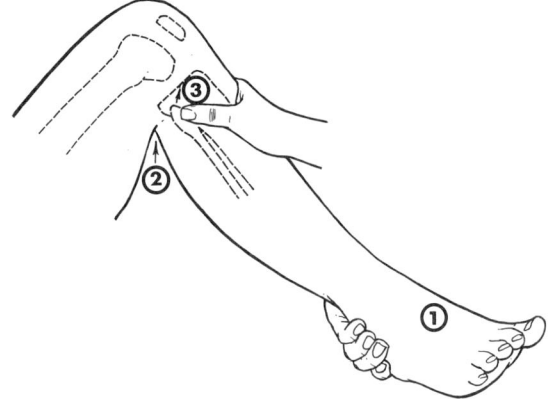

Subsequent Management

The knee should be immobilized for three weeks in a long leg cast with the ankle dorsiflexed.

A fair number of these patients (50 per cent or more) when treated with closed reduction will experience recurring symptoms of pain and instability. This injury is best treated by surgical excision of the proximal fibula.

ACUTE TRAUMATIC HEMARTHROSIS

REMARKS

Knee effusion occurs with many significant internal injuries, although some, such as cruciate tears, will cause greater hemarthrosis than others, such as meniscal injuries.

Any knee that is acutely swollen after injury should be carefully investigated to identify the cause. Beside meniscal and ligamentous injuries, common causes include articular fracture, patellar dislocation, and fat pad injury.

Nontraumatic causes of acute effusion, particularly infection such as gonococcal arthritis, must also be considered if the history of trauma is vague.

Acute, symptomatic, and palpable effusion should be removed by arthrocentesis. This relieves the discomfort from the joint capsule distension and also allows analysis of the joint fluid to distinguish traumatic from nontraumatic causes.

Blood cell counts and joint fluid cultures may be necessary, particularly with persistent or recurrent effusions.

Joint fluid from traumatic hemarthrosis should have a straw color, or should appear bloody or xanthochromic. It may contain visible fat droplets with an intra-articular fracture or, occasionally, some cartilage debris. Cell counts include less than 2,000 white blood cells but many red blood cells.

Accumulation of fluid within 2 hours of an injury indicates hemarthrosis, but fluid that accumulates 12 to 24 hours after injury usually is an irritative synovial effusion.

Joint swelling may be absent with significant injury because of extravasation into surrounding soft tissue rather than into the joint itself. Quite frequently the area of localized swelling also indicates the area of soft tissue disruption about the joint.

MANAGEMENT OF TRAUMATIC HEMARTHROSIS

Aspirate the joint.

Apply an elastic compression bandage.

Immobilize the leg on a posterior plaster splint; elevate the leg and surround the knee with bags containing ice.

Repeat the aspiration after 1 or 2 days if necessary.

After 7 to 10 days of complete rest institute graduated quadriceps exercises.

Now allow partial weight bearing with crutches.

After 10 to 14 days discard the posterior plaster splint, permit full weight bearing, and step up the quadriceps and joint exercises.

Always search for and correct the primary cause of hemarthrosis, using arthrography and arthroscopy as necessary. Dehaven, among others, has shown that an acute knee injury with hemarthrosis is one of the best indications for the use of arthroscopy.

Aspiration of the Knee Joint

Perform the procedure with strict aseptic precautions.

1. Raise an intradermal wheal, using 1 per cent procaine and a fine hypodermic needle, on the outer aspect of the knee just above the superior pole of the patella.

2. After two to five minutes, pass into the joint cavity a large-bore needle at a right angle to the skin.

Aspiration of joint fluid is aided by massaging the suprapatellar pouch.

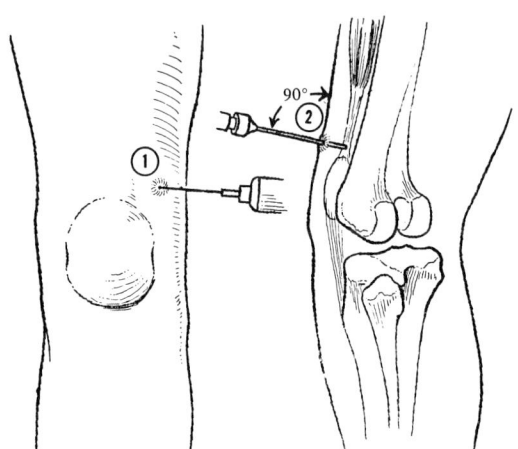

Immobilization

1. Apply a sheet of foam rubber over the anterior and posterior aspects of the knee joint.

2. Make firm, even compression with a circular cotton elastic bandage.

3. Rest the limb on a posterior plaster splint extending from the upper thigh to just above the malleoli; secure the splint with a 7-cm cotton elastic bandage.

Note: Encourage active exercise while the knee is immobilized and reevaluate carefully if the hemarthrosis and symptoms are not improved within one week.

Occasionally, intra-articular cortisone injection may be effective in relieving recurrent traumatic synovitis without underlying meniscal or other cause.

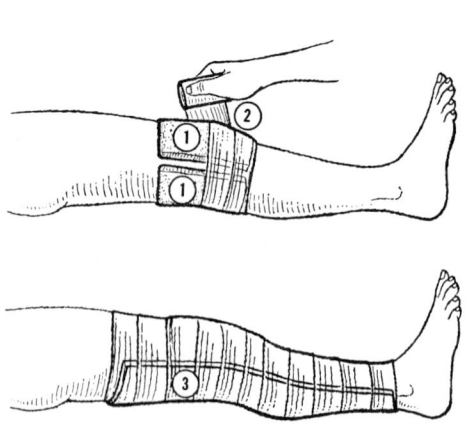

OPEN JOINT INJURIES

REMARKS

The knee is by far the joint most susceptible to open injuries. Penetrating gunshot wounds, open fractures, or lacerations may enter the knee joint.

The potential complications occurring in open knee injuries are major and care should be taken to determine if the joint is involved by any laceration, penetrating wound, or open fracture.

Methods that are helpful in making the diagnosis include palpating an opening into the joint, visualizing air in the joint on x-ray, or extravasating irrigation solution from the joint into the wound.

When in doubt about whether the joint is involved by an open wound, the wisest approach is exploratory arthrotomy.

Cultures of the wound should be made preoperatively and intraoperatively and broad-spectrum antibiotics should be given until cultures indicate which is the most appropriate antibiotic.

Surgical irrigation and removal of contaminated tissue should be thorough. The open joint injury should be closed primarily without using devices such as irrigation-suction tubes.

Ballard and coworkers have pointed out that in management of extremely contaminated or infected joint injuries, the most adequate method of evacuating the joint is by leaving it open and allowing active mobilization rather than immobilization. Articular cartilage is not adversely affected by this open method, whereas it can be rapidly destroyed by infected synovial fluid that has not been adequately drained.

Types of Injuries Requiring Arthrotomy

1. Puncture wound into the suprapatellar pouch.

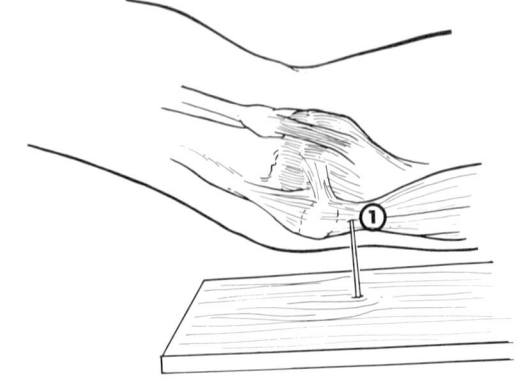

OPEN JOINT INJURIES

Types of Injuries Requiring Arthrotomy (Continued)

2. Open fracture of the patella.

Note: These open joint injuries should be treated by surgical exploration and cleansing and primary closure. Broad-spectrum antibiotic treatment is continued until the wound is healed.

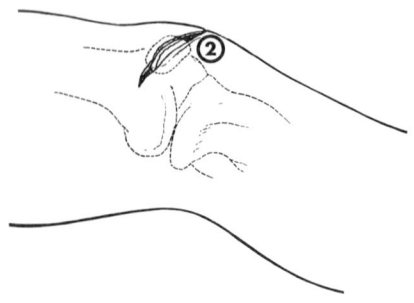

MANAGEMENT OF GROSSLY CONTAMINATED OPEN KNEE INJURIES

Some grossly contaminated open knee injuries should be treated as already septic joints.

This method of management is also useful for suppurative arthritis and postoperative knee joint infections.

Types of Injuries Requiring Open Treatment

1. A grossly contaminated open gunshot wound should be treated as a septic knee joint.

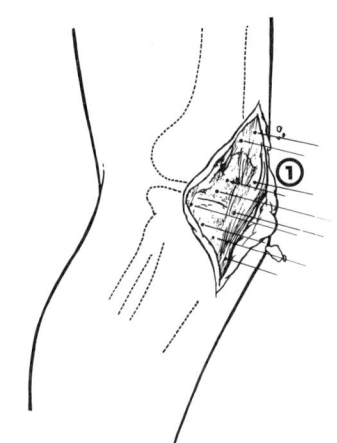

Operative Technique

1. The joint is explored from both medial and lateral incisions extending from the superior pole of the patella to approximately 1 cm below the tibial plateau.

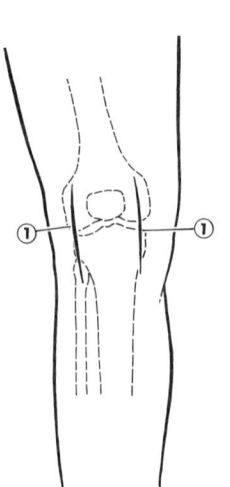

1694

2. The joint is thoroughly irrigated with saline-and-antibiotic solution and all blood clots, foreign matter, and loose bone fragments are removed.

Note: Avoid removing the menisci or fat pad unless they are grossly damaged or infected.

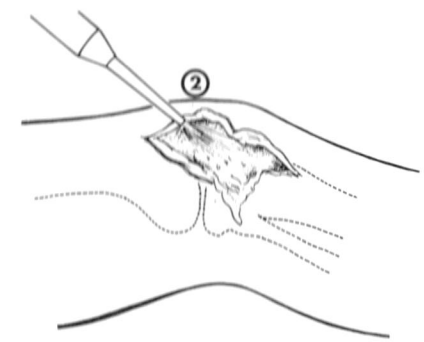

Postoperative Management

1. Both wounds are left wide open and the knee is immobilized for 24 hours in a bulky dressing. Subsequently, whirlpool treatment is started and patient is encouraged to actively exercise the knee while it is in the whirlpool.
2. Wire skin sutures may be used merely as support sutures to prevent wide retraction of the skin edges.

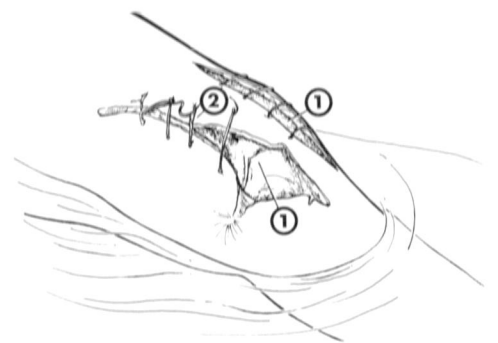

Subsequent Management

Whirlpool treatment is continued on a daily basis and the patient is encouraged to exercise the knee actively when it is not in the whirlpool.

Usually within the first postoperative week, the exudate will decrease sufficiently to require only a small dressing on the knee.

The wounds are allowed to close by formation of granulation tissue and by gradual tightening of the wire sutures.

Wound closure may require 4 to 6 weeks or longer.

If knee motion does not exceed 70 degrees after several weeks of active exercise, the knee should be manipulated under anesthesia, provided there is no associated patellar fracture or other injury contraindicating manipulation.

FRACTURES OF THE CONDYLES OF THE TIBIA

REMARKS

Fractures of the tibial condyles have been called car bumper fractures because the lateral plateau is particularly exposed in auto-pedestrian accidents.

The most common cause, however, is a fall that exerts a sudden valgus and compressive loading on the knee, driving the prominent anterior part of the lateral femoral condyle like a wedge into the lateral plateau.

Other common mechanisms are direct blow to the knee of a car occupant and crushing blow to the knee by a heavy weight such as a falling tree or log.

Approximately 60 per cent of these fractures involve only the lateral condyle, 20 to 25 per cent involve both condyles, and 10 to 15 per cent involve only the medial condyle.

The types of plateau fracture can be most simply classified as undisplaced, depression, and split-depression fractures.

If the force of the compression loading is severe, the proximal fibula may also be fractured, but in most instances the fibula remains intact to provide some stability to the plateau fracture.

The diagnosis of an undisplaced fracture may be subtle, and oblique views as well as standard x-rays are required to detect a fracture associated with the painful hemarthrosis.

Radiographic assessment should include a tibial plateau view to compensate for the 15-degree angle the plateau makes with the tibial crest. This permits consistent evaluation of the depth of depression of the plateau surface.

The surface area of a condylar depression is extremely difficult to measure on the x-ray. The most effective technique of estimating damage is with single-contrast arthrography, which can be done after the hemarthrosis is aspirated. Single contrast injection also is helpful to demonstrate any significant ligamentous rupture, which occurs in approximately 10 per cent of these fractures (see page 1559).

Despite the alarming radiographic appearance of lateral plateau fracture, the clinical result is usually quite good. This is in contrast to most compression fractures of weight-bearing surfaces in the ankle, in which

FRACTURES OF THE CONDYLES OF THE TIBIA

traumatic arthritis is quite common. The reason for the good results with lateral tibial plateau fractures appears to be that the fracture rarely in-involves the weight-bearing surface. Walker has demonstrated on cadaver knees that loads up to 150 kg are carried almost entirely on the lateral meniscus. Load distribution on the medial compartment is equally shared by the medial meniscus and the exposed articular cartilage. This may explain why fractures in the medial tibial plateau lead more often to traumatic arthritis than do the more common lateral plateau fractures.

The valgus mechanism producing a lateral plateau fracture consistently spares the lateral meniscus and fractures the weaker cartilage of the lateral plateau. The lateral meniscus should not be removed during any surgical repair of the fracture because it serves as an effective load carrier and protects the healing articular fracture.

Role of Menisci in Weight Bearing (Walker)

With loading of up to 150 kg across the knee,

1. Contact on the medial side is evenly distributed between the medial meniscus and the articular surface.
2. Contact on the lateral side is almost entirely carried by the lateral meniscus.

Note: The valgus compression mechanism that produces lateral plateau fractures is applied to the surface that is ordinarily not bearing weight.

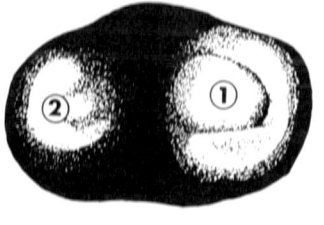

LATERAL   MEDIAL

Types of Lateral Plateau Fractures

1. Undisplaced fracture.
2. Depression fracture.

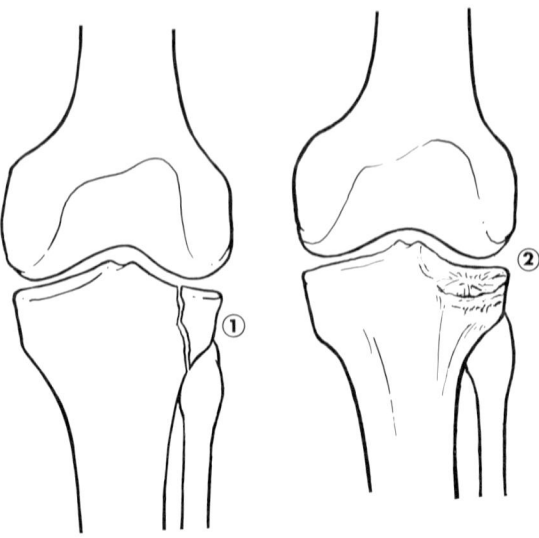

Types of Lateral Plateau Fractures (Continued)

3. Split-depression fracture with intact fibula.
4. Split-depression fracture with fractured fibula.

Note: Fractures produced by compression-valgus load should be distinguished from fractures of the rim of the joint, which are caused by the avulsion of the lateral capsule (see page 1585).

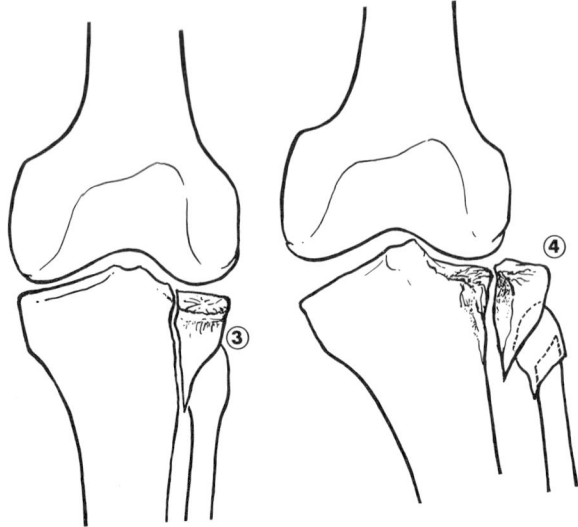

Other Types of Tibial Condylar Fracture

1. Bicondylar fracture with or without an intact fibula.
2. Medial spinotuberosity fracture.

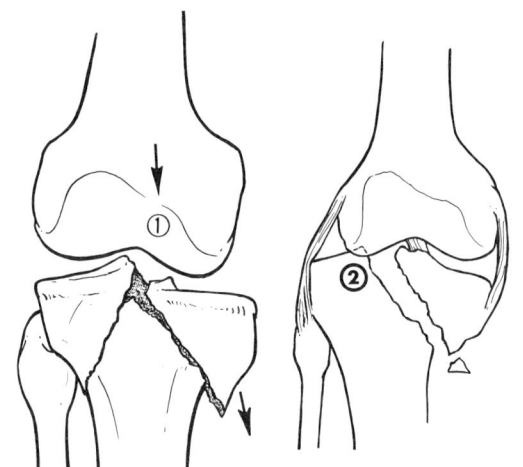

3. Lateral spinotuberosity fracture.

Note: Spinotuberosity fracture, which is essentially a fracture-dislocation, must be distinguished from the usually more stable tibial condylar fracture.

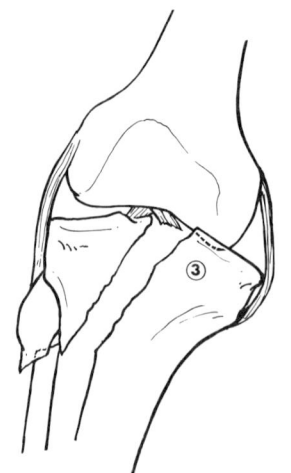

THE INFLUENCE OF THE FIBULA ON TIBIAL PLATEAU FRACTURE (SARMIENTO)

REMARKS

Most lateral tibial plateau fractures are associated with an intact fibula, which supports the fracture during weight bearing and prevents further collapse.

Fracture of the lateral plateau with a proximal fibular fracture may collapse further with weight bearing. This should be kept in mind during treatment.

Fracture of both condyles does not lead to significant further collapse if the proximal fibula is fractured. Weight-bearing stresses appear to be equally distributed through both condyles in this situation.

If the fibula is intact with a bicondylar or medial condylar fracture, the medial condyle may collapse into a varus deformity.

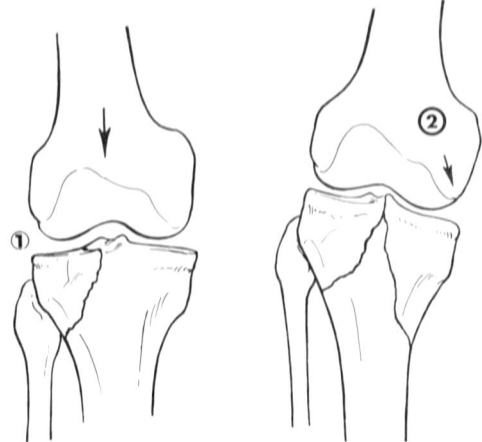

1. An intact fibula supports the lateral plateau fracture against collapse.
2. An intact fibula tends to produce varus deformity with bicondylar or medial plateau fracture.

RADIOGRAPHIC EVALUATION OF TIBIAL PLATEAU FRACTURE

REMARKS

Anteroposterior x-rays tend to overemphasize the degree of condylar collapse, since they are not usually taken parallel to the joint surface. An angled view is necessary to visualize the sloping articular surface of the tibia properly.

Single-contrast arthrogram may also be used to demonstrate the depth and area of surface involvement and to visualize ligamentous injuries that are often associated with plateau fracture (see page 1559).

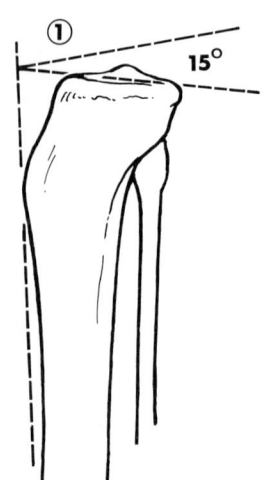

1. Tibial plateau views should accommodate for the normal 15-degree tilt of the joint surface relative to the tibial cortex.

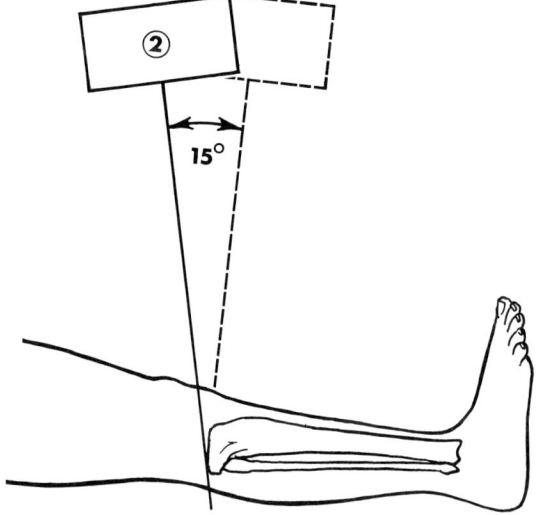

2. A tibial plateau view should be an anteroposterior view angled at 105 degrees.

MANAGEMENT

REMARKS

The treatment of these fractures should restore the joint as close to normal anatomy and stability as possible. Prolonged (more than four to six weeks) immobilization of the injured knee should be avoided.

Undisplaced tibial plateau fractures warrant symptomatic treatment, including knee joint aspiration and partial weight bearing with crutches for six to eight weeks. Ordinary loading during knee motion does not risk displacement of these fractures, and cast immobilization is unnecessary for most patients with undisplaced fractures.

Displaced fractures of either the depression or the split-depression type can be effectively treated by closed reduction that applies a varus load to the joint. This tightens the capsular attachment to the periphery of the plateau and thereby elevates the fracture fragments underneath the lateral meniscus. Centrally depressed fractures are unloaded by the varus position of the knee, and over a period of six to eight weeks, the healing process reconstitutes the plateau.

The technique of varus reduction depends on adequate fibular support and soft tissue attachment. It may not be effective with a split-depression fracture down through the fibula, which should be treated by closed reduction. The possibility of open reduction should, however, be explained to the patient.

Early active protected knee motion is an important part of therapy. Motion is vital to joint surface nutrition and serves to reconstitute a new articular surface after fracture much as it does after joint arthroplasty.

In most instances closed reduction is effective and can be maintained using a cast-brace device. Knee hinges are applied so as to maintain a varus load on the knee while still allowing flexion and extension during the healing process. The addition of the cast-brace to closed reduction treatment has significantly diminished the indication for internal fixation in order to permit knee motion of these intra-articular fractures.

Closed reduction with cast-brace immobilization is preferable to operative fixation of most of these injuries. Results are at least comparable, and significant complications of septic arthritis, peroneal nerve palsy, or avascular necrosis of subchondral bone, which can follow open treatment, are avoided with closed treatment.

Fracture of the Lateral Tibial Condyle without Fragmentation or Depression

REMARKS

A large proportion of these fractures, particularly in elderly patients, are undisplaced or minimally displaced.

Treatment should include aspiration of hemarthrosis to relieve discomfort and application of a soft tissue compression dressing.

Prereduction X-Ray

Fracture of the lateral condyle without displacement and with an intact fibula.

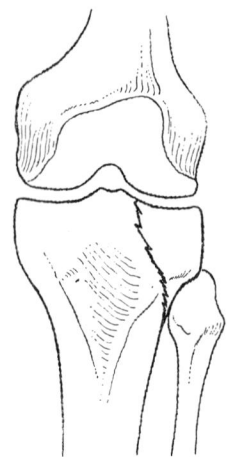

Immediate Management

1. Aspirate the knee.
2. Apply a soft tissue compression dressing or Jones' type dressing with compression bandages and an ace wrap.

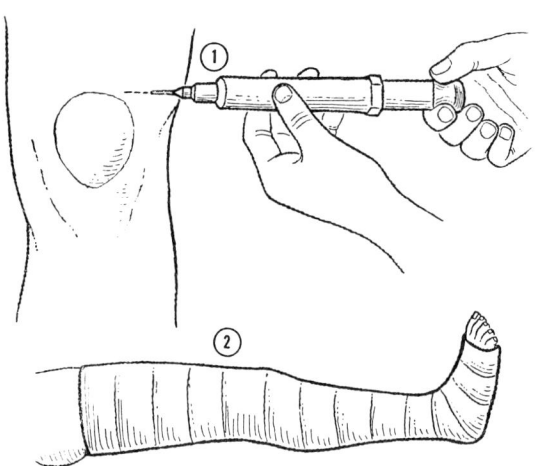

Subsequent Management

Allow the patient to walk with crutches and bear minimal weight on the fractured limb. Institute quadriceps exercises immediately.

In most instances, cast immobilization of these undisplaced fractures in elderly patients is unnecessary and adds to disability. However, the fracture should be radiographed within the first week after the patient is walking with crutches.

After six to eight weeks with adequate quadriceps strength, weight bearing may be increased progressively and the patient may gradually discard crutches in favor of a cane.

All external support can generally be discarded by eight to ten weeks, depending on the symptoms and the recovery of muscle strength about the knee.

Closed Reduction and Cast-Brace Immobilization for Displaced Lateral Plateau Fracture

REMARKS

Preoperative evaluation of this injury should include anteroposterior, lateral, and oblique x-rays as well as 105-degree tibial plateau view (see page 1700).

Prior to reduction, the knee joint should be aspirated and a bulky compression should be applied with plaster splints for immobilization until reduction can be accomplished.

Several days after the injury, under light general anesthesia, the reduction is carried out.

Prereduction X-Rays

SPLIT-DEPRESSION FRACTURE

1. There is a split-depression fracture with depression of as much as 10 mm in some areas of the plateau.
2. The lateral margin and lateral meniscus remain elevated.
3. The fibula is not fractured.

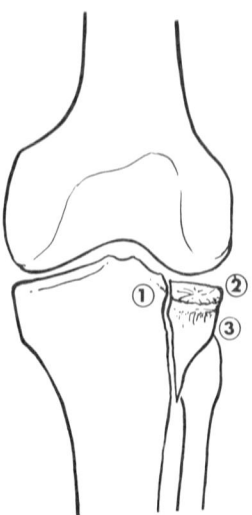

FRACTURES OF THE CONDYLES OF THE TIBIA

Prereduction X-Rays (Continued)

CENTRAL DEPRESSION FRACTURE

1. The tibial plateau view shows a central depression in some areas of at least 20 mm.
2. The peripheral meniscal region remains intact.

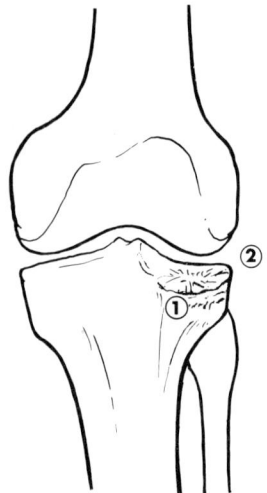

Reduction by Traction and Manipulation

Note: If the joint is distended, always aspirate the blood before proceeding with the reduction.

1. Fasten the patient's feet to the foot pieces of the fracture table.
2. The knees are extended.
3. Make moderate mechanical traction of the affected limb.

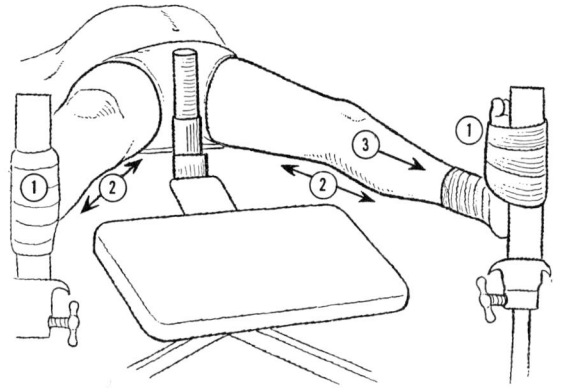

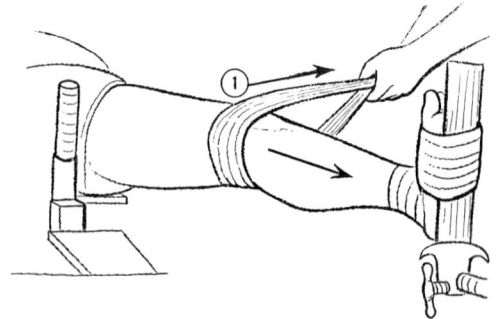

1704

FRACTURES OF THE CONDYLES OF THE TIBIA

1. While traction is maintained an assistant makes manual lateral traction on the knee, using a muslin sling.
2. Traction and varus manipulation elevate the plateau fracture by the pull of the soft tissue attachments.

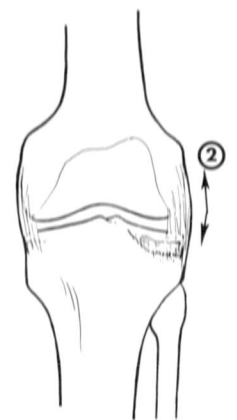

1. Now firmly compress the tibial tuberosity with the heels of the hands or
2. If necessary, the plateau may be compressed by a padded C clamp.

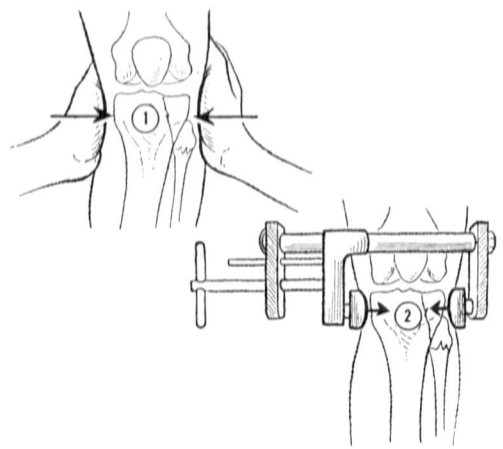

Immobilization

1. While traction is maintained, a cast-brace is applied.
2. The hinges are incorporated to exert a continued varus loading on the knee joint.

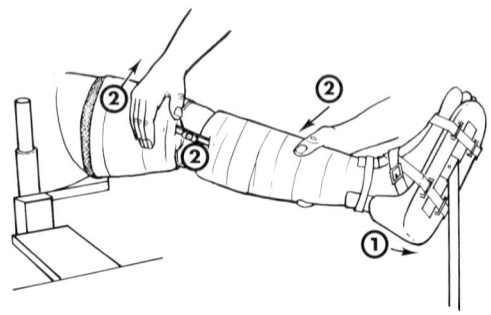

Immobilization *(Continued)*

1. The cast should be applied well down over the femoral condyles and
2. Well up over the tibial plateau to protect against valgus loading.

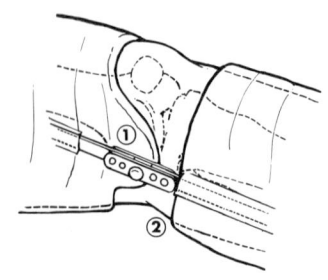

Postreduction X-Rays

SPLIT-DEPRESSION FRACTURE

1. The depressed fragment has been elevated close to a normal anatomic position by the pull of the attached soft tissue.
2. The widening of the plateau surface is diminished.

Note: Even if reduction does not completely elevate the bone fragments to the level of the functional plateau, the varus reduction will permit healing of the plateau without significant depression.

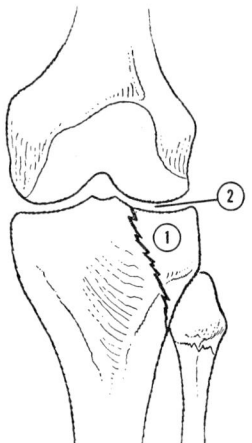

CENTRAL-DEPRESSION FRACTURE

1. Central depression of 5 to 10 mm may be accepted, provided that
2. The weight-bearing meniscal region is intact.

Note: Drennan and co-workers have demonstrated that central depression fractures can reconstitute the tibial plateau surface and heal with excellent results despite incomplete reduction.

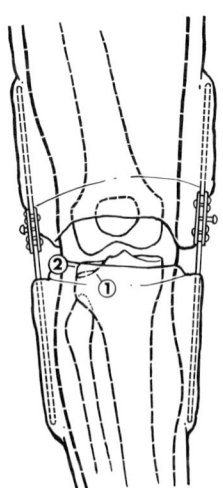

Postreduction Management

Begin active range-of-motion exercises on a regular schedule for at least five minutes out of every hour.

Encourage the patient to do straight-leg raising with gradually increasing loads.

Partial weight bearing with crutches may be allowed because redisplacement of the fracture is prevented by the varus position of the knee joint.

The cast-brace may be removed after eight weeks, when x-ray should show adequate healing of this cancellous bone fracture.

Continue crutch-protected weight bearing for six weeks longer until the patient has full active control of the knee.

Internal Fixation for Displaced Lateral Plateau Fracture and Other Tibial Condylar Fractures

REMARKS

Operative fixation is usually unnecessary except in occasional fractures that cannot be reduced by traction and varus manipulation techniques.

Drennan and coworkers have pointed out that results from closed varus reduction of a plateau fracture are more likely to be unsatisfactory in a severe split-depression fracture than in a central-depression fracture. Operative treatment should be reserved mainly for failure to reduce the split-depression fracture.

Lateral plateau fractures associated with proximal fibular fractures may lose sufficient stability to prevent closed reduction or to make them unstable with a cast-brace technique.

Spinotuberosity fracture, which includes the tibial spine and tuberosity, is frequently associated with subluxation of the proximal tibia.

Operative fixation is necessary for this unstable fracture-dislocation, which should be distinguished from plateau fractures.

Approximately 10 per cent of these fractures demonstrate disruption of the medial capsular structures when they are studied by arthrography or stress x-ray. Closed reduction and cast-brace immobilization can be used effectively to promote healing of the medial capsular tears and simultaneously the tibial plateau fracture. On long-term follow-up of displaced lateral plateau fractures, Moore and coworkers found no significant incidence of residual ligamentous instability.

Unstable Tibial Condylar Fractures

Rarely operative reduction is necessary for:
1. A split-decompression fracture associated with
2. A fractured fibula.

Note: The loss of both soft tissue and fibular support may prevent adequate closed reduction and necessitate open reduction and internal stabilization.

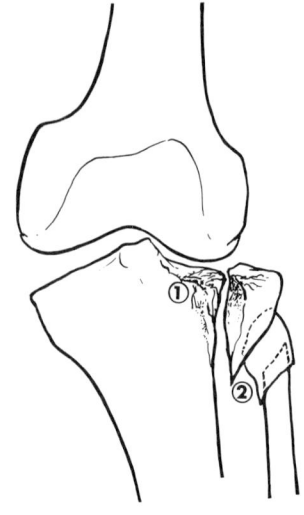

Lateral Spinotuberosity Fracture

1. The fracture involves the tibial spine and cruciate ligament.
2. The fibula is fractured.
3. Medial tibial subluxation results.

Note: These are not true plateau fractures but are actually disruptions of the major stabilizing elements of the knee joint and should be treated by internal fixation.

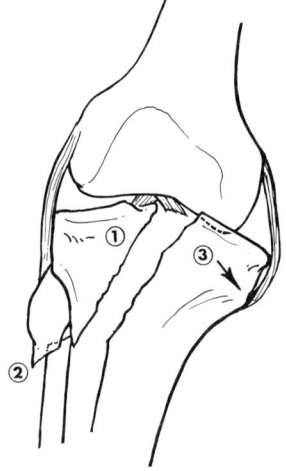

Operative Procedure

Apply a tourniquet around the upper third of the thigh.
1. The skin incision begins just anterior to the lateral collateral ligament immediately above the joint line. It curves gently downward and forward to the lateral margin of the patellar tendon, then continues downward parallel to the margin of the tendon and terminates at the level of the distal end of the tibial tubercle.

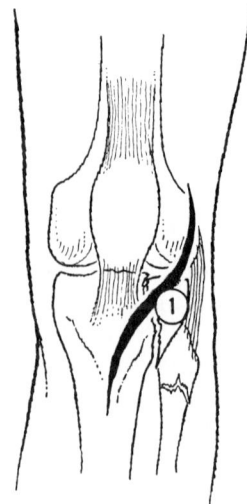

2. Divide the aponeurosis along the line of the skin incision.

3. Open the capsule in the line of the upper arm of the skin incision.

Note: The lateral meniscus should not be removed because it serves an important weight-bearing function and protects the fractured surfaces. If it is partially detached anteriorly, it should be repaired rather than removed.

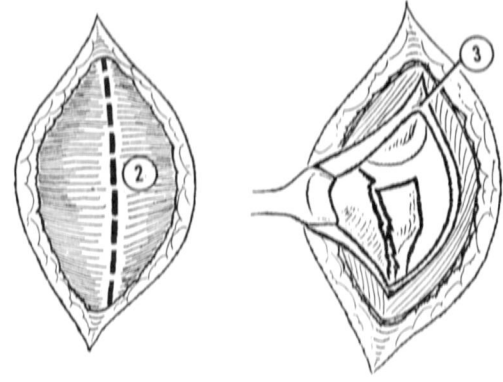

1. After flushing the wound with normal saline, elevate the tibial tuberosity into its anatomic position, using a stout curette.

2. While the corrected position is maintained (a compression clamp may be used), transfix the fragment with two pins that pierce the cortex of the opposite tibial condyle. Use Knowles or Haggie pins.

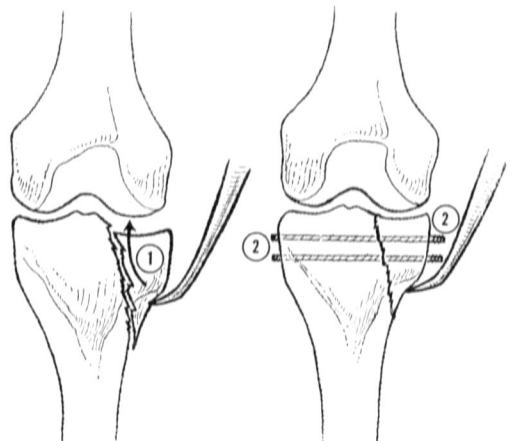

Alternate Procedure: Circumferential Wire Technique (Rassmussen)

The fracture is reduced on a fracture table with the knee extended (see page 1716).

For unstable comminuted plateau fractures:

1. Drill two holes from the lateral to the medial side and use a drill with a perforated end or wire loops to pass 20-gauge soft wire from the medial to the lateral surface.

2. Tighten the wire medially to compress the condyles and hold the reduction.

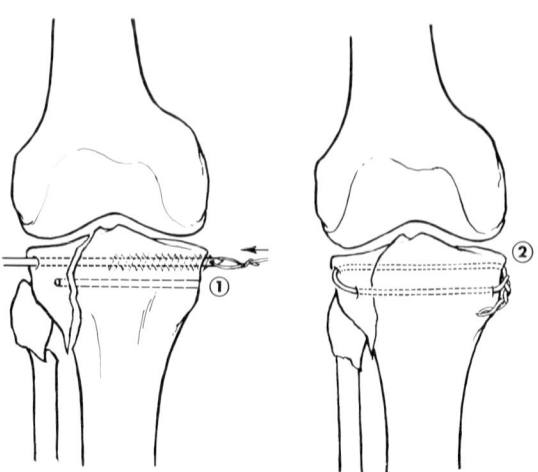

Immobilization

1. Apply a cast-brace while maintaining traction on the fractured limb.
2. The hinges are incorporated to exert a varus loading on the knee joint.

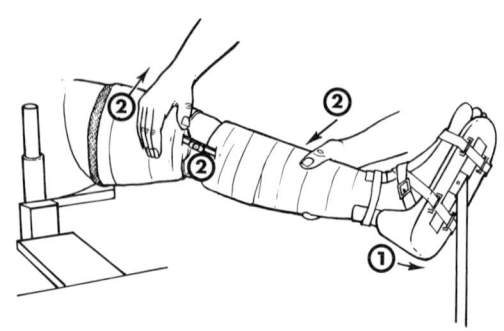

1. The cast should be applied well down over the femoral condyles and
2. Well up over the tibial plateau to protect against valgus loading.

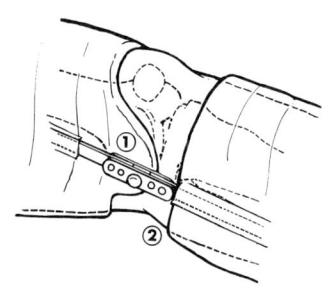

Note: Always observe the patient carefully for anterior compartment syndrome following any operation in this area. The tourniquet should be released and hemostasis should be obtained prior to closure.

The early signs of impending muscle ischemia are restlessness and severe pain as the patient recovers. These indicate a need to remove the cast and investigate muscle compartments carefully (see page 67).

Postoperative Management

Begin active range-of-motion exercises to the knee joint as soon as the postoperative pain and swelling subside.

Encourage the patient to do straight-leg raising with gradually increasing loads.

Partial weight bearing with crutches may be allowed because redisplacement of the fracture is prevented by the varus position of the knee and the internal fixation.

The cast-brace may be removed after eight weeks, when x-rays should show adequate healing of this cancellous bone fracture.

Continue crutch-protected weight bearing for six weeks longer, until the patient has full active control of the knee.

Bone Grafting for Split-Depression Fractures

REMARKS

This type of fracture is relatively uncommon.

Drennan and coworkers have shown that the split-depression fracture is associated with an unsatisfactory objective result and residual valgus angulation in about 20 per cent of patients treated by closed methods. However, most of the patients with unsatisfactory objective results had no pain or functional disability and were in the relatively older age group.

Operative treatment of these fractures should be extremely selective and probably limited to young individuals because even the unsatisfactory results from closed reduction and cast-brace method are better than those from operative fixation.

If it proves impossible to achieve adequate closed reduction or fixation by simple methods such as circumferential wire, bone grafting supplementation may rarely be necessary.

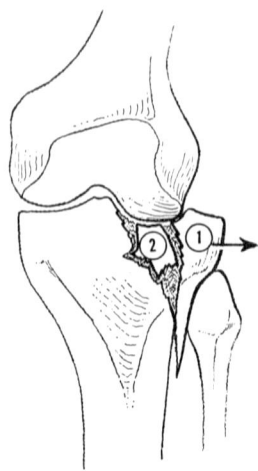

Prereduction X-Ray

1. The tuberosity is split and displaced laterally.
2. A large fragmented portion of the tibial plateau is depressed into the tibial condyle.

Operative Reduction

Apply a tourniquet around the upper end of the thigh.

1. The skin incision begins just anterior to the lateral collateral ligament immediately above the joint line. It curves gently downward and forward to the outer margin of the patellar tendon 1 cm below the articular surface of the condyle; then it continues downward parallel to the tendon and terminates at the level of the distal end of the tibial tubercle.
2. Divide the aponeurosis along the line of the skin incision.
3. Open the capsule in the line of the upper arm of the skin incision.

Note: The lateral meniscus should not be removed because it serves an important weight-bearing function and protects the fractured surfaces.

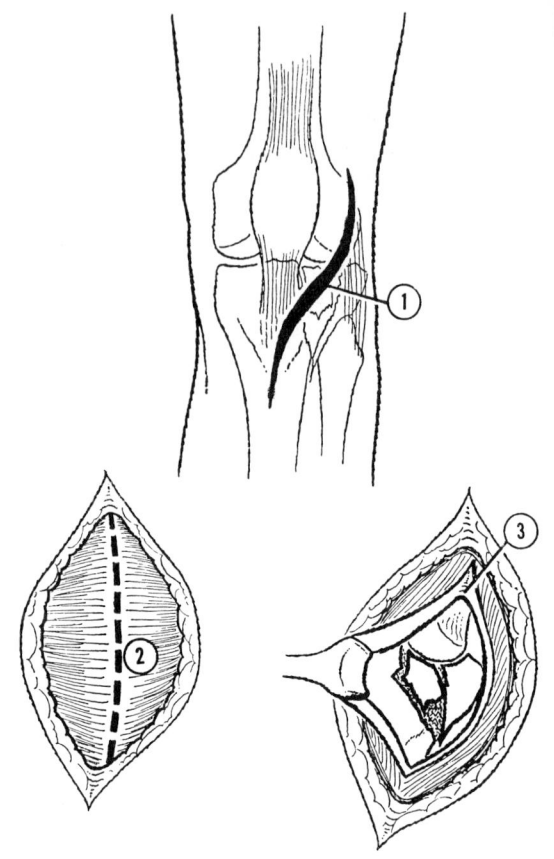

1. After flushing out the joint cavity with normal saline solution, elevate the depressed fragment into place, using a curette.
2. Elevate and compress the displaced outer fragment into its normal position.
3. While the corrected position is maintained (a compression clamp may be used), traverse the marginal fragment and the opposite tibial tuberosity with two threaded pins that are parallel to the articular surface and pierce the cortex of the inner tuberosity. Use Knowles pins or circumferential wire fixation.
4. Pack the remaining defect with cortical bone struts long enough to support the central fragment.

Note: Bone-bank bone is quite suitable to fill in the large gaps associated with these cancellous fractures.

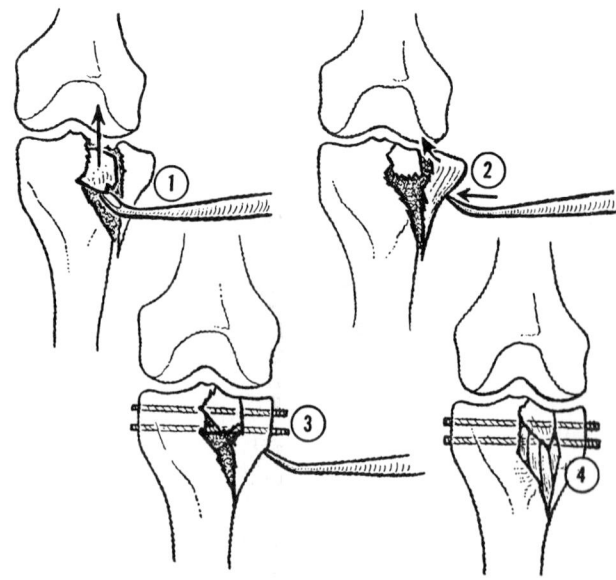

Immobilization

1. Apply a plaster cast from the groin to the toes.
2. The knee is extended.
3. The foot is dorsiflexed 90 degrees.

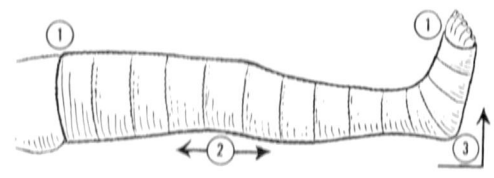

Note: Always observe the patient carefully for anterior compartment syndrome following any operation in this area. The tourniquet should be released and hemostasis should be obtained prior to closure.

The early signs of impending muscle ischemia are restlessness and severe pain as the patient recovers. They indicate the need to split the cast and investigate the muscle compartment carefully (see page 67).

Postreduction X-Ray

1. The central fragment is elevated.
2. The congruity of the articular surface is restored.
3. Pins traverse both tuberosities.

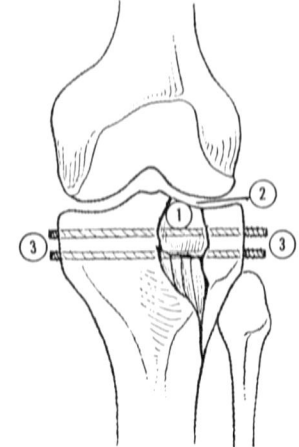

Postoperative Management

Have the patient begin quadriceps exercises on a regular schedule on the first postoperative day.

Progress to straight-leg raising exercises with some resistance.

Remove the postoperative cast by the second or third week, and when the swelling has subsided, apply a cast-brace holding the knee in slight varus position (see page 1710).

The patient should work on vigorous range-of-motion exercises and quadriceps strengthening while in the cast-brace.

All external cast support may be removed by the end of eight weeks, when these cancellous fractures are usually healing well.

Continue protective crutch walking for six weeks longer until the knee is completely healed clinically and radiographically.

The Knowles pins or wires may need to be removed by the end of twelve weeks if they are causing irritation to the soft tissues.

Bicondylar and Spinotuberosity Fractures of the Tibia

REMARKS

Fractures of both condyles of the tibia do not collapse further if the fibula is fractured. The fractured fibula allows for appropriate transfer of weight bearing forces through both condyles of the tibia. If the fibula is intact, the tendency is for the fracture to develop varus angulation.

Spinotuberosity or displaced condylar fracture involving the tibial spine is frequently unstable and can be considered a fracture-dislocation. The separated spinotuberosity fragment maintains a normal relationship with the femur while the remaining tibial surface dislocates or subluxates either laterally or medially.

The instability of these fractures may not be appreciated, and displacement can occur in a plaster cast.

Bicondylar fractures with a varus tendency due to an intact fibula or condylar fractures with involvement of the tibial tuberosity and spine (spinotuberosity fractures) frequently require internal fixation. A circumferential wire loop applied as described by Rasmussen after a closed reduction is effective in achieving stability of the condyles but should be supplemented by external cast-brace support.

Bicondylar Fracture with Involvement of the Fibula

1. Weight bearing is equally distributed on both condyles and an angulatory deformity does not result.

2. A fracture of the fibula with a bicondylar fracture is beneficial because it prevents varus angulation.

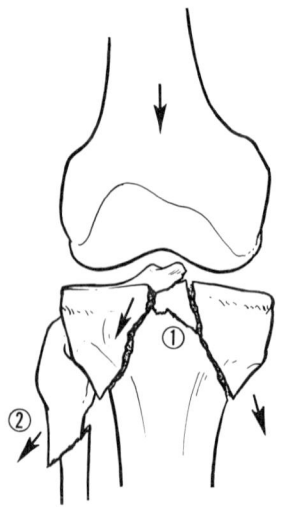

Bicondylar Fracture without Involvement of the Fibula

1. Varus angulation is frequently due to the force exerted by the intact fibula.

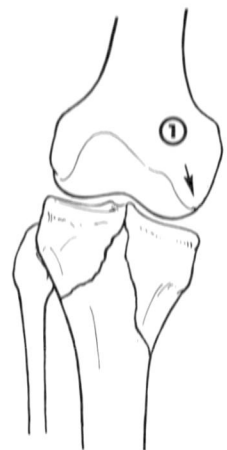

Internal Spinotuberosity Fracture (Duparc and Filipe)

1. The medial tibial plateau displaces internally while maintaining its normal relationship with the femur.
2. The remaining tibial surface displaces laterally and superiorly.

Note: This fracture may displace sufficiently to be considered a fracture-dislocation (see also page 1626).

Displacement of this type will result in a varus knee deformity unless the fracture is reduced and held with internal fixation.

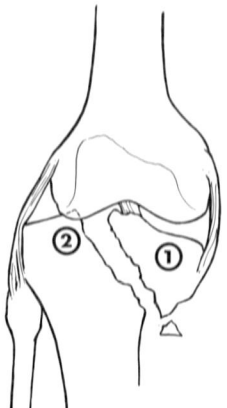

External Spinotuberosity Fracture

1. The lateral tibial plateau displaces laterally with the femoral shaft.
2. The fibula is also fractured and laterally displaced.
3. The remaining tibial surface displaces medially and superiorly.

Note: This is less common than the internal spinotuberosity fracture but is frequently unstable enough to require internal fixation.

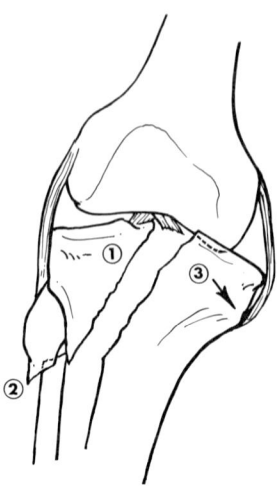

FRACTURES OF THE CONDYLES OF THE TIBIA

Technique of Closed Reduction and Circumferential Wire Fixation (Rasmussen)

Note: If the joint is distended, always aspirate the hemarthrosis before proceeding with reduction.

1. The patient's feet are supported on the fracture table.
2. The knees are extended.
3. Heavy traction is applied to the fractured limb.

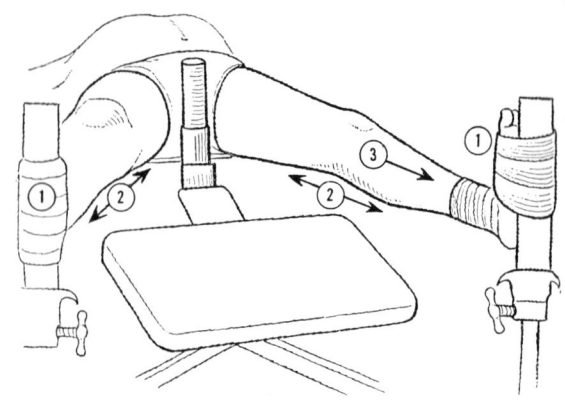

1. The widened condyles may be reduced by direct manual pressure or
2. By using a compression clamp.

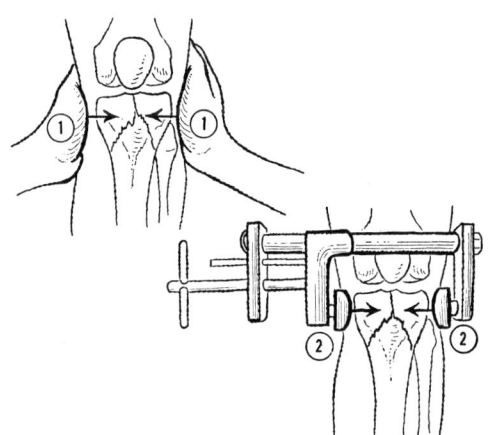

When x-ray confirms satisfactory closed reduction:

1. Through a small lateral incision drill two 3-mm drills with perforated ends from the lateral side through the plateaus, paralleling the joint space.
2. The location of the drill should be parallel to the joint surface as verified by image-intensified fluoroscopy. The peroneal nerve should be protected during insertion of the posterior drill.
3. A second incision is made medially and a 20-gauge stainless steel wire is passed through both drill holes using a perforated tip as a carrier for the wire.
4. The free ends of the wire are pulled and twisted tightly together and are buried in a drill hole through the cortex on the medial side.

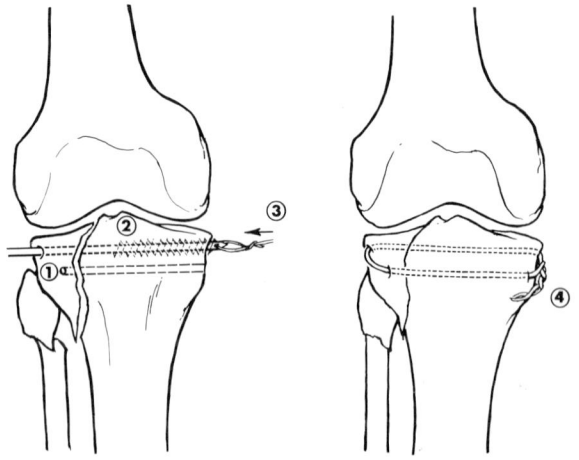

FRACTURES OF THE CONDYLES OF THE TIBIA

After the wound is closed:

1. Apply a cast-brace with the hinges loading the knee into a varus or valgus position depending on the initial instability. An internal spinotuberosity fracture should be immobilized with the knee in valgus. An external spinotuberosity fracture should be held in moderate varus.

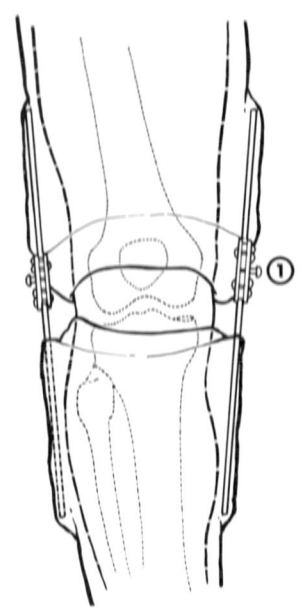

2. The cast-brace should allow full extension and 45 degrees of flexion but should protect against varus and valgus strain.

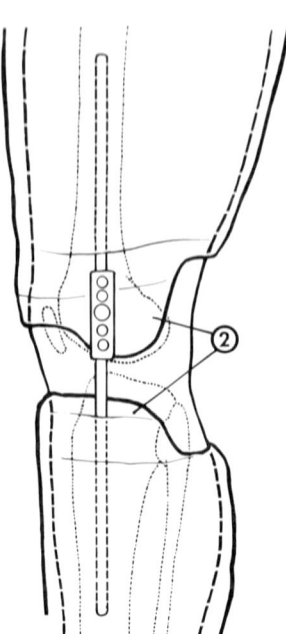

Subsequent Management

For the immediate postoperative period, apply ice to the knee and elevate the leg until the swelling subsides.

Subsequently, the patient may be up walking with crutches and toe-touch weight bearing but should avoid full weight bearing on the unstable knee joint.

The reduction should be radiographed periodically for several weeks after the operation, and if the fracture remains stable the patient can gradually increase weight bearing.

Cancellous bone fractures of this type heal by 8 to 10 weeks, after which the cast-brace may be removed and partial weight bearing may be continued with crutches.

The patient may discard the crutches by 12 to 18 weeks but should continue with a cane until good strength and motion have been regained in the knee joint.

The circumferential wire need not be removed; it will not irritate the soft tissues if it has been buried in the cortex of the bone.

SUMMARY: PITFALLS AND COMPLICATIONS OF KNEE INJURIES

One of the most common pitfalls in managing a knee injury is failure to analyze the problem systematically. The history should be taken attentively and the physical examination should be done thoroughly and on the basis of accurate anatomic perceptions.

A history of a painful snap, pop, or tearing sensation should always be considered an indication of serious problems. The football player who feels such a sensation after being hit from the posterolateral aspect is highly likely to have disrupted the deep and superficial medial capsular structures. The basketball player who feels something pop after landing off balance is likely to have torn the lateral capsular structures.

Knee injuries should not be dismissed because of an unimpressive history of trauma. The patient's ability to walk on the leg without significant pain does not rule out the possibility of severe ligamentous damage. Systematic physical examination is essential for proper evaluation of the knee, as it is for the heart or any other body system.

Instability of the knee in full extension most often indicates the need for prompt surgical repair. Injury to the lateral joint structures must also be considered a prime indication for prompt surgical intervention.

The significance of anterior cruciate ligament injuries remains debatable. Operative repair of an isolated cruciate injury appears to be inappropriate unless combined with repairs of the meniscotibial and other capsular structures responsible for anteroposterior stability.

The massive posterior cruciate ligament is the prime stabilizer against straight mediolateral instability in extension. Repair of this structure and any associated injury to the posterior capsule is essential but it can be overlooked in surgical management.

The importance of the deep capsular or meniscofemoral and meniscotibial ligaments to knee stability should also be recognized during surgical repair. Meniscectomy should be avoided, if at all possible, in repairing an acute ligamentous injury so as to maximize the contribution of the meniscofemoral and meniscotibial ligaments. Removal of a "loose" meniscus has proven to be a common pitfall that frequently only adds to the instability of the acutely injured knee.

Dislocation inflicts a serious disruption on the knee joint and is fraught with complications, particularly from neurovascular injuries associated with the ligamentous rupture. Distal circulation must be carefully assessed before and after reduction. Operative repair of ligamentous injuries, particularly the posterior capsule and cruciate ligaments, is generally indicated but should be delayed until the distal circulation is assured. Except for occasional posterolateral dislocation, reduction of a knee dislocation is relatively easy. Managing and avoiding the complications from neurovascular and ligamentous injury may be quite difficult.

Fractures of the patella are common injuries that may be unduly complicated if one fails to keep in mind the primary objective, which is to restore function to the extensor mechanism. The fractured patella can be repaired rather than excised and the extensor strength can be restored sufficiently to allow prompt functional knee exercises.

Among the most commonly unrecognized but significant injuries are those involving the extensor apparatus, particularly patellar instability or quadriceps rupture. The patient's ability to extend the knee actively and the mediolateral stability of the patella should be carefully assessed in any physical examination. Otherwise the pain and instability associated with extensor apparatus disruption are all too frequently taken as signs of ligamentous injury.

Dislocation and subluxation of the proximal tibiofibular joint is a rare injury but one that can be confused with internal derangement of the knee unless properly evaluated. Recurrent or chronic symptoms of tibiofibular instability are best managed by simple resection rather than fusion of the joint.

Open joint injuries can be fraught with complications unless they are adequately assessed and promptly drained. A high index of suspicion of intraarticular involvement with any penetrating wound or open laceration about the knee will help avoid tragic complications from joint sepsis.

Fractures of the tibial condyles frequently create the pitfall in which the radiographic appearance is treated more than the anatomic and real problem. The objective of treatment is to restore an adequate weight-bearing surface, which on the lateral side of the joint is primarily the lateral meniscus. Closed reduction with varus manipulation of the knee effectively reduces the majority of lateral plateau fractures and permits early flexion-extension motion with the aid of cast-brace support. The unusual split-depression condylar fracture or spinotuberosity fracture that causes instability and subluxation of the tibial surface is the prime candidate among these fractures for internal fixation.

In caring for the patient with injury to ligamentous and bony structures of the knee, we must carefully determine what are the real anatomic problems and critically question what are the realistic objectives of treatment.

REFERENCES

Arnoczky, S. P., Rubin, R. M., and Marshall, J. L.: Microvasculature of the cruciate ligaments and its response to injury. J. Bone and Joint Surg., 61-A:1221, 1979.

Ballard, A., Burkhalter, W. E., Mayfield, G. W., et al.: The functional treatment

REFERENCES

of pyogenic arthritis of the adult knee. J. Bone and Joint Surg., 57-A:1119, 1975.

Brown, G. A., and Sprague, B. L.: Cast brace treatment of plateau and bicondylar fractures of the proximal tibia. Clin. Orthop., 119:184, 1976.

Chick, R. R., and Jackson, D. W.: Tears of the anterior cruciate ligament in young athletes. J. Bone and Joint Surg., 60-A:970. 1978.

Cirincione, R. J., and Baker, B. E.: Tendon ruptures with secondary hyperparathyroidism. J. Bone and Joint Surg., 57-A:852, 1975.

Cofield, R. H., and Bryan, R. S.: Acute dislocation of the patella: Results of conservative treatment. J. Trauma, 17:526, 1977.

Daniel, D., and Rice, T.: Valgus-varus stability in a hinged cast used for controlled mobilization of the knee. J. Bone and Joint Surg., 61-A:135, 1979.

Dehaven, K. E.: Diagnosis of acute knee injuries with hemarthrosis. Am. J. Sports Med. 8:9–14, 1980.

Dehne, E., and Torp, T. P.: Treatment of joint injuries by immediate mobilization. Clin. Orthop., 77:218, 1971.

Donelson, R. G., and Tomaiouli, M.: Intra-articular dislocation of the patella. J. Bone and Joint Surg. 61-A:615, 1979.

Drennan, D. B., Locher, F. G., and Maylahn, D. J.: Fractures of the tibial plateau. J. Bone and Joint Surg., 61-A:989, 1979.

Duparc, J., and Filipe, G.: Fractures spino-tuberositaires. Rev. Chir. Orthop., 61:705, 1975.

Ecker, M. L., Lotke, P. A., and Glazer, R. M.: Late reconstruction of the patellar tendon. J. Bone and Joint Surg., 61-A:884, 1979.

Ellsasser, J. C., Reynolds, F. C., and Omohundro, R.: The non-operative treatment of collateral ligament injuries of the knee in professional football players. J. Bone and Joint Surg., 56-A:1185, 1974.

Ferguson, A. B., Brown, T. D., Fu, F. H., et al.: Relief of patellofemoral contact stress by anterior displacement of the tibial tubercle. J. Bone and Joint Surg., 61-A:159, 1979.

Fetto, J. F., and Marshall, J. L.: Medial collateral ligament injuries of the knee: A ratonale for treatment. Clin. Orthop., 132:206, 1978.

Green, N. E., and Allen, B. L.: Vascular injuries associated with dislocation of the knee. J. Bone and Joint Surg., 59-A:236, 1977.

Hughston, J. C.: A surgical approach to the medial and posterior ligaments of the knee. Clin. Orthop., 91:29, 1973.

Hughston, J. C., Andrews, J. R., Cross, M. J., et al.: Classification of knee ligament instabilities. Part I: The medial compartment and cruciate ligaments. J. Bone and Joint Surg., 58-A:159, 1976.

Hughston, J. C., Andrews, J. R., Cross, M. J., et al.: Classification of knee ligament instabilities. Part II: The lateral compartment. J. Bone and Joint Surg., 58-A:173, 1976.

Hughston, J. C., Bowden, J. A., Andrews, J. R., et al: Acute tears of the posterior cruciate ligament. J. Bone and Joint Surg., 62-A:438, 1980.

Hughston, J. C., and Eilers, A. F.: The role of the posterior oblique ligament in repairs of acute medial (collateral) ligament tears of the knee. J. Bone and Joint Surg., 55-A:923, 1973.

Insall, J., and Salvati, E.: Patella position in the normal knee joint. Diag. Radiol. 101:101, 1971.

Kennedy, J., and Fowler, P.: Medial and anterior instability of the knee. J. Bone and Joint Surg., 53-A:1257, 1971.

Lieb, F. J., and Perry, J.: Quadriceps function. J. Bone and Joint Surg., 53-A:749, 1971.

Maquet, P.: Advancement of the tibial tuberosity. Clin. Orthop., 115:225, 1976.

Marshall, J. L., Reeber, R. M., Wang, J. B., et al.: The anterior cruciate ligament. Orthop. Rev. 7:35–46, 1978.

Matthewson, M. H., Dandy, D. J.: Osteochondral fractures of the lateral femoral condyle. J. Bone and Joint Surg., 60-B:199, 1978.

REFERENCES

Meyers, M. H., and Harvey, J. P.: Traumatic dislocation of the knee joint. J. Bone and Joint Surg., 53-A:16, 1971.

Meyers, M. H., Moore, T. M., and Harvey, J. P.: Follow-up notes on articles previously published in the Journal. Traumatic dislocation of the knee joint. J. Bone and Joint Surg., 57-A:430, 1975.

Mooney, V.: Cast bracing. Clin. Orthop., 102:159, 1974.

Moore, T. M., and Harvey, J. P.: Roentgenographic measurement of tibial-plateau depression due to fracture. J. Bone and Joint Surg., 56-A:155, 1974.

Moore, T. M., Meyers, M. H., and Harvey, J. P.: Collateral ligament laxity of the knee. J. Bone and Joint Surg., 58-A:594, 1976.

Ogden, J. A.: Subluxation and dislocation of the proximal tibiofibular joint. J. Bone and Joint Surg., 56-A:145, 1974.

Patzakis, M. J., Dorr, L. D., Ivler, D., et al.: The early management of open joint injuries. J. Bone and Joint Surg., 57-A:1065, 1975.

Price, C. T., and Allen, W. C.: Ligament repair in the knee with preservation of the meniscus. J. Bone and Joint Surg., 60-A:61, 1978.

Quinlan, A. G., and Sharrard, W. J.: Postero-lateral dislocation of the knee with capsular interposition. J. Bone and Joint Surg., 40-B:660, 1958.

Rasmussen, P. S.: Tibial condylar fractures. J. Bone and Joint Surg., 55-A:1334, 1973.

Rorabeck, C. H., and Bobechko, W. P.: Acute dislocation of the patella with osteochondral fracture. J. Bone and Joint Surg., 58-B:237, 1976.

Sarmiento, A.: Fractures of the proximal tibia and tibial condyles. Clin. Orthop. 145:136–143, 1979.

Siwek, K. W., and Rao, J. P.: Bilateral simultaneous rupture of the quadriceps tendons. Clin. Orthop., 131:252, 1978.

Slocum, D. B., Larson, R. L., and James, S. L.: Late reconstruction of ligamentous injuries of the medial compartment of the knee. Clin. Orthop., 100:23, 1974.

Taylor, A. R., Arden, G. P., and Rainey, H. A.: Traumatic dislocation of the knee. J. Bone and Joint Surg., 54-B:96, 1972.

Torg, J. S., Conrad, W., and Kalen, U.: Clinical diagnosis of anterior cruciate ligament instability in the athlete. Am. J. Sports Med. 4:84–93, 1976.

Torisu, T.: Isolated avulsion fracture of the tibial attachment of the posterior cruciate ligament. J. Bone and Joint Surg., 59-A:68, 1977.

Trillat, A., De Jour, J., and Couette, A.: Diagnostic et traitement des subluxations récidivantes de la rotule. Rev. Chir. Orthop., 50:813, 1964.

Walker, P. S., and Erkman, M. J.: The role of the menisci in force transmission across the knee. Clin. Orthop., 109:184, 1975.

Wang, J. B., and Marshall, J. L.: Acute ligamentous injuries of the knee. Single contrast arthrography — a diagnostic aid. J. Trauma, 15:431, 1975.

Wang, J. B., Rubin, R. M., and Marshall, J. L.: A mechanism of isolated anterior cruciate ligament rupture. J. Bone and Joint Surg., 57-A:411, 1975.

Weber, M. J., Janecki, C. J., McLeod, P.: Efficacy of various forms of fixation of transverse fractures of the patella. J. Bone and Joint Surg., 62-A:215, 1980.

Wilkinson, J.: Fracture of the patella treated by total excision. J. Bone and Joint Surg., 59-B:352, 1977.

FRACTURES OF THE TIBIA AND FIBULA

FRACTURES OF THE SHAFT OF THE TIBIA

REMARKS

Fractures of the tibia are the most common of long bone fractures that fail to heal. Recent studies indicate that tibial fractures constitute 70 per cent or more of nonunions treated by electrical stimulation.

These fractures can be a much more benign condition if the biologic processes as well as the mechanics of fracture management are always kept in mind.

Mechanisms and Mechanics of Tibial Fractures

REMARKS

Fractures of the tibia result from direct, indirect, and fatigue mechanisms.

Direct Mechanisms

1. This causes a bending fracture, characteristically transverse across the long axis of the bone but frequently

2. A segmental fracture.

Note: Direct mechanisms involve a break across the haversian systems and cause significant microscopic disruption to the haversian canal structure of the bone.

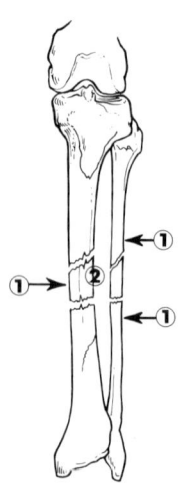

Indirect Mechanism

An indirect torsional mechanism causes:

1. A spiral oblique fracture that tends to cross between the haversian systems along the path of least resistance.

The resultant disruption of haversian canal blood supply is considerably less with these fractures than with direct mechanisms and the healing response is quite prompt following indirect injury.

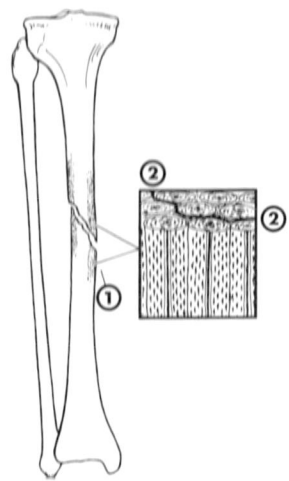

Fatigue Fractures

1. Fatigue fractures of the tibia and fibula are failures of bone from repetitive loading, e.g., from jogging.

2. They are usually undisplaced transverse fractures, which are problems more of correct diagnosis than of treatment.

Note: Fatigue fractures have sometimes been confused with more serious problems such as osteoblastic osteosarcoma.

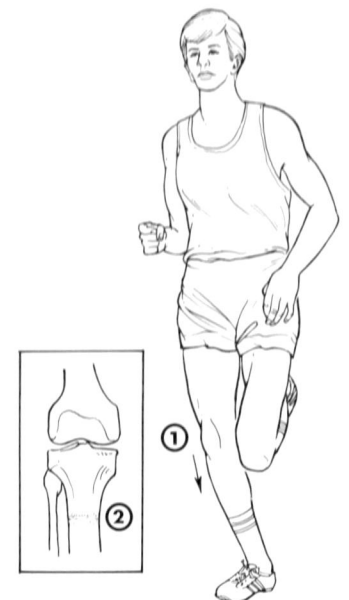

Biomechanics of Torsional Fractures

Indirect torsional loading consistently produces a fracture that is determined by the direction of twist (see also page 1464).

1. External torsional loading, which is most common, produces a fracture line that begins first in the distal medial tibial cortex and then

2. Spirals upward to the proximal lateral tibial cortex and

3. Fractures the fibula proximal to the tibia.

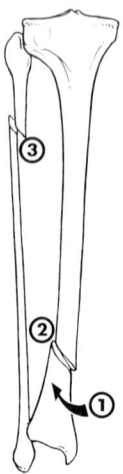

Biomechanics of Torsional Fractures (Continued)

INTERNAL TORSIONAL FRACTURES

These are less common. Characteristically, the mechanism causes

1. Failure first in the distal fibula, then
2. Fracture through the distal lateral tibial cortex and
3. Spiral upward through the proximal medial cortex.

Note: Recognizing the mechanism is important for reducing the fracture and preventing internal-torsional (varus) or external-torsional (valgus) malalignment.

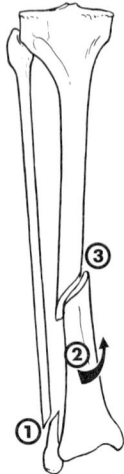

Biomechanics of the Fibula

REMARKS

The fibula has been shown by Lambert to carry at least one sixth of the static loading on the leg, mostly through its articulation with the talus.

The contribution of the fibula to stability of the leg becomes particularly important following a tibial fracture. The presence of an intact fibula indicates significantly less trauma in either a closed or an open tibial fracture and a significantly improved prognosis for prompt healing.

The intact fibula can also be a deforming factor, since it tends to act as a spring and rotates the tibial fracture internally, leading to a varus (internal-torsional) deformity in the healed fracture. This is particularly likely with fractures in the distal or proximal third of the tibia.

Fracture of the tibia associated with a fibular fracture tends to develop a valgus (external-torsional) deformity, which must be considered and prevented during treatment.

Comminuted, open distal tibial fractures can be effectively stabilized by fixing the adjacent fibula with an intramedullary rod, thereby avoiding direct surgical invasion of the fragmented tibia.

Stabilization by fibulotibial synostosis can be an effective method of supporting a tibial fracture with extensive bone loss.

Resection of the fibula has been recommended for surgical exposure during fasciotomy and in treating delayed union of the tibia. This can add to tibial instability and necessitates internal stabilization of the fractured tibia.

The fibula should be considered a valuable adjunct rather than an obstruction to the management of a tibial fracture.

Weight-Bearing Function of the Fibula (Lambert)

1. The talus always has an oblique articulation that maintains firm contact with the fibula in all positions of flexion and extension.

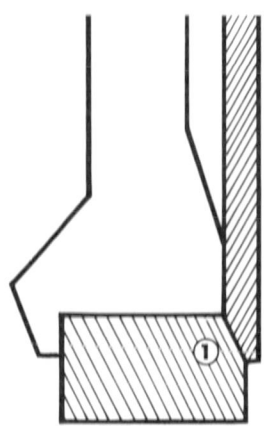

The articulation between the fibula and the talus causes the fibula to function:
1. As a lateral stabilizing structure and
2. As an axial load-carrying structure.

Note: Direct measurements indicate that the fibula carries at least one sixth of the static load on the leg. This proportion increases significantly with pathologic conditions such as fractures of the tibia.

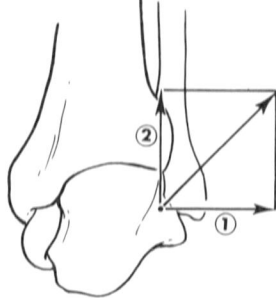

Ankle instability may also result from loss of distal fibular stability. Hsu and coworkers have reported considerable valgus growth deformity in children after loss of distal fibular support.

THE STABILIZING EFFECT OF THE FIBULA AND THE INTEROSSEOUS MEMBRANE ON TIBIAL FRACTURES (Sarmiento and Latta)

REMARKS

If the fibula is intact, the mechanism of injury producing the tibial fracture was of lesser violence. Even an open tibial fracture with intact fibula heals more readily than one with fibular fracture. If the fibula is fractured the interosseous membrane can still provide important stability if it is not torn.

Because of the stabilizing effect of the fibula and the interosseous membrane, most tibial fractures shorten no more than the amount seen at the time of the initial injury, provided that external stabilization of the limb is adequate.

FRACTURES OF THE SHAFT OF THE TIBIA

1. The fibula is fractured at the same level as the tibia; the interosseous membrane remains intact.

2. Even with severe initial displacement, these fractures remain stable owing to interosseous ligament support.

3. If the fibula is fractured at a distance from the tibial fracture,

4. Severe displacement occurs only with complete disruption of the interosseous membrane. This indicates significant loss of intrinsic fracture stability.

Influence of the Fibula on Tibial Fracture Deformity

1. Unstable fracture of the tibia with a bone gap will demonstrate

2. Rotation of the fibula and of the distal tibial fragment as much as 30 degrees around the proximal fibulotibial joint.

3. Synostosis of the fibula to the tibia effectively stabilizes the tibial defect.

1. In fracture of the distal tibia with an intact fibula, internal torsion-varus deformity often develops.

2. This should be anticipated and should be prevented by immobilizing the fracture in external rotation.

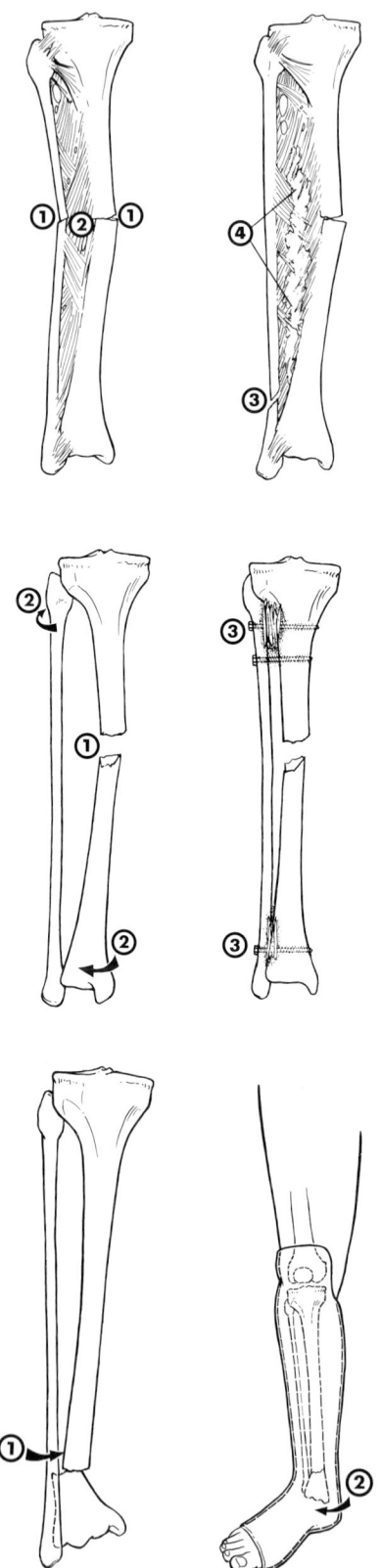

FRACTURES OF THE SHAFT OF THE TIBIA

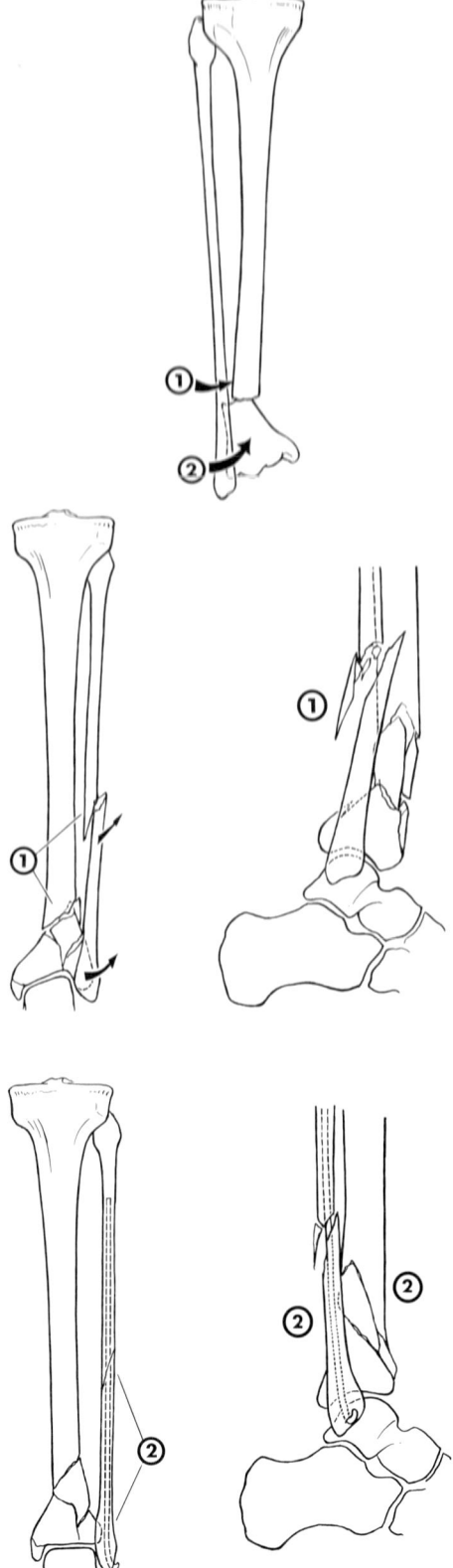

1. In proximal tibial fracture of varus torsional deformity develops if
2. The fibula is intact.

Note: An osteotomy of the fibula may be necessary to correct a torsional tibial fracture deformity before the fracture heals in a malunited position. The intact fibula may act as a torsional spring angulating the tibia.

1. Fracture of the distal tibia associated with fracture of the fibula, leads to valgus (external-torsional) deformity.

Note: This should be anticipated and should be prevented by immobilizing the fracture in internal rotation. Stabilization of the fibula may also be necessary.

2. This open comminuted fracture of the distal tibia is effectively stabilized by fixing the adjacent fibula.

Biology of Tibial Fracture Healing and the Effect of Fracture Management

REMARKS

The biologic effect of a tibial fracture, particularly the relationship of the healing response to blood supply, is dramatically displayed in the tibia. Trueta has shown that the tibia has one of the richest vascular areas in bone tissue in its upper metaphysis and one of the poorest in the distal part of the shaft. The tibia is also lacking in soft tissue attachment and extraosseous blood supply anteriorly and medially. External callus and early union must be derived from soft tissue laterally and posteriorly.

Trueta's work has also indicated that the pumping action of muscles surrounding the fracture enhances bone vascular flow and the process of new bone formation.

In the distal tibia, which is almost entirely surrounded by tendons rather than richly vascularized muscle, intramedullary callus formation predominates (see also page 13).

Rhinelander has shown that the contribution of extraosseous circulation to fracture healing is only temporary and that by six to eight weeks the majority of the fracture is supplied, as the normal bone is, by medullary circulation.

Early functional treatment within the first six weeks following injury is the most effective technique of maximizing the contribution of muscular or extraosseous circulation to the healing process. After six weeks fracture revascularization and healing are almost entirely dependent on intramedullary vessels and callus formation.

1. Treatment by intramedullary nail inhibits medullary bridging callus, which must be compensated for by
2. External callus formation.

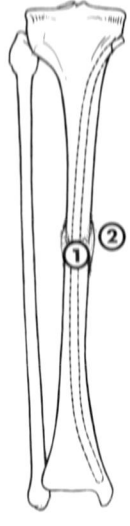

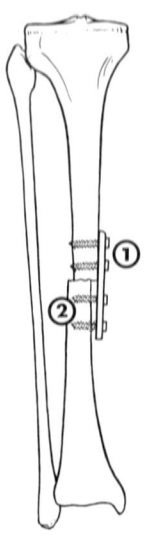

1. Rigid plate fixation of the tibia inhibits external callus formation but does allow intramedullary callus.
2. If loosening occurs, the benefit of immobilization is lost and both external and internal callus are impaired, so fibrocartilage fills the gap.

1. Cerclage wires applied loosely around the fracture site may be of value to stabilize an open fracture after wound debridement.
2. The wires should not be applied so tightly that they absorb the weight-bearing stresses; they should allow stresses to be transmitted from fragment to fragment.

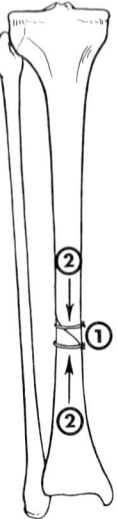

1. Proximal and distal pin transfixion may effectively immobilize the fracture, but
2. The pins should not distract or enlarge the fracture gap.
3. Pins through the muscle and surrounding soft tissue inhibit functional exercise and diminish circulation to the external callus.

Note: Transfixion pins should be considered only temporary immobilization, and should be removed in two to three weeks to allow functional weight-bearing treatment.

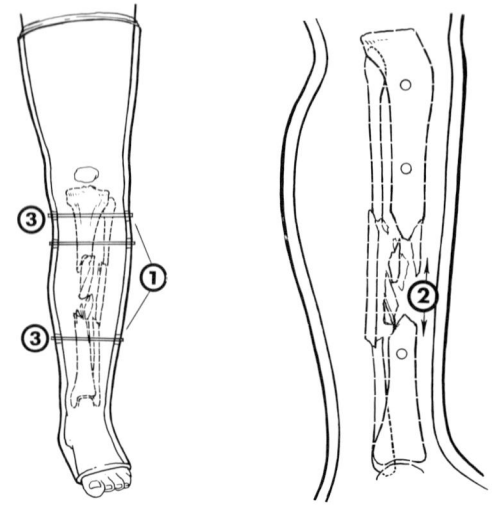

1. Closed reduction and early functional weightbearing treatment maximize external callus response.
2. Stability results from the relatively incompressible soft tissues, which do not permit shortening when
3. Combined with the resistance provided by the walls of the cast.

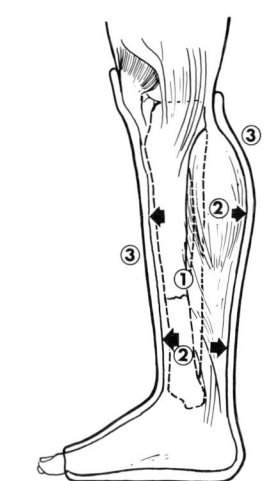

RATIONALE OF CLOSED TREATMENT

REMARKS

No other fracture in the body provokes more controversy between biologically and mechanically oriented surgeons than a tibial fracture. Its accessibility and convenient architecture have made the tibia a prime target for both plate and intramedullary nail fixation. The bone demonstrates an admirable capacity to heal despite these techniques rather than because of them.

Traditional concepts regarding management of these fractures have been revised or disproved by evidence accumulated over the past 30 years. The concept that rigid fixation is necessary for osteogenesis has been proved untenable. Slight, controlled fracture motion associated with functional weight bearing provokes early callus response most beneficially.

The concept that closed treatment demands absolute immobilization of the joints proximal and distal to the fracture has also been disproved, particularly by the work of Sarmiento. The evidence abounds that functional motion rather than forced immobilization is most compatible with effective healing.

The results of operative treatment, even in the most experienced hands, may come close but they never quite equal those of closed functional management.

The surgeon who elects to perform open reduction of a fractured tibia assumes, or causes the patient to assume, risks that are unnecessary in the majority of fractures.

OBJECTIVES OF CLOSED TREATMENT

REMARKS

Anatomic reduction is ideal, but the major objective in treating the tibial fracture is to obtain union without distorting joint alignment. The x-ray after reduction should always include the knee and ankle on one film in order to assess this alignment.

Shortening of 1 to 1.5 cm is quite acceptable and, in fact, desirable for comminuted fractures.

Closed reduction can usually achieve the objectives of restoring joint alignment and minimizing shortening.

If fracture shortening or angulation cannot be corrected by the usual closed techniques, fixation of the proximal and distal fragments by transverse pins will permit accurate alignment. Transfixion pins should be removed within three weeks so as to avoid fracture distraction and permit functional weight-bearing treatment.

Before embarking on treatment, always discuss the advantages and complications of both open and closed options for the patient. Most patients will readily accept the limited risk of slight shortening from closed treatment rather than choose the larger risk of infection and chronic osteomyelitis from internal fixation.

TECHNIQUE OF CLOSED REDUCTION

Initial Cast Application (Dehne, Brown and Coworkers)

An initial cast should be applied as soon as possible after injury. A posterior splint or other temporary splint is inadequate and should be avoided.

FRACTURES OF THE SHAFT OF THE TIBIA

If patients are given adequate explanation and reduction is done gently, most will tolerate cast application without anesthetic or narcotics.

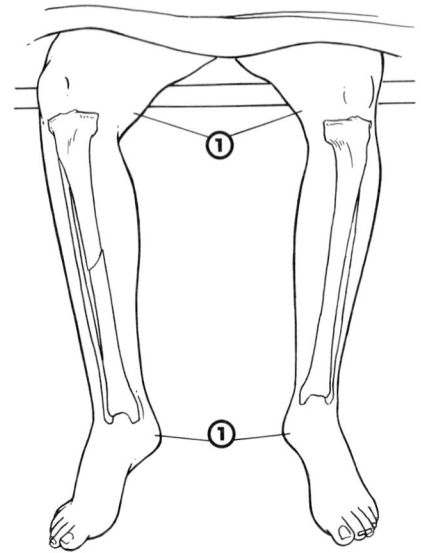

1. The patient sits on the edge of a table with the legs hanging down to allow fracture realignment and correction of any malrotation detected by comparison of the fractured leg with the unfractured leg.

Note: If general anesthetic is required, the cast is best applied with the fractured leg hanging from the edge of the table. This allows gravity to work for fracture reduction rather than against it.

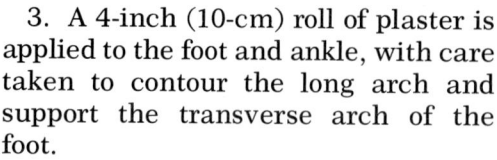

2. Two layers of cast padding or bias stockinette are rolled from the toes to above the knee.

3. A 4-inch (10-cm) roll of plaster is applied to the foot and ankle, with care taken to contour the long arch and support the transverse arch of the foot.

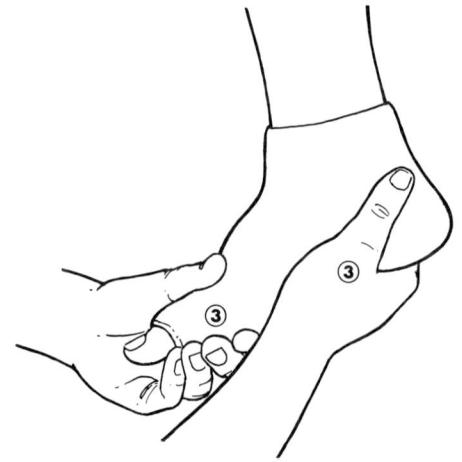

4. A 6-inch (15-cm) roll of plaster is rolled from the foot cast to the knee. The fracture is aligned by molding the plaster to correct any varus or valgus tendency.

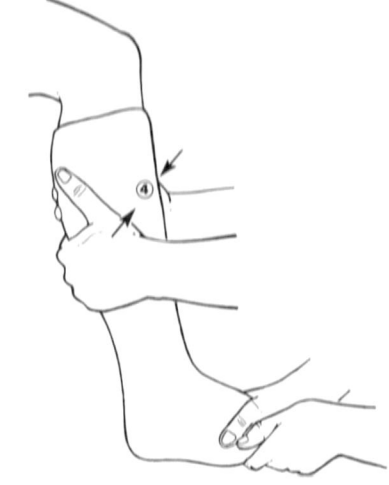

5. When the lower leg plaster has hardened, the knee is extended and the cast is applied above the knee to immobilize the knee in the fully extended position.

Note: Avoid immobilizing the knee in flexion. This adds to the patient's discomfort and exaggerates the tendency of the limb to swell.

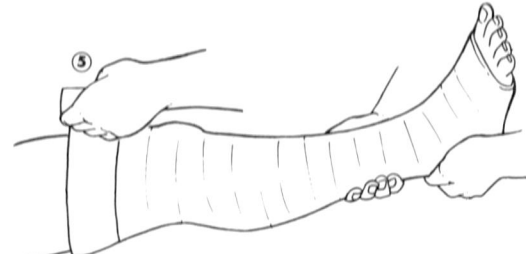

Subsequent Management

1. Always elevate the fracture by an overhead suspension.

Note: Do not rely on pillows for elevation; they are ineffective.

2. The patient actively works on toe extension and isometric leg muscle exercises.

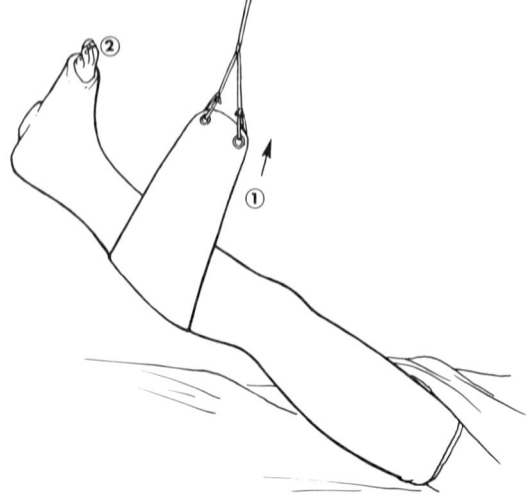

Start three-point weight bearing with crutches the day following cast application.

Advise the patient that he will feel some discomfort or possibly some motion at the fracture for the first few weeks.

The patient may be out of bed and walking but he should not sit or stand. Whenever he is not walking, the leg should be elevated to avoid swelling within the cast. This preventive regimen must be continued for five to seven days until swelling is no longer likely. After one week the cast may be changed to a short leg patellar-tendon-bearing (PTB) cast or the long leg cast may remain on the leg, depending on the skills of the surgeon and the activity of the patient.

The major advantage of a short leg PTB cast is that it allows the patient to return readily to work or school and restores his sense of being able to function normally.

The PTB cast must be applied according to Sarmiento's principles or it will allow angulation of an unstable fracture.

If the surgeon has any doubt about his ability to apply a short leg cast properly, it is safer by far to continue with the long leg cast technique until union is assured.

Technique of Applying Patellar-Tendon-Bearing (PTB) Cast (Sarmiento)

By seven to ten days the initial cast has usually loosened and fracture discomfort has diminished sufficiently to permit cast change.

1. The patient sits on the table with his legs hanging over the edge, and alignment of the fracture is evaluated by comparison with the opposite limb.

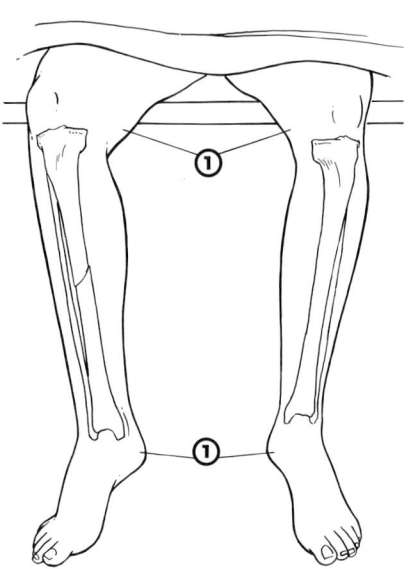

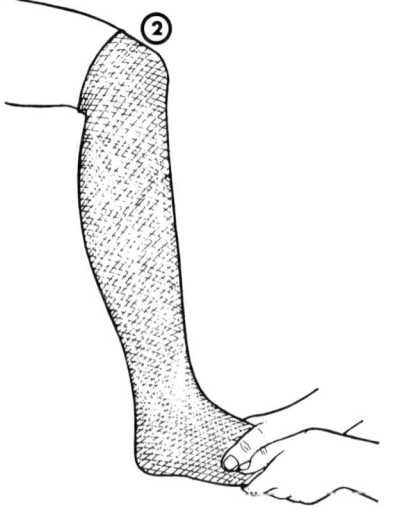

2. A double-layered stockinette is applied from the toes to 5 cm above the patella.

3. A 4 inch (10-cm) roll of plaster is applied around the foot directly over the stockinette. The longitudinal and transverse arches are carefully molded.

Note: Take care to avoid wrinkles in either the stockinette or the plaster, particularly at the ankle.

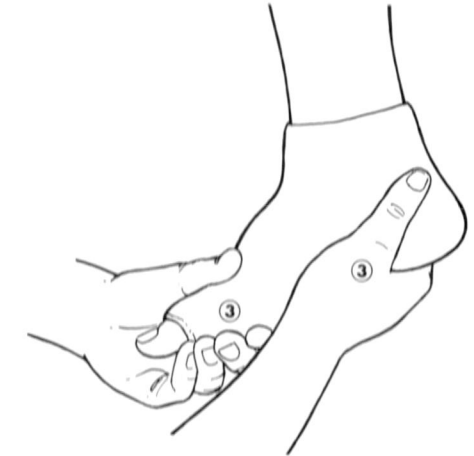

4. While the foot and ankle portion is drying, the cast is extended to the tibial tuberosity. Mold the cast firmly along the anterior tibial surface and in the peroneal and calf muscle region. An assistant supports the toes during this application.

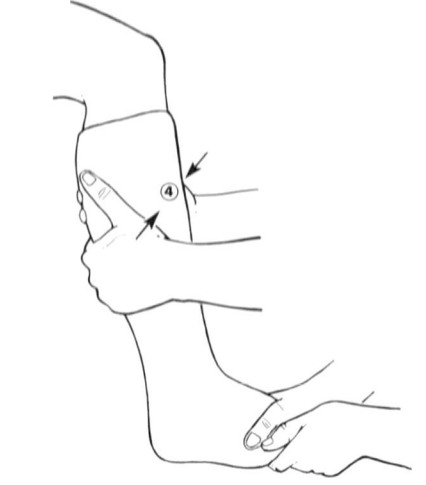

5. The final portion is applied with the knee held at 45 degrees to relax the patellar tendon. The cast is molded over the patellar tendon and the popliteal space.

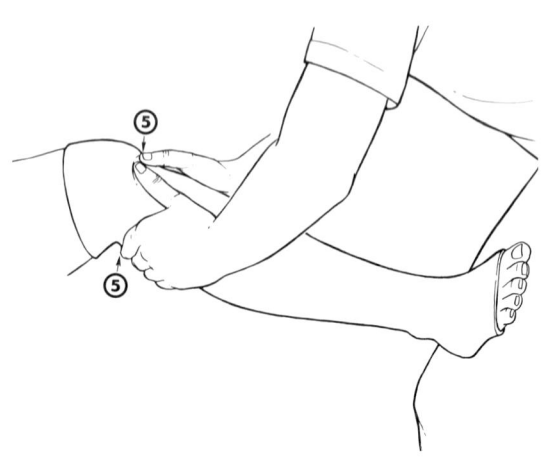

Technique of Applying Patellar-Tendon-Bearing (PTB) Cast (Sarmiento) (Continued)

6. The cast is trimmed to resemble a PTB prosthesis. The lateral wings should fit snugly over the femoral condyles to enhance rotational stability. The anterior portion should allow full extension, and the posterior portion should relieve the hamstrings sufficiently to permit full knee flexion.

Note: The cast distributes most of the weight load to the posterior calf and the tibial flare, not to the patellar tendon.

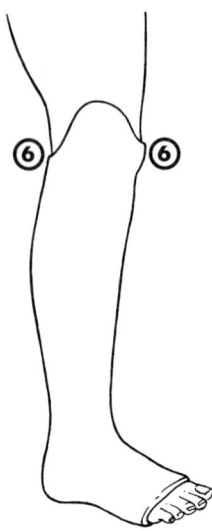

Postreduction X-ray

The x-rays should be taken to show alignment of the knee and ankle on the same cassette.

The cassette may have to be placed diagonally for tall patients in order to visualize the critical alignment of the proximal and distal joints.

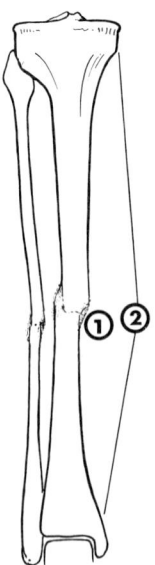

In all types of tibial fractures, the following signs should be checked by x-ray.

ANTEROPOSTERIOR VIEW

1. Shortening should be kept at 1 cm. or less, if at all possible.
2. The knee and ankle axes should be correctly realigned.

Lateral View

1. Avoid anterior angulation of proximal fracture fragments, which can slough skin entrapped between the hard bone and the cast.
2. Anterior angulation is corrected by allowing slight recurvatum of the fracture.

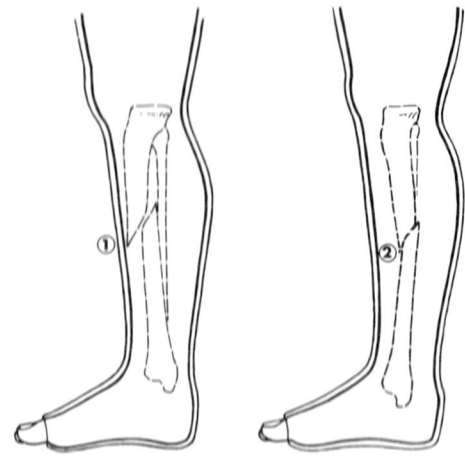

1. Posterior angulation of distal fracture fragments is corrected by
2. Allowing slight equinus position of the foot.

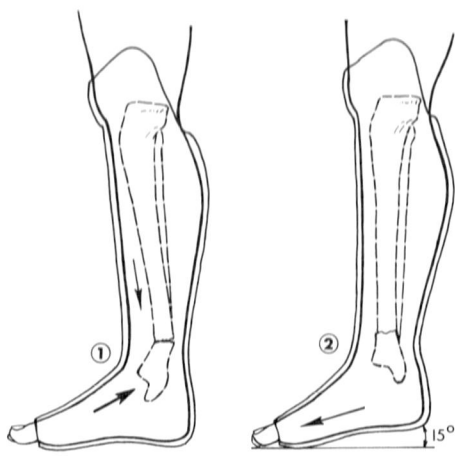

Subsequent Management

After 24 hours, partial weight bearing with crutches is encouraged but not forced.

Most patients are able to walk without external support within 2 weeks, when they can return to work or school.

Weekly follow-up x-rays should be done for the first several weeks to detect any changes in alignment or loosening of the cast.

By 6 weeks the cast generally needs to be replaced. Some patients will be able to continue with the initial cast until the fracture heals. The average healing time with fractures treated in this manner is 15 weeks.

The patient should be reminded that the cast does not provide rigid fracture immobilization but does permit some translation or pistoning motion in the early weeks of weight-bearing treatment. Since this motion, which takes place during the early phases of repair, is the result of function, it is not detrimental to healing.

Objectives of Treatment: Three-Dimensional Fracture Management

REMARKS

Bones are three-dimensional structures. After fracture they tend to deform naturally in three dimensions.

X-rays are, at best, two-dimensional interpretations of these three-dimensional deformities. Unfortunately, we physicians have become so conditioned to rely on x-rays that we frequently forget the importance of longitudinal alignment or alignment in the third dimension.

Ultimately, it is the three-dimensional clinical appearance and the functional length of the healed fracture that are most important to the patient, not arbitrary radiographic criteria based on two-dimensional thinking.

The most reliable method of evaluating the three-dimensional fracture alignment is by clinical inspection. This is true of all long-bone and short-bone fractures, whether in the fingers or in the femur (see pages 1238, 1461, and 1779).

The major use of radiographic evaluation should be to insure that joint alignment is not altered during treatment. The alignment of the knee and ankle joints should be reviewed more critically on postreduction x-rays than the relative position of the fracture fragments.

The length of the fractured limb should be maintained, if at all possible, but shortening of 1.0 to 1.5 cm. may frequently be accepted and may actually be necessary in comminuted fractures. This slight amount of shortening is not functionally significant to the patient and usually does not indicate the need for open reduction.

FRACTURES OF THE SHAFT OF THE TIBIA

THREE-DIMENSIONAL FRACTURE ALIGNMENT

First example

Prereduction X-Ray

1. A comminuted distal tibial fracture associated with
2. An intact fibula tends to produce internal torsion of the distal fragment and distortion of ankle alignment.

Note: This may be interpreted as a varus angulation on x-rays but is primarily an internal torsional problem.

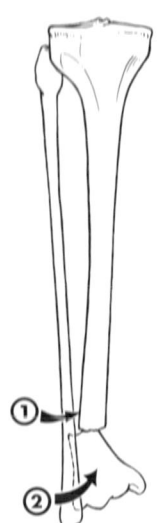

Results After Functional Treatment

1. The distal tibial fracture has been reduced by external torsional correction.
2. Healing is evident at 16 weeks.
3. Alignment of the knee and ankle joints is satisfactory.

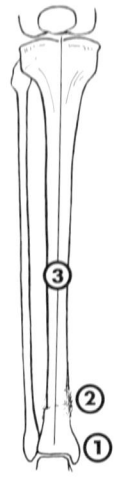

Second example

Prereduction X-Ray

1. A transverse tibial fracture with
2. A fracture of the fibula. This tends to produce a three-dimensional external torsional deformity, which on x-ray is interpreted as a valgus angulation.

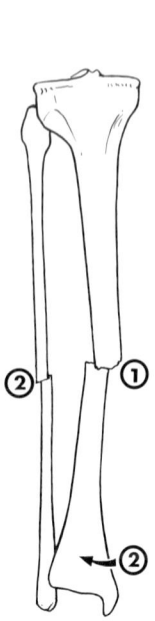

1741

FRACTURES OF THE SHAFT OF THE TIBIA

Prereduction X-Ray (Continued)

RESULTS AFTER FUNCTIONAL TREATMENT

1. The fracture has healed at 16 weeks.
2. The ankle alignment has been maintained by internally rotating the distal fragment.

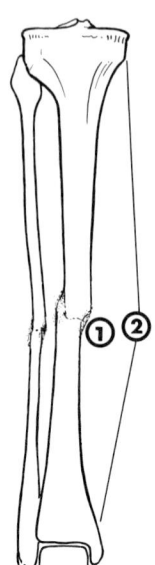

FUNCTIONALLY ACCEPTABLE FRACTURE SHORTENING

Segmental Fractures

PREREDUCTION X-RAY

1. Segmental fracture of the tibia and fibula.
2. Shortening of up to 1.5 cm may be acceptable for this type of fracture.
3. The knee and ankle alignment must be corrected.

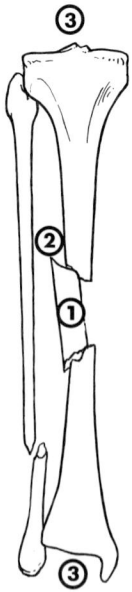

FRACTURES OF THE SHAFT OF THE TIBIA

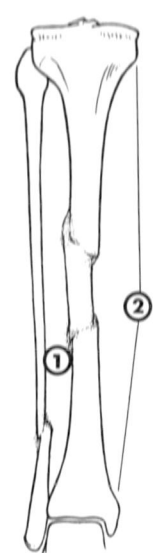

RESULTS AFTER 20 WEEKS OF
FUNCTIONAL CAST TREATMENT

1. Segmental fractures have both healed primarily by external callus formation.
2. The knee and ankle alignments have been maintained.

BILATERAL FRACTURES

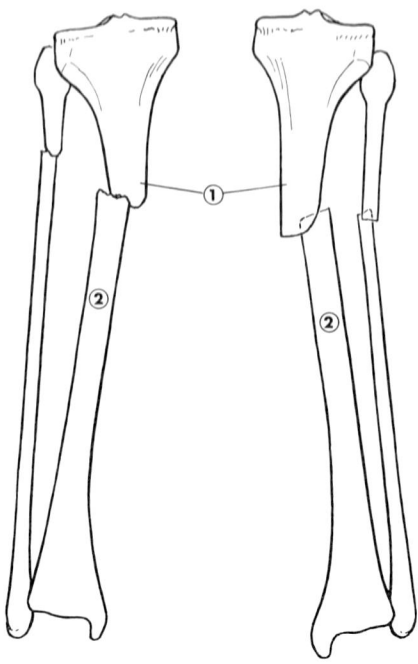

PREREDUCTION X-RAY

1. Bilateral fractures of the tibia and fibula.
2. Slight (10 mm) overriding may be accepted but it should not increase with weight-bearing treatment. Angulation of the fracture must be corrected.

RESULTS AFTER 16 WEEKS OF
FUNCTIONAL TREATMENT

1. Both fractures have healed by external callus.
2. Alignment achieved at initial reduction has been maintained until healing.

Note: If reduction is not achieved by closed means, either because joints remain malaligned or the fracture shortens excessively, transfixion pins incorporated in plaster are most useful for temporary stabilization.

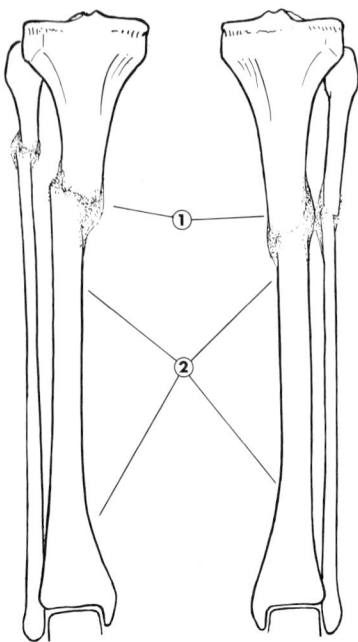

Management of Unstable Fractures by Cast and Transfixing Pins (Pins-in-Plaster Treatment)

REMARKS

Most tibial fractures can be reduced and held quite satisfactorily by the closed techniques described above. Comminuted or segmental fractures occasionally and open fractures frequently require a brief period of pin transfixion. This allows the surrounding soft tissues to heal sufficiently to provide intrinsic hydraulic stability when the cast is applied.

Anderson and Hutchins have demonstrated the technique of transfixion pins to be extremely effective in preventing excessive shortening and in eliminating the risks of and need for open reduction and internal fixation.

This method is more reliable and considerably simpler than other current popular external fixation techniques. Cast support immobilizes the foot and surrounding soft tissues as well as the fracture. Other

FRACTURES OF THE SHAFT OF THE TIBIA

external fixation techniques ignore the importance of such support for soft tissue healing.

By the end of three weeks the surrounding soft tissues have usually healed sufficiently that the pins may be removed and ambulatory cast treatment (as previously described) may be started.

Use of transfixion pins for longer than six weeks may produce fracture distraction and may result in either delayed union or nonunion.

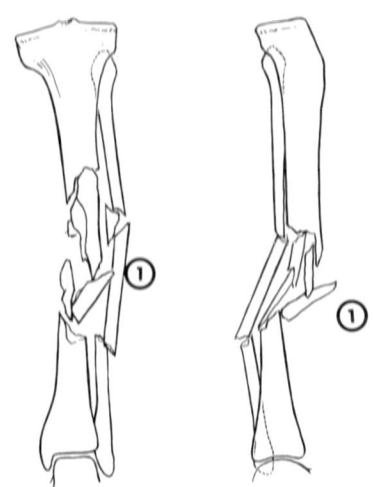

Preoperative X-Ray

1. Unstable segmental tibial and fibular fractures cannot be adequately stabilized in a cast.

TECHNIQUE OF CLOSED REDUCTION AND PIN TRANSFIXION

General or spinal anesthesia is preferable to permit insertion of the pins and to relax the surrounding muscles to allow fracture reduction.

Avoid distracting the fracture. The pull of gravity is all the traction necessary for most fractures.

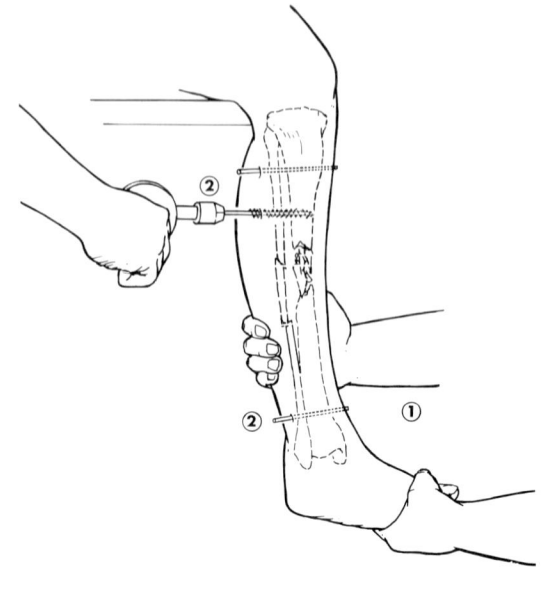

1. The surgeon reduces and holds the reduction while

2. An assistant inserts two 3-mm threaded Steinmann pins in the proximal fragment and one in the distal fragment using sterile technique. The pins should be inserted at least 3 to 4 cm from the fracture using a hand-powered rather than a motor-driven drill.

FRACTURES OF THE SHAFT OF THE TIBIA

CAUTION

1. A single pin may cause the proximal fragment to pivot, which may cause pressure necrosis of the skin over the fracture site.
2. Avoid using a power drill, which overheats the bone and causes necrotic ring sequestra.
3. Relieve all skin tension produced by the percutaneous pins.

Note: The pins are cut off with bolt cutters 2.5 cm from the skin, dressed with Betadine ointment, and covered with corks to prevent erosion through plaster.

Then the pins are incorporated in a long leg plaster cast.

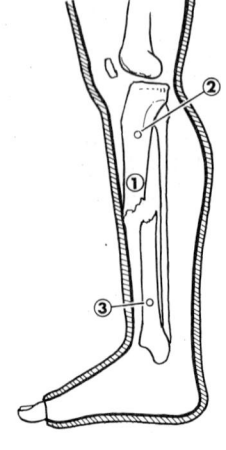

Postreduction X-Ray

Immediate postreduction x-ray should show:
1. Correct alignment of the joints proximal and distal to the fracture site and
2. Restoration of fracture length without distraction of the fracture.

Note: Slight shortening of 5 to 10 mm may be accepted.

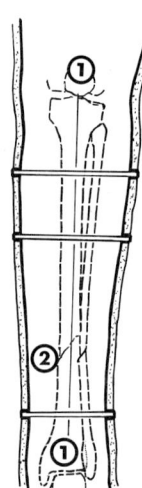

CAST WEDGING

REMARKS

Correction of angulatory deformities but not of torsional deformities is still possible after pins-in-plaster technique.

It is important to use a wedging technique that does not become a distracting lever on the fracture fragments. A closing rather than an opening wedge technique is required.

X-ray Before Cast Wedging

1. Films after transfixion pins show residual valgus and angulation.

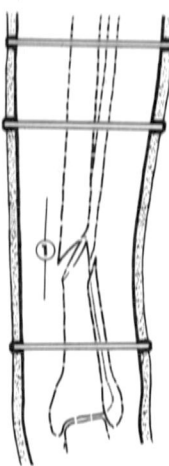

Closing Wedge Technique

1. A wedge is cut on the side toward which the foot and distal fragment are to be carried.
2. Leave two 2-cm hinges intact on opposite sides of the cast to prevent distracting the fracture.
3. Make a linear cut on the side opposite the wedge, extending from one hinge to the other.

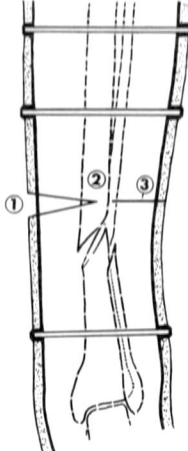

X-Ray after Cast Wedging

1. The wedge is partially closed. The opposite wedge is maintained in an open position with small blocks, and the area is rewrapped with plaster.
2. The angulatory deformity has been corrected.
3. Fracture length has been maintained without distracting the fracture site during the wedging.

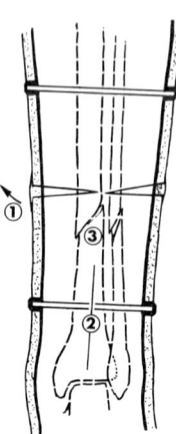

Subsequent Management

The pins-in-plaster technique should not interfere with the important management of the soft tissue injury. The open wound can be redebrided and cleansed in the operating room in two to four days and as often as necessary thereafter.

The patient is allowed crutch walking with toe-touch weight bearing for three to four weeks. After this, the transfixion pins can generally be removed.

After pin removal, apply a snug long leg walking cast, as previously described.

Using the pins-in-plaster technique for longer than six weeks tends to produce fracture distraction and a higher incidence of delayed union or nonunion. These complications can be avoided by removing the pins as soon as the surrounding soft tissues have healed enough to permit stabilization of the fracture in a snug weight-bearing cast.

OPEN TIBIAL FRACTURES

Principles of Management

REMARKS

Although the surgeon cannot control the degree of initial violence producing an open tibial fracture, he or she can, by following basic biologically oriented principles, minimize the risks of infection and nonunion.

Four of the most important principles to follow are:
1. Leave closed fractures closed.
2. Open and debride all open fractures.
3. Leave open fractures open.
4. Assume that initial debridement is incomplete, and plan a second look.

LEAVE CLOSED FRACTURES CLOSED

A major cause of open fracture is the surgeon. Even simple internal fixation carries the risk of significant infection with a tibial fracture.

In view of the excellent results from functional treatment of tibial fractures, closed fractures should remain closed.

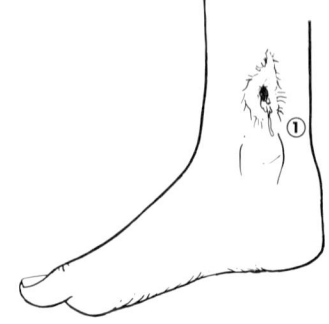

1. Chronic osteomyelitis has disabled this patient for eight years after screw fixation of a torsional distal tibial fracture. These fractures heal quite effectively without surgical intervention.

OPEN AND DEBRIDE ALL OPEN FRACTURES

Open fractures may result from the fracture pushing through the skin so as to "compound from within."

These wounds may appear deceptively innocuous but can be significantly contaminated by foreign material.

1. A small puncture wound may or may not have been produced by bone fragments pushing outward. Operative cleansing and debridement are necessary even with relatively "minor" open fractures. Do not undertreat the real problem of the open fracture while observing the patient for injuries elsewhere.

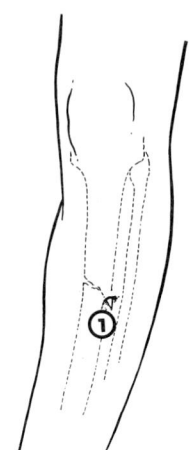

LEAVE OPEN FRACTURES OPEN

Violent injury to both soft tissue and bone demands complete wound cleansing, particularly to remove necrotic muscle and foreign material.

Even after the most "meticulous" surgical cleansing, one is virtually assured to have left behind some potentially infected tissue.

Most open fractures should be regarded more as abscesses than as clean surgical wounds. Closing an abscess of this nature is antithetical to the biologic treatment of wounds.

1. Leaving the wound open allows free drainage of the contaminated fracture site. This permits the body's homeostatic mechanisms to heal the soft tissue wound from below.
2. Closing a contaminated wound promotes abscess formation and eventual involvement of the bone. This produces sequestered harbors for chronic infection.

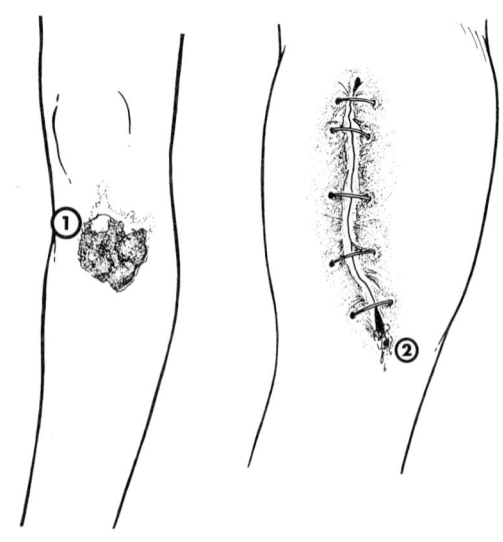

ASSUME THAT THE INITIAL DEBRIDEMENT IS INCOMPLETE AND PLAN A SECOND LOOK

Plan to reexplore and have a second look at the open fracture in the operating room within two to four days after initial wound treatment.

Do not rely on inspection through a cast window, which is inadequate. Anticipate that foreign material has been left in unexplored areas.

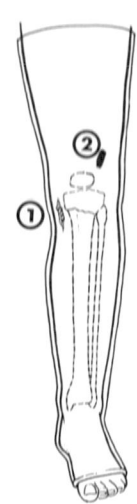

1. This postoperative x-ray after "thorough debridement" of a medial open tibial fracture showed
2. A metal fragment from the victim's motorcycle bike lodged in the suprapatellar pouch.

Note: A planned reexploration of the contaminated fracture in the operating room allows the surgeon a second chance to excise necrotic tissues and remove foreign material. The clean wound may be closed secondarily. When in doubt, the wound should be left open to heal by intussusception.

Cultivation of Healing: The Ultimate Biologic Principle

WOUND HEALING BY SPONTANEOUS INTUSSUSCEPTION

REMARKS

The ultimate principle of open fracture management is that healing cannot be imposed; it can only be cultivated.

Although many epigrammatic statements may be found in the literature to the effect that open fractures must be converted to closed ones as soon as possible, most heal best by spontaneous closure. Vigorous attempts at secondary closure or local or cross-leg flaps frequently impede rather than improve soft tissue and skeletal healing.

Spontaneous wound closure occurs through the process of wound intussusception, or shrinkage. This reliable biologic process was well known to most surgeons in antiquity, who never closed wounds. Unfortunately, this knowledge appears to have been lost to many modern surgeons, who believe that wounds cannot heal without their contributions.

The Greeks and Romans recognized that spontaneous shrinkage of a wound resulted from asymmetric migration of the wound edges.

Carrel has demonstrated that contractile forces reside in the granulation tissue that fills the wound.

The nature of this force has been clearly defined by modern electron microscope studies. Gabbiani and others have confirmed that the contractility of wound edges is due to the differentiation of fibroblasts into myofibroblasts. These cells, which are akin to smooth muscle cells, then contract to pull the wound edges centripetally.

In addition to removing all potential wound contaminants and avoiding the wound abscesses likely after premature closure, the surgeon can contribute most effectively to biologic wound healing with continuous cast support. The mechanical support of the cast aids wound intussusception. The moist occlusive dressing that the cast provides promotes epithelial coverage of the shrinking wound edges.

1. Characteristically in wound contraction the wound edge closest to the center migrates most rapidly, thereby altering the contour of the scar.

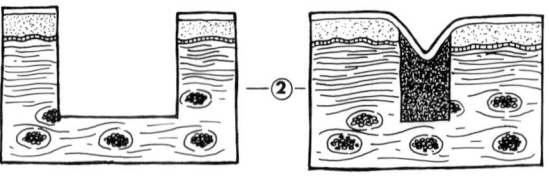

2. Use of continuous cast immobilization supports the mechanical process of wound contraction and

3. The moist dressing from the cast aids epithelialization over the contracting wound edges.

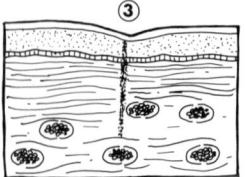

THE FATE OF EXPOSED BONE

REMARKS

One justification for elaborate and frequently destructive attempts at closure is to cover bone, which for some reason is thought to die if left exposed to air.

The illogicality of this belief has been demonstrated by Paul Brown and others, who repeatedly and convincingly have shown that bone exposed in the fracture site requires neither local flaps nor pedicle flaps from a distance.

Contamination of the open wound does not mean that infection is present, as long as the drainage is outward. The host defense mechanisms readily cope with the bacterial contaminants, which find no place to lodge.

An understanding of the circulatory patterns of the healing response is necessary to appreciate how bone remains viable despite exposure to air.

1. The blood supply to exposed bone in a fracture comes centrifugally from the medullary canal, not from the periosteum. This flow of nutrients maintains the viability of bone, which may appear nonviable on gross inspection.

2. The major circulatory response for tibial fracture healing comes from the posterior and lateral soft tissue attachments. These are effective even if the anterior and medial cortices remain exposed.

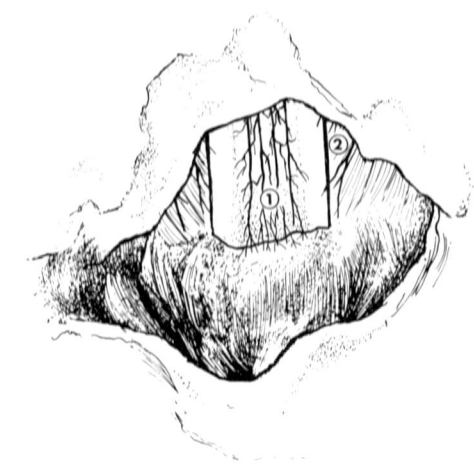

3. Bone that is exposed is rapidly covered by contractile wound edges, provided that bacteria are not permitted to sequester in dead or damaged soft or hard tissue.

4. Epithelialization is promoted by the moist environment within the cast dressing.

Note: Splint-skin grafting may occasionally be useful to provide a biologic dressing and to diminish serous wound drainage. Ultimate wound healing is generally better when skin grafting is avoided.

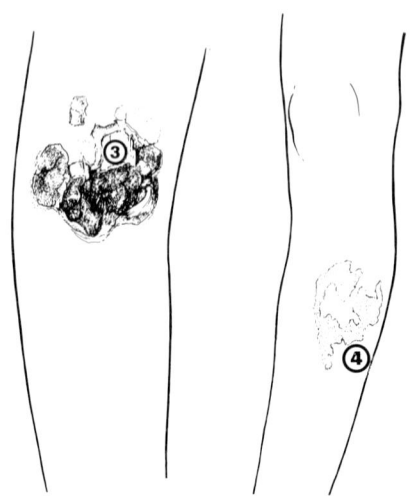

ANTIBIOTIC MANAGEMENT IN OPEN FRACTURES

REMARKS

Bacterial contamination is inevitable with open fractures but is not equivalent to bacterial infection.

The organisms found are likely to be both gram-positive and gram-negative. Currently, most prove to be sensitive to cephalothin sodium or oxacillin, either of which should be given promptly and intravenously in the emergency room following initial culture.

Parenteral antibiotics are administered every six hours for three days or until the second debridement insures adequate healing of the wound.

Antibiotic coverage should be considered as an aid in but not as a definitive means of treating open fractures. The major drawback of antibiotic use is that it can be overemphasized by some as a primary treatment rather than as an aid to adequate debridement.

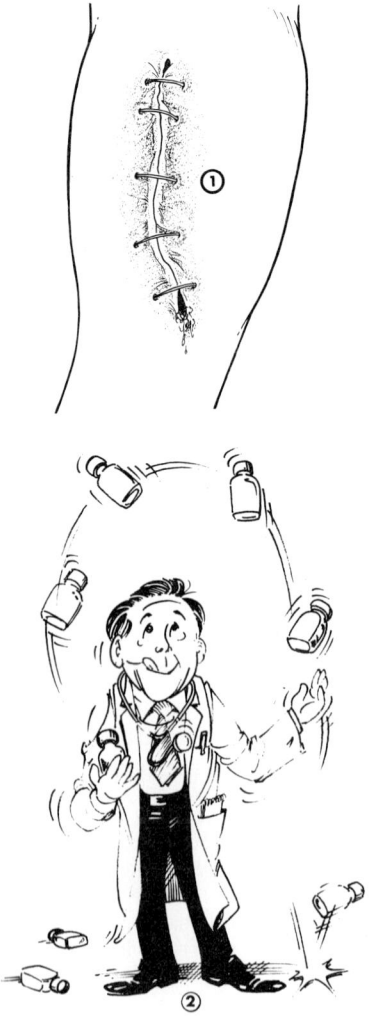

1. Antibiotic coverage can mask abscesses forming at the fracture site after primary closure.

2. Juggling antibiotic coverage is no substitute for redebridement and recleansing of contaminated open fractures. This may have to be done frequently, every two to four days, to insure freedom from osteomyelitis.

GAS GANGRENE IN OPEN FRACTURES

REMARKS

Tibial fracture is by far the fracture most commonly associated with clostridial myonecrosis. In Brown and Kinman's studies of civilian injuries, more than half of open fractures complicated by gas gangrene occurred in the tibia.

Some patients may have severe associated injuries to the chest, head, or abdomen. The open fracture may then be cared for in the emergency room under the misassumption that time can be saved taking care of the "less severe wound" while the patient is being prepared for treatment of the more serious injuries.

Characteristic symptoms of restlessness, increasing pain, fever, drainage, and tachycardia become manifest within 36 to 48 hours after injury, and the infected fracture rapidly becomes life-threatening.

Gas gangrene infection occurs despite antibiotic prophylaxis.

This complication may also follow secondary closure of a wound after initial open treatment. When in doubt, always leave the wound open.

Do not depend on antibiotic manipulation or even hyperbaric oxygenation in patients with symptomatic evidence of clostridial myonecrosis. Complete debridement of necrotic muscle, with amputation as necessary, is the only lifesaving procedure once this extremely toxic infection develops.

The incidence in civilian injuries of clostridial infection, which is a life-threatening complication, exceeds that in military casualties, which are traditionally considered the usual victims. The basic principle learned in the military but still to be learned in civilian medicine is to avoid primary closure of open fractures. Consistently, the overwhelming majority of gas gangrene problems develop *after* primary closure of open fractures or other extensive soft tissue wounds.

For further discussion of this complication, which is still prevalent and particularly likely to follow tibial fractures, see pages 130–132.

WHIRLPOOL THERAPY FOR SOFT TISSUE WOUNDS COMPLICATING TIBIAL FRACTURES

REMARKS

In grossly contaminated or infected fractures, a pulsating stream of fluid provides safe mechanical cleansing postoperatively. A whirlpool bath, to which an agent such as Betadine or chlorox is added, serves this purpose effectively.

Whirlpool therapy is especially useful in the first one to two weeks after the injury or infection.

Many techniques of external fixation are available to immobilize the fracture during whirlpool therapy. The simplest and least expensive but most effective method is to use a water-resistant cast that allows ingress of the whirlpool solution through a cast window.

At the end of seven to ten days the wound will show healthy granulation tissue and the whirlpool therapy can be discontinued.

Whirlpool treatment should be considered only as an aid. It should not be prolonged so that it interferes with functional weight-bearing treatment of the fractures.

1. An infection in the wound is evident one week after primary closure of an open tibial fracture.

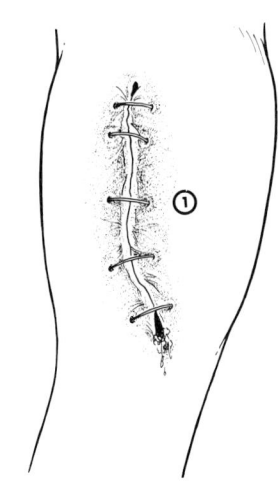

1. The surgical wound is opened widely and is thoroughly cleansed in the operating room.

2. The fracture is then immobilized postoperatively in a water-resistant plaster cast.

3. A window over the wound allows inflow of the pulsating whirlpool fluid.

Note: The casted limb is immersed in the whirlpool for 15 minutes twice a day. Following this, the limb and the cast are allowed to air dry and the wound is covered by a sterile dressing.

After ten days the wound should be clean and should be starting to fill in with granulation tissue. At this point a functional weight-bearing cast can be applied and the healthy wound is allowed to heal by natural intussusception.

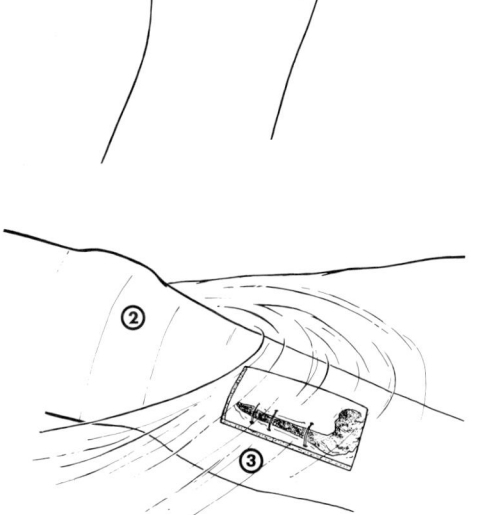

Results at Six Months

1. Soft tissue healing and
2. Fracture healing have occurred simultaneously during functional cast treatment.

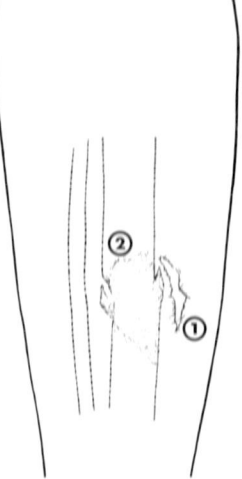

Bone Defects with Open Tibial Fractures

REMARKS

One of the most difficult problems to manage is the open fracture with bone loss due to either initial injury or ill-conceived surgical excision.

For a review of the technique of wound debridement, see page 125.

Keep in mind Learmonth's verse:

> From the edge of the skin,
> Take a piece very thin.
> The tenser the fascia,
> The more you should slash 'er;
> Of muscles much more,
> 'Til you see fresh gore,
> And bundles contract,
> At the least impact,
> Hardly any bone,
> Only bits alone.

MANAGEMENT OF DETACHED (LOOSE) BONE FRAGMENTS

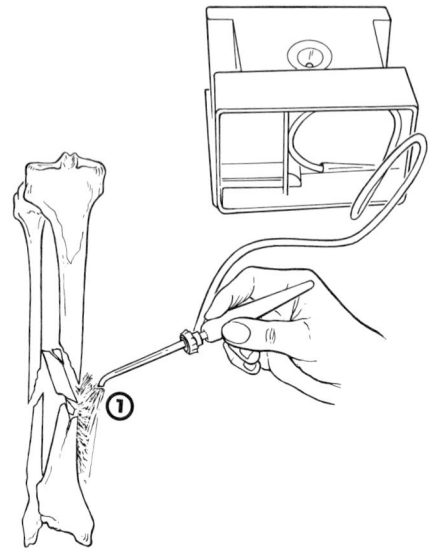

1. Every attempt should be made to salvage bone. Irrigation with pulsed pressure systems effectively removes debris and dirt attached to the bone fragments.

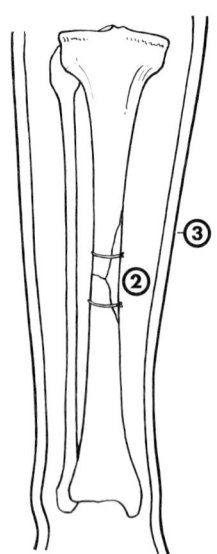

2. Large butterfly fragments completely detached from soft tissues should not be removed. They can be stabilized with cerclage wire, which does not impair revascularization of the cortical fragment.

3. Immobilization depends on external cast support and not on the wire, which is being used only to hold the butterfly fragment in the bone gap.

MANAGEMENT OF EXTRUDED DIAPHYSEAL FRAGMENTS

REMARKS

Hansen and coworkers have demonstrated by radiography, scintiscanning, and microscopic examination that even large extruded diaphyseal fragments can be reincorporated into the tibia. Infection must be avoided and the surrounding soft tissues must be preserved to permit reincorporation.

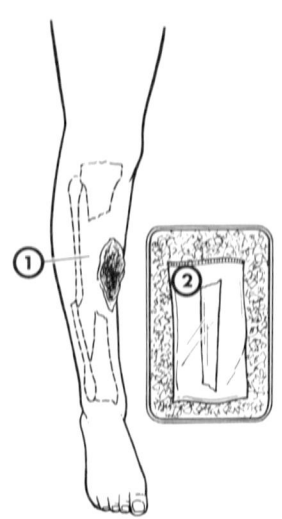

1. Preoperative appearance of a 15-cm diaphyseal tibial defect after a motorcycle injury.
2. The diaphyseal fragment was brought in to the hospital with the patient.

Note: The extruded bone fragment should be managed initially as an amputated digit or limb. The bone should be wrapped in a plastic bag and kept on ice. Avoid soaking the bone in saline or other fluids that may be cytotoxic.

X-ray One Year After Reimplantation

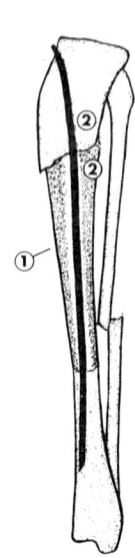

1. The reimplanted diaphyseal segment is fixed with an intramedullary rod.
2. The variations in bone density in the different areas of the tibia indicate that healing has occurred by revascularization proximally and distally and around the periphery of the reimplanted fragment. The major portion of the fragment is still not revascularized. Structurally, this "dead bone" is almost as strong as living bone.

OPEN TIBIAL FRACTURES

EARLY FIBULAR BYPASS PROCEDURES FOR MASSIVE BONE LOSS

REMARKS

Dehne has shown that in the presence of a tibial defect, the proximal fibulotibular joint becomes a pivot around which the distal part of the limb can swing 30 degrees or more.

When part of the tibial bone has been irretrievably lost, the fibula can be made an effective stabilizer by synostosing it to the tibia. This may be a very effective early salvage procedure, particularly when the tibial fracture gap has become infected.

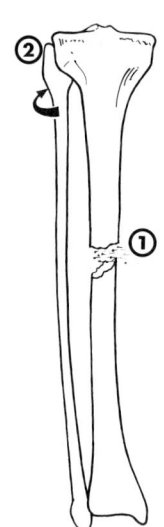

Preoperative X-ray

1. A gunshot injury to the tibia has caused significant fracture gap from bone loss.
2. Mobility at the proximal fibulotibial joint allows the distal fragment to rotate with the fibula as much as 30 degrees.

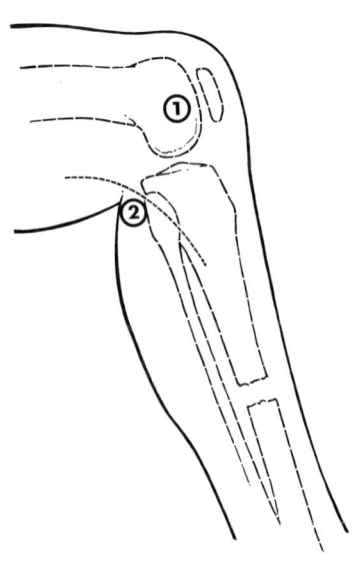

Fibulotibial Synostosis

1. The patient is positioned with the knee flexed to protect the peroneal nerve.
2. The incision is made beginning at 2 cm above the fibula, extending down to the neck, and then curving anteriorly to the crest of the tibia.

1. The common peroneal nerve is identified and protected.
2. The fibula is osteotomized beneath the nerve and moved anteriorly and medially to contact the tibia.
3. Two screws are used to fix the fibula to the tibia, and synostosis is further encouraged by cancellous bone graft laid between the fibula and tibia.

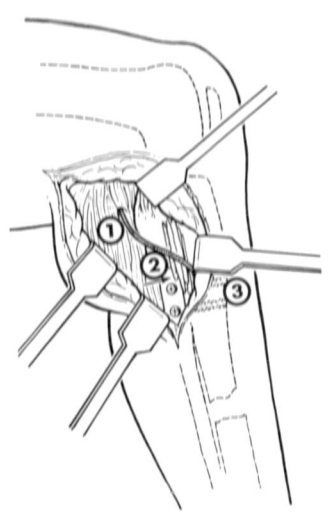

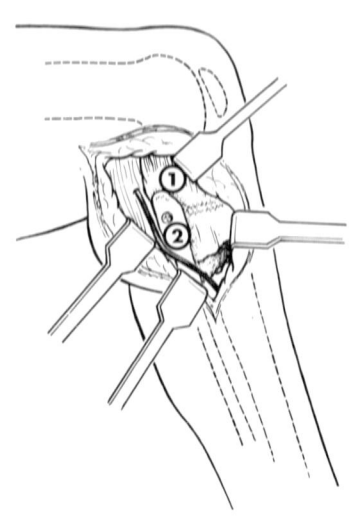

Alternate Procedure

For higher tibial defects,
1. The cartilage is excised from the upper tibiofibular articulation and a cavity is gouged out of the tibia.
2. The entire proximal fibula is fixed to the tibia with lag screws.

Note: Avoid excessive narrowing of the foramen for the anterior tibial artery. Always release the tourniquet after the procedure to ensure adequate distal circulation.

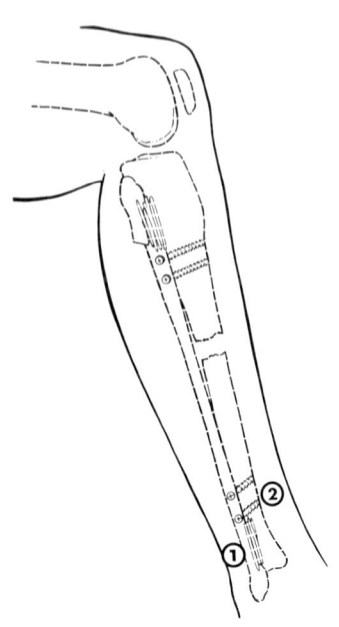

1. A second incision is made over the distal fibula, and the fibula is osteotomized obliquely.
2. The tibial surface is gouged to accommodate the osteotomized fibula and the fibular fragment is fixed to the tibia with two screws.

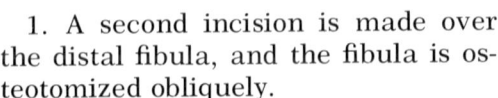

OPEN TIBIAL FRACTURES

X-Ray Two Years After Injury

1. There is good tibiofibular synostosis.
2. The fibula has hypertrophied to carry full weight without external protective support.

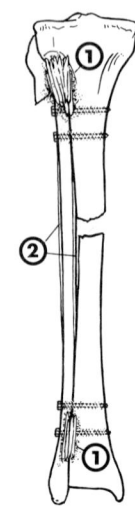

PROXIMAL AND DISTAL PIN TRANSFIXION AND EARLY AUTOGENOUS BONE GRAFTING

REMARKS

Massive direct injuries causing bone loss require multiple debridements to insure freedom from infection.

Distal and proximal pins in plaster can be used to maintain length and ankle joint alignment for four to six weeks until soft tissue healing is in progress.

Early autogenous matchstick-size bone grafts may then be used to fill in large defects.

Clinical Appearance

1. An open fracture with extensive bone loss has resulted from a power takeoff injury.

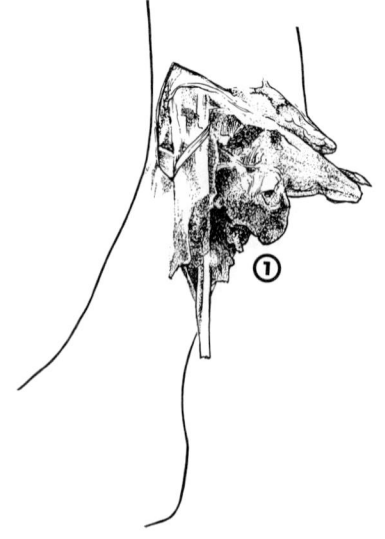

Preoperative X-Ray

1. Bone loss of 4 cm. is evident on anteroposterior and lateral views.
2. The fibula is still present and may be used for tibial graft.

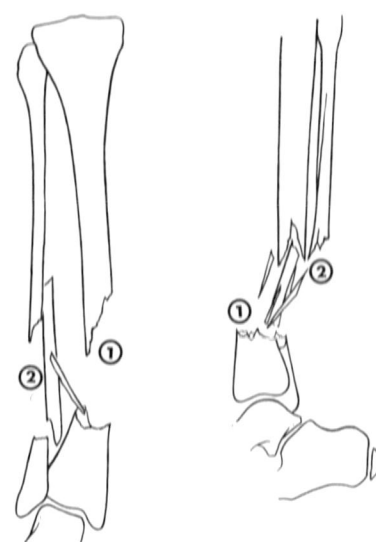

Operative Procedure

1. After multiple debridement to insure freedom from infection, the wound is left open.
2. The length of the limb and the ankle joint alignment are maintained by proximal and distal pins incorporated in plaster.

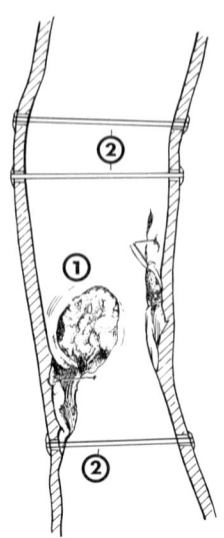

Operative Procedure (Continued)

1. Autogenous bone grafting is done at six weeks when the soft tissues are healing.
2. The pins may be removed prior to bone grafting, when the surrounding soft tissue and soft callus are sufficient to stabilize the fracture.

Note: The soft tissue wound need not be completely closed to permit bone grafting.

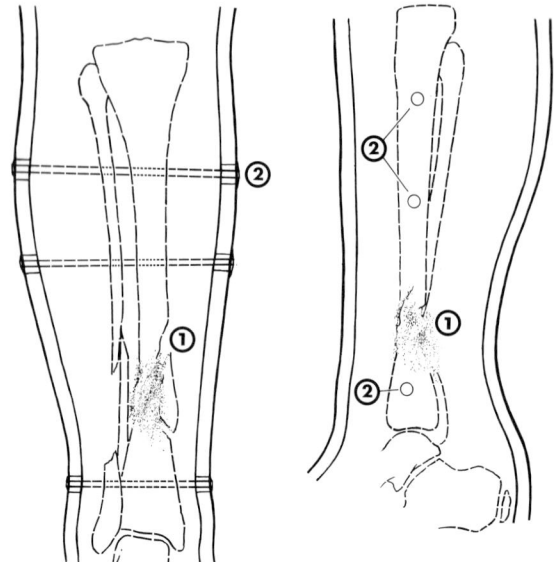

Pitfalls of Treating Open Tibial Fractures

REMARKS

Besides the initial problems relating to the severity of injury, tibial fractures may lead to management-induced complications, which rapidly transmute the patient into an appendage of his limb.
The most common problems are:
Surgical "assembly lines."
Bone defects.
Infected plate fixation.
Fracture distraction.
There are other causes, but the four listed above predominate. The physician choosing any form of fracture management is wise to anticipate its potential pitfalls as well as its technical advantages.

Surgical "Assembly Lines"

The history of failure when surgical intervention preempts functional weight-bearing treatment has been convincingly detailed by Dehne. The surgical mission frequently proposed is to obtain a healthy field at the fracture site for subsequent reconstructive bone grafting. The sequence, which averages ten surgical procedures and at least four years of morbidity, is as follows:

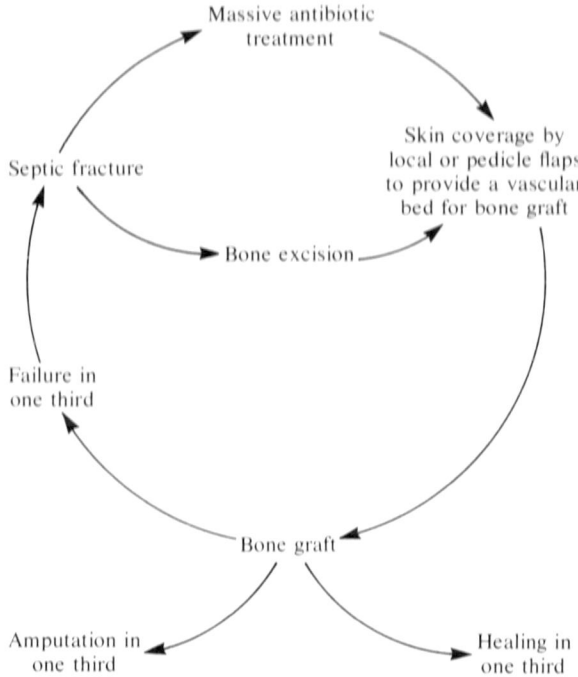

Note: The priorities of functional weight-bearing treatment are, first, union of the fracture and, second, soft tissue healing. Once these priorities are satisfied the "infection" proves most often to be a self-limiting contamination. Use biologic rather than mechanistic techniques in order to avoid the surgical assembly line pitfall.

Bone Defects

1. Loose bone fragments, even when completely detached, should be left at the fracture site to fill gaps and to induce new bone.

2. Surgical excision of bone leads to an infected nonunion with frequently insurmountable defects, as illustrated by this fracture after surgical excision.

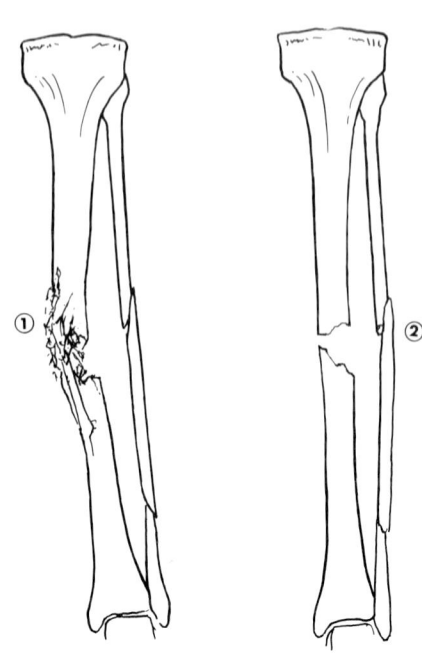

Infected Plate Fixation

1. The tibial fracture seems admirably suited for plate fixation.
2. Soft tissue necrosis occurring over the plate causes an infected nonunion, particularly after application of a plate to the medial cortex.

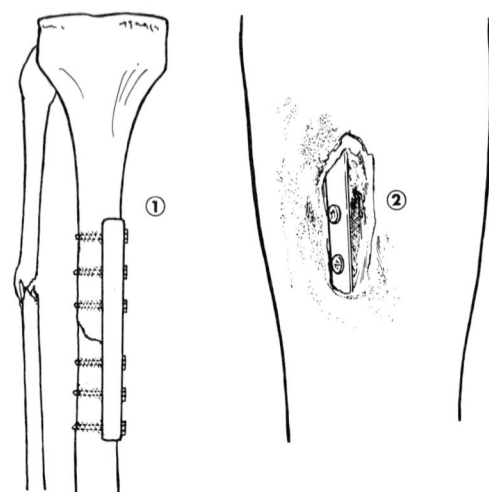

Fracture Distraction

1. Significant fracture gap can be created inadvertently by external fixation devices that distract the fracture. Necrosis of the bone fragments proximal and distal to the fracture may also contribute to fracture "gaposis."
2. Removing the transfixion pins when the soft tissues are healing at three to four weeks allows the fracture to be impacted with functional weight-bearing treatment.

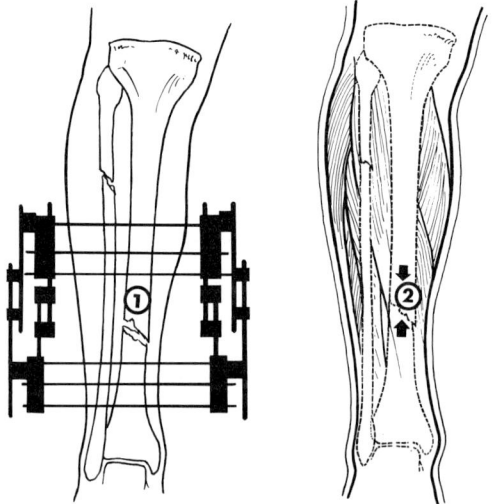

OTHER PROBLEMS IN TIBIAL FRACTURE

Segmental Fractures

REMARKS

This unstable fracture can be treated by closed functional cast method in most instances.

Reduction must be particularly directed at adequate knee-ankle alignment rather than anatomic restoration of the tibial segments. Slight shortening and overriding of the fracture fragments are desirable.

Reduction and maintenance of satisfactory alignment can be difficult, but this fracture will unite satisfactorily with functional weight-bearing treatment (see page 1742).

Rarely, if closed reduction proves inadequate, particularly in a patient with multiple injuries, internal fixation is indicated. The most effective stabilizing technique is usually intramedullary nailing, by either closed or open method. This achieves the necessary fracture fixation with minimal soft tissue and skeletal trauma.

OPERATIVE TECHNIQUE: CLOSED LOTTES NAILING (BLIND NAILING)

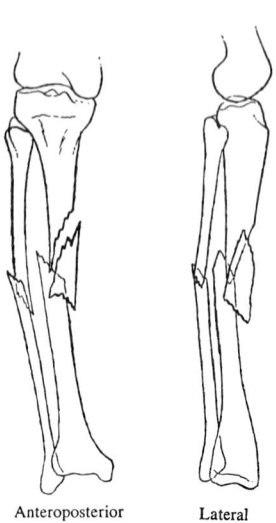

Anteroposterior   Lateral

Prereduction X-Ray

A segmental fracture associated with an adjacent fibular fracture may prove particularly unstable for closed reduction.

Operative Procedure

The patient lies on a fracture table:
1. The knee is flexed 90 degrees.
2. The hip is flexed 50 degrees.
3. The foot and ankle are draped separately.

Note: Adequate radiography, preferably with image-intensified fluoroscopy, is important to perform blind nailing effectively.

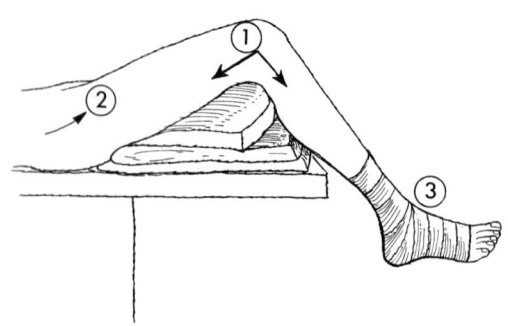

1. While an assistant exerts downward traction on the foot,
2. Manipulate the fragments into anatomic alignment.
3. Make a skin incision on the anteromedial aspect of the tibia 2 cm medial to the most prominent part of the tibial tubercle; extend it proximally to the medial side of the inferior margin of the patella.
4. Deepen the incision to the bone, but do not open the knee joint.

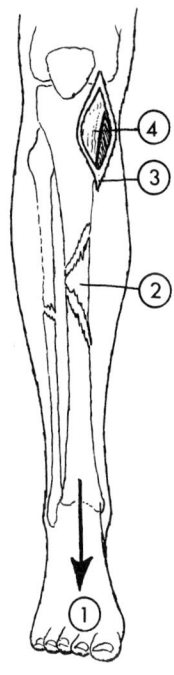

1. With a 9-mm drill make a hole in the tibia at the level of the middle of the tibial tubercle; first perforate the tibial cortex, holding the drill at right angles to the bone.
2. Then aim the top of the drill at the crest of the tibia at the point of juncture of the middle and distal thirds. While drilling the channel, slowly depress the drill handle until it is almost parallel to the shaft of the tibia.

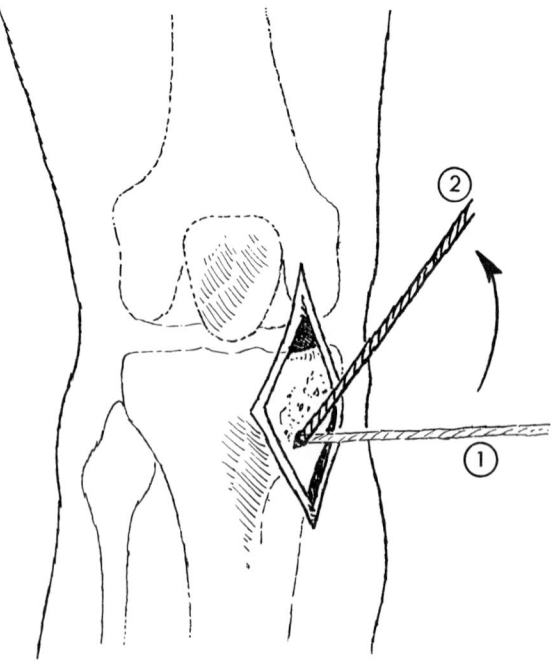

Determining the Length of the Nail

1. Measure the distance from the medial malleolus to the tibial tubercle of the unaffected side.
2. Use a Lottes nail 9 mm in diameter.

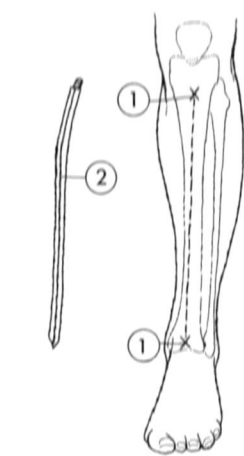

Insertion of the Nail

1. Insert the Lottes nail and align the tip with the juncture of the middle and distal thirds of the tibia.
2. Its dorsal fin points forward.
3. Tap the nail until it strikes the posterior cortex of the tibia.

Note: To prevent maceration of the skin and soft tissues while driving the nail, place a metal shield between the nail and the soft tissues in front of the knee.

4. Then with the palm of the hand depress the middle of the nail so that it almost parallels the longitudinal axis of the tibia. (This advances the tip of the nail.) As the nail is driven into the canal, maintain downward pressure until it actually dents the skin over the knee.
5. As the nail advances, check its progress with image-intensified fluoroscopy.

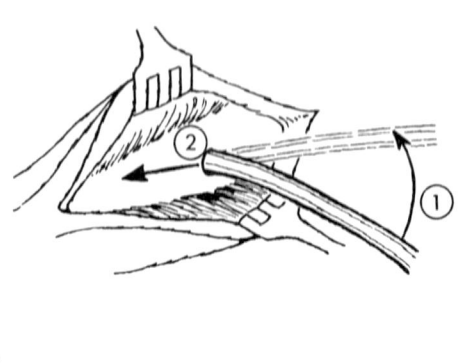

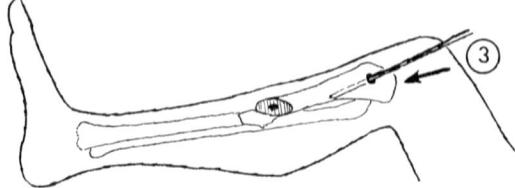

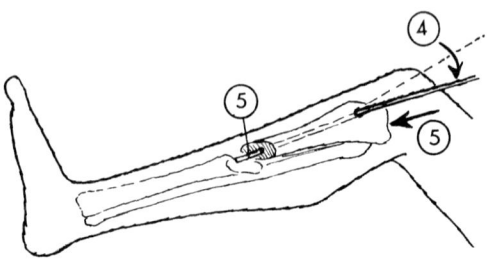

Insertion of the Nail (Continued)

1. When the level of the fracture site is reached by the tip of the nail,
2. Check the alignment of the fragments and correct any rotational deformity.
3. Drive the nail across the fracture site for 5 to 6 cm.

Note: Check the stability of the fragments. Obvious instability means that the nail has not engaged the distal fragment. If this is the case, withdraw the nail and reinsert it.

4. Now drive the nail into the distal fragment.

Note: Before seating the nail, take x-rays to determine the position of the fragments and the relationship of the tip of the nail to the ankle joint.

5. If the position of the fragments and the level of the tip of the nail are satisfactory, drive the nail in until the driver strikes the cortex. (The threaded portion of the nail remains above the level of the cortex so that it can be extracted later.)

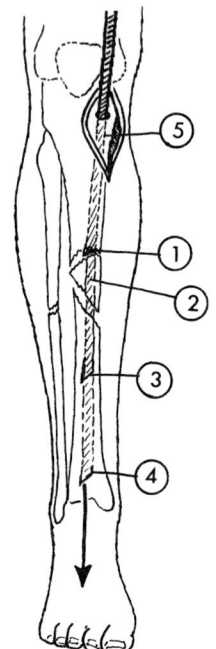

Postreduction X-Ray

1. The fragments are in normal position.
2. The tip of the nail is well above the distal articular surface of the tibia.

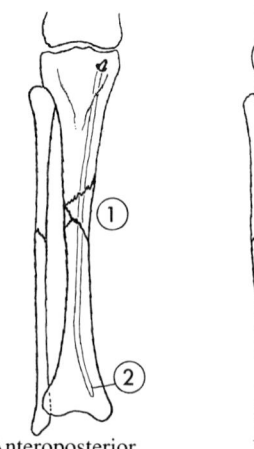 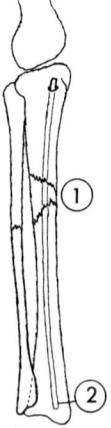

Anteroposterior   Lateral

Immobilization

1. Apply a long leg cast with the knee in extension.

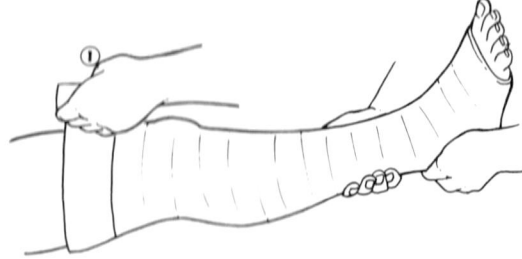

Postreduction Management

1. Always elevate the fracture by an overhead suspension.

Note: Do not rely on pillows for elevation; they are ineffective.

2. The patient actively works on toe extension and isometric exercises of the muscles of this leg.

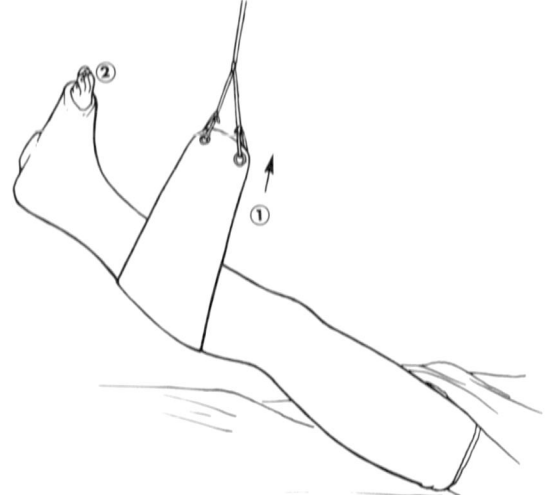

Start three-point weight bearing with crutches within one to two days after operation.

The patient may be out of bed and walking but he should not sit or stand. Whenever he is not walking, the leg should be elevated to avoid swelling within the cast. This preventive regimen must be continued for 5 to 7 days until swelling is no longer likely.

After 1 week the cast may be changed to a short leg PTB or the long leg cast may be kept, depending on the skills of the surgeon and the activity of the patient.

Lottes nailing should be considered an internal splint rather than a rigid immobilizing method. The rate of union is not accelerated by this method.

After 14 to 16 weeks, the external cast support may be removed and fracture stability may be evaluated clinically and radiographically.

The patient should continue with protected weight bearing using crutches for 6 to 8 weeks longer, until union is assured.

The nail is not removed until the fracture lines are completely obliterated on x-ray.

OTHER PROBLEMS IN TIBIAL FRACTURE

OPEN METHOD OF INTRAMEDULLARY NAILING

Prereduction X-Ray

Segmental fractures of the tibia with fracture of the adjacent fibula may result in marked instability.

Note: When there has been bone lost or union has been delayed, intramedullary nailing should be supplemented by cancellous bone grafting.

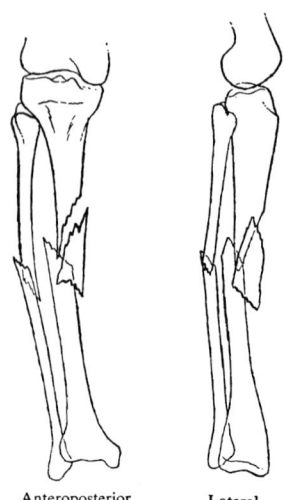

Anteroposterior   Lateral

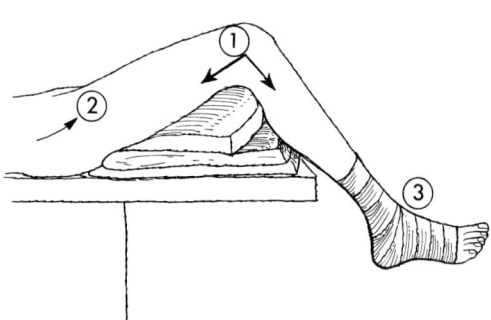

Open Reduction

The patient lies on a fracture table.
1. The knee is flexed 90 degrees.
2. The hip is flexed 50 degrees.
3. The foot and ankle are draped separately.

1. Make the incisions just lateral to the tibial crest.
2. By sharp dissection expose the tibial crest and incise the periosteum longitudinally.

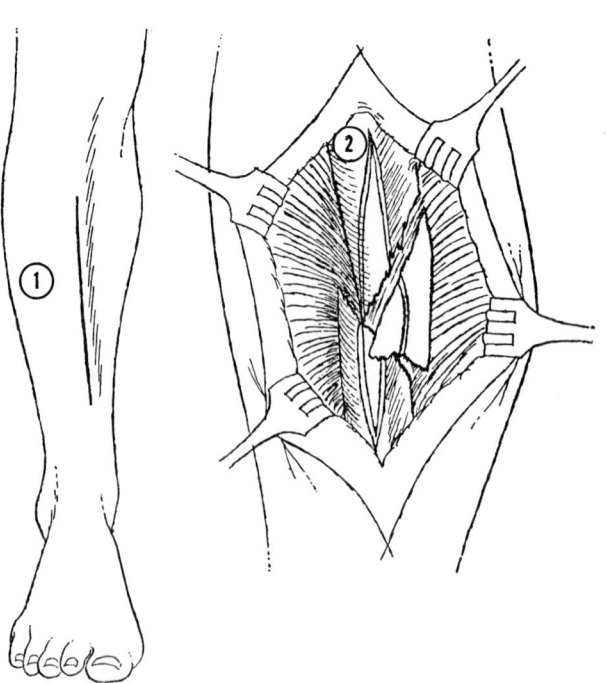

1. By subperiosteal dissection expose the ends of the fragments just enough to permit reduction and application of cancellous bone grafts across the fracture sites.

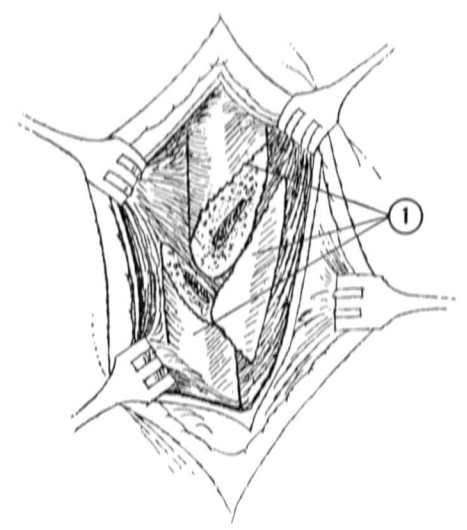

1. Make a short longitudinal incision 2 cm. medial to the tibial tubercle; it extends proximally to the inferior margin of the patella.
2. By subperiosteal dissection expose the bone at the inferior portion of the incision.
3. With a 9-mm. drill for a Lottes nail, first perforate the tibial cortex.
4. Then aim the tip of the drill at the crest of the tibia at the juncture of its middle and lower thirds.

Note: While drilling the channel, depress the drill handle slowly and continuously until it is almost parallel to the shaft of the tibia.

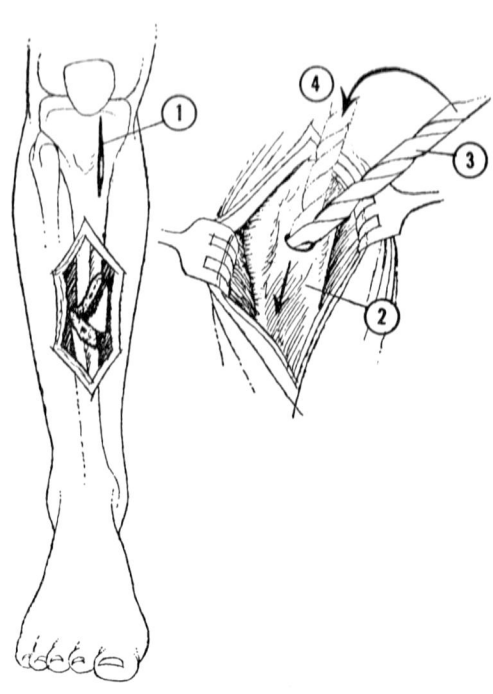

Determining the Length of the Nail

1. Measure the distance from the medial malleolus to the tibial tubercle of the unaffected side.
2. Use a Lottes nail 9 mm. in diameter, or larger as necessary to achieve adequate fixation. Two nails may be necessary for a tibia with a wide medullary canal.

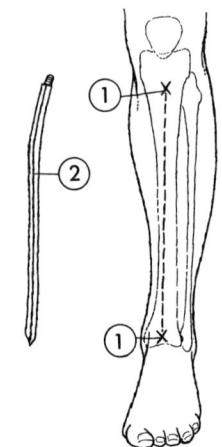

Insertion of the Nail

1. Insert the Lottes nail and align the tip with the juncture of the middle and lower thirds of the shaft.
2. Its dorsal fin points forward.

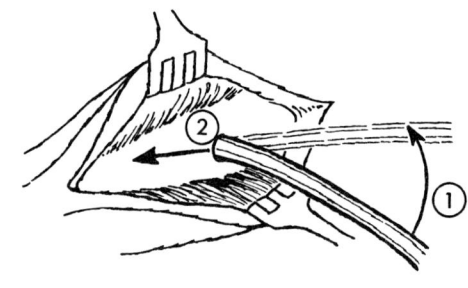

3. Tap the nail until it strikes the posterior cortex.

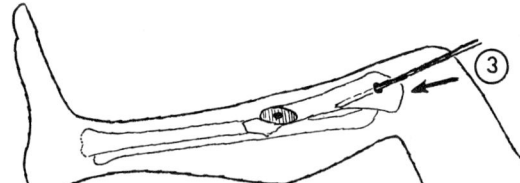

4. Then with the palm of the hand depress the middle of the nail so that it lies almost parallel with the longitudinal axis of the tibia.
5. Drive the nail until the tip appears through the medullary canal of the proximal fragment.

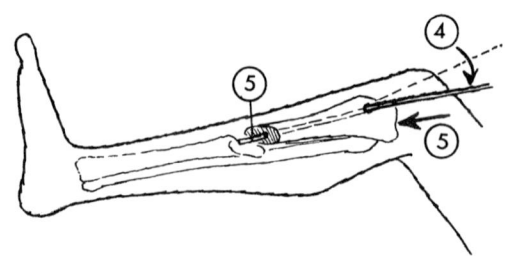

1. An assistant exerts traction on the lower end.
2. He aligns the great toe with the patella.
3. With a curette lever the fragments into their normal anatomic position.
4. Drive the nail into the medullary canal of the middle fragment.

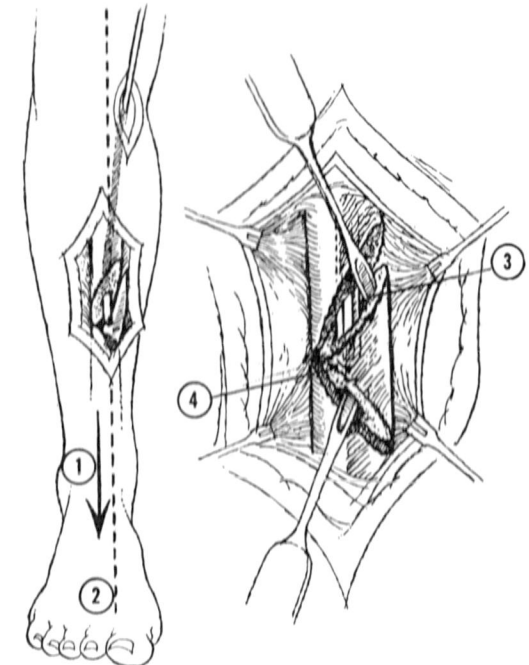

1. Drive the nail until it appears through the medullary canal of the middle fragment.
2. Again exert traction; correct the rotational deformity and with a curette lever the fragments into their normal position; now drive the nail across the fracture site.
3. Finally drive the nail further in until the driver strikes the cortex.
4. Tap the sole of the foot with the palm of the hand to impact all fragments.

Note: At this point check the reduction and the position of the nail by x-ray; if it is satisfactory, proceed.

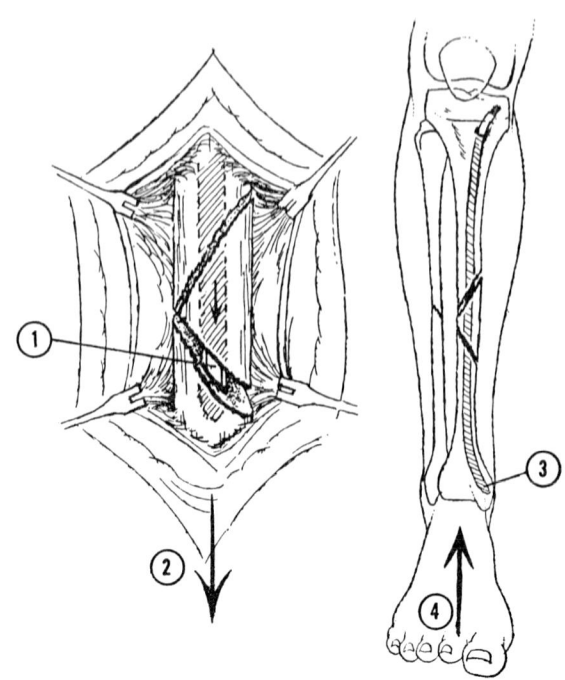

Cancellous Bone Graft

Pack slabs of cancellous bone (previously removed from the anterior crest of the ilium) around the fracture site.

Note: One or two supplemental cerclage wires may add useful internal stability without disrupting soft tissue blood supply to the fracture site (see page 1731).

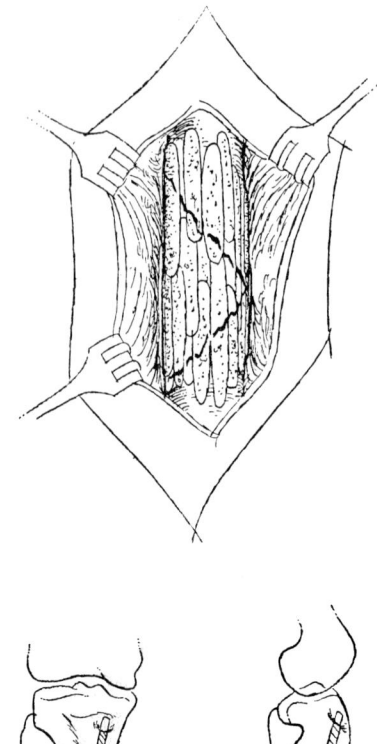

Postreduction X-Ray

1. The nail is in correct position and is of proper length.
2. The fragments are in normal alignment.
3. Cancellous bone slabs surround the fracture site.

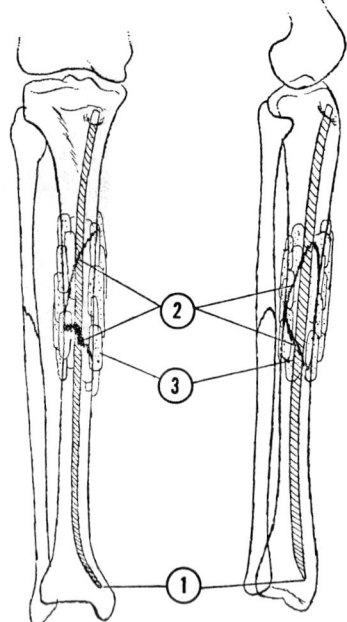

Anteroposterior   Lateral

Immobilization

1. Apply a long leg cast with the knee in extension.

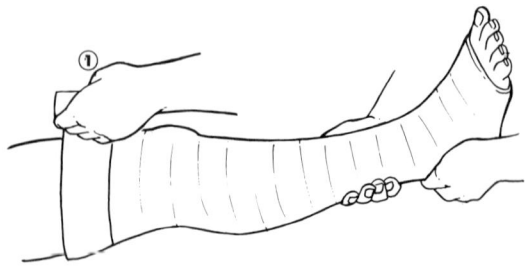

Malunion, Delayed Union, and Nonunion

MALUNION

REMARKS

Malunion occurs when the fracture heals in a position that distorts knee and ankle joint alignment. This is most frequently a problem with distal third fractures, which tend to rotate externally. The result is a shift of the axis of the ankle joint away from and out of the weight-bearing line. The importance of approaching these fractures with a three-dimensional understanding has been discussed on page 1740.

A fracture in the distal third of the tibia with an intact fibula tends to rotate internally. This also shifts the axis of ankle motion inward from the weight-bearing line and causes the patient to walk on the outside of his foot.

Both internal and external torsional deformities can cause ankle pain and may require derotational osteotomy to relieve symptoms.

Shortening after a tibial fracture is rarely sufficient to impair function. Shortening of 1.0 to 1.5 cm. is not perceptible to most patients. Greater shortening should be avoided, but if it occurs because of fracture comminution, it can usually be accommodated with a heel lift. More frequently the patient simply alters his gait and walks with his foot in slight equinus to accommodate. Shortening after the tibial fracture is not nearly as disabling as is torsional malalignment of the ankle.

1. The weight-bearing line normally falls slightly medial to the hip and knee and lateral to the ankle axis.
2. An external rotational deformity after a distal tibial fracture shifts the ankle axis laterally and
3. Orients the axis of motion away from the weight-bearing line.

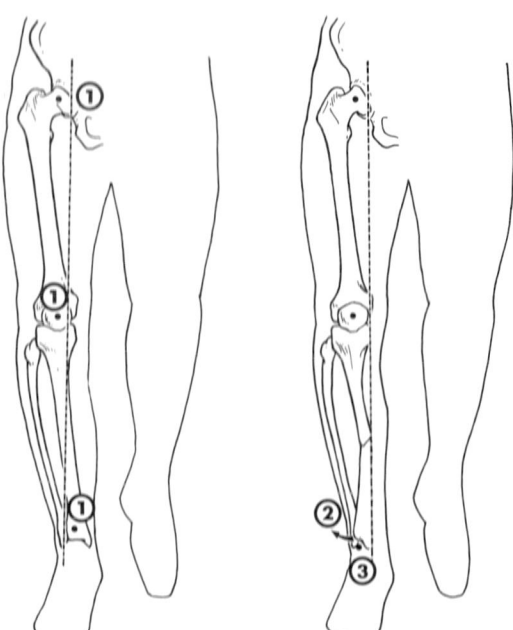

1. Internal rotation of the distal fracture shifts the axis of motion medial to the weight line and
2. Rotates the ankle mortise, causing the patient to walk on the outside of the foot.

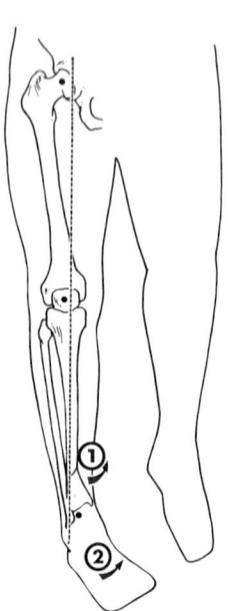

Proximal Tibial Malunion (Sarmiento)

1. An oblique medial condylar or bicondylar fracture may develop varus deformity if the fibula is intact.
2. Osteotomy of the proximal fibula may be necessary to prevent malunion.

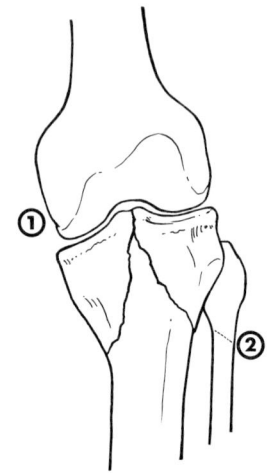

VALGUS DEFORMITIES OF FRACTURES OF THE UPPER TIBIAL METAPHYSIS IN CHILDREN (WEBER)

REMARKS

It has been noted by Jackson and Cozen that relatively undisplaced proximal tibial metaphyseal fractures in children can produce significant valgus angulation with growth.

Weber has indicated that this frequently may be the result of a fibrous interposition of the pes anserinus muscle insertion into the fracture site. This alters the effect of muscle pull on the proximal tibial metaphysis and results in overgrowth on the medial side of the physis.

1. Valgus growth deformity may follow upper tibial metaphyseal fracture in a child.
2. Fibrous interposition of the pes anserinus and periosteal fibers has been found by Weber. If this occurs it should be removed surgically to prevent resistant and previously unexplainable valgus growth deformity after such a relatively minor fracture.

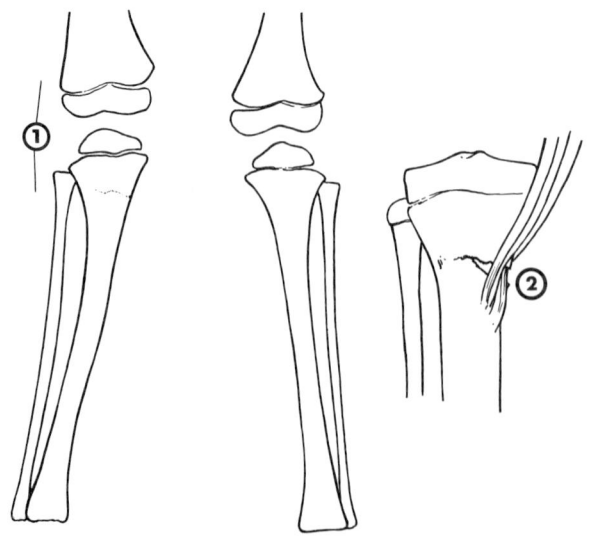

NONUNION AND DELAYED UNION

REMARKS

Tibial fractures are notoriously prone to result in nonunion. Present-day studies of all types of nonunion after long-bone fractures indicate that 70 per cent or more occur in the tibia. As many as 25 per cent of open tibial fractures have resulted in nonunion in some series. Ischemia of soft tissue and bone adds significantly to this liability.

One should be careful to distinguish the fairly common problem of a tibial fracture in which radiographic union is delayed from a fracture that is truly nonunited clinically.

Most tibial fractures should be well on their way to union by 12 weeks. Any painful motion evident at the fracture after 16 weeks warrants treatment to expedite fracture healing.

In the past physicians have delayed 10 to 12 months on the average before treating nonunion by standard bone-grafting techniques. With newer, relatively simple and effective methods of electrical osteogenesis that are currently available, treatment of the nonunited fracture can be instituted within 5 to 6 months after injury.

For fractures with extensive bone loss, prompt tibiofibular synostosis, posterior bone grafting, or autogenous onlay graft with internal fixation may be indicated.

DIAGNOSIS OF NONUNION

REMARKS

The diagnosis of nonunion is quite frequently dependent on the physician's subjective opinion based on the failure of external callus formation.

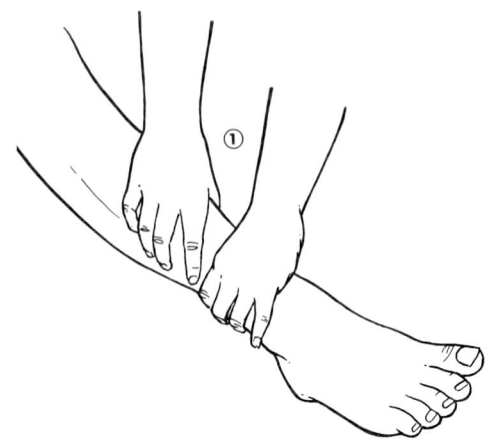

The radiographic impression of a nonunited fracture must be confirmed by:

1. Pain in the fracture site with stress.

Subsequent Management

Electrical stimulation is continued for twelve weeks.

The cast should be left unchanged if at all possible, since removing the cast may inadvertently also remove the electrodes.

After twelve weeks the electrodes are taken out and the fracture is protected for six to eight weeks longer, until union is complete.

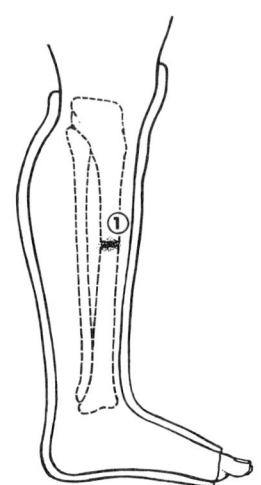

X-Ray after 16 Weeks of Treatment

1. The nonunion is filling in by intramedullary callus in the region of electrode insertion.

AUTOGENOUS BONE GRAFTING AND INTERNAL FIXATION OF UNSTABLE NONUNION

REMARKS

Autogenous onlay bone grafting has been an effective technique to stimulate tibial fracture union. The method is rapidly being replaced by electrical stimulation, which does not require removal of the patient's bone for the graft. However, a nonunion with gross instability requiring internal fixation should also receive the benefit of autogenous bone grafting.

Autogenous bone grafting promotes bone union by introducing viable bone-forming cells, as well as by providing a matrix across which vessels may bridge the fracture site.

The technique of internal fixation suitable for most unstable tibial fractures is intramedullary nailing. Reaming of the medullary canal is necessary to allow insertion of the nail.

Unstable fractures in the distal third may require plate fixation, with the plate applied to the convex surface of the deformity.

Preoperative X-Ray (Unstable Nonunion)

Note: This x-ray was taken 11 months after injury.

1. There is a short oblique fracture of the midthird of the tibia that is grossly unstable on stress x-ray. The fibula, which has been osteotomized adjacent to the tibia, no longer contributes support to the fracture site.
2. The bone ends are sclerotic and smooth.
3. The medullary canal is closed and will require reaming for intramedullary nailing.

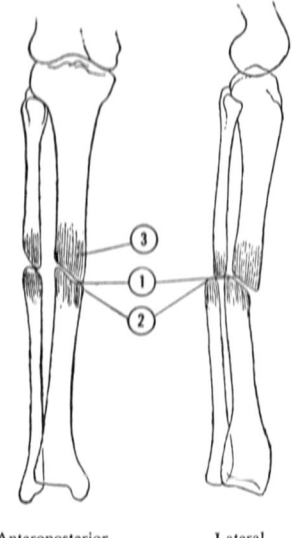

Anteroposterior Lateral

Technique of Intramedullary Nailing and Autogenous Bone Grafting

1. Make a 12-cm incision on the lateral surface of the tibia centered over the fracture site.
2. By sharp dissection expose the fracture site and open the periosteum longitudinally.

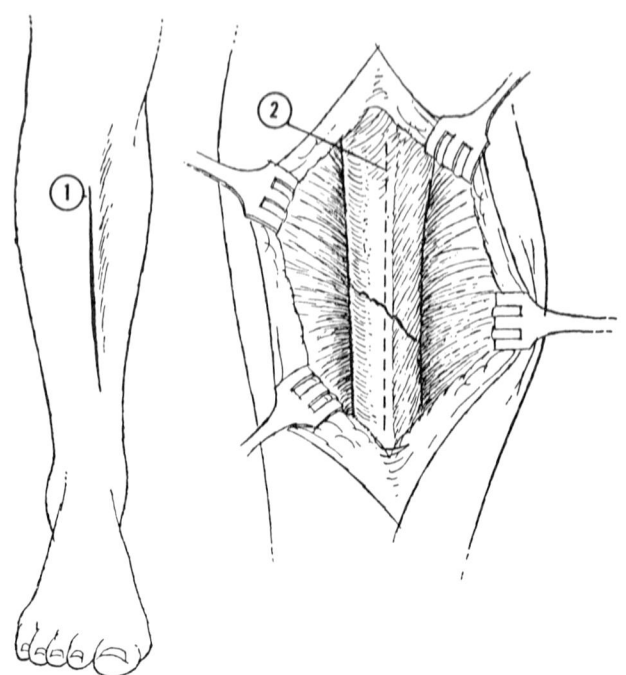

Postoperative Immobilization

1. Apply a long leg cast with the knee in complete extension. The cast is elevated for the first three to five days with an overhead suspension.

2. The patient is encouraged to actively exercise the toe and leg muscles as well as the quadriceps and hamstrings while the leg is in the cast.

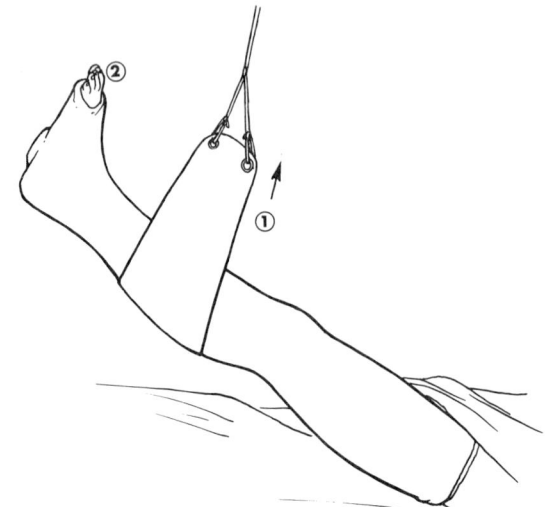

Subsequent Management

Start three-point weight bearing using crutches the day following cast application.

Advise the patient that he will feel some discomfort and possibly some motion at the fracture for the first few weeks.

The patient may be out of bed and walking but he should not sit or stand. Whenever he is not walking, the leg should be elevated to avoid swelling within the cast. This preventive regimen must be continued for 5 to 7 days, until swelling is no longer likely. After 1 week the cast may be changed to a short leg patellar-tendon-bearing (PTB) cast or the long leg cast may be kept, depending on the skills of the surgeon and the activity of the patient.

The major advantage of a short leg PTB cast is that it allows the patient to return readily to work or school and restores his sense of being able to function normally.

The PTB cast must be applied according to Sarmiento's principles or it will allow angulation of unstable fractures.

If the surgeon has any doubt about his or her ability to apply a short leg cast properly, it is safer by far to continue with the long leg cast until union is assured.

INFECTED NONUNION

REMARKS

This is the most common and most serious complication of open or opened tibial fractures.

The frequency of infected nonunion ranges from less than 1 per cent in series treated by closed, functional cast methods to as high as 35 per cent with plate fixation of open fractures. This contrast is so marked that it must be attributed to the technique and not merely to differences in degree of initial injury.

If infected nonunion occurs, the best method of fracture immobilization becomes an important consideration.

For infected nonunions with bone gap, fibulotibial synostosis may be the best answer (see page 1760).

If internal fixation has already been achieved by intramedullary nail, infection control may be possible without removing the nail.

Usually when infection follows plating, the fixation device must be removed. Frequently, the plate has become loose and the bone beneath the plate has become sequestered, to serve as a source of bacterial refuge. Open drainage and cast immobilization are then necessary after plate removal to permit infection control and future bone graft.

The most effective way of managing the infected nonunion, once the acute infection subsides, is by posterolateral autogenous bone grafting. This avoids the infected anteromedial area of the tibia by inserting the bone graft into the well-vascularized posterior and lateral muscle compartments around the fracture site.

Preoperative X-ray

1. A fracture has resulted from a high-energy impact, leaving a defect in the proximal tibia.
2. The fibula has not healed.
3. There is persistent drainage from the anteromedial tibial surface.

Note: The primary indication for the posterolateral grafting is the infected nonunion in which drainage persists despite other treatment. Antibiotics are used as appropriate, depending on results of wound cultures. Obvious sequestra and loose internal fixation devices should be removed before the bone grafting but not at the time of bone grafting. Intramedullary rods do not usually have to be removed.

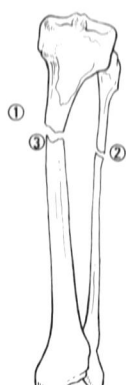

Operative Procedure for Posterolateral Bone Grafting

1. The fracture is approached in most instances through a posterolateral incision 18 cm in length along the posterolateral border of the fibula. Rarely, depending on the nature of the wound and fracture location, a posteromedial approach may be useful.

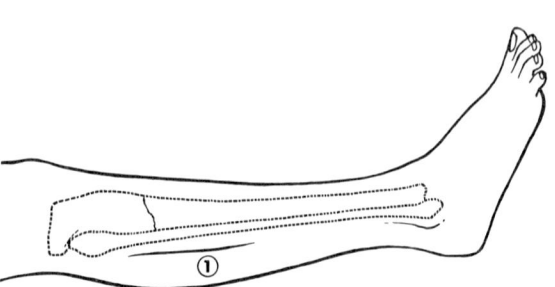

Typically, there is tenseness between the tibia and the triceps surae in the distal medial aspect of the leg with posterior compartment involvement.

The compartment syndromes should be readily distinguishable from nerve injury and major arterial injury as well as from thrombophlebitis. Do not mistake rapid swelling of the calf after a fracture for phlebitis; it is most often indicative of acute or chronic (false aneurysm) injury of the artery.

Direct measurement of intramuscular compartment pressure may be helpful in deciding about the need for fasciotomy (see page 65). Photoplethysmographic techniques, as described recently by Bendick and coworkers, provide noninvasive detection of vascular compromise.

Patients with clinical symptoms and physical findings of compartment compression syndrome require prompt fasciotomy decompression. Matsen and Clawson have shown that decompression of the entire constricted compartment by fasciotomy and epimysiotomy as necessary, within 12 hours after onset of the syndrome, usually has satisfactory results.

FOUR-COMPARTMENT PARAFIBULAR DECOMPRESSION (MATSEN AND COWORKERS)

Note: All four compartments of the leg should be decompressed if one of them is involved in an acute compression syndrome. The fibula should not be removed in order to perform the fasciotomy, because its removal would cause a significant increase in the instability of the tibial fracture.

Operative Procedure

1. An incision is made from the fibular neck to the lateral malleolus.
2. The lateral compartment is open.

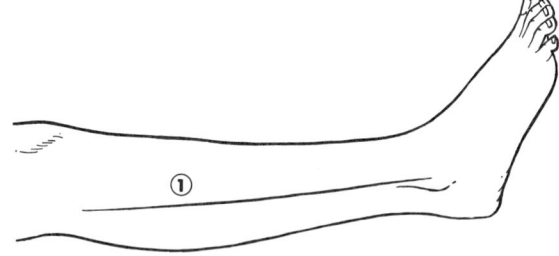

3. Retracting the anterior skin exposes the fascia of the anterior compartment, which is then opened with care taken to avoid the superficial peroneal nerve.

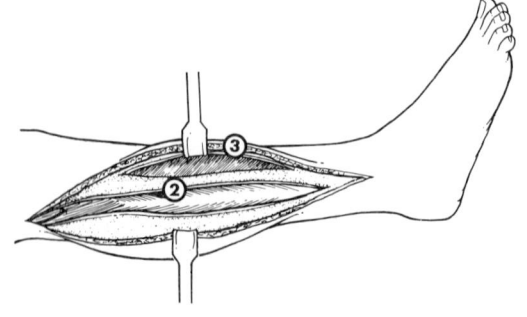

4. The posterior skin is retracted to expose the fascia of the superficial posterior compartment, which is opened.

5. The soleus is released from the fibular shaft and retracted posteriorly to allow decompression of the deep posterior compartment.

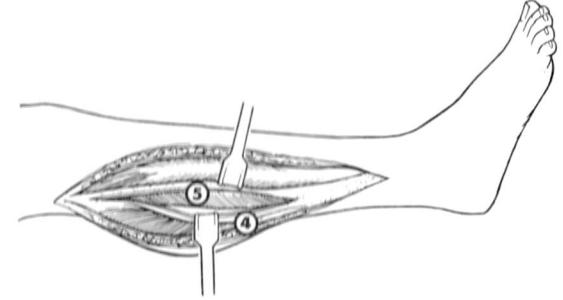

Subsequent Management

After surgical decompression of ischemic muscle compartments associated with a fractured limb, intramedullary nail fixation provides necessary stability for maintaining alignment and allowing inspection of the wound.

The wide open wound may be slowly closed by progressive wound edge approximation using sterile paper tapes applied to the wound each day. This allows rapid reduction of the width of the skin defect to a relatively thin scar and is preferable to skin grafting.

DEFORMITIES FROM COMPARTMENT SYNDROMES

An unrelieved compartment syndrome can cause permanent functional loss and infection in necrotic muscle.

Residual deformities from a posterior compartment syndrome associated with a tibial fracture include:
  1. Cavus of the entire foot.
  2. Adduction of the forefoot.
  3. Claw toes.

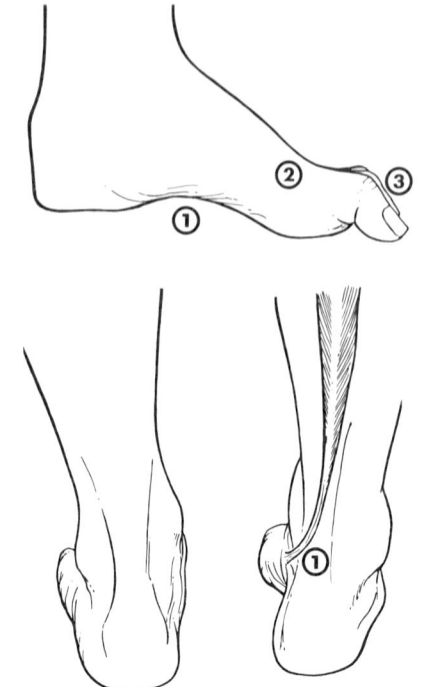

1. Contracture of the posterior tibial muscle particularly contributes to the cavovarus deformity.

Note: Karlstrom has pointed out that when no weight bearing is allowed in treating a fracture, there is no natural counterforce to the pull of the contracted tibialis posterior muscle. Functional weight-bearing treatment serves to stretch out contracture of this muscle.

Slight equinus position in the cast may also be helpful to prevent increased pressure in the posterior compartment with tibial fracture.

SUMMARY: COMPLICATIONS AND PITFALLS OF MANAGING TIBIAL FRACTURES

The diagnosis of a tibial fracture, which is usually obvious, may be missed if it is a fatigue injury or is associated with injuries elsewhere, particularly in the ankle. Always radiograph the entire leg with any ankle injury to rule out the possibility of proximal injury to the tibia, fibula, or both.

Initial assessment should include direct inspection of the leg to determine whether the tibial fracture is open or closed. Palpation and CMS (circulation, motor, and sensory function) testing should be conditioned into any initial evaluation to detect active or impending compartmental syndromes promptly.

In assessing the fracture one should also consider the status of the fibula, which affects the tibial fracture significantly. An intact fibula indicates a relatively stable tibial fracture that is likely to develop a varus (internal torsional) deformity. A fibular fracture is more often associated with a valgus (external torsional) deformity, particularly in distal tibial fracture. Reduction of a tibial fracture should be done with these potential joint deformities always in mind. The major objectives of treatment are to achieve prompt union and to restore knee and ankle alignment. Most often these objectives are best achieved by closed functional cast treatment.

Cast application requires as much skill as proper surgical technique. The physician using functional weight-bearing cast treatment should follow closely the techniques described. Complications from a cast that is either too loose or too tight can then be safely avoided.

The major pitfall of managing tibial fractures is nonunion. Early functional treatment has a definite benefit in diminishing the chance of nonunion by maximizing the external callus process. Newer techniques of electrical osteogenesis also affect biologic processes and stimulate intramedullary callus. Consequently, tibial fracture management is best based on biologic rather than mechanistic principles.

Should the fracture be unsuited for standard closed methods, transfixion pins in plaster work quite effectively as temporary stabilizing techniques. Internal fixation, if necessary, is best accomplished by intramedullary nailing, which minimizes trauma to the already damaged surrounding soft tissue.

Infected nonunion is a major complication of an open tibial fracture or a fracture that has been opened. A systematic approach to the common problems of the open tibial fracture should include thorough and repeated wound debridement and should avoid primary closure. Antibiotics should be used only to supplement adequate surgical debridement, not to replace it.

Once infected nonunion has occurred, bypassing the infected anteromedial surface with a posterior bone graft or a tibiofibular synostosis may be necessary to rescue both the patient and the surgeon from the pitfall.

The contribution that the fibula and intraosseous membrane make to tibial fracture stability is significant. The fibula can actually be made an effective substitute for the tibia by synostosis or posterior bone graft. Osteotomy or removal of the fibula adds to tibial instability and necessitates internal fixation of the unstable tibial fracture. Save the fibula!

Major instances in which management tends to add to the patient's fracture disease occur with the surgical "assembly line," deficits created by bone excision, infected plate fixation, and bone "gaposis" from fracture distraction. Treatment that relies more on the biology than on the mechanics of fracture healing will avoid these pitfalls.

Concepts of tibial fracture management have changed considerably over the past 20 years. Dictums that proximal and distal joint immobilization or rigid fracture fixation is essential for adequate healing have been supplanted by new information. A major pitfall to avoid is the inability to accommodate to new but valid and effective methods of fracture management.

References

Abraham, E. A., McMaster, W. C., Krijger, M., and Waugh, T. R.: Whirlpool therapy for the treatment of soft tissue wounds complicating extremity fractures. J. Trauma, 14:222–226, 1974.

Anderson, L. D., Hutchins, W. C., Wright, P. E., and Disney, J. M.: Fractures of the tibia and fibula treated by casts and transfixing pins. Clin. Orthop., 105:179–191, 1974.

Bendick, P. J., Mayer, J. R., Glover, J. L., and Park, H. M.: A photoplethysmographic technique for detecting vascular compromise: A preliminary report. J. Trauma, 19:398–402, 1979.

Brighton, C. T., Friedenberg, Z. B., Zemsky, L. M., and Polles, P. R.: Direct current stimulation of non-union and congenital pseudarthroses. J. Bone and Joint Surg., 57A:368–377, 1975.

Brown, P. W.: The early weight-bearing treatment of tibial shaft fractures. Clin. Orthop., 105:167–178, 1974.

Brown, P. W.: The fate of exposed bone. Am. J. Surg., 137:464–469, 1979.

Brown, P. W.: The open fracture. Clin. Orthop., 96:254–265, 1973.

Brown, P. W., and Kinman, P. B.: Gas gangrene in a metropolitan community. J. Bone and Joint Surg., 56A:1445–1451, 1974.

Campanacci, M., and Zanoli, S.: Double tibiofibular synostosis (fibula pro tibia) for non-union and delayed union of the tibia. J. Bone and Joint Surg., 48A:44–56, 1966.

Connolly, J. F.: Perils and pitfalls of open tibial fractures. Am. Fam. Physician, 11:64–72, 1975.

Connolly, J. F.: Torsional fractures and the third dimension of fracture management. South. Med. J., 73:884–891, 1980.

ANATOMIC FEATURES AND MECHANISMS OF INJURIES

REMARKS

Injuries to the ankle produce the most common of joint instability problems, particularly in young active individuals.

Depending on the mechanism, the ankle injury may cause either a sprain or a fracture. Sprains are commonly the result of inversion mechanisms, whereas excessive eversion or external torsion of the ankle produces fractures.

The reason for these differences can be best explained by a review of the functional anatomy of the ankle joint.

Functional Anatomy of the Ankle Joint

BONY COMPONENTS

The bony configuration of the ankle joint provides inherent stability; essentially it is a hinge joint capable of movement in one plane — flexion and extension.

The mortise of the joint is formed on one side by the distal end of the tibia, the internal (medial) malleolus, and on the other side by the distal end of the fibula and the external (lateral) malleolus; the moving component projecting into the mortise is the talus, which fits very tightly.

The malleoli, which hug the sides of the talus, are of unequal length and shape; the medial malleolus is a short, stubby pyramidal structure whose tip extends only halfway down on the body of the talus; the lateral malleolus is rectangular and extends almost to the level of the talocalcaneal joint.

The body of the talus is not symmetrical; its anterior portion is much wider than its posterior, so that when the foot is dorsiflexed the anterior portion abuts firmly against the two malleoli, creating a very stable situation.

Close has shown that as dorsiflexion of the ankle takes place the malleoli separate in fairly regular increments up to as much as 1.5 mm. This allows the articular surfaces of the malleoli to remain closely applied to the sides of the talus throughout the range of ankle motion.

Bony Configuration of the Ankle Joint

1. The articular surface of tibia forms the top of the mortise.
2. The internal and external malleoli form the sides of the mortise.
3. Note the length of the internal malleolus compared with
4. The length of the external malleolus, which flanks the entire side of the talus.

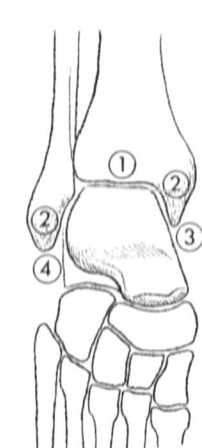

Body of the Talus

1. The anterior portion of the body is wider than
2. The posterior portion of the body.

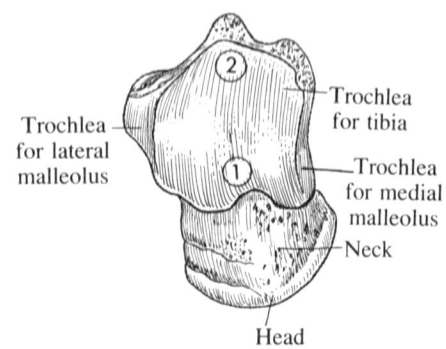

WIDENING OF THE MORTISE WITH ANKLE FLEXION AND EXTENSION

Despite its wedge shape the talus does not lousen in the ankle joint mortise during plantar flexion of the foot.

The articular surfaces of the malleoli remain in close contact with the sides of the talus throughout the total arc of motion.

As dorsiflexion takes place, the malleoli separate in regular increments up to 1.5 mm. This is accomplished by a medial rotation of the tibia on the talus and a relatively lateral rotation of the fibula with respect to the tibia.

1803

Ligaments on the Medial Aspect of the Ankle Joint

The deltoid ligament is a complex structure consisting of:
1. A tibiocalcaneal portion,
2. A posterior tibiotalar portion,
3. An anterior tibiotalar portion, and
4. A tibionavicular portion.
5. To repair the posterior tibial portion of the deltoid, the tendon of the tibialis posterior must be retracted forward.

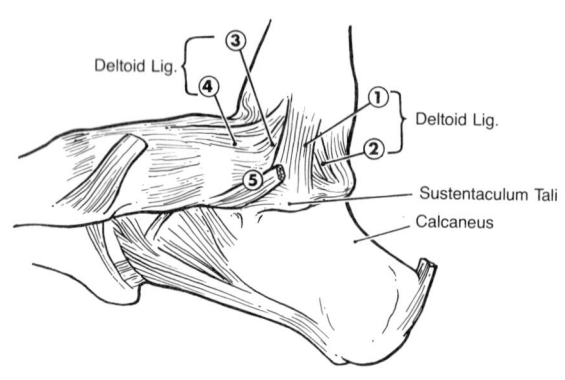

Ligaments on the Lateral Aspect of the Ankle Joint

1. The anterior tibiofibular ligament is relatively elastic to permit slight rotation of the tibia and fibula during dorsiflexion.
2. The anterior talofibular ligament is a relatively weak structure and most subject to injury with forceful inversion. When this ligament is torn, anterior instability is evident clinically.
3. The calcaneofibular ligament may also be torn along with the talofibular ligament, resulting in tilting of the talus in the mortise.
4. Tearing of the talocalcaneal ligaments will produce further instability of the subtalar joint.
5. Rarely, the posterior talofibular ligament will also be torn by inversion with the ankle in dorsiflexion.

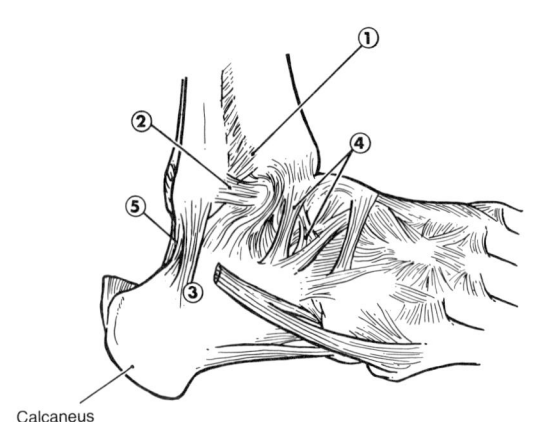

Mechanisms of Ankle Sprains

REMARKS

The bony articulations of its mortise make the ankle quite resistant to failure in the mediolateral direction; i.e., in abduction or adduction.

Most ankle injuries are produced by torsional overloading.

Because of the anatomy with the elongated lateral malleolus, ankle sprains are primarily injuries to the lateral ligaments produced by inversion and internal rotation.

External rotation or eversion injuries most characteristically cause malleolar fractures.

Internal Torsion Mechanism

Internal torsional injuries occur
1. After the heel strikes with the ankle plantar flexing.

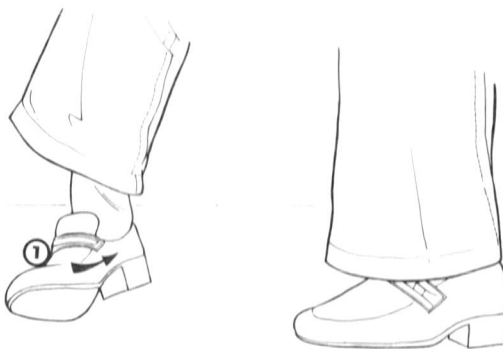

2. The fibula quickly abuts against the distal anterior tibial tubercle of the groove.
3. The resultant strain is absorbed primarily by the weak anterior talofibular ligament.

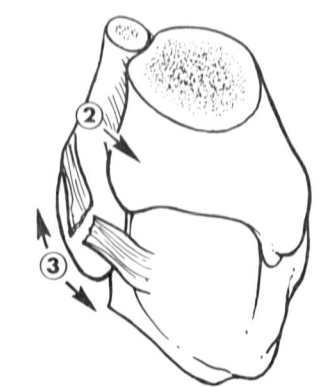

Continued inversion overloading during stance phase leads to:
1. Disruption of the calcaneofibular ligament and
2. Disruption of the talocalcaneal ligaments.

Note: Chrisman and Snook have shown that both the anterior talofibular and the calcaneofibular ligaments must be torn for gross inversion instability to be evident on stress x-rays.

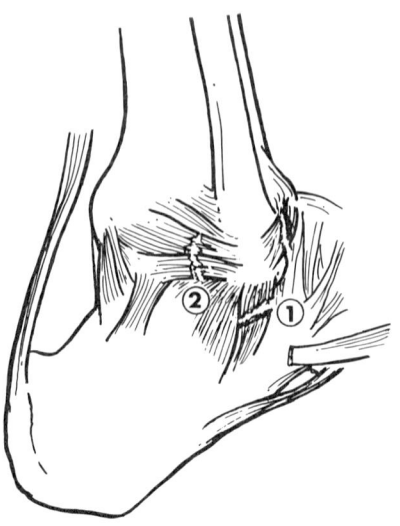

EVALUATION AND MANAGEMENT OF ACUTE ANKLE SPRAINS

REMARKS

Ankle sprain represents one of the most frequent injuries to the musculoskeletal system treated by primary care physicians, surgeons, orthopaedists, and athletic trainers. Dameron estimates one significant ankle sprain occurs daily per 10,000 population, with the exact proportion depending on the population's enthusiasm for sports such as basketball.

By far the majority of sprains prove to be partial Grade I injuries to the talofibular ligament with excellent prognosis for prompt recovery. These are best managed symptomatically by minimal external support and early mobilization exercises.

Approximately one in four patients with acute injuries will suffer recurrent episodes of instability. Too frequently these are ignored or the patient is considered psychoneurotic despite anatomic disruption.

Young athletic individuals are particularly handicapped by ankle instability, but even relatively sedentary patients can be inconvenienced by it.

Lateral ankle instability for 10 years or longer has been shown by Harrington to cause degenerative arthritis of the ankle in approximately 80 per cent of the cases. Most patients with long-standing lateral instability will notice worsening of pain in the anterior or medial part of the joint aggravated by walking. Clearly such a patient would be benefitted by early operative repair or reconstruction to stabilize the ankle prior to arthritic changes.

Rarely, anterior instability may cause chronic problems. Suspect disruption of the anterior support structures in any patient with bimalleolar ankle sprain.

INITIAL EVALUATION

The initial evaluation should consider any history of ankle instability as well as the potential future demands the individual will make on the ankle.

Ligamentous damage should be carefully assessed by directly palpating the areas of maximum tenderness anteriorly, posteriorly, and occasionally anteromedially.

Stress testing of the ankle can be done without anesthesia within a few hours after the injury. This should include testing for anteroposterior instability, the most common finding, as well as for inversion instability from talofibular and calcaneofibular injury.

The presence or absence of pain on stress testing is significant. Complete ligamentous tears are rarely accompanied by much pain on stress testing. All testing must be based on a comparison with the opposite, uninjured ankle rather than on any absolute radiographic measurement.

By careful assessment, one can usually categorize the injury as Grade I, with only a few ligamentous fibers involved, or Grade III, with severe and complete double tears, i.e., both the talofibular and calcaneofibular ligaments.

The gray zone, or Grade II injury, overlaps these categories. Fortunately, most such injuries are closer to Grade I than Grade III. When in doubt, proceed conservatively.

In addition to assessment for ligamentous injuries, x-rays of a sprained ankle should be scrutinized carefully for osteochondral or facet fractures of the talus, which are frequently associated injuries.

Clinical Tests

1. The ankle is carefully palpated to locate any areas of tenderness laterally or medially.
2. Dorsiflexion and plantar flexion are tested to determine if injury is in the anterior capsule.
3. The heel is carefully palpated and adducted to determine if injury involves the calcaneofibular or talocalcaneal ligaments.

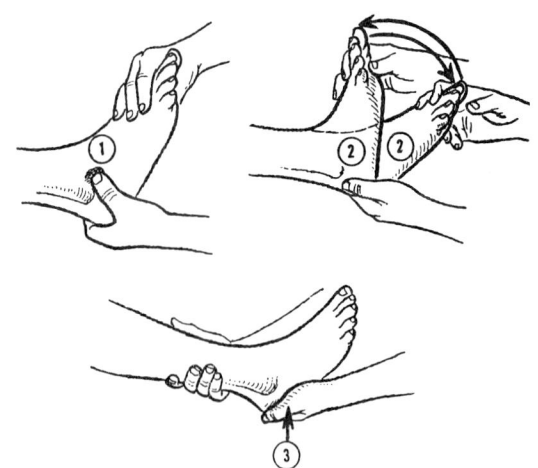

Stress Testing

This can usually be done in the acutely injured ankle without anesthesia.

ANTERIOR DRAWER SIGN

1. The injured ankle should be tested at a right angle — not in plantar flexion, which would tighten the injured ligaments.
2. The examiner's hand stabilizes the distal tibia and palpates the anterior ankle joint.
3. The other hand is placed behind the heel and pushes the talus forward out of the joint.

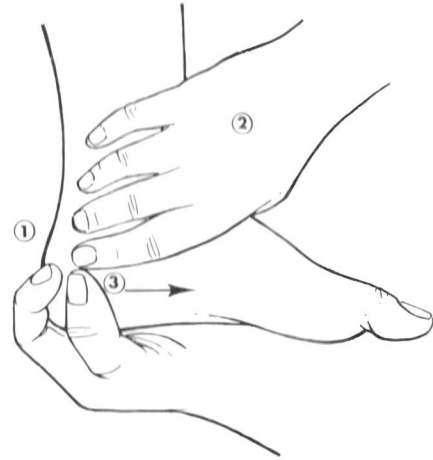

Abnormal drawer test result is indicated by:
1. Anterior displacement of the talus from 4 to 16 mm more than the opposite side as evidenced by direct palpation or by x-ray.

Note: Bimalleolar ankle sprains should be carefully assessed for this displacement.

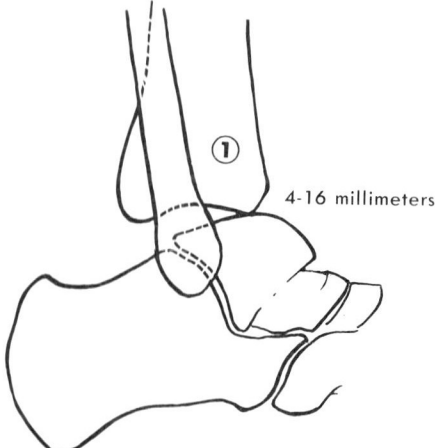

4-16 millimeters

Stress Testing (Continued)

INVERSION STRESS TESTING

1. The ankle is held in neutral.
2. The examiner supports the distal tibia while palpating the anterolateral joint space.
3. Forceful inversion is applied by pushing on the talus and calcaneus.

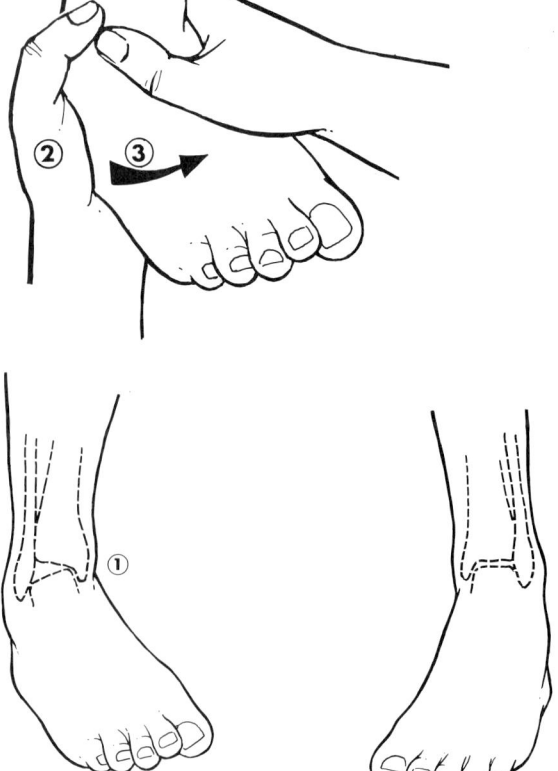

Positive inversion stress instability is indicated by:

1. Tilting of the talus 10 degrees more than the opposite side as indicated either by palpation or by x-ray.

Note: X-rays of the ankle should also be evaluated for evidence of avulsion fractures or osteochondral fractures of the talus indicating more extensive injury.

Arthrography has been employed to assess ligamentous injury but in most instances does not appear to be any more useful than careful palpation and stress testing of the ankle within a few hours after injury.

Selection of Treatment According to Grade

GRADE I INJURIES

If the tenderness is primarily over the anterior talofibular ligament and there is no tenderness over the calcaneofibular or posterior talofibular ligament, and if the talus is stable on anteroposterior drawer and inversion stress tests, early mobilization treatment is warranted.

1. The ankle is wrapped with an elastic bandage.
2. A full role of 1 inch (2.5-cm) tape is applied over the bandage with the ankle everted. Tape strips are applied mainly over the lateral and medial aspects of the ankle.

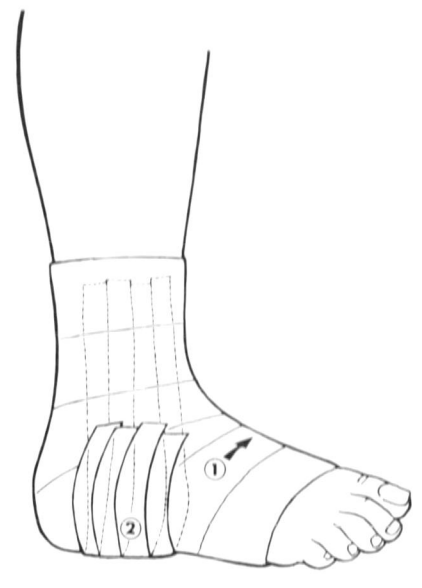

3. The ankle should be free to move in flexion and extension but limited in inversion.

Note: The wrapping is primarily for the patient's comfort. If swelling or irritation of the ankle occurs, the patient should be advised to relieve the taping with scissors. Non–weight-bearing ambulation using crutches tends to produce a symptomatic tight heel cord, which should be avoided. Encourage the patient to bear partial weight with crutches.

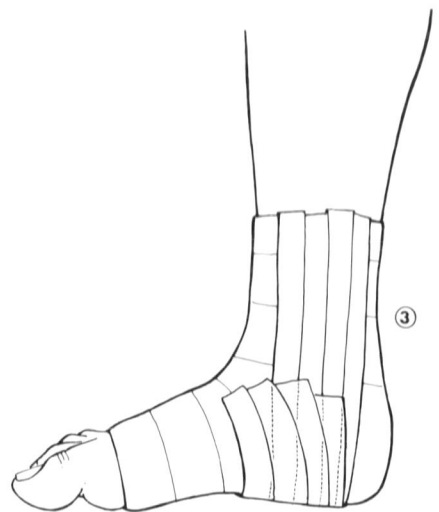

CAUTION

Avoid wrapping the acutely sprained ankle with tight, circumferential dressing, e.g., Unna boot. This may cause a posterior compartment syndrome (see page 1793).

1. The ankle is elevated for three to five days, and ice is applied whenever the patient is not walking with crutches.

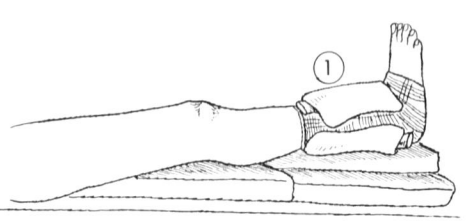

Subsequent Management

Freeman and coworkers have shown that functional instability of the foot after ankle injury may be due to loss of afferent nerve fibers injured in the capsular disruption. Exercises should be designed to develop coordination of the calf muscles to overcome the proprioceptive deficits after the ankle injury.

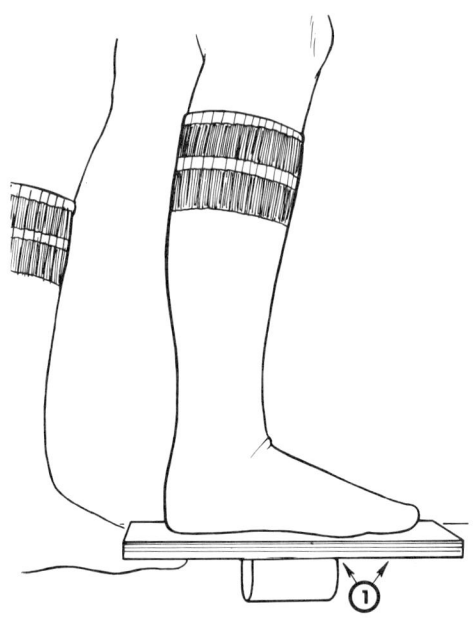

When pain has subsided at three to five days, the patient begins balancing exercises.

1. The patient stands on a board that has a block on its undersurface and functions as a seesaw.

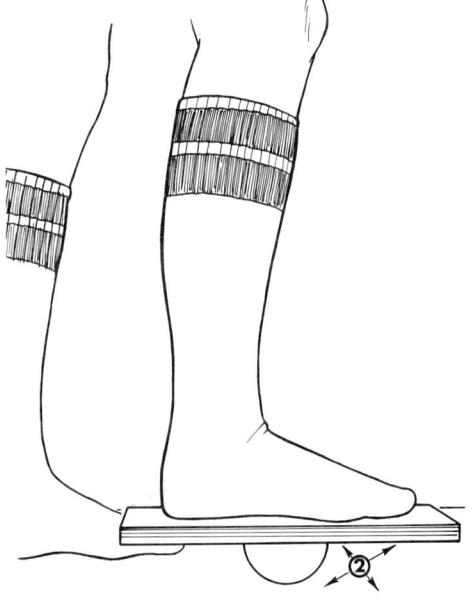

2. Subsequently, the patient exercises on a second board with the undersurface on a sphere.

The treatment is designed to control swelling, to help the patient regain full range of movement, and to develop coordination of the calf muscles.

Most patients require, on the average, five treatments before they are able to balance with the injured leg on the moving surface.

GRADE II (GRAY ZONE) INJURIES

REMARKS

Patients with Grade II injuries have diffuse ankle tenderness, including the region of the calcaneofibular ligament posteriorly and frequently the medial deltoid region. There is usually some demonstrable anterior instability but no instability on inversion stress testing.

Pathology of Grade II Injuries

1. A complete tear of the anterior talofibular ligament allows anterior instability.
2. If the injury is produced by forceful plantar flexion, the anterior deltoid ligament may be damaged and the patient presents with a bimalleolar ankle sprain.
3. The major portion of the calcaneofibular ligament is intact and prevents inversion instability.

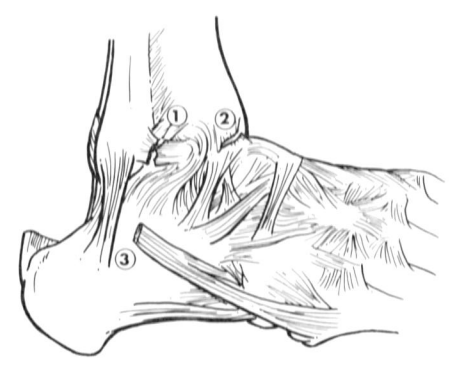

Management

Most of these "gray zone" injuries can be treated as Grade I sprains by taping and early mobilization (see page 1812).

Rarely, a short leg walking cast may be necessary for the individual requiring firmer support than that provided by taping.

A practical means of distinguishing the rare patient in need of operative repair is the degree of pain on stress testing. When stress testing causes little pain despite evidence of anterior or inversion instability, the ligaments are usually completely torn and require operative repair, particularly in active young individuals.

Extreme pain preventing forceful stressing indicates a partial ligamentous disruption, which can be effectively treated by closed means.

Failure to distinguish the complete injury can still be remedied by a delayed ligamentoplasty or reconstruction of the capsule for persistent symptoms. These procedures do not require a great deal more operating time than the initial surgical repair. The only shortcoming is the time lost in waiting to see the outcome.

GRADE III INJURIES

REMARKS

In a Grade III, or complete, injury there is significant anterolateral tenderness over the anterior talofibular ligament, posterior over the calcaneofibular ligament, and sometimes over the posterior talofibular ligament. Lateral tilting as well as anterior instability is demonstrably increased in comparison with the opposite ankle.

Characteristically, in complete tears there is relatively little pain on stress testing in comparison with incomplete tears in which stress testing causes significant pain.

These severe injuries frequently are seen in active young athletes such as basketball players or in individuals with a history of recurrent ankle instability. Such injuries are best managed by prompt operative repair. Injuries in individuals who are less active and have had no previous problems with ankle instability may be treated as Grade II sprains despite evidence of complete ligament tear. Staples reported a series in which only three of nine patients with arthrographic evidence of double ligament rupture treated nonoperatively developed some functional instability.

Operative repair provides the best chance for anatomic stability and total functional recovery in young active patients. It should be recommended for active athletes with Grade III injuries. Any individuals with recurrent problems of instability and Grade III injuries should also be offered operative repair, since long-standing ankle instability leads to degenerative arthritis.

Other indications for primary operative repair are Grade III injuries associated with small avulsion fractures, particularly with osteochondral fracture of the talus. These may be subtle fractures produced by impaction of the lateral talus against the fibula during the inversion injury. If unrecognized, these fractures can cause persistent ankle pain and instability.

Pathology of Grade III Injuries to the Lateral Ankle Ligaments

1. The injury occurs most often in an active young adult who twists the ankle while jumping.
2. Complete rupture of the anterior talofibular ligament occurs.

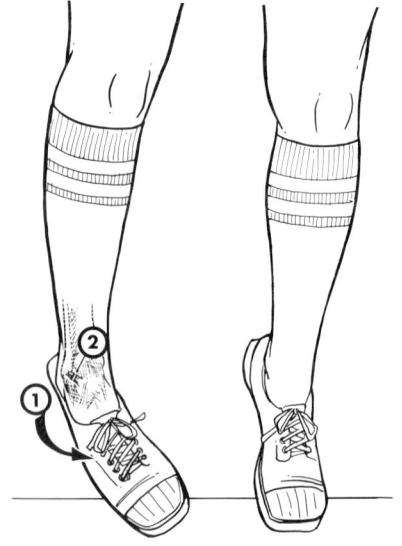

3. Continued inversion of the ankle as it starts to dorsiflex.
4. Disrupts the calcaneofibular ligament and occasionally the posterior talofibular ligament.

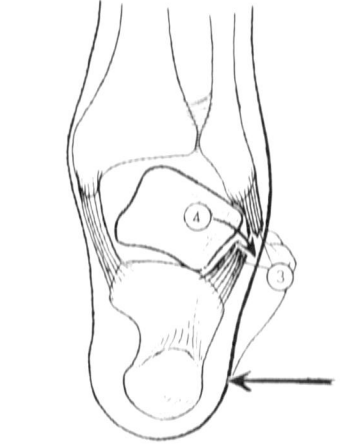

Clinical Tests

1. Tenderness is located both over the talofibular ligament and
2. Over the calcaneofibular ligament.
3. On inversion stress testing, the ankle is relatively painless and excessively mobile in comparison with the opposite side.

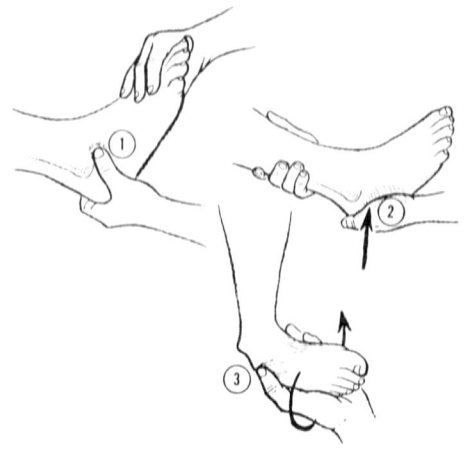

4. Anterior drawer sign is also evident.

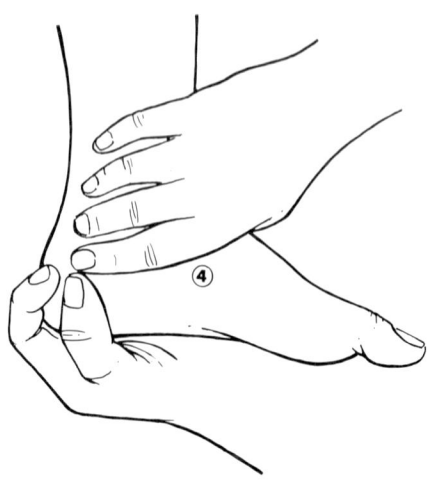

Appearance on X-Ray

1. After initial injury, stress testing of the ankle will demonstrate increased tilting of the talus, at least 10 degrees more than is evident on the opposite, uninjured side.

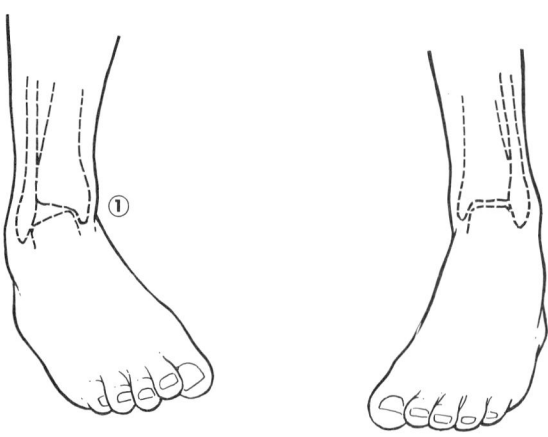

2. Osteochondral fractures of the lateral talus may be associated with 5 per cent of sprained ankles and should be carefully looked for (see page 1958).

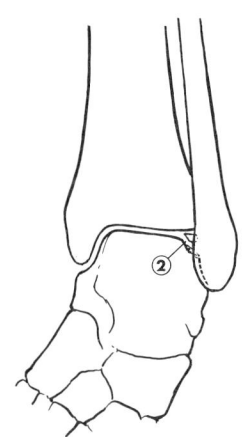

3. Fractures of the posterior facet of the talus may be missed or may be confused with ankle sprains (see page 1974).

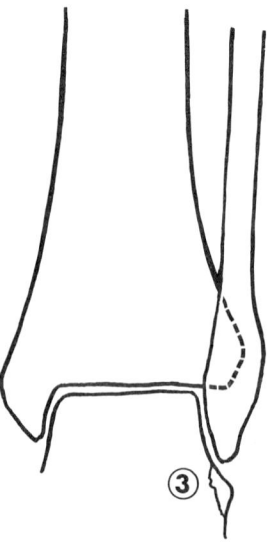

X-Ray of long-standing ankle instability

1. X-rays after many episodes of recurrent instability of 10 or more years' duration will show narrowing of the medial joint space and arthritic changes.

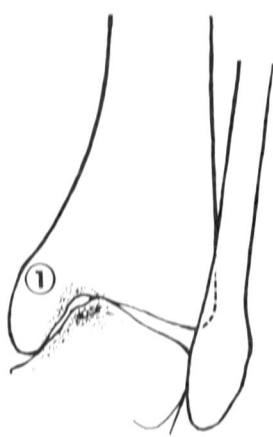

CAUTION

There may be fractures associated with ankle sprains.
1. Frequently, x-rays are coned diligently to visualize what is assumed to be only an ankle sprain,
2. Fractures of the proximal tibia or
3. Fractures of the proximal fibula are missed.

Note: Careful physical examination is necessary to rule out missed fractures proximal to the area of x-ray.

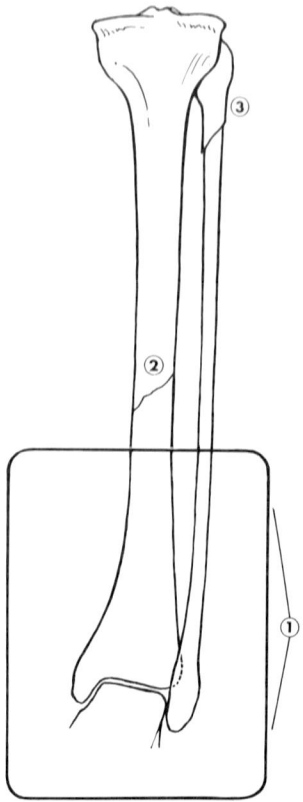

Operative Repair of Grade III Injuries

1. The exact placement of the incision is important. It begins 5 cm proximal to the distal end of the fibula and runs distally, parallel to the bone and 1.5 cm anterior to its margin.
2. The incision then curves posteriorly, distal to the fibula, to run to a point halfway between the tip of the fibula and the posterior plantar surface of the heel.
3. Carefully identify and preserve the lateral branches of the superficial peroneal nerve and
4. The sural nerve.

Note: As many veins as possible should also be preserved to minimize the chance of necrosis of the wound margin.

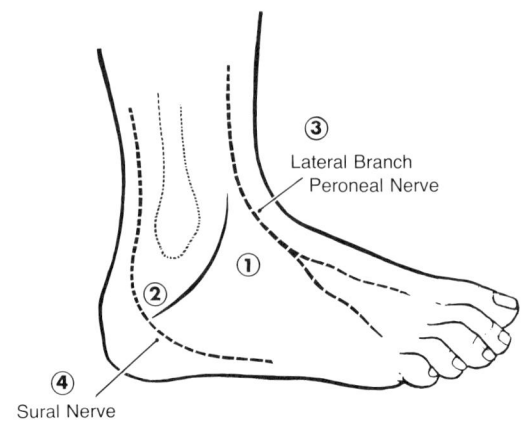

1. The aponeurotic tissue overlying the tibiofibular ligament and joint capsule is opened.
2. The tears of the capsule of the joint and the anterior talofibular ligament can then be palpated.

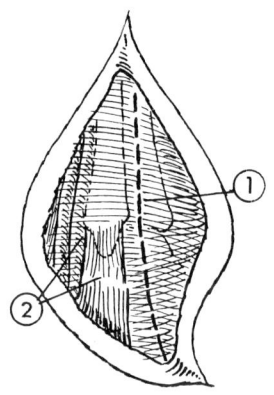

3. To expose the calcaneofibular ligament and the posterior portion of the talofibular ligament, the peroneal tendon sheath is opened and the peroneal tendon is retracted.

Note: Frequently the tears allow visualization of the tibiotalar joint and often the talocalcaneal joint. The stability of these joints should be tested before and after repair.

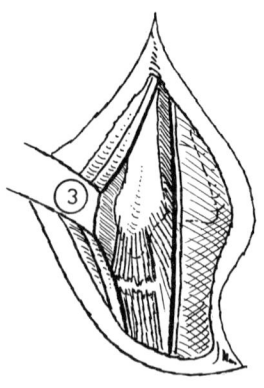

1. If the ligaments are avulsed from bone, they should be reattached by two holes drilled in the bone.
2. Heavy 0 nonabsorbable suture is used to repair ligaments torn in their substance.

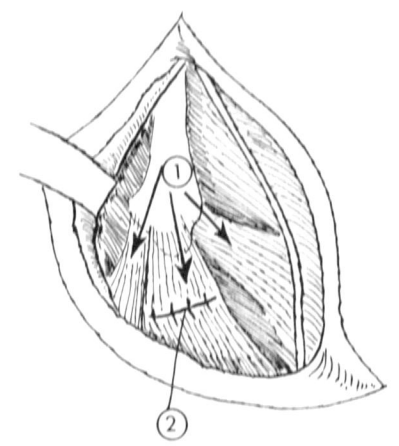

3. Allow the peroneal tendons to return to their normal positions.
4. Approximate the edges of the fascia over the tendons.

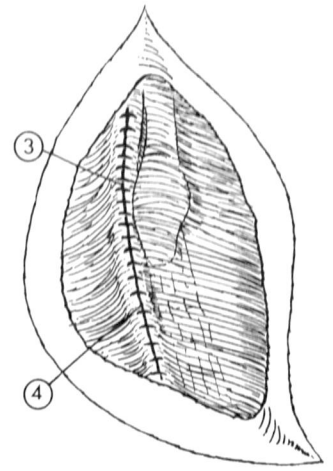

CAPSULAR "SNUGGING":
LIGAMENTOPLASTY PROCEDURE

For generalized laxity or a delayed repair when definition of the injury is difficult:
1. Cut a triangular flap sharply in the capsule.
2. The capsular flap is then tightened and sutured to repair the anterior talofibular and the calcaneofibular support structures.

Note: Always test stability of the repair following completion of the suturing.

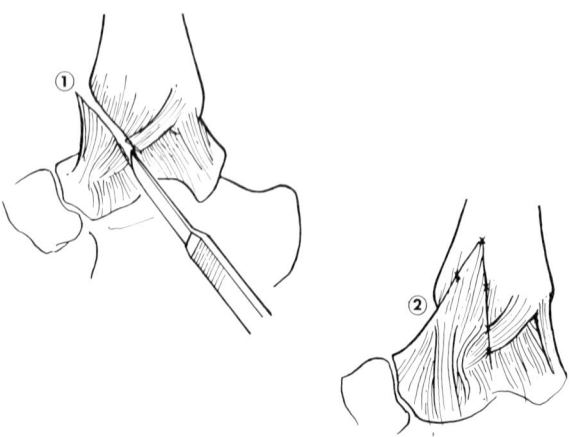

Immobilization

Apply a compression bandage and a posterior plaster splint.

1. The foot is at a right angle with the leg.
2. The foot is slightly everted.

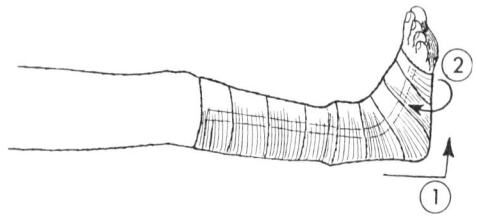

Postoperative Management

Allow the patient to sit for 30 to 60 seconds every half hour on the second day; when this is tolerated well, crutch walking is started.

The initial postoperative splint and bandage are changed after 7 to 10 days and a walking cast is applied.

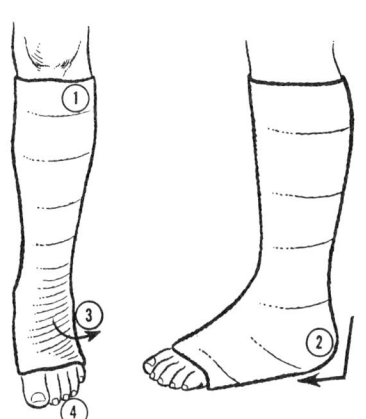

1. The cast extends from the toes to just below the knee.
2. The foot is at a right angle to the leg.
3. The heel is slightly everted.
4. The toes are free.

After three weeks remove the cast and begin balancing exercises.

1. The patient stands on a board that has a block on its undersurface and functions as a seesaw.

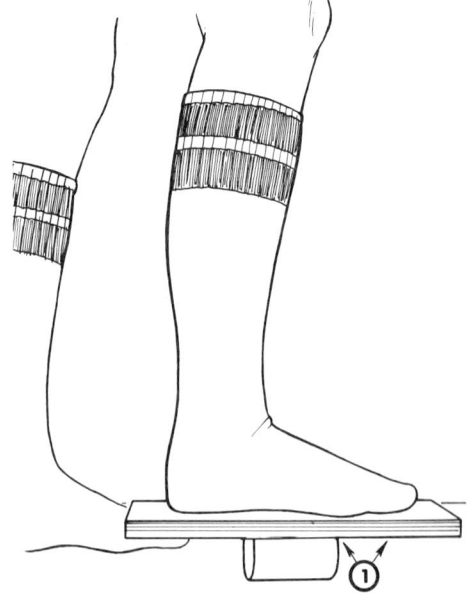

2. Subsequently, the patient exercises on a second board with the undersurface on a sphere.

The treatment is designed to encourage full range of motion and coordination of calf muscles. Most patients require on the average of five treatments before they are able to balance with the injured leg on a moving surface.

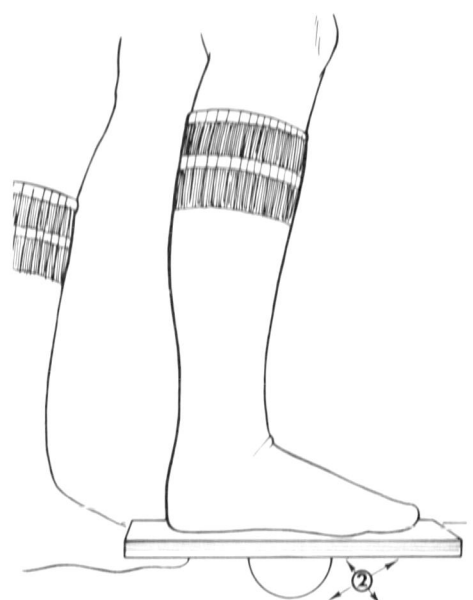

Cast Treatment for Grade III Injuries

If a nonoperative method is chosen for a severe Grade III injury, the patient may be more comfortable with cast immobilization.

Put the limb at complete rest and elevation for 24 to 48 hours.

Apply a compression bandage and ice.

After the swelling has subsided, in 24 to 48 hours, apply a walking cast.

1. The cast extends from below the knee to the toes.
2. The foot is at a right angle to the leg.
3. The heel is slightly everted.
4. The toes are free.

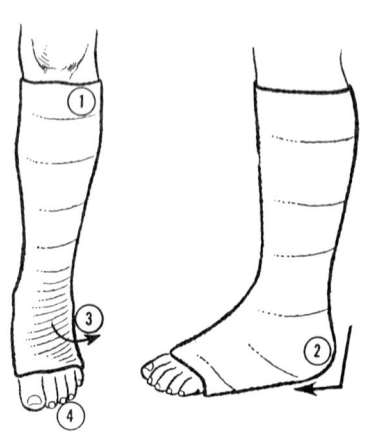

Cast Treatment for Grade III Injuries (Continued)

The cast is removed after three weeks and balancing exercises are begun as described above.

If the ankle is still tender after cast removal, it may be wrapped and taped as described on page 1813.

1. Support the ankle to prevent inversion injury.
2. Elevate the heel with a 6.4-mm outer heel wedge to hold the ankle in slight eversion.

Note: The patient should be followed closely and advised that recurrent episodes of ankle instability can and should be corrected by operative repair. Approximately one in four patients with Grade III injuries treated nonoperatively will have recurrent ankle instability and may need reconstruction of the lateral supports.

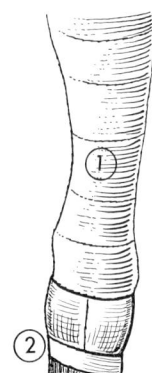

Treatment of Other Ligamentous Injuries

DELTOID LIGAMENT INJURIES

REMARKS

Significant isolated injuries to the deltoid do not occur. This is due to the key stabilizing role of the lateral malleolus.

Yablon and coworkers have demonstrated that the talus faithfully follows the lateral malleolus. Injury sufficient to displace the talus laterally occurs only with displaced fractures of the lateral malleolus.

Staples has pointed out that even after complete excision of the deltoid ligament, i.e., after an open fracture, a stable ankle is possible provided that the lateral malleolus remains intact.

The cause of any lateral talar displacement must be carefully sought and corrected because it is a prime factor in unsatisfactory results after ankle injuries (see page 1841).

Occasionally a plantar flexion injury disrupts the anteromedial deltoid as well as the anterior talofibular ligament and produces anterior ankle instability. The patients who present with bimalleolar rather than isolated deltoid sprains can usually be treated by cast support (see page 1823).

Lateral talar displacement does not result from an isolated deltoid ligament tear.

1. An avulsion injury of the deltoid ligament is evident on x-ray.
2. The talus is shifted laterally, as indicated by widening of the medial joint space.
3. A subtle angulated fracture of the lateral malleolus is the basic cause of the talar shift and needs to be corrected.

Note: Repair of deltoid ligament tears associated with lateral malleolar fracture is discussed on page 1850.

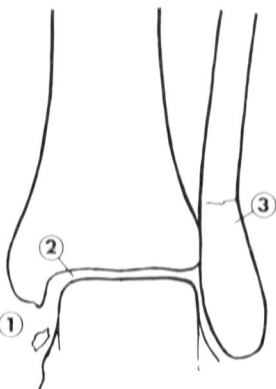

TEAR OF THE DISTAL TIBIOFIBULAR LIGAMENT

REMARKS

This lesion rarely occurs as an isolated injury. It is usually produced by external rotation of a supinated ankle, which proceeds rapidly to fracture of the ankle (see page 1838).

The wide anterior portion of the body of the talus forces the fibula way from the tibia, especially when an external rotation force is acting.

The clinical findings are mild. There is no abnormal lateral motion and no pain when the lateral ligaments are stressed.

Motion is not painful.

There is some pain on extreme dorsiflexion of the foot. Pressure in the interval between the tibia and fibula, anteriorly and posteriorly, causes pain.

X-ray examination is normal.

These ligamentous injuries can be treated as Grade I or Grade II sprains with ankle taping. Occasionally injuries to the distal tibiofibular joint produce stiffening or synostosis (see page 1883).

1. The ankle is wrapped with an elastic bandage.

2. A full roll of 1 inch tape is applied over the bandage with the ankle everted. Tape strips are applied mainly over the lateral and medial aspects of the ankle.

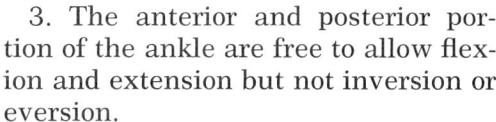

3. The anterior and posterior portion of the ankle are free to allow flexion and extension but not inversion or eversion.

Note: The wrapping is primarily for the patient's comfort. If swelling or irritation of the ankle occurs, the patient should be advised to relieve the taping with scissors.

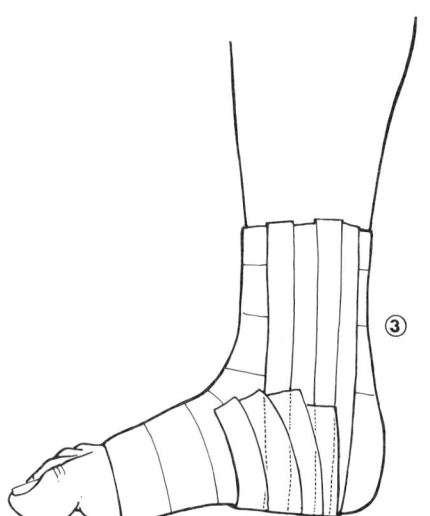

CAUTION

Avoid wrapping the acutely sprained ankle with a tight, circumferential dressing, e.g., Unna boot. This may cause a posterior compartment syndrome (see page 1793).

1. The ankle is elevated and ice is applied for three to five days when the patient is not walking with crutches. Taping should be removed or changed by no later than five days.

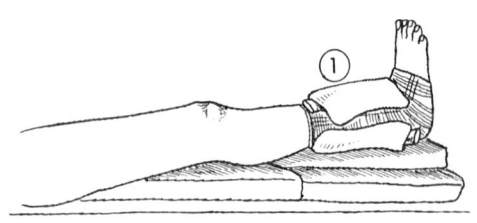

Subsequent Management

When the pain has subsided at three to five days the patient should begin balancing exercises (see page 1822). This treatment is designed to control swelling and to regain full range of motion and develop coordination of calf muscles.

RECURRENT INSTABILITY OF THE LATERAL LIGAMENTS

REMARKS

Persistent ankle instability is a well-known disability of athletes as well as active adults.

The evaluation of ankle instability by x-ray is subject to several difficulties, including a definition of what amount of talar tilt evident on stress x-rays of the ankle is normal. In general, more than 10 degrees of tilt in comparison with the opposite ankle can be considered evidence of significant lateral instability.

Stress x-rays do not demonstrate subtalar instability which can be a significant cause of problems for some patients.

Chrisman and Snook have pointed out that the stress x-rays of a clinically unstable ankle are like myelography in the diagnosis of a ruptured intervertebral disc. The results are not always reliable but are a useful adjunct.

More important than radiographic studies in diagnosis of recurrent instability are:

1. A history of recurrent sprain or "giving way" during mild activity and
2. A palpable sulcus in the anterolateral aspect of the ankle joint on inversion.

ARTHRITIC CHANGES ASSOCIATED WITH LONG-STANDING LATERAL LIGAMENT INSTABILITY

Harrington has shown that long-standing (for 10 years or more) lateral instability results in unbalanced loading and frequently in osteoarthritic changes. Patients with this instability characteristically develop increased ankle pain and radiographic evidence of degenerative arthritis of the medial half of the tibial and talar surfaces.

These changes may be only minimally apparent unless weight-bearing x-rays are made.

Weight-bearing X-rays of Early Degenerative Changes

Anteroposterior view

1. There is early grooving of the medial tibial palfond and
2. Spurring of the medial aspect of the talus and medial malleolus.

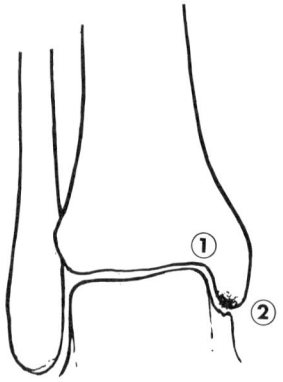

Lateral view

1. Anteroposterior stress instability secondary to chronic anterior talofibular disruption and
2. Anterior tibial spurring are evident.

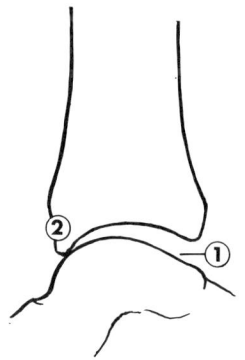

Weight-bearing X-ray of Advanced Arthritis in a Symptomatically Lax Ankle

1. The medial joint space is narrowed. There is sclerosis of the subchondral bone in the medial half of the joint.

Note: Operative reconstruction of the lateral ligaments can relieve symptoms in the mildly-to-moderately arthritic ankle and possibly can reverse changes that are already manifest.

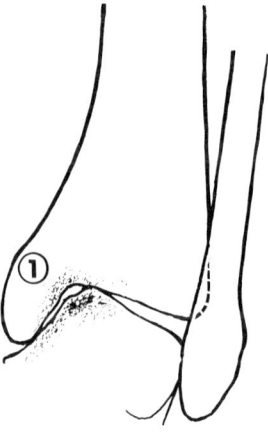

Reconstruction of Lateral Ligament Instability (Chrisman and Snook)

This procedure is simple and effective but can cause 15-degree to 30-degree limitation of foot inversion.

It employs a split portion of the peroneus brevis tendon to replace the anterior talofibular ligament as well as the anterior talocalcaneal ligament.

The operation, therefore, repairs both of the important ligaments but preserves the eversion function of the peroneus brevis.

1. A curved incision is made paralleling the peroneus brevis tendon from 8 cm above the tip of the fibula to the base of the fifth metatarsal.
2. The brevis tendon is split from its insertion up to its musculotendinous junction, and the longer half is detached from the muscle belly and pulled distally under
3. The intact superior retinaculum of the pulley at the fibular groove.

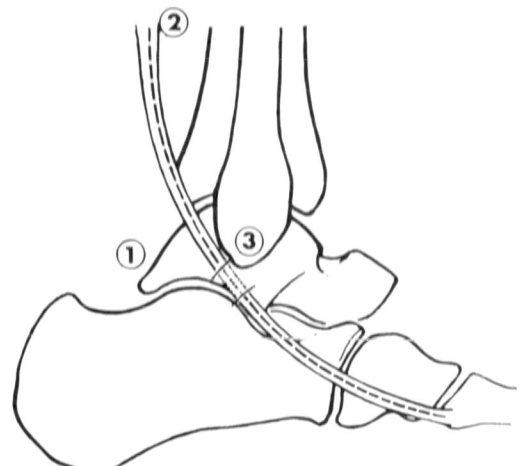

1. A horizontal hole parallel to but not compromising the articular surface is drilled in the distal part of the fibula.
2. The mobilized half of the tendon is threaded through the anterior talocalcaneal ligament and then through the hole in the fibula.
3. With the ankle everted, the tendon is fixed under moderate tension to the talocalcaneal ligament and to any remnants of the talofibular ligament and at both ends of the tunnel.

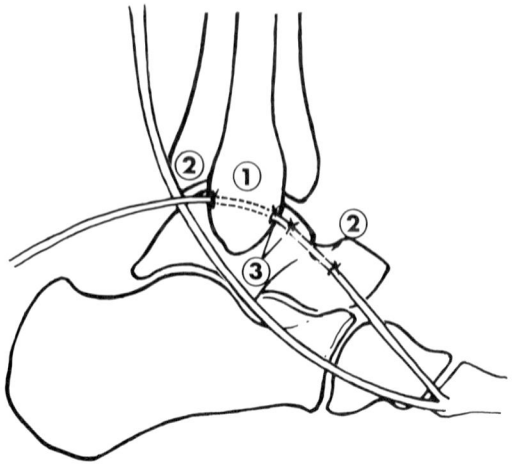

Reconstruction of Lateral Ligament Instability (Chrisman and Snook) (Continued)

1. The remaining portion of the tendon is pulled downward to the calcaneus and passed through a 2.5 cm tunnel drilled in the bone.
2. The tendon is sutured in place under moderate tension.
3. Any remaining end of the tendon is sutured distally near its insertion on the fifth metatarsal or into the anterior calcaneofibular ligament.

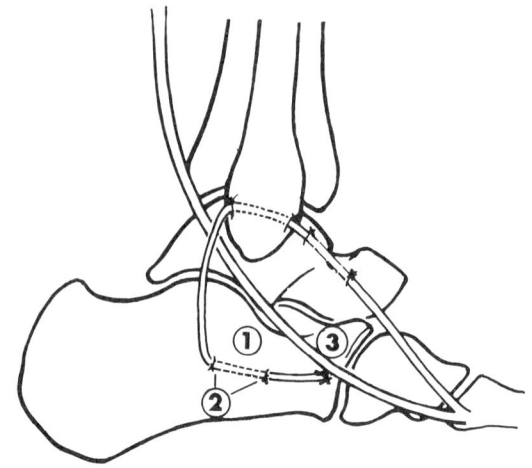

Postoperative Management

The incision in this area may be slow to heal. The sutures should be left in place for at least three weeks.

A below-knee cast is applied and partial weight bearing with crutches is continued for eight weeks.

After eight weeks the cast is removed and the patient is allowed to walk in a shoe with a heel wedge.

Six to seven months after operation, the shoe may be discarded and the patient may be allowed to wear normal shoes.

ANTERIOR ANKLE INSTABILITY

REMARKS

Post-traumatic anterior talar instability is much more common after a sprain than either inversion or eversion tilting of the talus.

Forced plantar flexion frequently disrupts the relatively weak anterior capsular structures. Most patients then present with bimalleolar ankle sprains (see page 1808).

All patients with pain and swelling over both malleoli should be carefully evaluated for positive anterior drawer instability.

1. The ankle is tested in a neutral position.

Note: If the ankle is allowed to plantar flex, the capsular ligaments tighten and prevent displacement. Also, the talus cannot move caudad, which is necessary in order for its dome to displace under the anterior tibial margin.

2. The examiner's hand stabilizes the distal tibia and then palpates the anterior ankle joint.
3. The examiner's other hand is placed behind the heel and pushes the talus forward out of the joint.

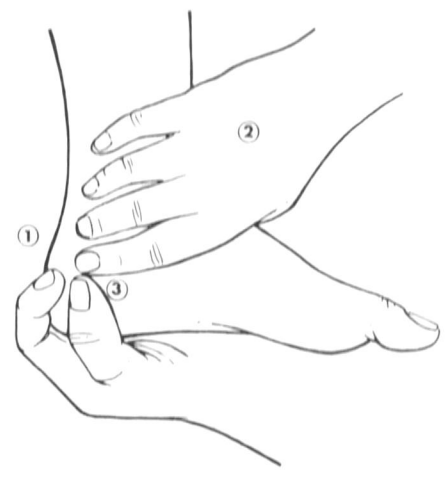

1. When the heel is pulled forward, an anteroposterior motion of the talus relative to the tibia is felt by the examiner and seen by the patient. Anterior displacement of 4 mm or more compared with the opposite ankle should be considered abnormal.

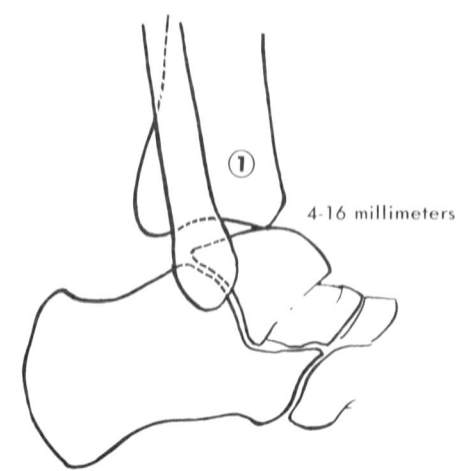

Nonoperative Treatment: Cast Immobilization

Since the cause of the instability is, in most cases, stretching of the anterior talofibular ligament and, in some cases, of the anterior deltoid fibers, cast immobilization is necessary.

1. The cast is applied from the toes to just below the knee.
2. The foot must be held at a right angle.
3. The heel is slightly everted.
4. The toes are free.

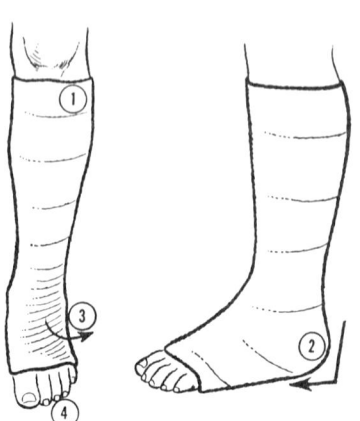

Subsequent Management

After two weeks remove the cast and begin balancing exercises.

1. The patient stands on a board that has a block on its undersurface and functions as a seesaw.

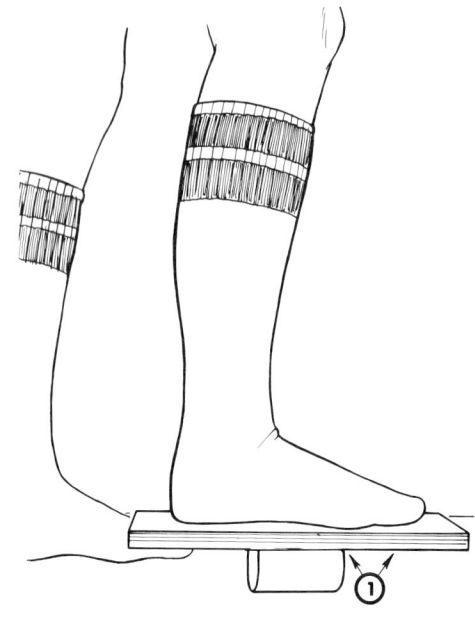

2. Subsequently the patient exercises on a second board with the undersurface on a sphere.

The treatment is designed to encourage full range of motion and coordination of calf muscles. Most patients require on the average of five treatments before they are able to balance with the injured leg on a moving surface.

The patient should be advised that recurrent episodes of ankle instability can occasionally be a problem but this condition can and should be corrected by operative repair.

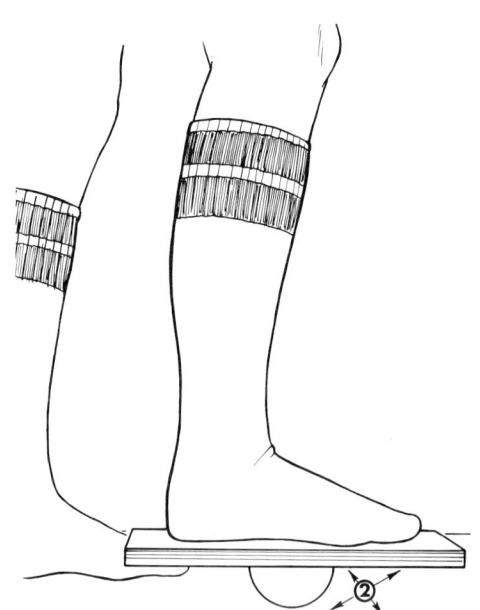

Operative Repair

If gross anterior instability exists with little or no pain on stressing the ankle, operative repair may be indicated. This is particularly true in an active young athlete or in any individual with a previous history of instability.

In occasional cases, there may also be an associated instability on inversion, but usually the tilt of the talus is not large.

Recurrent anterior ankle instability is less likely to be a problem to the patient than recurrent lateral or inversion instability (see page 1827).

Surgical procedure

1. The exact placement of the incision is important. It begins 5 cm proximal to the distal end of the fibula and runs distally parallel to the bone and 1.5 cm anterior to its margin.
2. The incision then curves posteriorly distal to the fibula to run a point halfway between the tip of the fibula and the posterior plantar surface of the heel.
3. Carefully identify and preserve the lateral branches of the superficial peroneal nerve and
4. The sural nerve.

Note: As many veins as possible should also be preserved to minimize the chance of necrosis of the wound margin.

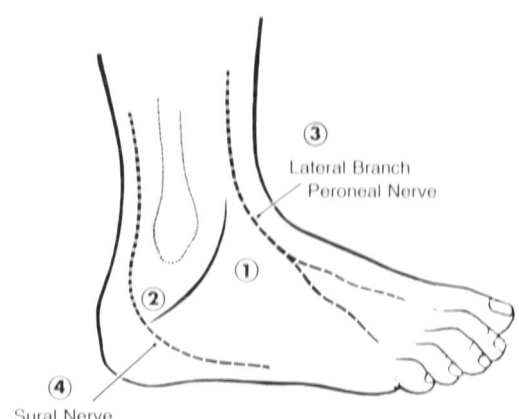

1. If the capsular injury cannot be precisely located, cut a triangular flap in the capsule.
2. The capsular flap is then sutured with the ankle dorsiflexed and everted in order to tighten the anterior talofibular and the calcaneofibular support structures.

Note: Always test stability of the repair following completion of suturing.

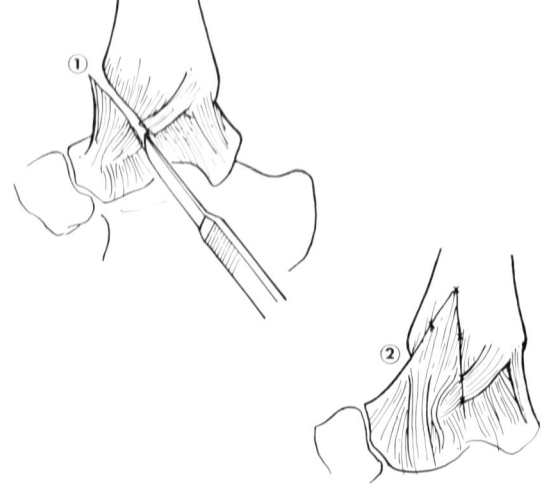

Immobilization

Apply a compression bandage and a posterior plaster splint.
1. The foot is at a right angle with the leg.
2. The foot is slightly everted.

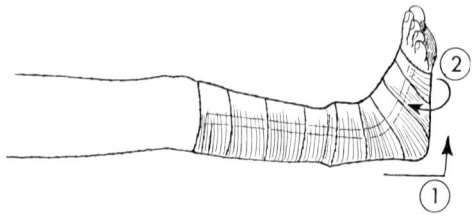

Subsequent Management

Allow the patient to sit for 30 to 60 seconds every half hour on the second postoperative day; when this is well tolerated, crutch walking is started.

The initial postoperative splint and bandage are changed after 10 days and a walking cast is applied.

After three weeks remove the cast and begin weight bearing with crutches. Progress to full weight bearing when symptoms and performance permits.

Achieving a normal gait and restoring strength and motion as quickly as possible are very important.

Specific exercises should be used to restore balance coordination and calf muscle strength (see page 1832).

FRACTURES OF THE ANKLE

REMARKS

Just as sprains result most often from internal torsion or inversion mechanisms, fractures of the ankle are produced by eversion or external torsional injuries. These displace the ankle in three dimensions, external, posterior, and lateral.

The anatomy of the distal tibiofibular joint, with the groove preventing anterior fibular displacement with internal rotation but allowing posterior fibular displacement with external torsion, has been discussed previously (see page 1804). This anatomic arrangement places the ligaments at risk with internal torsion but the bony supports of the ankle at risk with external torsion.

Less frequently, pure pronation-abduction injuries or supination-adduction injuries will fracture the ankle without torsional displacement.

The most complete and applicable system classifying ankle fractures according to mechanism is that of Lauge-Hansen, as reviewed by Yde. This classification is well worth reviewing in order to select appropriate treatment and evaluate results.

Lauge-Hansen Mechanistic Classification of Ankle Fractures (Yde)

REMARKS

This classification should be based on adequate x-rays, including mortise views with the foot internally rotated as well as lateral and oblique studies.

The first word in this classification takes into consideration the position of the foot at the time of the injury, and the second word refers to the direction of the injury force on the talus.

Between 50 and 60 per cent of ankle fractures occur when the foot is supinated and external rotational force is applied to the talus (S-EX fracture).

Twenty per cent result from pure supination-adduction mechanisms (S-AD fracture).

Pronation and abduction (P-AB) or pronation and external rotation (P-EX fracture) mechanisms cause the remaining 20 per cent.

The distribution of these types vary in many series, but the predominance of the S-EX types is evident in all reports.

The characteristics of the fibular fracture, when present, indicate the nature of the mechanism.

1. Supination–external rotation (S-EX) fracture is characterized by a spiral oblique fracture of the fibula that runs from the anterior distal margin up to the posterior superior cortex below the level of the syndesmosis.

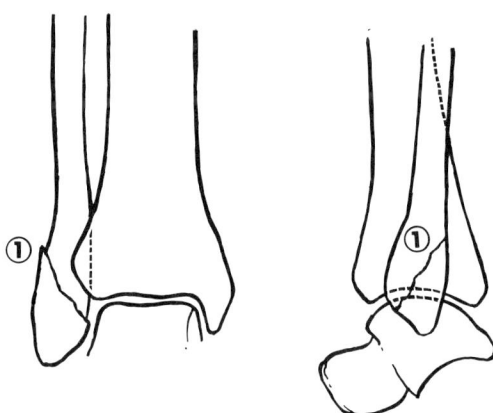

SUPINATION EXTERNAL ROTATION

2. Pronation–external rotation (P-EX) fracture involves the fibula above the syndesmosis and is associated with diastasis of the tibiofibular joint. The fracture of the fibula runs from the superior anterior cortex down to the posterior inferior cortex. The location of this fracture varies but never is less than 2.5 cm above the tibiotalar joint.

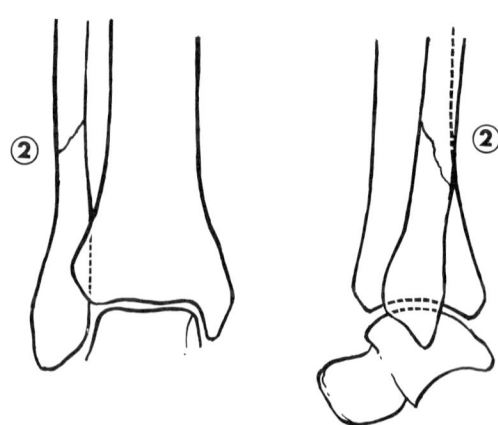

PRONATION EXTERNAL ROTATION

3. Supination-adduction (S-AD) fracture is a characteristic transverse fibular fracture slightly distal to the mortise, or occasionally an avulsion fracture of the tip of the fibula.

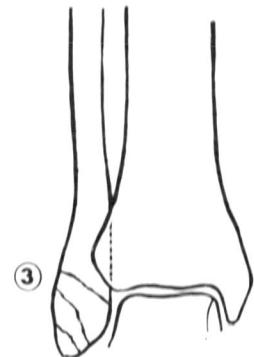

SUPINATION

4. Pronation-abduction (P-AB) fracture is characterized by low, transverse or slightly oblique supramalleolar fracture of the fibula running from the inferomedial cortex to the lateral cortex.

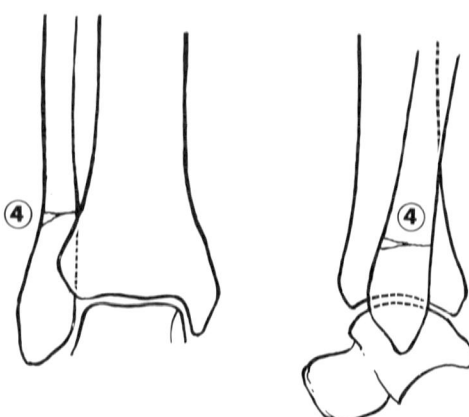

PRONATION

Note: No categorization is perfect. Pankovich, for example, has pointed out that fibular fractures above the syndesmosis may be seen with a supination-external rotation or pronation-abduction mechanism depending on the degree of supination or pronation at the time of injury (see page 1863).

OTHER TYPES OF ANKLE FRACTURES

Approximately 95 per cent of ankle fractures can be categorized according to Lauge-Hansen's method.

Other types include those produced by:

1. Pronation-dorsiflexion mechanism resulting in a displaced fracture of the distal tibial articular surface.

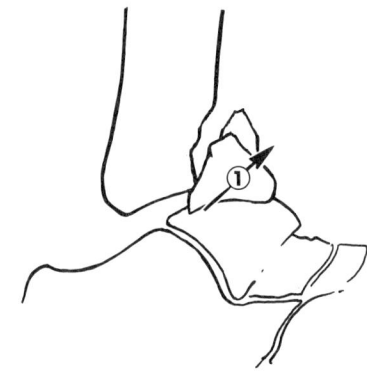

2. Avulsion fracture of the posterior tibial margin produced by a mechanism such as tripping over a curbstone.

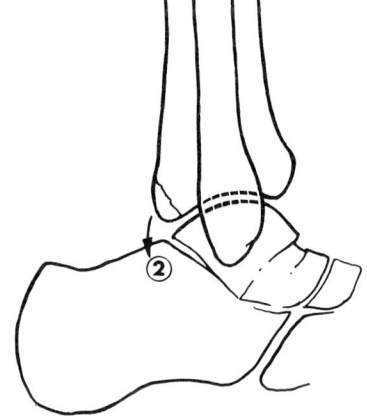

STAGES OF MALLEOLAR FRACTURES (LAUGE-HANSEN)

The severity of an ankle fracture depends on the stage to which the injury has advanced as well as on the mechanism.

This staging may seem unduly complex but it is quite logical and important to understand in order to anticipate what combination of bone and ligamentous injuries is likely.

Stages of Supination–External Rotation (S-EX) Fractures

Forceful external rotation of the ankle with the foot supinated causes the following sequence of injuries to the structures about the ankle:

Stage I produces an injury to the anterior part of the anterior tibiofibular ligament (ATFL) or an avulsion fracture of its attachment to either the fibula or the tibia.

Stage II results in a typical spiral fracture of the lateral malleolus running from the anterior margin in a dorsoproximal direction and including the Stage I injury.

Stage III produces a fracture of the posterior tibial margin and includes Stages I and II.

Note: It is not necessary to have a fracture of the posterior margin before the injury advances to a Stage IV fracture.

Stage IV produces a fracture of the medial malleolus or rupture of the deltoid ligament and includes Stages I and II and sometimes Stage III.

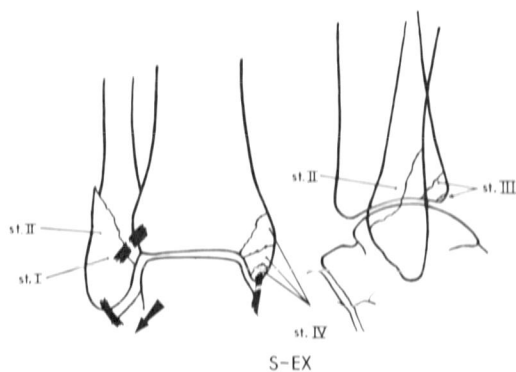

Stages of Supination-Adduction (S-AD) Fractures

An adduction injury to the supinated foot produces the following stages of damage to the bone and ligamentous structures of the ankle.

Stage I is a fracture of the lateral malleolus at or distal to the level of the tibiotalar joint or a rupture of the anterior talofibular or calcaneofibular ligament.

Stage II results in a fracture of the medial malleolus and includes Stage I. Most of these fractures are oblique or vertical but some may be transverse. Frequently the fracture includes the posteromedial tibial surface.

Note: Supination-adduction fracture is the only type associated with medial displacement of the talus. All the other types tend to displace the talus laterally or posterolaterally.

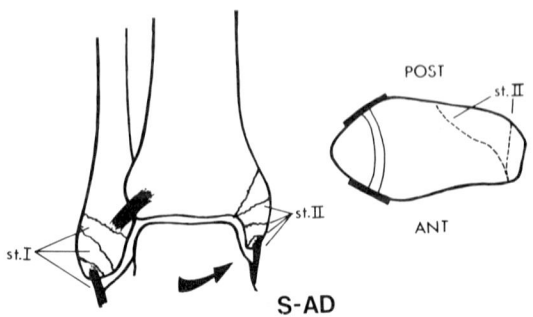

Stages of Pronation-Abduction (P-AB) and Pronation–External Rotation (P-EX) Fractures

Abduction or external rotation injuries to the pronated foot tend to produce the same initial stages of injury. They differ primarily in the type of fibular fracture that results.

Stage I is a fracture of the medial malleolus or rupture of the deltoid ligament. These are identical for both P-AB and P-EX injuries.

Stage II is a rupture of the distal tibiofibular syndesmosis and includes Stage I. Occasionally, avulsion fracture of the posterior tibial tubercle or the anterior tibial tubercle may be found at this stage in both mechanisms.

The difference between P-AB and P-EX fractures is determined by the type of fibular fracture produced at this stage. Characteristically, P-AB mechanism causes a low transverse supramalleolar fracture of the fibula and also includes Stages I and II.

P-EX fracture at Stage III is characterized by a high supramalleolar fracture of the fibula and includes Stages I and II. The level of the fracture varies, but no fracture is less than 2.5 cm. above the tibiotalar joint. Characteristically the fracture line runs from the anterior fibular margin in a distal direction.

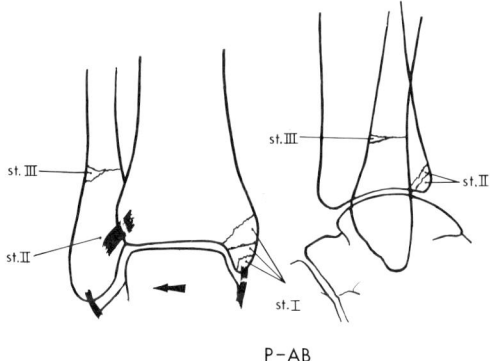
P-AB

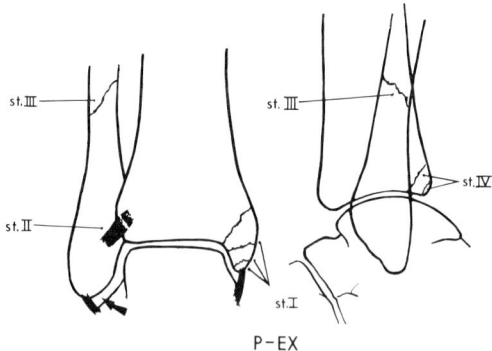
P-EX

P-EX Stage IV is an avulsion fracture of the posterior tibial margin, most often involving more than 25 per cent of the surface.

P-AB mechanisms produce avulsions of the posterior tibiofibular ligament rather than fractures of the tibia.

Note: Lauge-Hansen found in his cadaver experiments that there was frequently a fracture of the posterior tibial margin following Stage III of the P-EX mechanism. However, Yde found clinically that fracture of the posterior tibial margin precedes fibular fracture and should be anticipated as part of Stage II of the injury.

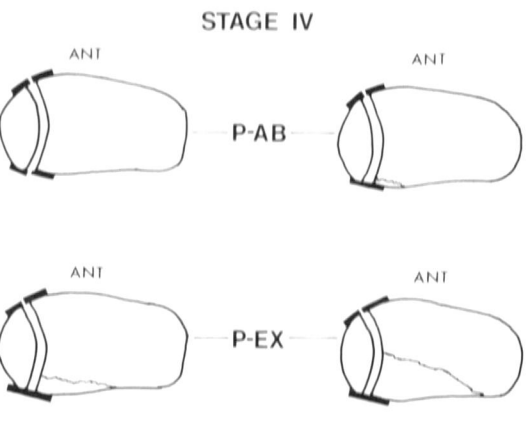

Management of Ankle Fractures

SIGNIFICANCE OF THE LATERAL TALAR SHIFT

REMARKS

The major concern in regard to managing ankle fractures is the degree of instability of the talus.

Most frequently the talus is displaced laterally or posterolaterally by the mechanism of the injury. Only with the supination-adduction mechanism is medial displacement of the talus likely.

Disruptions of the lateral bony support and of either the medial ligamentous or the medial bony support are necessary to cause the common problem of a lateral shift of the talus.

The degree of talar displacement is best measured on a mortise view taken with the foot internally rotated.

Identifying the mechanism by the characteristics of the fibular fracture helps to separate the stable from the unstable injury. Once lateral displacement occurs, the tibiotalar contract area is altered rapidly. Ramsey and Hamilton have demonstrated a 42 per cent decrease in contact area with 1 mm of lateral talar shift. Since the stress on the talus per unit area increases as contact area decreases, talar displacement of even 1 mm should be corrected to minimize chances of an unsatisfactory result.

The position of the talus in the ankle mortise is best assessed by a mortise view.

Mortise View of the Ankle

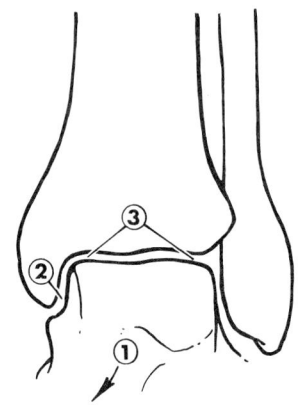

1. The x-ray is taken with the ankle internally rotated 20 degrees
2. The medial joint space should be approximately the same as
3. The superior joint space.

Changes in Tibiotalar Contact Caused by Lateral Shift

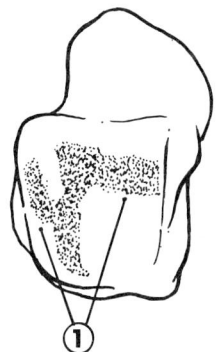 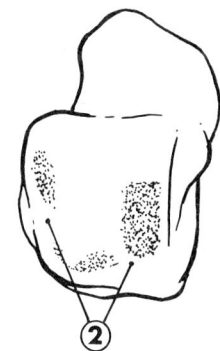

1. In the normal articulation, the tibiotalar contact extends across the breadth of the talus and is wide on the lateral side and narrow on the medial side.
2. Once the talus displaces laterally 1 mm, contact occurs only on the medial and lateral prominences of the talus. No contact occurs in the midportion.

Note: The key to correcting lateral talar shift is to restore the bony support provided by the lateral malleolus.

EVALUATION OF REDUCTION AND RESTORATION OF THE ANKLE MORTISE: THE TALOCRURAL ANGLE

REMARKS

Sarkisian and Cody have shown that the reduction of the ankle mortise can be best evaluated by carefully measuring the talocrural angle on the fractured side in comparison with the uninjured side. A difference greater than 2 degrees indicates failure to restore the ankle mortise to normal and an increased likelihood of a poorly functioning joint.

This talocrural measurement is based on the fact that the fibular side of the joint is the key to reduction. Rotational as well as longitudinal alignment of the fibular fracture must be exact in order to maintain the integrity of the mortise.

During the heel-strike and foot-flat phases of gait, the force of rotation is absorbed in the tibiofibular syndesmosis as the talus is stressed laterally against the fibula. If the fibular fracture is rotated and shortened, the talus will rotate excessively and produce pain and eventually ankle arthritis (see page 1804).

The talocrural angle is formed by the intersection of two lines,
1. One drawn parallel to the tibial articular surface and
2. One drawn between the tips of the two malleoli on the mortise view.
3. The ankle control measurement varies between 8 and 15 degrees.

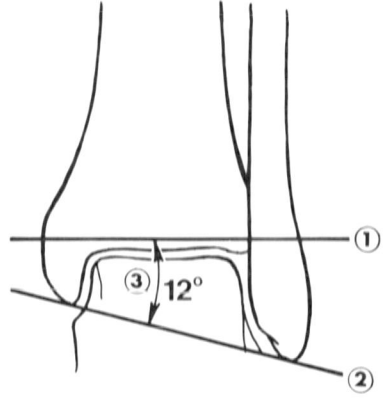

4. Variation of 2 degrees or more between the fractured and the unfractured ankles indicates incomplete restoration of the ankle mortise due to shortening or malrotation of the fibula.

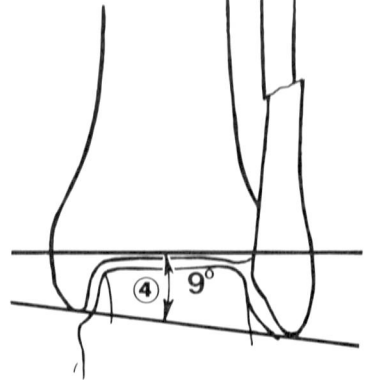

MANAGEMENT OF ANKLE FRACTURES BASED ON CLASSIFICATION AND STAGING

REMARKS

Comprehending the mechanisms producing common ankle fractures is important for proper management. If one recognizes the type and stage of the fracture, other associated injuries will be detected and repaired as necessary.

The end result of treatment depends to a certain extent on the type of initial injury as well as the degree of initial displacement. It is particularly dependent on the success of reduction. To achieve successful reduction, all injured structures contributing to the ankle instability should be restored as closely to normal as possible by either closed or open means.

FRACTURE OF THE LATERAL MALLEOLUS WITHOUT OR WITH LATERAL DISPLACEMENT

REMARKS

The key to classifying the type of ankle fracture is the pattern of the lateral malleolar fracture (see page 1836).

Reduction of the lateral malleolus also is the key to restoring ankle stability. Yablon and coworkers have demonstrated that incomplete reduction of the lateral malleolus leads to talar displacement and late degenerative arthritis. Anatomic repositioning of the talus is possible only when the lateral malleolus is accurately reduced. Displacement of the talus faithfully follows that of the lateral malleolus.

A large percentage of lateral malleolar fractures are undisplaced S-EX injuries. Care should be taken, however, to rule out the potential problems of instability.

When both the medial and lateral sides of the ankle have been injured, displacement of the talus is likely and internal fixation is generally indicated.

X-rays of ankle fractures can be analyzed to determine the mechanisms of injury and appropriate treatment.

FRACTURE OF THE LATERAL MALLEOLUS WITHOUT LATERAL DISPLACEMENT

Appearance on X-Ray

A. 1. Spiral fracture of the lateral malleolus (displacement is insignificant).
   2. The talus has not shifted.
   3. The tibiofibular joint is not widened.
B. 1. Avulsion of the lateral malleolus (transverse fracture).
   2. No shift of the talus.
   3. No tibiofibular diastasis.

Note: These x-rays may indicate either S-EX or S-AD mechanisms.

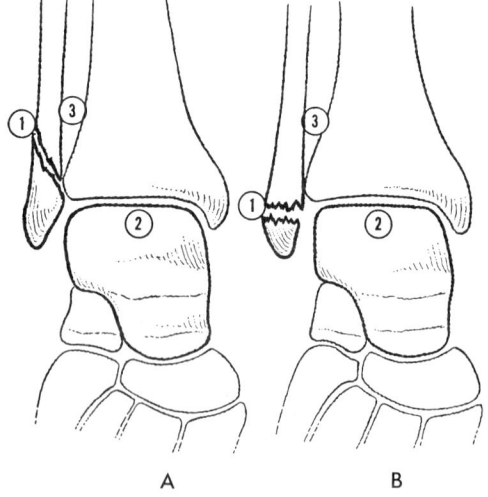

Staging of Injury

LAUGE-HANSEN (S-EX) STAGE II FRACTURE

The mechanism of supination–external rotation injures the ankle as follows:

Stage I is a tear of the anterior tibiofibular ligament in its substance or from its bony attachment.

Stage II is a spiral oblique fracture of the fibula that is undisplaced and continues to support the talus.

Note: Always examine carefully for injuries to the posterior tibial margin or to the medial deltoid ligament associated with Stage II of this mechanism and indicative of greater instability than is evident on initial x-ray (see page 1881).

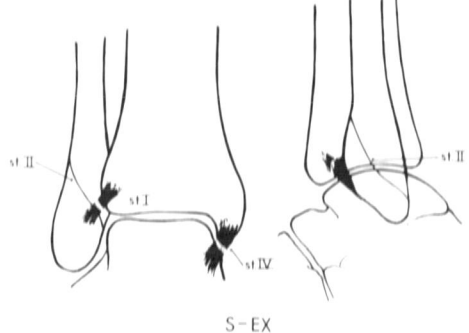

LAUGE-HANSEN (S-AD) STAGE I FRACTURE

Supination-adduction mechanism injures the ankle as follows:

Stage I is an avulsion fracture of the lateral malleolus distal to the level of the tibiotalar joint. This may or may not be associated with a tear of the anterior talofibular ligament.

Note: These are both stable injuries because only the lateral support of the ankle is injured.

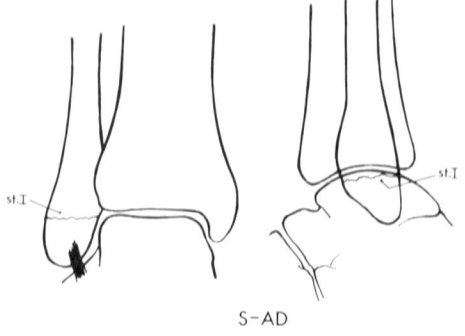

Management

1. Apply a below-knee, well-fitting, nonpadded plaster walking cast.
2. The toes are free.
3. The foot is at a right angle to the leg.
4. The foot is in a neutral position.

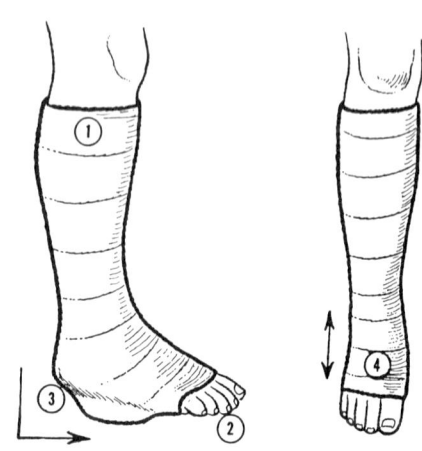

Subsequent Management

Allow weight bearing as tolerated when the cast hardens.

Remove the case in three to five weeks.

Encourage range-of-motion exercises to the ankle and therapy to improve proprioception and balance as for a Grade III ankle sprain (see page 1822).

FRACTURE OF THE LATERAL MALLEOLUS WITH LATERAL DISPLACEMENT

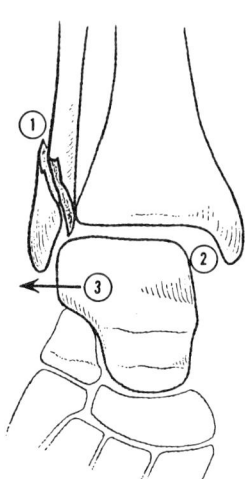

Prereduction X-Ray

ANTEROPOSTERIOR VIEW

1. Spiral fracture of the lateral malleolus.
2. Widening of the interval between the medial malleolus and the talus.
3. Lateral shift of the talus.

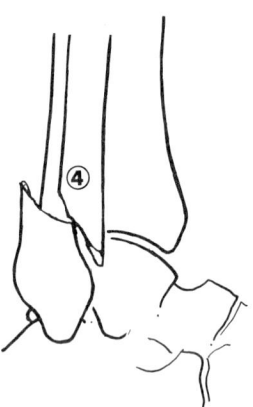

LATERAL VIEW

4. The fibular fracture is locked in a shortened and externally rotated position, preventing closed reduction.

Staging of Injury: Lauge-Hansen (S-EX) Stage IV Fracture

The mechanism of supination–external rotation injures the ankle as follows:

Stage I is disruption of the anterior talofibular ligament.

Stage II is the spiral oblique fracture of the lateral malleolus.

Stage III is an injury to the posterior tibiofibular ligament or fracture of the posterior articular margin.

Note: It is not necessary to have a fracture of the posterior margin before the injury advances to a Stage IV.

Stage IV is a fracture of the medial malleolus or in this instance a disruption of the deltoid ligament.

Note: In contrast to the S-EX Stage II and S-AD Stage I injuries illustrated on page 1845, this injury to both the medial and lateral support structures is unstable and generally requires operative fixation.

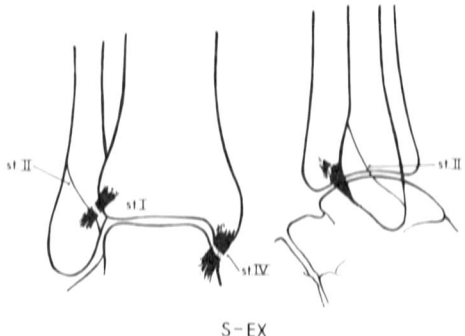

S-EX

OPERATIVE TREATMENT

REMARKS

Operative treatment is usually necessary to restore the malleolus to its proper length and rotational alignment, and thereby to correct lateral talar displacement.

The talofibular ligament may not require repair unless it is torn extensively, as visualized through the lateral incision.

The deltoid ligament should be repaired through a separate medial incision, with care taken to reconstruct both the anterior or superficial portion and the deep or posterior portion.

Surgical repair of all the damaged medial and lateral structures permits early postoperative joint exercises and good functional recovery.

Reduction and Fixation of the Fracture of the Lateral Malleolus

1. Make a vertical incision beginning just distal to the top of the lateral malleolus and extending directly upward on the center of the bone.
2. Divide the deep fascia and retract its margins with the skin flaps.
3. Divide the periosteum longitudinally, and by subperiosteal dissection expose the fibula and the fracture site.

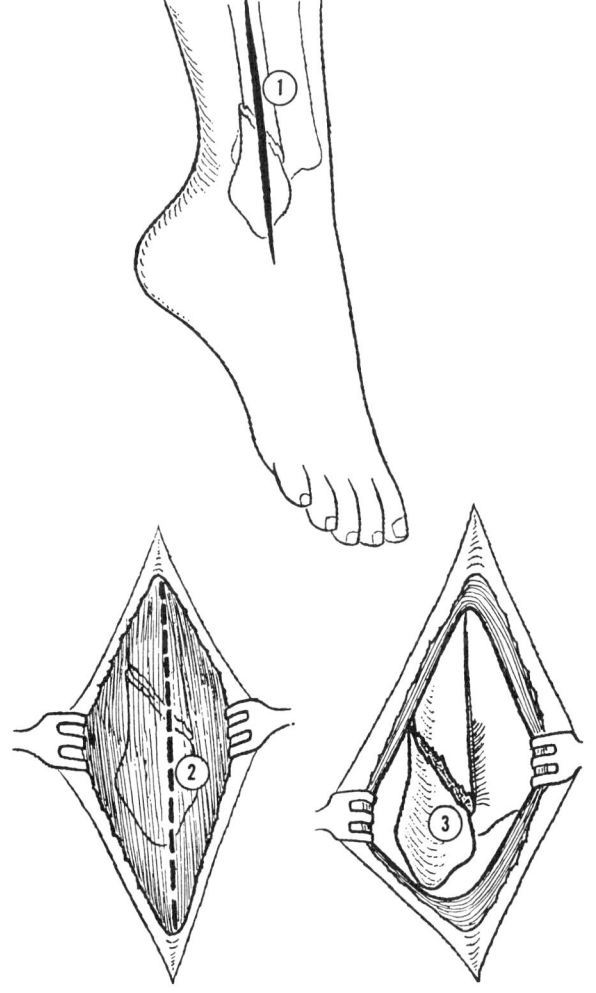

1. Reduce the malleolus to proper length and rotational alignment and hold it with a towel clip.

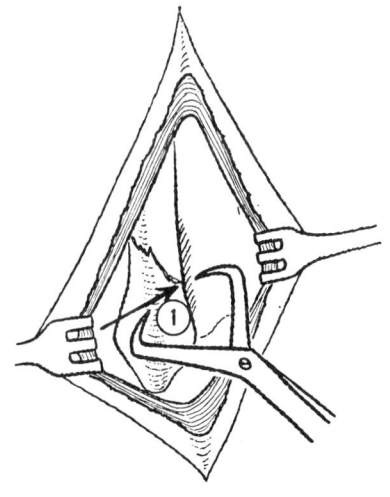

2. Secure the fixation with one or two screws drilled across the fracture site or

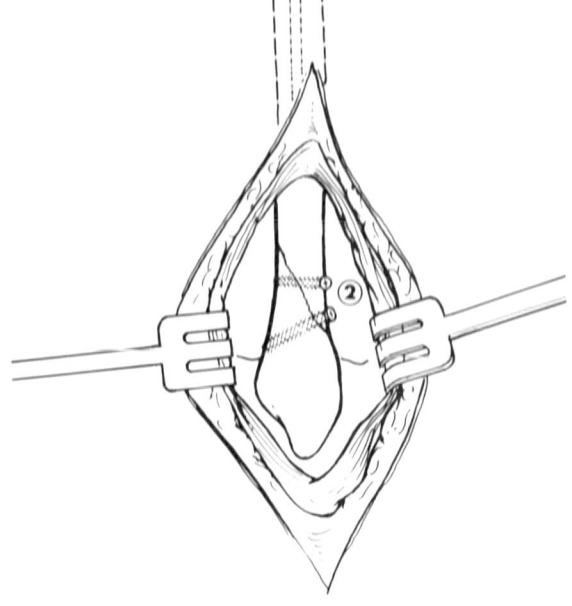

3. With a Rush pin introduced through the medullary canal.

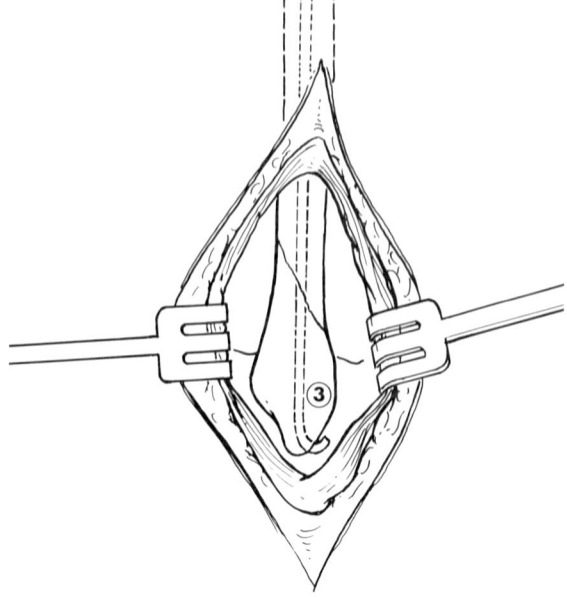

Repair of the Deltoid Ligament

1. Make a 10-cm curved incision beginning posterior to the malleolus, extend it distally and anteriorly about 2 cm distal to the tip of the malleolus, and terminate it on the tuberosity of the navicular.

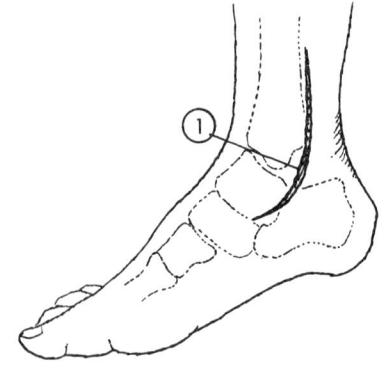

2. Reflect the skin flaps and
3. Visualize the tear in the deltoid.

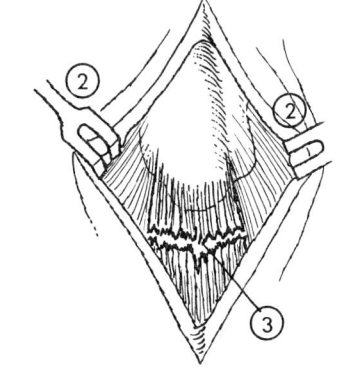

4. Inspect for hematomas or defects in the posterior deltoid.
5. Repair all damaged portions of the deltoid with interrupted sutures.

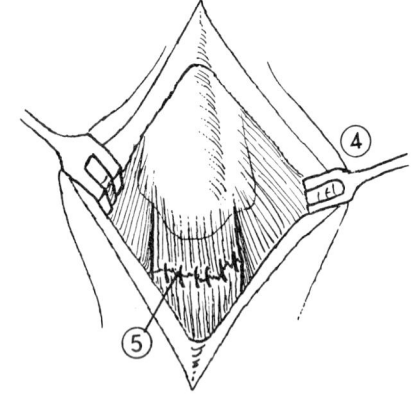

6. If the deep posterior deltoid ligament is torn, it can be exposed by retracting the posterior tibial tendon forward.

Note: Always obtain intraoperative x-rays to insure adequate reduction and position of the internal fixation device.

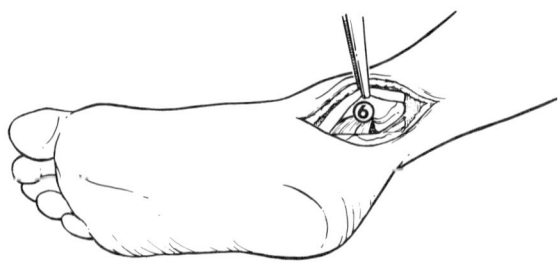

Postreduction X-Ray

1. The preoperative loss of fibula length and rotational alignment should be corrected.
2. The screws (or Rush Pin) should be adequately fixing both proximal and distal fragments.
3. The talus should be restored to its normal position in the mortise.

Note: The reduction can be most accurately evaluated by comparing the talocrural angle of the fractured and unfractured ankles (see page 1843).

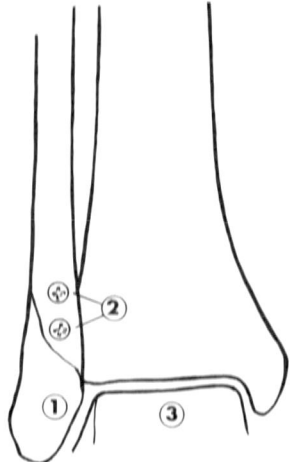

Postoperative Management (Burwell and Charnley)

A bulky postoperative dressing is applied until the initial swelling has subsided and the foot of the bed is elevated.

After three days the postoperative dressing may be changed to a lighter dressing and the patient should be encouraged to do ankle and foot exercises for five minutes every half hour throughout the day. These exercises are not painful because the medial and lateral support structures are repaired, and the range of motion will gradually increase.

When the patient has regained adequate motion, usually within ten days, the stitches are removed, and a cast is applied from the toes to below the knee.

Immobilization

1. Apply a short leg, unpadded plaster cast.
2. The toes are free.
3. The foot is at a right angle to the leg.
4. Mold the plaster well around the malleoli.
5. The foot is in a neutral position in regard to inversion and eversion.

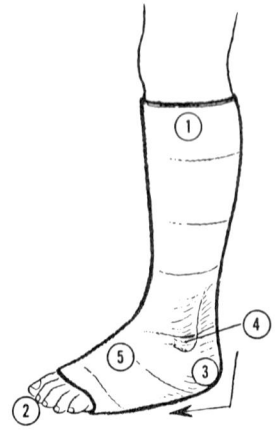

FRACTURES OF THE ANKLE

Subsequent Management

After the cast is applied the patient is allowed out of bed to walk with two crutches.

The cast may be removed, on the average, within five weeks.

After removal of plaster, the patient generally regains normal range of motion in the ankle promptly.

Removal of the screws is usually unnecessary unless they are causing pain or discomfort.

NONOPERATIVE TREATMENT OF DISPLACED FRACTURES OF THE LATERAL MALLEOLUS

REMARKS

This should not be the primary choice of treatment. It should be employed if there are definite contraindications precluding surgical treatment.

Manipulative Reduction

1. The limb hangs over the end of the table.
2. Place one hand over the medial aspect of the leg and
3. The other over the lateral aspect of the foot and the lateral malleolus.
4. Push the foot strongly inward.

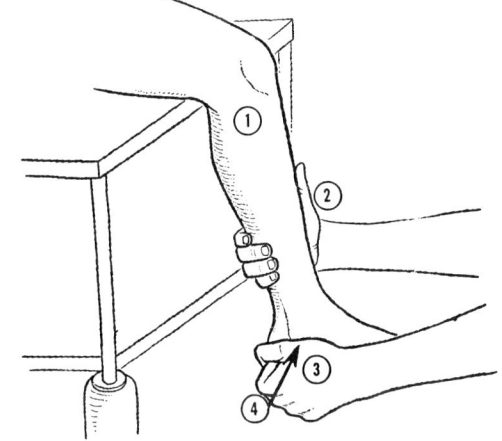

1. While the foot rests on the surgeon's knee,
2. A below-knee plaster cast is applied.

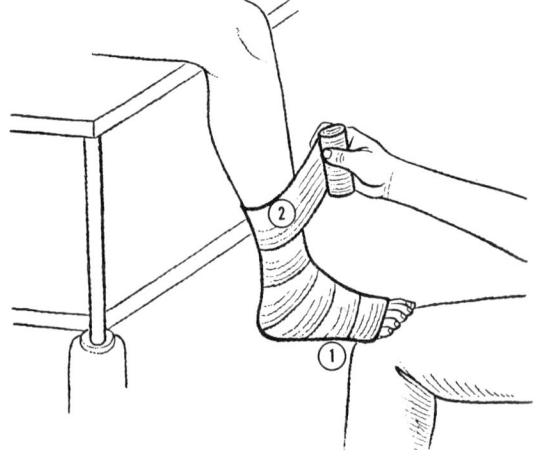

1. While the plaster is setting, the limb is steadied with one hand on the medial aspect of the leg.
2. The other hand makes steady strong pressure inward over the lateral malleolus and foot.
3. The plaster is molded well over and around the malleoli.

Note: Inward pressure should be maintained until the plaster has set.

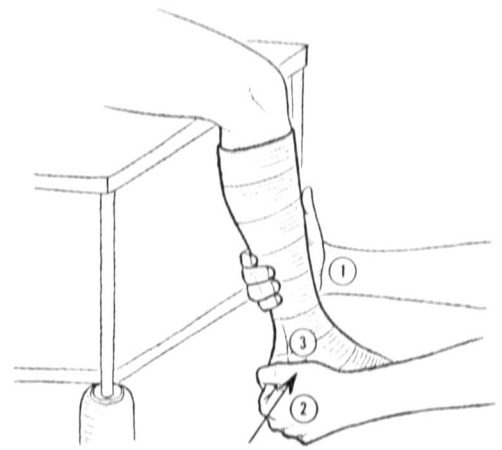

Closed Reduction of Supination–External Rotation Fractures with Quigley's Traction

Early operation is preferable for most displaced S-EX fractures.

Occasionally there may be severe swelling of the ankle requiring elevation of the leg well above the heart level.

An excellent method elevating the limb to diminish the swelling and sometimes to achieve reduction of S-EX fractures is with Quigley's traction.

1. A long leg stockinette is rolled over the fractured limb, which has been prepared with benzoin.
2. The foot of the fractured ankle is suspended by balanced weights. The knee is supported by a sling to prevent hyperextension.
3. The force of gravity and the inverted position of the ankle reduce the fracture while allowing the edema to subside.

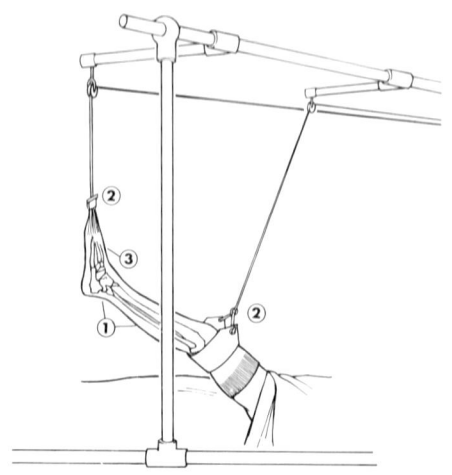

Postreduction X-Ray

1. The talus occupies its normal position in the mortise.
2. The lateral malleolus has been corrected.

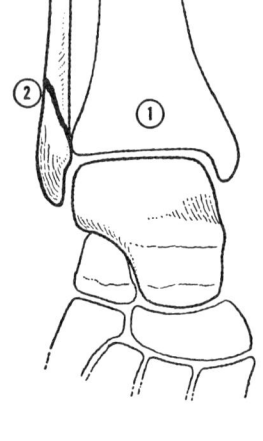

3. Always check reduction on lateral x-ray to insure that the posterior displacement of the malleolus has been corrected.

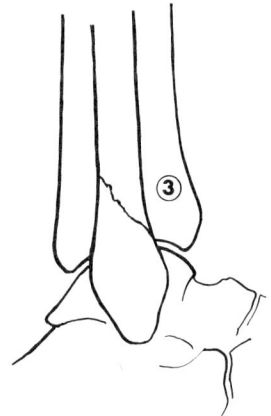

CAUTION

The key to reduction is to restore the fibula to proper length and rotational alignment (see page 1842).

1. Occasionally, repositioning of the talus can be achieved by the forceful internal rotation of the ankle but without
2. Complete reduction of the fibula.
3. This only stretches the lateral capsule and may lead to redisplacement of the talus.

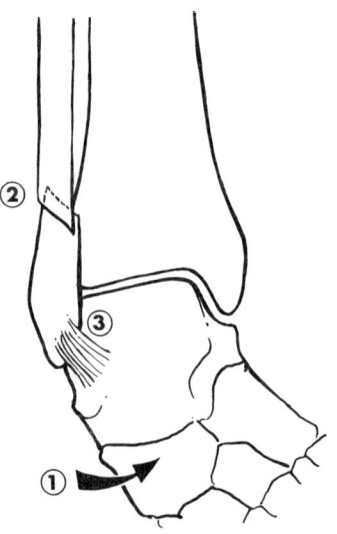

Immobilization

If reduction is satisfactory in Quigley's traction,

1. Apply a long cast with the foot held in the inverted position.

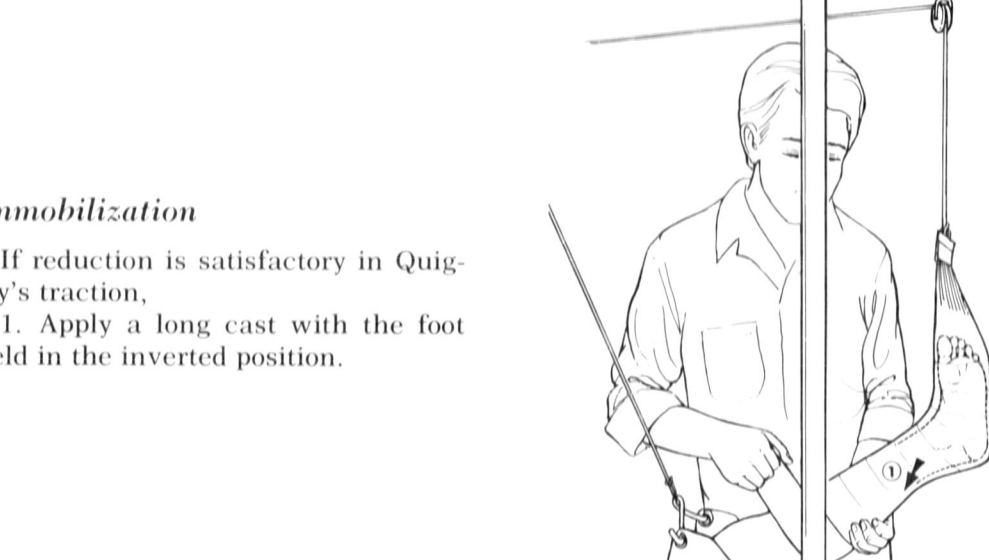

Management After Closed Reduction

The patient may be allowed to walk on crutches without bearing weight on the fractured leg.

Reevaluate the reduction by x-ray within the first week. If reduction of the ankle mortise is lost at any time, open reduction should be carried out.

Avoid repeated manipulations, which are most likely to result in poor ankle function.

The cast is changed at four weeks and the foot is taken out of the inverted position. Reevaluate by x-rays at that time to be sure that the reduction of the lateral malleolus is maintained.

The cast can be removed eight weeks after fracture and the patient can be started on active exercises and physical therapy to restore ankle motion.

ISOLATED FRACTURES OF THE MEDIAL MALLEOLUS

REMARKS

Isolated fractures of the medial malleolus are characteristically Stage I lesions from a pronation-abduction or pronation–external rotation mechanism.

The mechanism may advance to Stage II and rupture the anterior tibiofibular ligament, but this would not be evident on x-ray.

Because of the intact fibular support, the talus does not displace.

Closed reduction is frequently successful provided that a reasonable approximation of the malleolar fragments is achieved.

The malleolar fracture heals slowly without periosteal callus; frequently, clinical stability precedes radiographic evidence of union by several months with closed treatment.

Operative fixation may be indicated for widely displaced fragments that are not reduced by closed manipulation.

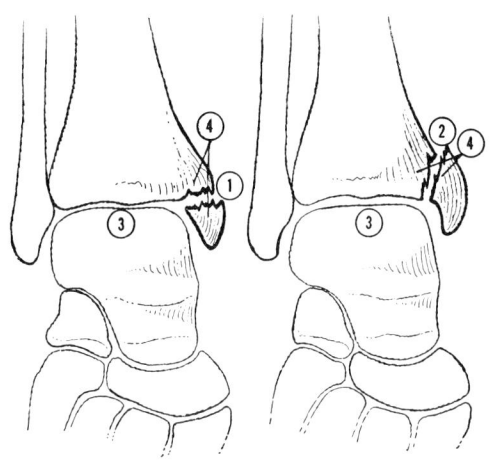

Appearance on X-Ray

1. Transverse fracture of the medial malleolus.
2. Oblique fracture of the medial malleolus.
3. The talus is in its normal position.
4. There is wide separation of malleolar fragments.

Staging of Injury: Lauge-Hansen P-AB or P-EX Fracture, Stage I or II

Pronation-abduction and pronation–external rotation mechanisms injure the ankle in the following stages:

Stage I avulses the medial malleolus or sometimes the deltoid ligament.

Stage II causes rupture of the distal tibiofibular syndesmosis, which may not be evident on x-ray.

Note: This injury involving only the medial support of the ankle is stable and can usually be treated by a closed method, provided that adequate reduction of the malleolus is achieved.

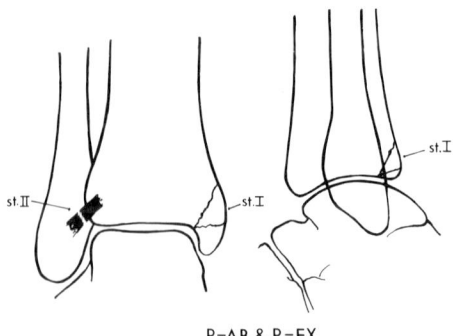

P-AB & P-EX

NONOPERATIVE TREATMENT

Closed reduction and cast application are usually successful for isolated medial malleolar fractures of this type and stage.

Technique of Closed Reduction

1. The limb hangs over the end of the table.
2. With both thumbs the surgeon manipulates the fragments into normal position.
3. Then with the heels of the hands, the surgeon compresses firmly both malleoli.

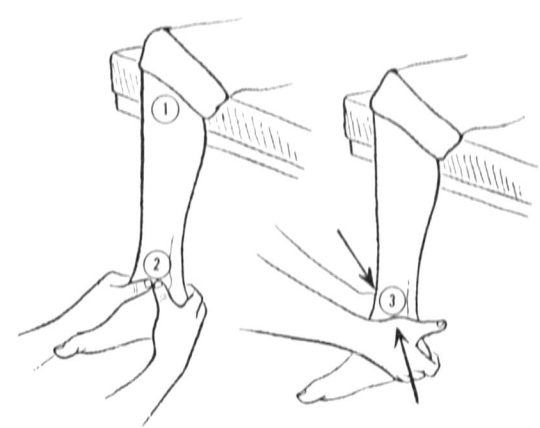

While the foot rests on the surgeon's knee:
1. A short leg plaster cast is applied.
2. The foot is at a right angle to the leg.
3. The foot is in a neutral position in regard to inversion and eversion.
4. While the plaster is setting, firm pressure is made over the medial malleolus, pushing it inward.

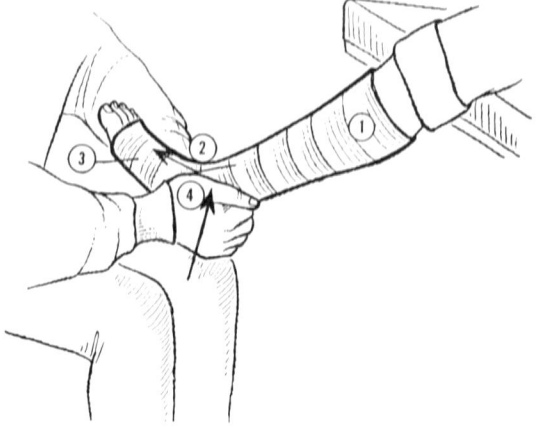

Postreduction X-Ray

1. The malleolus is restored to its normal position.

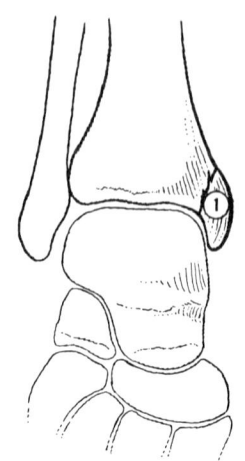

Immobilization

1. A plaster cast extends from below the knee to behind the metatarsal heads.
2. The foot is at a right angle to the leg.
3. The foot is in a neutral position.
4. A heel for walking is incorporated in the cast.

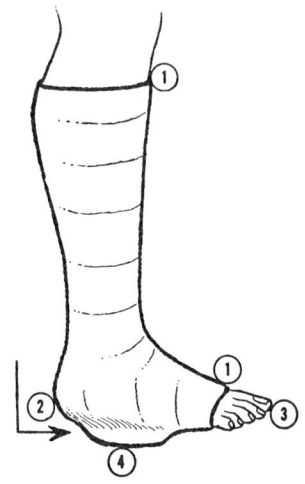

Management

Allow weight bearing.
Insist on active exercises for the toes.
Remove the cast at the end of six weeks.
Institute active exercises to restore ankle and foot movements.

SURGICAL TREATMENT

REMARKS

Failure to restore the malleolar fragment to its anatomic position justifies surgical intervention.

In some instances a periosteal flap lying between the fragments precludes manipulative reduction; it must be removed under direct vision.

Always check for avulsion fractures of the posterior tibial surface. This may occur in Stage II of a P-EX injury, and requires fixation if more than 25 per cent of the joint surface is involved (see page 1841).

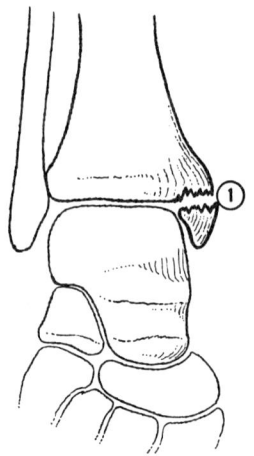

Preoperative X-Ray

1. Wide separation of malleolar fragments (manipulative measures failed in this case).

Operative Reduction

In general this method must be resorted to for most displaced fractures.

1. Make a 7-cm incision beginning 2.5 cm distal to the tip of the malleolus; the incision extends directly upward over the center of the bone.
2. Reflect the skin flaps and divide the deep fascia.
3. Visualize the fracture site and the displaced malleolar fragment.
4. Remove the periosteal flap interposed between the fractured surfaces.

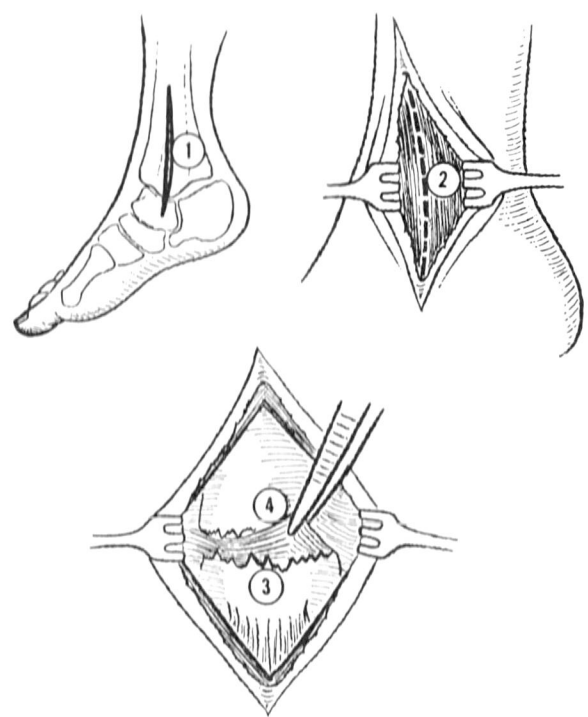

1. Insert a small elevator anterior to the fracture and inspect for any tears of the anterior deltoid or capsule. If these structures are torn, they should be sutured back to the distal tibia.

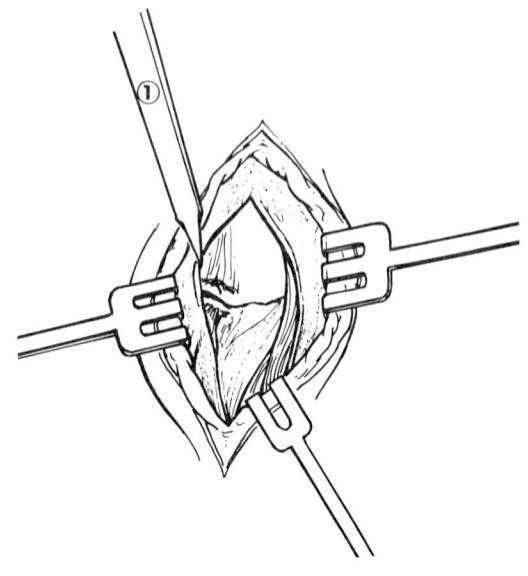

Operative Reduction (Continued)

After cleaning out the fracture site with a fine curette:

1. Grasp the malleolar fragment with a towel clip and secure it in its anatomic position.
2. Make a small longitudinal incision through the fibers of the deltoid ligament to expose the tip of the malleolus.
3. Drive a 5-cm screw obliquely through the malleolar fragment, taking care to avoid the articular surface.

CAUTION

Avoid compression screws for malleolar fractures; they are unnecessary and tend to split the small fragment if overly compressed.

If the medial malleolar fragment is too small to be fixed with the screw, use two Kirschner wires.

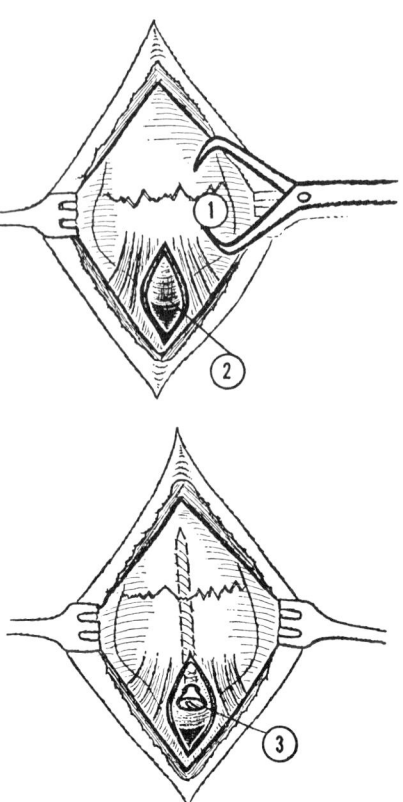

Postoperative X-Ray

1. The malleolar fragment is in perfect anatomic position.
2. There is a transfixion screw across the fracture in the medial malleolus.

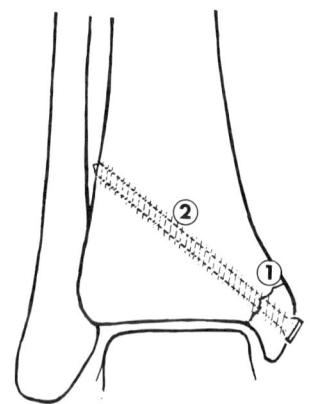

Postoperative Management

A bulky postoperative dressing is applied until the initial swelling has subsided, and the foot of the bed is elevated.

After three days the postoperative dressing may be changed to a lighter dressing and the patient may be encouraged to do ankle and foot exercises for five minutes every half hour throughout the day. These exercises are not painful because the medial and lateral support structures are stable, and the range of motion will gradually increase.

When the patient has regained adequate motion, usually within ten days, the stitches are removed and a cast is applied from the toes to below the knee.

Immobilization

1. Apply a short leg unpadded cast.
2. The toes are free.
3. The foot is at a right angle to the leg.
4. Mold the plaster well around the malleolus.
5. The foot is in a neutral position as to inversion and eversion.

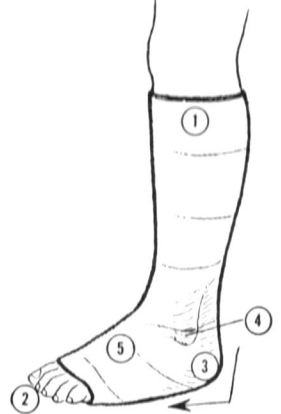

Subsequent Management

After the cast is applied the patient is allowed out of bed to walk with two crutches.

Subsequently the cast may be removed, on the average within five weeks.

After removal of plaster, the patient generally regains normal range of motion in the ankle promptly.

Removal of the screws is usually unnecessary unless they are causing pain or discomfort.

FRACTURE OF THE MEDIAL MALLEOLUS WITH RUPTURE OF THE LATERAL LIGAMENT

REMARKS

This combination is the result of a supination-adduction mechanism. It is the only mechanism that will displace the talus medially, and it can result in an unstable mortise.

Since both the medial and the lateral support structures are lost, operative fixation is desirable to restore mortise stability.

Appearance on X-Ray

1. There is an oblique fracture of the medial malleolus.
2. The talus is tilted and displaced medially.
3. The joint space is widened laterally and is consistent with a tear of the talofibular ligament.

Note: A fracture of the lateral malleolus may also occur.

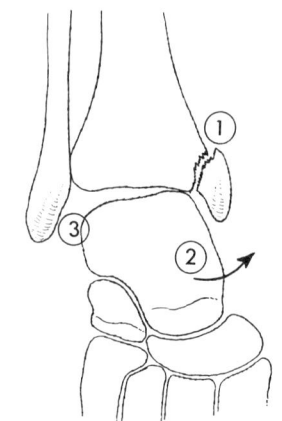

Staging of Injury: Lauge-Hansen S-AD Fracture Stage II

A supination-adduction injury to the ankle produces the following stages of injury:

Stage I injures the anterior talofibular and calcaneofibular ligaments.

Stage II fractures the medial malleolus, most characteristically with an oblique fracture line. Frequently the fracture also involves the posteromedial tibial surface.

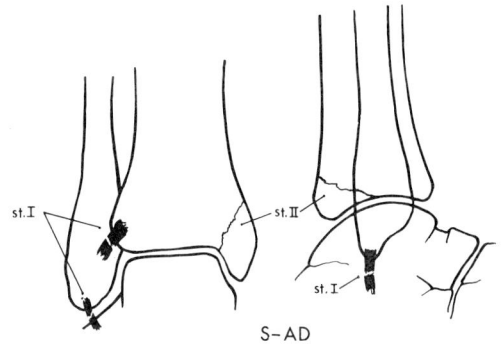

Closed Reduction Technique

The techniques of reduction and immobilization for this injury are the same as those described for isolated fractures of the medial malleolus (see page 1856).

Operative Management

1. The medial malleolus is fixed with a screw (for technique see page 1859).
2. The lateral ligament is repaired (for technique see page 1820).

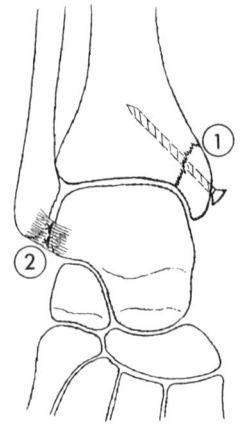

FRACTURE OF THE FIBULA PROXIMAL TO THE TIBIOFIBULAR SYNDESMOSIS

REMARKS

These injuries, according to the Lauge-Hansen classification, are produced most often by P-EX mechanisms. However, Pankovich has shown that, depending on the position of the foot at the time of injury, an S-EX or P-AB mechanism may also fracture the fibula above the syndesmosis.

The specific mechanism may be identified by the characteristics of the fibular fracture (see page 1836).

Identifying the mechanism is helpful in selecting treatment, because the fibular fracture produced by supination may not have associated medial injuries and can be treated closed. Fibular fracture resulting from pronation mechanisms always has associated disruption of the medial support structure and generally requires internal stabilization.

In order for the fibula to be fractured above the syndesmosis, the tibiofibular ligaments and the intraosseous membrane are usually disrupted. The key to reduction, however, is to stabilize the fibular fracture because the distal talofibular ligament remains intact and the talus faithfully follows the fibula.

The syndesmosis can be repaired by direct suture but fibulotibial screw fixation should be avoided because it restricts the rotation in the syndesmosis necessary to allow dorsiflexion (see page 1804).

Stages of Supination–External Rotation (S-EX) Fracture of the Fibula Proximal to the Syndesmosis (Pankovich)

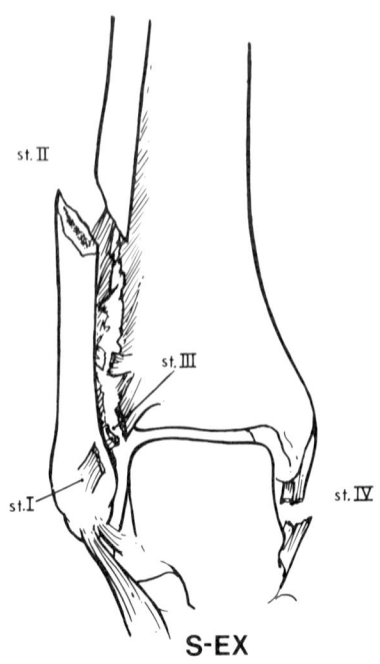

Because the deltoid ligament is relaxed in supination, a fracture of the fibula occurs before medial disruption.

Stage I is a rupture or avulsion of the anterior tibiofibular ligament associated with rupture of the intraosseous ligament.

Stage II is a fracture of the fibula above the syndesmosis. This is characterized by a typical spiral fracture extending from the anterior edge in a posterosuperior direction.

Stage III is a rupture of the posterior tibiofibular ligament or a fracture of the posterior tubercle of the tibia.

Stage IV is a rupture of the deltoid ligament or a fracture of the medial malleolus.

Stages of Pronation-Abduction (P-AB) Fracture of the Fibula Proximal to the Syndesmosis

With the foot in pronation the deltoid ligament ruptures first followed by complete diastasis of the syndesmosis and then a fracture of the fibula.

Stage I is a rupture of the deltoid ligament or a fracture of the medial malleolus.

Stage II is rupture of all of the ligaments of the syndesmosis or avulsion fractures of their bony insertions.

Stage III is a fracture of the fibula proximal to the syndesmosis.

The fracture is characterized as a transverse or slightly oblique line running from the lateral surface in an inferomedial direction.

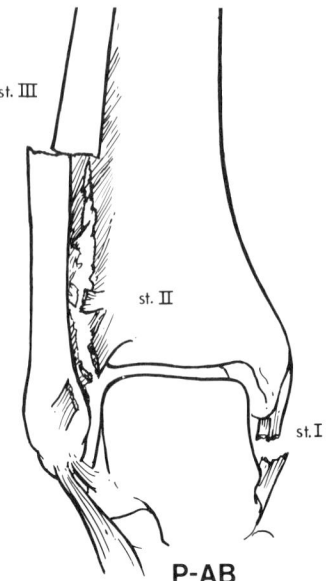
P-AB

Stages of Pronation–External Rotation (P-EX) Mechanisms Producing Fractures of the Fibula Proximal to the Syndesmosis

This mechanism applies strong tension to the deltoid ligament or medial malleolus and then continues to disrupt the tibiofibular and intraosseous ligaments, frequently fracturing the posterior tibial attachment of the ligament, and finally fracturing the fibula.

Stage I is a fracture of the medial malleolus or a rupture of the deltoid ligament.

Stage II is a rupture of the anterior tibiofibular ligament or its bony insertion associated with rupture of the intraosseous ligament.

Stage III is a fracture of the fibula above the syndesmosis. This is characterized by a fracture line that runs from the anterior edge in a posteroinferior direction.

Stage IV is a fracture of the posterior tubercle of the tibia or a rupture of the posterior tibiofibular ligament. This injury frequently involves a large portion of the posterior articular surface.

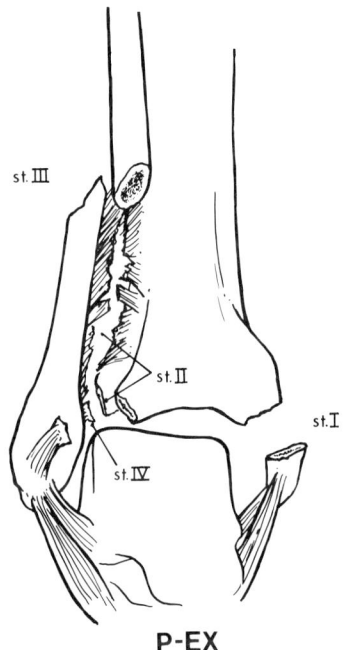
P-EX

Appearance on X-Ray

P-EX FRACTURE STAGE IV

1. Wide separation of the talus from the medial malleolus indicates disruption of the deltoid.
2. Gross posterolateral displacement of the fibula indicates disruption of the tibiofibular ligament and intraosseous ligament.
3. The fibular fracture line runs from the anterior cortex in a posteroinferior direction, characteristic of the P-EX mechanism.
4. The talus displaces posterolaterally with the fibula.

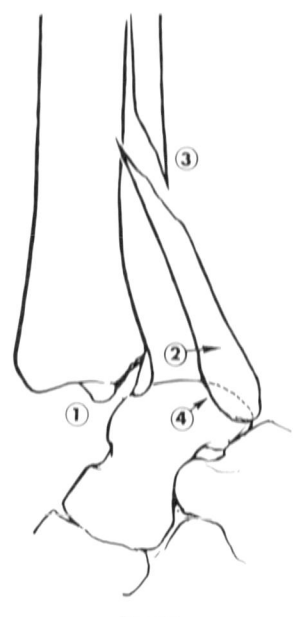

P-EX

P-AB FRACTURE STAGE III

1. Widening of the medial joint space indicates deltoid ligament rupture.
2. Diastasis of the syndesmosis.
3. The fibular fracture line characteristically runs transversely or slightly obliquely from the lateral cortex in an inferomedial direction.

Note: These injuries to the medial and lateral support structures are sufficiently unstable to require operative fixation.

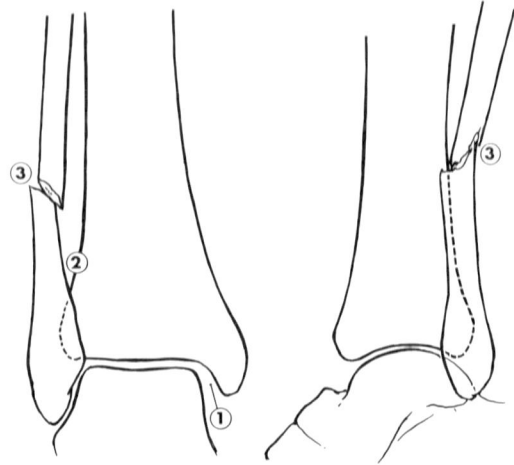

Appearance on X-Ray
(Continued)

S-EX FRACTURE STAGE II

1. Slight widening of the syndesmosis.
2. Characteristically, the fibular fracture line spirals from the anterior edge of the cortex in a posterosuperior direction.
3. The medial joint space is normal.

Note: This injury involves the lateral ankle support structure and is usually stable. It most often may be treated closed. One must carefully evaluate for clinical signs of medial ligament pain, progressive increase in the medial clear space, or shortening of the fibula, any of which is indicative of more advanced stage requiring operative fixation.

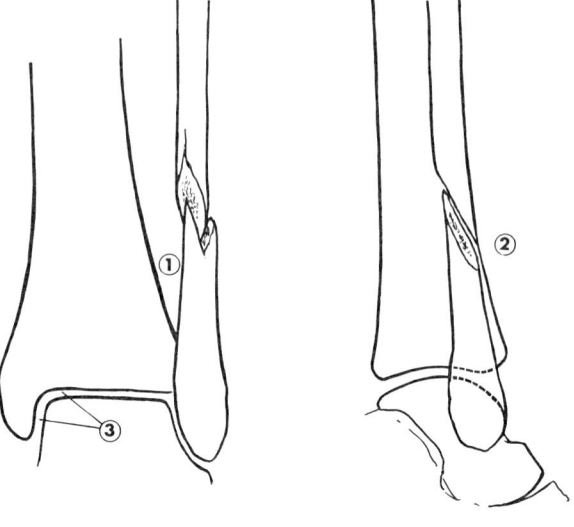

MANAGEMENT OF FIBULAR FRACTURES PROXIMAL TO THE SYNDESMOSIS

REMARKS

S-EX Stage I, II, or III injuries are stable provided that the fibula does not shorten and the medial joint space is normal. They may be treated by cast immobilization. Be certain that the fibular fracture is restored to length by the closed reduction. Shortening of the fibula results in tilting of the talus and an unsatisfactory result (see page 1842).

S-EX Stage IV injuries are unstable because the medial as well as the lateral support of the ankle is disrupted. These generally require internal fixation of both the medial and lateral structures to insure satisfactory ankle support.

P-AB and P-EX injuries are unstable, since both the medial and lateral support structures are involved. Operative fixation is usually the treatment of choice with these injuries.

The key to stabilizing the ankle mortise is to restore the fibula to normal length and alignment.

The intraosseous ligament can be repaired by direct suture. Transosseous screw fixation across the fibula into the tibia should be avoided because this decreases rotation in the syndesmosis necessary for normal ankle dorsiflexion (see page 1804).

P-EX mechanisms are particularly likely to produce large posterior tibial articular surface fractures involving more than 25 per cent of the joint surface. These require internal fixation to stabilize the posterior articular surface (see page 1841).

Operative Reduction and Internal Fixation

The sequence should be to stabilize the fibula first and then the tibiofibular syndesmosis through the same incision.

The medial malleolus is then fixed through a separate incision. If necessary, any avulsion fracture of the posterior tibial surface can be fixed by screws inserted from anterior to posterior through the medial incision.

1. The incision runs over the anterior cortex of the fibula from the area of fracture down to the ankle joint to expose the tibiofibular syndesmosis.
2. The incision should avoid the superficial peroneal nerve anteriorly and
3. The sural nerve posteriorly.

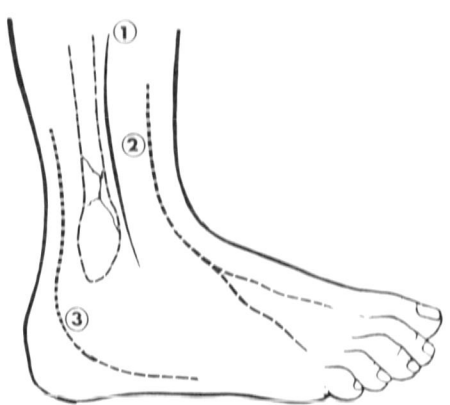

1. The fibular fracture is reduced and stabilized with a semitubular five-hole plate.
2. The reduction should restore the normal length of the lateral malleolus on the fractured side (compared with the unfractured side—see page 1842).

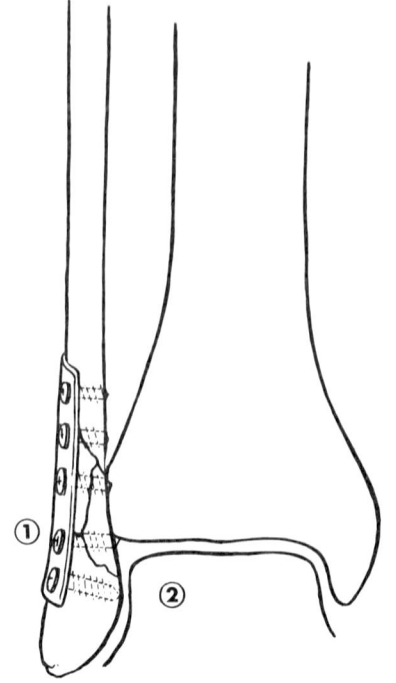

Operative Reduction and Internal Fixation (Continued)

1. The tibiofibular syndesmosis is then explored and stability is tested.

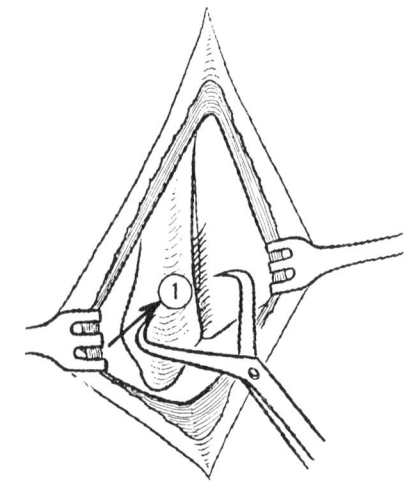

2. If the distal fibula is unstable, the tibiofibular ligament is sutured, *or*

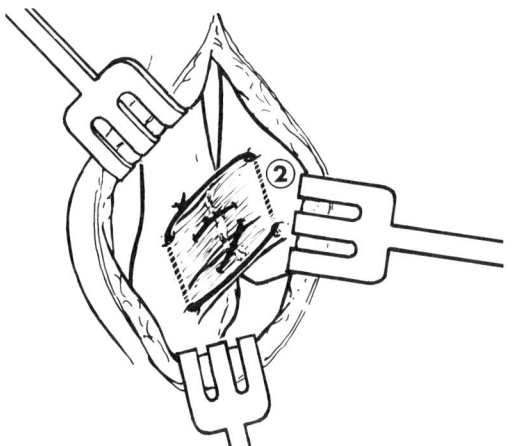

3. If there is an avulsion fragment from the bony attachment, it is reattached with a screw.

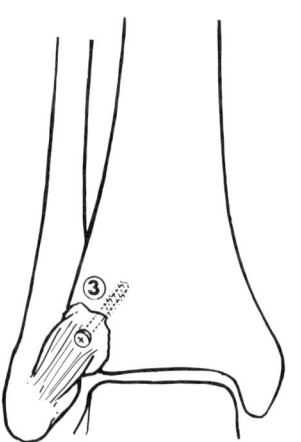

1. A second incision is made over the anteromedial tibia beginning 2 cm distal to the tip of the malleolus and extending upward 7.5 cm over the fracture site.
2. Reflect the skin flaps and divide the deep fascia.
3. Visualize the fracture site and the displaced malleolar fragment.
4. Remove the periosteal flap interposed between the fractured surfaces.

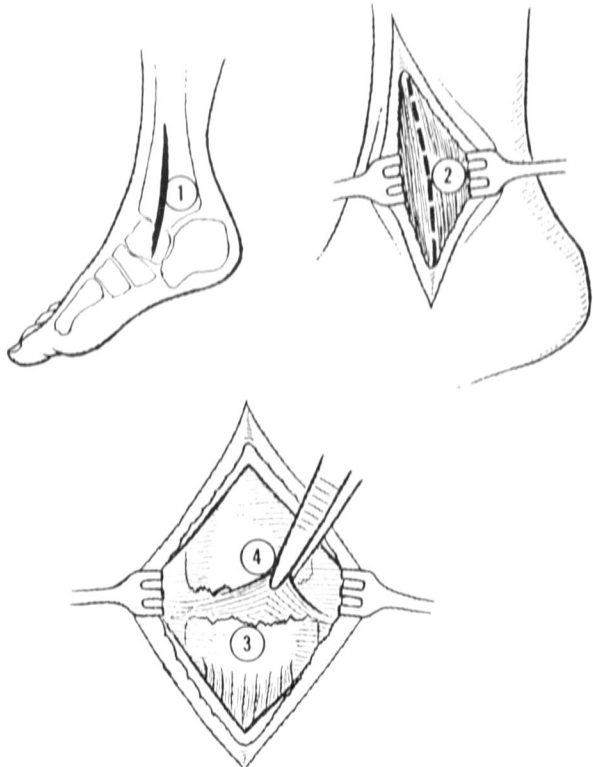

1. Visualize the anterior capsule by inserting a small elevator anteriorly to determine if there is any rupture of the deltoid or capsular structures, which should be repaired to bone. The posterior deep deltoid ligament is also visualized, if necessary, by retracting the posterior tibial tendon forward (see page 1850).

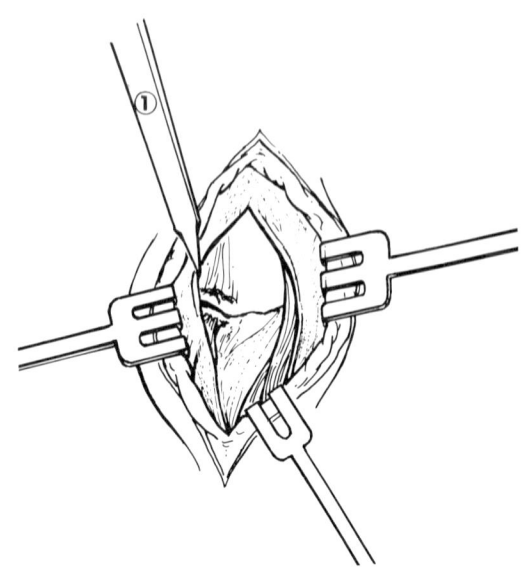

Operative Reduction and Internal Fixation (Continued)

After cleaning out the fracture site with a fine curette,

1. Grasp the malleolar fragment with a towel clip and secure it in its anatomic position.
2. Make a small longitudinal incision through the fibers of the deltoid ligament to expose the tip of the malleolus.
3. Drive a 5-cm screw obliquely through the malleolar fragment and upward into the tibia.

Note: Avoid using compression screws, which tend to split the malleolar fragment.

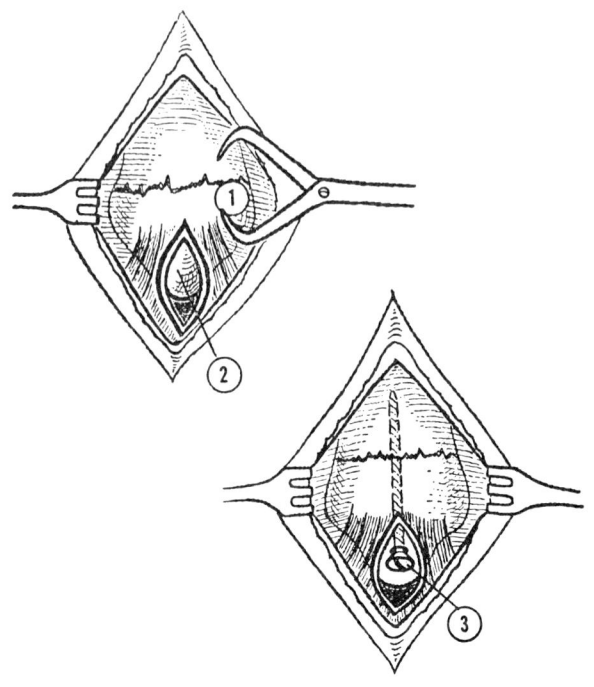

FIXATION OF POSTERIOR TIBIAL ARTICULAR FRACTURE

If the fragment off the posterior tibial articular surface involves more than 25 per cent of the surface, it should be stabilized. This can be done from front to back.

1. Reduction is achieved using Weber's reduction forceps.
2. Two cancellous screws are inserted at slightly different levels using a lag screw effect.

Note: This technique eliminates the need for a posterior approach but may not allow an exact reduction. Fixation is satisfactory to permit early postoperative range-of-motion exercises.

If reduction is not satisfactory by this method, a posterolateral exposure via Henry's approach will permit direct visualization of the fracture. The patient must, however, be prone for this exposure (see page 1893).

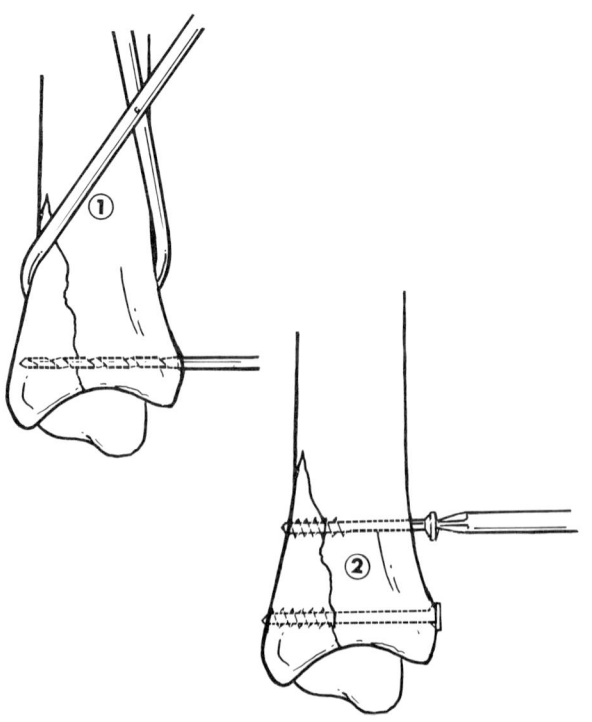

Postreduction X-Ray

P-EX FRACTURE WITH FRACTURE OF THE POSTERIOR ARTICULAR SURFACE

1. The fibula is stabilized by the plate.
2. The distal tibiofibular syndesmosis has been restored by direct suture of the tibiofibular ligament.
3. Restoration of fibula length and alignment has restored the talus to its normal position.
4. The medial malleolus is reduced anatomically and fixed with a screw.
5. The posterior tibial fragment is fixed by a screw inserted from anterior to posterior.

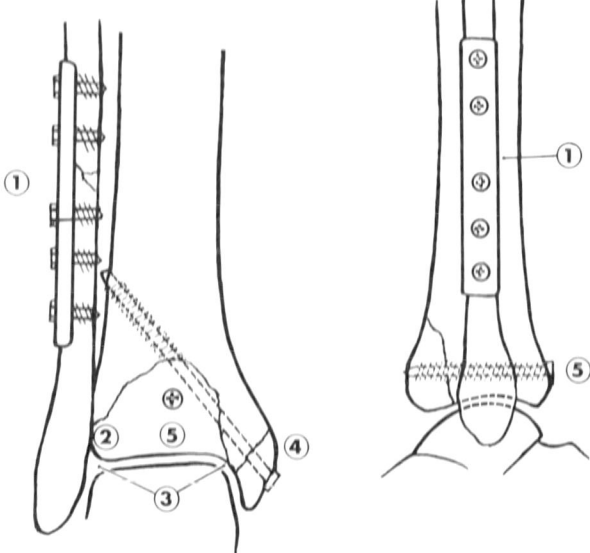

P-AB FRACTURE WITH DISRUPTION OF THE SYNDESMOSIS

1. The fibula has been fixed with a semitubular plate.
2. Avulsion fracture of the tibiofibular ligament is fixed with a screw.
3. The talus has been restored to proper position.
4. The medial malleolar fragment is fixed with a screw.

Note: Reduction can be most accurately evaluated by comparing the talocrural angles in the fractured and unfractured ankles (see page 1843).

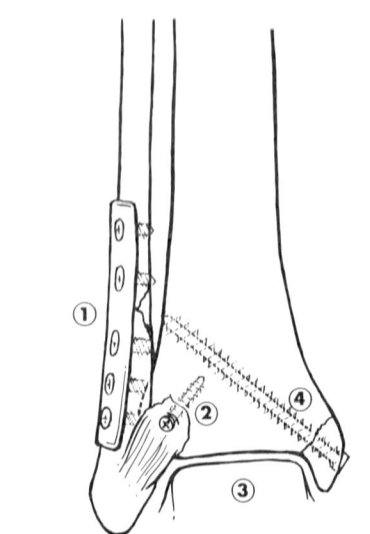

Postoperative Care

1. The ankle is immobilized in a well-padded short leg splint and elevated until the swelling subsides.

By the fourth or fifth day the splint may be removed to begin active movement of the ankle, and by seven to ten days full range of motion is usually regained.

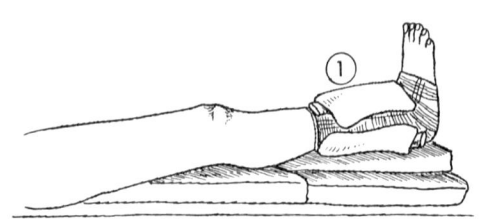

Postoperative Care (Continued)

After full range of motion is achieved the sutures are removed and:
1. A short leg cast is applied.
2. The toes are free.
3. The ankle is at a right angle.
4. The malleoli are well molded.
5. The ankle is in a neutral position in regard to inversion or eversion.

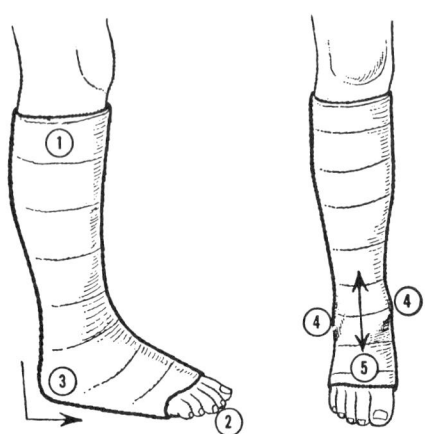

Subsequent Management

The period of cast immobilization depends on the degree of initial injury and the rigidity of fixation achieved by the surgery.

In most instances the patient is able to discard the plaster by six to eight weeks but should continue on crutches for six weeks longer.

Most ankle fractures have healed satisfactorily by the end of twelve weeks, and the patient should be regaining close to normal motion.

The internal fixation need not be removed unless it is causing symptoms.

BIMALLEOLAR FRACTURES

REMARKS

Fractures of both malleoli result most commonly from supination–external rotation (S-EX) mechanisms.

Pronation-abduction (P-AB) mechanisms also produce fractures of both malleoli at or below the level of the syndesmosis.

Both S-EX and P-AB mechanisms cause lateral displacement of the talus.

Supination-adduction (S-AD) mechanisms also cause bimalleolar fractures but tend to produce medial displacement.

Closed reduction is possible with bimalleolar fractures produced by P-AB or S-AD mechanisms without torsional deformity.

S-EX fractures are frequently associated with impingement of the lateral malleolus on the proximal fibula that prevents the talus from resuming its normal anatomic position. Consequently, open reduction of the lateral malleolus is indicated to restore fibular alignment and return the talus to its normal articulation.

The fibular fracture can be stabilized by screws, plates, intramedullary pins, or tension-band wiring.

The medial malleolar fracture should also be stabilized in order to permit early functional ankle exercises.

In all bimalleolar fractures the posterior articular surface of the tibia should be evaluated on x-ray to determine whether it is fractured or injured enough to cause ankle instability.

Fractures of Both Malleoli With Lateral Displacement of the Talus

Prereduction X-Ray

S-EX MECHANISM STAGE IV

1. An oblique spiral fracture of the lateral malleolus runs from the anterior margin in a dorsal proximal direction.
2. The fractures of the medial malleolus and
3. The talus are displaced laterally.
4. The anteromedial clear space of the joint is widened.

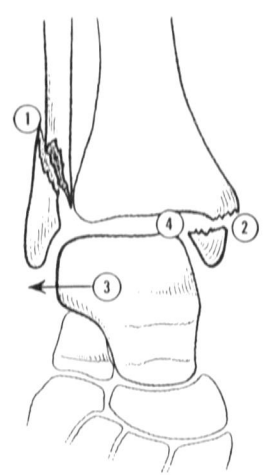

P-AB MECHANISM

1. Fracture of the medial malleolus.
2. Low-transverse supramalleolar fracture of the fibula.
3. The talus is shifted laterally.
4. The anteromedial clear space is widened.

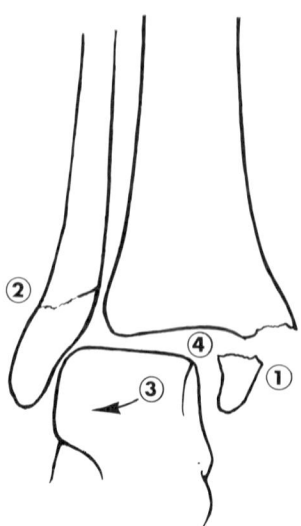

Staging of Injury

Pronation-abduction mechanism produces injury to the ankle in the following stages:

Stage I is a fracture of the medial malleolus or a rupture of the deltoid ligament.

Stage II is a rupture of the distal tibiofibular syndesmosis.

Stage III includes the fracture in the supramalleolar region of the fibula. The fracture is characteristically transverse or slightly oblique and extends in an inferomedial direction.

Note: P-AB mechanisms may rupture the posterior tibiofibular ligament but rarely produce significant fractures of the articular surface.

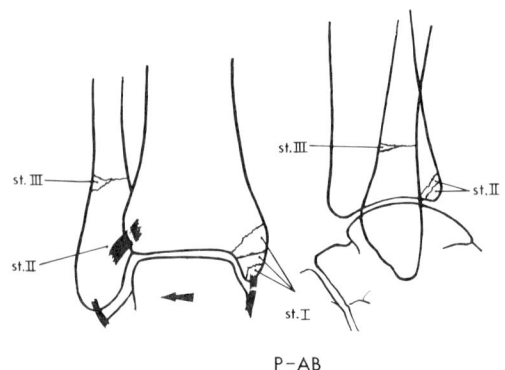

P-AB

Supination-external rotation mechanisms produce injury to the ankle in the following stages:

Stage I is avulsion of the anterior tibiofibular ligament.

Stage II is an oblique spiral fracture of the lateral malleolus running from the anterior edge to the posterosuperior cortex.

Stage III is a fracture of the posterior tibial margin.

Note: It is not necessary for this fracture to occur before the injury advances to a Stage IV fracture.

Stage IV is a fracture of the medial malleolus.

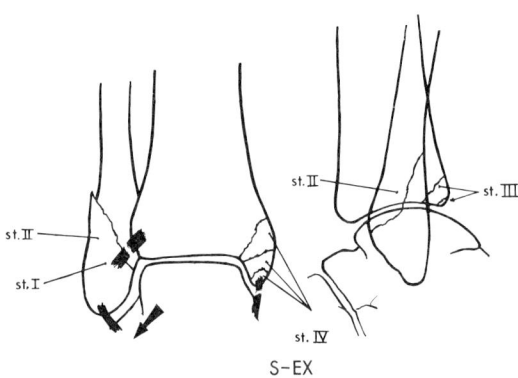

S-EX

FRACTURE OF BOTH MALLEOLI WITH MEDIAL DISPLACEMENT OF THE TALUS: SUPINATION-ADDUCTION (S-AD) FRACTURE

REMARKS

The S-AD mechanism is the only type of ankle fracture producing medial displacement of the talus.

This mechanism may occur in children and cause a type IV epiphyseal fracture.

The resultant asymmetric growth arrest and varus ankle deformity have been discussed on page 251.

Since the tendency is medial displacement, the key determinant of the reduction is the medial malleolus. If this is not satisfactorily returned to normal position, operative fixation is indicated.

Prereduction X-Rays

1. The talus is displaced medially as a result of the mechanism.
2. The medial malleolus has a characteristic shearing fracture.
3. The lateral malleolus is avulsed.

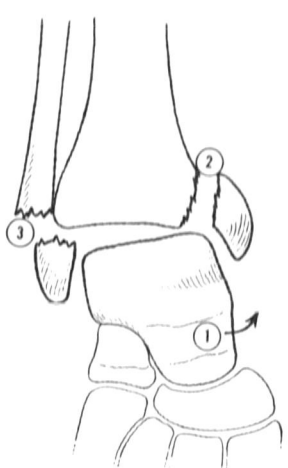

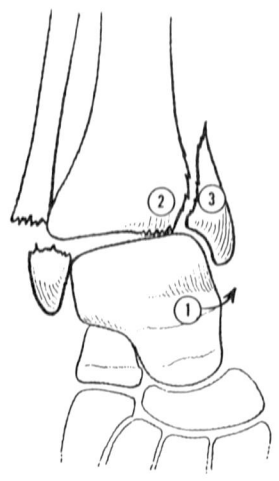

1. The talus is tilted and displaced medially.
2. The fracture line is comminuted and extends around posteriorly.
3. The medial malleolar fragment includes part of the posteromedial articular surface.

S-AD FRACTURE IN A 12-YEAR-OLD BOY

This lesion may cause premature arrest of growth on the medial side of the tibial epiphysis (see page 251).

1. The talus is displaced medially.
2. The medial side of the epiphyseal plate is crushed.
3. The lateral malleolus is avulsed.

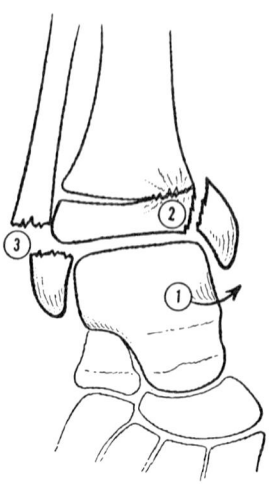

Staging of S-AD Fracture

Stage I includes a fracture of the lateral malleolus at or distal to the level of the tibiotalar joint.

Stage II includes a fracture of the medial malleolus. This may extend posteriorly to involve the articular surface.

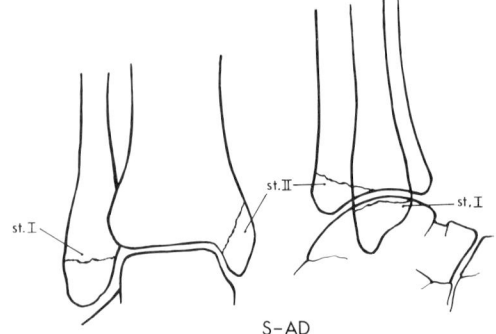

Operative Treatment

Both malleoli should be fixed internally to permit early postoperative range-of-motion exercises.

For a laterally displaced talus, the stability of the fibula is key. For a fracture with medial talar shift, the medial malleolus is of prime concern.

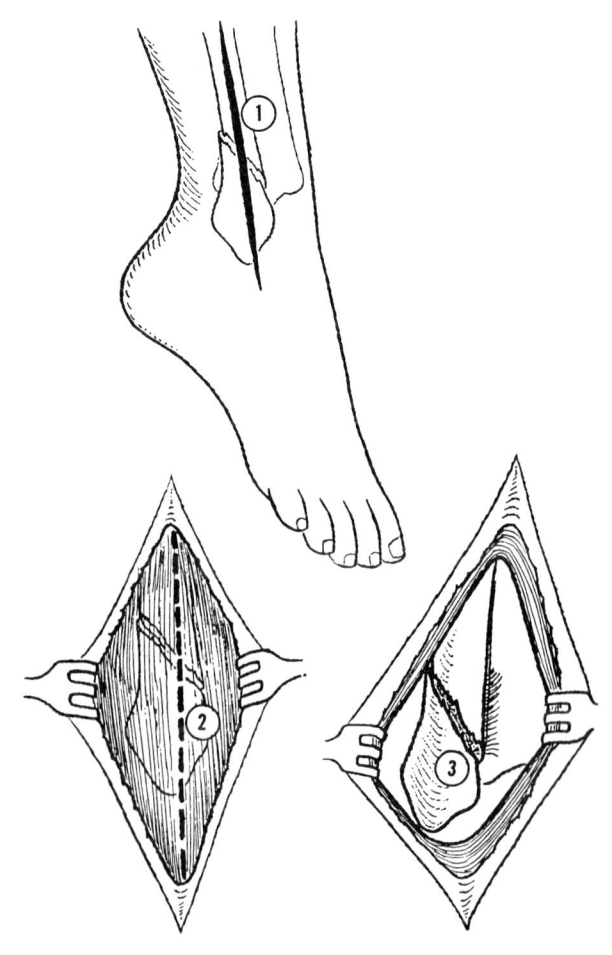

1. Make a vertical incision centered over the fibular fracture, taking care to avoid the superficial peroneal nerve anteriorly and the sural nerve posteriorly.

2. Divide the deep fascia and retract its margins with the skin flaps.
3. Divide the periosteum longitudinally, and by subperiosteal dissection expose the fibula and the fracture site.

1. The distal lateral malleolar fracture is stabilized with a towel clip.

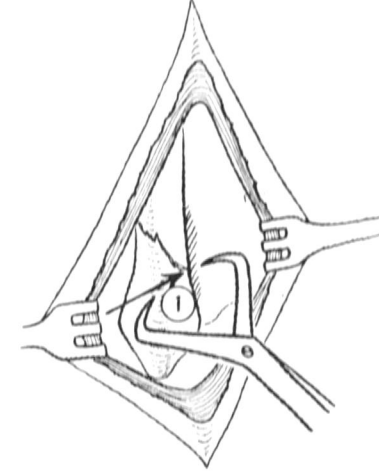

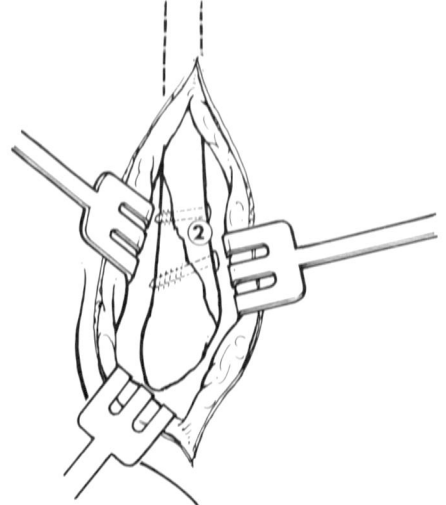

2. The fracture is fixed with two screws or

3. With a five-hole plate with screws or

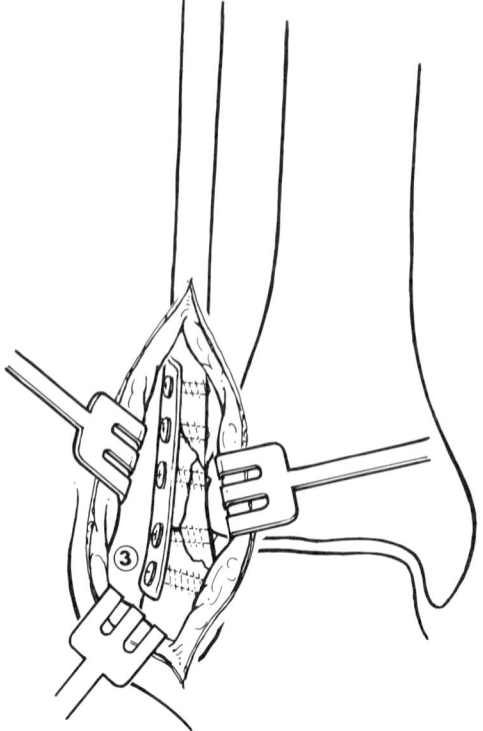

FRACTURES OF THE ANKLE

Operative Treatment *(Continued)*

4. For low fibular fractures, with Kirschner wires and a tension-band wire.

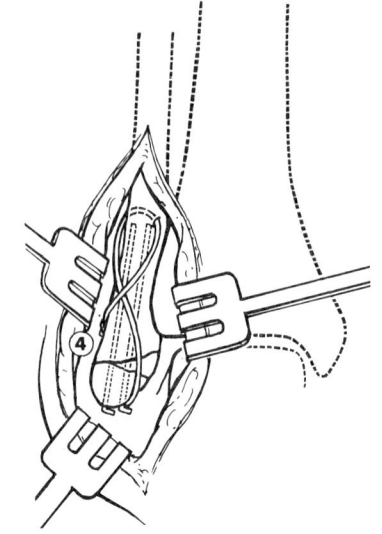

1. If the anterior tibiofibular ligament is disrupted, it should be sutured in its substance or

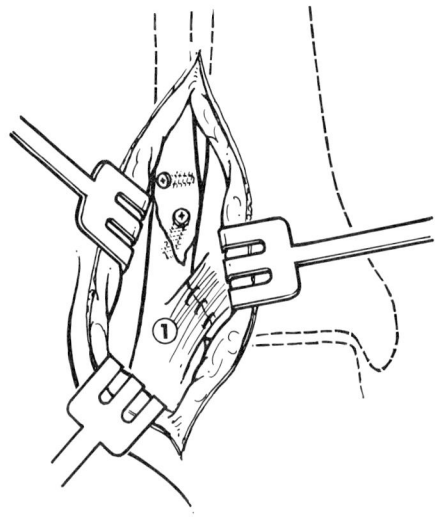

2. At its bony attachment.

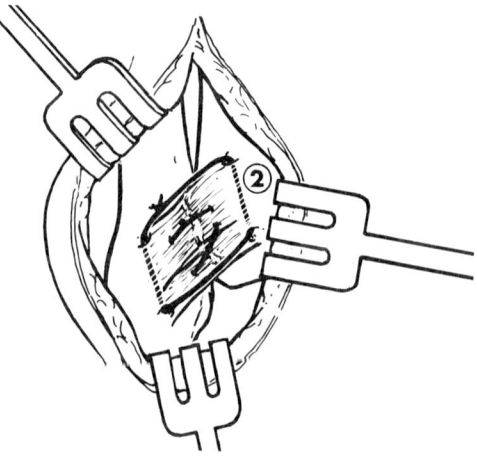

1. Reattachment of the ligament to bone is preferable and can be done by making oblique drill holes in the tibia and fibular cortices.

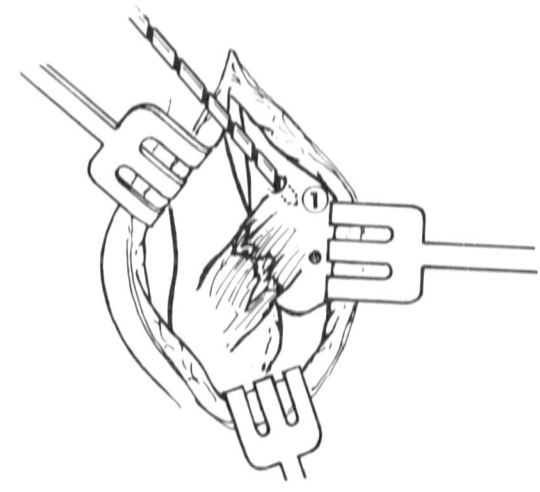

2. After enlarging the hole with a towel clip, the suture is passed through the cortex using a curved needle.

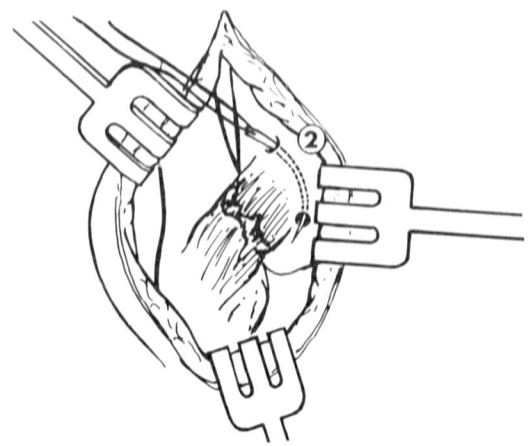

3. Suturing ligament to bone gives a stronger repair than does suturing within the ligament itself.

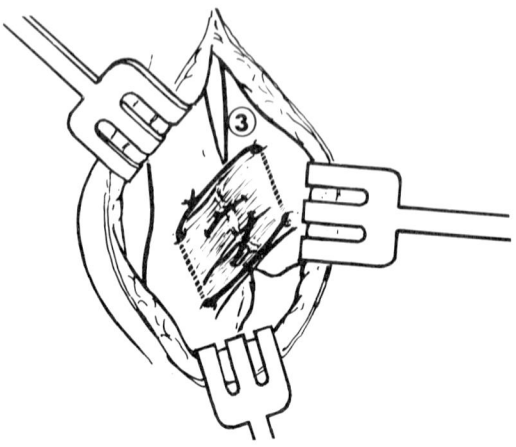

Operative Treatment (Continued)

OPERATIVE REDUCTION OF THE MEDIAL MALLEOLAR FRACTURE

1. Make an anterior incision beginning 2 cm distal to the medial malleolus and extending proximally across the fracture site or
2. If the fracture involves the posterior medial cortex, the incision should be placed posteriorly.

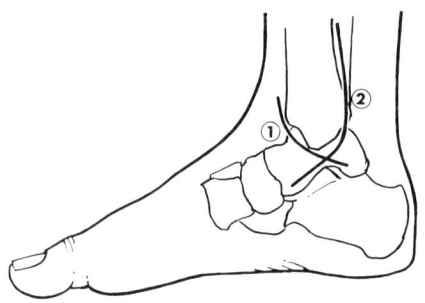

3. Reflect the skin flaps and divide the deep fascia.

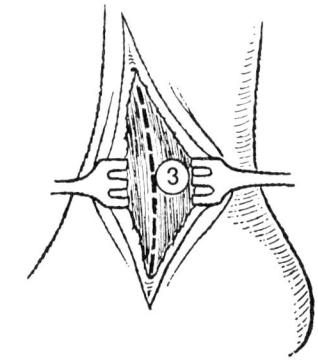

4. Visualize the fracture site and the displaced malleolar fragment.
5. Remove the periosteal flap interposed between the fractured surfaces.

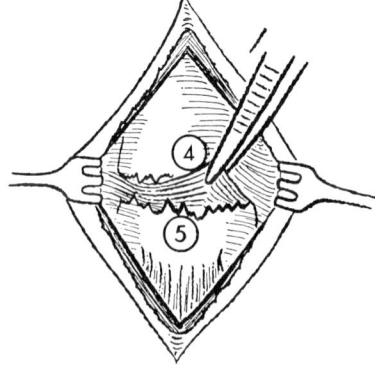

1. Inspect the anterior capsule by inserting a small elevator anteriorly to determine if there is any anterior rupture of the deltoid or capsular structure, which should be repaired to bone.

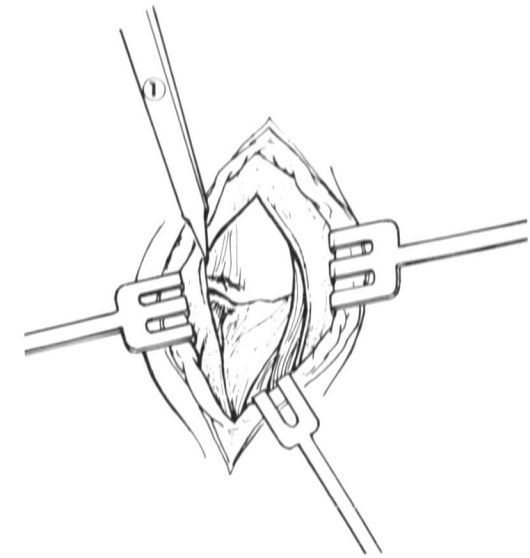

After cleaning out the fracture site with a fine curette:
1. Grasp the malleolar fragment with a towel clip and secure it in its normal anatomic position.
2. Make a small longitudinal incision through the fibers of the deltoid ligament to expose the tip of the malleolus.

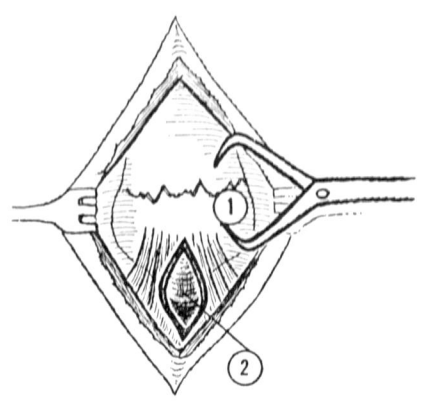

3. Drive a long screw obliquely through the malleolar fragment and the lower end of the tibia.

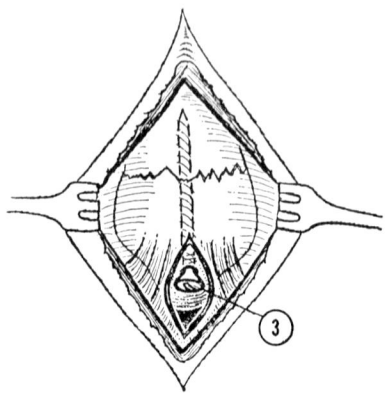

Postreduction X-Ray

1. The medial malleolus is in its normal position and transfixed with a screw.
2. The lateral malleolus has been restored to length and anatomic alignment and is held with two screws.
3. The talus occupies its normal position in the mortise.

Note: Reduction can be most accurately evaluated by comparing the talocrural angles in the fractured and unfractured ankles (see page 1842).

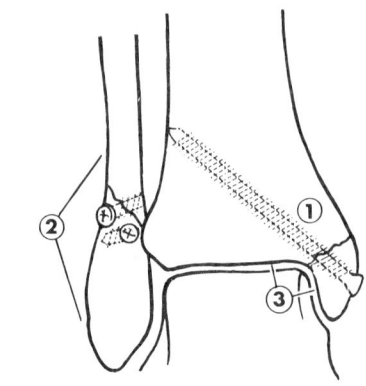

Postoperative Management

1. The ankle is immobilized in a well-padded short leg splint and elevated until the swelling subsides.
2. By the fourth or fifth day the splint may be removed to begin active movement of the ankle, and by seven to ten days full range of motion is usually regained.

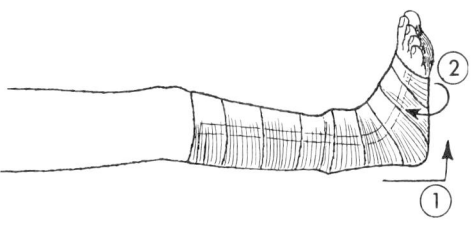

After full range of motion is achieved the sutures are removed and:

1. A short leg cast is applied.
2. The toes are free.
3. The ankle is at a right angle.
4. The malleoli are well molded.
5. The ankle is in a neutral position in regard to inversion or eversion.

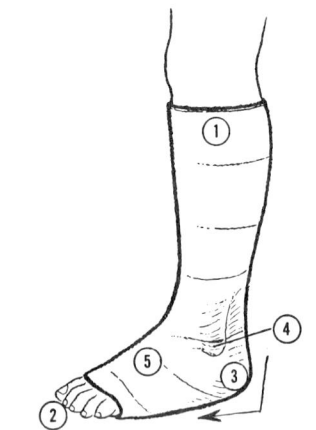

Subsequent Management

The period of cast immobilization depends on the degree of initial injury and the rigidity of fixation achieved by the surgery.

In most instances the patient is able to discard the plaster by six to eight weeks but should continue on crutches for six weeks longer.

Most ankle fractures have healed satisfactorily by the end of twelve weeks and the patient should be regaining full motion.

The internal fixation need not be removed unless it is causing symptoms.

Significance of Injuries to Distal Tibiofibular Ligaments

Injury to the tibiofibular ligaments may cause diastasis but rarely produces symptoms of ankle instability. The anterior tibiofibular ligament must be mobile in order to permit tibial rotation, which is necessary during ankle dorsiflexion (see page 1804).

If diastasis is associated with lateral talar shift, the talus must be reduced. This can be done most effectively by stabilizing any fracture of the fibula and directly suturing the torn anterior tibiofibular ligament.

Avoid fixing the interosseous space with a tibiofibular screw as has been advocated to correct diastasis. This frequently results in loss of ankle motion.

Occasionally, external torsional injuries will produce a diastasis of the ankle associated with a Maisonneuve fracture of the proximal fibula. Even with the severe types of this injury, it is primarily the lateral displacement of the talus, not the ankle diastasis, that causes problems and must be corrected. This can be done most effectively by internal fixation of the fibula and direct suture of the injured ligaments rather than by transosseous screw fixation.

Occasionally, transosseous screw fixation is necessary for a chronic malunited ankle, in which it is the only method of correcting lateral talar displacement.

A fairly common source of disability from injuries to the distal tibiofibular syndesmosis occurs with ankylosis and loss of mobility rather than diastasis.

1. Bony ankylosis from an injury to the distal tibiofibular syndesmosis causes ankle stiffness and pain with prolonged walking.

Note: These ankle symptoms can be relieved by excision of the bony ankylosis and interposition of a free fat graft between the distal fibula and tibia in order to restore ankle mobility.

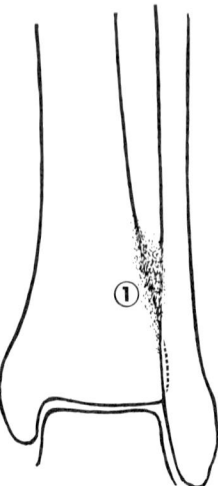

CHRONIC DIASTASIS AND MALUNION TREATED WITH TRANSOSSEOUS SCREW FIXATION

Preoperative X-Ray

1. A chronic malunion of an ankle injury has resulted from fibular shortening and
2. Lateral displacement of the talus with the fibula.

Note: In order to correct the lateral displacement of the talus, the fibula must be repositioned and fixed internally. Fibula and tibia screw fixation can aid in repositioning the talus in its normal articulation with the tibia (see also page 1841).

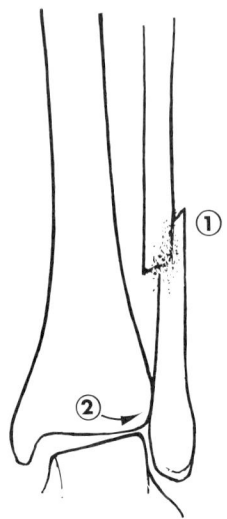

Postoperative X-Ray

1. The fibula has been osteotomized and is held with a plate.
2. Additional support is achieved by a screw between the fibula and tibia.
3. Correct realignment of the talus and the mortise has been achieved.

Note: The transosseous screw should be removed at eight to ten weeks to allow normal rotation of the distal tibiofibular joint during ankle motion and to avoid breakage of the screw.

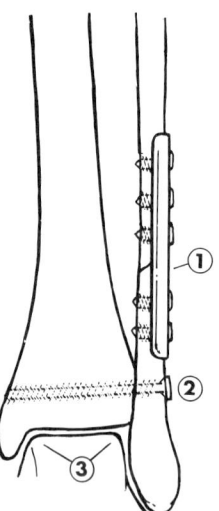

MAISONNEUVE FRACTURE OF THE PROXIMAL FIBULA BY DIASTASIS OF THE ANKLE

According to Pankovich, this injury is more common than generally appreciated. Forceful external rotation of the foot produces the lesion in five stages.

1. Rupture of the anterior tibiofibular ligament or avulsion of its bony insertion, usually associated with rupture of the interosseous ligament.
2. Fracture of the posterior tibial tuberosity or rupture of the posterior tibiofibular ligament.
3. Rupture of the anteromedial joint capsule or avulsion fracture of its bony insertion.
4. Fracture of the fibula in its proximal third.
5. Rupture of the deltoid ligament or fracture of the medial malleolus.

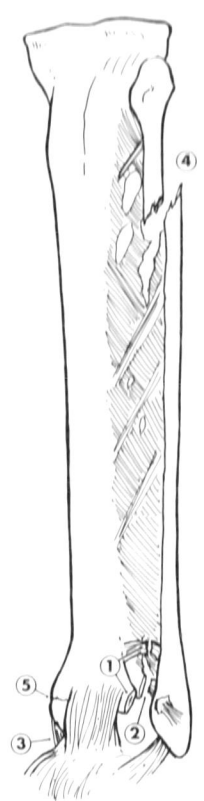

Clinical Evaluation

The Maisonneuve fracture may be easily overlooked.

The examiner should look carefully for a lesion of the proximal fibula if there is: (1) an isolated fracture of the posterior tibial tubercle, particularly with associated anteromedial capsular tenderness; (2) deltoid ligament rupture or fracture of the medial malleolus without a fracture of the lateral malleolus; or (3) tenderness over the syndesmosis and anteromedial capsule.

Management

Most Maisonneuve fractures of the proximal fibula with diastasis of the ankle can be treated by cast immobilization for three weeks.

For the more advanced stages of this lesion, particularly if there is wide diastasis and instability of the ankle, operative fixation is indicated.

The lateral support should be restored first by repairing the tibiofibular ligament. The intraosseous ligament may also be sutured, but transosseous screw fixation should be avoided. It is usually unnecessary if adequate ligamentous suturing is accomplished.

Following repair of the lateral ligaments, the anteromedial capsule is repaired by a separate incision.

Preoperative X-Ray

1. A Maisonneuve fracture of the proximal fibula associated with
2. Wide diastasis of the distal tibiofibula syndesmosis and
3. Avulsion of the deltoid ligament.

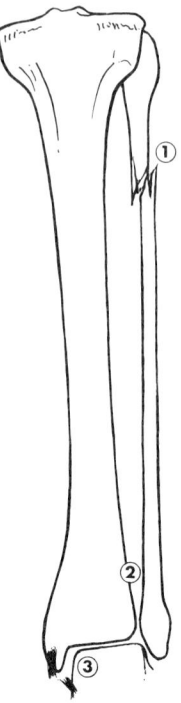

Postoperative X-Ray

1. The widening of the distal tibiofibular joint has been reduced by repair of the anterior ligament and
2. Repair of the deltoid ligament.
3. The anteromedial clear space of the mortise has been restored to normal.
4. The proximal fibula fracture need not be stabilized.

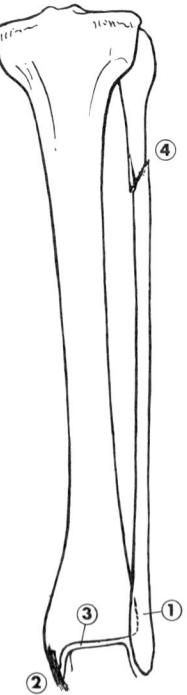

POSTERIOR DISLOCATION OF THE FOOT WITH POSTERIOR MARGINAL FRACTURE OF THE TIBIA

REMARKS

Posterior marginal fractures most often result from external torsion whereby the posterior tibiofibular ligament is avulsed with its tibial attachment. The resultant fracture is off the posterolateral portion of the articular surface.

The mechanisms that produce these posterior marginal fractures are the supination–external rotation (S-EX), the pronation–external rotation (P-EX), and the supination-adduction (S-AD) types.

Most often with the S-EX mechanism, the fragment is fairly small, i.e., less than 25 per cent of the surface, and does not usually produce ankle instability.

With a P-EX mechanism, the posterior tibial fracture is likely to involve more than 25 per cent of the surface and to contribute to instability.

In adolescents, the P-EX mechanism will produce a two-fragment epiphyseal fracture in which the lateral fragment includes part of the epiphysis and the posterior tibial metaphysis, which displace posterolaterally. The medial malleolar portion of the epiphysis remains in continuity with the tibial shaft.

Infrequently, the posterior marginal fracture may result from an S-AD mechanism, which characteristically involves the posteromedial surface. This fragment is part of the medial malleolar fracture and can be fixed in the process of the malleolar fixation.

In most instances, stable fixation of the posterior articular surface can be achieved with screws inserted from anterior to posterior at the time of fixation of the lateral malleolus. Reduction of the lateral malleolus helps to stabilize the posterior fragment still attached by the posterior tibiofibular ligament.

If the posterior fragment requires direct visualization, the posterior approach of Henry allows excellent exposure but requires that the patient be in the prone position.

Types and Mechanisms

S-EX MECHANISM STAGE IV

Prereduction X-Ray

1. The spiral oblique fracture of the lateral malleolus is characteristic of the S-EX mechanisms.
2. The medial malleolus has been avulsed.
3. The talus is shifted laterally and posteriorly with the lateral malleolus.
4. The posterior marginal fracture and
5. The talus have both displaced posteriorly.
6. The articular surfaces of the talus and the tibia are not congruous.

Staging of Injury

The supination–external rotation mechanism injures the ankle in the following stages:

Stage I is a disruption of the anterior tibiofibular ligament.

Stage II is the oblique spiral fracture of the lateral malleolus running from the anterior margin in the dorsal proximal direction at the level of the tibiotalar joint.

Stage III is a fracture of the posterior tibial margin. This is usually the result of avulsion by the posterior tibiofibular ligament, whcih remains attached to the lateral malleolus.

Note: Only about 14 per cent of posterior fracture fragments associated with S-EX mechanisms involve more than 25 per cent of the joint surface and produce instability.

Stage IV is the fracture of the medial malleolus or, sometimes, a rupture of the deltoid.

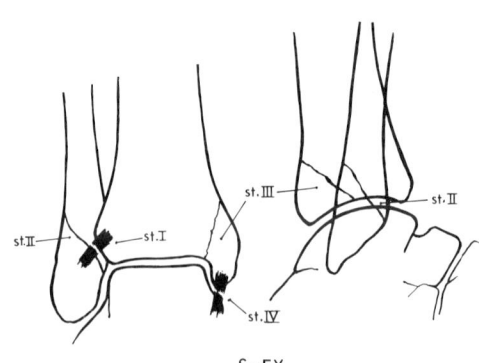

S-EX

P-EX MECHANISM STAGE III

Prereduction X-Ray

1. Avulsion of the medial malleolus.
2. Fracture of the shaft of the fibula above the syndesmosis running obliquely from anterior edge in a posteroinferior direction.
3. Lateral displacement of the talus.
4. The fracture of the fibula at the high level indicates rupture of the tibiofibular ligament; diastasis of the tibiofibular joint results.
5. Posterior marginal fracture of the tibia.
6. Posterolateral displacement of the talus, which follows the displaced lateral malleolus.

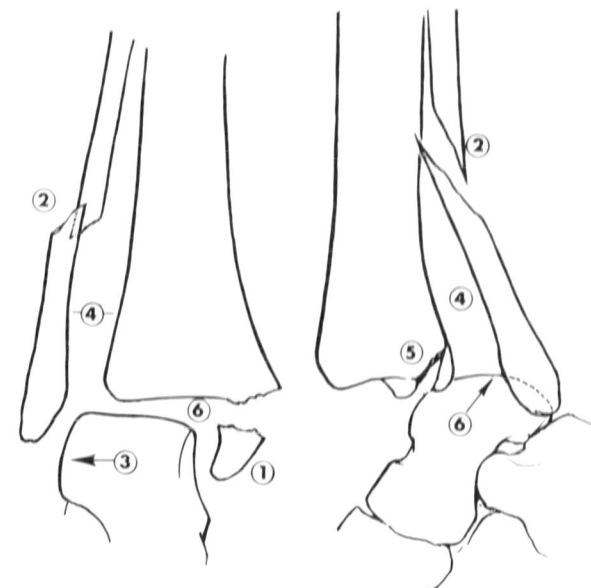

Staging of Injury

P-EX mechanisms produce the following stages of injury:

Stage I is a fracture of the medial malleolus or rupture of the deltoid.

Stage II is rupture of the distal tibial syndesmosis. Stage II also is associated with a fracture of the posterior tibial margin due to avulsion by the tibiofibular ligament. In many instances this involves more than 25 per cent of the joint surface and causes posterolateral instability.

Stage III produces a high fracture of the fibula above the syndesmosis, which characteristically runs from the anterior fibular margin in a dorsal-distal direction.

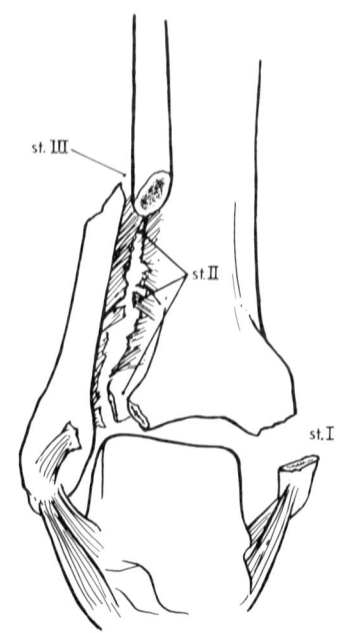

P-EX EPIPHYSEAL FRACTURE IN AN ADOLESCENT

Prereduction X-Ray

1. Anteroposterior tomogram shows a fracture through the epiphysis with displacement.
2. The medial malleolar portion remains in continuity with the tibial shaft.
3. The lateral portion of the epiphysis displaces externally.

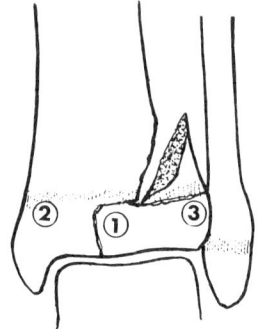

4. On lateral x-ray, the medial malleolus displaces anteriorly with the shaft, and
5. The lateral fragment, including the remainder of the epiphysis and a portion of the posterior metaphysis, is displaced posteriorly.
6. The fibula is usually intact but may be fractured and angulated anteriorly.

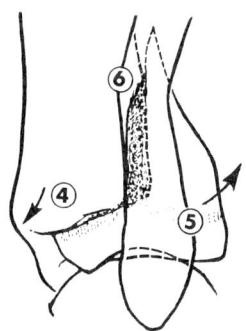

Staging of Injury

Pronation and external rotation in an adolescent leads to a different sequence from that in adults.

Stage I is a rupture of the anterior tibiofibular ligament.

Stage II is a type III epiphyseal fracture.

Stage III is a fracture up through the posterior metaphysis with posterior displacement of the lateral epiphyseal fragment, the metaphyseal fragment, and the fibula.

Stage IV is a greenstick fracture of the fibula with anterior angulation due to the posterior displacement of the fragment.

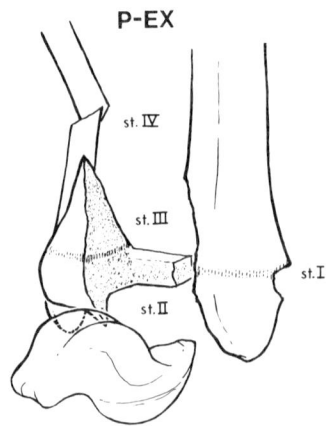

S-AD MECHANISM STAGE II

Prereduction X-Ray

1. Avulsion of the lateral malleolus.
2. Shearing of the medial malleolus.
3. The talus is displaced medially.

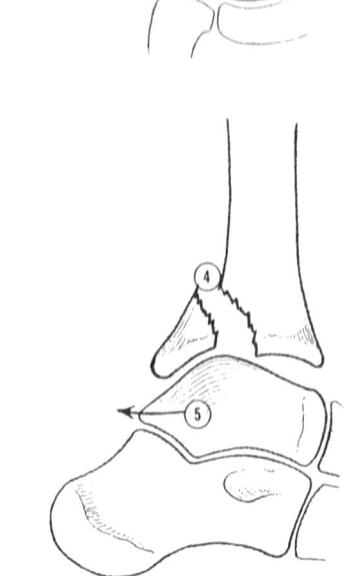

4. Posterior marginal fracture of the tibia.
5. Posterior displacement of the talus.

Staging of Injury

Supination-adduction mechanism injures the ankle in the following stages:

Stage I is a fracture of the lateral malleolus at or distal to the level of the tibiotalar joint, or rupture of the anterior talofibular and calcaneofibular ligaments.

Stage II is a fracture of the medial malleolus, usually of an oblique nature. The S-AD mechanism involves the posteromedial articular surface rather than the posterolateral articular surface.

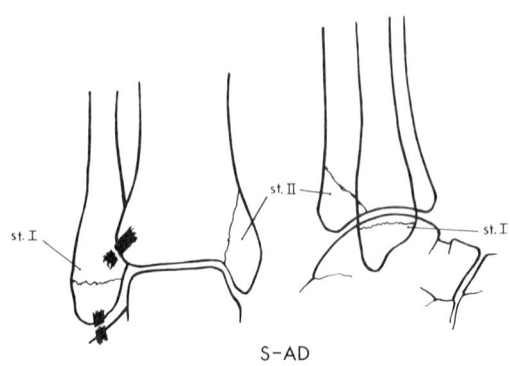

Operative Reduction for Posterior Marginal Fractures

Indications

The majority of these fractures with posterior dislocation of the talus are unstable and require fixation of the posterior marginal fracture for adequate stability of the ankle.

The distal epiphyseal fracture in the adolescent may generally be treated by a closed method, but the reduction should be anatomic. If the epiphyseal fracture is associated with a fibular fracture, operative reduction is usually necessary.

The fractures of the lateral and medial malleoli are fixed first as described on page 1866. Stabilization of the fibula frequently adds stability to the posterolateral articular fragment because the posterior tibiofibular ligament remains intact.

The posterolateral articular fracture may then be fixed with two screws inserted from the anteromedial cortex.

If adequate reduction is not possible by this method, the posterolateral fracture may be exposed via Henry's posterolateral approach. The patient, however, must be positioned prone for this approach.

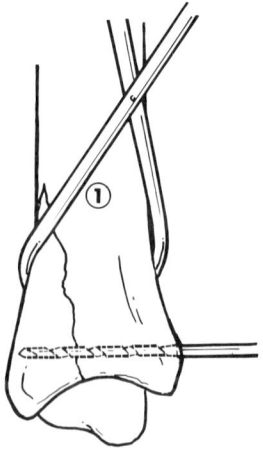

Operative Technique

Note: The medial and the lateral malleoli are fixed under direct vision as described on page 1866.

1. Reduction of the posterolateral fragment is achieved using Weber's reduction forceps.

2. Two cancellous screws are inserted at slightly different levels from the anteromedial cortex using the lag screw effect.

Note: If reduction by this method is not satisfactory, the posterolateral exposure by Henry's approach will permit direct visualization of the fracture.

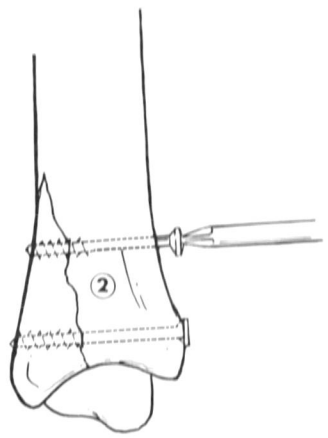

Alternate Procedure: Henry Approach

The patient lies in a prone position. Place a sandbag under the foot.

1. Make a 9-cm incision just lateral to the Achilles tendon; begin the incision at the level of the lateral malleolus.

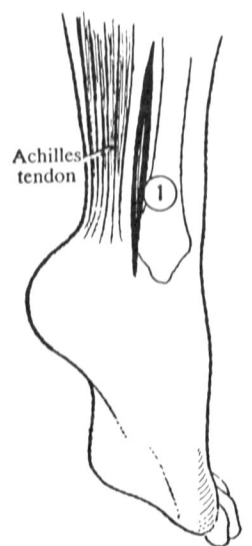

2. Divide the fascia and retract it with skin flaps, exposing the peroneal tendons and the flexor hallucis longus muscle.
3. Divide longitudinally the fascia covering the flexor hallucis longus muscle.
4. Make a longitudinal incision through the lateral fibers of the flexor hallucis longus and the periosteum of the tibia.
5. By subperiosteal dissection expose the distal end of the tibia and the fracture site.
6. Retract the tendon of the flexor hallucis longus and the Achilles tendon medially.

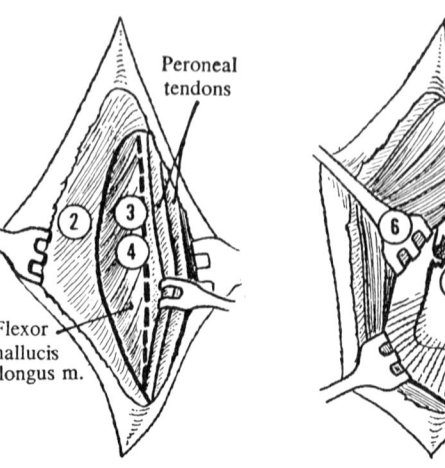

Alternate Procedure: Henry Approach (Continued)

To expose the fibular fracture:
1. Dissect laterally, taking care to avoid the sural nerve.
2. Retract the peroneal tendons posteriorly to visualize the fracture.
3. Apply a five-hole plate to the fracture.

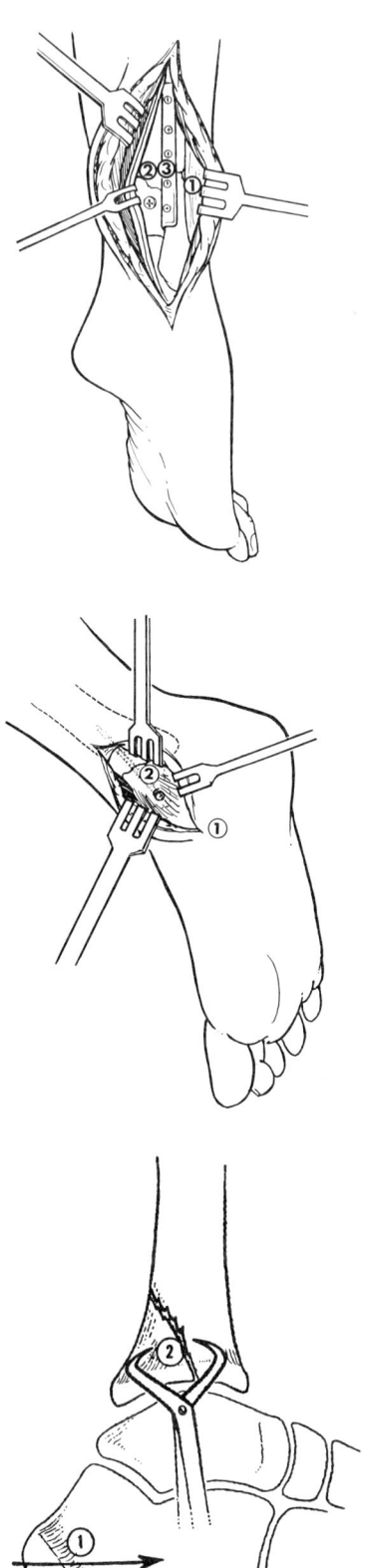

To expose a medial malleolar fracture:
1. Make a second incision over the medial fracture site.
2. Reduce and fix the medial malleolus with a 5-cm screw.

After fixation of the lateral and medial fractures,
1. Reduce the posterior dislocation of the talus by forward traction on the foot.
2. Grasp the posterior marginal fragment with a towel clip and pull it into its normal position.

1. Hold the fragment in position and
2. Fix the fragment with one or two screws directed anteromedially into the tibial shaft.

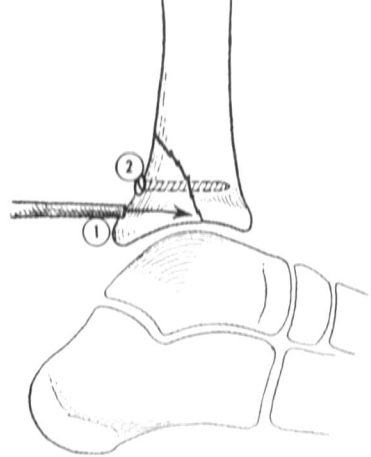

Postreduction X-Ray

Lateral view

1. The posterior fragment is restored to its anatomic position.
2. The talus fits accurately under the tibia.
3. The articular surfaces of the talus and the tibia are congruous.

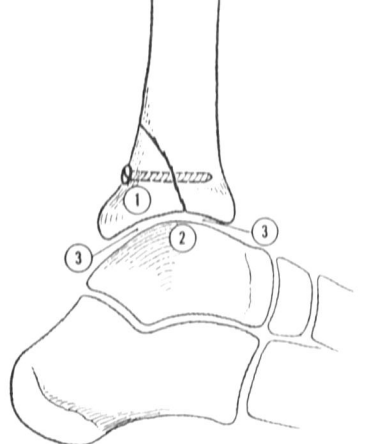

Anteroposterior view

1. The fibular fracture has been stabilized with the plate.
2. The medial malleolar fracture is fixed with a screw.
3. The talus is in its normal position in the mortise.

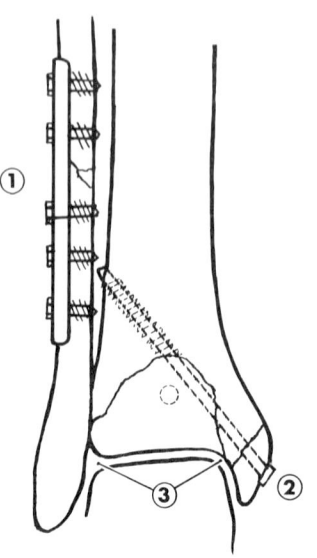

Postoperative Care

1. The ankle is immobilized in a well-padded short leg splint and elevated until the swelling subsides.
2. By the fourth or fifth day the splint may be removed to begin active movement of the ankle, and by seven to ten days full range of motion is usually regained.

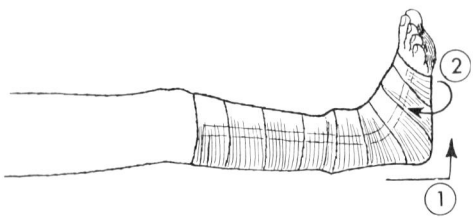

After full range of motion is achieved, the sutures are removed and:
1. A short leg cast is applied.
2. The toes are free.
3. The ankle is at a right angle.
4. The malleoli are well-molded.
5. The ankle is in a neutral position in regard to inversion and eversion.

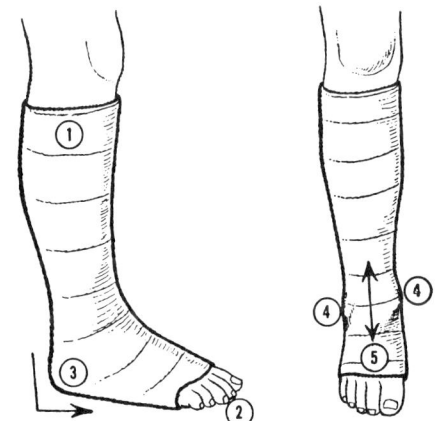

Subsequent Management

The period of cast immobilization depends on the degree of initial injury and the rigidity of fixation achieved by the surgery.

In most instances the patient is able to discard the plaster by six to eight weeks but should continue on crutches for six weeks longer.

Most ankle fractures have healed satisfactorily by the end of twelve weeks and the patient should be regaining full motion.

The internal fixation need not be removed unless it is causing symptoms.

Two-Fragment Fracture of the Distal Tibial Epiphysis in Adolescents

REMARKS

This injury results from the common pronation–external rotation mechanism in an adolescent with a partially fused distal tibial epiphysis (see page 1890).

Characteristically there is a two-fragment fracture, which consists of:
1. A medial fragment including the tibial shaft, the medial malleolus and anteromedial part of the epiphysis, and
2. The lateral fragment including the remainder of the epiphysis and the posterior tibial metaphysis with the attached fibula.

Reduction

This fracture, which results from external torsional mechanisms, can frequently be reduced by internally rotating the ankle.

As with the adult injury, it is particularly important that the articular surface be restored to normal.

If the fibula has been fractured or angulated, closed reduction may not be possible. Open reduction and screw fixation of the lateral tibial epiphyseal fracture then become necessary.

Prereduction X-Ray

1. A widely displaced two-fragment fracture in a 14-year-old boy.
2. The greenstick fracture of the fibula with anterior displacement of the tibial shaft and medial malleolus makes closed reduction difficult.

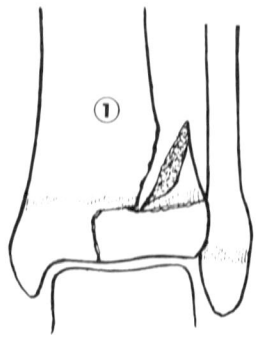
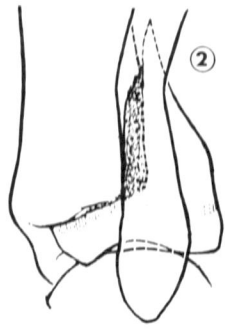

Postreduction X-Ray

1. The epiphyseal fracture has been reduced under direct vision and
2. Is fixed with screws inserted transversely across the bony epiphysis in the younger adolescent or
3. From the anterolateral cortex to the posteromedial cortex in the older adolescent with a closing epiphyseal plate.

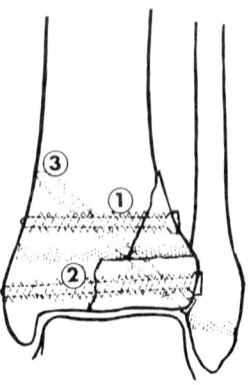

PRONATION-DORSIFLEXION INJURIES

Anterior Marginal Fractures with Anterior Subluxation of the Talus

REMARKS

These fractures are invariably produced by forceful dorsiflexion of the ankle as in a fall from a height or in an automobile collision.

If the foot is pronated at the time of dorsiflexion injury, the talus acts as a wedge against the anterior and medial articular surfaces. Lauge-Hansen described this as an additional mechanism of pronation and dorsiflexion that is characterized by a large fragment torn from the anterior tibial lip with forward subluxation of the talus and a fracture of the base of the medial malleolus.

These injuries, although infrequent, can be among the most difficult ankle fractures to manage. The fracture tends to explode the articular surface, so that traumatic arthritis is the common sequela.

In selecting management, one should distinguish pronation-dorsiflexion fractures from other types of comminuted distal tibial fractures, particularly those produced by external or internal torsion. These other injuries are entirely different from the pronation dorsiflexion injury both in mechanism and in prognosis.

Pathology

Pronation-dorsiflexion injuries occur in four stages:

Stage I is fracture of the medial malleolus (1).

Stage II is avulsion of a large fragment from the anterior lip of the tibia (2).

Note: Because of this fracture the lateral tibial plafond remains attached to the fibula and displaces with it. This is in contrast to the usual fibular fracture proximal to the syndesmosis, which is associated with diastasis of the fibulotibial articulation (see page 1863).

Stage III is a supramalleolar fracture of the fibula. Characteristically the fibula angulates posteriorly as the talus displaces anteriorly (3).

Stage IV is a transverse fracture of the tibia at the level of the proximal margin of the anterior tibial fragment (4).

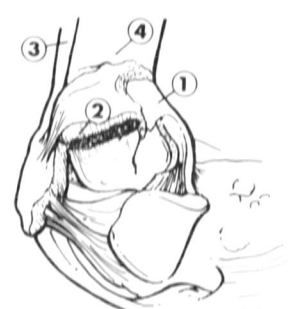

Appearance on X-Ray

1. Fracture of the medial malleolus.
2. Comminuted fracture of the anterior margin of the tibia.
3. Forward displacement of the talus with the marginal fracture.
4. The lateral tibial cortex remains attached to the fibula.
5. The fibula angulates posteriorly as the talus displaces anteriorly.

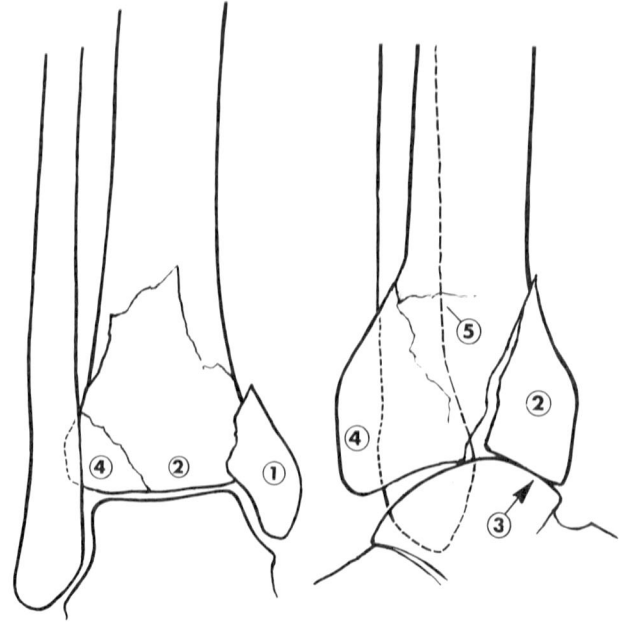

Appearance on X-Ray (Continued)

In children the mechanism produces:
1. A type II fracture of the distal tibial epiphysis with
2. An anterior marginal fracture from the tibial metaphysis and
3. A greenstick fracture in the supramalleolar region of the fibula with posterior angulation.
4. An impacted or torus fracture of the distal tibial metaphysis.

Note: These fractures in children heal uneventfully by closed reduction techniques. In adults, the key to reduction is to reduce and hold the anterior marginal fracture of the tibia, which is allowing anterior subluxation of the talus.

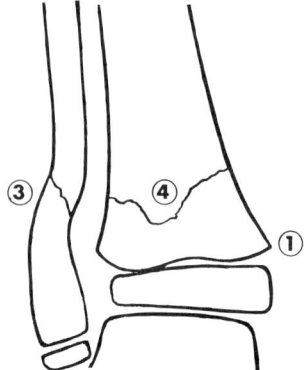

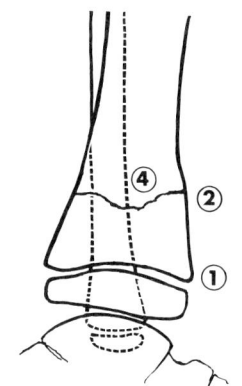

DIFFERENTIAL DIAGNOSIS OF PRONATION-DORSIFLEXION FRACTURES

REMARKS

A pronation-dorsiflexion injury should be distinguished from fractures of the distal tibia produced by external or internal rotation mechanisms.

With these injuries the talus displaces with the fibula. This is in contrast to pronation-dorsiflexion injuries in which the talus displaces anteriorly with the cortical fracture of the articular surface of the tibia.

Pronation — External Rotation Fracture of the Distal Tibia

Prereduction X-Ray

1. Fracture of the medial malleolus or avulsion of the deltoid ligament.

2. Compression fracture of the lateral palfond of the distal tibia rather than an avulsion of the tibiofibular ligament.

Note: In this fracture the lateral tibial plafond remains attached to the fibula and displaces with it. Consequently the talus rotates posterolaterally with the fibula rather than anteriorly with the anterior cortical margin. This displacement also contrasts with the usual fibula fracture proximal to the syndesmosis associated with diastasis of the tibiofibular articulation (see page 1863).

3. Fracture of the fibula above the syndesmosis is characterized by an oblique pattern running from the posteroinferior to the anterosuperior cortex.

4. Fracture of the tibial metaphysis above the level of the articular surface fracture.

Note: The key to reducing this fracture is to restore and stabilize the fibula to length.

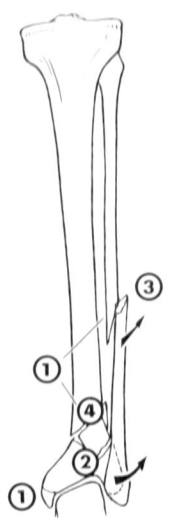

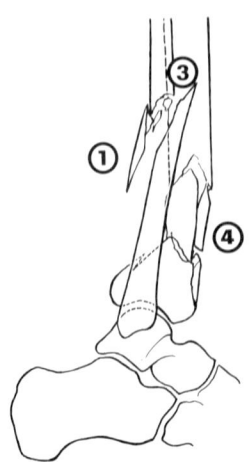

X-Ray After Stabilization

1. Intramedullary pin fixation of the fibula restores length and rotational alignment to the lateral support of the ankle.
2. The lateral plafond fracture, which is still attached to the fibula, is reduced by reduction of the fibula.
3. The talus is restored from its displaced position by reduction of the fibula.
4. The metaphyseal fracture of the tibia can be treated by closed means.

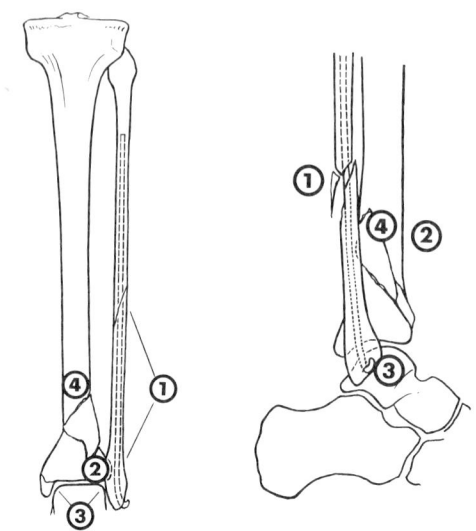

INTERNAL ROTATION FRACTURE OF THE TIBIA

Other comminuted fractures of the distal tibial shaft that can be confused with pronation-dorsiflexion injuries are those resulting from internal torsional mechanisms.

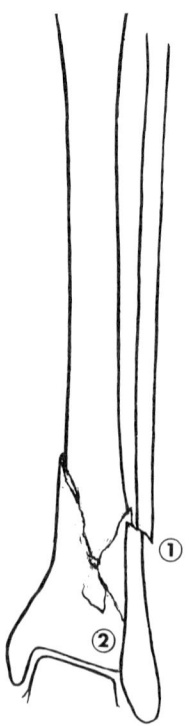

Prereduction X-Ray

1. Fracture of the fibula at or below the level of the tibia or, occasionally, an intact fibula.
2. A comminuted fracture of tibia running from the distal lateral to proximal medial cortex.

Note: These fractures, which are produced by internal torsional mechanism, are reduced by external rotation of the distal fragment. Stabilization of the fibular fracture will not aid in reduction and may frequently promote "varus drift" of the fracture.

Postreduction X-Ray

Comminuted fracture of the distal tibia produced by internal torsional mechanisms is reduced closed by externally rotating the distal fragment.

1. Reduction and cast immobilization with the foot externally rotated prevents "varus drift" of the fracture.
2. The fibular fracture need not be fixed internally.

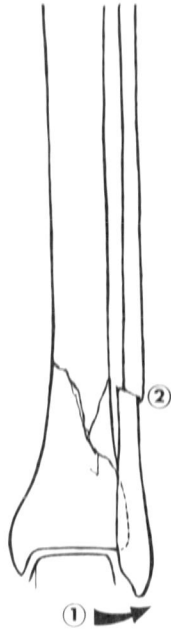

MANAGEMENT OF PRONATION-DORSIFLEXION EXPLOSION INJURIES

REMARKS

The intra-articular fractures of the distal tibia described on page 1898 are among the most difficult to treat surgically.

Skin sloughing is common after open reduction in these injuries because of the significant associated soft tissue swelling. Elevation of the limb from an overhead frame for several days may be wise prior to any operation.

Before embarking on operative intervention, carefully analyze the x-ray to determine the degree of fracture comminution. Tomograms are quite helpful for this purpose.

The major objective of operative fixation is to stabilize the key fragments within the mortise and not necessarily any of the tibial shaft fracture. Bone grafting may be added to fill in any large defect resulting from crushing of the metaphysis.

If the fibula is intact the chance for adequate stabilization of the tibial fracture is improved. An intact fibula generally indicates that both the posterior and lateral cortices of the tibia are also intact.

Operative Management

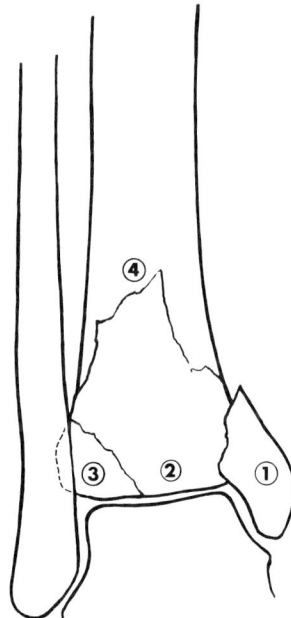

Preoperative X-Ray

1. Fracture of the medial malleolus.
2. Anterior cortical fragment allowing anterior subluxation of the talus.
3. The lateral tibial plafond remains attached to the fibula.
4. Metaphyseal fracture without fracture of the posterior tibial cortex.

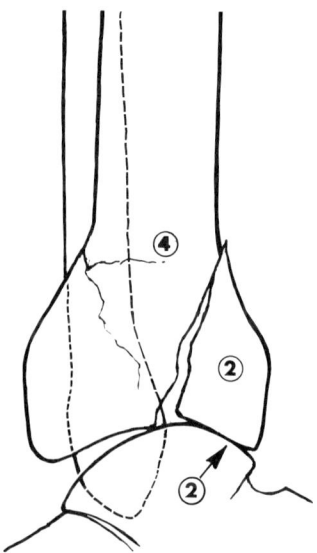

Postoperative X-Ray

1. The small fragments on the anterior cortex are fixed first with Kirschner wires.
2. Major fragments from the anterior cortex and the medial malleolus are fixed with screws.
3. Fixation of the metaphyseal fracture is not necessary once the key fragments have stabilized. Occasionally, cancellous bone grafting may be necessary to fill in defects in the metaphysis.

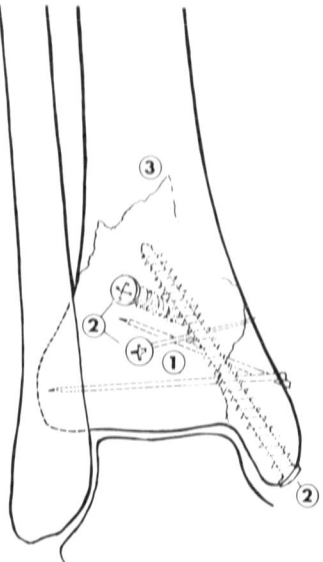

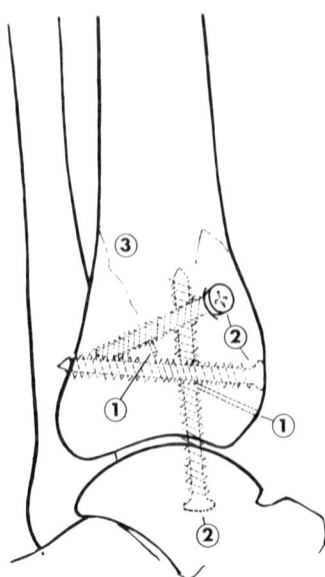

Supplemental Fixation with Skeletal Traction

If the stability of the articular surface is insecure after internal fixation, do not traumatize or disrupt the circulation to the bone fragments by further attempts at fixation. This only adds to the likelihood of ischemic necrosis and collapse of the metaphyseal support.

Skeletal traction can be applied postoperatively using a pin inserted into the os calcis. This supplements the operative fixation of the mortise and allows a guarded range of motion exercise program postoperatively.

Postoperative Skeletal Traction

1. A skeletal pin is inserted through the calcaneus.
2. A Salvatori* traction bow is hinged so as to allow ankle motion without torquing the pin.

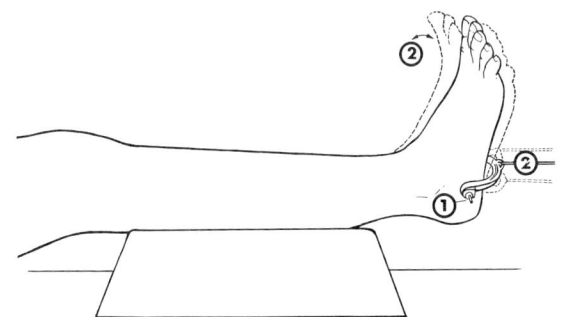

Postoperative Management

The fracture is suspended in traction immediately postoperatively and the patient is allowed to start guarded range-of-motion exercises by the third or fifth postoperative day.

After one to two weeks of postoperative exercises, traction may be discontinued.

A short leg PTB cast is then applied, but the leg is kept non–weight bearing for approximately four to six weeks. The PTB cast is then removed and a walking cast is applied for six weeks longer. The prognosis, even with adequate reduction of these fractures, is guarded because risk of traumatic arthritis is dependent on the injury sustained by the talus as well as by the articular surface of the tibia.

The patient who remains free of symptomatic traumatic arthritis after the first year is likely to have a satisfactory result.

ALTERNATE METHOD: CLOSED REDUCTION

In most intances, internal fixation is necessary for these unstable injuries.

Rarely, closed reduction may be possible using cast immobilization or, for severely comminuted fractures, os calcis traction with range-of-motion exercises.

---

*Available from Wright Manufacturing, Memphis, Tennessee.

Prereduction X-Ray

1. The anterior marginal fragment is displaced upward.
2. The talus is displaced forward.
3. The articular surfaces of the talus and the tibia are not congruous.

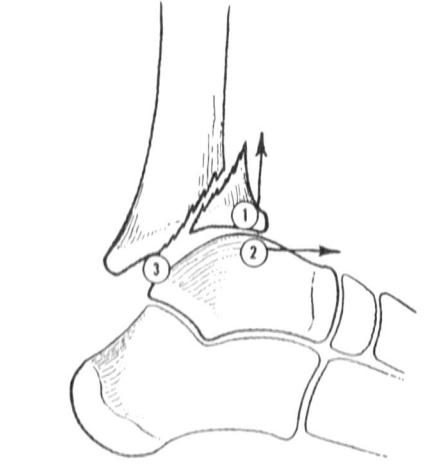

Manipulative Reduction

1. The patient's leg hangs over the edge of the table.
2. The operator grasps the forefoot with one hand and the heel with the other.
3. The operator makes strong traction downward and, at the same time,
4. Forcibly plantar flexes the foot.

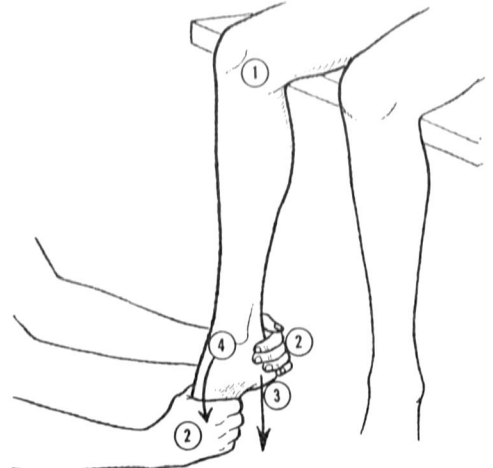

1. While the operator maintains downward traction and plantar flexion of the foot,
2. An assistant makes direct pressure on the fragment with both thumbs, molding the fragment into place.

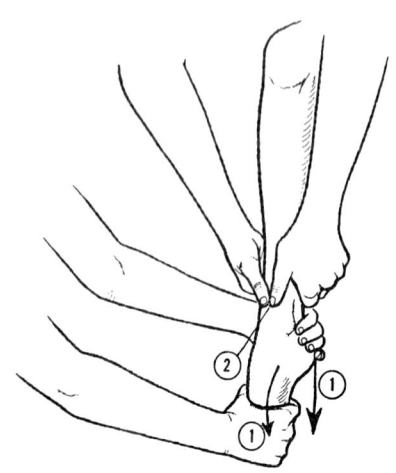

Manipulative Reduction
(Continued)

1. While the position of plantar flexion is maintained,
2. A lightly padded below-knee plaster cast is applied,
3. The plaster is molded well over the front of the ankle and around both malleoli.

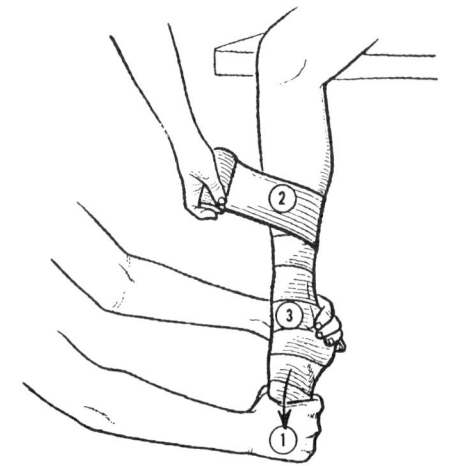

Postreduction X-Ray

1. The anterior marginal fragment is restored to its anatomic position.
2. The articular surfaces of the talus and the tibia are congruous.
3. The forward displacement of the talus is corrected.

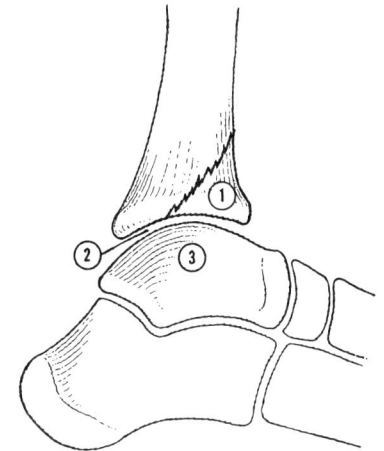

Postreduction Management

Check reduction with x-rays immediately after the application of the plaster cast.

After three weeks apply a new cast and reduce the amount of plantar flexion.

Six weeks after the reduction remove the second cast and bring the foot to a right angle with the leg.

Permit weight bearing in plaster at the end of ten weeks.

Remove the last cast at the end of twelve weeks.

Now institute active exercises and physical therapy to restore normal movements of the ankle and tarsal joints.

Severe Comminution of the Inferior Articular Surface of the Tibia (Explosion Fracture)

REMARKS

With severe compression violence the entire lower end of the tibia may be disrupted. A fracture of the fibula also may occur.

The talus is driven into the substance of the lower end of the tibia.

Fracture of one or both of the malleoli may be concomitant lesions.

Restoration of a normal articular surface is impossible by the usual closed or open methods.

In this unusual instance, os calcis traction, which allow the patient to exercise the ankle and remodel the fracture, offers the best chance for a satisfactory joint and relatively normal function.

Prereduction X-Ray

1. Severe comminution of the articular surface of the tibia.
2. Fracture of both malleoli.
3. The talus is displaced upward and
4. Forward.

Note: Attempted operative intervention in this severely comminuted fracture would probably be unsuccessful and might increase the potentials for wound necrosis or infection.

Initial Treatment: Os Calcis Traction

1. Insert a 2-mm threaded Steinmann pin through the os calcis.
2. Elevate the limb on a frame or pillows.
3. Apply 5 kg (11 lb.) of traction using a Salvatori* traction bow.
4. The bow is designed to allow joint motion without torquing the pin.

*Available from Wright Manufacturing, Memphis, Tennessee.

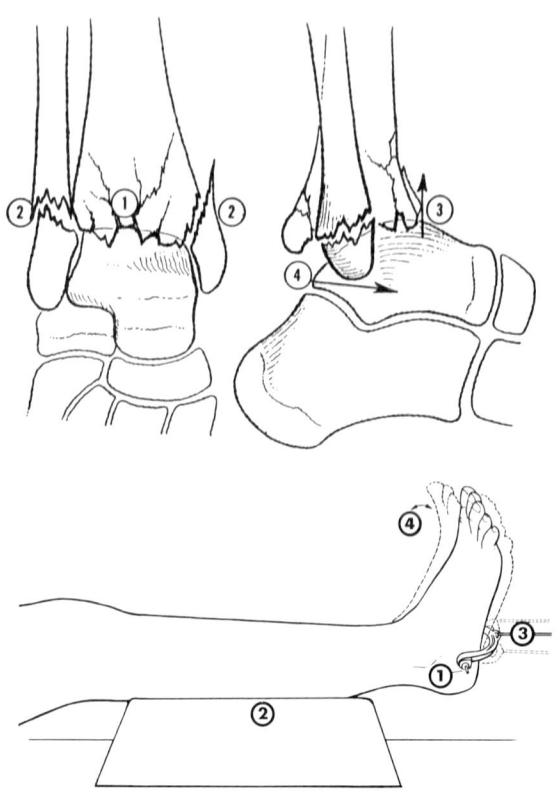

Postreduction X-Ray after Two Days of Traction

1. The articular fragments are still incompletely reduced but the position is improved.
2. The joint space is widened owing to the traction.

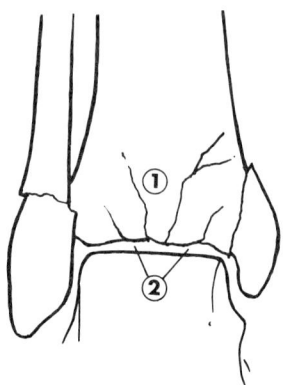

3. The talus is no longer displaced forward and upward.

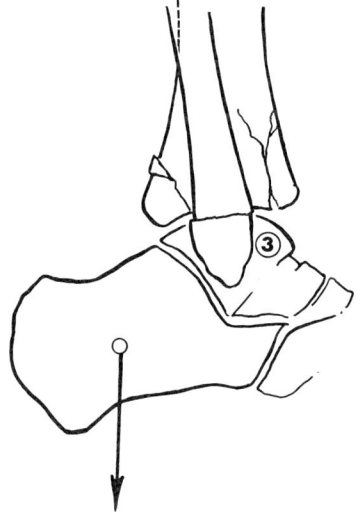

Subsequent Management

The patient is kept in traction and is encouraged to actively exercise the ankle on an hourly basis for four to six weeks.

After six weeks, the traction is removed and a snug, well-molded short leg cast is applied.

The patient is allowed up on crutches with toe-touch weight bearing for six weeks, after which time the cast is removed.

The patient should continue on crutches until the leg can bear weight fully without discomfort.

The prognosis in these injuries should be guarded, because the chance of osteoarthritis is dependent on the amount of damage to the tibial articular surface as well as to the talus.

The patient who is free of symptomatic osteoarthritis after the first year has a good prognosis. However, if painful arthritis occurs and prevents weight bearing, joint arthrodesis should be performed.

ARTHRODESIS OF THE ANKLE FOR EXPLOSION FRACTURES

REMARKS

Primary arthrodesis should be avoided even with the severely comminuted distal tibial fracture because the degree of radiographic changes of arthritis may not correlate with the degree of clinical symptoms.

After careful observation for six to twelve months following the ankle fracture, if the patient has persistent pain and inability to bear weight satisfactorily, an arthrodesis should be carried out.

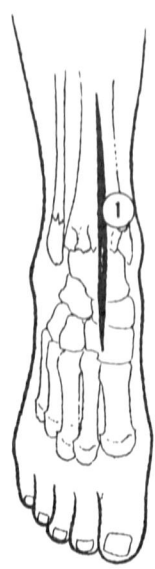

1. Make a vertical incision on the anterior aspect of the ankle joint; it begins 10 cm above and terminates 3 cm below the ankle joint.

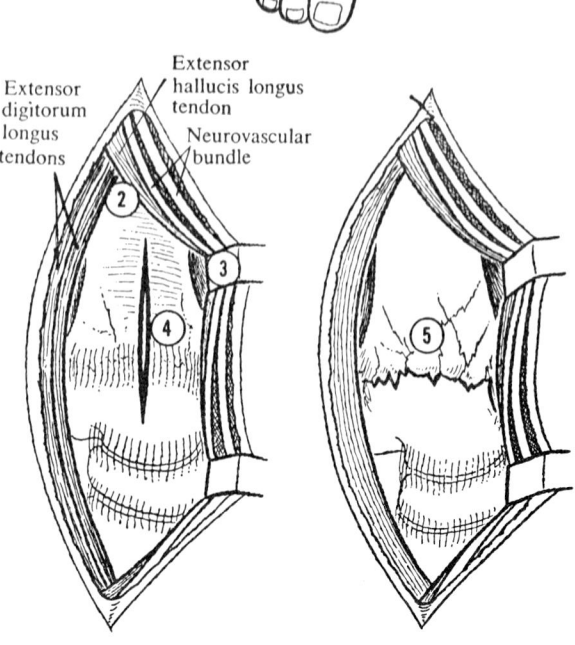

2. Divide the deep fascia longitudinally and develop the interval between the extensor digitorum longus and the extensor hallucis longus tendons.

3. Identify the neurovascular bundle and retract it medially with the extensor hallucis longus.

4. Incise the periosteum and capsule.

5. Expose the anterior surface of the tibia and the ankle joint by sharp subperiosteal and subcapsular dissection.

1. Plantar flex the foot.
2. With a thin-bladed osteotome and a fine curette remove the cartilage of the articular surface of the tibia and of the superior articular surface of the talus.
3. Remove the cartilage from the articular surfaces of the medial and lateral malleoli and the lateral surfaces of the talus.

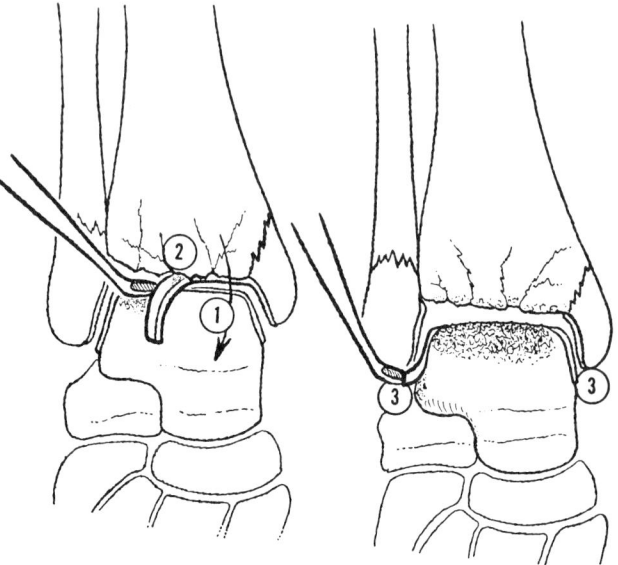

1. Align the talus accurately under the tibia.
2. With a motor saw remove a full thickness of cortical graft 2.5 cm wide and 8 cm long from the tibia immediately above the joint surface.
3. With a thin-bladed osteotome make a slot of suitable dimensions on the anterior portion of the body and on the superior surface of the neck of the talus.

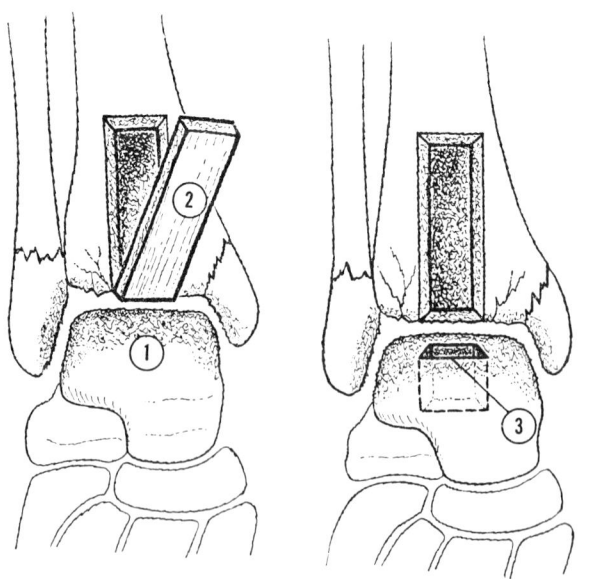

1. Slide the tibial graft into the slot in the talus and impact it firmly in position with an impactor.
2. Fill the spaces between the lateral surfaces of the talus and the malleoli and between the talus and the tibia with cancellous bone chips. (Obtain them from the medullary canal of the tibia.)

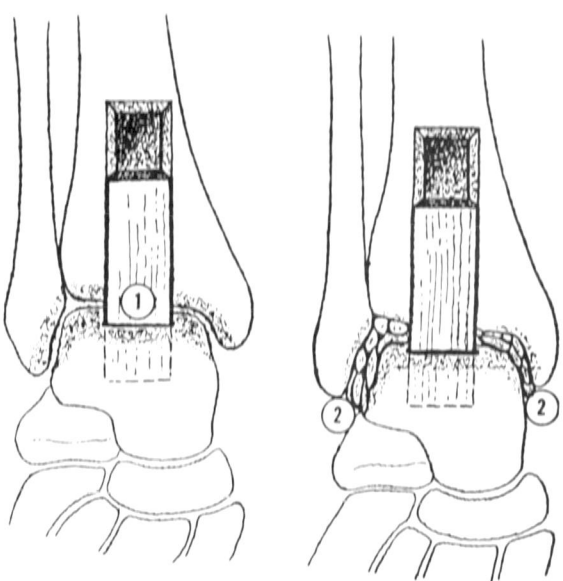

Note position of foot in relation to the tibia:

In men the position of the foot should be at a right angle to the leg.

In women the position of the foot should be plantar flexed 5 degrees.

1. Drive heavy cancellous screws from the medial to the lateral surfaces in a posterior direction to support the talus in the selected position.

Note: Compression arthrodesis using the Charnley apparatus may also be employed for the purpose of rigidly fixing the ankle (see page 1946).

Immobilization

1. Apply a circular cast from behind the metatarsal heads to the midthigh.
2. The knee is flexed 30 degrees.
3. In men the foot is at a right angle.
4. In women the foot is plantar flexed 5 degrees.
5. The foot is in a neutral position in regard to inversion and eversion.

Note: X-rays taken at the operating table permit accurate assessment of ankle position.

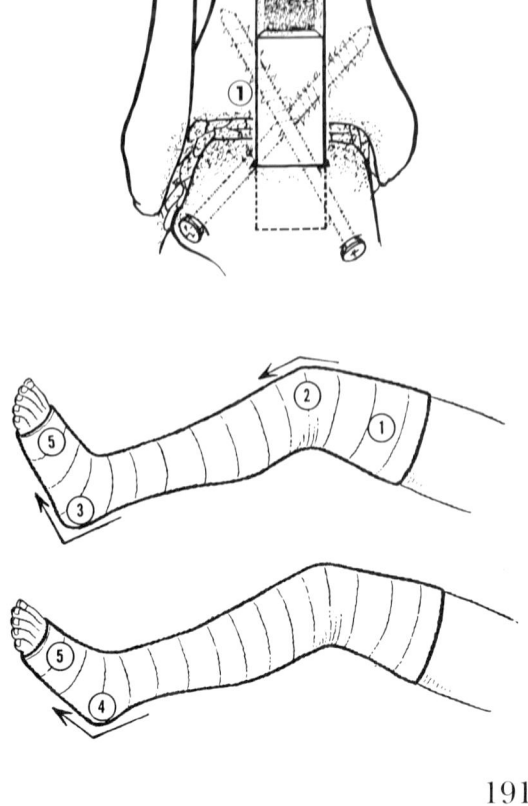

Postoperative Management

Apply a snug-fitting, long leg plaster cast at the end of three weeks.

Apply a walking, non-padded, below-the-knee cast at the end of eight weeks.

Now permit weight bearing with crutches.

The cast immobilization is discontinued only when radiographic examinations reveal complete consolidation.

It may require four to six months for consolidation to be complete.

Isolated Posterior Articular Fracture of the Tibia from Avulsion Injury (Curbstone Fracture)

REMARKS

Isolated fractures may occur from sudden avulsion injury when the individual strikes his dorsiflexing toe during swing phase. Most often this is done by stumbling over a curbstone.

The considerable force generated by the foot, which is accelerating at this point up to 4 G, is quite sufficient to avulse the posterior articular surface of the tibia.

Typically this is an undisplaced fracture and requires only symptomatic treatment, usually with cast support for three weeks.

Mechanism of Injury

1. The foot strikes the curbstone while accelerating during swing phase.

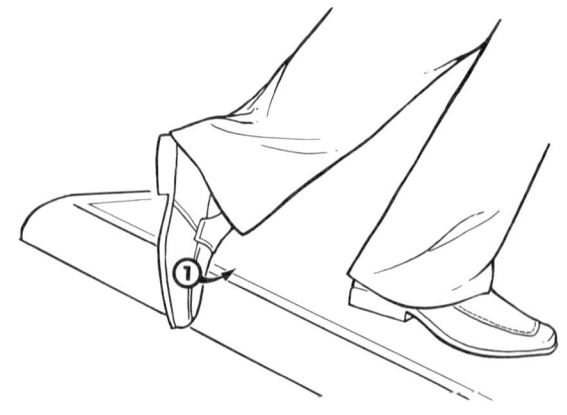

2. The pull of the posterior capsule avulses the posterior articular fragment. This is usually less than ten per cent of the joint surface.
3. The remaining medial and lateral articular structures are undamaged.

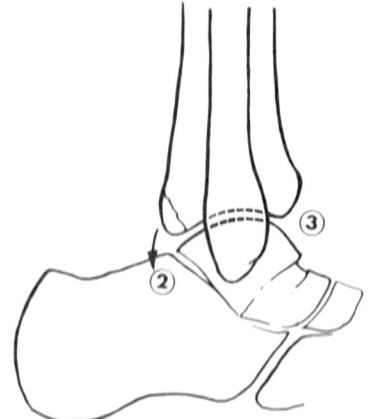

Management

Treatment should be symptomatic to relieve the discomfort in the ankle.

Most frequently the patient is comfortable with a short leg walking cast maintained for three weeks.

Immobilization

1. Apply a circular plaster cast from the base of the toes to just below the knee.
2. The foot is in 10 degrees of plantar flexion.
3. The foot is in neutral position in regard to inversion and eversion.
4. The plaster is molded well around the heel, in front of the foot, and around the malleoli for the patient's comfort.

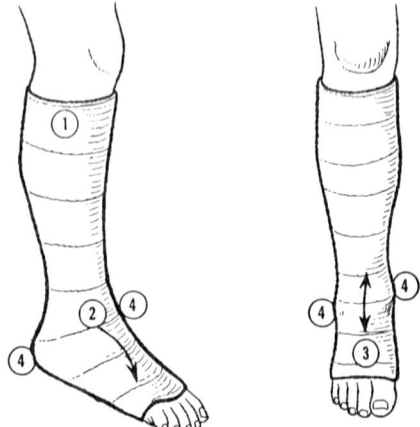

Subsequent Management

The patient may walk on the cast for three weeks using either a cast walker or walking boot. After this time the cast is removed.

Subsequently the ankle is treated as a Grade II sprain and exercises are started to regain normal range of motion (see page 1812).

DISLOCATIONS OF THE ANKLE JOINT

Posterior Dislocation of the Ankle Joint

REMARKS

Although this lesion is rare it is the most common of all dislocations of the ankle joint.

The lesion is the result of severe plantar flexion of the foot with a strong forward thrust of the leg.

In most instances the dislocation is accompanied by a fracture of one or both malleoli or posterior marginal fracture of the tibia.

Prereduction X-Ray

1. The tibia and the fibula are displaced forward.
2. The talus, with the foot, is displaced backward.

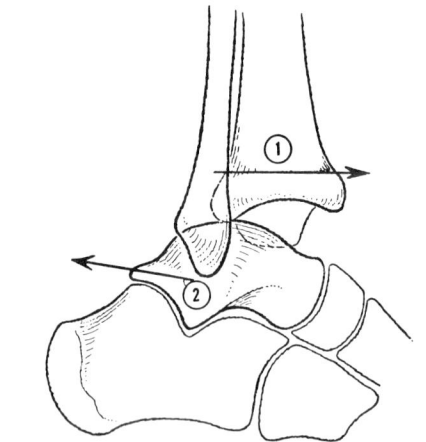

Manipulative Reduction (Under General Anesthesia)

1. The knee is flexed.
2. The assistant makes counter traction on the leg.
3. Grasp the forefoot with one hand and the heel with the other.
4. The foot is slightly plantar flexed.

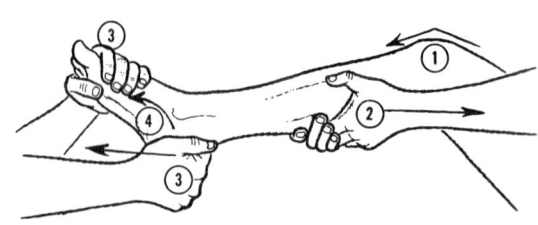

1. Make straight downward traction on the plantar flexed foot; then,
2. Pull the foot forward while
3. A second assistant makes counter pressure on the front of the lower leg.

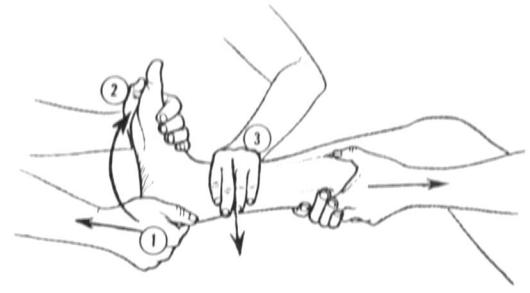

Postreduction X-Ray

1. The talus is in correct relationship to the tibia.
2. The articular surfaces of the talus and the tibia are congruous.

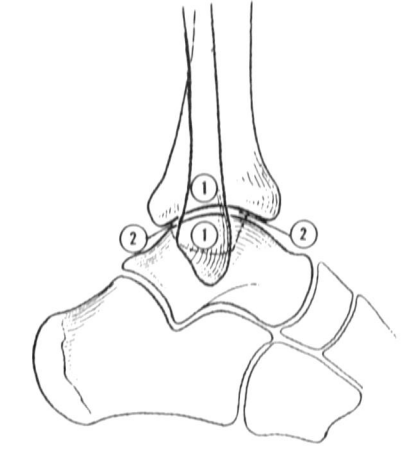

Immobilization

1. Apply a circular plaster cast from the base of the toe to just below the knees.
2. The foot is dorsiflexed 90 degrees.
3. The foot is in a neutral position in regard to inversion and eversion.
4. Mold the plaster well around the heel and the front of the foot and the malleoli.

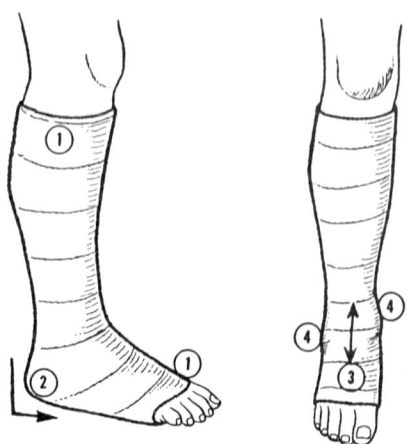

Postreduction Management

The patient can be ambulatory on crutches immediately.
The cast is reapplied at the end of three weeks.

The second cast is removed six weeks after reduction and weight bearing, at first on crutches, is permitted.

Physical therapy and active exercises are instituted to restore normal ankle and foot movements (see page 1822).

Note: If associated fractures of the malleoli are present, the dislocation is reduced first and then the fractures are treated as previously described, by open reduction and internal fixation.

Anterior Dislocation of the Ankle Joint

REMARKS

This lesion is indeed rare, and when it occurs it is frequently accompanied by a fracture of the anterior margin of the tibia.

The lesion is produced by forcible dorsiflexion of the foot or a fall on the heel with the foot in dorsiflexion.

Fracture of one or both malleoli may be concomitant lesions.

In this lesion the anterior capsule may be separated from the neck of the talus.

Prereduction X-Ray

1. Backward displacement of the tibia and the fibula.
2. Forward displacement of the talus.
3. Small marginal fracture of the anterior tip of the tibia.

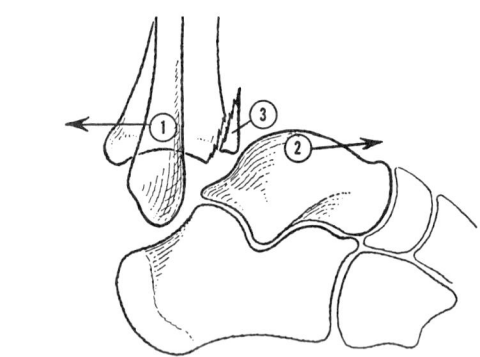

Manipulative Reduction (Under General Anesthesia)

1. The knee is flexed.
2. The operator grasps the forefoot with one hand and the heel with the other.
3. Dorsiflexion of the foot is slightly increased (to disengage the talus).
4. An assistant makes counter traction on the leg.

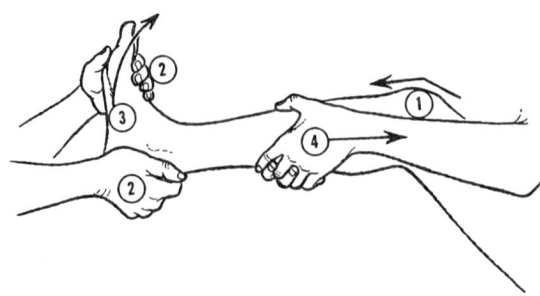

1. Straight downward traction is made.
2. Then the foot is pushed directly backward while
3. A second assistant makes counter traction on the back of the lower leg.

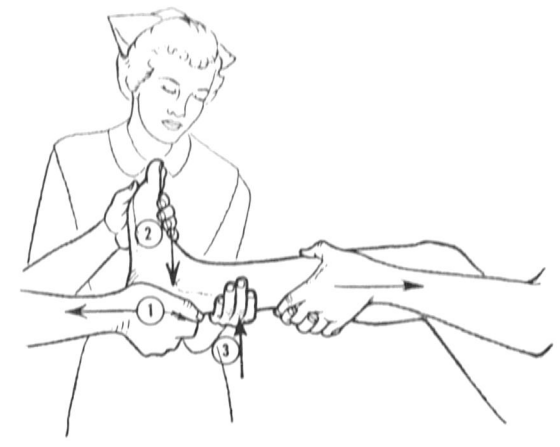

Postreduction X-Ray

1. The talus is in normal relation to the tibia.
2. The articular surfaces of the talus and the tibia are congruous.
3. The small anterior marginal fragment is in its anatomic position.

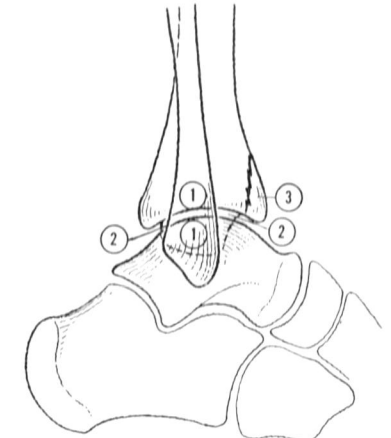

Immobilization

1. Apply a circular plaster cast from the base of the toes to just below the knee.
2. The foot is slightly plantar flexed.
3. The foot is in a neutral position in regard to inversion and eversion.
4. Mold the plaster well around the heel, the front of the foot, and the malleoli.

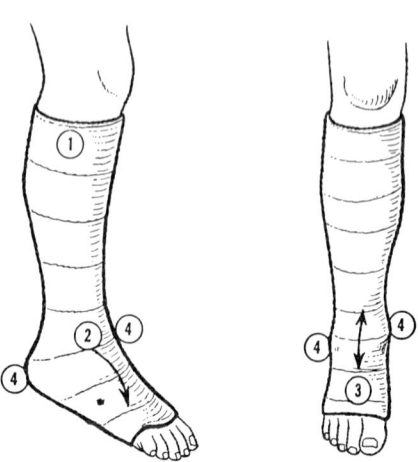

Postreduction Management

The patient should be ambulatory on crutches immediately without bearing weight on the affected limb.

The plaster cast is replaced at the end of three weeks with the foot in 90 degrees of dorsiflexion.

The second cast is removed six weeks after reduction, and weight bearing on crutches is permitted.

Physical therapy and active exercises are instituted to restore normal movements of the ankle and foot (see page 1822).

Note: If concomitant fractures of the malleoli are present, dislocation is reduced first and then the fracture is treated as previously described, by open reduction and internal fixation.

Upward Dislocation of the Talus

REMARKS

This rare lesion is commonly complicated by marked comminution of the lower end of the tibia and a fracture of the fibula.

There is complete disruption of the distal tibiofibular joint with upward displacement of the talus between the tibia and the fibula.

Internal fixation of the tibiofibular joint with repair of the deltoid ligament is the procedure of choice.

Prereduction X-Ray

1. Wide separation of the tibiofibular joint.
2. Upward displacement of the talus.
3. Slight comminution of the lateral portion of the tibial articular surface.

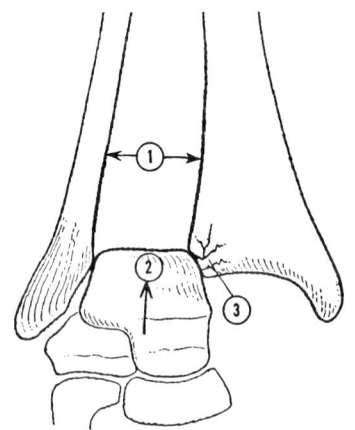

Treatment and Postoperative Management

After reduction of the dislocation by strong downward traction on the foot and counter traction on the leg, the diastasis of the ankle joint is reduced and stabilized by a screw driven through the fibula and the tibia, and the deltoid ligament is repaired (see page 1850).

Postreduction X-Ray

1. The talus fits accurately under the tibia and in the ankle mortise.
2. The fibula is secured to the tibia with a transfixion screw.
3. The fibula fits snugly against the tibia.

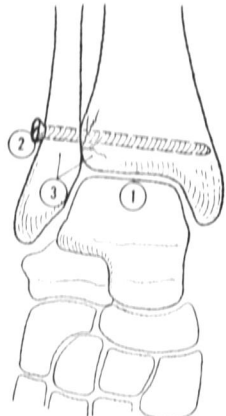

Lateral Dislocation of the Ankle Joint

REMARKS

This lesion is always associated with fractures of the malleoli and may be the result of violent inversion or eversion mechanisms.

Often the lesion is an open one.

Prereduction X-Ray

1. Fracture of the medial and lateral malleoli.
2. Lateral and upward displacement of the talus.

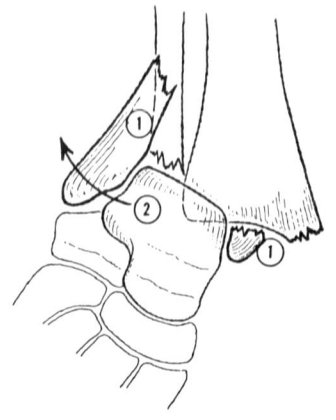

Treatment and Postreduction Management

After reduction by traction and manipulation the subsequent plan of treatment is the same as for fractures of the malleoli with lateral or medial displacement of the talus; these techniques have been described previously.

Postreduction X-Ray

1. The talus is in its normal position in the mortise.
2. The lateral malleolus is secured by screws.
3. The medial malleolus is secured by a screw.
4. The articular surfaces of the talus and the tibia are congruous.

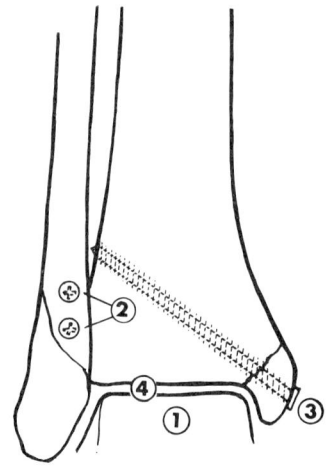

Irreducible Fractures of the Lateral Malleolus

REMARKS

In rare instances widening of the ankle mortise may not be corrected entirely by reduction of the lateral malleolus.

It may be the result of rupture of the medial ligament or avulsion of the medial malleolus with displacement of the posterior tibial tendon or posterior tibial artery and nerve between the intact portion of the medial malleolus and the talus.

Always suspect such a possibility when, in a fracture of the lateral malleolus with lateral displacement of the talus, the talus cannot be accurately reduced.

Pathology

1. The posterior tibial tendon is trapped between the medial malleolus and the talus.
2. The talus is displaced laterally.
3. There is a fracture of the lateral malleolus.
4. There is an avulsion of the tip of the medial malleolus.

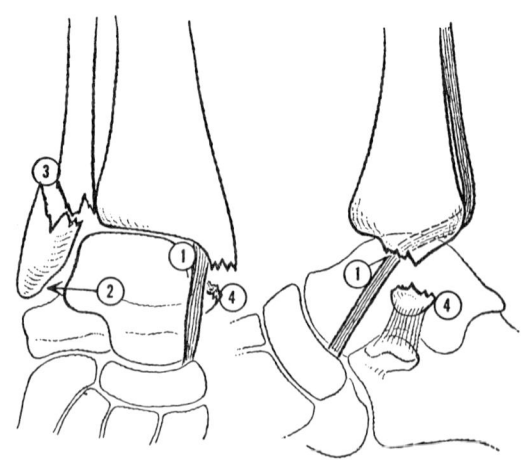

Prereduction X-Ray

1. Fracture of the lateral malleolus.
2. Lateral shift of the talus.
3. Avulsion of the tip of the medial malleolus.

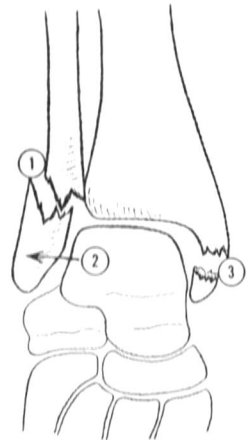

Operative Reduction

1. Make an 8-cm incision along the posterior margin of the medial malleolus; the incision curves forward just below the tip of the malleolus for 5 cm more.

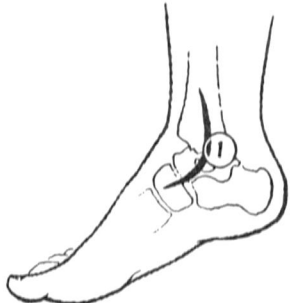

2. Divide the deep fascia, exposing

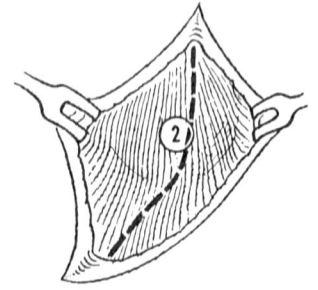

3. The avulsed medial malleolus and
4. The medial ligament.
5. Identify the posterior tibial tendon between the intact portion of the malleolus and the talus.

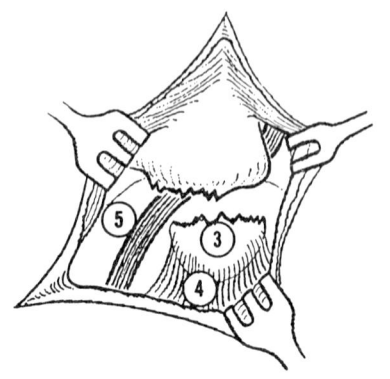

Operative Reduction (Continued)

1. With a hook replace the posterior tibial tendon in its normal position.

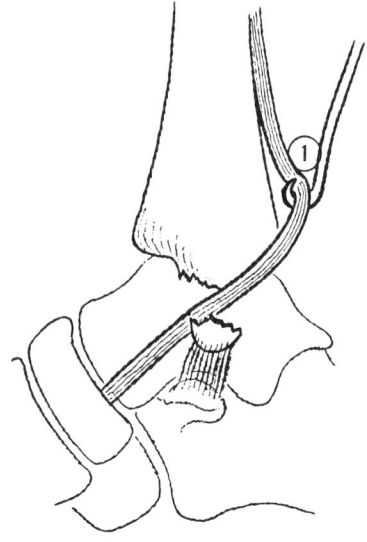

2. Secure the avulsed tip of the medial malleolus to the tibia with a screw.

Note: The fracture of the lateral malleolus with displacement is reduced and fixed as previously described on page 1848.

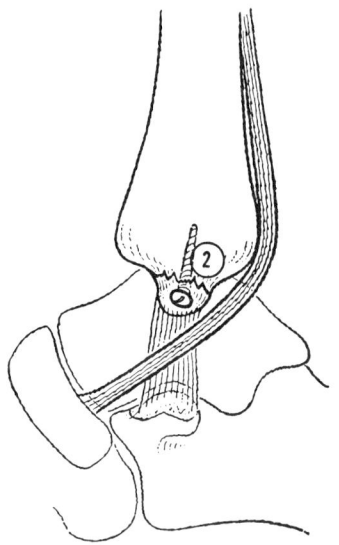

IRREDUCIBLE POSTERIOR FRACTURE-DISLOCATION OF THE ANKLE JOINT (BOSWORTH FRACTURE)

REMARKS

Occasionally in posterior fracture-dislocations the proximal end of the fractured fibula becomes displaced behind the tibia and locked there.

The usual mechanism is a severe external rotational injury, which forces the talus back out of the mortise. The fibula generally sustains a characteristic supination-external rotation fracture with the fracture line running from the distal anterior cortex to the proximal posterior cortex. The fibula may sometimes remain intact and become dislocated behind the tibia.

Most often the proximal fibular fragment becomes entrapped, either in the posterolateral ridge of the tibia with a posterior malleolar fracture, or in the interosseous membrane.

Once the fibula is freed from its entrapment, it will snap back into correct position.

Owing to the extreme rotation of the foot, the x-ray may be misleading. The anteroposterior x-ray may be mistaken for the lateral, or vice versa. The relationship of the tibia to the proximal fibular fragment may be considered normal or due to improper positioning. Correct orientation, particularly if the knee joint is included on the x-ray, will prevent the physician's being misled by the position of the fibula, malleolus, and talus.

Mayer and Evarts have shown that with correct diagnosis, closed reduction is possible using traction and medial rotation of the foot while pressing laterally on the fibular shaft.

If closed reduction fails, a lateral approach to the fractured fibula is sufficient to allow adequate reduction and internal fixation of the injury.

Prereduction X-Ray

LATERAL VIEW

1. Medial malleolus.
2. The lateral malleolus is rotated externally and is not superimposed on the medial malleolus as it should be in a normal lateral.
3. The distal end of the fibular shaft is entrapped posteriorly.
4. A typical oblique fracture of the fibula (S-EX mechanism).
5. The position of the patella aids in proper orientation of the x-ray.

ANTEROPOSTERIOR VIEW

1. Medial malleolus.
2. Lateral malleolus and fibular shaft are displaced posteriorly.
3. The foot is rotated externally.

Note: If true anteroposterior and lateral views are not used, the overlap may not be demonstrated on the anteroposterior view, and the posterior displacement may not be demonstrated on the lateral view.

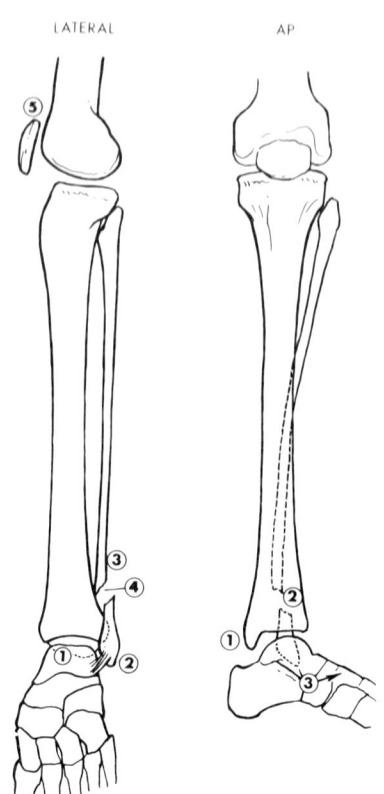

Technique of Closed Reduction (Mayer and Evarts)

Under adequate anesthesia:
1. The surgeon's right hand is used to apply axial traction and to internally rotate the foot.
2. The heel of the surgeon's left hand applies an anterolaterally directed force to the fibula.

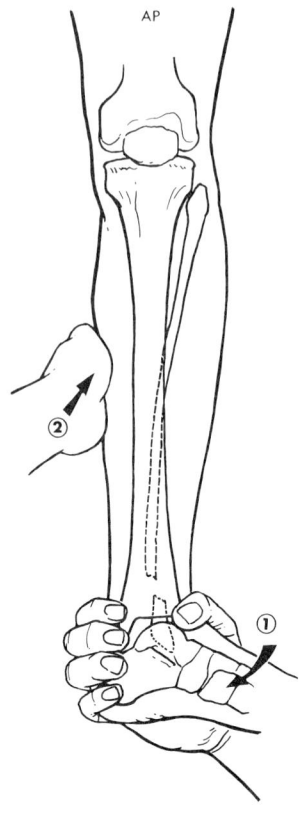

A snap is heard as the ankle reduces; usually the joint returns to a stable and acceptable position.

If a fracture of the fibula or medial malleolus remains displaced, internal fixation should then be carried out.

Subsequently, a long leg cast is applied and the injury is treated as previously described (see page 1848).

If closed reduction is not possible, open reduction should be performed via a lateral approach.

VASCULAR IMPAIRMENT RESULTING FROM POSTERIOR FRACTURE-DISLOCATION OF THE ANKLE

Tipton and D'Ambrosia have reported that the dorsalis pedis artery can be entrapped by the extensor retinaculum with posterior dislocation of the fibula. This is especially serious if there is also a simultaneous injury to the posterior tibial artery.

Prompt reduction of the fibula releases the entrapped vessel and restores distal arterial flow.

Prereduction Relationship

1. Posterior dislocation of the fibula
2. Tightens the extensor retinaculum and
3. Entraps the dorsalis pedis artery. Closed reduction should be done promptly as described on page 1926.

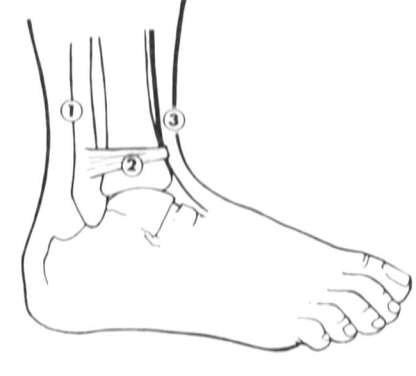

Postreduction Relationship

1. The fibula is restored to normal position.
2. The extensor retinaculum is no longer tight.
3. Release of the dorsalis pedis artery restores distal flow to normal.

Note: If the posterior fibular dislocation cannot be reduced by closed manipulation, perform operative reduction promptly.

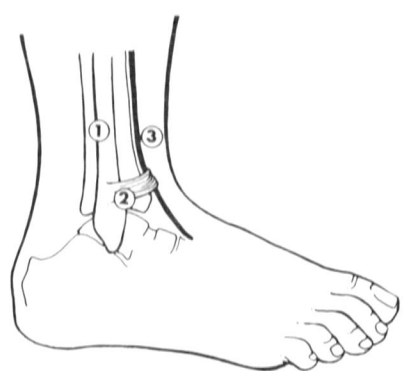

Operative Reduction of Irreducible Posterior Fracture-Dislocation of the Ankle

1. Make an incision 10 to 12 cm long on the lateral aspect of the leg beginning just distal to the tip of the lateral malleolus.
2. Divide the deep fascia; retract the flaps and expose the fractured end of the distal fragment.
3. Locate the distal end of the proximal fibular fragment behind the tibia.

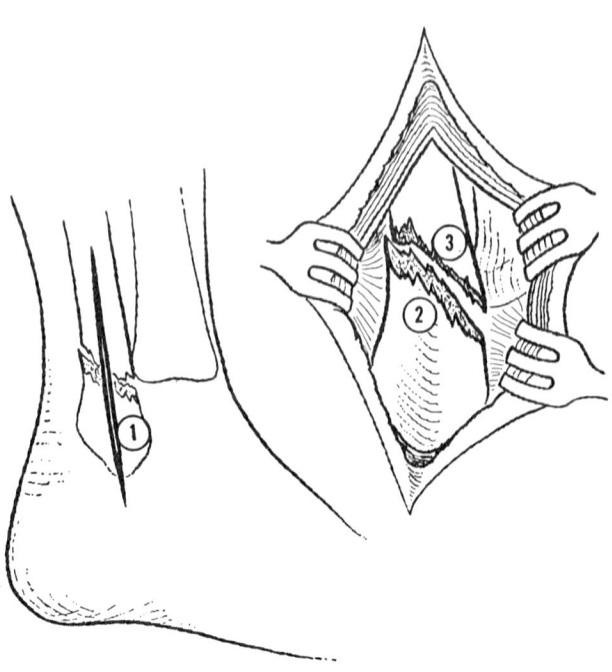

Operative Reduction of Irreducible Posterior Fracture-Dislocation of the Ankle (Continued)

1. Place a pry or curette between the fibular fragment and the tibia, and apply strong leverage on the displaced fragment.

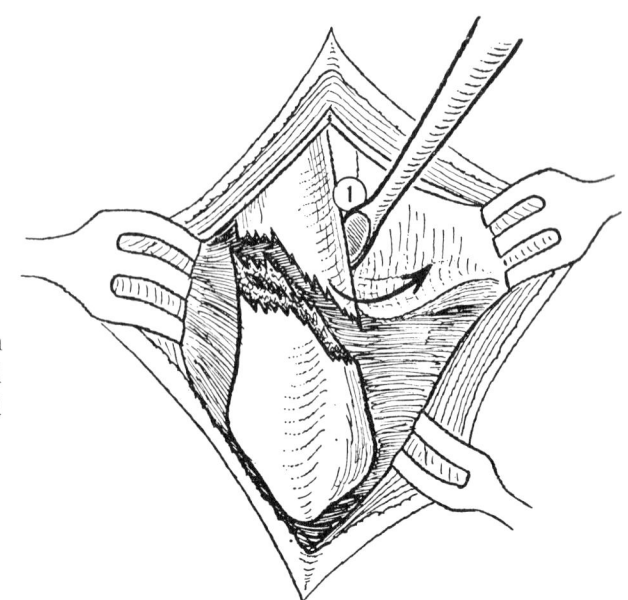

1. The fibular fragments are in alignment.
2. Transfix the fragments with a small screw or
3. Pass a wire through the distal fragment and into the medullary canal of the proximal fragment.

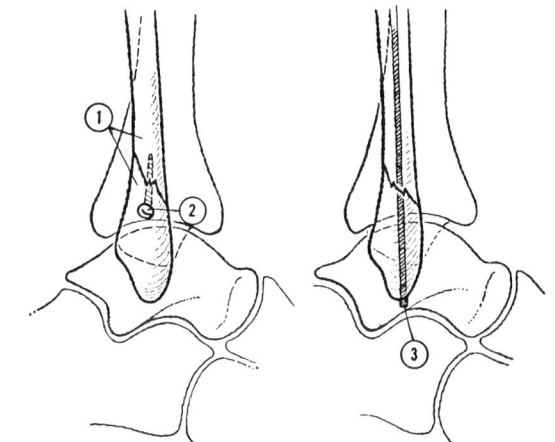

Subsequent Management

Treatment and postreduction management of the fracture of the lateral malleolus and lateral displacement of the talus is described on page 1851.

Rotational Displacement of the Distal Tibial Epiphysis With or Without Fibular Fracture
(Henke and Kiple)

REMARKS

This is an extremely rare lesion, but it does occur with forceful external rotation injuries in children and adolescents.

The injury is similar to the Bosworth fracture except that the rotational malalignment occurs through the epiphysis rather than through the ankle joint itself.

The key to the diagnosis is an x-ray of the entire leg showing the relationships of the knee and ankle.

Reduction is usually accomplished readily by traction and internal rotation in a manner similar to the reduction for Bosworth's fracture.

Since bony bridge formation between the epiphysis and the metaphysis is to be expected after this injury, growth arrest from the epiphysiodesis is the usual sequela.

Prereduction X-Ray

ANTEROPOSTERIOR VIEW

1. The anteroposterior x-ray looks like a normal lateral view because of the posterior displacement of the fibula behind the tibia.
2. The fibula may or may not be fractured.
3. The rotational deformity has occurred through the distal tibial epiphysis.

LATERAL VIEW

1. The fibula has displaced and locked posterolaterally.
2. The epiphyseal displacement is evident.

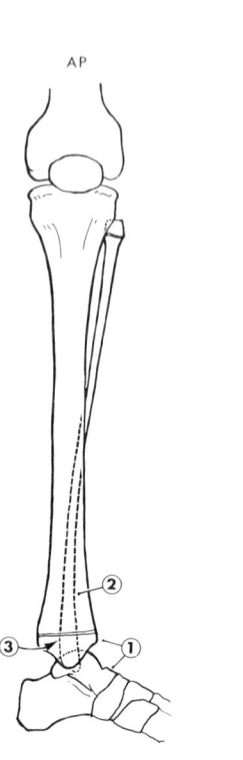
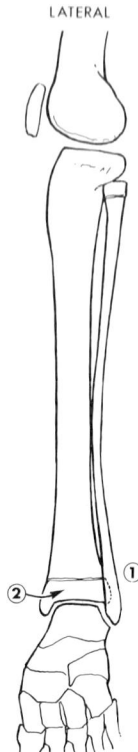

Postreduction X-Ray

After reduction by traction and internal rotation of the foot (see page 1926),

1. The alignment of the knee and ankle has been restored.
2. The fibula is in normal relationship to the distal tibia.

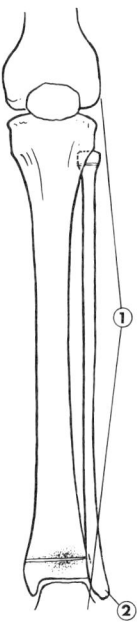

Subsequent Management

The leg should be supported in a long leg cast for approximately three to four weeks. After this time the epiphyseal injury has usually healed satisfactorily and the cast may be discontinued.

If the fibula is fractured, cast immobilization should be continued for six weeks until radiographs show evidence of union.

The patient and parents should be advised that this injury in all likelihood has disrupted growth of the ankle. The degree of shortening that can be anticipated is usually minimal. Many patients with this injury are in the adolescent age group and close to bony maturity.

OPEN FRACTURES AND FRACTURE-DISLOCATIONS OF THE ANKLE JOINT

REMARKS

Because of the superficial position of the malleoli, marked displacement of the foot to one side or the other frequently causes rupture of the soft tissues and skin on the side opposite the displacement.

A fall from a height may drive the ends of the tibia and the fibula through the skin.

Circulation to the skin in this area is frequently tenuous, particularly in older patients. Further skin loss or excision should be avoided during wound management.

The principles of management for open ankle fractures are the same as those outlined for open tibial fractures (see page 1749). After thorough irrigation and cleansing of the contaminated wound, the injury should be left open and drained adequately.

Prophylactic broad-spectrum antibiotics are indicated as an adjunctive measure but should not be substituted for thorough wound cleansing. Repetition of debridement and cleaning of the ankle fracture should be planned within two to three days postoperatively.

If the ankle itself is unstable, internal fixation may be utilized on the side opposite from the open wound.

Occasionally, fixation by proximal and distal pins in plaster or by a transarticular pin driven vertically up from the heel may be needed to stabilize the open fracture. These unusual measures are useful, particularly if there is excessive skin loss or contamination.

Open ankle fractures carry a poorer prognosis for healing and restoration of ankle function than do similar closed fractures; however, if infection is avoided and adequate ankle stability is achieved, one may anticipate satisfactory results.

OPEN FRACTURES AND FRACTURE-DISLOCATIONS OF THE ANKLE JOINT

Typical Case

1. Ragged open wound on the outer aspect of the ankle.
2. The foot is markedly inverted.
3. The fractured end of the fibula and the articular surface of the tibia are exposed.

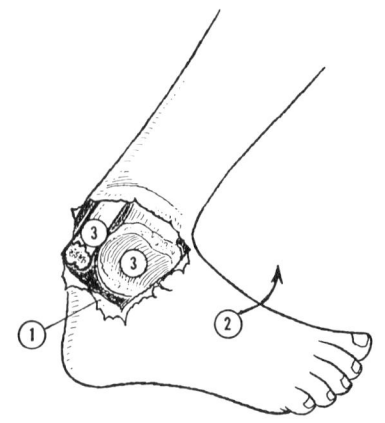

Prereduction X-Ray

1. The talus is displaced upward and inward.
2. The medial and lateral malleoli have followed the talus.
3. Exposed end of the proximal fragment of the fibula.

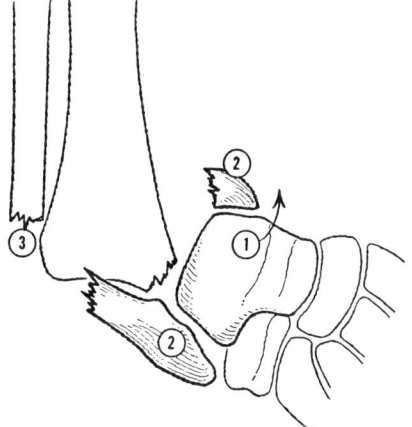

Preparation of the Area

1. Initial irrigation should be with copious amounts of water to cleanse the leg of all dirt accumulated at the time of injury. This is purely a mechanical washing requiring 10 to 15 liters of fluid.

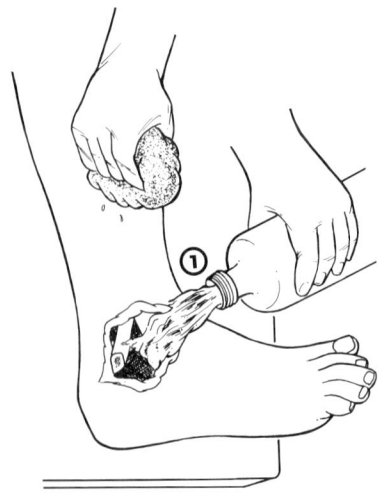

2. A pressure irrigation system such as a Water Pik is helpful to remove dirt fixed in deep tissue and bone after the injury.

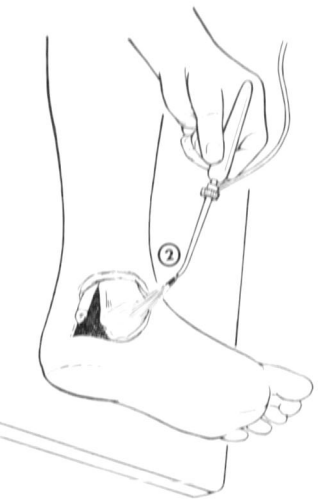

1. After thorough mechanical cleansing of the leg, the wound is prepped with Betadine solution.

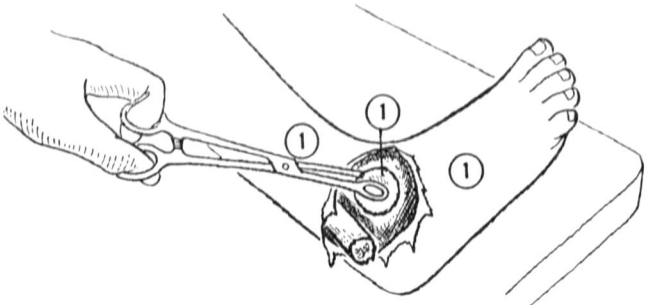

2. The field is draped in a sterile manner.
Surgeon and assistant change gowns and gloves before the next step of the procedure.

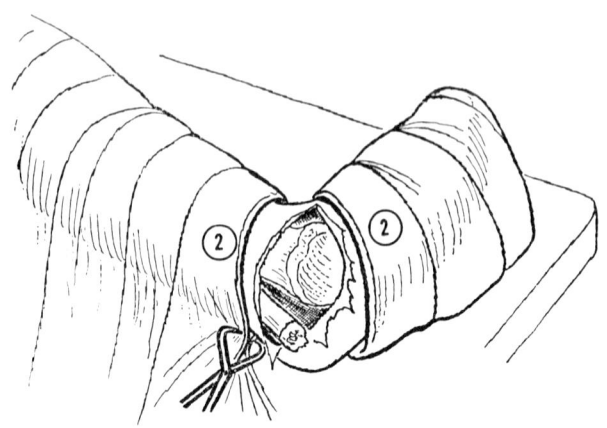

Preparation of the Area (Continued)

1. Excise the skin edges but spare as much skin as possible.
2. Excise all devitalized soft tissue.
3. Bone excision should be minimal. Remove only loose small bits and pieces. Large loose fragments should be thoroughly cleansed and reinserted into the fracture site to help in stabilization.
4. Remove contaminated dirty ends of bone with a rongeur or a sharp curette.

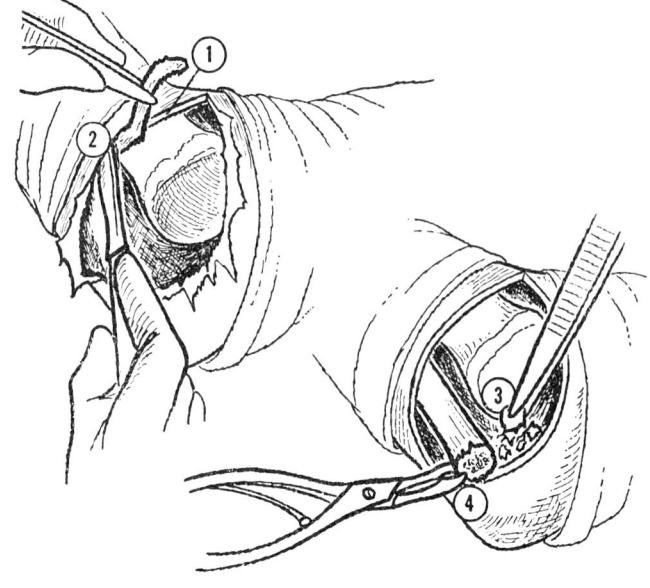

1. Before reducing the fracture, flush the wound again with 8 to 10 liters of saline followed by an antibiotic solution containing broad-spectrum antibiotics.

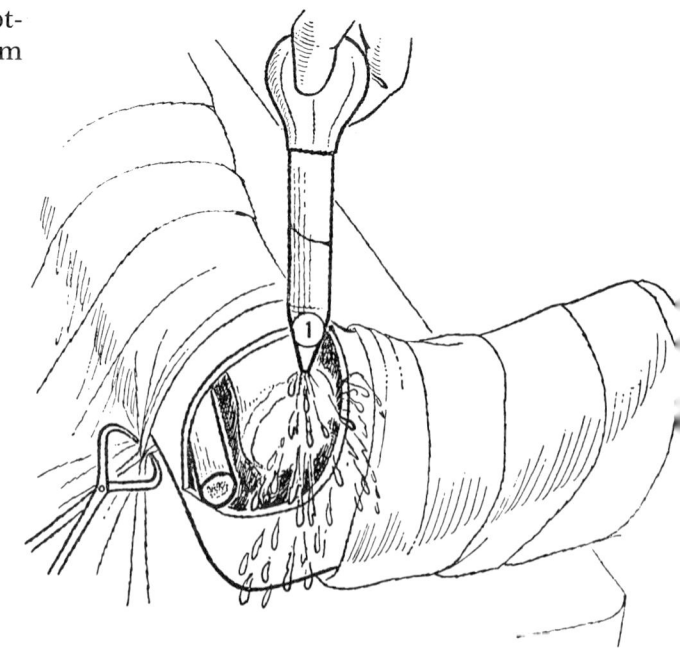

Reduction

Depending on the type of dislocation or fracture-dislocation, employ the same methods depicted for the closed lesions of the same types.

Always give preference to methods without use of internal fixation if at all possible.

After reduction,

1. The wound over the ankle is left open but held with 3-0 stainless steel wire suture to prevent retraction of the wound edges.
2. A Penrose drain is inserted into the ankle wound to encourage adequate drainage.

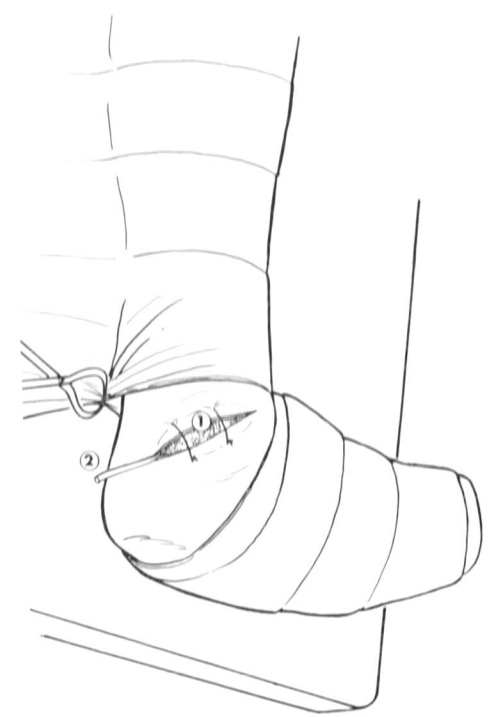

Immobilization

1. Apply a circular cast from behind the metatarsal heads to the upper thigh.
2. The foot is in a neutral position and at right angle to the leg.
3. The knee is flexed 30 degrees.

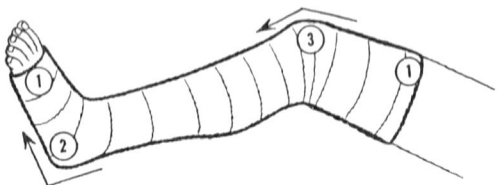

Postoperative Management

Elevate the limb on pillows.

Surround the operative site with ice bags.

Prescribe a broad-spectrum antibiotic; continue the drug until the wound heals by secondary intention.

Check constantly for evidence of circulatory embarrassment or infection.

If no complications arise, the subsequent treatment is the same as for closed lesions of the same type.

REDUCTION AND STABILIZATION OF UNSTABLE OPEN ANKLE FRACTURES

This may be accomplished by:
1. Proximal and distal pin transfixion (Laskin),
2. Vertical transarticular pin fixation (Childress), or
3. Delayed internal fixation of the fracture when the soft tissue wound is healed.

Technique of Steinmann Pin Fixation (Laskin)

The fracture is manipulated and x-rays are taken in the operating room after wound treatment to show adequate reduction of the fracture: Then,

1. A 3-mm smooth Steinmann pin is inserted into the proximal tibia just distal to the tibial tuberosity.

2. A second pin is inserted 2 cm distal and 2 cm posterior to the tip of the lateral malleolus transversely through the calcaneus.

3. Two-cm-square felt pads are placed about the exit points of each pin.

4. A cast is applied incorporating the Steinmann pins while holding reduction of the fracture.

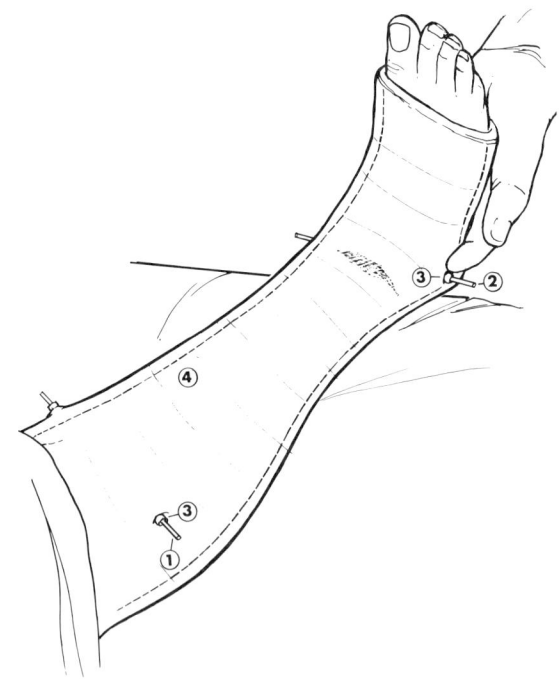

Alternate Method: Vertical Transarticular Pin Fixation (Childress)

Note: This technique should be restricted to injuries with extensive skin loss.

1. The fracture-dislocation of the ankle is reduced and the foot is placed in slight equinus. This aids in directing the pin toward the posterior portion of the talus.
2. A Kirschner wire is drilled 10 cm upward through the calcaneus into the talus but does not cross the ankle joint. This pin is aimed toward the center of the tibia and should contact the inferior region of the calcaneus about 2.5 cm. posterior to the calcaneocuboid joint.

Note: X-rays in two planes are then made to determine the adequacy of the reduction and the location of the wire. If it is decided to use the vertical pin, the Kirschner wire is used as a guide and a 3-mm Steinmann pin is inserted using an air-powered drill.

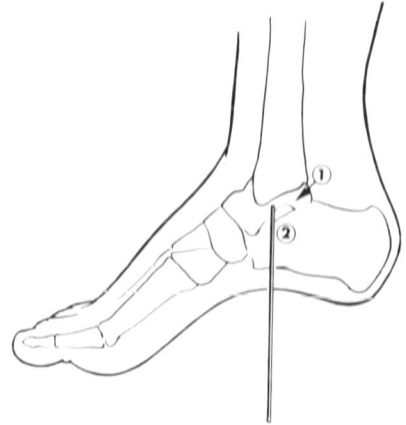

1. The Steinmann pin is driven into the distal tibia and
2. The pin is allowed to protrude 2.5 cm. through the skin; this is bent at a right angle.

Note: The transarticular pin should not be incorporated in the plaster, and all weight bearing should be prevented until the pin is removed.

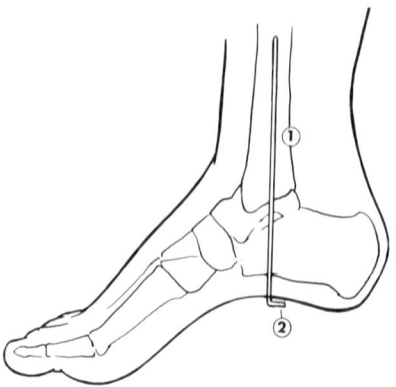

Subsequent Management After Transverse or Vertical Steinmann Pin Fixation

The Steinmann pins are removed six weeks after their insertion.
The fracture is then immobilized for four to six weeks longer in a short-leg walking cast. The patient is allowed to bear weight as tolerated.

OPEN FRACTURES AND FRACTURE-DISLOCATIONS OF THE ANKLE JOINT

Alternate Method: Delayed Internal Fixation

In most open ankle fractures, the wound should be healing sufficiently in seven to ten days to permit delayed internal fixation on the side opposite the open wound.

This technique may be employed if the soft tissue wound allows and the closed reduction method proves inadequate.

Postreduction X-Ray

1. The ankle has been stabilized by screw fixation of the medial malleolus and cast support of the lateral malleolar fracture.
2. The talus is in the normal position in the mortise.

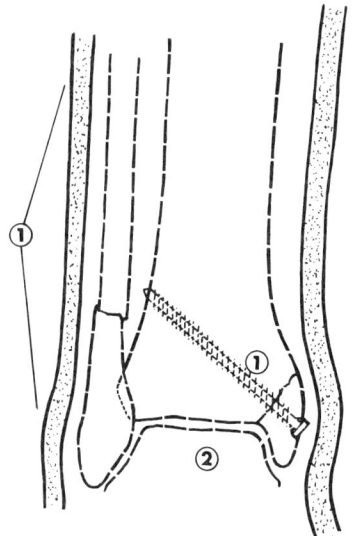

Subsequent Management after Delayed Internal Fixation

A long leg cast is applied for six weeks.

The cast is then changed and a short leg walking cast is applied for from four to six weeks, depending on the radiographic evidence of union.

MALUNITED FRACTURE-DISLOCATIONS OF THE ANKLE

REMARKS

The end result is related to the amount of initial talar displacement, the type of fracture, and the presence or absence of a deltoid ligament injury. Joy and coworkers have found that P-EX mechanisms produced a higher frequency of poor results and that P-EX and S-EX mechanisms associated with torn deltoid ligament were also likely to lead to poor results.

Despite factors resulting from the type and degree of initial injury, adequate reduction does correlate with good clinical result, and anatomic restoration should be the goal of treatment.

Fractures that are discovered to be healing or that heal in a malunited position should be considered for corrective osteotomy. This is particularly indicated in the patient for whom weight bearing produces symptoms without radiographic evidence of traumatic arthritis.

The degree of arthritis evident on x-ray does not necessarily correlate with the patient's clinical symptoms. However, the patient with both significant clinical pain and radiographic changes of arthritis after an ankle fracture should be offered an ankle arthrodesis as an effective solution to the problem.

EXAMPLES OF MALUNITED FRACTURE-DISLOCATION REQUIRING CORRECTIVE OSTEOTOMY

Note: The recommendation for corrective osteotomy must be strictly tailored to the needs of the patient. The results after the osteotomy are not as good as after primary anatomic reduction of the fracture. A relatively pain-free ankle in an older patient may be made worse by attempted anatomic restoration. The active young adult with symptomatic malunion is a primary candidate for corrective osteotomy.

First Example

Appearance on X-Ray

1. Shortening of the fibula allowing lateral displacement of the talus.
2. Diastasis of the tibiofibular joint.
3. Eversion of the ankle resulting from the shortening of the fibula and causing symptoms on weight bearing.
4. Widening of the medial clear space.

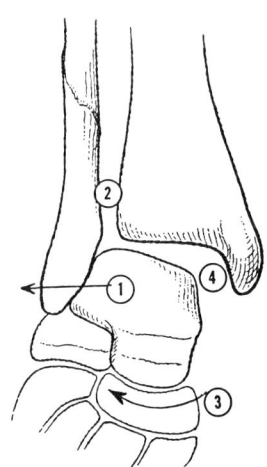

Postreduction X-Ray

1. The fibula has been restored to length by an osteotomy. The osteotomy is fixed with a plate.
2. The distal tibiofibular syndesmosis is supported with a screw.
3. The ankle mortise has been restored to normal.

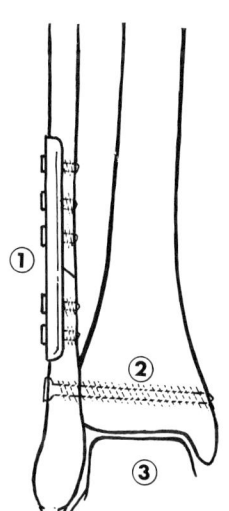

Second Example

Appearance on X-Ray

1. Lateral displacement of the talus resulting from
2. Shortened and malunited fracture of the external malleolus.
3. Incongruity of the articular surface of the talus and tibia.
4. Widening of the ankle mortise.

Note: Correct reduction and realignment of the fibula is key to restoring the ankle mortise to normal. This can be accomplished by principles of fracture fixation outlined in this chapter.

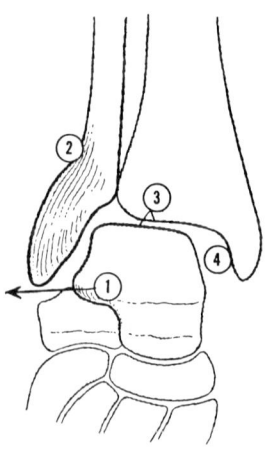

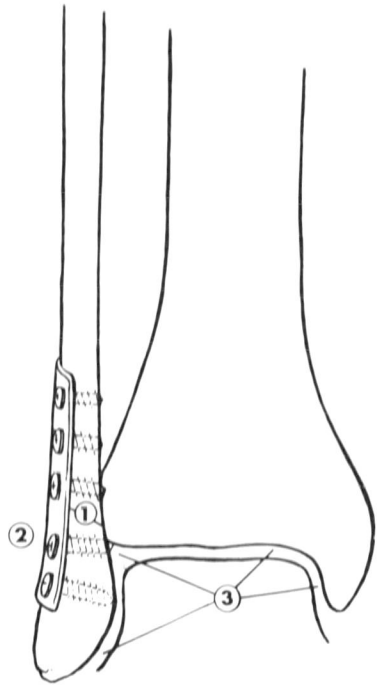

POSTREDUCTION X-RAY

1. The fibula has been osteotomized and restored to correct alignment.
2. Fixation is accomplished by a plate.
3. Correct reduction of the fibula has restored the talus to normal position of the mortise.

EXAMPLES OF MALUNITED FRACTURE-DISLOCATION REQUIRING ARTHRODESIS

Prereduction X-Rays

FIRST EXAMPLE

1. Healed fracture of the posterior articular surface.
2. The talus is chronically dislocated posteriorly.
3. There is concentrated wear on the articular surface owing to incongruity of the talus and tibia.

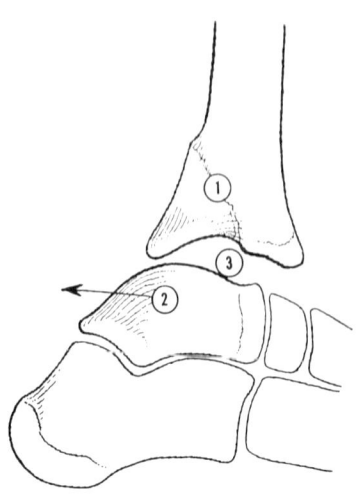

Prereduction X-Rays (Continued)

SECOND EXAMPLE

1. Marked incongruity of the articular surface of the talus and tibia.
2. Irregularity and wearing out of the joint surface is evident.
3. The posterior joint space is lost.
4. There is posterior displacement of the talus.

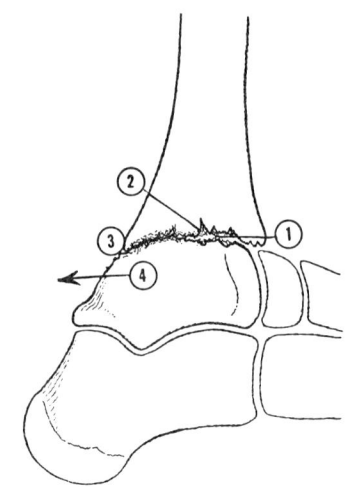

ARTHRODESIS OF THE ANKLE JOINT (ANTERIOR METHOD)

Operative Procedure

1. Make an incision on the anterior aspect of the ankle joint beginning 10 cm above and terminating 2.5 cm below the ankle joint.

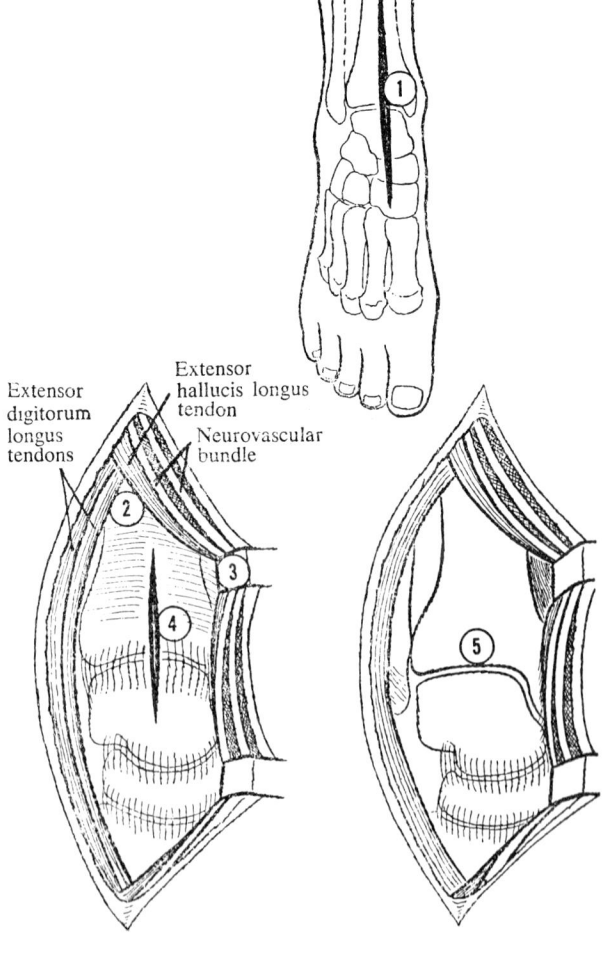

2. Divide the deep fascia in the line of the skin incision and develop the interval between the extensor hallucis lungus and the extensor digitorum longus tendons.
3. Retract the neurovascular bundle medially.
4. Incise the periosteum, capsule, and synovium in the line of the skin incision.
5. By subperiosteal dissection expose the anterior surfaces of the tibia, the talus, and both malleoli.

1. With a thin-bladed, sharp osteotome remove the articular cartilage of the tibia, the talus, and the fibula.

Note: Correct any medial or lateral deviation of the talus by removing a larger wedge of bone from the inner or outer side of the talus or of the tibia.

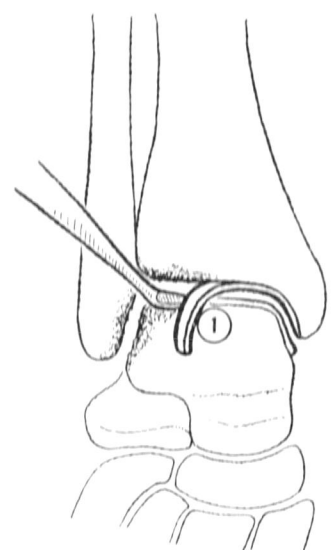

1. Remove a full thickness cortical graft 2.5 by 8 cm from the anterior surface of the tibia immediately above the joint.
2. Cut a slot in the anterior portion of the body and the superior surface of the neck of the talus.

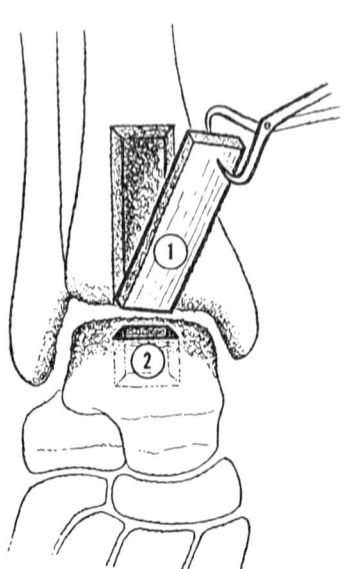

Operative Procedure (Continued)

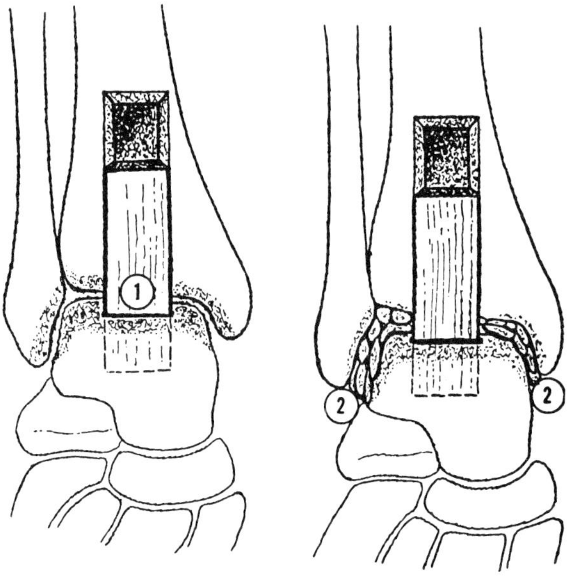

After aligning the talus in the desired position in relation to the tibia,

1. Slide the cortical graft into the slot in the talus and countersink its distal end into the slot.
2. Pack bone chips into the space between the talus and the tibia and fibula. Use medullary bone from the tibia.

Note: In men, place the foot at a right angle; in women, in 5 degrees of plantar flexion.

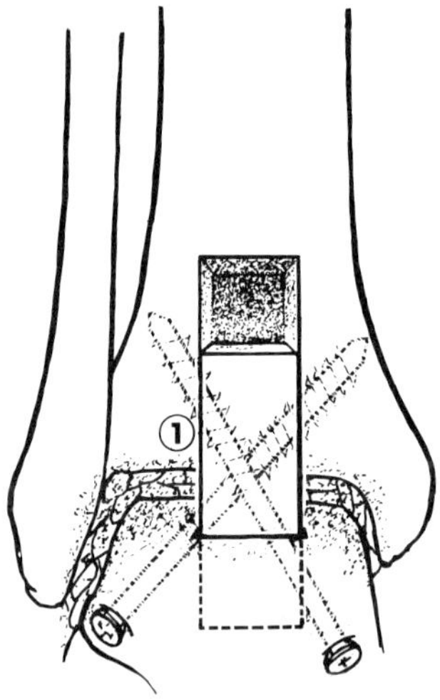

1. The position of the talus is maintained by transarticular cruciate lag screw fixation.

Note: Alternate method of maintaining the position is with a Charnley arthrodesis technique.

Immobilization

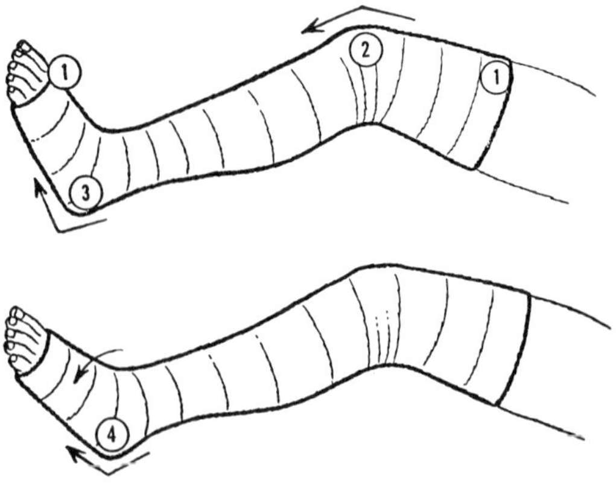

1. Apply a circular plaster cast from behind the metatarsal heads to the midthigh.
2. The knee is slightly flexed.
3. In men the foot is at a right angle.
4. In women the foot is plantar flexed 5 degrees.

Note: X-rays taken at the operating table allow accurate assessment of ankle and foot position.

Postoperative Management

Elevate the limb on pillows.

Apply ice bags around the operative site.

After four weeks remove the long leg cast and apply a short leg, skintight plaster cast with a walking heel.

Now permit weight bearing with crutches.

Take x-rays every four weeks to check progress.

Discontinue the plaster immobilization when consolidation is complete (usually 12 to 16 weeks).

ALTERNATE METHOD: COMPRESSION ARTHRODESIS OF THE ANKLE (CHARNLEY)

Operative Procedure

1. Make a 10-cm longitudinal incision over the subcutaneous surface of the distal end of the fibula ending 2 cm distal to the lateral malleolus.

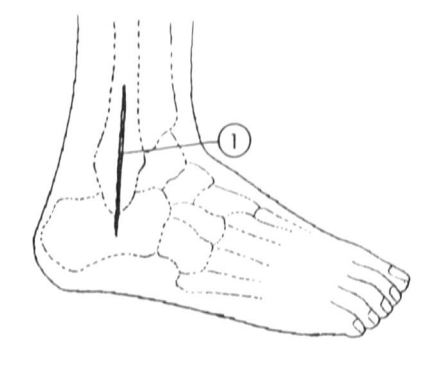

2. Expose the fibula at the upper end of the wound and, with a sharp osteotome, divide it.
3. By sharp dissection free the fibula from all soft tissue attachment except along its posterior aspect.

4. Reflect the fibula downward.

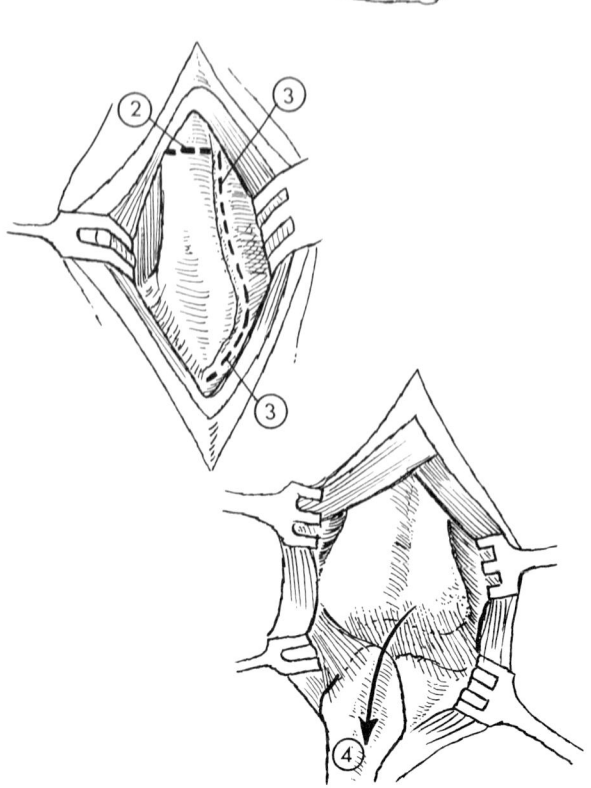

Operative Procedure (Continued)

1. Divide the capsule and ligaments on the anterior and lateral aspects of the ankle joint and expose the articular surfaces of the tibia and talus.
2. Open up the ankle joint like a book, with the hinge medial.
3. Resect the articular surfaces of the tibia and talus so that there is good contact between the raw surfaces when the ankle is in 5 degrees of plantar flexion.

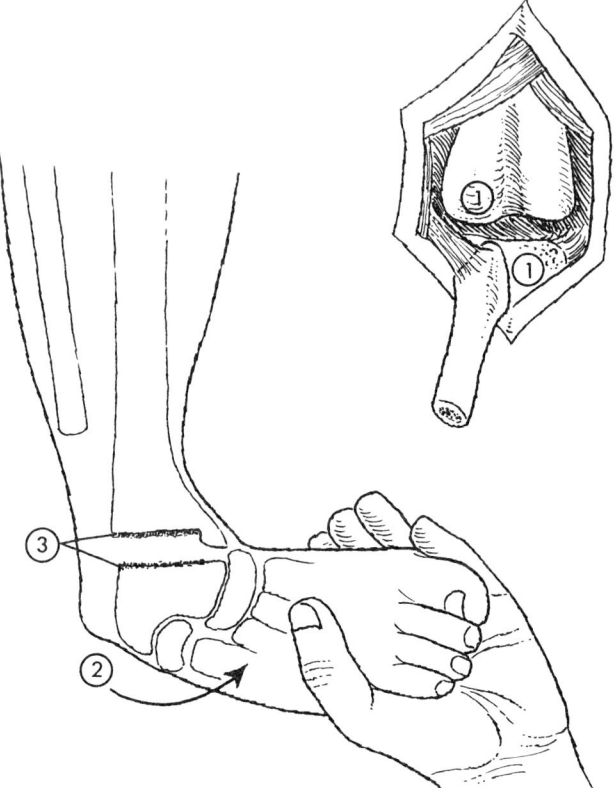

1. Split the fibula longitudinally; the medial half can now be used for chips to pack around the site of arthrodesis.
2. With a sharp osteotome make a level surface on the lateral aspect of the tibia and talus.
3. Pass a Steinmann pin through the talus anterior to its transverse axis.
4. Apply the compression clamps to the distal pin and to a second pin inserted in the tibia above the ankles.

Note: Postoperative management is similar to that described for anterior ankle joint arthrodesis.

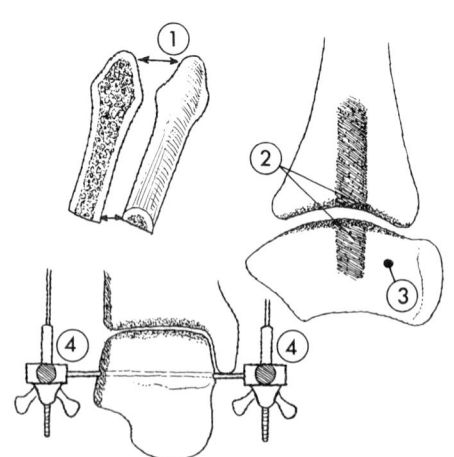

SUMMARY: PITFALLS IN MANAGING ANKLE INJURIES

These common injuries are usually straightforward and uncomplicated. Like all such "usually uncomplicated" injuries, they tend to be underappreciated and are sometimes undertreated.

The common ankle sprain does not require intense diagnostic evaluation but does require thoughtful clinical and radiographic assessment in order to grade the degree of injury. Take care to rule out possible associated injuries such as osteochondral fractures of the talus or fracture of the proximal fibula or tibia.

Treatment should be based not only on the degree of ankle sprain but also on the needs of the patient. The usual first or second degree injury is best treated symptomatically by minimal external support and early exercise therapy to regain range of ankle motion and calf muscle coordination.

The young active individual with a Grade III injury should be offered operative repair, particularly if there is a history of ankle instability. Operative repair of an acute injury is not mandatory because reconstruction of the unstable ankle gives equal satisfactory results.

A common pitfall with chronic or recurrent ankle instability is to dismiss the symptoms as minor because of lack of specific radiographic evidence of talar tilting. A history of recurrent pain or giving way during mild activity and a palpable sulcus in the anterolateral aspect of the ankle confirm the diagnosis. The results of stress x-rays are not always reliable but can be a useful adjunct. Reconstructive procedures, such as the Chrisman-Snook operation, are quite effective in relieving symptoms of ankle instability and preventing osteoarthritic changes. Operative corrections should not be denied these patients because of overconservatism or placing too much emphasis on arbitrary radiographic criteria.

Fractures of the ankle are as common as ankle sprains and are also commonly subject to both undertreatment and overtreatment. Understanding the mechanism of the injury and recognizing the pattern of the fibular fracture associated with various mechanisms aids appropriate selection of treatment.

The detrimental effect of lateral talar shift on ankle load distribution and the importance of fibular length and alignment for ankle stability are the conceptual benchmarks for treatment. Treatment by either closed or open methods should restore the position of the talus in the mortise by means of accurate reduction of the fibula. Accepting even minimal lateral displacement of the talus can produce an unsatisfactory outcome.

In contrast to the real problem of lateral talar displacement, disruption of the distal tibiofibular syndesmosis does not usually cause long-term symptoms.

Overemphasis on the distal tibiofibular diastasis leads to transosseous fibulotibial screw fixation and loss of ankle dorsiflexion. This can be avoided by recognizing and repairing the specific anatomic structures involved, particularly the anterior tibiofibular ligament as well as the fibula.

Posterior marginal fractures may cause posterior instability of the talus. This potential complication should be anticipated particularly in pronation–external rotation mechanisms and should be prevented by adequate internal fixation.

Anterior marginal fracture with anterior subluxation of the talus is among the most difficult of ankle fractures to manage. This injury which is produced by a pronation-dorsiflexion mechanism should be distinguished from comminuted fracture of the articular surface produced by pronation–external rotation mechanism. In the latter instance stabilization of the fibula is helpful for reduction of the talus. For the pronation-dorsiflexion injuries the key fragments of the anterior articular surface must be fixed in order to restore stability of the talus. Attempting to fix all the components of the fracture rigidly may prove disastrous. Fixing the metaphyseal fracture frequently causes distraction of the fracture and subsequent nonunion.

Skeletal traction is an effective method of restoring ankle congruity and ankle motion after a comminuted articular fracture. It should be used in preference to accepting traumatic arthritis and early ankle fusion as inevitable because of intimidating changes on the x-ray. Avoid the pitfall of inordinate dependence on radiographs. The ultimate decision regarding ankle arthrodesis should be based on clinical symptoms rather than arbitrary radiographic criteria.

REFERENCES

Burwell, H. N., and Charnley, A. D.: The treatment of displaced fractures at the ankle by rigid internal fixation and early joint movement. J. Bone and Jt. Surg., 47-B:34, 1965.

Charnley, J.: Compression arthrodesis of the ankle and shoulder. J. Bone and Jt. Surg., 33-B:180, 1951.

Childress, H. M.: Vertical transarticular pin fixation for unstable ankle fractures. Impressions after 16 years of experience. Clinical Orthop., 120:164, 1976.

Chrisman, O. D., and Snook, G. A.: Reconstruction of lateral ligament tears of the ankle. J. Bone and Jt. Surg., 51-A:904, 1969.

Close, J. R.: Some applications of the functional anatomy of the ankle joint. J. Bone and Jt. Surg., 38-A:761, 1956.

Cooperman, D. R., Spiegel, P. G., and Laros, G. S.: Tibial fractures involving the ankle in children. J. Bone and Jt. Surg., 60-A:1040, 1978.

Dameron, T. B.: Management of acute ankle sprains. So. Med. J. 70(10):1166, 1977.

REFERENCES

Eventov, T., Salama, R., Goodwin, D. R. A., et al.: An evaluation of surgical and conservative treatment of fractures of the ankle in 200 patients. J. Trauma, 18:271, 1978.

Freeman, M. A. R.: Treatment of ruptures of the lateral ligament of the ankle. J. Bone and Jt. Surg., 47-B:661, 1965.

Freeman, M. A. R., Dean, M. R. E., and Hanham, I. W. F.: The etiology and prevention of functional instability of the foot. J. Bone and Jt. Surg., 47-B:678, 1965.

Harrington, K. D.: Degenerative arthritis of the ankle secondary to long-standing lateral ligament instability. J. Bone and Jt. Surg. 61-A:354, 1979.

Hawkins, L. G.: Fracture of the lateral process of the talus. J. Bone and Jt. Surg., 47-A:1170, 1965.

Henke, J. A., and Kiple, D. L.: Rotational displacement of the distal tibial epiphysis without fibular fracture. J. Trauma, 19:64, 1979.

Joy, G., Patzakis, M. J., and Harvey, J. P.: Precise evaluation of the reduction of severe ankle fractures. J. Bone and Jt. Surg., 56-A:979, 1974.

Kellam, J. F., and Waddell, J. P.: Fractures of the distal tibial metaphysis with intra-articular extension. The distal tibial explosion fracture. J. Trauma, 19:593, 1979.

Landeros, O., Frost, H. M., and Higgins, C. C.: Post-traumatic anterior ankle instability. Clinical Orthop., 56:169, 1968.

Laskin, R. S.: Steinmann-pin fixation in the treatment of unstable fractures of the ankle. J. Bone and Jt. Surg., 56-A:549, 1974.

Lauge-Hansen, N.: Fractures of the ankle. Arch. Surg., 67:813, 1953.

Lauge-Hansen, N.: Fractures of the ankle. Arch. Surg. 60:957, 1950.

Mayer, P. J., and Evarts, C. M.: Fracture dislocation of the ankle with posterior entrapment of the fibula behind the tibia. J. Bone and Jt. Surg., 60-A:320, 1978.

Morrey, B. F., and Wiedman, G. P.: Complications and long-term results of ankle arthrodesis following trauma. J. Bone and Jt. Surg., 62A:777, 1980.

Pankovich, A. M.: Fractures of the fibula proximal to the distal tibiofibular syndesmosis. J. Bone and Jt. Surg., 60-A:221, 1978.

Pankovich, A. M.: Maisonneuve fracture of the fibula. J. Bone and Jt. Surg., 58-A:337, 1976.

Quigley, T. B.: A simple aid to the reduction of abduction–external rotation fractures of the ankle. Am. J. Surg., 97:488, 1959.

Ramsey, P. L., and Hamilton, W.: Changes in tibiotalar area of contact caused by lateral talar shift. J. Bone and Jt. Surg., 58-A:356, 1976.

Sarkisian, J. S., and Cody, G. W.: Closed treatment of ankle fractures: A new criterion for evaluation — A Review of 250 cases. J. Trauma, 16:323, 1976.

Staples, O. S.: Injuries to the medial ligaments of the ankle. J. Bone and Jt. Surg., 42-A:1287, 1960.

Staples, O. S.: Ruptures of the fibular collateral ligaments of the ankle. J. Bone and Jt. Surg., 57-A:101, 1975.

Tipton, W. W., D'Ambrosia, R. D.: Vascular impairment as a result of fracture-dislocation of the ankle. J. Trauma, 15:524, 1975.

Wilson, F. C., and Skilbred, L. A.: Long-term results in the treatment of displaced bimalleolar fractures. J. Bone and Jt. Surg., 48-A:1065, 1966.

Yablon, I. G., Heller, F. G., and Shouse, L.: The key role of the lateral malleolus in displaced fractures of the ankle. J. Bone and Jt. Surg., 59-A:169, 1977.

Yde, J.: The Lauge-Hansen classification of malleolar fracture. Acta Orthop. Scand, 51:181, 1980.

FRACTURES AND FRACTURE-DISLOCATIONS OF THE BONES OF THE FOOT

FRACTURES AND DISLOCATIONS OF THE TALUS

REMARKS

The talus is subject to injury by mechanisms that can be attributed to extremes of the motion ordinarily occurring between the foot and the leg. These include hyperextension, hyperflexion, inversion, eversion, and compression loading.

Understanding these mechanisms is helpful for both prompt diagnosis and appropriate treatment.

Hyperextension Injuries

Hyperextension mechanisms produce fracture at the junction of the long, exposed talar neck and body.

Peterson and Romanus have demonstrated that this fracture results from hyperextension loading on a plantar flexing foot. Most commonly this occurs when the victim pushes the foot downward against the floor of a motor vehicle or aircraft in preparing to crash.

The common denominator in all these injuries is the application of force to the plantar surface of the tarsometatarsal area of the foot.

1. The brake pedal impacts against the arch of the plantar flexed foot.
2. The extension loading is absorbed entirely by the exposed talar neck, causing it to fracture.
3. Impaction against the articular surface of the tibia is not necessary to produce talar fracture. Usually the tibia is undamaged.

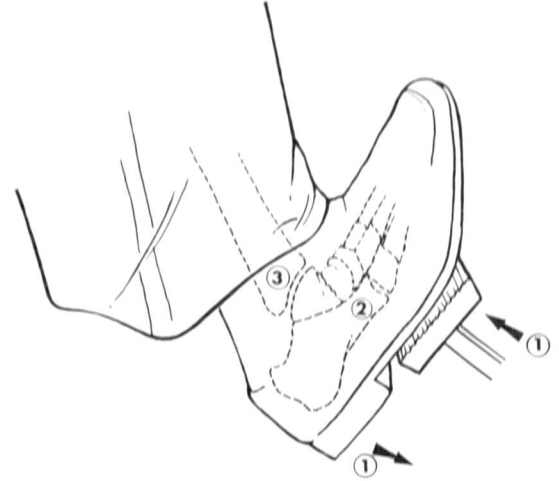

TYPES OF TALAR NECK FRACTURE FROM HYPEREXTENSION INJURY

This injury may be one of four basic types, depending on the severity of the fracture and the displacement of head and neck fragments.

Type I: Undisplaced Fracture

1. The vertical neck fracture of the talus is undisplaced.
2. The subtalar joint is normal.

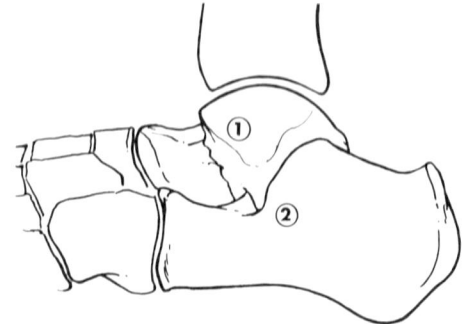

Type II: Displaced Fracture With Subtalar Dislocation or Subluxation

1. Displaced vertical neck fracture.
2. The body displaces, dislocates, or subluxates posteriorly and into equinus.
3. The calcaneus and the remaining portion of the foot subluxate anteriorly with the head fragment.

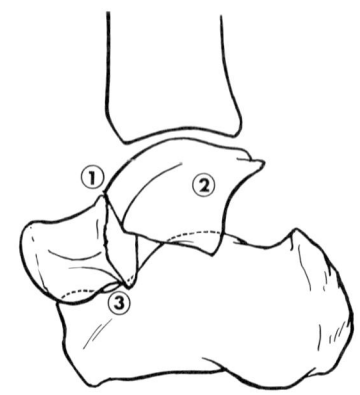

Type III: Displaced Fracture With Complete Dislocation of Body Out of Ankle Mortise

1. The vertical neck fracture is displaced.
2. The body of the talus has dislocated out of the subtalar joint and out of the ankle mortise.

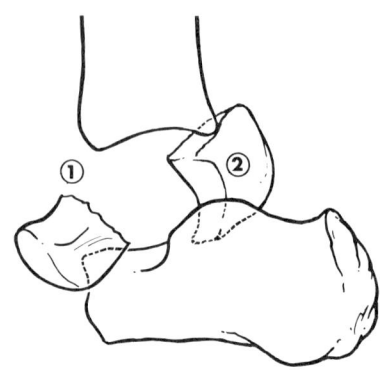

Type IV: Fracture of the Talar Neck With Dislocation of the Body and Dislocation or Subluxation of the Head

1. Grossly displaced vertical fracture of the neck.
2. The neck fragment is dislocated out of the talonavicular joint.
3. The body fragment subluxates from the subtalar joint or may completely dislocate out of the ankle.

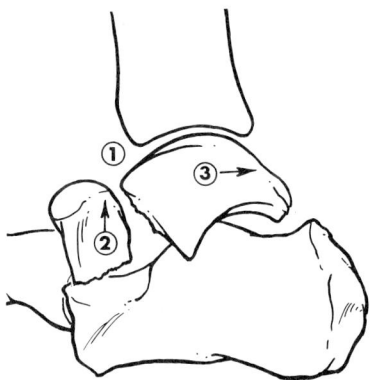

Other Fractures from Hyperextension Injuries: Fractures of the Lateral Process of the Talus

These are the second most common type of talar fractures as reported by Hawkins.

The most plausible mechanism is severe hyperextension of an inverted foot. This causes the lateral facet of the calcaneus to shear off the posterior or lateral process of the talus.

This is usually an undisplaced fracture and frequently is not recognized or is confused with an ankle sprain (see page 1818).

1. On the anteroposterior view, a transverse fracture of the lateral process may be obscure.
2. The fracture may be evident only on a lateral view.

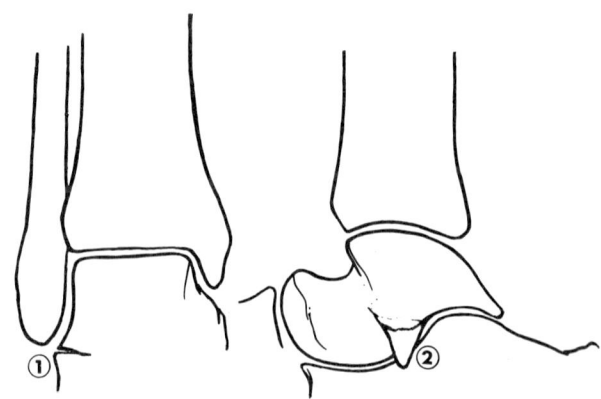

Hyperflexion Injuries

REMARKS

Flexion injuries occur when the force is applied to the heel of the foot behind the posterior tubercle of the talus.

This is a fairly common injury sustained by an athlete while jumping or kicking.

In plantar flexion, a blow to the back of the heel wedges the talus between the posterior calcaneal facet and the posterior tibial margin.

The result is either:

1. A fracture of the posterior talar body or

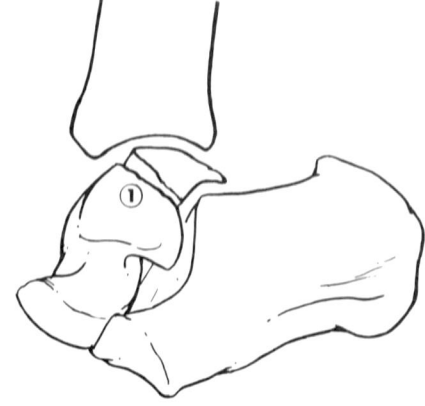

2. A fracture of the posterior talar tubercle.

Note: This undisplaced fracture may be confused with an os trigonum, which can be ruled out by views of the opposite, uninjured ankle.

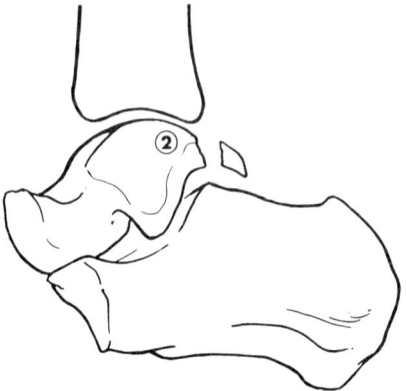

Inversion Injuries

Forced inversion produces injuries such as:

1. Sprain of the calcaneofibular, subtalar, or tibiocalcaneal ligament.

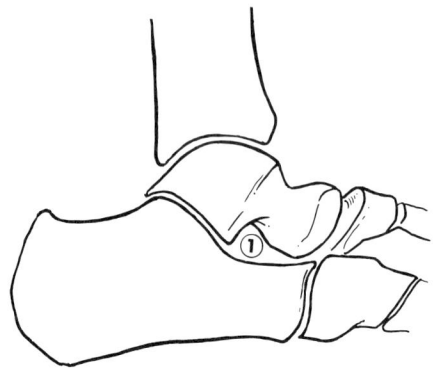

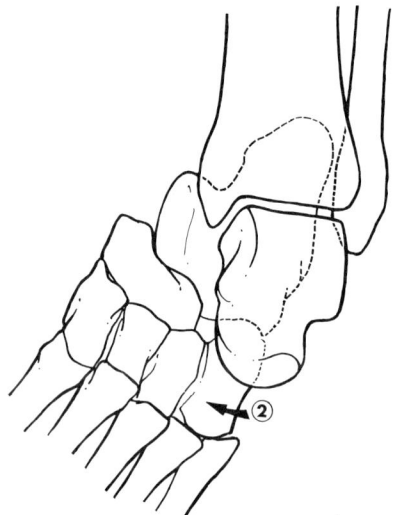

2. Medial dislocation of the subtalar joint.

3. Complete anterior dislocation of the talus.

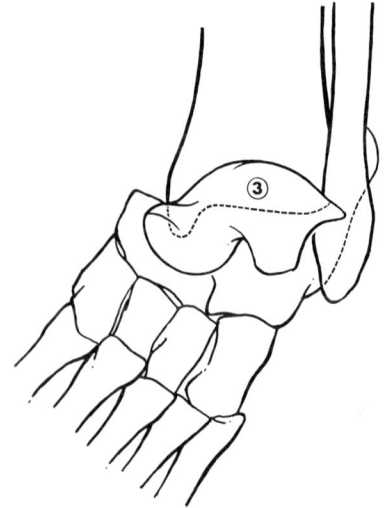

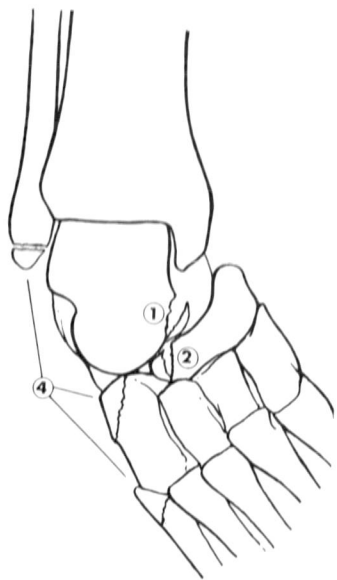

Fractures Resulting From Inversion Injury and Associated With Subtalar Dislocation

1. Vertical shear fracture off the talar head or neck.
2. Fracture of the navicular.
3. Fracture of the posterolateral talus resulting from avulsion by the posterior talofibular ligament.
4. Fracture of fifth metatarsal, cuboid, or fibula.

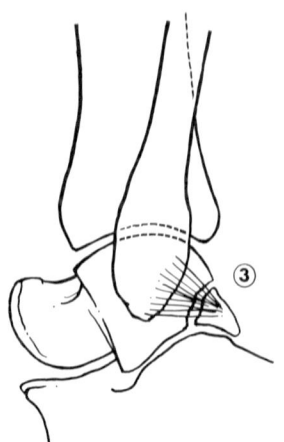

Osteochondral Fractures of the Dome of the Talus Resulting From Inversion Mechanisms

Forced inversion, or inversion with hyperextension loading, can produce:

1. Fracture of the anterolateral surface of the talus.

2. Fracture of the medial surface of the talus is believed to be produced by inversion and loading in plantar flexion. It may also represent a form of spontaneous osteochondritis dissecans.

Note: Osteochondral fractures of the talus are frequently confused with ankle sprain because the mechanism of the injury and the symptoms are similar (see page 1818).

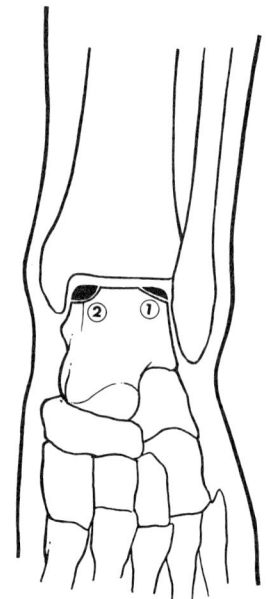

Eversion Mechanisms

REMARKS

Eversion infrequently causes injury to the talus owing to the structural limitations built into the subtalar joint to resist eversion.

The occasional injury resulting from eversion mechanisms include:
1. Lateral subtalar dislocation.

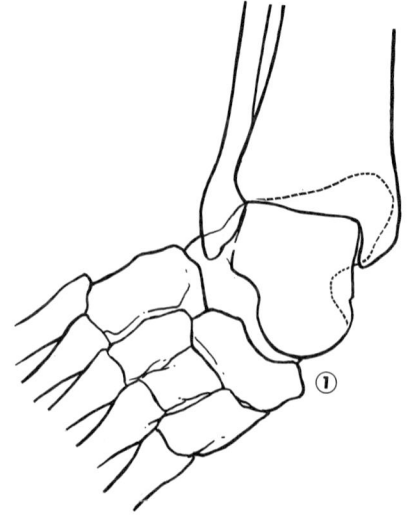

2. Fractures of the lateral malleolus, the navicular, or the cuboid associated with lateral subtalar dislocation.

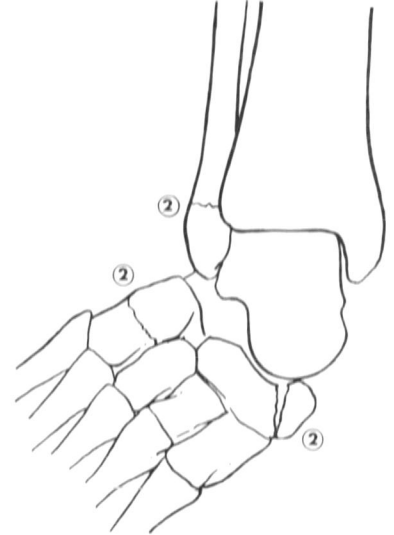

3. Avulsion of the medial side of the posterior talar tubercle produced by the pull of the posterior tibiotalar ligament.

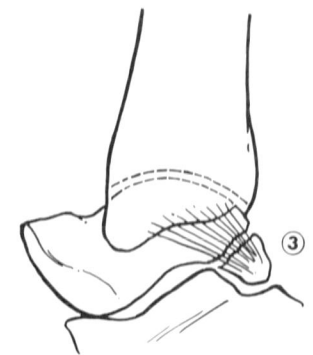

Injuries from Compression or Mixed Mechanisms

REMARKS

Extreme compression loading of the talus causes serious structural damage to both the talus and the surrounding articulations. The result is generally a combination of injuries and mechanisms.

Additional forces may occur in rapid sequence, causing both inversion and eversion injuries.

These might include:

1. Comminuted fracture of the talus from hyperextension and compression.

2. Oblique fracture of the medial malleolus resulting from adduction of the ankle.

3. Lateral dislocation of the foot from an eversion mechanism.

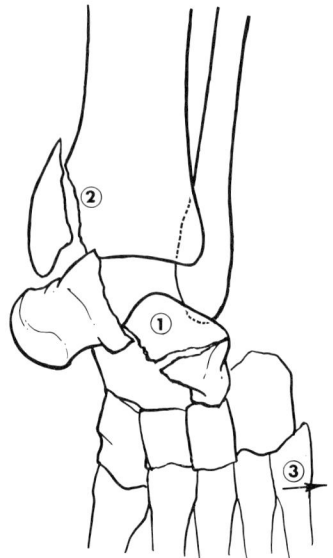

Management of Hyperextension Injuries

TYPE I INJURIES: UNDISPLACED FRACTURE OF THE NECK OR BODY OF THE TALUS

This type of fracture should be carefully assessed by true lateral views as well as anteroposterior views with the foot in plantar flexion.

The lateral view helps particularly to detect subtalar dislocation or dorsal displacement of the head-and-neck fragment.

The anteroposterior view with the foot in maximum plantar flexion enables one to detect any rotational or varus deformity of the head-and-neck fragment.

Technique of Anteroposterior X-Ray (Canale and Kelly)

1. The ankle is placed in maximum equinus position (this is the usual position for reduction of all fractures of the talar neck).
2. Flexion of the hip and knee aids in plantar flexion of the ankle.
3. The foot is plantar flexed 15 degrees.
4. The tube is directed cephalad at a 75-degree angle from the table top.

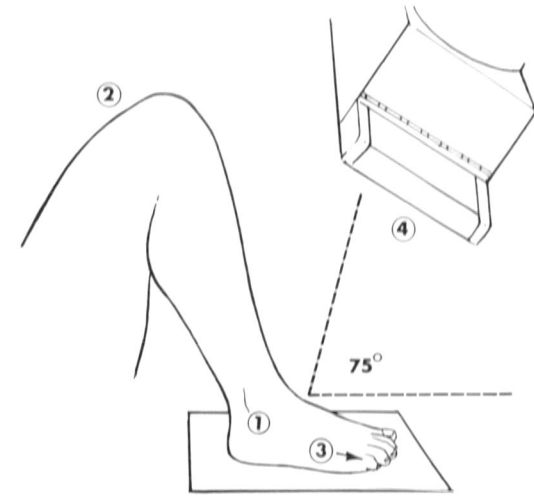

Prereduction X-Rays

ANTEROPOSTERIOR VIEW

1. The head-and-neck fragment is aligned with the body fragment without torsional or medial displacement.
2. The forefoot is in normal relation with the hindfoot.

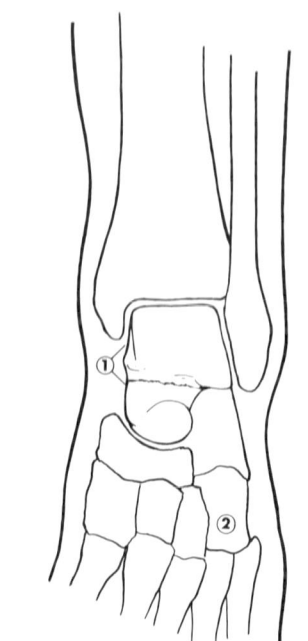

LATERAL VIEW

1. The vertical fracture through the neck of the talus is evident without dorsal displacement of the head and neck fragment.
2. The subtalar joint is not subluxated or dislocated.

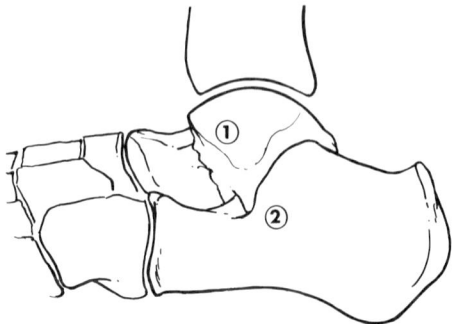

Immobilization

1. Apply a circular plaster cast from behind the metatarsal heads to the midthigh.
2. The knee is flexed 30 degrees.
3. The foot is in slight plantar flexion.

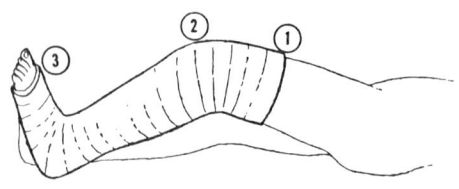

Management

The patient may walk on crutches but must not bear weight on the injured limb.

The cast is changed at the end of four weeks.

The foot is brought out of plantar flexion during the cast change at the end of four weeks.

CAUTION

Avoid dorsal displacement of the neck fragment during cast change.

1. When the foot is brought out of equinus, the distal fragment may be displaced dorsally.
2. The result can be a dorsal beak on the talus, which causes painful ankle motion and may require excision.

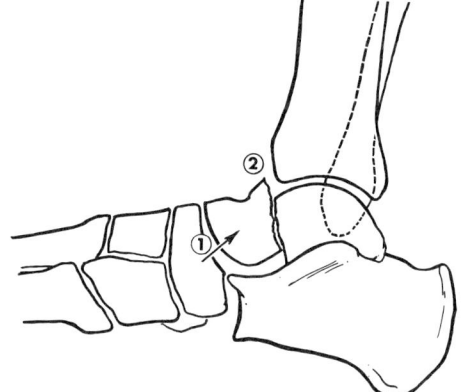

Subsequent Management

The cast can be discarded at the end of eight weeks, but the patient should continue partial weight bearing with crutches.

Institute exercises to restore normal motion in the ankle and joints of the foot.

Full weight bearing is generally possible at the end of twelve weeks.

Advise the patient that complications such as avascular necrosis and arthritis are rare but still possible with this type of fracture.

Follow the patient clinically and by x-ray for six months or longer after the injury to detect any signs of these complications (see page 1993).

TYPE II INJURIES: FRACTURE OF THE NECK OF THE TALUS WITH SUBLUXATION OF THE SUBTALAR JOINT

REMARKS

Any displacement of the fractured talus or subluxation of the subtalar joint is a general indication for accurate open reduction and internal fixation.

Closed reduction may rarely be successful. It may sometimes be indicated in the patient with multiple injuries that preclude prompt operative fixation of the talus and reduction of the subtalar joint.

The subtalar joint must be carefully assessed on a true lateral x-ray. Fracture alignment in the frontal plane is best evaluated by an anteroposterior x-ray taken with the foot in plantar flexion, as described on page 1961.

Prereduction X-Ray

LATERAL VIEW

1. Displaced vertical fracture through the neck of the talus.
2. The body of the talus is displaced into equinus and posteriorly.
3. The os calcis is displaced anteriorly with the neck and body of the talus.

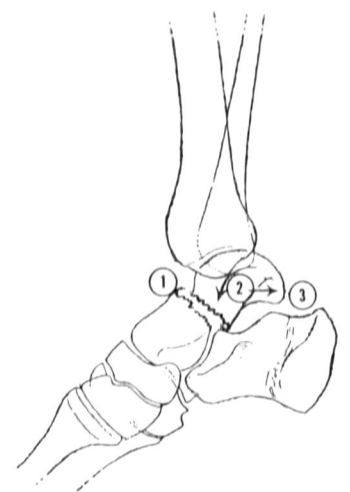

ANTEROPOSTERIOR VIEW IN PLANTAR FLEXION

1. The head-and-neck fragment is rotated internally.
2. The forefoot rotates inward with the head-and-neck fragment.
3. The fibula rotates internally with the talus.

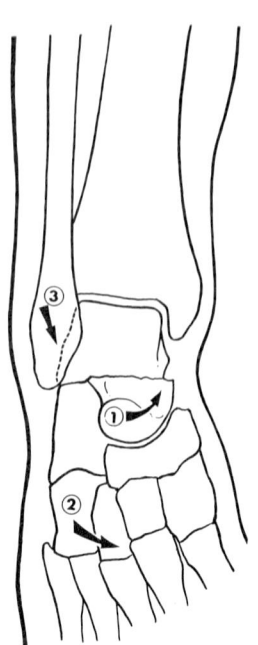

Manipulative Reduction

Note: This should be restricted to individuals in whom operative fixation is contraindicated.

1. The leg hangs over the end of the table with the knee flexed 45 degrees; an assistant steadies the lower leg.
2. The operator grasps the heel with one hand and the forefoot with the other hand.
3. The operator strongly plantar flexes the foot and at the same time
4. Pushes the foot backward and
5. Everts the foot.

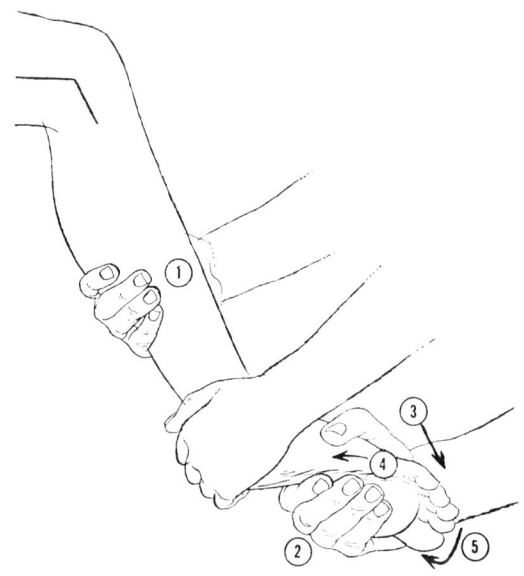

Postreduction X-Ray

Lateral view

1. The neck and body are in normal position.
2. The articular surfaces of the body and calcaneus are now congruous.

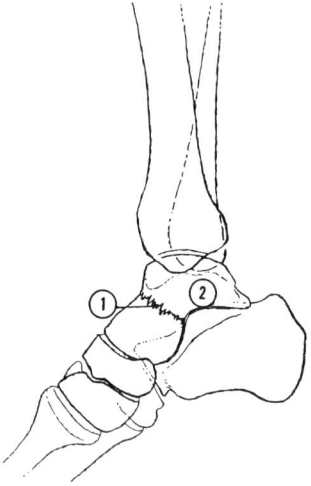

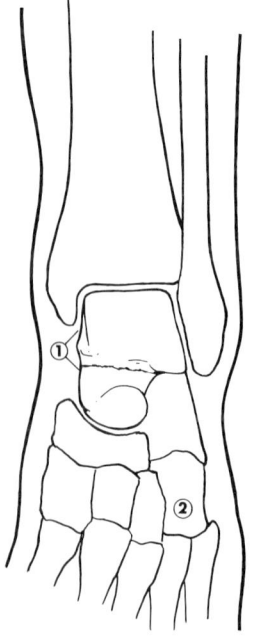

Anteroposterior view in plantar flexion

1. The torsional displacement of the distal head-and-neck fragment has been corrected.
2. The forefoot is in normal relation with the hind foot.

Immobilization

1. Apply a circular cast from behind the metatarsal heads to the midthigh.
2. The knee is flexed 30 degrees.
3. The foot is plantar flexed and everted.

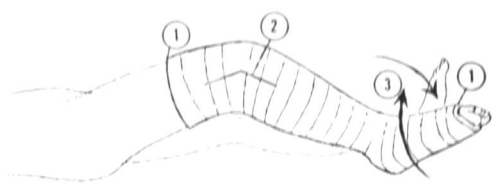

Postreduction Management

Allow the patient to walk on crutches without bearing weight on the injured limb.

The cast is changed at the end of four weeks and the foot is brought out of the plantar flexed everted position.

CAUTION

Avoid dorsal displacement of the neck fragment during the cast change.

1. When the foot is brought out of equinus, the distal fragment may be displaced dorsally.
2. The result can be a dorsal beak on the talus, which causes painful ankle motion and may require excision.

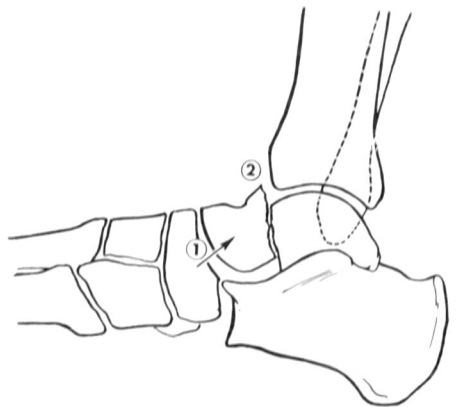

PREFERRED METHOD: CLOSED REDUCTION AND SCREW FIXATION USING A POSTERIOR APPROACH (TRILLAT AND COWORKERS)

REMARKS

Lemaire and Bustin recently reported good to excellent results with this technique, which was originally described by Trillat and coworkers.

The method permits internal fixation of displaced talar fractures without adding further to the risk of avascular necrosis. Good reduction and secure internal fixation avoid joint incongruity or malrotation and secondary osteoarthritis. The method avoids the need to immobilize the foot in equinus and eliminates the risk of displacing the fracture when the foot is dorsiflexed. Fixation of the talus from front to back compresses the fracture line, and the consequent rigid fixation frequently shortens the period of postoperative immobilization.

If adequate closed reduction is not possible or if the talus is completely dislocated (Type III or Type IV), open reduction of the fracture is usually necessary to achieve adequate internal fixation.

The Trillat method does not give complete protection against avascular necrosis. No weight should be borne on the fracture side until at least well after the signs of revascularization and healing are seen on x-ray (see page 1995).

Prereduction X-Ray

1. Displaced vertical fracture through the neck of the talus.
2. The body of the talus is displaced into equinus and posteriorly.
3. The os calcis is displaced distally with the neck and body of the talus.

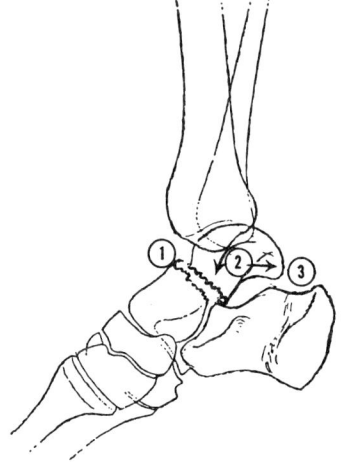

Technique of Closed Reduction and Posterior Screw Insertion

The patient is placed prone on the operating table and the injured limb is prepared and draped with a tourniquet at thigh level.

The fracture has been manipulated and reduced as described on page 1964.

In Type II fractures, anatomic alignment is usually possible, but in Type III or IV fracture-dislocations, open reduction is usually necessary.

When reduction is ascertained by x-ray in both the anteroposterior plantar flexion view and the lateral view, a screw is inserted from the posterolateral aspect of the talus.

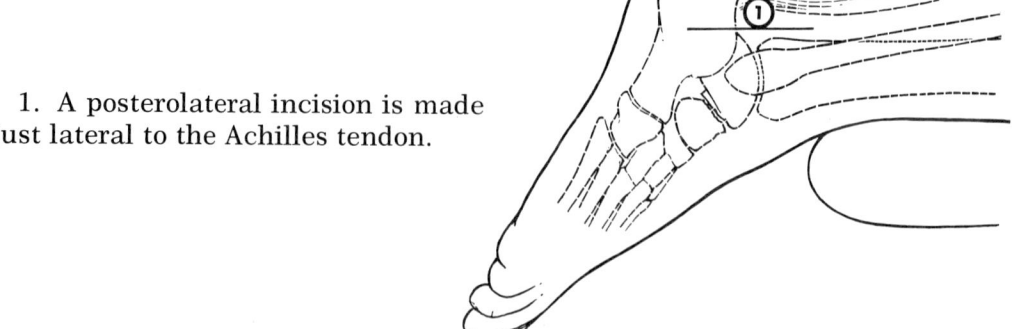

1. A posterolateral incision is made just lateral to the Achilles tendon.

2. A Kirschner wire is introduced under fluoroscopic guidance from the posterior tubercle along the longitudinal axis of the talus as perpendicular as possible to the fracture line.

3. In the frontal plane, the wire should be placed slightly off center and should be left as a guide for drilling and inserting the screw.

4. With the Kirschner wire in place, the posterior tuberosity is drilled and tapped, and a cancellous bone lag screw is inserted.

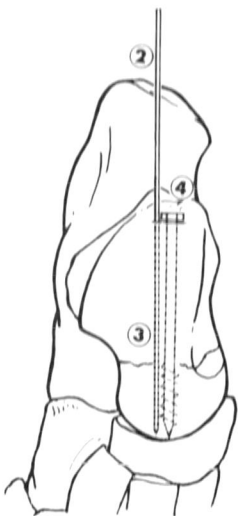

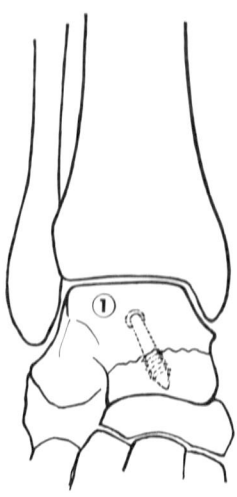

Postreduction X-Rays

The position of the screw should be satisfactory on both:

1. Anteroposterior and
2. Lateral views.

Note: If satisfactory reduction is not achieved by closed manipulation, open reduction under direct vision should be carried out.

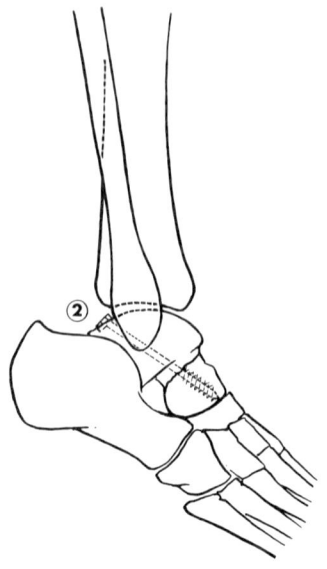

Alternate Technique: Operative Reduction under Direct Vision

1. Make an 8-cm incision on the anteromedial aspect of the ankle; it begins in front of and above the medial malleolus, curves forward and then downward, and terminates on the inner aspect of the navicular.
2. By sharp dissection expose the head and neck of the talus.
3. Retract the posterior tibial tendon out of the field.

Note: Avoid damaging the artery to the tarsal canal (see page 1994).

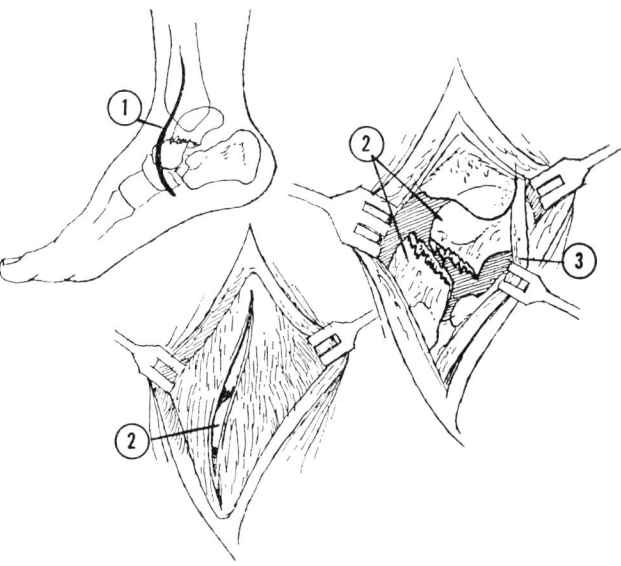

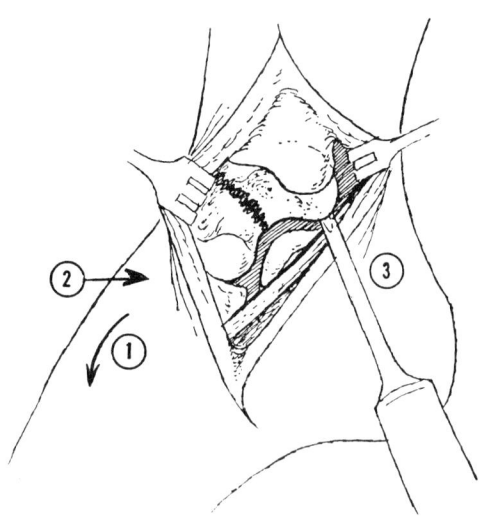

Reduce the fracture-dislocation:
1. Plantar flex the foot.
2. Push the foot backward.
3. Lever (if necessary) the body into apposition with the neck of the talus.

1. Grasp and hold both fragments with a tenaculum.
2. On the medial aspect of the neck just proximal to the articular surface drill a hole directed obliquely posteriorly and laterally through the neck and body and secure the fragments with a screw of proper length.

Note: Always obtain an intraoperative anteroposterior view of the foot in plantar flexion and a lateral view to insure the adequacy of reduction.

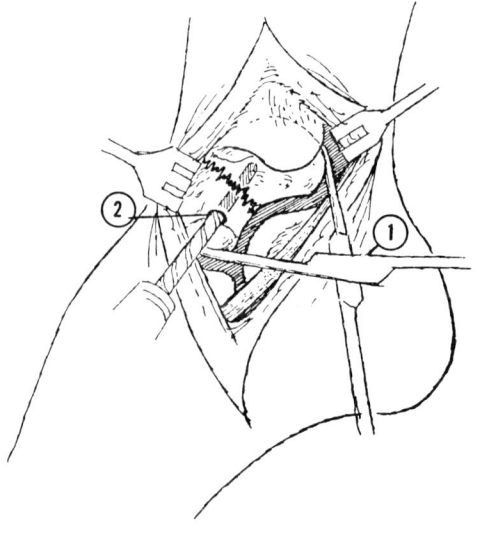

Intraoperative X-Rays

ANTEROPOSTERIOR VIEW IN PLANTAR FLEXION

1. The torsional alignment of the distal fragment has been correctly restored.
2. The forefoot is in proper relationship with the hindfoot.

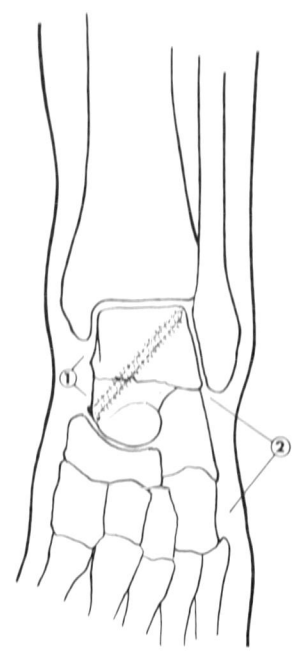

LATERAL VIEW

1. The body of the talus and calcaneus are in normal relationship.
2. The screw is transfixing both fragments.

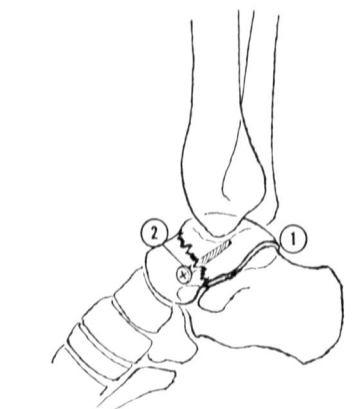

Postoperative Immobilization

1. Apply anterior and posterior splints to allow for the postoperative swelling.
2. The knee is flexed 30 degrees.
3. The ankle is at a right angle.
4. The foot is neutral in regard to eversion and inversion.

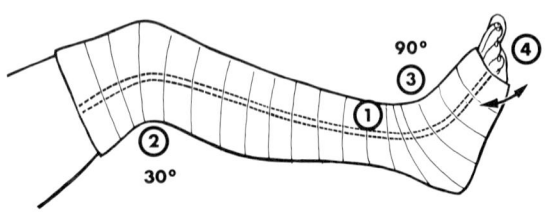

The sutures and splints are removed at the end of 10 to 14 days and a circular plaster cast is applied.

Plaster cast immobilization is continued for 4 to 6 weeks and then the cast is discarded.

Weight bearing can generally be resumed 2 months after injury if there is evidence of revascularization and subchondral bone atrophy (see page 1995).

If there is any question about the possibility of avascular necrosis, weight bearing should be delayed and the ankle should be protected (see page 1996).

TYPE III AND TYPE IV INJURIES: DISPLACED FRACTURES OF THE NECK WITH DISLOCATION OF THE HEAD OR BODY OF THE TALUS

REMARKS

A large percentage of these injuries, which are produced by extreme violence, are open and require prompt operative wound treatment and associated internal fixation.

Operative reduction and internal fixation are also indicated for closed Type III or IV injuries.

Early attempts at manipulation may be necessary to relieve skin tension or to improve temporarily the position of the talus while the patient is being treated for life-threatening injuries.

A satisfactory result from closed management is highly unlikely with injuries displaced to this degree. Nonunion or malunion is the rule with closed treatment, and adequate operative reduction and internal fixation is the preferred method.

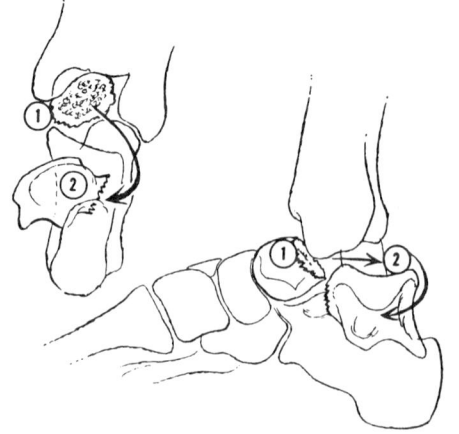

Prereduction X-Ray

1. Vertical fracture through the neck of the talus with some comminution.
2. The body of the talus is displaced backward and is rotated.

Manipulative Reduction (Under General Anesthesia)

1. Place a canvas sling around the distal end of the thigh; the sling is suspended from an overhead cross bar on the fracture table.
2. The knee is flexed 90 degrees.
3. The operator grasps the heel with one hand and the forefoot with the other.
4. The operator pulls the foot forward and forces it into marked dorsiflexion.

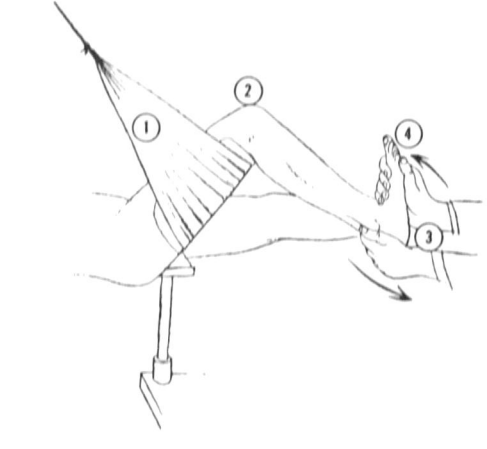

While the forward pull on the foot and dorsiflexion are maintained,
1. The operator strongly everts the foot; this maneuver unlocks the sustentaculum tali.

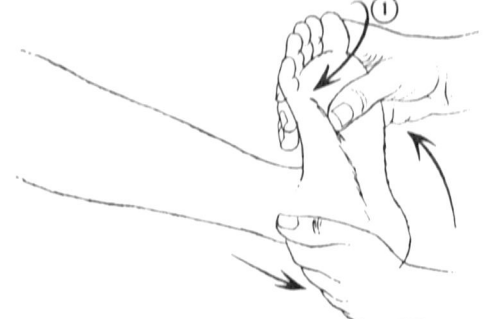

1. While an assistant makes firm pressure behind the ankle on either side of the Achilles tendon,
2. The operator plantar flexes the foot.

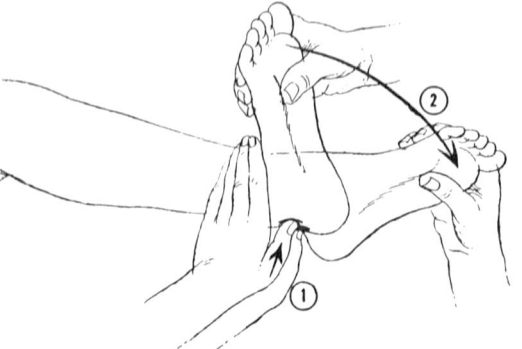

PREFERRED METHOD: OPEN REDUCTION AND SCREW FIXATION

Because of the extreme amount of soft tissue damage usually associated with this injury, wide surgical dissection should be avoided.

After the dislocated body is replaced, the fracture can be reduced in plantar flexion and held by a cancellous screw inserted from the body into the head-and-neck fragment.

If the head-and-neck fragment is also dislocated, a second incision may be required to permit reduction and minimize disruption of the blood supply to the talus.

If at all possible, the talus should be salvaged despite the virtual certainty of avascular necrosis. Reconstitution of the talus by creeping substitution is possible following adequate reduction and fixation.

If the talus is so comminuted that adequate reduction is impossible or if bone fragments have been lost, stabilization of the foot by a tibiocalcaneal or tibiotalar (Blair) fusion should be considered (see page 2001).

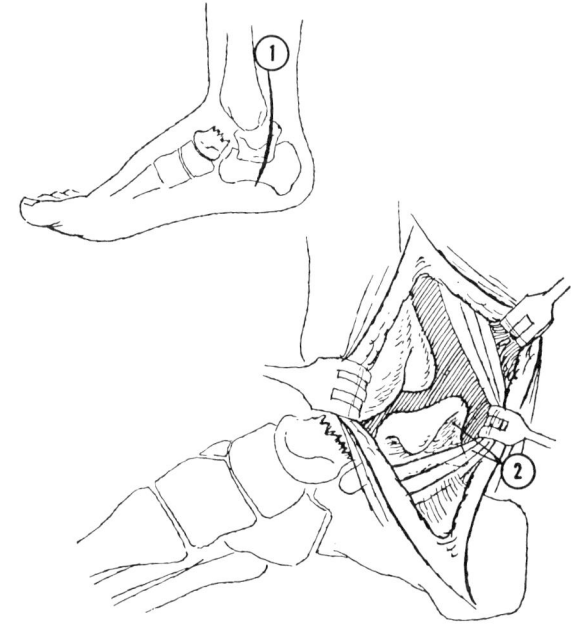

Operative Procedure

1. Make a 10-cm vertical incision over the posteromedial aspect of the ankle joint.
2. Expose the body of the talus and the posteromedial aspect of the calcaneus.

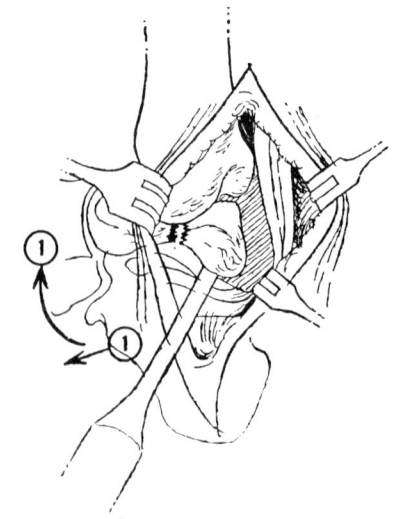

1. With the foot pulled forward and dorsiflexed, lever the body into the tibiofibular mortise.

2. Finally, plantar flex the foot to complete the reduction.

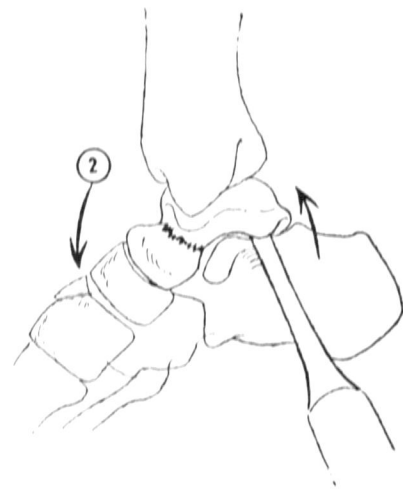

1. Insert a smooth Kirschner wire from the posterior tuberosity of the talus into the head-and-neck fragment.
2. In the frontal plane, the wire should be placed slightly off center and left as a guide for drilling and inserting the screw.
3. With the Kirschner wire in place, the posterior tuberosity is drilled and tapped, and a cancellous bone lag screw is inserted.

Postreduction X-Rays

The position of the screw should be satisfactory on both:
1. Anteroposterior and
2. Lateral views.

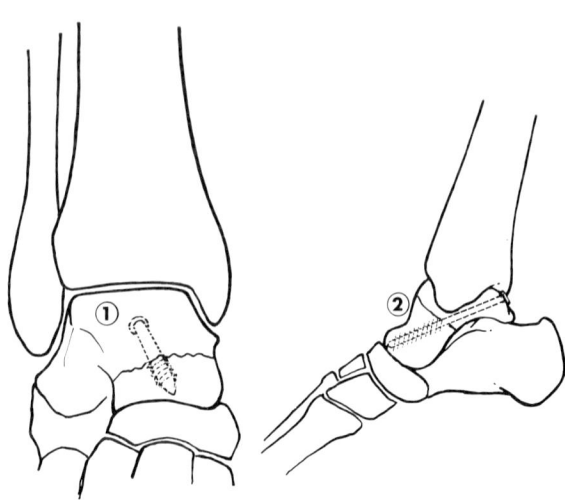

Immobilization

1. Apply anterior and posterior plaster splints to allow for the usual postoperative swelling.
2. The knee is flexed 30 degrees.
3. The ankle is held at 90 degrees.
4. The foot is slightly pronated.

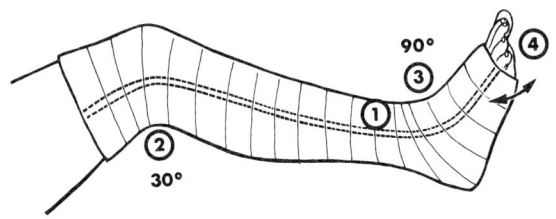

Postoperative Management

Keep the limb elevated and apply ice packs to the foot and ankle.

Check the circulation distally on an hourly basis for evidence of circulatory embarassment.

By the end of 10 to 14 days the sutures and splints are removed and a short leg cast is applied with the foot in a position of slight plantar flexion and pronation.

The cast is changed in 4 weeks and the foot is brought up to neutral position.

Healing is usually complete and the plaster can be discontinued by the end of 12 to 14 weeks. The patient is advised to continue on crutches and to bear no weight on the leg but to actively exercise the ankle and foot.

Radiographic changes of avascular necrosis should be expected after this significant injury, and the patient should be advised to continue to protect the ankle from loading by either remaining on crutches or using specific braces (see page 1996).

FRACTURES OF THE LATERAL PROCESS OF THE TALUS

REMARKS

Hawkins has pointed out that after talar neck fracture, fracture of the lateral process is the second most common fracture of the talus.

The initial diagnosis is frequently missed owing to the sometimes subtle radiographic findings. The patient is then treated for a sprain and has persistent symptoms.

Unexplained and persistent pain about the lateral side of the ankle following a forced dorsiflexion-inversion injury should be carefully evaluated for a fracture of the lateral process of the talus.

Prereduction X-Ray

1. On the anteroposterior x-ray the fracture may be obscure.

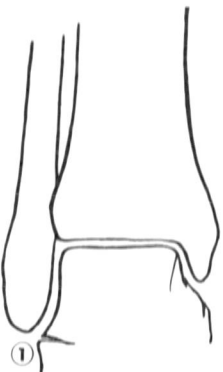

2. The lateral x-ray usually shows a chip off the lateral process.

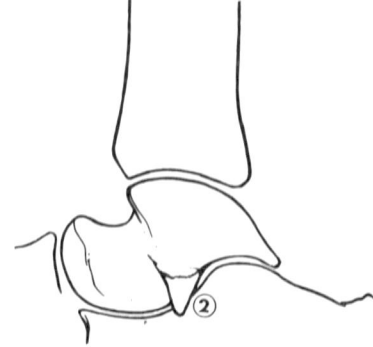

Initial Management

If the fracture is diagnosed promptly, treatment by a short leg, partial weight bearing cast is most effective.
1. Apply a below-the-knee plaster cast with
   2. Walking heel.
   3. The foot is at a right angle and
   4. in neutral rotation

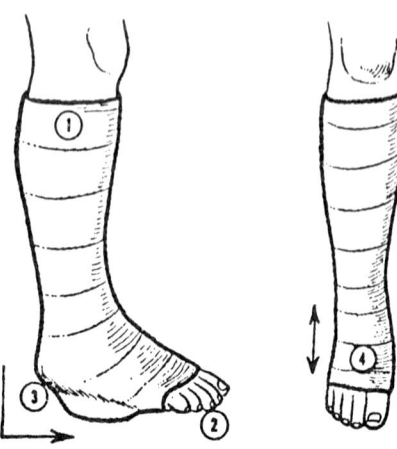

Subsequent Management

The patient bears partial weight on the leg and remains in the cast for four weeks; then the cast is removed.

Progressive weight bearing is allowed until the leg is pain free.

Management of Displaced or Unrecognized Fractures

1. For initially displaced or unrecognized fractures or

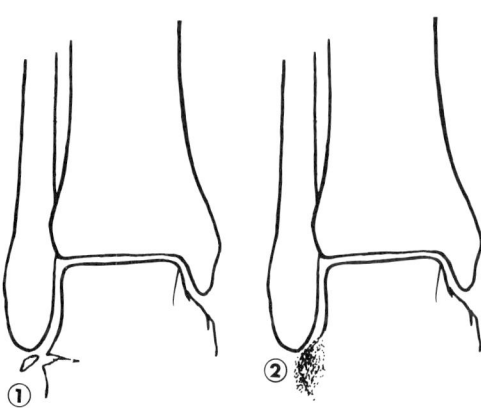

2. Fractures that heal with symptomatic overgrowth,

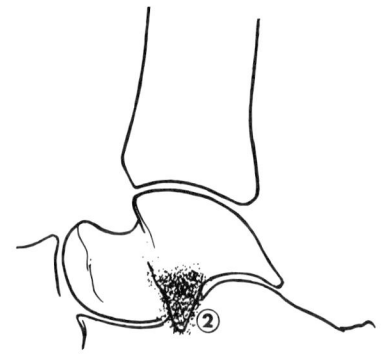

3. Treatment is by excision of the fragment.

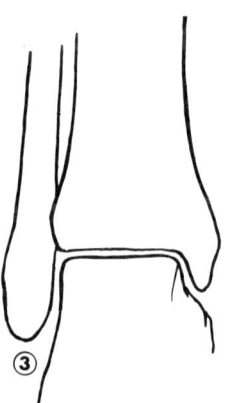

Management of Hyperflexion Injuries

FRACTURE OF THE POSTERIOR PROCESS OF THE TALUS

REMARKS

These injuries frequently occur in an athlete such as a basketball player who sustains a plantarflexion injury while jumping.

The posterior talar body is wedged between the os calcis and the posterior tibia, resulting in a fracture of the posterior tuberosity of the talus.

An alternate mechanism is an avulsion from forced inversion or eversion (see pages 1957 and 1959).

Smaller fracture fragments must be distinguished from os trigonum (accessory bones). Comparison x-rays of the opposite ankle are helpful to distinguish sesamoid bones from fracture fragments.

Quite frequently, confusion of the undisplaced posterior talar fracture with an os trigonum results in prolonged disability for the patient.

Treatment with a plaster cast is usually sufficient for the injury when recognized early.

For the unrecognized and symptomatic injury or the fracture that heals with excessive callus and impaired function of the flexor hallucis longus tendon, surgical excision is indicated.

X-Ray of the Acute Injury

1. A posterior tuberosity fracture has occurred from a blow to the plantar flexed heel of a basketball player.

Note: Comparison x-rays of the opposite ankle show that this is a fracture rather than an os trigonum.

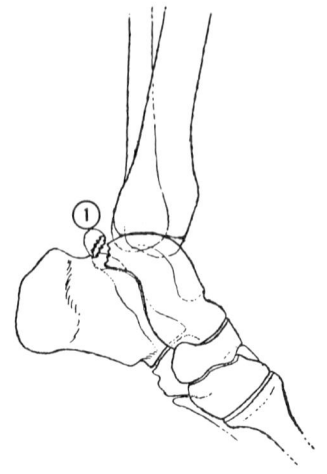

Manipulative Reduction

The patient is in the prone position with the knee flexed 90 degrees.

1. An assistant strongly dorsiflexes the foot while
2. The operator makes deep downward pressure on either side of the Achilles tendon directly over the displaced fragment.

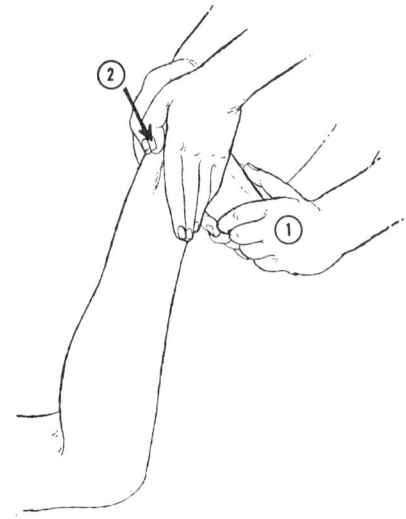

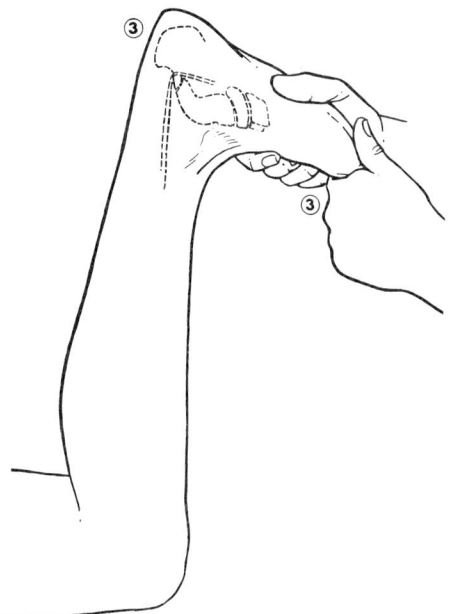

3. Dorsiflexing the big toe aids reduction by pulling on the flexor hallucis longus tendon, which runs behind the fragment.

Postreduction X-Ray

1. The posterior process of the talus is in apposition to the body of the talus.

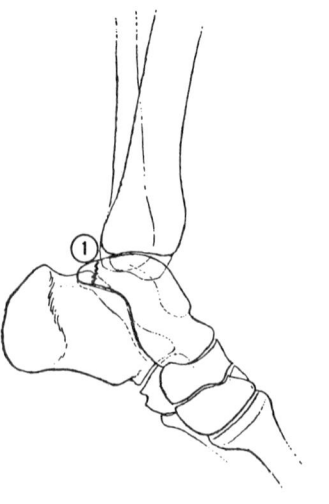

Immobilization

1. Apply a circular plaster cast from behind the toes to midthigh.
2. The foot is slightly dorsiflexed.
3. The knee is flexed 30 degrees.

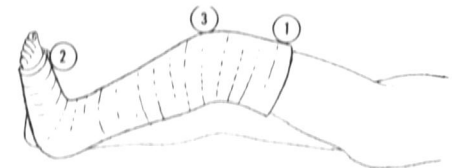

Postreduction Management

Allow immediate ambulation on crutches with no weight borne on the affected foot.

Remove the cast at the end of four weeks.

Now permit weight bearing.

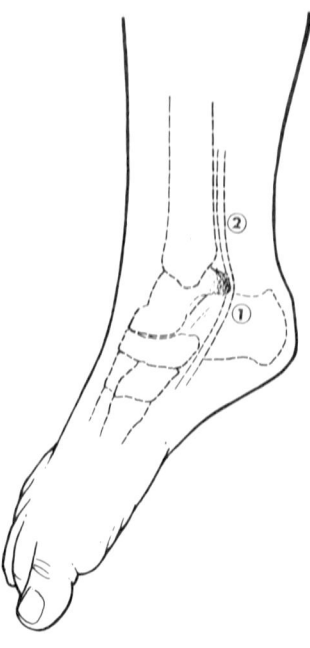

Indications for Surgical Excision of the Fragment

1. The displaced fracture that heals with excessive callus, causing painful impairment of the flexor hallucis longus tendon.
2. Unrecognized fracture of the posterior tuberosity that causes persistent pain due to impingement of the fragment against the posterior tibia.

X-Ray After Excision of the Fragment

1. The impingement symptoms from the fracture have been relieved.
2. The subtalar joint is unaffected by the excision.

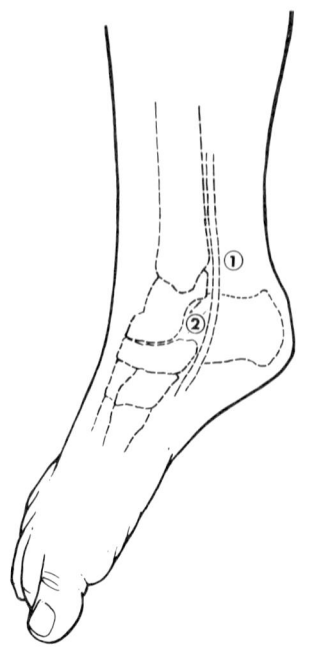

Management of Inversion Injuries

REMARKS

The most common dislocation of the talus is a medial subtalar dislocation produced by inversion.

Complete dislocations of the talus out of the mortise is fortunately infrequent but it can occur with severe inversion.

Inversion mechanisms produce injuries such as:
1. Sprain of the subtalar ligaments.
2. Medial subtalar dislocation.
3. Complete dislocation of the talus.
4. Osteochondral lesions of the talus.

Inversion injuries may also produce fractures associated with subtalar dislocation, including:
1. Shear fracture of the head of the talus.
2. Shear fracture of the navicular.
3. Avulsion fracture of the posterior talus.
4. Avulsion of the base of the fifth metatarsal.
5. Avulsion of the cuboid.
6. Avulsion of the lateral malleolus.

Management

Treatment for acute subtalar sprain is similar to tibiotalar sprain. (see page 1812). Operative repair may be necessary for the recurrent problem of instability of the subtalar joint, as described by Chrisman and Snook (see page 1829).

Subtalar dislocation as well as complete dislocation of the talus requires prompt reduction in order to avoid pressure necrosis of the skin and subsequent infection.

Occasionally reduction may be prevented if the talar head is entrapped by the extensor digitorum brevis or other soft tissue structures on the anterolateral aspect of the ankle. Shear fracture of the talus or the navicular can also lock and prevent reduction of the foot.

MEDIAL SUBTALAR DISLOCATION

Prereduction X-Ray

1. The talus is held in the tibiofibular mortise.
2. The foot is displaced medially at the subtalar and talonavicular joints.
3. The talus is in equinus owing to the loss of inferior and anterior support.

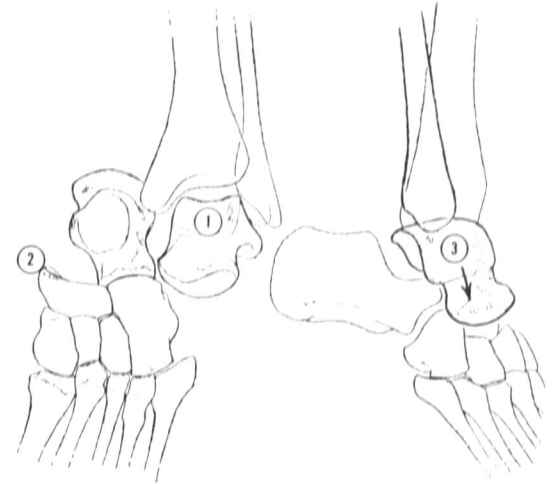

Manipulative Reduction

Note: Reduction should be performed promptly. If it is done within a few hours, morphine analgesia is satisfactory. In other cases, general anesthesia may be necessary.

1. Place a well-padded canvas sling under the distal end of the thigh and suspend it from an overhead cross bar on the fracture table.
2. The knee is flexed 90 degrees to relax the gastrocnemius.

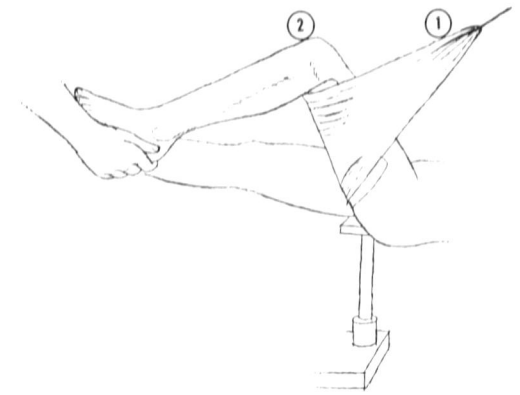

1. The assistant holds and steadies the lower leg.
2. The operator grasps the heel with one hand and the forefoot with the other.
3. The foot is first strongly plantar flexed; then
4. The foot is everted and abducted.

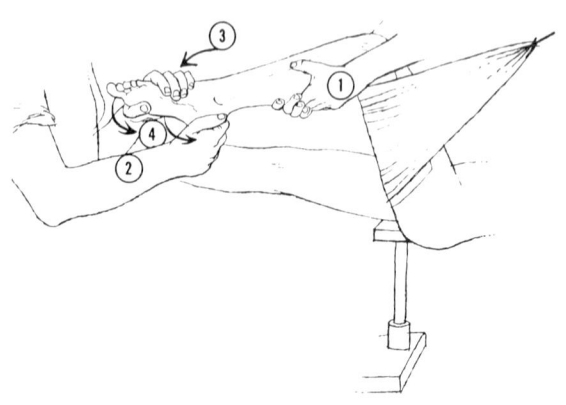

Postreduction X-Ray

1. The subtalar and talonavicular dislocations are reduced.
2. The talus is in its normal relation to the navicular, calcaneus, and tibia.

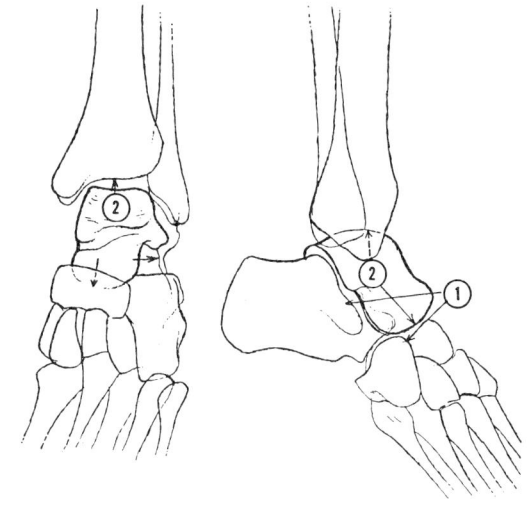

Obstacles to Reduction

Although most subtalar dislocations reduce promptly, Leitner found that approximately 8 per cent of medial subtalar dislocations are irreducible because of:

1. Entrapment of the head of the talus in the surrounding soft tissues or
2. Impaction of the fractures of the head of the talus or navicular.

Note: Occasionally the obstacles may be removed by grasping the heel and applying manual traction on the foot while alternating dorsiflexion and plantar flexion manipulation. This should be done carefully, and further fracture of the talus should be avoided. In most instances operative reduction should be carried out if the subtalar joint is not reduced promptly by careful manipulation (see page 1990).

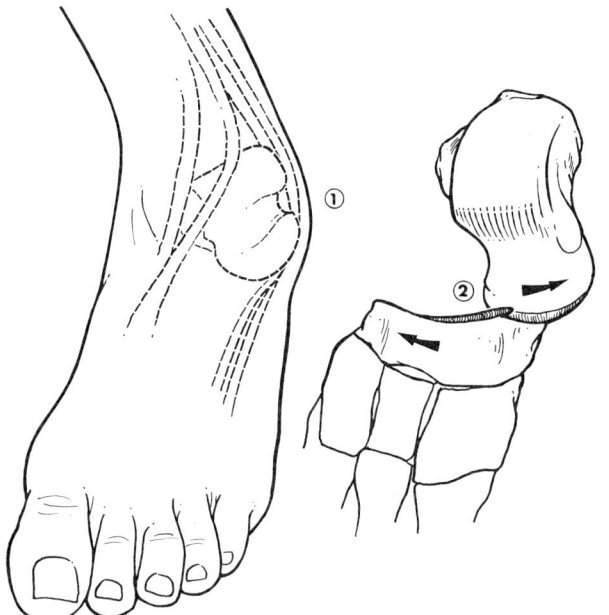

Immobilization

1. Apply anterior and posterior splints to allow for swelling of the foot after reduction.
2. The knee is flexed 30 degrees.
3. The foot is dorsiflexed 90 degrees.
4. The foot is in slight eversion.

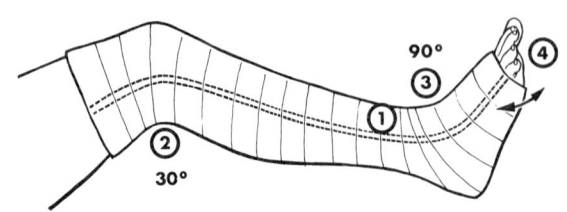

Postreduction Management

Elevate the limb on pillows.
Surround the foot with ice bags.
Check the toes frequently for circulatory impairment.

Christensen and coworkers have pointed out that the long-term prognosis after subtalar dislocation may be more serious than previously assumed. Symptomatic arthritis of the subtalar joint occurs in more than half these injuries. Pantalar arthritis occurs in 5 to 10 per cent.

The stability of the foot should be carefully evaluated after reduction to insure that subluxation does not persist or recur. Most subtalar dislocations are stable and do not require immobilization for more than two to three weeks. Early mobilization rather than prolonged immobilization is indicated to prevent fibrosis and stiffness in the subtalar as well as the other joints of the foot.

Changes of avascular necrosis do not usually complicate this injury. However, if an x-ray shows increased bone density, a period of protective weight bearing is indicated (see page 1995).

TOTAL DISLOCATION OF THE TALUS

REMARKS

Total dislocation of the talus represents the ultimate inversion injury to the ankle.

The talus dislocates out of its normal position in the ankle mortise and subtalar joint and displaces anteriorly to the lateral malleolus. Rarely, eversion injuries will produce total dislocation with medial displacement of the talus.

Prereduction X-Ray

1. The body of the talus is in front of the external malleolus.
2. The head of the talus is directed medially.
3. The talus is rotated in its longitudinal axis so that its inferior articular surface faces posteriorly.

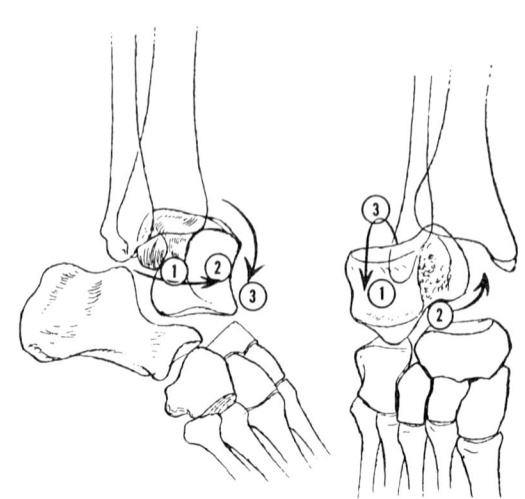

Manipulative Reduction

Note: In most instances closed reduction is unsuccessful. It may be attempted if other injuries preclude immediate open reduction of the dislocation. Operative reduction of the total dislocation is done in the same way as described for fracture-dislocation of the talus (see page 1972).

1. Place the limb in a padded canvas sling suspended from an overhead cross bar on a fracture table.
2. The knee is flexed 90 degrees.
3. An assistant grasps the heel with one hand and the forefoot with the other.

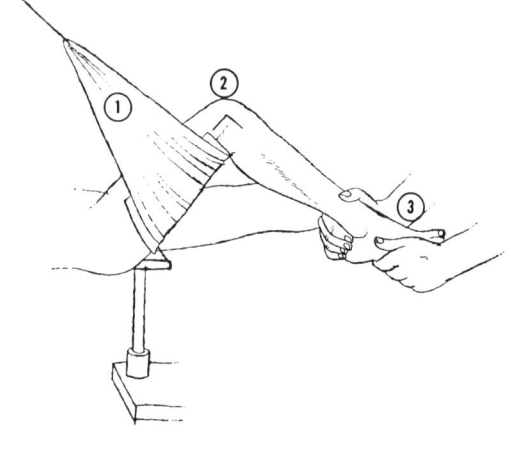

1. An assistant makes downward traction on the plantar flexed foot and at the same time
2. The foot is forcefully inverted.
3. While the position of inversion and plantar flexion is maintained, the surgeon's thumbs make firm pressure on the posterior portion of the talus.
4. The pressure is directed inward and backward, and at the same time
5. The talus is rotated around its longitudinal axis.

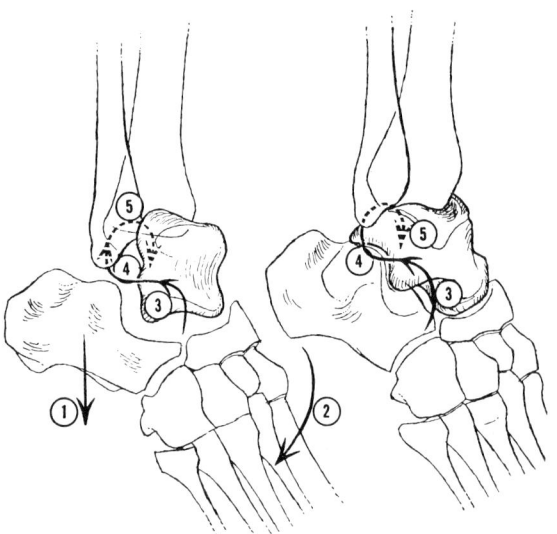

Postreduction X-Ray

1. The talus is in normal relation to the navicular.
2. The talus is accurately seated in the tibiofibular mortise.
3. The talus is in normal relation to the tibia, calcaneus, and navicular.

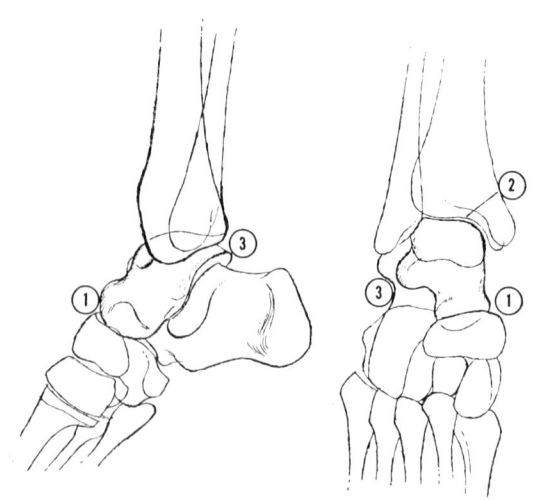

Immobilization

1. Apply anterior and posterior splints to allow for swelling of the foot after reduction.
2. The knee is flexed 30 degrees.
3. The ankle is held at a right angle.
4. The foot is in neutral position in regard to inversion and eversion.

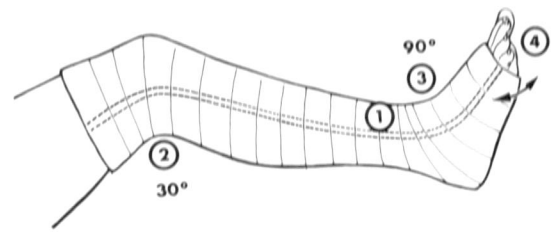

Postreduction Management

Elevate the limb on pillows.
Surround the foot with ice bags.
Check the toes frequently for circulatory impairment.
Replace the splints with a short leg cast when the swelling has subsided, by five to seven days.
Continue the cast immobilization for at least six to eight weeks, until circulatory status of the talus becomes evident.
Avascular necrosis is almost inevitable after complete dislocation of the talus. However, protective immobilization with specific braces is indicated to give the talus an opportunity to reconstitute itself prior to recommending any arthrodesis of the ankle (see page 1996).

ALTERNATE METHOD: SKELETAL TRACTION

REMARKS

This method is employed when manipulative measures fail to achieve reduction. Os calcis traction is frequently necessary even with open reduction in order to allow replacement of the talus back into the mortise.

Reduction by Skeletal Traction and Manipulation

1. Place the distal end of the thigh in a canvas sling suspended from a cross bar on the fracture table.
2. The knee is flexed 90 degrees.
3. Pass a Steinmann pin through the calcaneus and secure it to the mechanical traction apparatus at the foot of the table.
4. Make steady downward traction to open the interval between the tibia and the calcaneus.

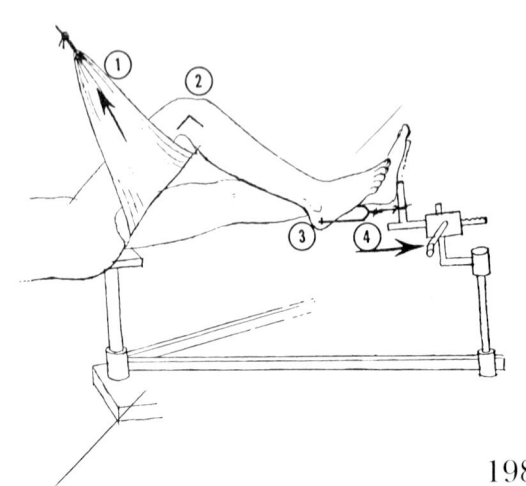

Reduction by Skeletal Traction and Manipulation (Continued)

1. An assistant makes strong inversion on the plantar flexed foot while
2. With both thumbs, the surgeon pushes the posterior portion of the talus inward and backward; at the same time
3. The surgeon attempts to rotate the talus around its longitudinal axis.

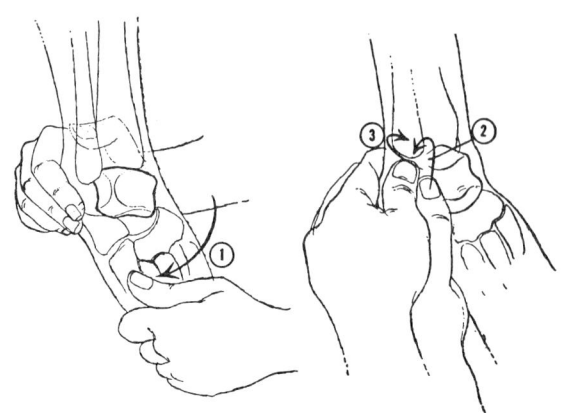

Immobilization and postreduction management are the same as described on page 1985.

Remove the pin from the calcaneus before the plaster cast is applied.

Note: In the event that the lesion is an open dislocation, excise the wound edges, flush the wound with copious quantities of saline solution, and proceed to reduce the dislocation as previously depicted (page 1972). Close the skin edges loosely and without tension after reduction is achieved.

Do not needlessly sacrifice skin.

Handle all soft tissues with great gentleness.

Do not sever the soft tissue attachments of the talus — its blood supply is already severely compromised.

OSTEOCHONDRAL LESIONS OF THE DOME OF THE TALUS

REMARKS

These injuries represent another condition that tends to be confused with a sprained ankle.

Inversion and dorsiflexion is most often the mechanism implicated.

The resulting lesion may be located either medially, laterally, or, rarely, centrally on the dome of the talus.

The shapes of the medial and lateral lesions are different on x-ray and at operation.

1. Lateral lesions are wafer-shaped and shallow, giving the appearance of being produced by shearing force.

2. Medial lesions are deep and cup-shaped. The depth of the crater is deeper than the width, suggesting that the etiology may be other than trauma.

Note: Lateral lesions tend to produce more persistent symptoms and more arthritic changes on x-ray.

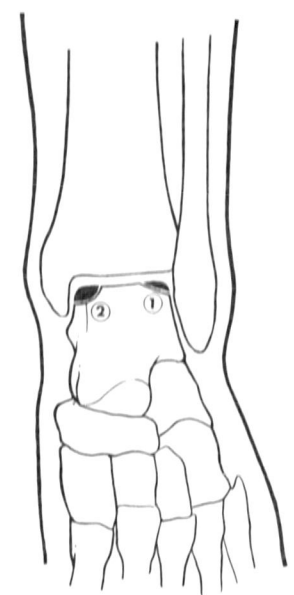

Stages of Osteochondral Lesions (Berndt and Harty)

1. Stage I involves a small area of subchondral compression.
2. Stage II is a partially detached fragment.

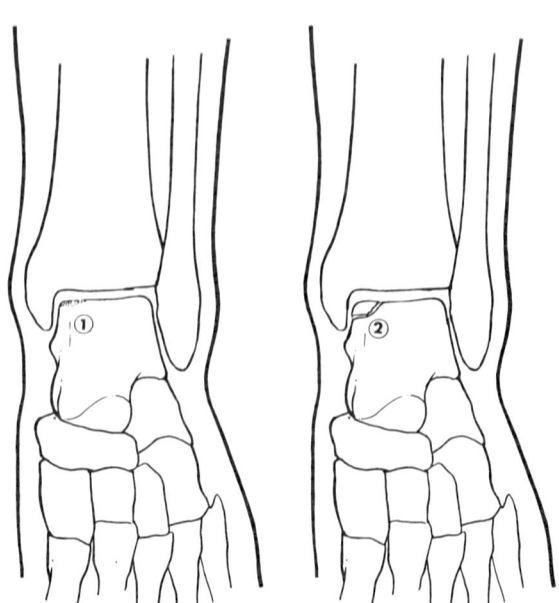

Stages of Osteochondral Lesions (Berndt and Harty) (Continued)

3. Stage III is a completely detached fragment remaining in the crater.
4. Stage IV is a fragment that is loose in the joint.

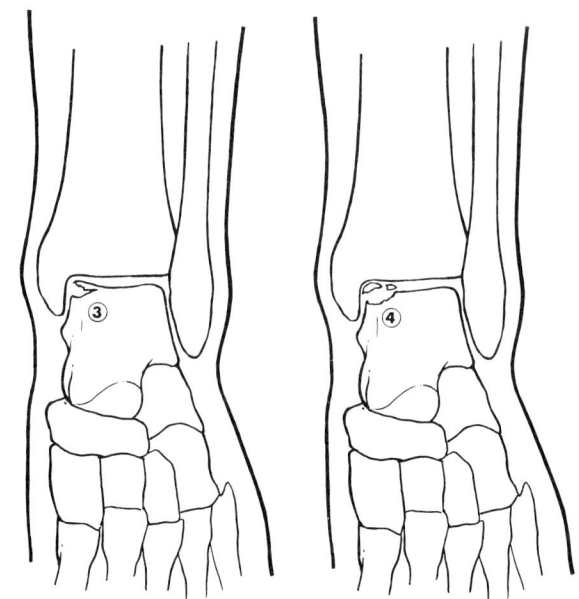

Management According to Stages (Canale and Belding)

1. Stage I and Stage II lesions regardless of location and Stage III medial lesions should be treated nonoperatively for at least four months. A brace, such as a patellar-tendon-bearing type, that unloads the ankle but still allows the ankle motion necessary for nourishment of the articular cartilage is ideal for this purpose.

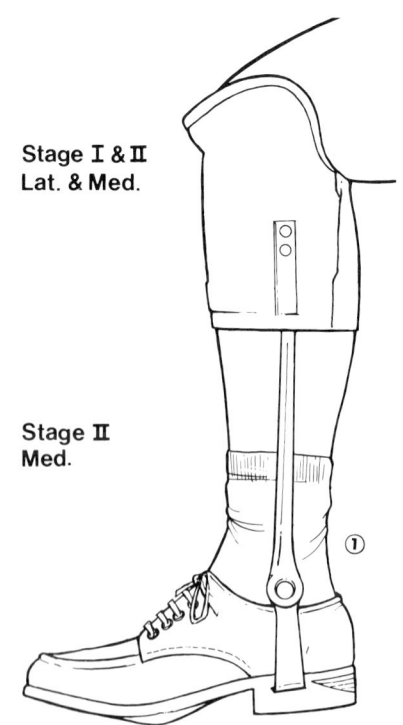

2. Stage III and IV lateral lesions and Stage IV medial lesions should be treated by surgical excision and curettage.

Note: Osteotomy of the medial malleolus is usually necessary to excise medial lesions.

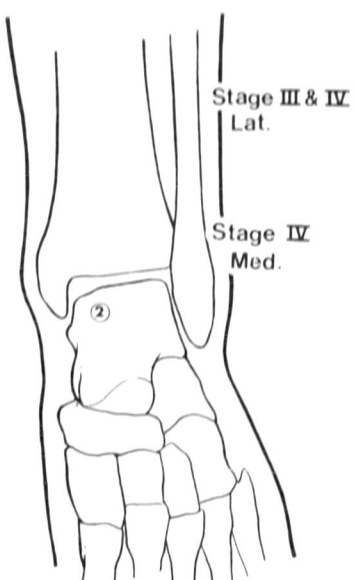

Any lesion in which symptoms persist after adequate (four to six months) nonoperative treatment should also have surgical excision and curettage. Long-term results indicate that few lesions unite when treated nonoperatively. Degenerative changes of the joint, both symptomatic and asymptomatic, are common (50 per cent of cases) regardless of treatment.

Management of Eversion Injuries of the Talus

REMARKS

Because of structural limitations to eversion in the subtalar joint, this mechanism infrequently causes a fracture or dislocation of the talus.

Eversion–external rotation injuries are most likely to fracture the ankle (see page 1839).

The most common injury to the foot with eversion is a lateral subtalar dislocation.

FRACTURES AND DISLOCATIONS OF THE TALUS

Occasionally fractures of the medial side of the posterior talar tubercle will also be produced by the pull of the posterior tibiotalar ligament during eversion.

Lateral subtalar dislocation is more likely than medial subtalar dislocation to be associated with obstruction to reduction. This is frequently due to the posterior tibial tendon becoming displaced dorsal and lateral to the neck of the talus.

Leitner and Böhler have described a method of closed manipulation for the locked lateral dislocation. If this technique fails, prompt open reduction is indicated.

Anteroposterior View: Lateral Subtalar Dislocation

1. The subtalar joint is displaced laterally as a result of the eversion injury.
2. The os calcis and foot are also displaced posteriorly.
3. Reduction is obstructed by the posterior tibial tendon wrapping dorsally over the lateral neck of the talus.

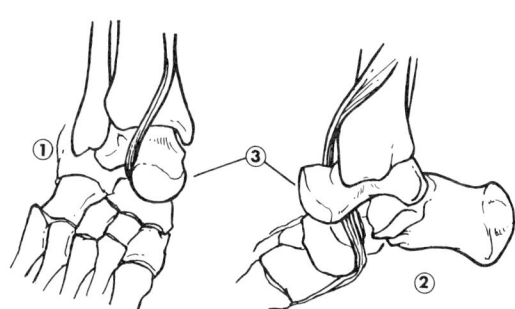

Technique of Closed Reduction (Leitner and Böhler)

1. The heel is grasped and the foot is pulled forward to correct posterior displacement.
2. The foot is then fully dorsiflexed to release the posterior tibial tendon.

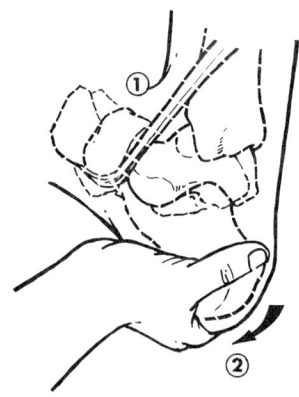

3. The foot is pushed medially and the reduction is completed with the tendon regaining its normal position.

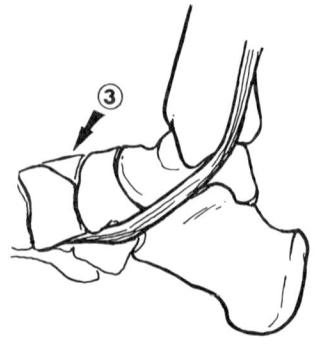

Subsequent Management

The foot is immobilized after reduction in a non–weight bearing short leg cast.

Elevate the leg for at least three to five days until the swelling has subsided.

The patient may then be up on crutches and should continue with non–weight-bearing crutch walking for two to three weeks.

The cast may then be removed and progressive weight bearing may be allowed.

Inversion and eversion are consistently limited after this injury but the end result may be quite satisfactory if avascular necrosis of the talus does not occur.

The patient should be followed by means of periodic x-rays for six months in order to detect signs of avascular necrosis (see page 1993).

Management of Compression Injuries of the Talus

REMARKS

Compression injuries can produce significant comminution and displacement of the talus and surrounding structures.

If possible, the talus should be reduced and fixed internally, but quite frequently this proves impossible.

In severely comminuted fractures of the talus a primary talectomy and tibiotalar arthrodesis may be indicated (see page 2000).

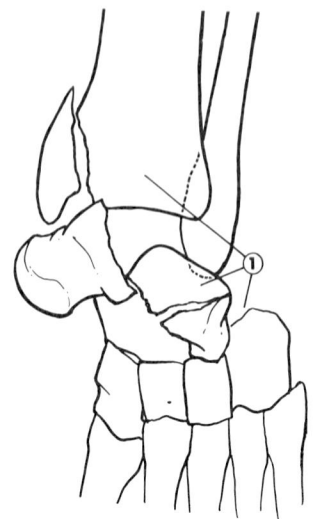

1. Compression injury has comminuted the talus, fractured the medial malleolus, and produced a subtalar dislocation.

2. Because of severe comminution preventing adequate reduction of the talus, the talus was removed and a tibiocalcaneal fusion was performed to stabilize the foot in a plantigrade position (see page 2000).

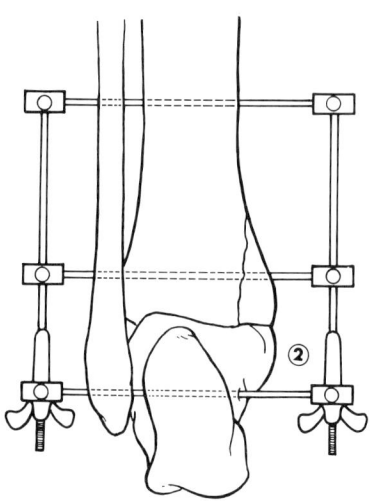

COMPLICATIONS OF FRACTURES AND FRACTURE-DISLOCATIONS OF THE TALUS

REMARKS

Undisplaced fractures of the talus generally heal rapidly without complication.

Displaced fractures or dislocations frequently result in significant problems, ranging from infection to malunion, avascular necrosis, and traumatic arthritis, all of which prolong the disability.

Avascular Necrosis

REMARKS

The most common complication following a fracture or dislocation of the talus is avascular necrosis produced by disruption of the blood supply to the talus.

Quite frequently this is of more significance radiographically than clinically, particularly if the condition is detected early and the ankle is protected.

The blood supply to the talus is quite diffuse and arises from three major arteries of the lower leg:
1. The posterior tibial artery.
2. The dorsalis pedis artery.
3. The peroneal artery.

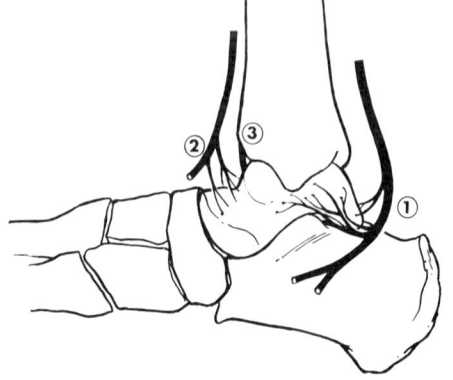

Blood Supply to the Posterior and Medial Talus

Mulfinger and Trueta have shown that there is a rich intraosseous blood supply to the talus, particularly through the tarsal sinus and tarsal canal.

1. The posterior tibial artery gives a branch to the posterior tubercle via its calcaneal branches.
2. These form a plexus over the posterior tubercle along with branches from the peroneal artery.
3. The artery of the tarsal canal arises from the posterior tibial artery 1 cm proximal to the medial and lateral plantar branches. The artery passes between the sheaths of the flexor digitorum longus and flexor hallucis longus into the tarsal canal.
4. A deltoid branch comes off the artery of the tarsal canal to supply the medial surface of the body. This vessel runs between the talotibial and talocalcaneal portions of the deltoid ligament.

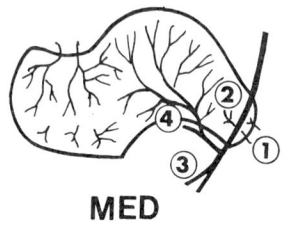

MED

Blood Supply to the Lateral Talus

5. The artery of the tarsal sinus starts from a loop formed between the dorsalis pedis and the lateral tarsal branch of the perforating peroneal artery.
6. The artery of the tarsal sinus gives branches to the head of the talus.
7. It enters the tarsal sinus to give blood supply to the body and
8. Anastomoses with the artery of the tarsal canal.

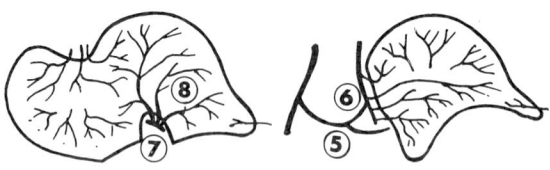

LAT

Effect of Injury on Blood Supply to the Talus

Most fractures of the neck of the talus do not cause avascular necrosis. The vessels entering the medial surface of the body and the anterolateral vessels as well as some of the vessels in the tarsal canal should remain intact.

The incidence of avascular necrosis rises sharply with dislocations and displaced fracture-dislocations of the body associated with extensive soft tissue detachment. Avascular necrosis is virtually inevitable after complete dislocation of the talus.

If the patient bears weight prematurely on the talus subject to avascular necrosis, subchondral collapse and secondary arthritis are likely. However, if weight bearing is prevented for the period necessary to allow the talus to reconstitute itself, avascular necrosis does not inevitably lead to traumatic arthritis.

Surgical approaches through the tarsal sinus obliterate the major blood supply to the talus from the artery of the tarsal sinus and tarsal canal. Wide medial facet removal will also add to the likelihood of avascular necrosis. This should be kept in mind during operative reduction or any surgical procedure in this area such as triple arthrodesis.

Diagnosis of Avascular Necrosis of the Talus

Avascular necrosis should be anticipated and suspected with any displaced fracture or dislocation of the talus.

Hawkins has pointed out that the time to recognize avascular necrosis is between the sixth and eighth week following the injury. By this time if the foot has not borne weight, disuse atrophy should be evident on the x-ray of the foot and distal tibia.

Subchondral atrophy evident on x-ray excludes the possibility of avascular necrosis and indicates the presence of healing revascularization.

Radiographic Signs of Normal Healing (Hawkins)

EARLY

1. X-rays of the ankle with the foot out of the cast show subchondral osteolysis of the dome, which indicates the presence of a revascularization response.

Note: Bone scans with isotopes such as sulfur colloid (see page 1452) may also be useful to determine the status of the blood flow to the talus. The significance of bone scans, however, is still under investigation.

LATER

2. As the contrast between dead bone of the body of the talus and the surrounding atrophic bone increases, the diagnosis of avascular necrosis can be made readily on lateral x-ray.

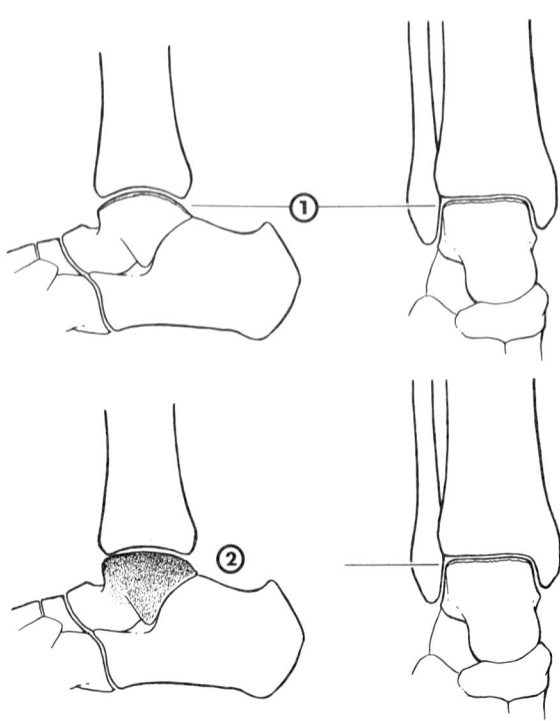

Management of Established Avascular Necrosis

No surgical procedure is effective in treating avascular necrosis once it occurs.

Protected walking with use of a brace is necessary to allow bony reconstitution and prevent the collapse of the talus and secondary osteoarthritis.

The most effective method of protecting the ankle after the fracture heals is with a patellar-tendon-bearing (PTB) orthosis.

1. The rigid ankle shifts the weight from the talus up to
2. The proximal tibia by means of the patellar-tendon-bearing design.
3. A rocker bottom and
4. SACH (solid ankle cushioned heel) allow some heel-toe gait despite the rigid ankle.

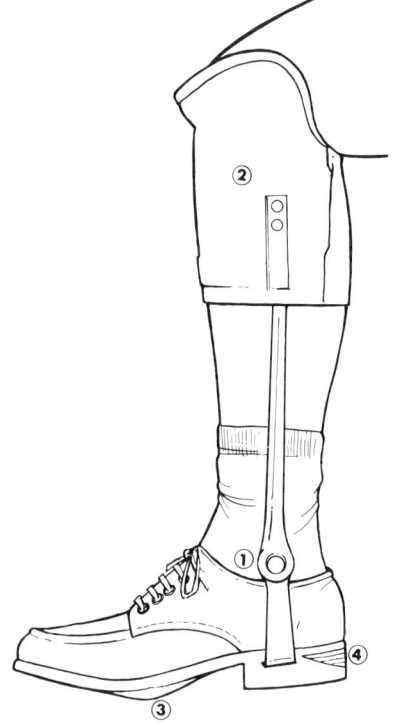

Subsequent Management

The ankle should be protected for a minimum of eight to twelve months after avascular necrosis is identified.

If there is no evidence of collapse of the talus one year after injury, the brace may generally be discarded.

The subtalar joint will have some arthritis and definite limitation of motion, but function of the limb may be quite satisfactory.

If symptomatic arthritis of the tibiotalar and subtalar joint occur, arthrodesis may be necessary. The tibiotalar as well as the subtalar joint should be fused because arthrodesis of only one of the symptomatic joints will worsen the symptoms in the other (see page 2000).

Keep in mind that clinical symptoms do not necessarily or consistently correlate with changes seen on x-ray.

X-Ray 15 Years After Avascular Necrosis

1. Anteroposterior and lateral x-rays show sclerosis and collapse of the talus.
2. Degenerative changes are evident in the ankle.

Note: This patient had been bearing weight fully on the foot and had been essentially asymptomatic from the time the fracture united.

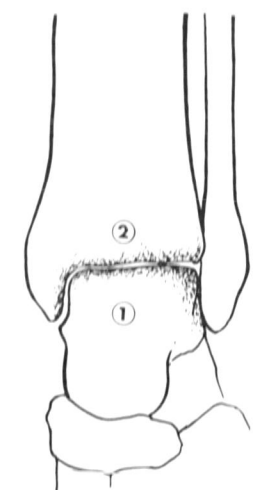

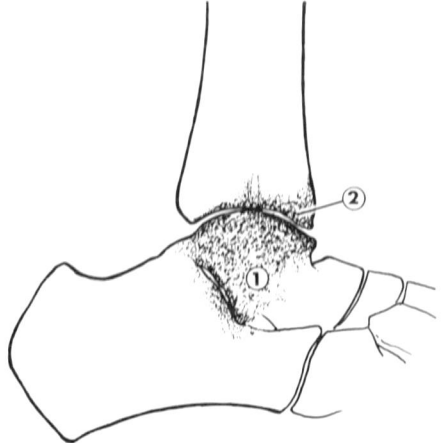

Nonunion and Malunion

REMARKS

Failure of the fractured talus to heal is infrequent, but delayed union requiring prolonged non–weight-bearing treatment is fairly commonly associated with closed management.

Early operative fixation is necessary for any displaced fracture of the talus, particularly when there is any question about the adequacy of the reduction on either the true lateral or the anteroposterior x-ray of the foot in plantar flexion.

The most common causes of malunion include:
1. Dorsal beaking of the talus.

Note: This frequently results when the cast is changed at about four to six weeks and the foot is taken out of a plantar flexed position of reduction.

2. Torsional malalignment.

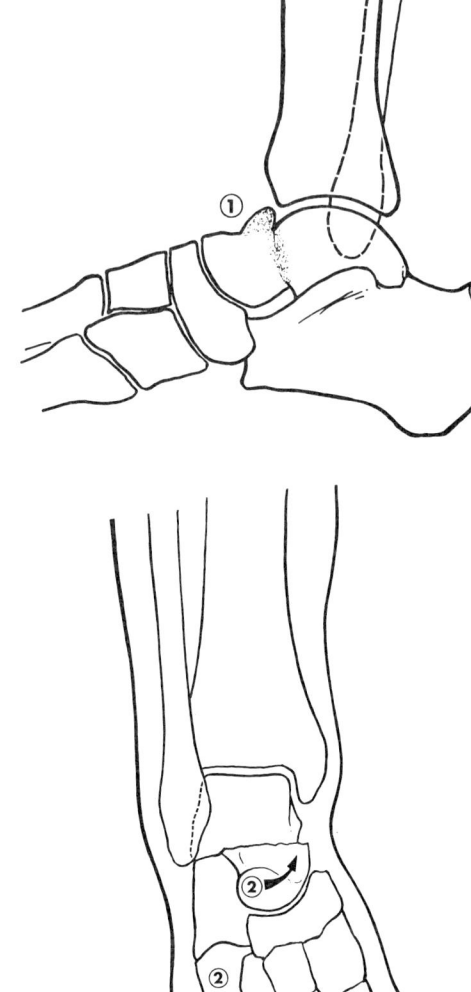

Torsional malalignment is the most common and most significant deformity.
1. Healing with the distal fragment internally rotated in relation to the head fragment produces
2. Inversion and varus position of the foot and causes the patient to walk on the lateral side of the foot.
3. Subtalar arthritis is common with torsional malalignment.

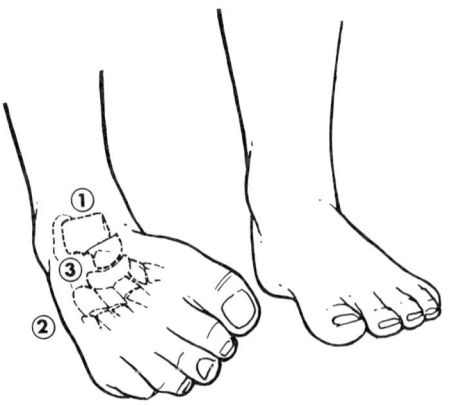

Management

FOR DORSAL BEAKING OF THE TALUS

1. Excision of the dorsal prominence relieves symptoms.

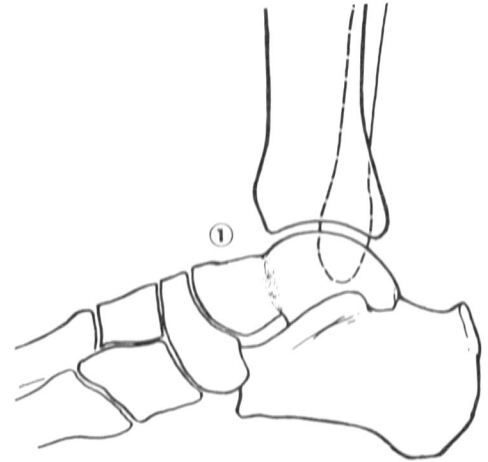

FOR TORSIONAL MALALIGNMENT

2. Triple arthrodesis of the hind foot is necessary to correct the position of the foot and relieve the symptoms of subtalar arthritis.

Note: Before performing an arthrodesis for painful, traumatic arthritis one should determine if the symptoms are also present in the ankle joint. An already arthritic ankle will be overstressed if the subtalar joint is fused.

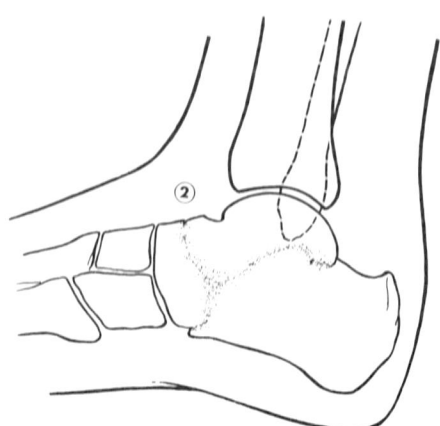

Infection

REMARKS

Because the talus is composed almost entirely of cancellous bone and because the injury frequently deprives the talus of its blood supply, infection is disastrous.

Repeated sequestrectomy or attempted excision of draining sinuses is futile for osteomyelitis of the talus.

Talectomy by itself gives unsatisfactory results because of painful instability.

The treatment of choice, once infection occurs after fracture or dislocation of the talus, is talectomy with tibiocalcaneal fusion. This removes the source of infection and still permits functional weight-bearing stability of the foot.

1. The talus is completely excised.
2. The articular cartilages of the calcaneus, the distal tibia, and the malleoli are removed.
3. The calcaneus is held in approximation against the tibia by transverse compression pins using the Charnley or external fixator technique for immobilization.

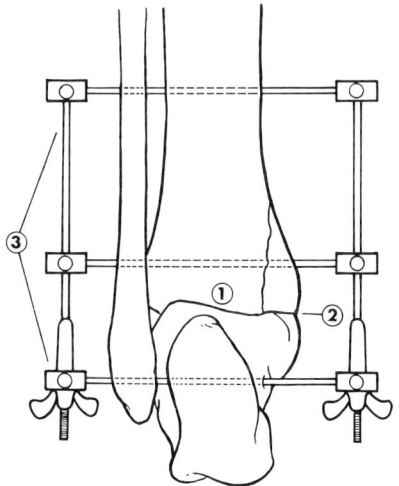

Note: Talectomy and tibiocalcaneal fusion are indicated only for infections or severely comminuted talar fractures. Even when complete avascular necrosis develops after a dislocated talus, the functional result is usually better if the talus is left in place and protected long enough for it to heal by creeping substitution. For symptomatic osteoarthritis without infection a Blair tibiotalar fusion may give better tibiopedal motion and less shortening of the foot than a tibiocalcaneal fusion (see page 2001).

Arthritis of the Subtalar and Tibiotalar Joints

REMARKS

Arthritis, particularly of the subtalar joint, develops in almost 50 per cent of talar fractures and in 60 to 70 per cent of fracture-dislocations. The incidence of arthritis appears to be related to the degree of initial injury, the degree of displacement, and the completeness of reduction. Rotational malalignment particularly leads to arthritis of the hindfoot.

Arthritic involvement of the tibiotalar as well as the subtalar joint may occur if there has been injury to the distal tibial articular surface or collapse of the talus secondary to avascular necrosis.

Not all patients with radiographic signs of arthritis will have significant subjective findings (see page 1997). Pain with strenuous activity or with walking on uneven ground may cause some of these patients to limp occasionally. Ten to 20 per cent will require triple arthrodesis for malunion (see page 1999).

Before performing an arthrodesis, keep in mind that instability of the subtalar joint may occasionally follow subtalar subluxation or dislocation as a result of ligamentous injury. If the patient's symptoms are more those of instability than of arthritis, the procedure of choice is a soft tissue reconstruction such as the Chrisman-Snook operation (see page 1829).

Should the arthritis result from talar collapse, symptoms arise primarily from the tibiotalar joint. If these symptoms warrant a reconstructive procedure, Dennis and Tullos have demonstrated that the Blair tibiotalar arthrodesis can give good or even excellent results. This is true for arthritis after avascular necrosis or after comminuted fractures of the talus or when part of the talus has been lost in the injury.

The Blair fusion has several advantages over other operations for complications of talar fracture-dislocations, e.g., tibiocalcaneal fusions. Normal appearance of the foot is retained, the alignment of the foot relative to the leg is almost normal, the foot is not shortened, the weight-bearing thrust is on normal tissue, and the fusion allows some flexion and extension of the foot and leg. With the Blair tibiotalar fusion, some motion of the subtalar joint as well as of the talonavicular joint is retained and allows almost a normal gait in patients with successful fusions.

BLAIR TIBIOTALAR FUSION

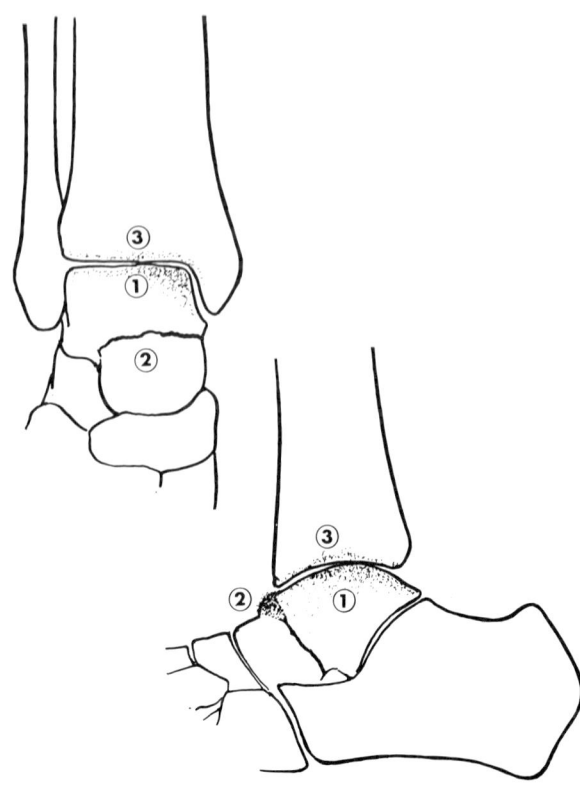

Preoperative X-Ray

1. Avascular necrosis and
2. Malunion of the talar fracture has resulted in
3. Tibiotalar arthritis six months subsequent to injury.

Operative Technique

1. An anterior approach is made via a longitudinal incision. The periosteum, capsule, and synovial membrane are incised in line with the skin incision.

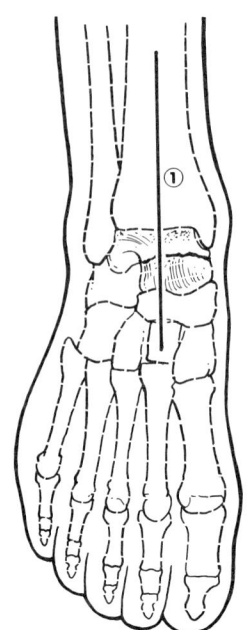

1. The foot is maintained in plantar flexion to protect the head and neck of the talus and to increase exposure of the ankle joint.
2. The body or remaining portion of the talus is removed with an osteotome or a large curette.

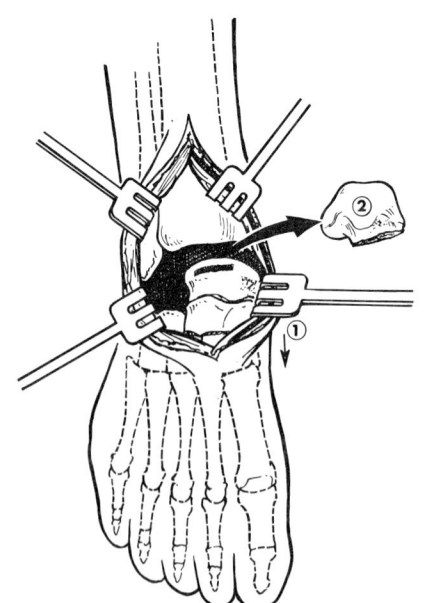

1. A rectangular graft, 2.5 cm by 5.0 cm, is prepared from the anterior aspect of the tibia using a power saw.
2. No cartilage is removed from the distal articular surface of the tibia.
3. A 2-cm slot is created in the neck of the talus. The graft should fit snugly into that slot.

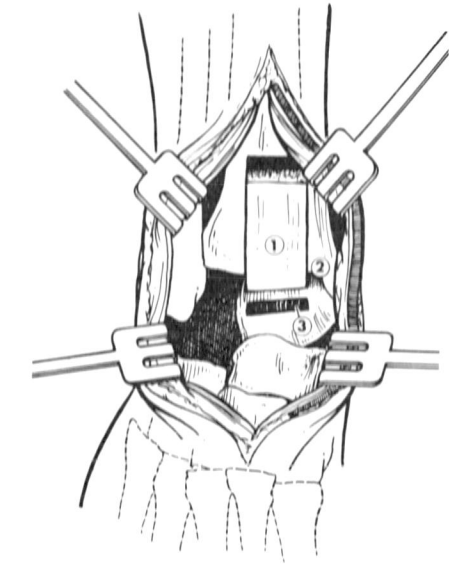

1. The foot is placed in 10 to 15 degrees of plantar flexion, and the graft is secured with a screw.
2. Cancellous bone from the tibial graft site is then curretted and packed about the graft.
3. Contact between the talar neck and the anterior edge of the tibia must be maintained.

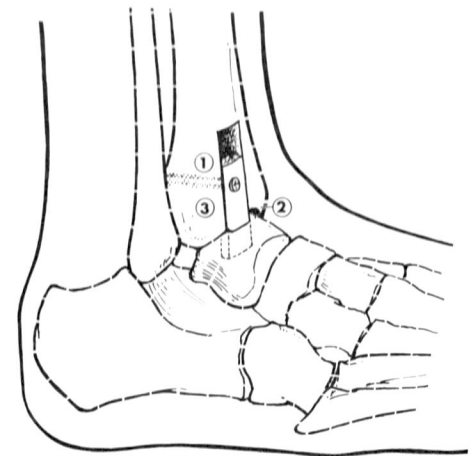

Immobilization

1. Apply anteroposterior splints to allow for postoperative swelling.
2. The knee is flexed to 30 degrees.
3. The foot is placed in 10 to 15 degrees of plantar flexion to maintain the position achieved in surgery.
4. The foot is in neutral in regard to inversion and eversion.

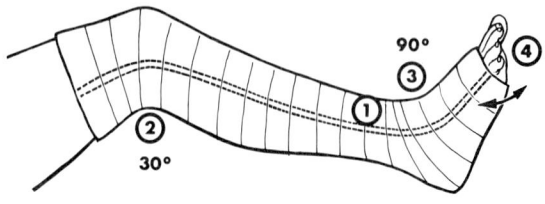

Subsequent Management

Elevate the limb on pillows. Surround the foot and ankle with ice bags.

The postoperative splints are changed to a long leg non-weight-bearing cast when the swelling has subsided, usually by five to seven days.

At the end of eight weeks a short leg, well-molded patellar-tendon-bearing cast with a walking heel may be applied (see page 1736).

Fusion should be complete at the end of 16 weeks, and the cast may be removed.

Even with pseudoarthrosis of the fusion, a satisfactory result is possible provided that at least 15 to 20 degrees of tibiopedal motion about the long axis of the tibia is maintained. This is the arch of motion between maximum dorsiflexion and maximum plantar flexion.

Postoperative X-Ray

1. A solid fusion is evident between the remnant of the talus and the tibia.
2. Motion is still possible in the subtalar joint and
3. Talonavicular joints

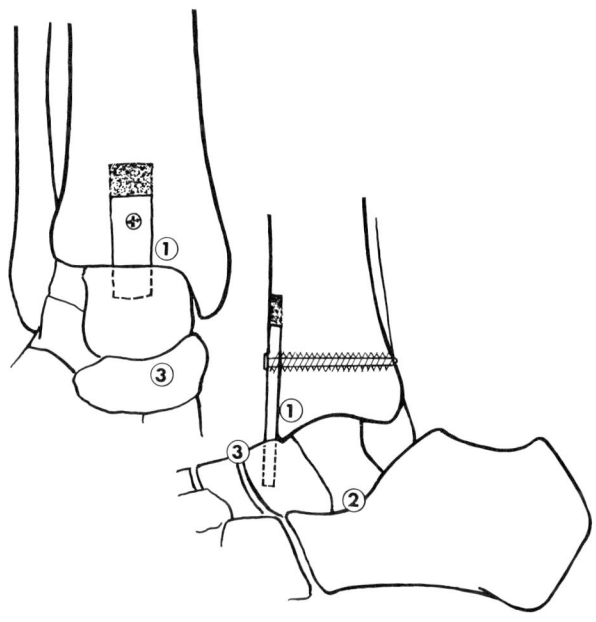

Clinical Result

1. The clinical appearance of the foot is good and
2. 15 to 20 degrees of tibiopedal motion are maintained.

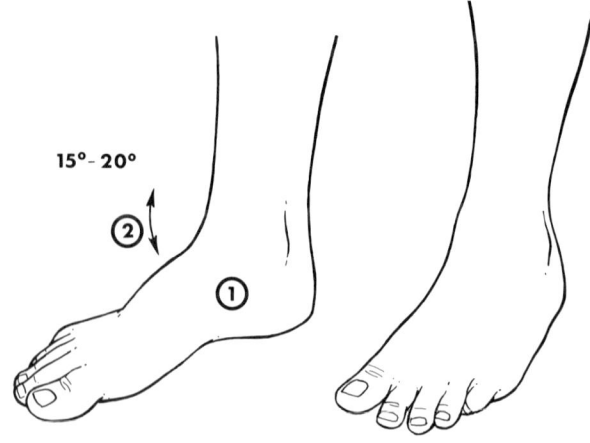

FRACTURES OF THE CALCANEUS

REMARKS

The calcaneus is the largest bone in the foot as well as the one most frequently fractured. The fracture may be incurred from a minor fall or from major violence.

Os calcis fracture is bilateral in 10 to 20 per cent of injuries. There are associated fractures of the spine, tibia, or ankle in 20 to 30 per cent of os calcis fractures. Every patient with an os calcis fracture should therefore be evaluated for fractures elsewhere.

The majority of these fractures extend into the subtalar joint and produce varying degrees of joint disruption. Less than 40 per cent involve only the nonarticular portion of the bone.

The treatment of fractures involving the nonarticular portion of the bone is mainly symptomatic. Cast immobilization is useful to relieve pain for a maximum of two to three weeks, after which the patient should be encouraged to start active range-of-motion exercises while protecting the injured foot with crutches.

Treatment of the more common fractures, which extend into the articular weight-bearing surface, is more problematic and should be based on detailed assessment of potential complications.

Isolated Fractures of the Calcaneus without Implication of the Subtalar Joint

REMARKS

Most of these fractures exhibit minimal or no displacement.

Vertical fractures occasionally show displacement of the medial tuberosity and some horizontal fractures show upward displacement of the fragment; these require manipulative reduction.

FRACTURES OF THE CALCANEUS

ISOLATED FRACTURES OF THE CALCANEUS REQUIRING NO REDUCTION

Appearance on X-Ray

1. Vertical fracture of the tuberosity without displacement.

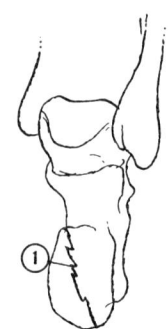

1. Fracture of the sustentaculum tali with minimal displacement.

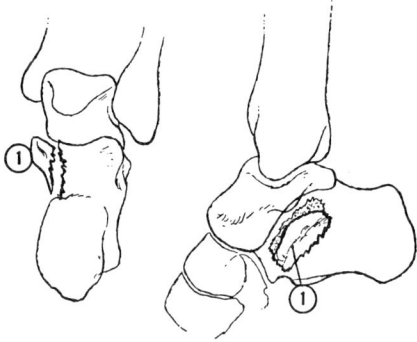

1. Horizontal fracture of the tuberosity without displacement.

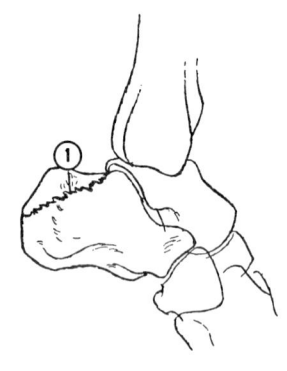

1. Minimally displaced fracture of the anterior process.

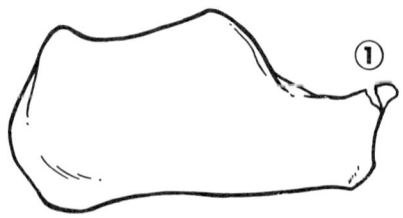

Immobilization

1. Apply a below-the-knee plaster cast with
2. Walking heel.
3. The foot is at a right angle and
4. In neutral in regard to inversion and eversion.

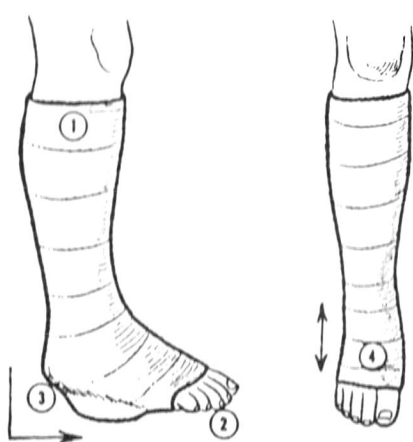

Subsequent Management

Permit weight bearing as tolerated.
Most of these fractures heal promptly, and disability, if any, is from some residual stiffness. Consequently, cast immobilization should be kept at a minimum and the cast can generally be removed at the end of two to three weeks.
Subsequently the patient is allowed to continue weight bearing with crutches and the crutches are discarded within two to three weeks after cast removal.
Apply an elastic ankle support to diminish edema the first three to five weeks after the cast is removed.

ISOLATED FRACTURES OF THE CALCANEUS REQUIRING REDUCTION

VERTICAL FRACTURE

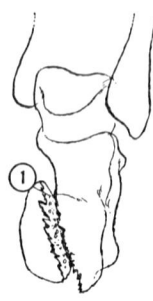

Prereduction X-Ray

1. Vertical fracture of the tuberosity with medial displacement of the medial process.

Manipulative Reduction

1. The patient's leg hangs over the edge of the table.
2. The forefoot rests on the operator's knee.

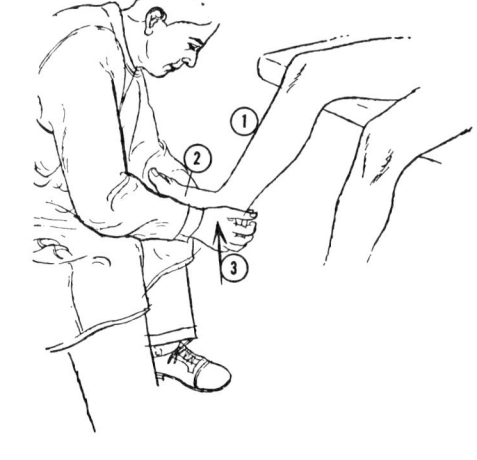

3. The operator compresses the heel with both hands while the plaster sets.
4. The molding of the plaster on the soft tissues and os calcis is sufficient to reduce the fracture.

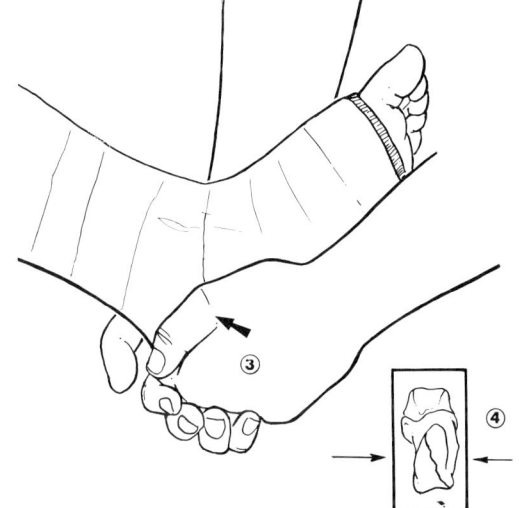

Immobilization

1. Apply a below-knee plaster cast with a
2. Walking heel.
3. The foot is at a right angle to the leg and
4. In neutral in regard to inversion and eversion.

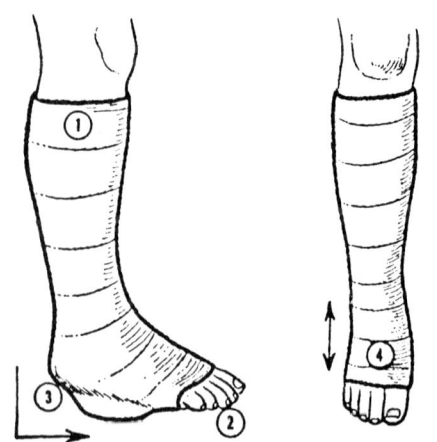

Management

Permit weight bearing immediately.
Replace the cast at the end of three weeks.
Remove the second cast six weeks after the injury.
Now apply an elastic cotton bandage around the foot and ankle for several more weeks.
Institute exercises to restore normal motion at the ankle, subtalar, and other joints of the foot.

HORIZONTAL FRACTURE OF THE CALCANEUS

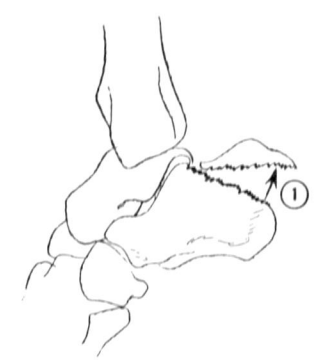

Prereduction X-Ray

1. Horizontal fracture of the tuberosity with upward displacement of the fragment.

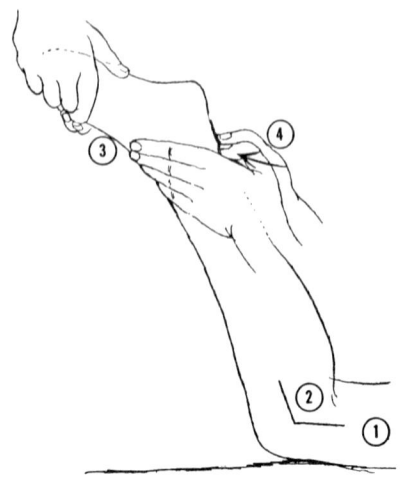

Manipulative Reduction

1. The patient is in the prone position.
2. The knee is flexed 70 degrees.
3. The foot is plantar flexed.
4. The operator places a thumb on each side of the Achilles tendon and makes firm downward pressure on the displaced fragment.

Immobilization

1. Apply a below-knee plaster cast with a
2. Walking heel
3. The foot is in slight plantar flexion.

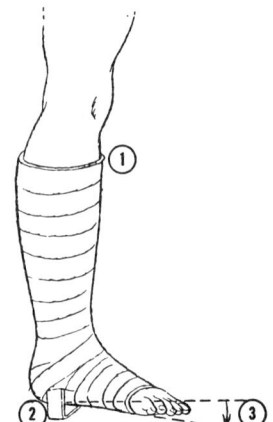

Management

Permit weight bearing immediately.
Replace the cast at the end of three weeks.
Remove the second cast six weeks after the injury.
Now apply an elastic cotton bandage around the foot and ankle for several more weeks.
Institute exercises to restore normal motion at the ankle, subtalar, and other joints of the foot.

Alternate Method: Open Reduction and Internal Fixation

Open reduction should be employed if the fragment is large or if manipulative methods fail.

Postreduction X-Ray

1. The fragment is in normal apposition to the rest of the calcaneus.
2. A cancellous lag screw is transfixing both fragments.

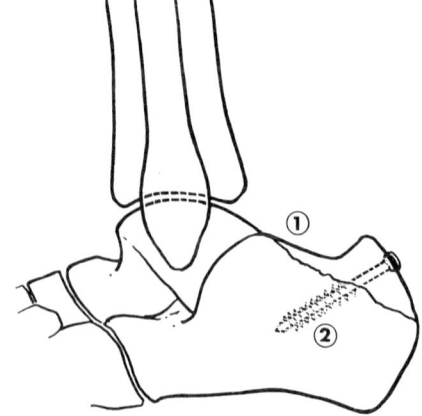

Immobilization

1. Apply a below-knee plaster cast with a
2. Walking heel.
3. The foot is in slight plantar flexion.

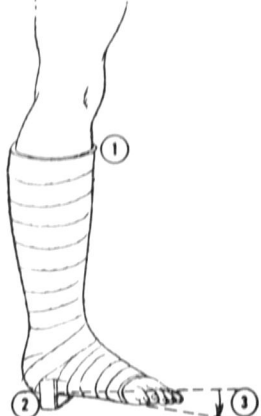

Subsequent Management

After four weeks the cast may be removed and the patient may start on range-of-motion exercises.

Continue the patient on crutches with partial weight bearing for three to four weeks after cast removal.

The screw need not be removed unless it is producing local symptoms.

Fracture of the Calcaneus with Implication of the Subtalar Joint

REMARKS

The majority of os calcis fractures (up to 70 per cent) cause varying degrees of damage to the articular surface of the subtalar joint.

There is a definite pattern to the fragments that is produced by the consistent pathomechanics of the injury as well as by the architectural relationships of the talus and the os calcis.

Normal Architecture of the Calcaneus

1. The tuberosity is offset laterally.
2. The sustentaculum is offset medially.

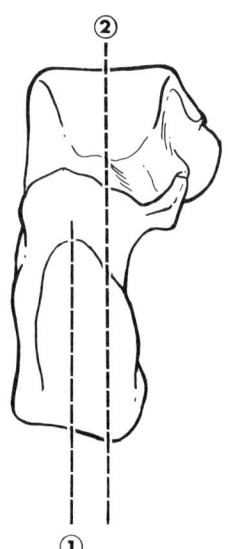

PATHOMECHANICS OF FRACTURES OF THE CALCANEUS

1. Downward force is transmitted by the talus to the subtalar joint.
2. The calcaneus is everted.
3. Spur on the lateral surface of the talus drives into the crucial angle of the calcaneus.

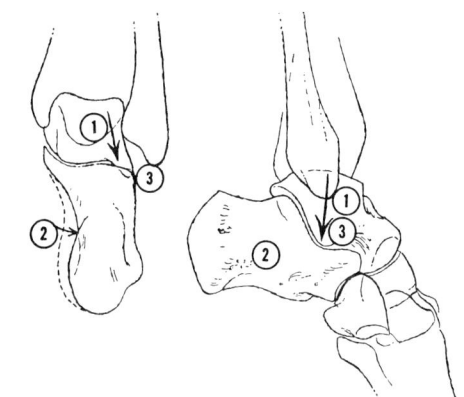

Patterns of Fracture

Burdeaux and coworkers, in biomechanical studies producing os calcis fractures in cadaver specimens, showed that consistently:

1. The fracture line runs between the sustentaculum tali and the tuberosity. It produces two major fragments that are seen on the axial view.

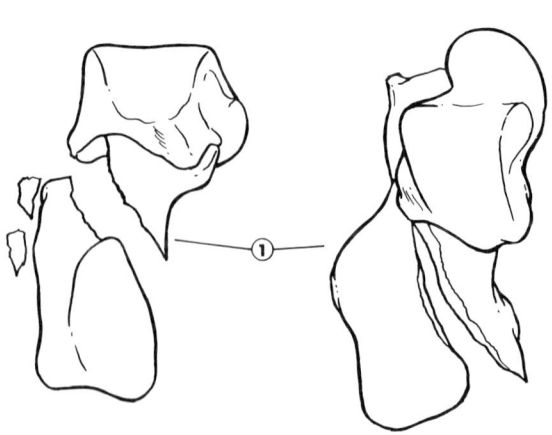

Axial View   Superior View

On the lateral view, the fracture may be:
1. Undisplaced.

2. Tongue type (Essex-Lopresti), or

3. Joint-depression type fracture (Essex-Lopresti).

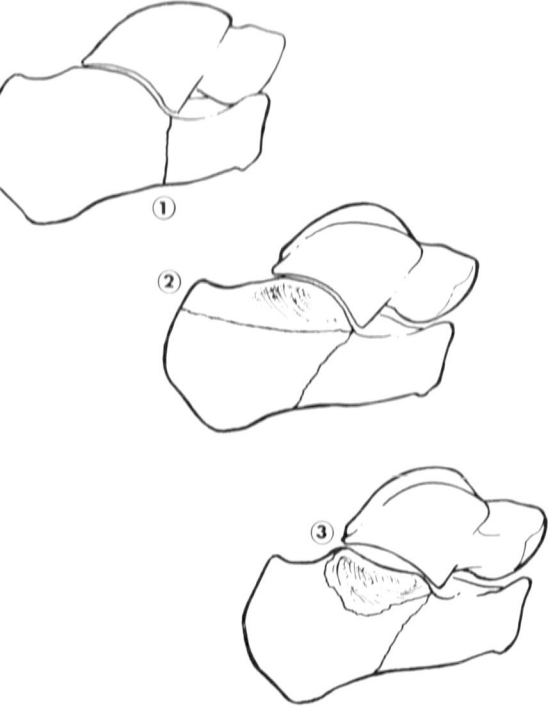

The main difference in these types is the size of the superolateral fragment.
1. In the tongue type there is a long fragment extending to the rear of the tuberosity.

2. In the joint depression type the fragment is short and extends back only to the end of the posterior facet.

Note: In both types, the fracture line separates the sustentaculum fragment from the tuberosity fragment.

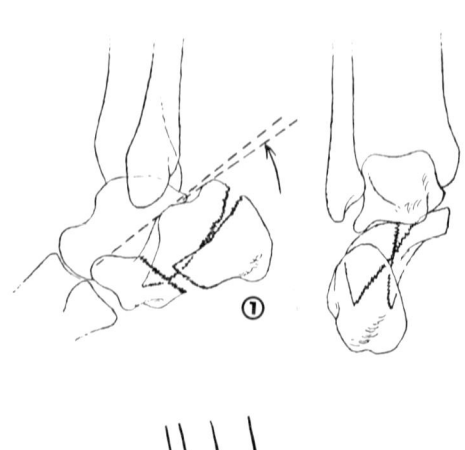

Basic Deformity in Both Tongue Type and Joint Depression Type

1. In a normal foot the angle formed by the line between the anterior and posterior facets and the line from the superior cortex of the body is normally 30 to 40 degrees (Böhler's angle).
2. Vertical compression of the calcaneus decreases this angle by driving the tuberosity upward and

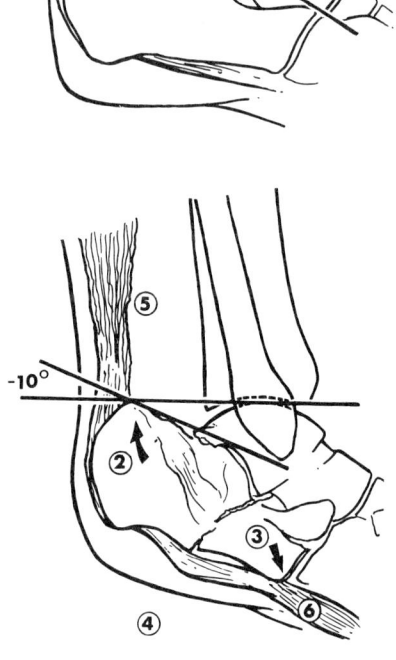

3. Driving the middle articular facet downward.
4. The plantar surface may become prominent.
5. The Achilles tendon is functionally lengthened.
6. The calcaneocuboid joint may also be involved.

Displacement on Axial View

1. In the normal foot the calcaneus should be in neither varus nor valgus position in relation to the ankle.
2. The peroneal tendon sheath is not compressed.

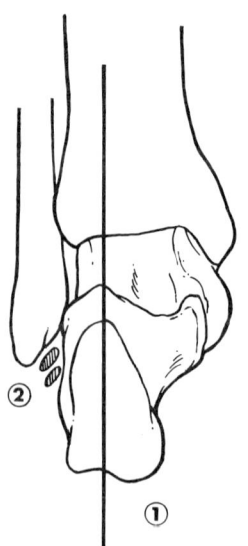

3. After fracture, the vertical fracture line consistently runs between the sustentaculum and the tuberosity fragment.

4. The tuberosity fragment is displaced laterally and usually into varus but sometimes into valgus.

5. The tuberosity is driven upward and laterally to impinge on the lateral malleolus and peroneal tendons.

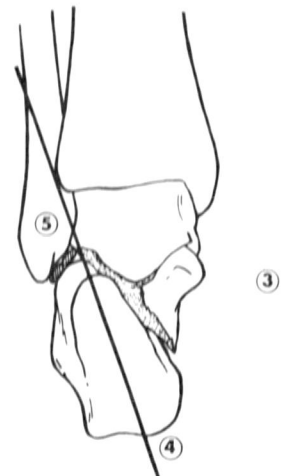

Displacement on Superior View

1. The sustentaculum fragment and talus are driven medially and downward. A characteristic spike of bone protrudes from the sustentaculum fragment medially.

2. The tuberosity fragment moves forward and laterally.

3. This produces shortening and widening of the heel, which is evident particularly when compared with

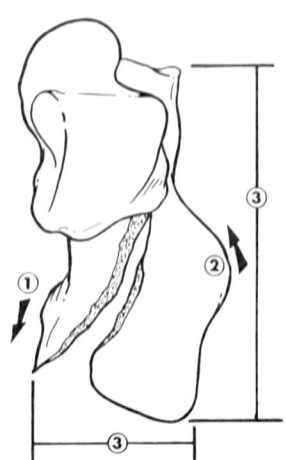

4. The normal relationship of the calcaneus to the talus.

Note: The displacement must be considered in three dimensions. The superolateral joint-depression or tongue type fracture involves the subtalar joint. The separation of the sustentaculum and tuberosity fragments causes the heel to be shortened and widened.

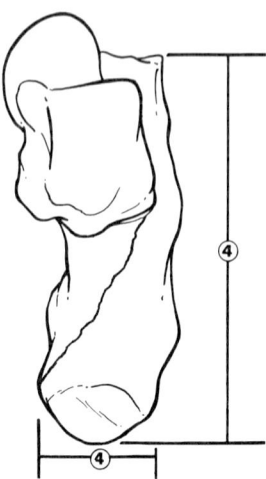

Radiographic Assessment

1. X-rays should include multiple oblique views increasing in 10-degree increments to show the calcaneal profile and the posterior articular facets.

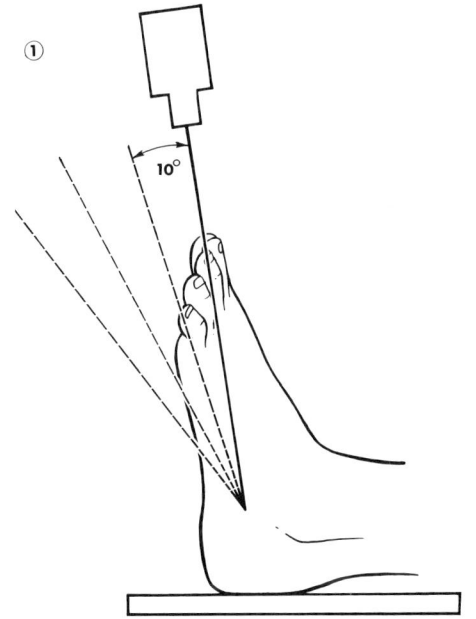

Management of Calcaneal Fractures Based on Assessment of All Potential Complications

REMARKS

The disability after os calcis fractures may range from minimal to severe.

The degree of subtalar joint disruption does not always correlate with the degree of residual symptoms. Paradoxically, the greater the degree of talocalcaneal involvement, the more likely is spontaneous ankylosis to occur and to eliminate pain from this region.

The subtalar joint is only one of numerous sources of pain likely to occur after a calcaneal fracture.

Consistently, the following problems can be anticipated in patients and kept in mind while selecting treatment.

Painful and Tender Hindfoot

1. This is most often located in the lateral peroneal region and results from impingement of the laterally displaced tuberosity fragment on the malleolus and soft tissue structures.

Note: McLaughlin has pointed out that unlike pain from the subtalar joint, which is most marked on inversion and eversion, this pain occurs most often with flexion and extension of the ankle.

2. A tender heel results from distortion of the plantar surface of the calcaneus causing either localized pain or
3. Diffuse plantar fasciitis.

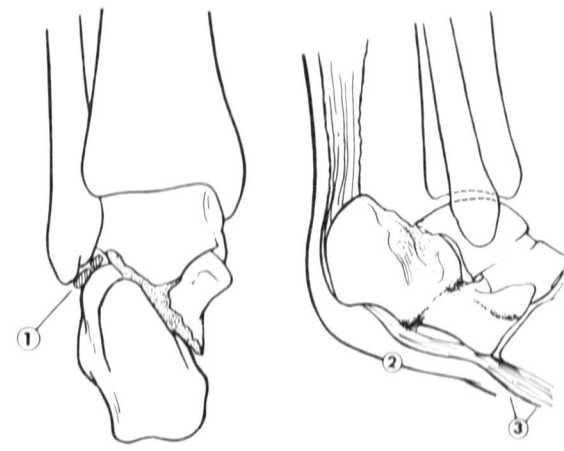

Stiffness of the Foot

1. This results from the edema of injury as well as from prolonged immobilization during treatment. The midtarsal joint, which can accommodate for loss of subtalar motion, is impaired by prolonged immobilization in non-weight-bearing treatment.

Note: Joint stiffness can be minimized by treatment that incorporates early mobilization of the foot.

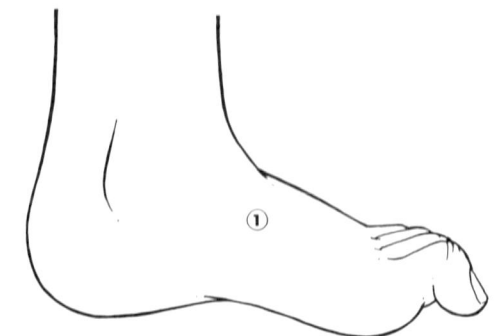

Peroneal Spastic Flat Foot

1. A chronic stenosing tenosynovitis of the peroneal tendon below and lateral to the fibula is likely to follow shortening and widening of the heel after fracture.

2. As a result of the tuberosity fragment, the peroneals contract and pull the forefoot into valgus. This results in lateral foot pain all along the region of the peroneal tendons.

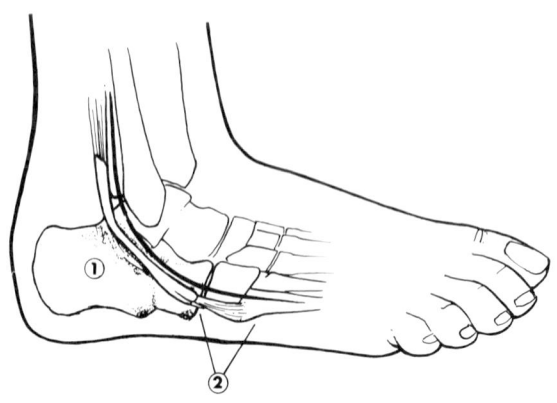

Abnormalities of Gait

A flatfooted (calcaneus) shuffling limp with inability to toe walk is common. This results from:
1. Upward displacement of the tuberosity and
2. Shortening of the heel, which impair

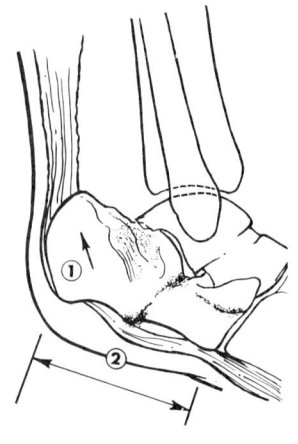

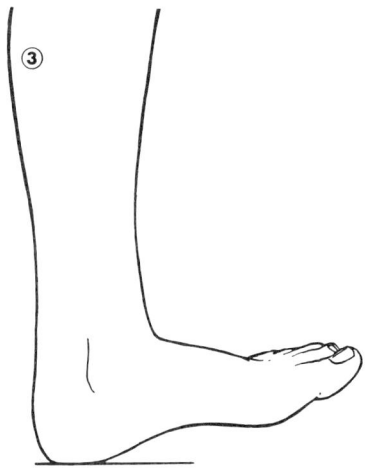

3. Calf muscle function particularly during pushoff.

Note: Treatment designed to restore length and reduce the tuberosity fragment is the only effective method of preventing the calcaneus gait. Once muscle impairment is established, there is little that can be done to correct this complication.

EARLY MOBILIZATION WITHOUT REDUCTION

REMARKS

Therapy advocated for these fractures has ranged from confirmed conservatism to intrepid intervention.

Most, but not all, can be treated nonoperatively by early mobilization methods. Even when reduction of the fracture is planned, mobilization techniques aid in diminishing edema and preventing stiffness of the joint.

The concept of early mobilization treatment is based on the fact that a fracture through a large cancellous bone such as the calcaneus achieves stability immediately by impaction of the fragments at the time of initial injury. To achieve fracture immobilization, the surgeon need only eliminate the weight-bearing stresses. It is not necessary to immobilize the foot by rigid external or internal fixation.

By emphasizing early mobilization, the surgeon can diminish fracture edema and minimize subsequent joint fibrosis and adhesion formation.

In many instances, no attempt at reduction is necessary because the initial deformity is compatible with good function. However, clinical deformity, particularly heel valgus or lateral bony prominences that might impinge on the peroneal tendons, should be corrected.

Subtalar motion is dependent on continuity between the posterior articular facets of the talus and the os calcis. Extreme displacement of Böhler's tuberosity angle (see page 2014) is not likely to yield a satisfactory result if treated by early mobilization without fracture reduction.

Weight bearing too early (sooner than eight weeks) or without plaster cast protection after early mobilization is also likely to lead to severe displacement and a poor result.

Lance and coworkers have found that the following criteria should be met in order to select candidates for early mobilization without fracture reduction:

1. Normal clinical appearance of the heel without peroneal tendon impingement.
2. X-rays that show involvement of the nonarticular portion of the talus or maintenance of reasonable congruity between the posterior articulating facets of the talus and calcaneus.
3. Age and general health status also influence the selection. For patients who are older than 60 years or who have been chronically ill, early active motion offers the swiftest and safest return to function.

Technique of Early Mobilization Management

X-rays of the foot to select patients for this technique should include lateral, oblique, and axial views in order to assess the degree of displacement, the shortening of the os calcis, and any incongruity of the posterior articular facets (see pages 2014 and 2016).

Patients should also be thoroughly assessed for other injuries and fractures, particularly of the spine and lower limb.

Early mobilization in treatment is important, even when reduction of the fracture is necessary.

1. The foot and ankle are padded generously with sheet wadding and wrapped with elastic bandage.

The fractured foot is elevated and ice is applied for five to seven days until the swelling has subsided.

Note: The bandage should be rewrapped several times daily to maintain compression.

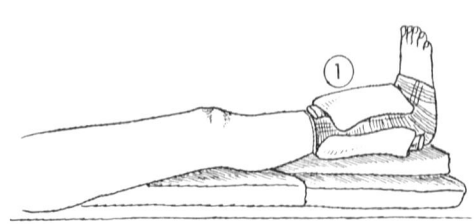

Subsequent Management

By day two or three the patient is encouraged to exercise the toes, tarsal joints, and ankle systematically on an hourly basis within the limits of pain.

By day three to five the patient may be up on crutches in order to go to the bathroom but should be cautioned against weight bearing or too much dependency of the foot.

At the end of one week, the foot should be reexamined for any clinical deformity or area of bony protrusion on the lateral or plantar surface. X-rays should be taken to determine the maintenance of fracture position. If heel widening or joint asymmetry is evident, reduction of the fracture should be carried out (see page 2022).

Weight bearing is deferred for six to eight weeks with linear fractures and ten to twelve weeks for fractures with comminution.

The presence or absence of pain is not an adequate criterion to determine the time for weight bearing because painless displacement of the fracture can occur with premature weight bearing. If, because of other fractures, the patient needs to put some weight on the side of the os calcis, a weight-bearing plaster cast molded well about the heel may be applied by seven to ten days, when the fracture swelling has completely subsided.

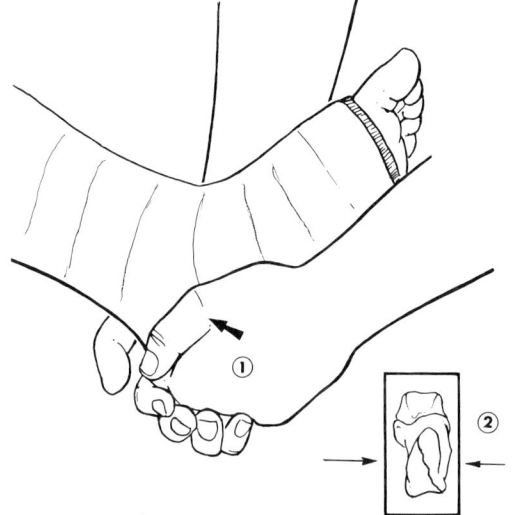

1. The cast is molded firmly about the fractured heel.
2. The heel is in a neutral position.

Example of Fracture Treated by Early Mobilization

1. A tongue-type fracture with Böhler's tuberosity angle depressed to 20 degrees.
2. Some displacement is evident but joint congruity is maintained.
3. The heel has not widened significantly and there is no significant bony protrusion on the lateral or plantar surface.

Note: There is no clinical deformity present except for some ecchymosis and slight swelling of the heel.

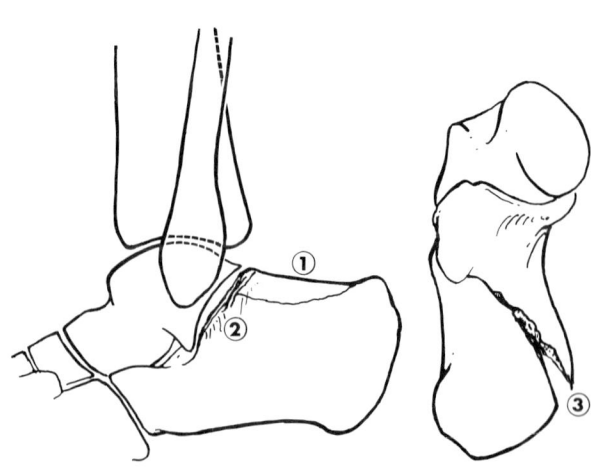

X-RAYS AFTER TREATMENT

1. There is good alignment of the articular surface, which correlates with the clinical appearance.
2. There is slight cortical prominence laterally but no impingement on the peroneal tendons.

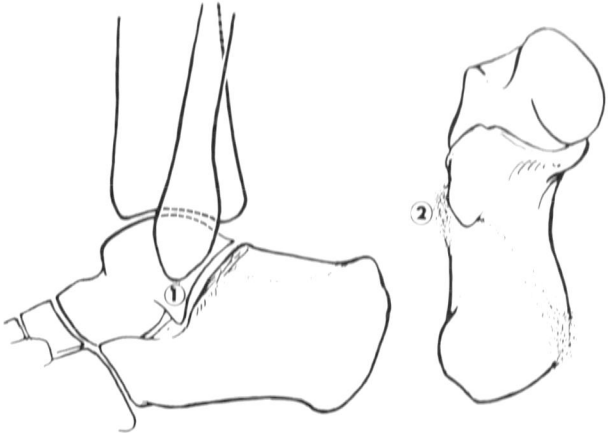

EARLY MOBILIZATION FOLLOWED BY CLOSED REDUCTION WITH SKELETAL TRACTION

REMARKS

Lance has estimated that 60 to 70 per cent of calcaneal fractures meet the clinical and radiographic criteria for treatment by early mobilization. The remaining fractures demonstrate sufficient incongruity of the subtalar joint surface to warrant reduction.

Displacement of the sustentaculum and tuberosity fragments produces shortening and widening of the heel, so that lateral and plantar bony prominences impinge on soft tissue.

Shortening of the heel will also produce gait abnormalities, particularly a calcaneus limp (see page 2018).

Although much emphasis has been placed on restoring the tuberosity angle to regain joint congruity, the key to reduction as described by McReynolds and demonstrated in biomechanical studies by Burdeaux is to restore the alignment of the tuberosity fragment with the medial sustentaculum and talus. These surgeons advocate operative reduction via a medial approach to realign these key fragments and thereby restore calcaneus length, reduce heel width, and return the tuberosity angle closer to normal.

This operative approach is effective for surgeons completely familiar with the technique.

However, the reduction can be achieved effectively by closed methods that employ longitudinal skeletal traction to align the tuberosity fragment with the sustentaculum and talus. A cast is then applied so as to maintain reduction.

Reduction by longitudinal traction should be done after five to seven days of elevation, when exercises have eliminated edema of the heel and encouraged motion in the uninjured tarsal joints.

Prereduction X-Ray

1. A central depression fracture of the calcaneus has depressed the tuberosity angle.
2. The plantar surface has developed a bony prominence.

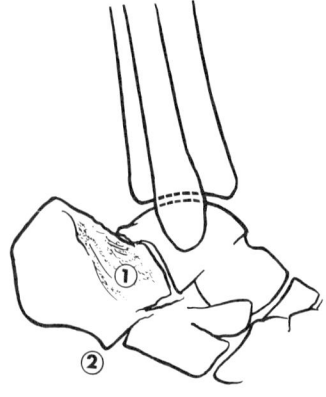

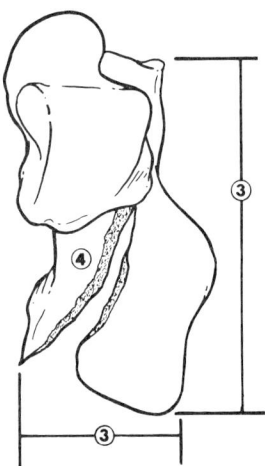

3. The heel has shortened and widened as a result of upward and lateral displacement of the tuberosity and
4. Downward and backward displacement of the sustentaculum talus.

Technique of Reduction by Longitudinal Traction

1. The foot is suspended by the toes by means of finger trap traction.
2. Under fluoroscopic guidance a 3-mm smooth Steinmann pin is inserted from the medial to the lateral side of the tuberosity fragment, with care taken to avoid the plantar neurovascular structures.
3. With a traction bow, the tuberosity is pulled downward and outward to correct its shortening and varus displacement.

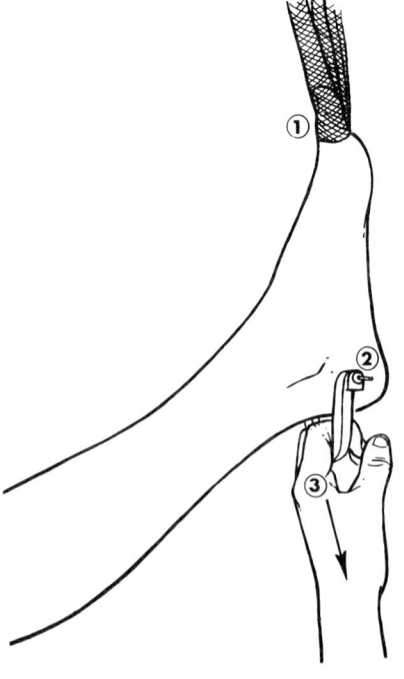

4. All the lateral and plantar bony prominences should no longer be palpable.

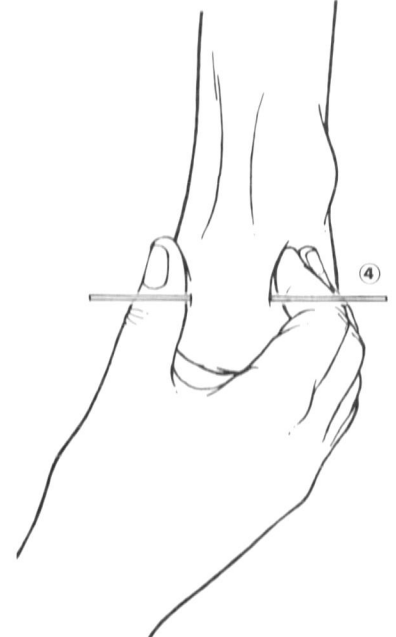

Postreduction X-Rays

1. The calcaneus has been restored to length and
2. Normal width.

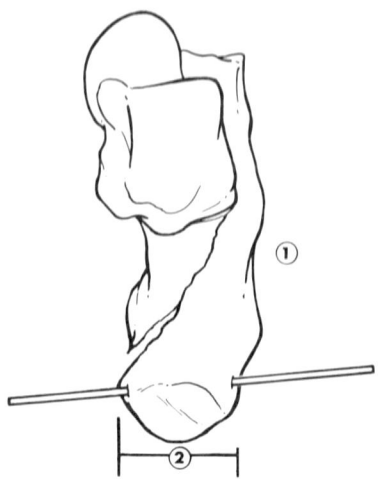

3. The tuberosity angle is corrected, although it has not returned to normal.
4. The plantar and lateral bony prominences have been dispersed.

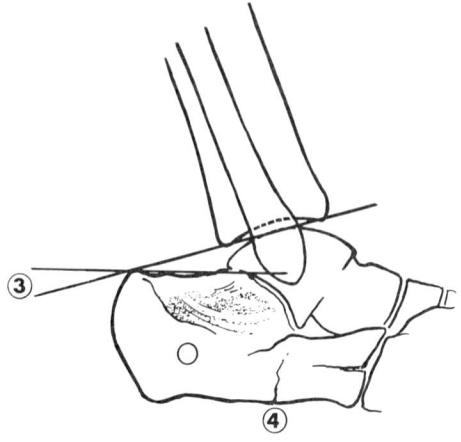

Immobilization

1. A short leg cast is applied while an assistant maintains traction.

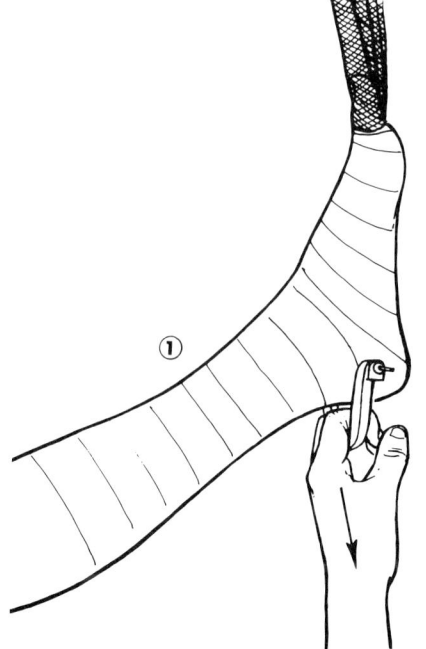

2. The heel is molded to maintain apposition of the tuberosity and the medial spike of the sustentaculum talus.
3. The pin is incorporated in plaster.

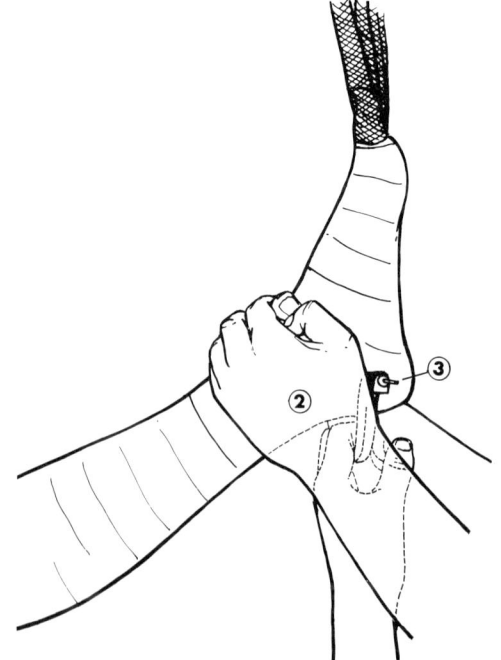

Subsequent Management

The foot is elevated for two to four days. Ice is applied to diminish swelling.

The pin is removed from the cast when the plaster is hardened, at the end of two days. Leaving the pin in longer than this is unnecessary to maintain reduction and may contribute to stiffening of the foot.

Note: It is important to use a smooth pin to allow easy removal through the plaster.

The patient may be up on crutches but should not bear weight on the fractured side.

The patient should continue to exercise his toes actively while in the plaster cast.

The cast is changed at the end of five to six weeks and a short leg walking cast is continued for one month longer.

The plaster may be discarded at the end of ten weeks, and progressive weight bearing may be allowed.

ALTERNATE REDUCTION TECHNIQUE FOR TONGUE-TYPE FRACTURES

Essex-Lopresti has shown this method to be effective for displaced tongue type fractures of the calcaneus.

The technique should be employed if the joint surface remains incongruous after one week of elevation and mobilization exercises, as described on page 2019.

Prereduction X-Ray

1. Primary fracture between the sustentaculum and tuberosity fragment.
2. Tongue-shaped fragment is depressed anteriorly and elevated posteriorly.
3. Secondary fracture line through the body of the calcaneus.
4. Loss of tuber angle. (The normal angle is 35 to 40 degrees.)

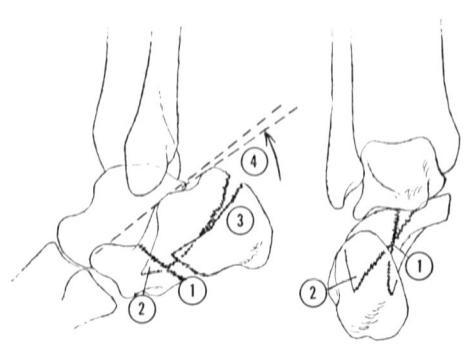

Manipulative Reduction and Pin Fixation

1. The patient is in a prone position.
2. Make a small incision over the calcaneus lateral to the Achilles tendon.
3. Insert a heavy Steinmann pin into the tongue fragment; the pin is directed in a longitudinal direction slightly to the lateral side.

Note: At this point check the position of the pin by x-ray.

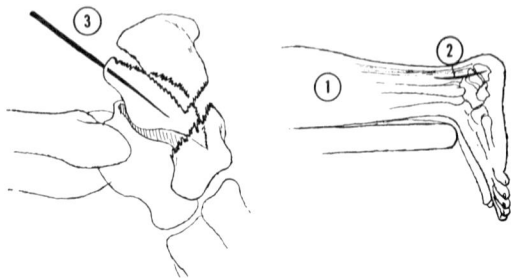

Manipulative Reduction and Pin Fixation (Continued)

1. Flex the knee 45 degrees.
2. Lift upward on the pin until the knee clears the table.

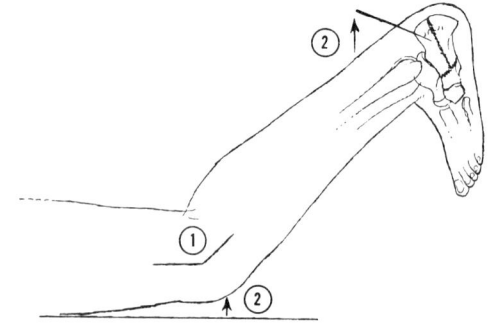

1. After measuring the exact thickness of the calcaneus of the normal foot, quickly compress the lateral walls of the fractured calcaneus with a Böhler clamp to the measurements of the normal calcaneus.
2. Drill the pin across the fracture site and into the anterior calcaneal fragment.

Note: Do not leave the clamp on too long because the skin may slough!

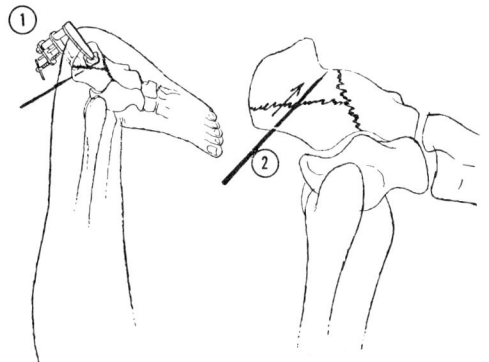

Postreduction X-Ray

1. The tuber angle has been restored.
2. The tongue fragment is elevated into normal position.
3. Articular surfaces of the subtalar joint are congruous.

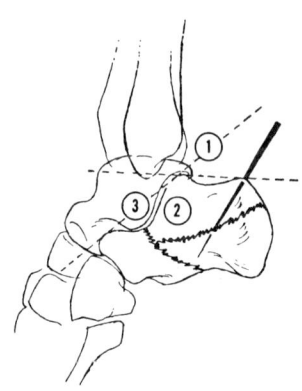

Immobilization

1. While the position is maintained by downward pressure on the pin,
2. Apply a below-knee plaster cast incorporating the pin.

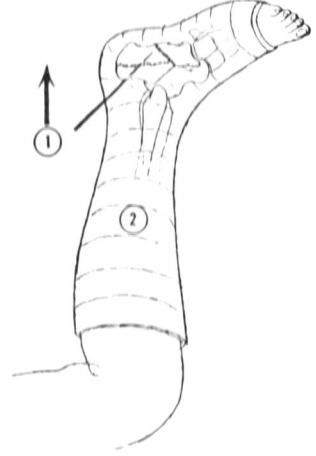

Subsequent Management

The foot is elevated for two to four days. Ice is applied to diminish swelling.

The pin is removed from the cast when the plaster is hardened, at the end of two days. Leaving the pin in longer than this is unnecessary to maintain reduction and may contribute to stiffening of the foot.

Note: It is important to use a smooth pin to allow easy removal through the plaster.

The patient may be up on crutches but should not bear weight on the fractured side.

The patient should continue to exercise the toes actively while in the plaster cast.

The cast is removed at the end of five to six weeks and a short leg walking cast is continued for one month longer.

The plaster may be discarded at the end of ten weeks and progressive weight bearing may be allowed.

Late Complications of Calcaneal Fractures

REMARKS

The majority of os calcis fractures heal promptly and with satisfactory functional results. This is particularly likely when the fracture can be treated by early mobilization without reduction.

The more complex the treatment rendered, the greater the disability likely to follow. This is particularly true after prolonged use of percutaneous pin fixation or operative reduction, as reported by most surgeons.

Many of initially painful sites will improve with time and forebearance. The surgeon must exercise the sharpest diagnostic acumen to locate the source of the pain and treat it promptly and appropriately by either nonoperative or operative methods.

The major complications to be anticipated and, if possible, prevented by initial treatment have been described on page 2016.

The most common longterm complaint is:

1. Lateral pain from the calcaneofibular abutment causing peroneal tenosynovitis.

Note: McLaughlin pointed out that this pain is aggravated by flexion and extension of the ankle, in contrast to the uncommon pain from the subtalar joint, which is aggravated by inversion and eversion of the foot.

2. Release of the peroneal tendon sheath and removal of the bony prominences can relieve these most common lateral pain symptoms after a calcaneal fracture.

Note: A free fat graft surrounding the tendon sheath can prevent recurrence of the bony mass and tendonitis.

3. The sural nerve may also be entrapped and therefore require decompression or removal.

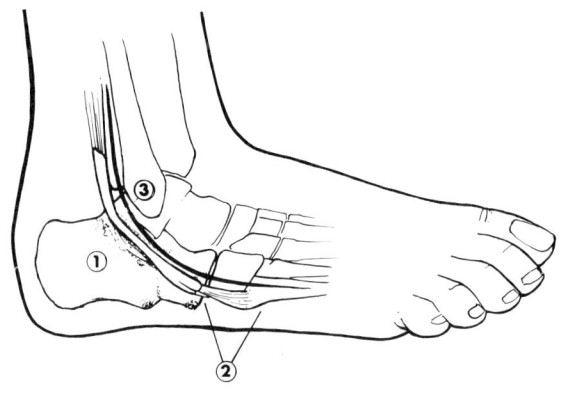

1. Distortion of the plantar surface due to upward displacement of the tuberosity fragment can produce a painful rocker-bottom prominence of the heel.

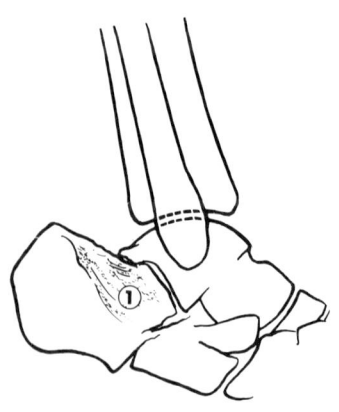

2. This can be relieved by soft heel cups* that protect the tender heel from pressure, or

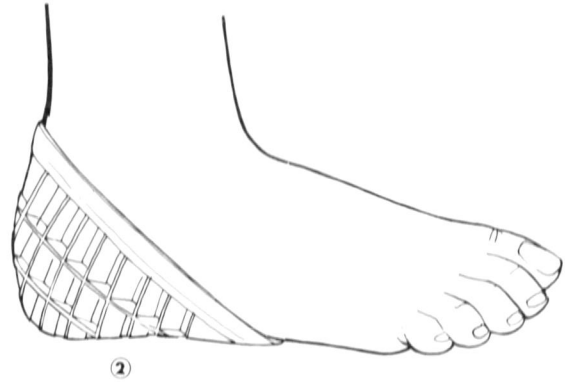

3. Surgical excision of the bony prominence may be required.

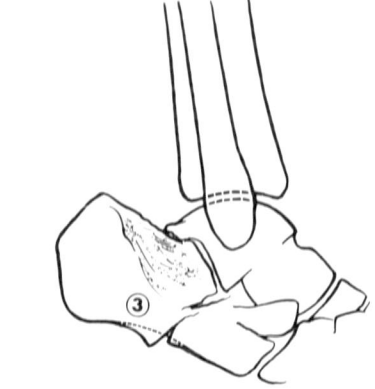

1. Stiffness of the foot, particularly the midtarsal area, may follow prolonged immobilization or operative treatment and be the cause of painful shuffling gait.
2. Orthopaedic shoes with well-fitted arch supports and cushioned soles may relieve this generalized foot discomfort.

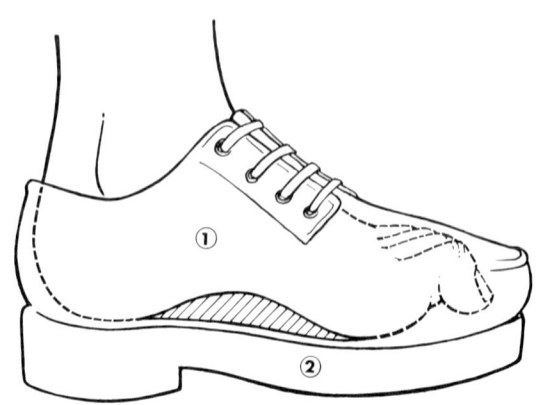

---

*Available from Tuli's, 5702 North 19th Avenue, Phoenix, Arizona 85015

Subtalar and Triple Arthrodesis

Severely displaced, crushed fractures of the calcaneus can cause considerable painful disability, particularly for patients who must earn their living by walking, standing, or climbing.

Arthrodesis is most effective if done within six to eight months after fracture, before the patient has developed chronic pain or causalgia-like symptomatology.

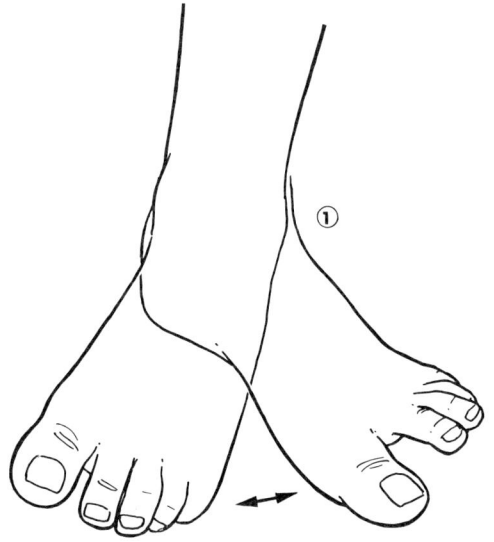

Subtalar arthrodesis by itself is notoriously ineffective in relieving this pain problem. Arthrodesis of all three joints of the hindfoot should be done if:

1. The patient has pain on inversion and eversion of the foot from the joints of the hindfoot and

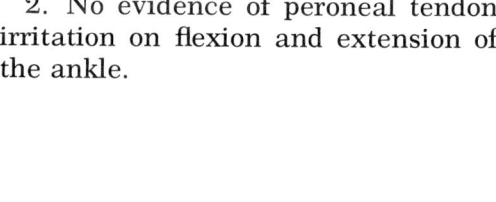

2. No evidence of peroneal tendon irritation on flexion and extension of the ankle.

3. Triple arthrodesis is most effective when done for persistent and significant joint pain within six to ten months after the fracture.

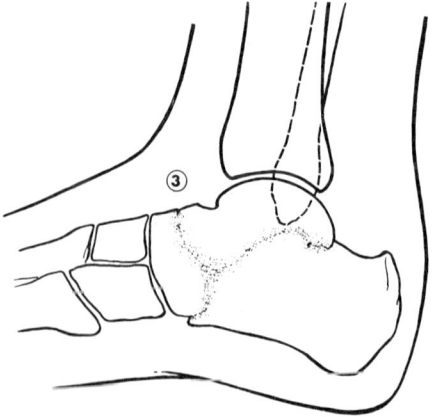

FRACTURES AND FRACTURE-DISLOCATIONS OF THE TARSAL NAVICULAR

REMARKS

The tarsal navicular is the keystone of the medial longitudinal arch of the foot and because of this position is subject to a number of injuries.

A fracture of the navicular is one of the most likely fractures of the foot to go unrecognized. What presents as a minor problem initially can leave the patient with the major disability of a painful foot.

Types of Fractures

Three types of injuries can produce these fractures.

The first is a relatively minor twisting of the foot that may cause no significant pain or swelling for several hours.

This represents the most common injury seen and occurs most often in women wearing high-heeled shoes.

1. Commonly there is an avulsion of the bone's cortex produced by its ligamentous attachment.

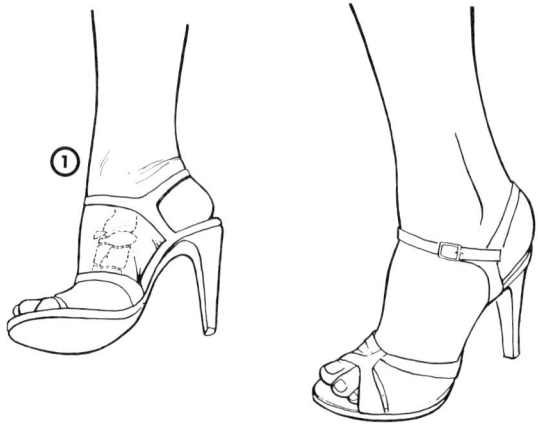

2. A second common fracture results from avulsion of the tuberosity of the navicular by the posterior tibial tendon or the deltoid and spring ligament complex.

Note: This may be mistaken for a sesamoid bone unless the x-ray is correlated with the clinical symptoms, which localize pain.

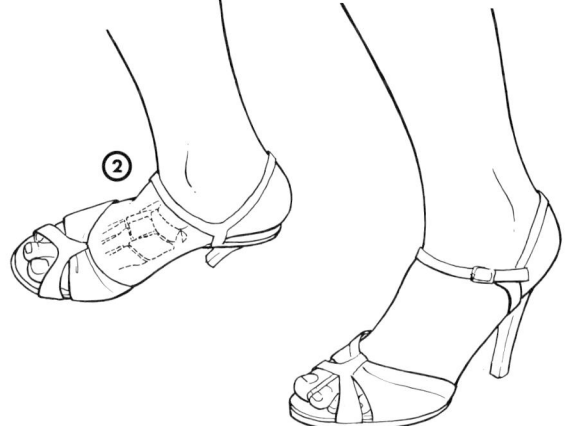

The third type of fracture results from forceful plantar flexion of the midfoot.

The naviculocuneiform ligaments tear first, producing:

1. A compression of the navicular by the medial cuneiform and fracture of the plantar surface.
2. If the talonavicular ligament fails, the bone will then dislocate dorsally.

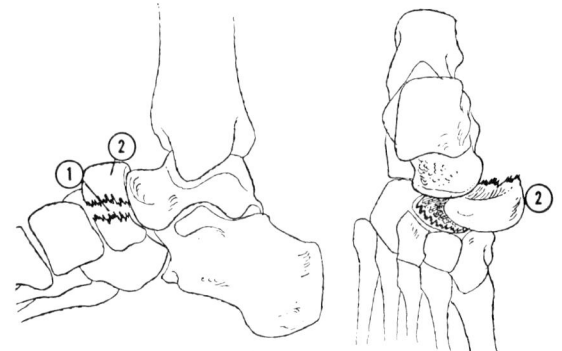

Diagnosis

Eichenholtz and Levine have reported that approximately one in four navicular fractures either will not be recognized on limited x-rays of the foot or will not be radiographed at all because of confusion with an ankle sprain.

1. Frequently, the fracture may only be visualized on a lateral projection. This view should always be included in any radiographic study of the injured foot.

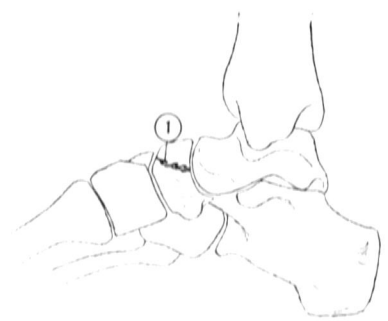

Management

Avulsion fractures of the cortex or tuberosity and undisplaced fractures of the body of the navicular can be treated symptomatically with a walking cast.

CAUTION

Avulsion fractures of the navicular associated with compression fractures of the cuboid result from midtarsal dislocation due to forceful abduction. This frequently requires fusion of the midtarsal joint to restabilize the longitudinal arch (see page 2039).

Displaced fractures in the navicular or fracture-dislocations generally require open reduction and internal fixation. Closed treatment may be attempted but the reduction should be anatomic to restore the keystone of the longitudinal arch.

If the navicular fracture is comminuted or a fracture-dislocation has gone unrecognized, fusion of the talonavicular and naviculocuneiform joints is generally necessary.

UNDISPLACED FRACTURE

Appearance on Lateral X-Ray

1. Fracture of the tuberosity of the navicular with minimal displacement.

Note: Distinguish this lesion from an accessory center of ossification frequently encountered at this site.

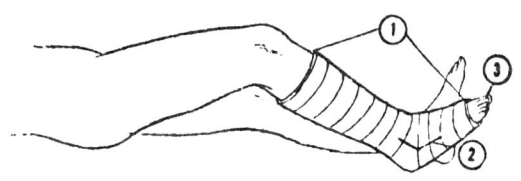

Immobilization

1. Apply a circular cast from behind the metatarsal heads to the tibial tubercle.
2. The foot is slightly plantar flexed.
3. The foot is in a neutral position in regard to inversion and eversion.

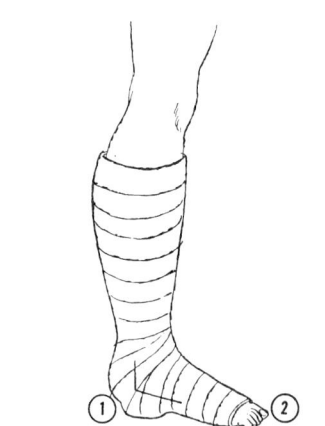

Subsequent Management

1. Apply a walking heel and permit weight bearing.
2. Have the patient exercise the toes actively.

For fractures of the dorsal tip of the navicular, remove the cast after four weeks.

For fractures of the tuberosity, remove the cast after eight weeks.

DISPLACED FRACTURES

Prereduction X-Ray

1. Fracture of the body of the navicular.
2. The dorsal fragment is displaced upward and medially.

Note: Closed reduction of the fracture-dislocation should be anatomic in order to restore the keystone function of the navicular to the longitudinal arch. In most instances this is impossible to accomplish by closed means, and open reduction is necessary.

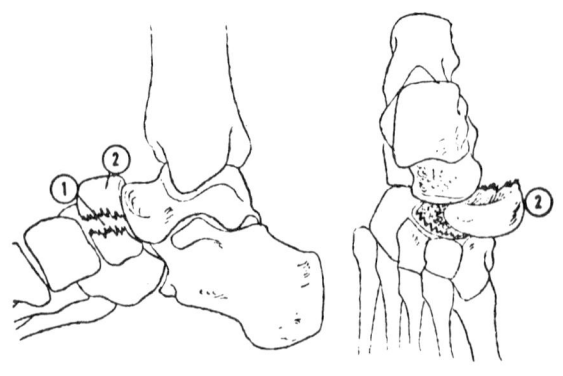

Manipulative Reduction (Under General Anesthesia)

1. The first assistant steadies the leg.
2. The second assistant makes strong traction while
3. The foot is plantar flexed and
4. The foot is everted.

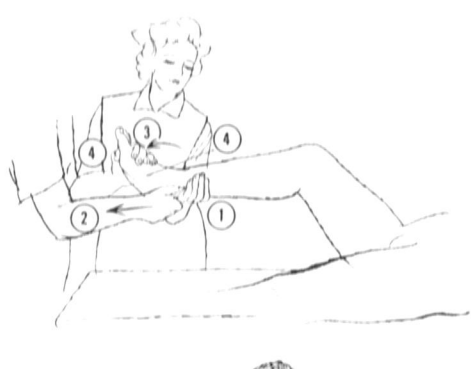

5. With the thumbs on the fragment the surgeon makes strong pressure downward.

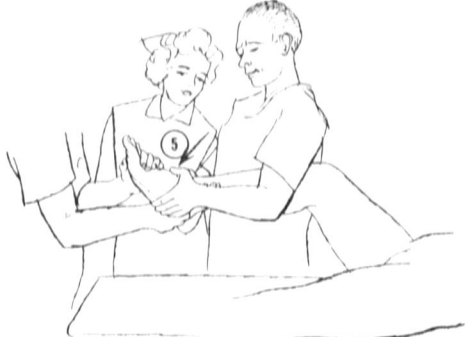

Immobilization

1. Apply a circular cast from behind the metatarsal heads to the tibial tubercle.
2. The foot is slightly dorsiflexed.
3. The foot is in a neutral position in regard to inversion and eversion.

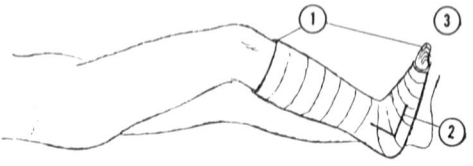

Subsequent Management

Allow the patient up on crutches without bearing weight on the affected foot after two or three days.

Change the cast at the end of ten days when the swelling has subsided. Add a walking heel and permit weight bearing.

In general, the plaster cast may be discontinued at the end of eight weeks and the patient may begin partial weight bearing with crutches.

Institute an active exercise program to restore normal movements of the ankle and tarsal joints.

In most instances closed reduction is incomplete and operative reduction is necessary.

Preferred Method: Open Reduction

Most displaced fractures and fracture-dislocations of the navicular are best treated by open and anatomic reduction with internal fixation using screws or Kirschner wires.

Operative Procedure

1. Make an 8-cm incision parallel to the lateral margin of the anterior tibial tendon centered over the talonavicular joint.
2. Divide the deep fascia and the transverse crural ligament above and the cruciate ligament below.
3. Make a linear incision through the fatty layer and capsule.
4. By sharp dissection expose the dorsal fragment and the talus above and the first cuneiform below.

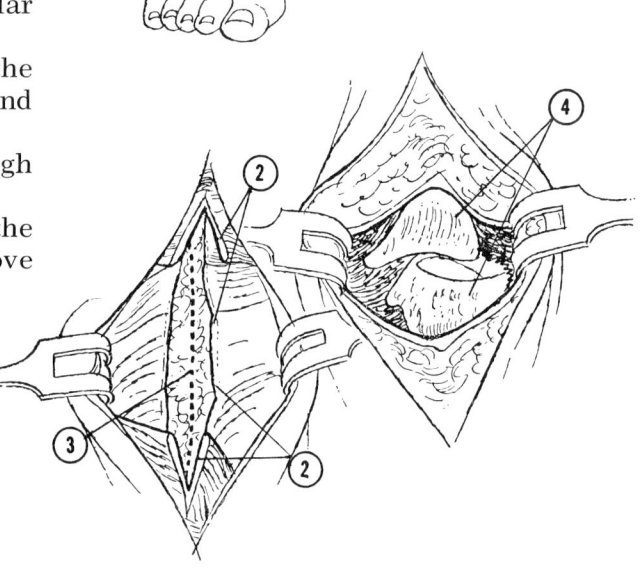

1. While the foot is plantar flexed and everted,
2. Make firm downward pressure on the dorsal fragment.

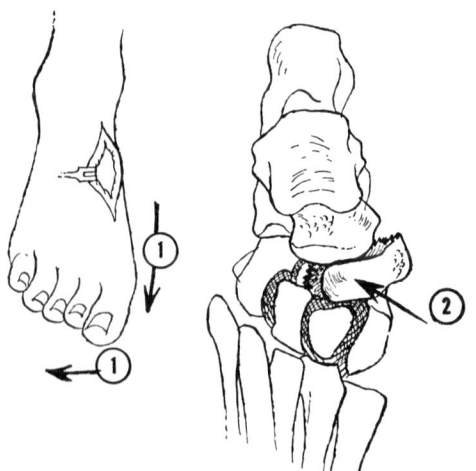

3. Fix the fracture fragments with a cancellous screw.

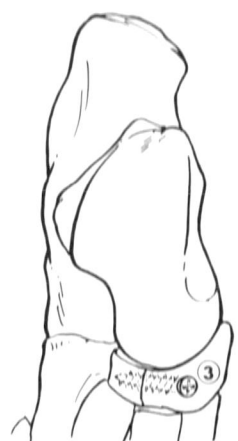

Alternate method

If the talonavicular or naviculocuneiform joint is unstable, use transarticular Steinmann pin fixation. A smooth Steinmann pin is preferable because threaded pins tend to distract the joint they traverse.
1. While the fragment is held in place,
2. Pass a 2-mm smooth Steinmann pin obliquely through the first cuneiform, the dorsal fragment of the navicular, and the head of the talus.
3. Cut the wire just below the level of the skin.

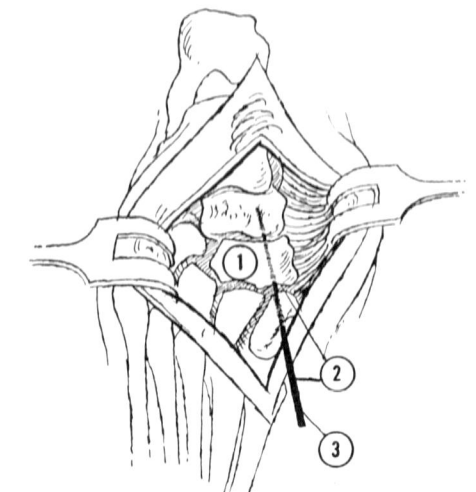

Postreduction X-ray

1. The dorsal fragment is in its normal relation to the talus and the cuneiform bone.
2. The Steinmann pin secures the fragment in its normal position.

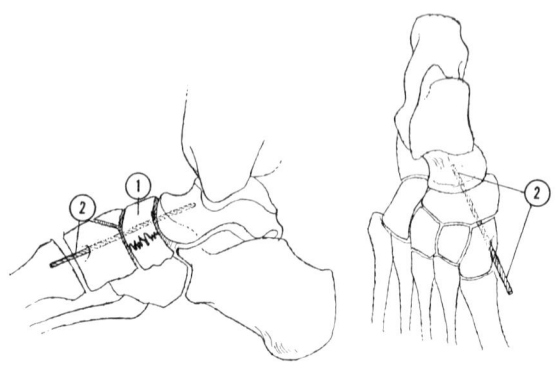

Immobilization

1. A below-knee plaster cast is applied.
2. The foot is slightly plantar flexed.
3. The foot is in neutral position in regard to inversion and eversion.
4. The cast is molded well under the longitudinal arch.

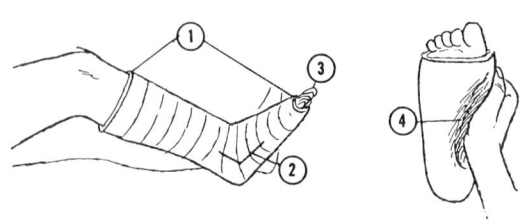

Postoperative Management

Allow the patient up on crutches without bearing weight on the affected foot.

Change the cast at the end of four weeks and remove the Steinmann pin.

In general, the plaster cast may be discontinued at the end of eight weeks and the patient may begin partial weight bearing with crutches.

Institute an active exercise program to restore normal movements of the ankle and tarsal joints.

MANAGEMENT OF A CHRONIC, UNRECOGNIZED FRACTURE-DISLOCATION

Approximately one in four fractures of the navicular may go unrecognized.

When the patient's symptoms of pain and swelling persist, the fracture or fracture-dislocation may be recognized only by means of x-rays taken several months after injury.

The patient's painful limp from chronic navicular injury can be relieved by fusion of the talonavicular joint and/or naviculocuneiform joint. If the subtalar joint is involved, triple arthrodesis may be necessary.

1. Nonunion with fracture-dislocation of the tarsal navicular eight months after original injury.
2. The keystone of the longitudinal arch is restored by fusion of the talonavicular and naviculocuneiform joints.

Note: The subtalar and calcaneocuboid joints are normal.

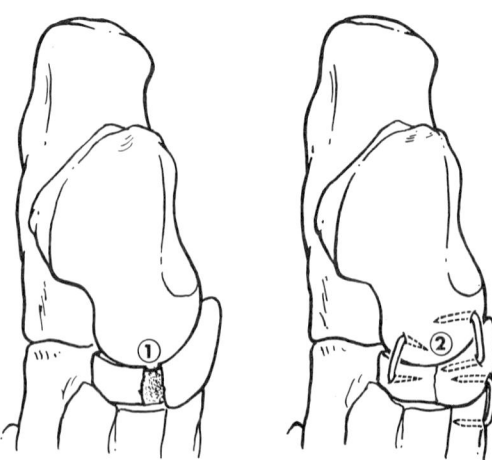

FRACTURES OF THE CUBOID AND CUNEIFORM BONES

REMARKS

Isolated injuries to these bones generally occur as the result of direct violence. As a rule there is little or no displacement of the fragments.

Indirect injuries to these bones occur most often from forced abduction or twisting of the foot while descending stairs. The result is actually a fracture-subluxation of the midtarsal joint.

This can be a treacherous and potentially disabling injury that masquerades as an innocent sprain of the ankle.

Pain and swelling on both sides of the midfoot should alert one to the associated subluxation and potentially unstable injury.

Commonly there is an avulsion of the navicular or cuneiform associated with a compression fracture of the cuboid.

If the initial x-rays are considered normal, the disability will persist unless the true nature of the tarsal instability is recognized and treated.

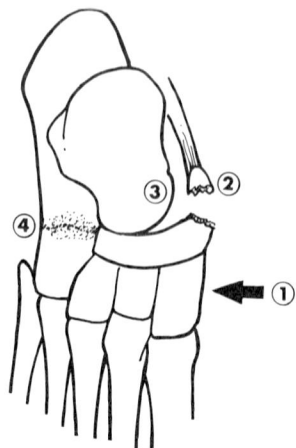

The mechanism is:
1. Forced abduction.
2. Avulsion of the tuberosity of the navicular.
3. Subluxation of the talonavicular joint.
4. Compression fracture of the calcaneocuboid.

UNDISPLACED FRACTURES FROM DIRECT INJURY

Appearance on X-ray

CUBOID FRACTURE

1. Comminuted fracture of the cuboid with minimal displacement.

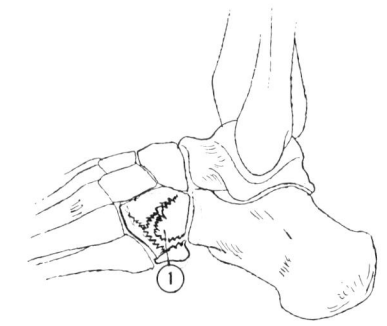

CUNEIFORM FRACTURE

1. Fracture of the second and third cuneiform bones with no displacement.

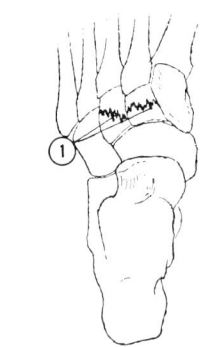

Immobilization

1. A circular plaster cast is applied from behind the metatarsal heads to the tibial tubercle.
2. The foot is in 90 degrees of dorsiflexion.
3. The foot is in a neutral position in regard to inversion and eversion.
4. The plaster is molded well under the longitudinal arch.

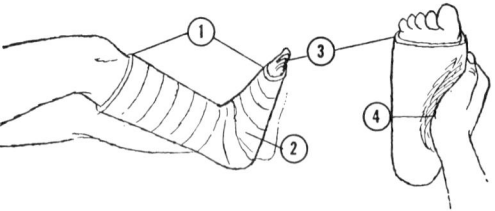

Management

Allow the patient up on crutches without bearing weight on the affected foot.

Remove the cast at the end of six weeks.

Fit the patient with a shoe with a Thomas heel and a longitudinal arch support.

OCCULT FRACTURE-SUBLUXATION OF THE MIDTARSAL JOINT FROM FORCED ABDUCTION

Appearance on X-ray

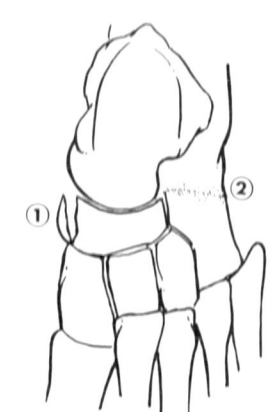

Note: These x-rays were originally interpreted as normal.

1. A small avulsion fracture of the navicular is evident. (This may be confused with a sesamoid bone.)
2. Oblique x-rays show a fracture of the cuboid including the calcaneocuboid joint.

Clinical Appearance

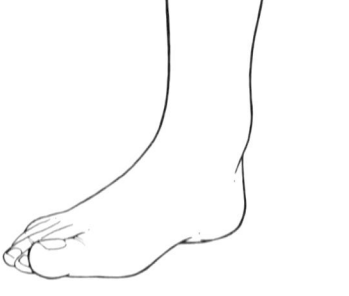
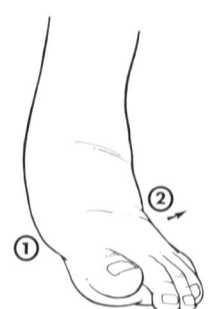

1. The deformity of the midtarsal subluxation produces pronation of the foot and
2. Abduction of the forefoot.

Management of Occult Fracture-Subluxation of the Midtarsal Joint

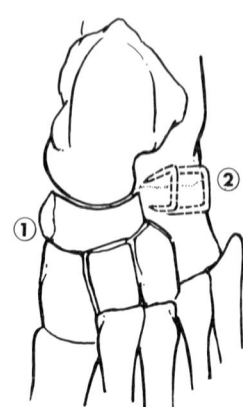

Treatment of these unstable injuries by plaster alone has resulted in persistent disability, as reported by Dewar and Evans. For fracture-subluxation, treatment should include:

1. Reattachment of the avulsed navicular fragment, repair of the talonavicular joint, and
2. Fusion of the calcaneocuboid joint.

OTHER OCCULT INJURIES TO THE MIDTARSAL JOINT

TOTAL DISLOCATION OF THE CUBOID WITHOUT FRACTURE

Drummond and Hastings have reported that complete dislocation of the cuboid is possible from forceful abduction of the foot.

This is an uncommon injury and may be missed on superficial clinical and radiographic examination.

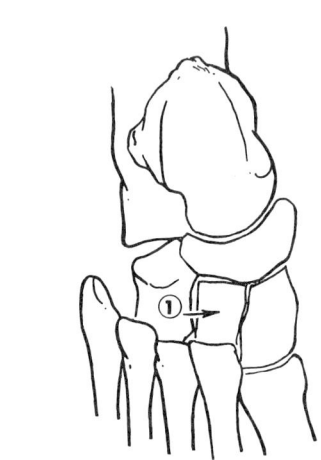

Appearance on X-ray

1. After a fall in which the victim lands on the inner side of the foot, the cuboid is displaced medially and

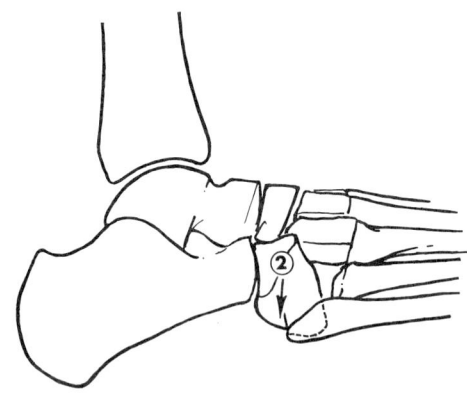

2. Downward.

Management

Operative reduction is necessary; it is achieved by inverting the foot to visualize and open the space normally occupied by the cuboid and then pushing the cuboid laterally back into the space.

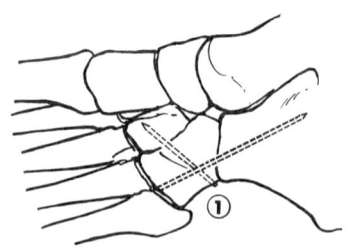

1. Kirschner wire fixation is usually necessary to maintain reduction because the ligaments surrounding the cuboid have been disrupted.

Subsequent Management

The foot is immobilized in a below-knee, non-weight-bearing cast for six weeks.

The cast and Kirschner wires are removed at the end of this time and the patient is gradually allowed to resume weight bearing on crutches.

ISOLATED DISLOCATION OF THE CUNEIFORM BONE

Schiller and Ray have reported that this rare injury is readily missed because of its deceptive radiographic appearance.

The injury is sustained from direct violence to the foot, and the edema of injury will mask any bony swelling or tenderness.

Careful assessment of a lateral x-ray is essential to detect the dislocation.

Prereduction X-ray

1. Except for overlapping of the navicular and medial cuneiform and
2. Rotation of the first metatarsal, the dislocation is not apparent on either the anteroposterior or the oblique x-ray.

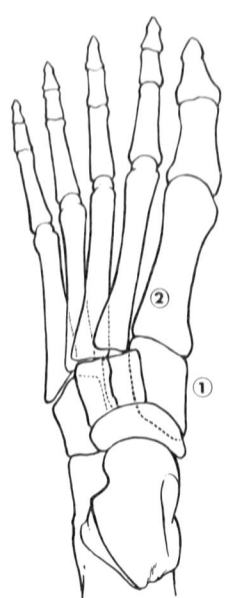

3. The plantar position of the medial cuneiform is obvious on lateral x-ray.

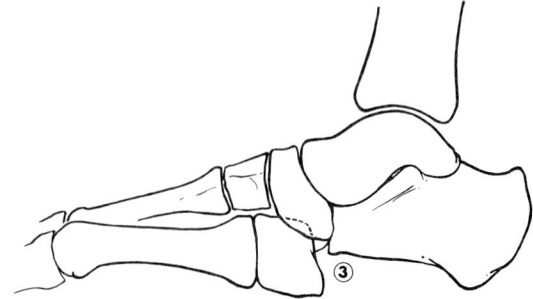

Management

In most instances, treatment is delayed either because of extreme swelling of the foot or because the diagnosis is not evident on initial x-rays.

The subsequent disruption to the medial longitudinal arch from this injury requires open reduction and arthrodesis of the reduced cuneiform to provide stability.

Postoperative X-ray

1. The dislocated cuneiform has been surgically reduced under direct vision.
2. Crossed Kirschner wires are used to stabilize the naviculocuneiform and first and second cuneiform joints.

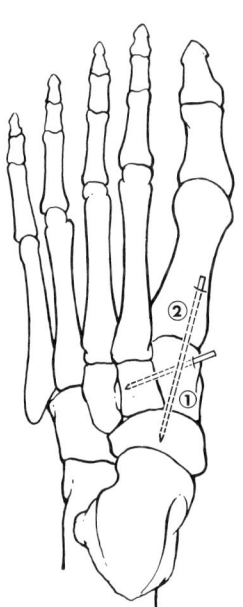

Subsequent Management

The foot is immobilized in a below-knee non-weight-bearing cast for eight weeks.

The pins and cast may be removed at the end of eight weeks and the patient may begin progressive weight bearing with crutches.

The crutches can be discontinued at the end of four to six weeks. The patient is encouraged to actively exercise the foot and ankle.

DISLOCATIONS AND FRACTURE-DISLOCATIONS OF THE MIDTARSAL JOINT

REMARKS

The midtarsal joint comprises the talonavicular and calcaneocuboid joints.

Dislocation is most often medial and is associated with a fracture of the navicular or cuboid. Fractures of these bones should not be treated without evaluation of the entire midfoot. Avulsion fractures may occur as isolated injuries but they may also mask significant injury and instability of the midtarsus (see page 2049).

Main and Jowett have also described a medial midtarasl dislocation without fracture, which is considered to be a swivel dislocation of the calcaneus under the talus. This is the result of an inversion mechanism that leaves the talocalcaneal ligament intact and therefore does not produce the usual complete subtalar dislocation with tilting of the calcaneus. The force is sufficient to dislocate the navicular medial to the talus but leaves the calcaneocuboid joint intact.

The midtarsal joint can also be dislocated as a result of a force applied to the plantar flexed foot. The injury may cause a fracture-dislocation of the navicular, as described on page 2032, or a plantar dislocation of both the talonavicular and calcaneocuboid components of the midtarsus. A plantar dislocation of the midtarsus is distinguished from a plantar subtalar dislocation by the maintenance of the normal subtalar joint space owing to the intact talocalcaneal ligament.

Lateral midtarsal dislocation results from forceful abduction causing an avulsion fracture of the navicular tuberosity and an impaction fracture of the lateral margins of the calcaneus or cuboid, as described on page 2039.

A lateral swivel dislocation may also occur at the midtarsal joint without a fracture.

Recurrent or persistent unrecognized instability of the midtarsus can follow from these injuries and requires arthrodesis of the talonavicular and calcaneocuboid joints. Hooper and McMaster reported bilateral recurrences that responded to midtarsal fusion.

Neurotrophic problems in the diabetic patient may also cause recurrent fractures and instability of the midfoot, but fusion may be difficult in this situation.

PREREDUCTION X-RAYS

Medial Midtarsal Dislocation with Fractured Cuboid

1. Inward displacement of the navicular and cuboid bones on the talus and calcaneus.
2. Tarsal bones at the level of the midtarsal joint are displaced upward.
3. Fracture of the cuboid bone with minimal displacement.

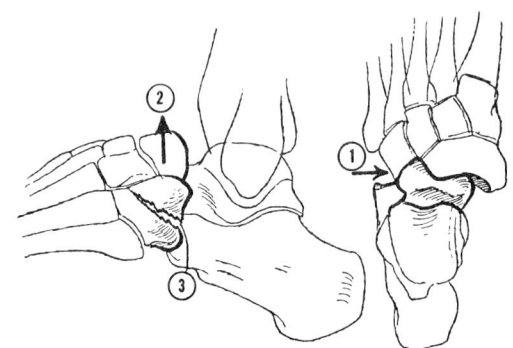

Medial Swivel Dislocation

1. The anteroposterior view shows dislocation of the talonavicular component.
2. The calcaneus swivels beneath the talus, maintaining articulation with the cuboid.
3. An oblique view shows that the calcaneocuboid component is intact and
4. The calcaneus is not tilted as it would be in a subtalar dislocation because the talocalcaneal ligament remains intact.

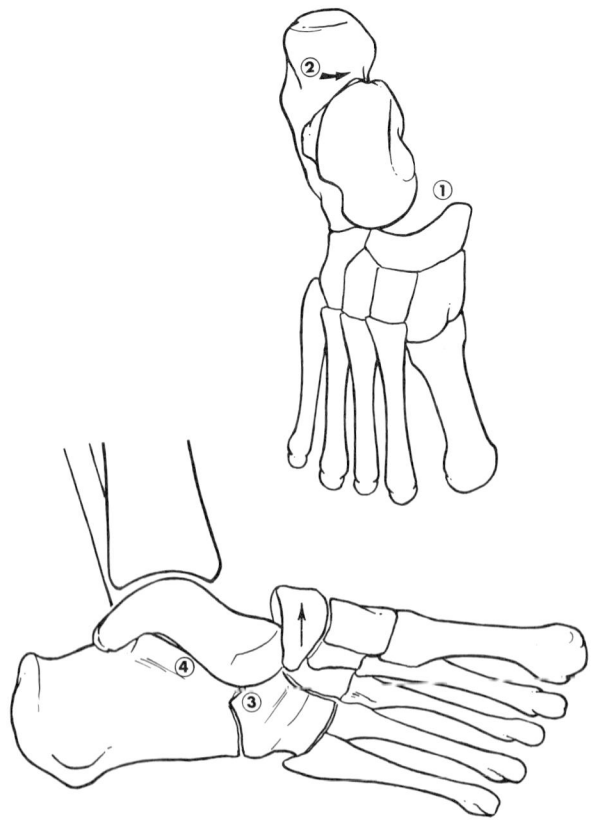

Plantar Dislocation

1. Lateral view shows dislocation of both the talonavicular and the calcaneocuboid components of the midtarsus.
2. The subtalar joint maintains its normal space because the talocalcaneal ligament remains intact.

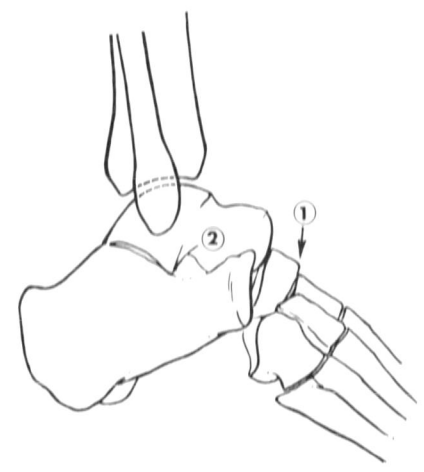

Lateral Swivel Dislocation

1. Anteroposterior view shows that the talonavicular joint has dislocated laterally.
2. The calcaneocuboid joint remains intact.
3. The hind foot does not evert but the os calcis has swiveled laterally owing to the intact talocalcaneal ligament.

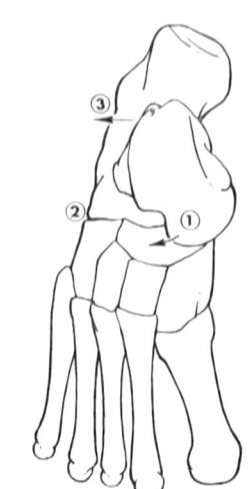

MANAGEMENT

Closed reduction is possible and it should restore the joint to anatomic normal. If there is any question about the adequacy of reduction, direct surgical exploration of the joint should be carried out.

Frequently the injury is unstable and should be supplemented by percutaneous Steinmann pin fixation of the midtarsus after reduction.

Fractures of the navicular or cuboid, particularly after abduction type injuries, require internal fixation as described on pages 2037 and 2041.

After reduction, test stability of the midtarsus by abduction and adduction, and if the joint proves unstable use percutaneous pin fixation.

Manipulative Reduction

1. One assistant fixes the ankle.
2. Another assistant grasps the forefoot and makes strong forward traction.
3. With the heels of the hands, the surgeon pushes the forefoot outward and the calcaneus inward; this reduces the inward displacement.
4. With the heels of both hands direct downward pressure is made on the anterior tarsal bone; this reduces the upward displacement.

Note: This same general pattern of manipulation is employed regardless of the direction of displacement.

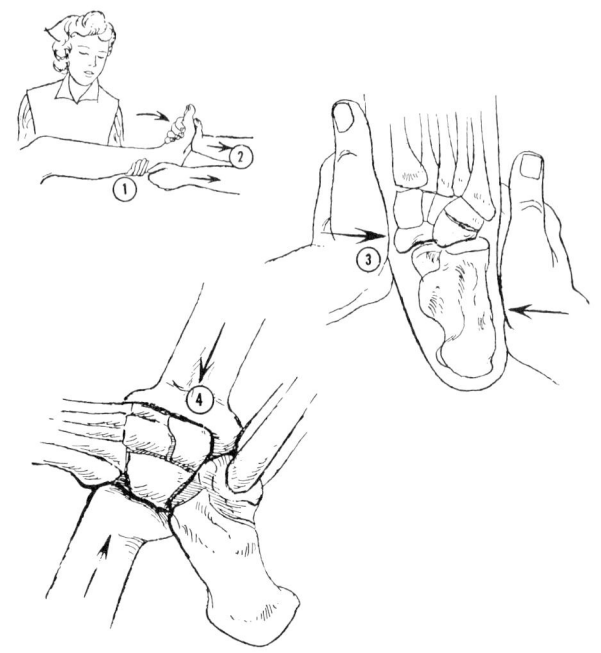

Postreduction X-Ray

1. The navicular and cuboid bones are in normal relationship to the talus and calcaneus.
2. Fracture of the cuboid bone.
3. If the midtarsus is at all unstable, it should be fixed with percutaneous Steinmann pins.

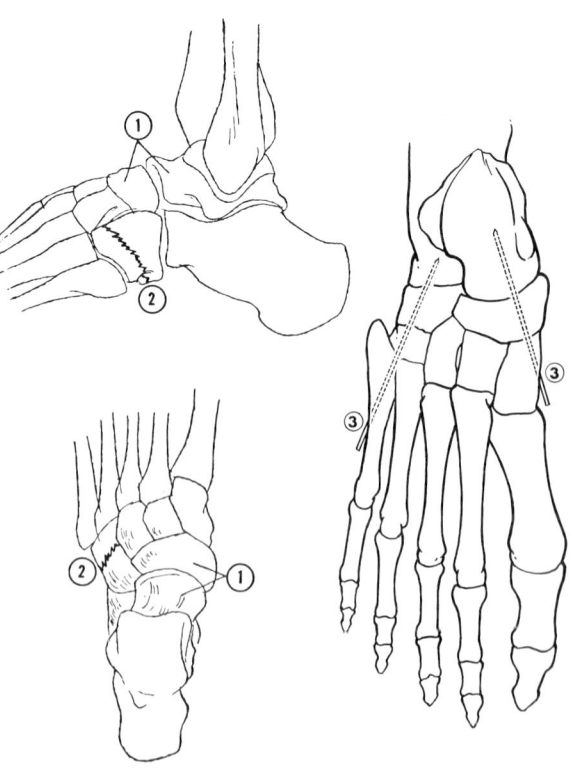

Immobilization

1. A circular plaster cast is applied from behind the metatarsal heads to the tibial tubercle.
2. The foot is in 90 degrees of dorsiflexion.
3. The foot is in a neutral position in regard to inversion and eversion.
4. The plaster is molded well under the longitudinal arch.

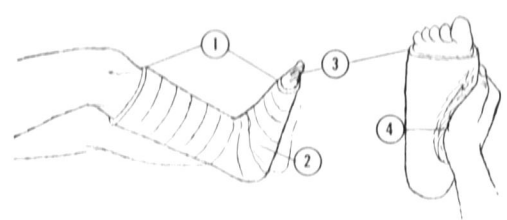

Postreduction Management

Allow the patient up on crutches without bearing weight on the affected foot.

Remove the cast and any percutaneous pins at the end of six weeks.

Fit the patient with a shoe with a Thomas heel and a longitudinal arch support.

Recurrent or Persistent Subluxation of the Midtarsus

Recurrent or persistent subluxation of the midtarsus is possible and may require fusion of the joint.

If the subtalar joint has developed arthritic changes a triple arthrodesis should be carried out.

1. Recurrent subluxation of the navicular and cuboid can occur with mild injury and can produce traumatic arthritis.

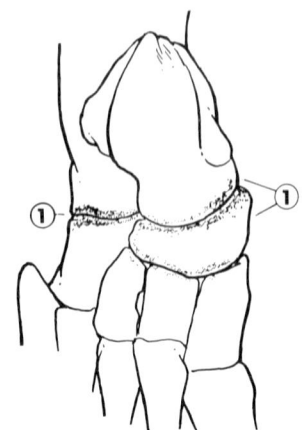

X-Ray After Fusion

1. The foot is stabilized by a fusion of the talonavicular and calcaneocuboid joints.

2. A triple arthrodesis is not necessary if the subtalar joint shows no arthritic changes.

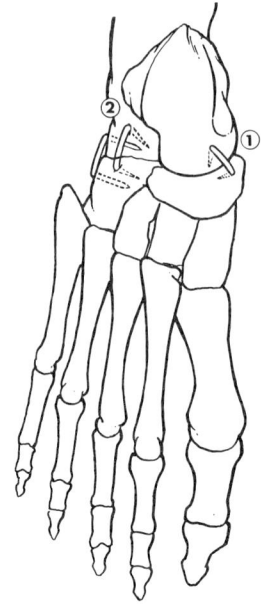

PERSISTENT AND CHRONIC DISLOCATION FROM A DIABETIC NEUROTROPHIC JOINT (CHARCOT FOOT)

1. Repeated injuries to the diabetic foot can cause chronic disruption of the midtarsus and persistent subluxation of the joint.

Note: This is the most common cause of Charcot joint today and should be treated by fusion of the midtarsal joint as described above. Fusion in the diabetic foot can be quite difficult but it can be done.

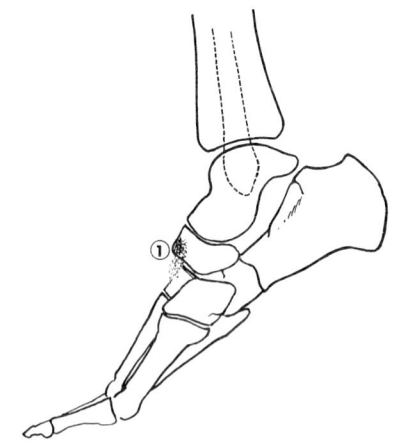

DISLOCATIONS AND FRACTURE-DISLOCATIONS OF THE TARSOMETATARSAL JOINT

REMARKS

Fractures and dislocations of the tarsometatarsal region are uncommon injuries and, unfortunately, are commonly unrecognized.

The classic mechanism dates back to the Napoleonic era, when in a cavalry accident a rider suffered the misfortune of his horse falling on his plantar flexed foot. It was for this injury that Lisfranc developed his amputation through the tarsometatarsal region.

Wiley has described both direct and indirect mechanisms of injury. The indirect mechanism is more common and less understood than the direct mechanism.

Visualizing the anatomy of this region is helpful to appreciate the mechanisms of injury.

Anatomy of the Tarsometatarsal Region

1. The ligamentous and bony articulations around the second metatarsal make this bone the keystone of the tarsometatarsal region.

2. The first metatarsal has no ligamentous attachment to the second and may be displaced in a divergent direction from the other metatarsals.

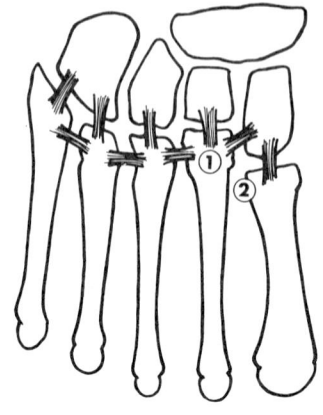

DIRECT MECHANISM

Direct mechanism results from a crushing injury that can produce varying degrees of fractures and dislocations.

As with any injury to the foot, adequate anteroposterior, lateral, and oblique x-rays are necessary in order to appreciate the extent of damage.

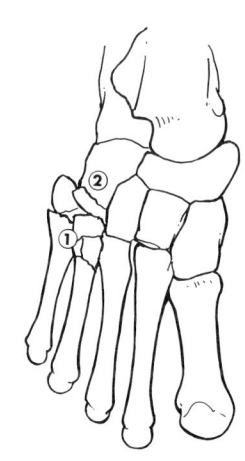

Typically, the injury follows a direct blow from a heavy weight dropping on the foot. This produces the following injuries:

1. Anteroposterior and oblique x-rays show multiple fractures of the fifth and fourth metatarsal and
2. Cuboid.

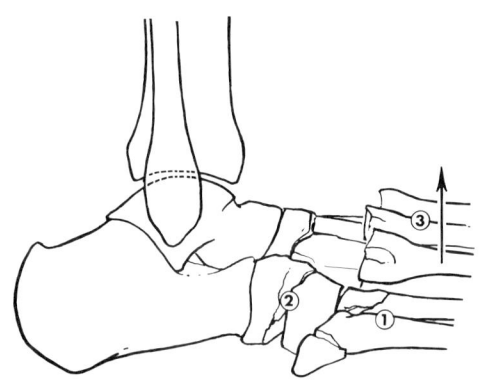

3. Lateral view shows dorsolateral dislocation not evident on anteroposterior view.

Divergent Dislocation

Direct injury between the first and second metatarsal may cause

1. Divergent dislocation, in which the first metatarsal moves medially while the remaining metatarsals move laterally.
2. Fracture of the navicular or cuneiform is common.

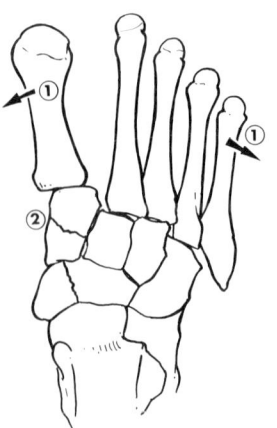

Note: Divergent dislocations are most likely to cause extensive swelling from disruption of the dorsalis pedis vessel. The possibility of vascular insult should always be kept in mind, particularly with violent direct mechanisms.

2052

INDIRECT MECHANISMS

These include both abduction and plantar flexion injuries as described by Wiley.

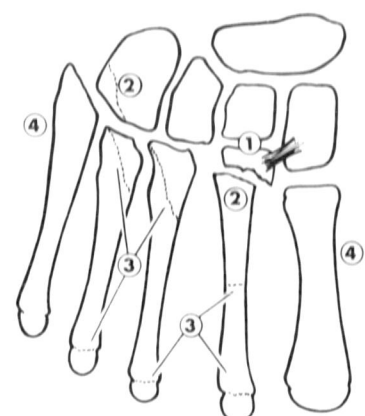

1. When the forefoot is violently abducted, the brunt of the strain is absorbed by the fixed base of the second metatarsal.
2. Fractures of the second metatarsal and of the cuboid are pathognomonic.
3. Other fractures of the metatarsal neck or bases may occur.
4. Fracture of the first or fifth metatarsal is uncommon.

Plantar Flexion Mechanism

Acute plantar flexion occurs in two ways.

The least common mechanism results from a violent blow to the heel in line with the axis of the foot while the toes are fixed. This was the classic injury sustained by a Napoleonic cavalryman when his horse fell on his foot.

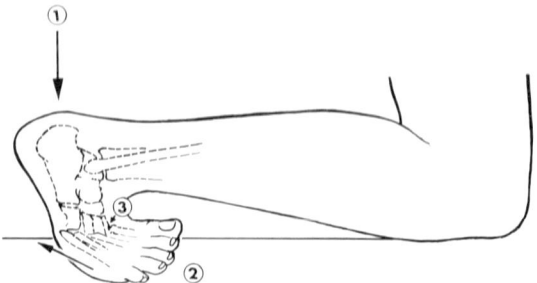

1. A violent force is applied to the heel in line with the axis of the foot.
2. The toes are fixed.
3. Direct heel-to-toe compression produces acute plantar flexion of the tarsometatarsal joint.

The second and more common indirect injury occurs with the ankle in acute plantar flexion or tiptoe position. This causes the foot to become a part of the entire lower leg.

The tarsometatarsal joint absorbs the brunt of forced plantar flexion and sudden deceleration.

Most commonly this occurs in a front-end automobile collision in which the outstretched foot is violently plantar-flexed and driven backward by the floorboard. Other mechanisms may be the result of trivial trauma such as stepping off a curbstone, falling from a stepladder, or inadvertently stepping into a deep hole.

Front-end Collision Mechanism

1. The foot and ankle are in maximum plantar flexion or tiptoe position at the time of injury.
2. Further plantar flexion dislocates the tarsometatarsal joint.
3. Rotation of the forefoot at the time of injury produces associated fracture of the metatarsal.

Note: The dislocated joints may reduce partially or completely after the injury. The fracture patterns of the tarsals and metatarsals then may be the only clue to the significant instability.

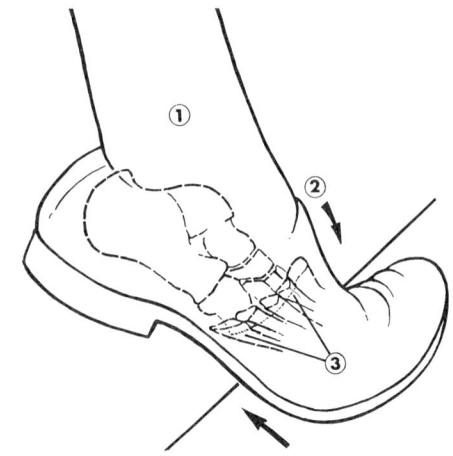

Management

REMARKS

Injuries from both direct and indirect mechanisms require prompt reduction and internal stabilization of the foot.

Direct injuries to the foot frequently cause an open wound or compromised circulation, both of which need to be managed in conjunction with reduction of the injury.

Even if a closed reduction is successful, the tarsometatarsal region is so unstable that percutaneous pin fixation of the joint is wise in order to avoid recurrent subluxation or dislocation despite cast immobilization.

MANIPULATIVE REDUCTION

Procedure

1. One assistant fixes the heel.
2. The second assistant makes strong steady traction on the forefoot.
3. While traction is maintained, the operator makes firm downward pressure on the bases of the metatarsal bones.

Note: The direction of the pressure is governed by the type of displacement; downward pressure is applied for upward displacement of the metatarsals and upward pressure for downward displacement.

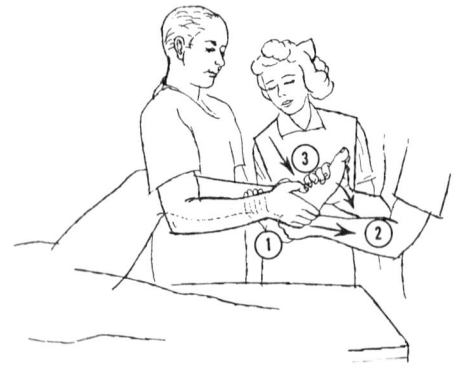

Postreduction X-Ray

1. The bases of the metatarsal bones are in normal relationship to the tarsal bones.

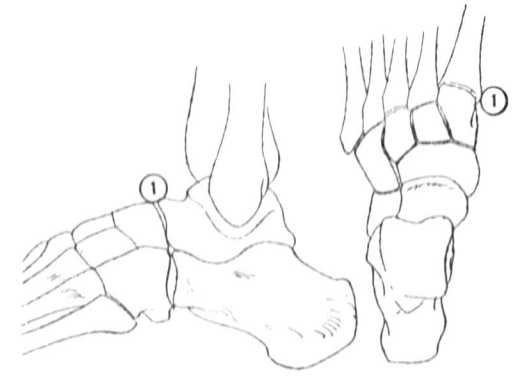

Percutaneous Pin Fixation

1. The reduction is stabilized by a 2-mm smooth Steinmann pin drilled through the first metatarsal into the navicular.
2. A second smooth pin is inserted through the fifth metatarsal into the cuboid.

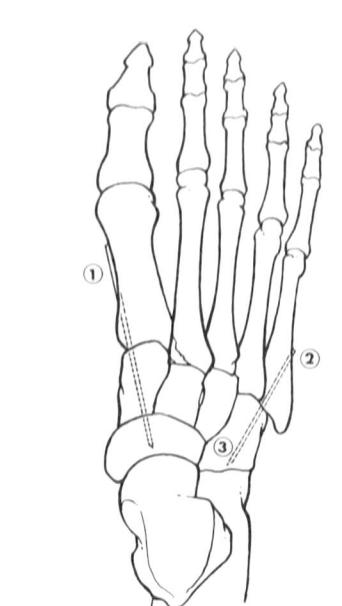

Immobilization

1. A padded circular cast is applied from the toes to below the knee joint.
2. The foot is at a right angle.
3. The foot is in neutral in regard to inversion and eversion.
4. The plaster is molded well under the longitudinal arch.

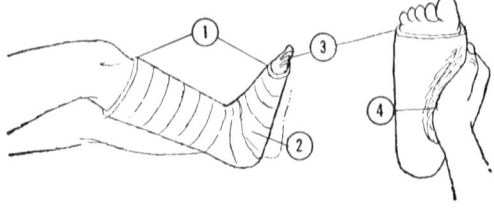

Postreduction Management

Elevate the limb on pillows.
Surround the foot with ice bags.
Check the circulation of the foot frequently.
After a few days allow the patient up on crutches without bearing weight on the affected foot.

Remove the cast and pins at the end of six weeks.

The patient is then allowed partial weight bearing on crutches for four weeks longer.

Subsequently the patient is permitted full weight bearing using a longitudinal arch support.

OPERATIVE REDUCTION

If manipulation is not successful or if dislocation recurs, open reduction and internal fixation should be performed.

The key to reduction is the fracture-dislocation of the second metatarsal.

Occasionally in dislocations that cannot be reduced by closed manipulation, the anterior tibial tendon may be interposed, particularly between the navicular and first cuneiform. This requires replacement of the tendon and reduction and fixation of the dislocation.

Operative Technique

1. A longitudinal incision is made lateral to the long axis of the first metatarsal. The first and second metatarsals are reduced under direct vision.

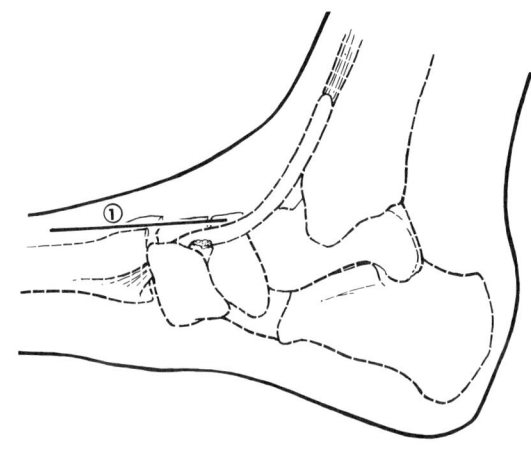

2. Occasionally, the anterior tibial tendon will have been displaced into the area of fracture-dislocation.

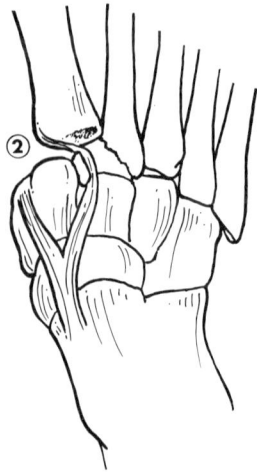

1. After reduction, the tarsometatarsal joint is stabilized by a percutaneous 2-mm Steinmann pin drilled from the first metatarsal into the navicular.

2. If the lateral metatarsals are not reduced, a second incision is made between the fourth and fifth metatarsals and the reduction is accomplished under direct vision. A second smooth Steinmann pin is inserted through the fifth metatarsal into the cuboid.

Note: These two pins produce stability of all of the metatarsals; fixation of the third or fourth metatarsal is not necessary.

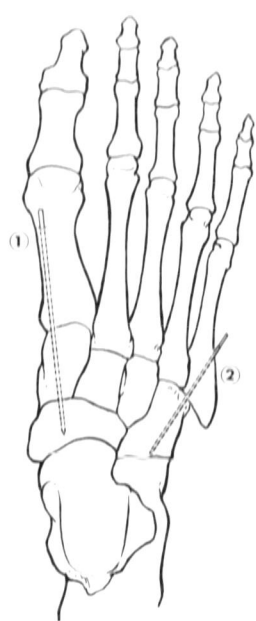

MANAGEMENT OF PERSISTENT OR UNRECOGNIZED DISLOCATIONS

When anatomic reduction is obtained by closed or open methods, excellent painless function is to be anticipated. Nevertheless, some arthritic changes may be evident even after ideal reduction.

Aitken and Poulson have pointed out that, although persistent or recurrent instability of the joint may cause obvious deformity, functional results can be quite good. The patient may lose pronation and the ability to stand on tiptoe, but complaints of pain or functional limitation may be minimal.

Accepting a persistent or recurrent deformity that is painless seems preferable to surgical fusion of Lisfranc's joint, but treatment must be tailored to the individual patient.

FRACTURES OF THE METATARSAL BONES

REMARKS

These lesions are usually the result of direct violent injuries; one or more bones may be involved.

Repeated stresses such as are produced by prolonged walking may cause a fracture in one or more metatarsal bones; usually the second or third metatarsal bone is involved. As a rule no displacement occurs. These are the so-called "march fractures."

Accurate reduction is essential in order to avoid serious disability of the foot; this is particularly true of fractures in the distal ends of the bones.

Most fractures can be treated by manipulative reduction; however, open reduction is justified if this method fails.

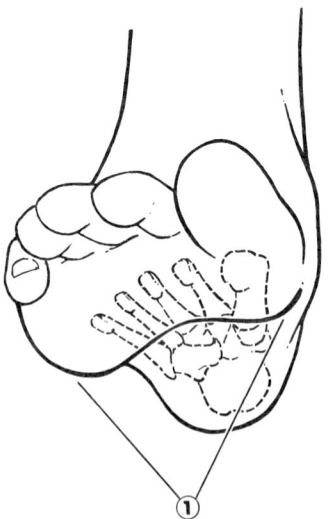

The reduction should correct and restore the normal transverse arch of the foot to avoid bony prominences in the weight-bearing surface.

1. The forefoot transverse arch is due to the architecture and relationship of the metatarsal heads which should not be disturbed by fracture displacement.

Fractures of the Metatarsal Bones without Displacement

Appearance on X-Ray

1. Fracture of the shafts of the second and third metatarsal bones with minimal displacement.

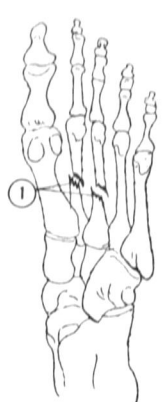

1. March fracture of the third metatarsal; only a faint fracture line is visible.
2. Same fracture three weeks after onset of symptoms; note marked callus formation.

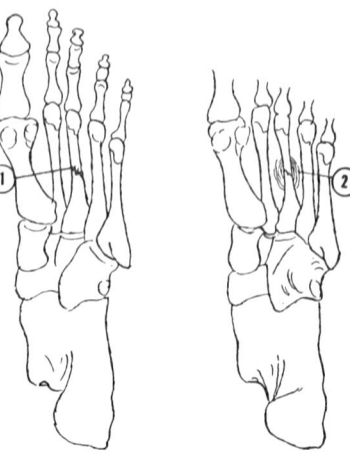

Immobilization

1. A circular plaster cast is applied from the toes to the tibial tubercle.
2. The foot is at a right angle.
3. The foot is neutral in regard to inversion and eversion.
4. The plaster is molded well under the longitudinal and transverse arches.

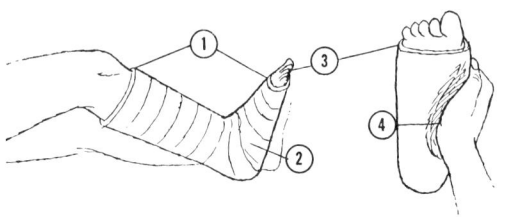

Management

Allow the patient to walk on crutches, bearing partial weight on the cast with a walking heel or cast shoe.

Three weeks of cast immobilization are adequate for most fractures of the metatarsals.

After removal of the cast, the patient should use a stiff-soled shoe with good support of the longitudinal and transverse arches.

Fracture of the Metatarsal Bones with Displacement

REMARKS

Accurate reduction of these fractures is essential in order to prevent prolonged disability.

Most such fractures can be reduced by manipulative maneuvers.

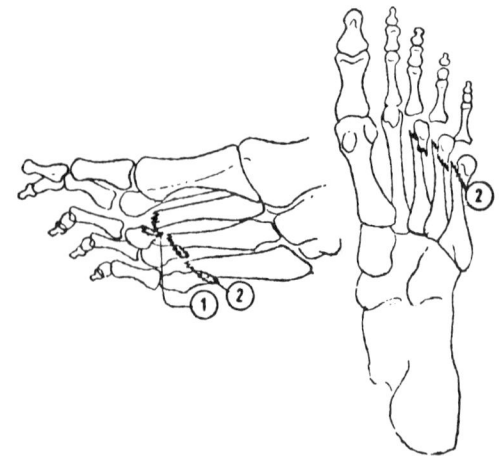

Prereduction X-Ray

1. Fracture of the neck of the third, fourth, and fifth metatarsals.
2. The distal fragments (heads of metatarsals) are displaced outward and downward.

MANAGEMENT

Manipulative Reduction

1. One assistant fixes the foot.
2. A second assistant makes steady traction on the toe by means of a loop of bandage around it.
3. The operator by direct pressure molds the fragments back into their anatomic position.

Note: This method is employed for each metatarsal fracture.

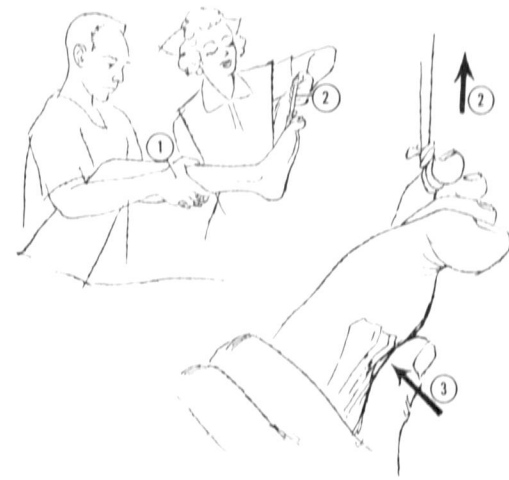

Postreduction X-Ray

1. The distal fragments of all three fractured metatarsals are in normal relation with the proximal fragments.

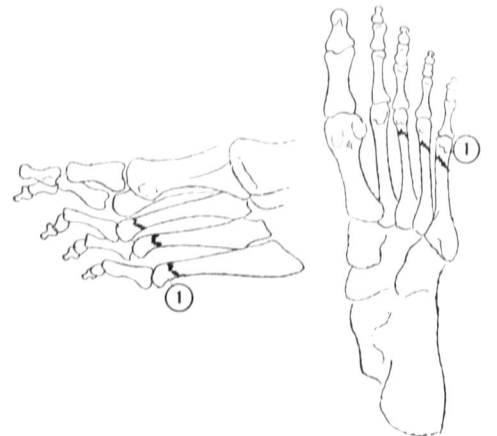

Immobilization

1. A circular plaster cast is applied from the toes to the tibial tubercle.
2. The foot is at a right angle.
3. The foot is in neutral in regard to inversion and eversion.
4. The plaster is molded well under the longitudinal and transverse arches.

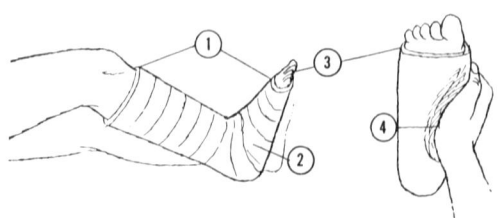

Subsequent Management

Allow the patient up on crutches without bearing weight on the affected foot.

After 10 to 14 days, when swelling and pain have subsided, remove the plaster cast and apply another short leg plaster cast with a walking heel; the patient may now bear weight on the foot.

Remove the second cast six weeks after injury.

Avoid early mobilization and weight bearing in order to prevent formation of exuberant callus at the fracture site.

After removal of the cast provide the patient with a stiff soled shoe with a support for the longitudinal and transverse arches.

ALTERNATE METHOD: OPERATIVE REDUCTION

Operative intervention is indicated when manipulative methods fail to achieve an accurate reduction.

Fractures just proximal to the heads are frequently difficult to maintain in normal alignment by conservative methods.

Prereduction X-Ray

1. Fractures of the shafts of the first, second, and third metatarsal bones.
2. The distal fragments are displaced downward and backward into the sole.

Note: In this instance manipulative methods failed to achieve an accurate reduction.

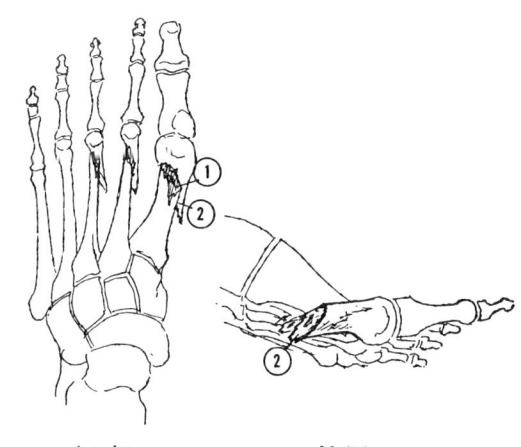

Operative Procedure

1. Make a 2.5-cm dorsal incision centered over the fracture site.
2. Expose the proximal and distal fragments by subperiosteal dissection.
3. With a small curette deliver the proximal end of the distal fragment into the wound.

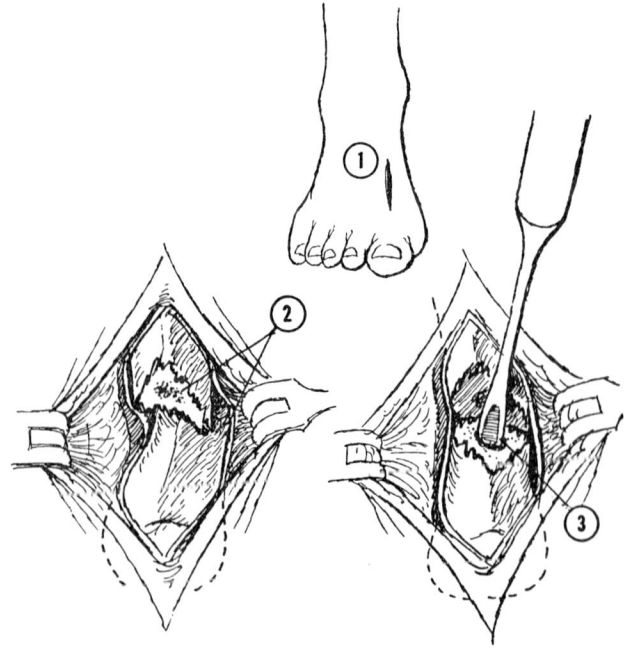

1. Dorsiflex the toe.
2. Pass a small Kirschner wire through the medullary canal of the distal fragment until it emerges from the skin.

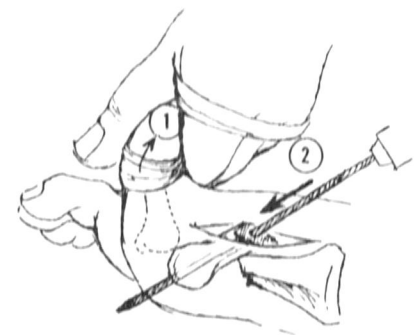

3. Reverse the drill and withdraw the wire until its proximal end is at the level of the fracture site.

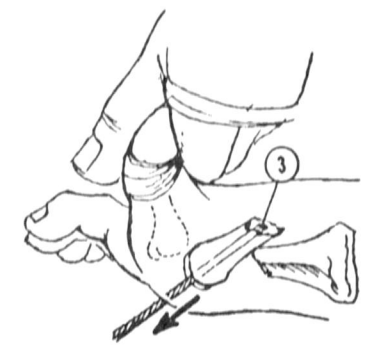

4. Appose the ends of the bone fragments.
5. Pass the wire proximally until its blunt end strikes the base of the metatarsal bone.
6. Cut the wire, leaving its end protruding 1 cm above the level of the skin.

Note: This procedure is executed for each metatarsal fracture.

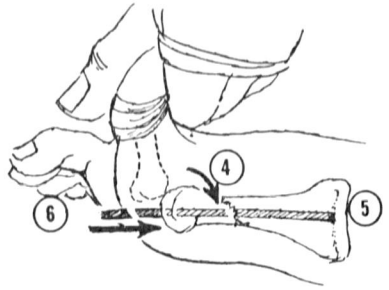

Postreduction X-Ray

1. All fragments are now in anatomic position.
2. A wire transfixes both fragments and maintains normal alignment.

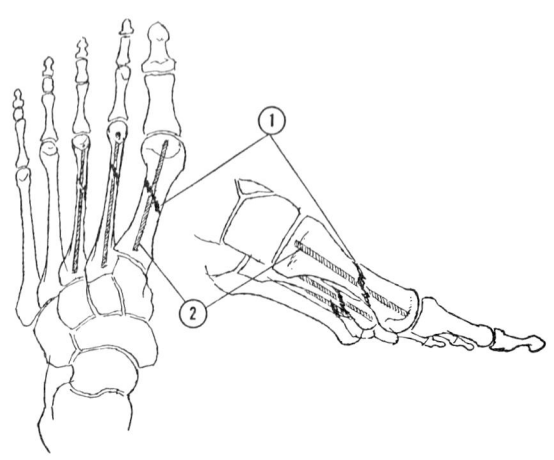

Immobilization

1. A circular plaster cast is applied from the toes to the tibial tubercle.
2. The foot is at a right angle.
3. The foot is in neutral in regard to inversion and eversion.
4. The plaster is molded well under the longitudinal and transverse arches.

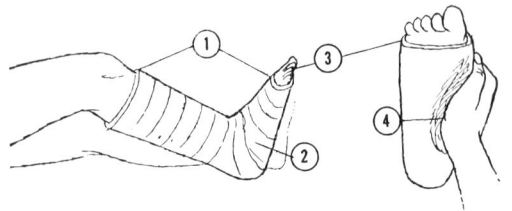

Postoperative Management

Elevate the foot on pillows.

Surround the foot with ice bags.

After three weeks remove the wire and apply a short leg plaster cast with a walking heel; again mold the plaster well under the longitudinal and transverse arches.

Six to eight weeks after operation remove the plaster cast and allow walking in a stiff-soled shoe with an arch support for the longitudinal and transverse arches.

Tuberosity and Proximal Shaft (Jones') Fractures of the Base of the Fifth Metatarsal

REMARKS

Dameron has pointed out that there are two types of fractures occurring in the proximal end of the fifth metatarsal.

The first and more common type is a fracture through the tuberosity, which is produced by inversion injury of the plantar flexed foot. These invariably heal with minimal treatment and without complication.

The tuberosity fracture must be distinguished from the less common fracture through the proximal portion of the shaft, which has been called the Jones' fracture. Sir Robert Jones reported sustaining such an injury himself while dancing around a tentpole.

Kavanaugh and coworkers have demonstrated this to be a stress fracture that occurs characteristically in basketball players and other young athletes. These have a much less favorable prognosis than tuberosity fractures.

Tuberosity fracture must also be distinguished from normal variations, particularly apophyses of the metatarsal. Dameron found apophyses radiographically visible in at least 22 per cent of children's feet. Most commonly this is seen between 9 and 11 years in girls and between 11 and 14 years in boys.

Other structures sometimes confused with tuberosity fractures are sesamoid bones in the peroneus longus or brevis tendon, found in approximately 15 per cent of foot x-rays. The smooth, sclerotic apposing surfaces of the sesamoid bone and the proximal portion of the base of the fifth metatarsal distinguish it from a fracture.

TUBEROSITY FRACTURE

Appearance on X-Ray

1. Avulsion fracture of the tuberosity is typically oblique in the region of the peroneus brevis insertion and results from inversion injury.

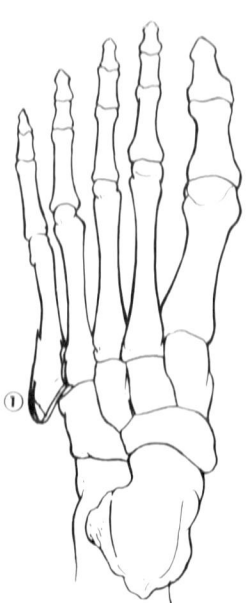

Tuberosity fracture must be differentiated from a normal apophysis.
1. The apophyseal line traverses the tubercle in a direction almost parallel to the long axis of the metatarsal.
2. It does not extend proximally into the metatarsal joint or medially into the joint between the fourth and fifth metatarsal.

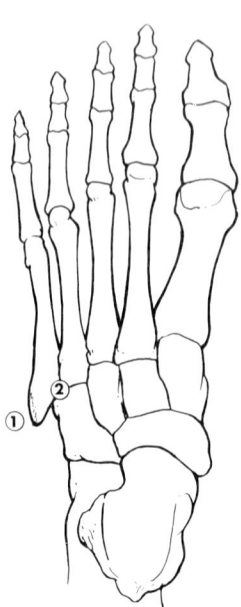

Management

The more common tuberosity fracture can be treated symptomatically, usually with a walking cast to relieve discomfort.

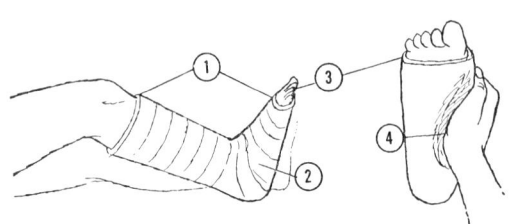

1. A circular plaster cast is applied from the toes to the tibial tubercle.
2. The foot is at a right angle.
3. The foot is in a neutral position as to inversion and eversion.
4. The plaster is molded well under the longitudinal and transverse arches.

Subsequent Management

The patient may bear weight on the cast as tolerated.

After 14 days the cast may be removed and the patient may begin walking with a hard-soled shoe.

In general, the patient need not be followed longer than three to four weeks, because radiographic and clinical union is almost inevitable.

JONES' FRACTURE

Appearance on X-Ray

1. A Jones' fracture is a transverse fracture occurring 0.5 cm distal to the splayed insertion of the peroneus brevis.
2. It has the characteristic of a stress fracture in that it appears to involve only the lateral cortex on the initial x-ray but later traverses the bone completely.

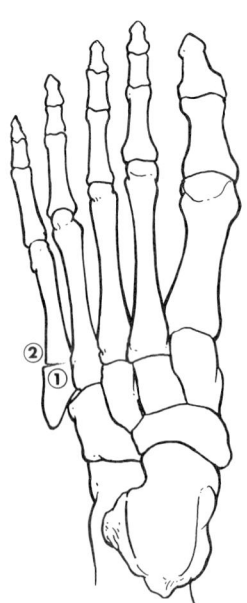

Mechanism

Kavanaugh and coworkers demonstrated this injury to be a fatigue or stress fracture resulting from a combination of
1. Vertical loading and
2. Mediolateral loading that is
3. Commonly sustained by a basketball player, who must constantly pivot or shift the direction of loading on the lateral border of the foot.

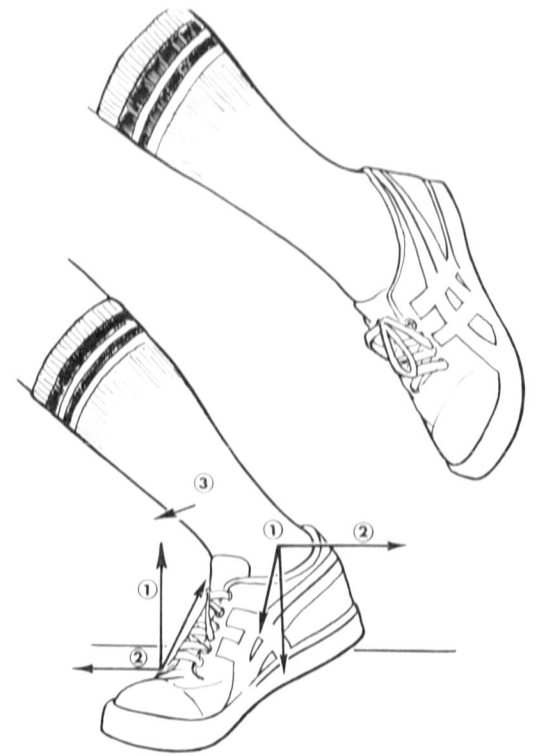

MANAGEMENT OF A JONES' FRACTURE IN THE NONATHLETE OR RECREATIONAL ATHLETE

A walking cast is applied as described for tuberosity fracture.

The cast should be continued for approximately four to six weeks, after which the patient may resume weight bearing with a hard-soled shoe.

The patient should be informed that delayed union is a possibility and that sports activities should be avoided until union is secure.

On the average this may take four months from the time of injury.

MANAGEMENT OF JONES' FRACTURE IN AN ACTIVE ATHLETE

This injury can be quite disabling in the athlete who is eager to return to competitive sports.

Immediate screw fixation as advocated by Kavanaugh and coworkers is the most effective method of managing this select group of patients.

Conservative treatment is likely to cause prolonged disability and recurrent fatigue fracture in individuals unwilling or unable to refrain from vigorous activities.

Screw fixation is also recommended for patients with recurrent fracture or nonunion.

Preoperative X-Ray

1. A typical transverse stress fracture in a basketball player.

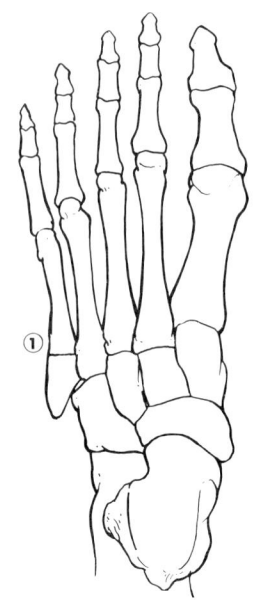

Operative Technique

1. The proximal end of the fifth metatarsal is exposed through a straight incision. Care is taken not to injure the terminal branches of the lateral sural nerve, which are usually present in this area.

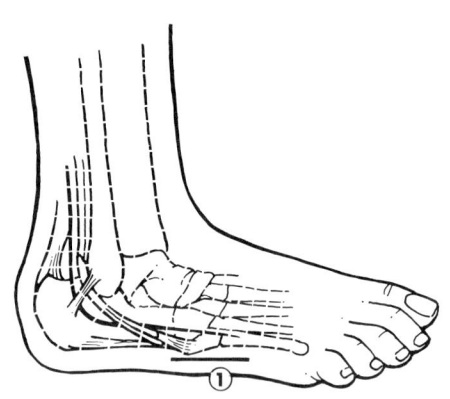

2. The peroneus brevis tendon is partially detached, exposing the underlying tuberosity.

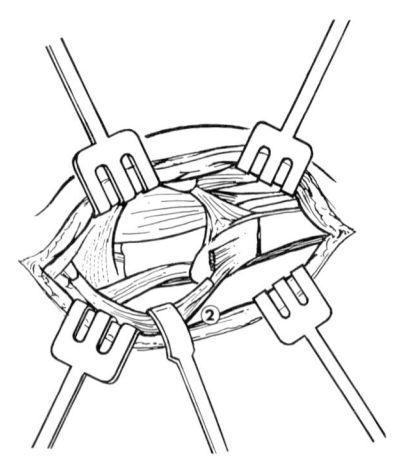

3. The intramedullary canal is drilled and x-rays are taken to confirm the position of the drill bit in the intramedullary canal.

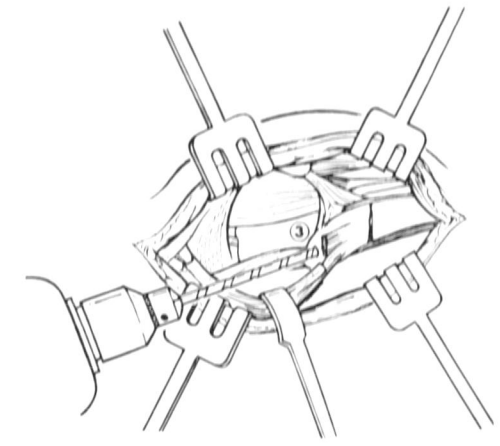

4. A malleolar type of cancellous bone screw is inserted across the fracture site.

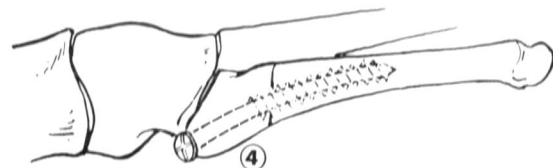

Postoperative X-Ray

1. The fracture has been stabilized by intramedullary screw fixation.

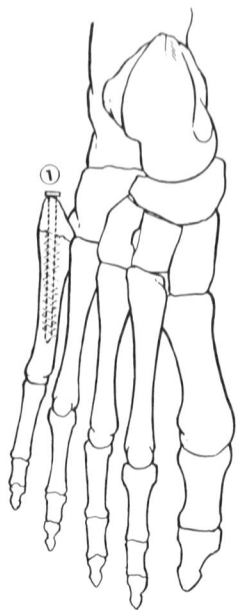

Postoperative Treatment

A compressive bandage is applied to the foot and the foot is kept non-weight-bearing with crutches for ten days.

Subsequently the dressing is removed and the foot is allowed to bear weight as tolerated in a hard-soled shoe.

Return to athletic competition is allowed six weeks postoperatively.

DISLOCATIONS OF THE METATARSOPHALANGEAL JOINTS

REMARKS

These are rare lesions; the great toe is most commonly involved.

Many are open lesions.

Immediate reduction is mandatory; a delay of several days may make it impossible to reduce the dislocation by closed methods.

These injuries are analogous to dislocations of the metatarsophalangeal joints of the hand and are subject to similar obstacles to reduction (see page 1177).

Typical Deformity

1. The proximal phalanx is displaced upward and backward in the vertical position.
2. The head of the metatarsal is prominent.
3. The distal phalanx is flexed.

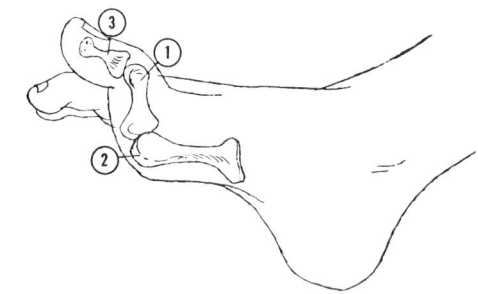

Prereduction X-Ray

1. The proximal phalanx rests on the dorsal aspect of the head of the metatarsal.
2. The distal phalanx is flexed.

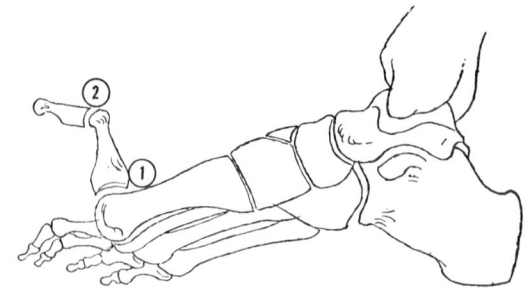

Manipulative Reduction

1. Pass a loop of bandage around the toe to make traction.
2. Make strong traction upward and backward (hyperextending the toe); this disengages the metatarsal head from the flexor tendons.

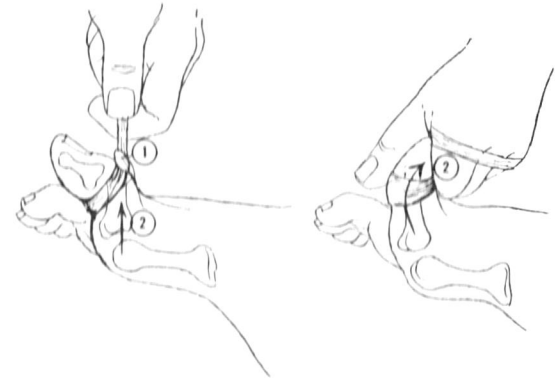

1. Now make traction upward and forward.
2. Place the thumb of the other hand behind the proximal end of the first phalanx and force the phalanx distally and downward over the metatarsal head.

Note: The key to reduction is to push, not pull, the proximal phalanx over the metatarsal head.

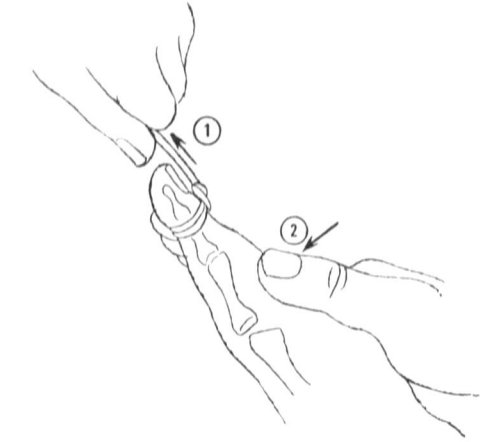

Immobilization

1. Apply a padded splint to the dorsum of the foot to prevent recurrent hyperextension of the metatarsophalangeal joint.
2. The toe is in neutral position.

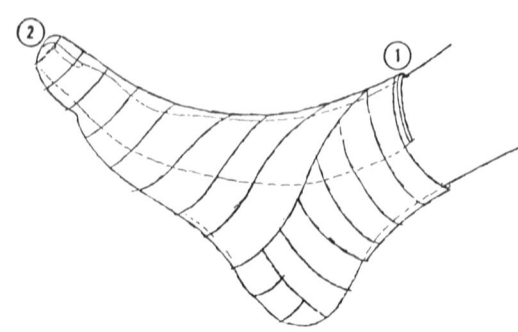

Management

Allow the patient up on crutches with no weight bearing on the affected foot.
Remove the plaster splint at the end of two weeks.
Provide the patient with a stiff-soled shoe.

Irreducible Dislocation of the Metatarsophalangeal Joints

Closed reduction may not be possible, particularly if multiple metatarsophalangeal joints are dislocated.

Operative reduction should be carried out promptly to relieve the obstruction from:

1. The capsule detached from the proximal phalanx and
2. The fibrocartilaginous plate flipped into the joint.

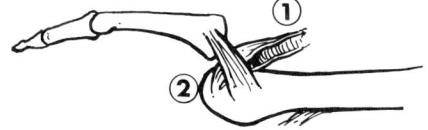

Note: A volar approach to the metatarsophalangeal joint allows visualization of these obstructions and permits release of the fibrocartilaginous plate and capsule, which form the main obstacles to reduction.

After reduction the joints are stable and do not require longer than two to three weeks of immobilization.

FRACTURES OF THE TOES

REMARKS

These lesions are usually the result of crushing injuries; the great toe is most often affected.
Comminution of the phalanx occurs relatively frequently.
Many fractures are of the open type.
As a rule displacement of the fragments is minimal.

Fractures of the Toes with Minimal or No Displacement

Appearance on X-Ray

PROXIMAL PHALANX OF FOURTH TOE

1. Oblique fracture of the proximal phalanx of the fourth toe with minimal displacement. (No reduction required.)

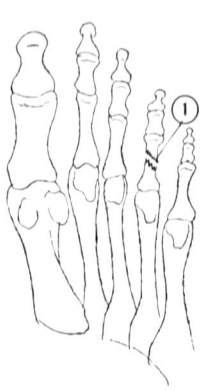

DISTAL PHALANX OF GREAT TOE

1. Comminuted fracture of the distal phalanx of the great toe.

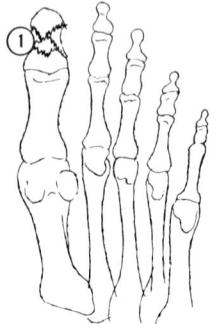

Immobilization for Fractures of the Outer Four Toes

1. Place a piece of felt between the toes.
2. Fix the fractured toe to the adjacent toe with strips of adhesive.
3. Shoe with top cut out and a bar on the sole placed behind the metatarsal heads allows full weight bearing.

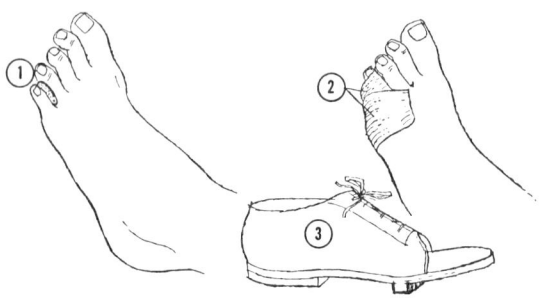

Immobilization for Fractures of the Great Toe

1. Place a piece of felt between the great toe and the second toe.
2. Bind the great toe to the second toe with strips of adhesive.

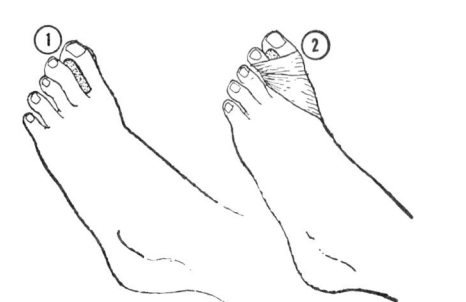

Management

For fractures of any of the toes allow the patient to bear weight in a shoe with a toe cap cut out and a metatarsal bar 1 cm high placed on the sole just behind the metatarsal heads.

In cases of severe swelling elevate the foot for two to three days before permitting weight bearing.

Remove the adhesive strapping after two to three weeks and provide the patient with a stiff-soled shoe.

Fractures of the Toes with Displacement

REMARKS

Generally displacement can be corrected by simple traction on the toe.

Fractures of the proximal phalanges may exhibit forward angulation of the fragments.

If reduction is not stable and the deformity recurs after traction is released, longitudinal pin fixation may be indicated.

Prereduction X-Ray

1. Fracture of the proximal phalanx of the great toe with forward angulation of the fragments.

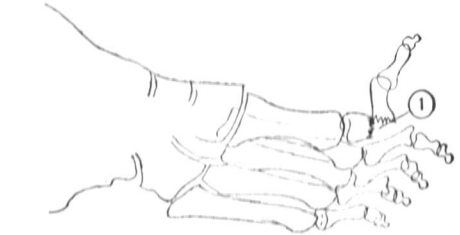

Manipulative Reduction

1. Pass a loop of gauze bandage around the toe.
2. Make direct traction upward and forward.
3. Place the thumb of the other hand over the apex of the angulation on the plantar aspect of the toe and make upward pressure.

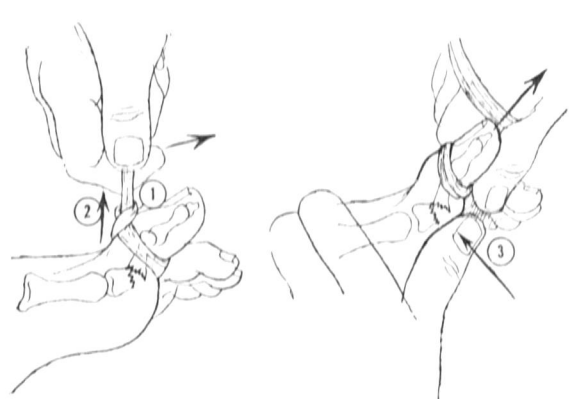

1. While traction is maintained flex the toe.

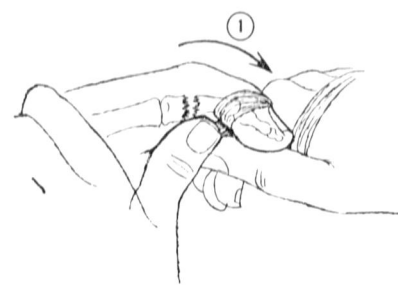

Immobilization

1. Place a piece of felt between the toes.
2. Bind the first toe to the second toe with strips of adhesive.

Note: If reduction is lost, insert a smooth Steinmann pin percutaneously through the long axis of the toe.

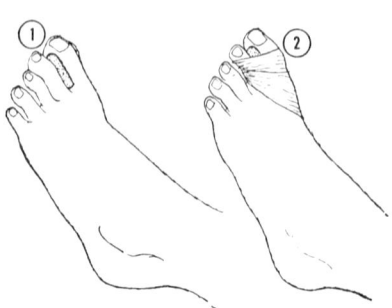

Subsequent Management

Maintain the splint immobilization for at least three weeks, after which time it may be discarded.

Subsequently the patient should protect the foot with a hard-soled shoe and bar under the metatarsal heads (see page 2074).

Fractures of the Sesamoid Bones of the Great Toe

REMARKS

These lesions are rare and are a result of direct trauma applied to the foot, crushing the sesamoids between the head of the metatarsal and the ground.

The inner sesamoid is involved more often than the outer.

Fracture must be distinguished from a bipartite or tripartite sesamoid. In the former the line of division is sharp and irregular; in the latter it is smooth and regular, and fragments are of equal size.

If pain and dysfunction persist after a period of immobilization and proper padding of the shoe, excision of the sesamoid is indicated.

Appearance on X-Ray

1. Fracture of the internal sesamoid.
2. The fragments are of unequal size.

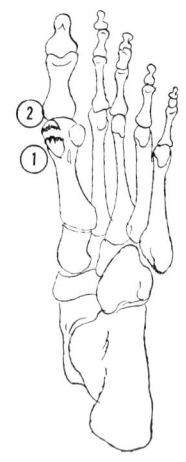

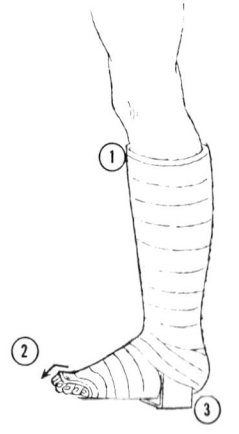

Immobilization

1. Apply a circular plaster cast from the toes to the tibial tubercle.
2. The great toe is moderately flexed.
3. A walking heel is incorporated in the cast.

Management

Remove the cast at the end of four weeks.

Permit weight bearing in a shoe with a 1-cm bar placed on the sole of the shoe just behind the metatarsal heads.

If pain persists after several months of adequate treatment, excision of the sesamoid is indicated.

Excision is also indicated in cases of old untreated fractures causing pain and dysfunction.

SUMMARY: PITFALLS AND COMPLICATIONS OF FRACTURES AND DISLOCATIONS OF THE FOOT

The potential pitfalls and complications of these injuries may be considered either diagnostic or therapeutic.

The diagnosis of most talar fractures or dislocations is usually straightforward. However, fractures of the lateral process and osteochondral fractures of the dome are frequently confused with ankle sprains. Avulsion fracture of the posterior tuberosity is mistaken for a sesamoid bone.

Treatment of talar fractures demands anatomic reduction. The incidence of delayed union or malunion after closed treatment of a displaced talar fracture is sufficiently high to require almost routine internal fixation. Preferably, the screw can be inserted from the posterior fragment into the head fragment to avoid vascular disruption. Avascular necrosis should be anticipated with most displaced talar fractures but by itself should not be considered an indication for fusion or other operation.

Diagnostic problems with calcaneal fractures arise from incomplete assessment of the three-dimensional components of the injury. X-rays should evaluate shortening and widening of the calcaneus as well as the amount of subtalar joint involvement. Pitfalls of treatment similarly arise from not considering all dimensions of the deformity. Restoration of normal articular congruity is important but many residual complications from calcaneal fractures are due to shortening and widening of the heel. Stiffness of the uninvolved tarsal joints also causes significant complications following treatment by either closed or open methods. Treatment techniques that emphasize active joint mobilization and restore normal heel length and width are most likely to yield good results.

Subtalar dislocations are readily reduced by closed manipulation and only infrequently require open reduction. Lateral dislocations, although less frequent than medial ones, are more likely to be associated with obstructions preventing reduction. The long-term prognosis or the complication rate after subtalar dislocation may be poorer than has been generally considered. Subtalar arthritis and even avascular necrosis of the talus may occur and may cause a painful symptomatic limp.

Fractures of the navicular, although infrequent, are among the most commonly unrecognized and undertreated injuries in the foot. The anatomy of the tarsal bones frequently obscures the navicular fracture on x-ray. Symptomatic instability of the midfoot then follows owing to damage to the keystone of the longitudinal arch. Painful symptoms on the medial side of the foot after what seems like a minor sprain should be carefully assessed by complete radiographic study for fracture of the navicular and other tarsal bones. Midfoot instability should also be looked for.

Fractures of the cuboid, particularly if associated with avulsion fractures of the navicular, are produced by forceful abduction and are frequently associated with midtarsal dislocation. Treatment of the midtarsal dislocation requires internal stabilization to prevent recurrent problems with instability.

Fractures and dislocations in the tarsometatarsal area, like injuries in the midtarsus, frequently may go unrecognized. Tarsometatarsal instability, however, does not produce the disability of midtarsal instability. Unstable fractures and dislocations of the tarsometatarsal joint require percutaneous pin fixation to restore medial and lateral stability. Failure to use pin fixation can result in displacement despite cast immobilization.

Fractures of the metatarsals are common and are usually uncomplicated, provided that treatment maintains the transverse arch of the foot. The most common fracture at the base of the fifth metatarsal is an avulsion fracture, which is generally uncomplicated. This should be distinguished from a stress fracture of the shaft of the fifth metatarsal, which is prone to complication by either nonunion or refracture, particularly in the active athlete.

As always, the physician who appreciates and anticipates the common diagnostic and therapeutic pitfalls is most likely to prevent them or minimize their significance.

References

Aitken, A. P., and Poulson, D.: Dislocations of the tarsometatarsal joint. J. Bone and Jt. Surg., 45A:246–260, 1963.

Berndt, A. L., and Harty, M.: Transchondral fractures (osteochondritis dissecans) of the talus. J. Bone and Jt. Surg., 41A:988–1020, 1959.

Burdeaux, W.: Calcaneal fractures. In *Foot Disorders*, (Gionnestras), Philadelphia, Lea and Febiger (to be published).

Canale, S. T., and Kelly, F. B.: Fractures of the neck of the talus. J. Bone and Jt. Surg., 60A:143–156, 1978.

Canale, S. T., and Belding, R. H.: Osteochondral lesions of the talus. J. Bone and Jt. Surg., 62A:97, 1980.

Christensen, S. B., Lorentzen, J. E., Krogsoe, O., et al.: Subtalar dislocation. Acta Orthop. Scand., 48:707–711, 1977.

Dameron, T. B.: Fractures and anatomical variations of the proximal portion of the fifth metatarsal. J. Bone and Jt. Surg., 57A:788, 1975.

DeBenedetti, M. J., Evanski, P. M., and Waugh, T. R.: The unreducible Lisfranc fracture. Clin. Orthop., 136:238–240, 1978.

Dennis, M. D. and Tullos, H. S.: Blair tibiotalar arthrodesis for injuries to the talus. J. Bone and Jt. Surg., 62A:103–107, 1980.

REFERENCES

Detenbeck, L. C., and Kelly, P. J.: Total dislocation of the talus. J. Bone and Jt. Surg., 51A:283–288, 1969.

Dimon, J. H.: Isolated displaced fracture of the posterior facet of the talus. J. Bone and Jt. Surg., 41A:275–281, 1961.

Drummond, D. S., and Hastings, E. E.: Total dislocation of the cuboid bone. J. Bone and Jt. Surg., 51B:716–718, 1969.

Eichenholtz, S. N., and Levine, D. B.: Fractures of the tarsal navicular bone. Clin. Orthop., 15:142–157, 1959.

Essex-Lopresti, P.: The mechanism, reduction technique, and results in fractures of the os calcis. Brit. J. Surg., 39:395–419, 1952.

Hawkins, L. G.: Fracture of the lateral process of the talus. J. Bone and Jt. Surg., 47A:1170–1175, 1965.

Hawkins, L. G.: Fractures of the neck of the talus. J. Bone and Jt. Surg., 52A:991–1002, 1970.

Hooper, G., and McMaster, M. J.: Recurrent bilateral mid-tarsal subluxations. J. Bone and Jt. Surg., 61A:617–619, 1979.

Kavanaugh, J. H., Brower, T. D., and Mann, R. V.: The Jones fracture revisited. J. Bone and Jt. Surg., 60A:776–782, 1978.

Kay, H. W.: Clinical applications of the Veterans Administration Prosthetics Center patellar-tendon-bearing brace. Artificial Limbs, 15:46–67, 1971.

Kenwright, J., and Taylor, R. G.: Major injuries of the talus. J. Bone and Jt. Surg., 52B:36–48, 1970.

Kleiger, B.: Injuries of the talus and its joints. Clin. Orthop., 121:243–260, 1976.

Lance, E. M., Carey, E. J., and Wade, P. A.: Fractures of the os calcis: A follow-up study. J. Trauma, 4:15–56, 1964.

Leitner, B.: Obstacles to reduction in subtalar dislocations. J. Bone and Jt. Surg., 36A:299–306, 1954.

Lemaire, R. G., and Bustin, W.: Screw fixation of fractures of the neck of the talus using a posterior approach. J. Trauma, 20:669–688, 1980.

McLaughlin, H. L.: Complex "locked" dislocation of the metacarpophalangeal joints. J. Trauma, 5:683–688, 1965.

McLaughlin, H. L.: Treatment of late complications after os calcis fractures. Clin. Orthop., 12:111–115, 1958.

Main, B. J., and Jowett, R. L.: Injuries of the midtarsal joint. J. Bone and Jt. Surg., 57B:89–97, 1975.

Mindell, E. R., Cisek, E. E., Kartalian, G., et al.: Late results of injuries to the talus. J. Bone and Jt. Surg., 45A:221–245, 1963.

Mulfinger, G. L., and Trueta, J.: The blood supply of the talus. J. Bone and Jt. Surg., 52B:160–167, 1970.

Peterson, L., Romanus, B., and Dahlberg, E.: Fracture of the collum taili — an experimental study. J. Biomechanics, 9:277–279, 1974.

Rowe, C. R., Sakellarides, H. T., Freeman, P. A., et al.: Fracture of the os calcis. JAMA, 184:92–93, 1963.

Schiller, M. G., and Ray, R. D.: Isolated dislocation of the medial cuneiform bone — a rare injury of the tarsus. J. Bone and Jt. Surg., 52A:1632–1636, 1970.

Wiley, J. J.: The mechanism of tarso-metatarsal joint injuries. J. Bone and Jt. Surg.: 53A:474–482, 1971.

Wilson, D. W.: Injuries of the tarso-metatarsal joints. J. Bone and Jt. Surg., 54B:677–686, 1972.

BIRTH FRACTURES AND PATHOLOGIC FRACTURES

REMARKS

Fracture union must be considered first a biological rather than a mechanical process. Nowhere is this more evident than in the contrasting problems of birth fractures and pathologic fractures.

This final section considers these two divergent problems and some of the present-day approaches to their management.

BIRTH FRACTURES OF LONG BONES

REMARKS

During a difficult birth (especially in breech presentations) the long bones of the extremities are not infrequently fractured.

The bones most commonly fractured, in order of frequency, are the shafts of the humeri, one or both clavicles, and the shafts of the femurs. Displacement of the epiphyses of the humerus and the femur also occur.

Skull fractures are exceedingly rare at birth even with severe intracranial damage. The wide open sutures and the extreme pliability of the skull provide adequate protection to the skull bones during delivery.

When skull fractures do occur they are of the depressed type of the parietal bones but require no treatment; as a rule the depressed area corrects itself spontaneously.

Generally fractures of the long bones are complete, with considerable displacement and angulation; large masses of callus form quickly, and union is rapid and complete within a short period.

Delayed union and nonunion are indeed rare.

Even severe angulatory deformities are removed completely during the first two or three years of life by the process of remodeling.

Upper Extremity

FRACTURES OF THE SHAFT OF THE HUMERUS

REMARKS

The fractures are usually transverse or spiral.

Lateral displacement and overriding are usually minimal.

Outward angulation may be pronounced.

Palsy of the musculospiral nerve may occur; check for this—it is usually a transitory lesion with full recovery in six to eight weeks.

Appearance on X-Ray

1. Fracture of the shaft of the humerus.
2. Outward angulation with no overriding.

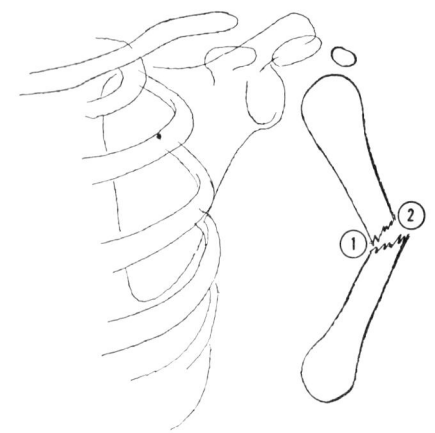

Management

1. Place a wad of soft cotton in the axilla to correct angulation.
2. Fix the arm to the chest with a bias-cut cotton bandage.
3. The hand is free.
4. A collar and cuff may be applied to support the limb.

Note: Remove the strapping after two-and-one-half to three weeks. Usually healing will occur with some outward angulation of the fragments. This deformity will correct within the first year through remodeling.

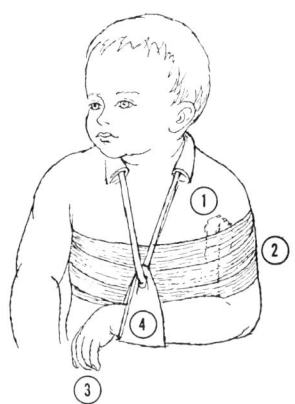

FRACTURE OF THE CLAVICLE

REMARKS

One or both clavicles may be affected.
This fracture often is not detected until two or three weeks after birth, when a mass of callus is very evident.
Generally the middle of the bone is fractured.
Occasionally, congenital pseudoarthrosis is mistaken for a fracture (see page 2109).

Appearance on X-ray

1. Fracture of the middle of the clavicle in an infant.
2. Inner fragment is displaced upward.
3. Outer fragment is displaced downward.

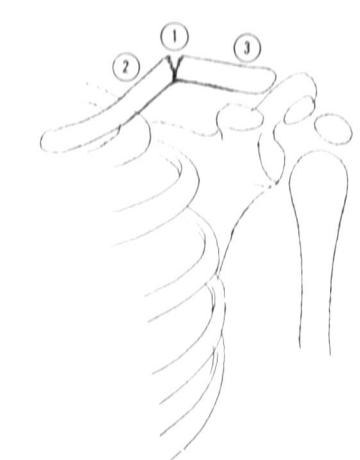

Management

If the fracture is two to three weeks old, no treatment is necessary.

If the fracture is recent:
1. Apply a wad of cotton in each axilla.
2. Apply a posterior figure-of-eight bandage around the shoulders. Use a soft bias-cut cotton bandage.

Note: Healing should be adequate at the end of two to three weeks, and the bandage may be removed.

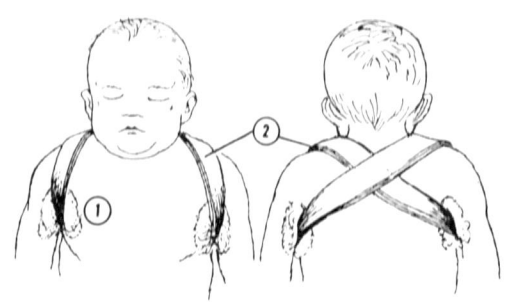

Lower Extremity

FRACTURES OF THE SHAFT OF THE FEMUR

REMARKS

This lesion usually is a transverse fracture of the middle third of the femur and is most often associated with difficult breech delivery.

Appearance on X-ray

1. Transverse fracture of the upper end of the femur.
2. Severe flexion deformity of the proximal fragment.

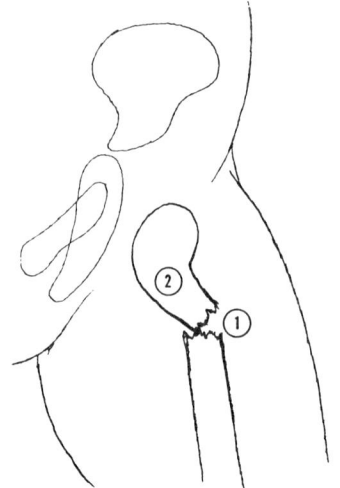

Reduction (Bryant Traction)

1. Apply skin traction to both legs (use strips of foam rubber for traction on the skin).
2. Make vertical traction; the feet are in a symmetrical position.
3. Use weights and pulleys; the buttocks must clear the mattress.
4. Hold child in a fixed position with a wide binder.

Note: Traction is removed after three weeks.

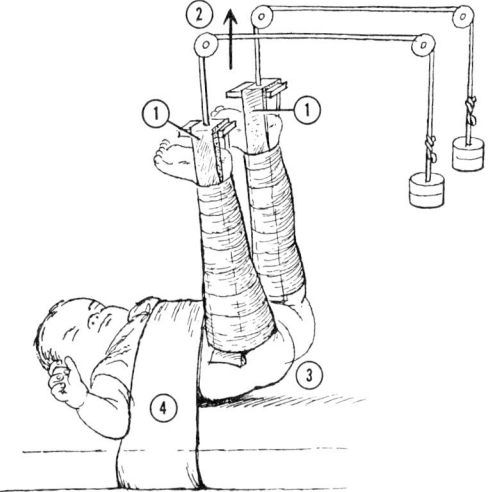

CAUTIONS

Check apparatus constantly.
Check periodically for evidence of circulatory disturbance.
Check for evidence of skin irritation.
Traction in infants and children may produce circulatory embarrassment. Any evidence of such a complication makes removal of the apparatus mandatory.

Other Causes of Birth Fractures

Among the more severe causes of birth fractures are osteogenesis imperfecta and congenital pseudoarthrosis.

If osteogenesis imperfecta is present at birth, the child is usually stillborn.

These congenital deficiencies are more often problems after birth and are therefore discussed as pathologic fractures associated with developmental abnormalities (see page 2100).

PATHOLOGIC FRACTURES

REMARKS

A pathologic fracture occurs in a bone that is weakened because of an underlying disease process.

The most common processes are metabolic, developmental, and tumor. Each of these types should be considered a possibility when assessing a fracture in a bone having an abnormal radiographic appearance.

Metabolic abnormalities include osteoporosis and osteomalacia, Paget's disease, and diseases of endocrine function.

The most common developmental abnormalities causing fracture are osteogenesis imperfecta, fibrous dysplasia, bone cysts, cortical defects, and congenital pseudoarthroses.

Tumors associated with fractures can be either "benign" or malignant. Among the more usual "benign" tumors associated with fractures are enchondroma of the hand, giant cell tumor of the wrist or knee, and eosinophilic granuloma located in the vertebral bodies, the diaphysis of a long bone, or the acetabular region.

The most common neoplasm arising primarily in bone (pathologic fracture) is multiple myeloma, which particularly involves the spine. Osteogenic sarcoma and other more slowly growing primary bone tumors such as reticulum cell sarcoma are more likely to present as pathologic fractures than the rapidly growing Ewing's sarcoma.

The most common pathologic fracture that the physician must treat today is that produced by metastatic cancer, particularly adenocarcinoma of the breast. Management of the pathologic fracture from metastatic cancer has become considerably more effective with recognition that the fracture need not be considered a death knell.

Metabolic Disorders That Cause Pathologic Fracture

OSTEOPOROSIS—SENESCENT AND OTHER TYPES

REMARKS

Senescent osteoporosis represents one aspect of the involutionary changes that take place throughout the body. The pathogenesis appears to relate to chemical and structural alterations in the matrix as well as to demineralization.

The condition is characterized by reduction of the amount of osseous tissue per unit of bone volume, by sparsity of spongy trabeculae, and by thinning and porosity of the cortices.

Osteoporosis may be combined with osteomalacia when there is deficiency of mineralization resulting from renal disease, malabsorption syndromes, or long-term anticonvulsant therapy.

The most common differential diagnoses for senescent osteoporosis are multiple myeloma and metastatic disease to the spine. These conditions are particularly to be suspected when an osteoporotic compression fracture occurs in a patient younger than 55 years. Before diagnosing senescent osteoporosis, particularly in the patient younger than 55, the physician should measure serum levels of calcium, phosphorus, alkaline phosphatase, and protein electrophoresis, which are normal in osteoporosis but are altered by the other two conditions.

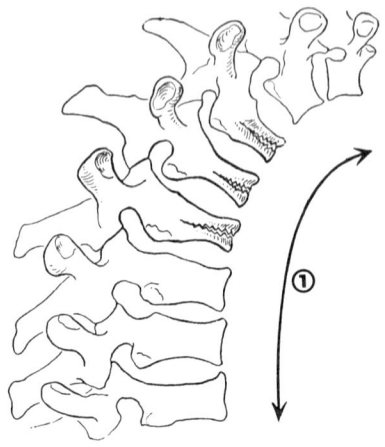

Typical senescent osteoporosis fractures include:
1. Multiple compression fractures of the vertebrae.

2. Femoral neck fracture.

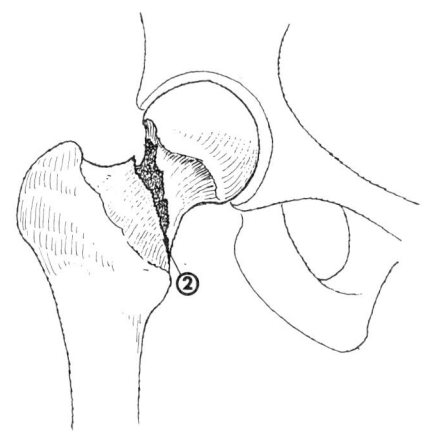

3. Fracture of the humeral neck.
4. Colles' fracture.

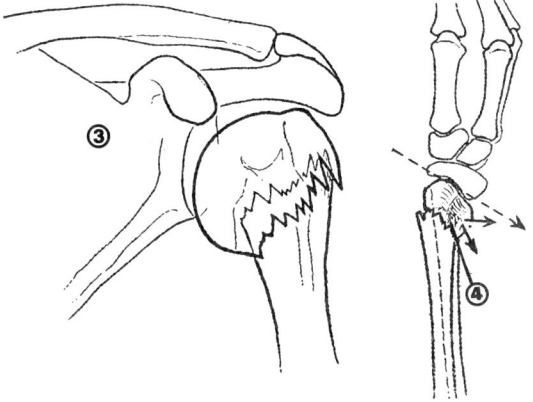

Multiple myeloma causes:
1. Complete collapse of a single vertebral body.

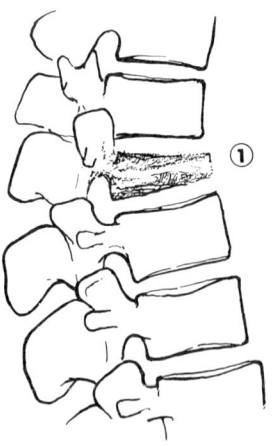

2. Punched-out lesions of the skull.

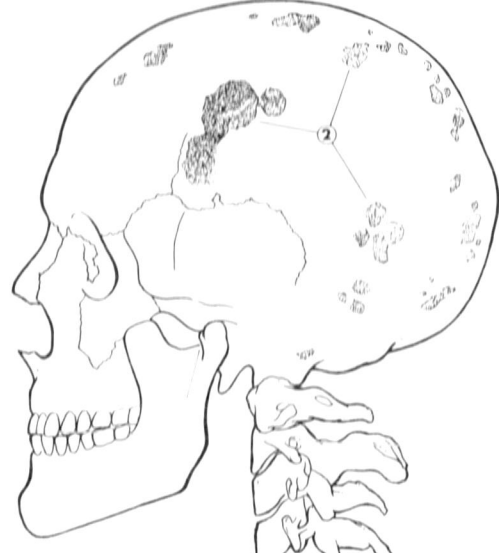

Fractures associated with osteomalacia, e.g., after renal disease, occur in:
1. The medial aspect of the femoral neck.
2. The diaphysis of the femur.
3. Pubic bones as Looser zones or fatigue-type fractures.

Note: Osteomalacia combined with osteoporosis may also result from malabsorption syndromes and long-term anticonvulsant therapy.

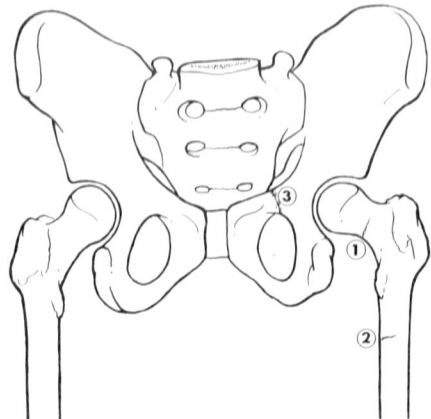

Management of Senescent Osteoporosis

Treatment of a fracture of a particular bone is discussed in the section of this book dealing with the part or bone affected (see, for example, Fractures of the Femoral Neck, page 1407).

Treatment should also incorporate therapy to correct the underlying metabolic abnormality.

Senescent osteoporosis may not be reversible but its progression can be altered by newer therapy. Lindholm and coworkers have reported that treatment with 1-alpha-hydroxyvitamin D_3 and calcium is beneficial in relieving clinical symptoms and chemical abnormalities. Further follow-up is necessary to evaluate this newer approach to the problem of osteoporosis.

PAGET'S DISEASE OF BONE (OSTEITIS DEFORMANS)

REMARKS

Paget's disease (osteitis deformans) is the second most common disease of bone metabolism after osteoporosis. The incidence has been reported to be as high as three per cent of population older than 40 years; most affected individuals remain asymptomatic. Its etiology may be viral but further investigation of this possibility is necessary.

Paget's disease begins as a localized area of bone resorption. As the disease progresses, rapidly alternating cycles of bone formation and resorption may be seen. The result is a gross alteration of normal bone architecture to a mosaic pattern of weak fiber and lamellar bone. When this disease is extensive, the serum alkaline phosphatase level is very high and there is increased urinary excretion of collagen degradation products as hydroxyproline-containing peptides.

A pathologic fracture is the most common complication of Paget's disease. The most common location for the fracture is in the proximal subtrochanteric region of the femur. It begins as a transverse or fatigue fracture resulting from repetitive loading. It progresses to a complete transverse fracture much like a broken piece of chalk or rotted wood.

Paget's disease is generally considered a polyostotic condition, but it may be monostotic and may present a diagnostic puzzle.

1. Monostotic Paget's disease in the vertebral body is dense or ivory in appearance.

2. Monostotic Paget's disease in the tibia presents as a flame-shaped area of osteolysis that begins at one end of the bone and works up into the diaphysis. The border between pagetic bone and normal bone is sharply demarcated.

Note: This is especially likely to occur after a period of immobilization.

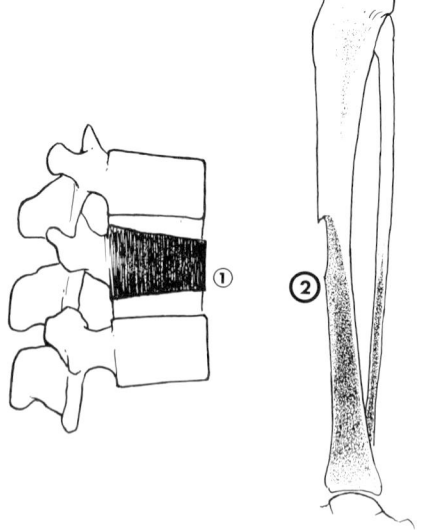

3. Over a period of years there is increased sclerosis.
4. Stress fractures,
5. Cortical enlargment and periosteal bone formation, and
6. Anterior bowing of the tibia characteristic of progressive Paget's disease.

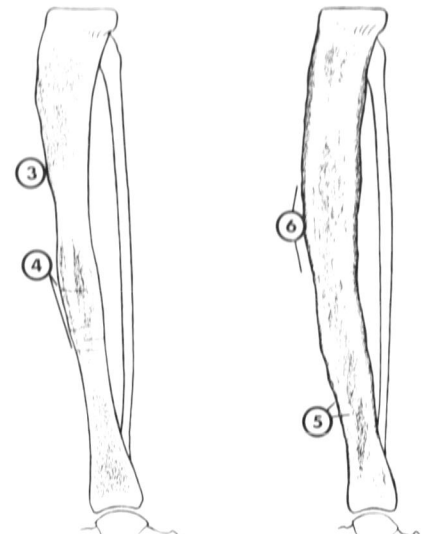

Diagnosis of Paget's Disease

The diagnosis can be made on the basis of the radiographic changes and elevation in levels of alkaline phosphatase and urinary hydroxyproline (HYP). The correlation between urinary HYP, reflecting bone degradation, and alkaline phosphatase, reflecting osteoblastic activity, indicates the coupling of bone formation and bone resorption in this disease.

Bone biopsy may be necessary, particularly to diagnose the process presenting in the osteolytic phase. However, biopsy should be avoided in weight-bearing bones such as the femur that are likely to fracture after diagnostic biopsy.

The most common condition from which Paget's disease must be differentiated on x-ray is metastatic carcinoma of the prostate, which produces similar bone changes, particularly in the pelvis. Marshall and Ling have described a useful radiographic sign, the pelvic brim sign, which is seen in 85 per cent of the patients with generalized Paget's disease and is not evident with osteoblastic or osteolytic metastasis to the pelvis.

1. Thickening of the pelvic brim or iliopectineal line is characteristic of Paget's disease. It probably is due to added stresses in this area resulting from destruction of the lamellae in the pelvis and the osteoblastic reaction.
2. Disease may be unilateral in a pagetic pelvis.

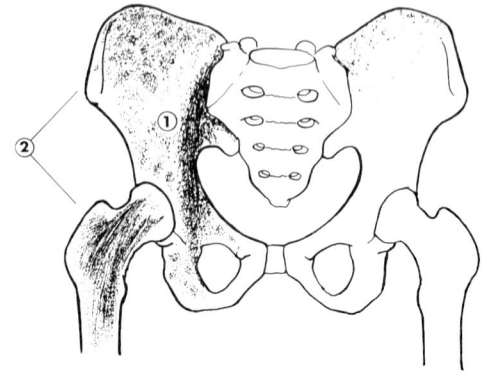

Malignant Degeneration of Paget's Disease

Malignant degeneration occurs in less than one per cent of patients with Paget's disease. However, approximately 20 per cent of all patients older than 40 years with bone sarcoma have associated Paget's disease. Malignant degeneration should be particularly suspected as an underlying condition in a pathologic fracture.

1. The tumors are destructive and create lytic changes in bone affected by Paget's disease.
2. A pathologic fracture may indicate the underlying malignant degeneration of Paget's disease.

Note: These tumors frequently contain tissue of different cell types, including osteosarcoma, chondrosarcoma, fibrosarcoma, and malignant giant cell tumor. The prognosis is extremely poor, possibly because the diagnosis of malignant degeneration in pagetic bone is delayed so frequently.

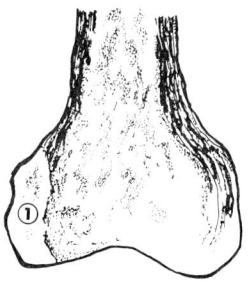 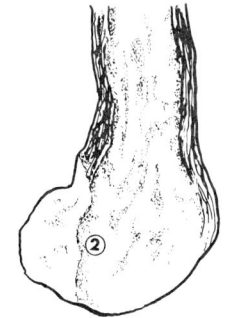

Management of Fractures Associated With Paget's Disease

REMARKS

The femur is the bone most commonly fractured in osteitis deformans.

Treatment in the past has been considered difficult and fraught with complications.

The most common complication is inadequate fixation of the fracture owing to the extreme softness of the diseased bone. Intramedullary fixation should be used whenever possible in order to avoid failure from loose plates or screws.

Troublesome bleeding may be encountered and should be anticipated, with adequate amounts of blood available for intraoperative transfusion. Preoperative treatment with calcitonin has been demonstrated by Meyers and Singer to decrease blood loss usually associated with operative treatment of pagetic bone.

Additional complications occur when the diseased bone is so dense that intramedullary fixation is difficult. This complication may be anticipated by preoperative radiographic assessment of the medullary canal.

Finally, prolonged postoperative immobilization of patients with Paget's disease can result in hypercalcemia, nephrolithiasis, and even renal failure. Open or closed treatment of a pathologic fracture in osteitis deformans should incorporate early mobilization of the patient to prevent these life-threatening sequelae.

Examples of femoral fracture problems associated with Paget's disease follow.

FRACTURES OF THE FEMUR

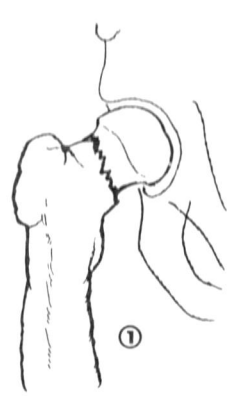

Preoperative X-Ray

1. Femoral neck fracture associated with osteitis deformans.

Note: Love has reported the incidence of nonunion with these fractures to be 75 per cent. The fracture should be managed by femoral prosthetic replacement.

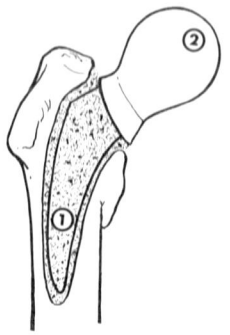

X-Ray After Cathcart Prosthesis

1. The Cathcart prosthesis has been cemented into the femoral canal.
2. The out-of-round design of the prosthesis permits synovial fluid to perfuse between the prosthesis and the acetabulum.

Note: If the acetabulum is diseased and weakened, protrusion of the prosthesis is likely. This can be prevented by total hip replacement.

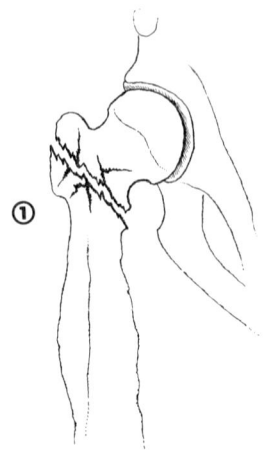

Preoperative X-ray

1. Intertrochanteric fracture in the femur with pronounced varus angulation.

PATHOLOGIC FRACTURES

Postoperative X-Ray

2. Fixation of the fracture has been accomplished by Ender rods.

Note: Because the major problem here is poor fixation due to soft bone, intramedullary technique is preferable to nail or plate fixation. Rarely, with extremely dense bone and obliteration of the medullary canal, a two-piece nail-plate device may be preferable.

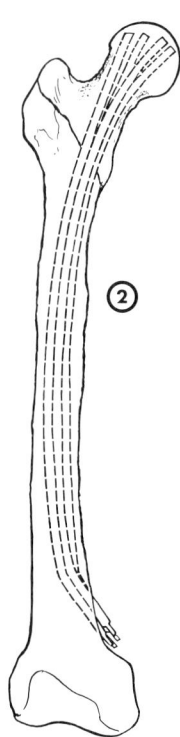

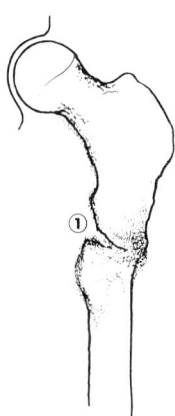

Preoperative X-ray

1. A subtrochanteric fracture has occurred with a severe varus deformity.

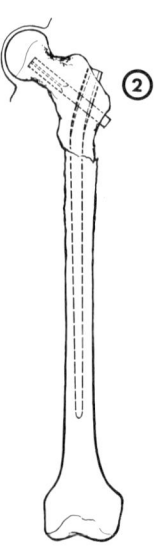

Postoperative X-Ray

2. A Zickel nail has been inserted after correction of the varus deformity.

PATHOLOGIC FRACTURES

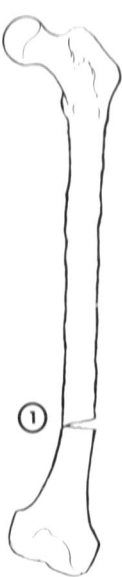

Prereduction X-Ray

1. Fracture of the distal femoral shaft.

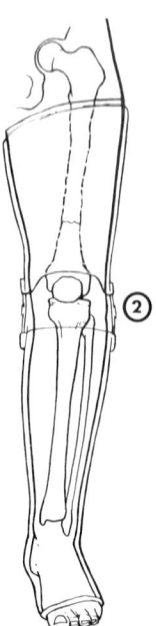

Postreduction X-Ray

2. Reduction has been accomplished and the fracture has been immobilized by a cast-brace. This permits the patient to be out of bed and avoids the complications of prolonged immobilization.

FRACTURES OF THE TIBIA

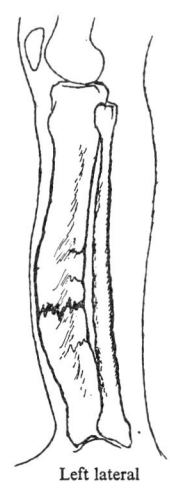
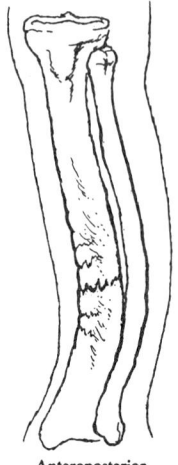

Left lateral   Anteroposterior

Prereduction X-Ray

Typical complete fracture of the tibia in a case of Paget's disease.

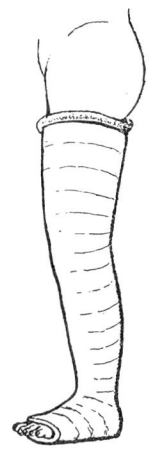

Postreduction Management

After correction of alignment apply a long leg cast from the groin to the toes.

Note: Meyers and Singer have shown that patients with tibia vara from Paget's disease may suffer marked difficulty in walking owing to osteoarthritis in the medial knee compartments.

If an adequate course of treatment with calcitonin does not relieve the pain, tibial osteotomy should be done to correct the tibia vara and knee joint symptoms. Adequate preoperative preparation with calcitonin decreases the inflammatory process of Paget's disease and diminishes perioperative bleeding.

HYPERCORTISONISM AND HYPERPARATHYROIDISM

REMARKS

The most common endocrine conditions associated with generalized weakening and fractures are hypercortisonism and hyperparathyroidism.

Prolonged cortisone treatment will produce bone changes similar to those of senescent osteoporosis, with similar resultant fractures.

Hyperparathyroidism may be primarily due to disease or tumor of the parathyroid, or it may be secondary to renal dysfunction. Primary hyperparathyroidism, with the wide-scale screening of serum levels of calcium and phosphorus done today, is usually diagnosed before the onset of bone signs and symptoms.

An elevated serum calcium level mandates that other conditions such as multiple myeloma, metastatic carcinoma, sarcoid, vitamin D poisoning, and milk-alkali type syndromes be ruled out.

Hyperparathyroidism is a relatively uncommon cause of bone demineralization and should not be confused with more common causes arising in bones or kidneys.

Bone lesions associated with hyperparathyroidism include the characteristic brown tumor with an old hemorrhagic, fibroblastic matrix and numerous giant cells. This can frequently be distinguished from a giant cell tumor only by correlating with blood chemistry.

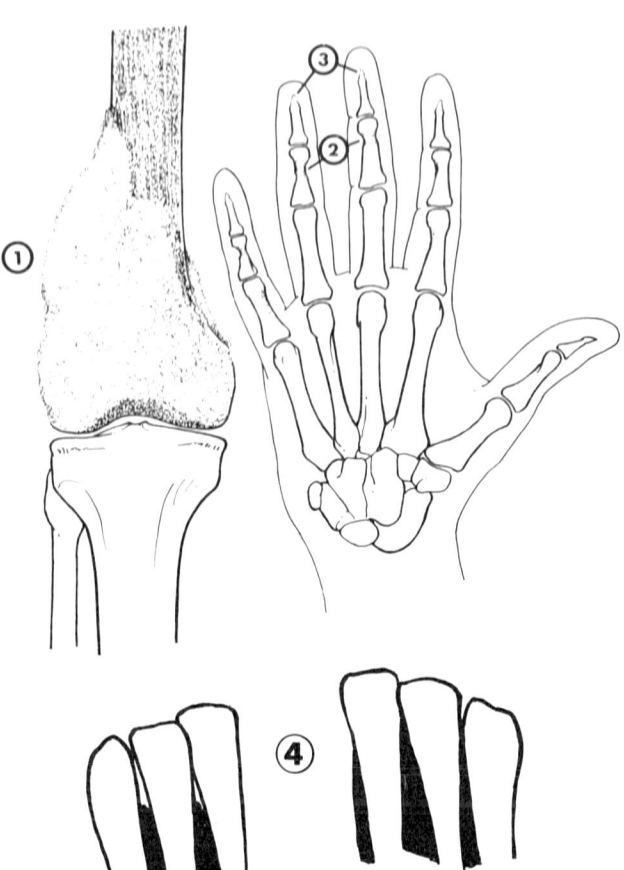

1. A large cystic area (brown tumor) of the femur with a cortical fracture produced by hyperparathyroidism. This can readily be confused with a giant cell tumor (see page 2121).

2. Extensive subperiosteal bone resorption in the phalanges.

3. Resorption of the tufts of the distal phalanges.

4. Resorption of the lamina dura around the teeth.

Management

Treatment is directed primarily at the parathyroid glands and the underlying disease.

The involved weight-bearing bones should be protected by bracing or cast until the underlying endocrine hyperfunction is corrected.

Abnormalities That Cause Pathologic Fracture

OSTEOGENESIS IMPERFECTA

REMARKS

Approximately 30,000 people are afflicted in the United States with brittle bone disease or osteogenesis imperfecta. This is an autosomal dominant alteration in the ability of mesenchymal cells, particularly osteoblasts and fibroblasts, to manufacture adequate and normal intercellular substance.

The condition results in multiple problems including thin skin and sclera, poor teeth, a tendency to macular bleeding, and hypermobile joints in addition to fragile bones.

The condition in its congenital form is usually fatal. A tarda form develops later in childhood and causes varying problems, among which is the tendency to increasing numbers of fractures and severe deformity.

The tendency to fracture eventually diminishes with maturity but the weakening of the skeletal structure can leave the patient with crippling deformities. This can be mitigated by treatment early in childhood.

The bone changes may not be apparent in the first few years of life. Enchondral ossification occurs normally and the length of cylindrical bones is not initially affected. Periosteal osteogenesis is disturbed, so the diameter of the bones is less than normal and the cortices are thin.

Radiographic Appearance

1. Normal-appearing epiphyseal growth centers.
2. Widened medullary canal.
3. Thin cortex.
4. Fatigue fracture of the distal tibia.

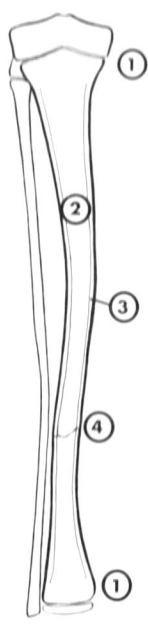

Changes after Three Years

1. Longitudinal growth has continued.
2. The diameters of the tibia and fibula have decreased.
3. Angulatory deformities have been produced by repeated fractures. This adds to the risk of refracture.

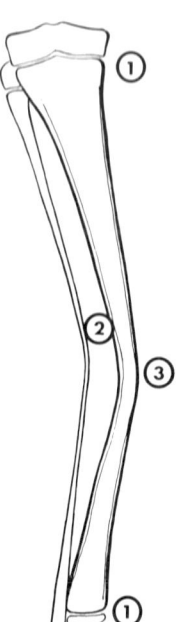

Progressive Changes in the Femur Associated with Osteogenesis Imperfecta

1. There is progressive anterior angulation and deformity from repeated fractures of the distal femur.
2. The callus formation is abundant.

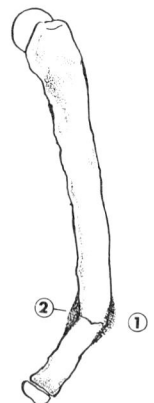

Progressive Changes in the Spine Associated with Osteogenesis Imperfecta

1. Vertebral collapse with compression fractures of the vertebrae is common.

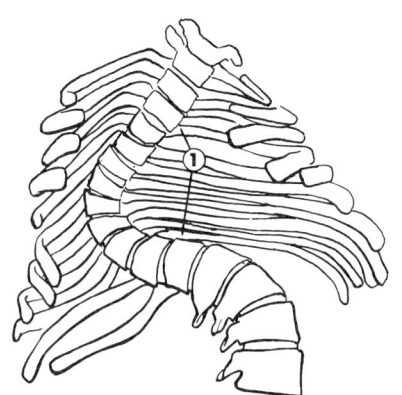

2. The pressure of the nucleus pulposus on the soft vertebral bodies causes the vertebrae to become biconcave (codfish vertebrae).
3. The patient is prone to develop severe kyphoscoliosis.

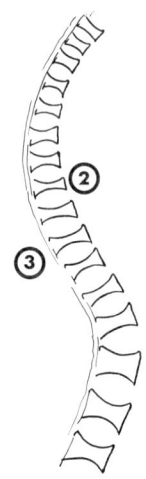

Management

Intramedullary fixation of weight-bearing bones after correction of structural deformities decreases the frequency of pathologic fractures and allows the patient to remain ambulatory. A telescoping nail has been developed by Bailey which allows fracture fixation but accommodates for growth of the bone. This technique is preferable to the repeated operations necessary as the child outgrows the length of a standard intramedullary nail.

The presence of scoliosis at a young age almost always leads to a predictable progression. External bracing (Milwaukee brace) usually fails to control the curvature and often deforms the ribcage. Spine fusion, with or without Harrington instrumentation, has been suggested by Benson and coworkers as a possible preferred treatment.

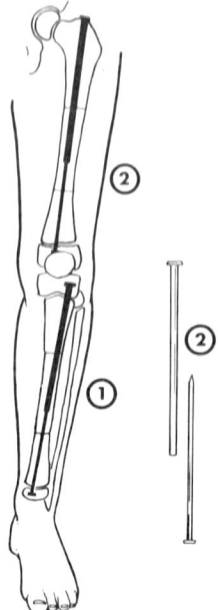

1. After multiple osteotomies, the deformed tibia, and
2. The deformed femur can be fixed with a Bailey telescoping rod, which allows maintenance of correction of the position during growth.

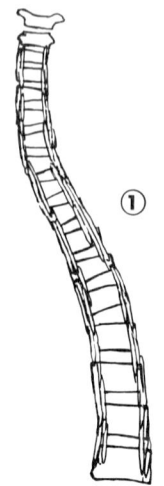

1. Kyphoscoliosis should be treated if at all possible by early fusion, with or without Harrington instrumentation.

PATHOLOGIC FRACTURES

FIBROUS DYSPLASIA

REMARKS

Fibrous dysplasia is a fairly common disease in which normal bone undergoing physiologic turnover is replaced by abnormal fibrous tissue and osteoid. The cancellous and cortical bone becomes eroded from within.

This condition is frequently confused with bone cysts, cortical defects, enchondromas, neurofibromas, and hyperparathyroidism.

Rarely, fibrous dysplasia will be associated with disturbance of skin pigmentation and of endocrine function (Albright's syndrome). Endocrine dysfunction is usually restricted to girls, except for occasional hyperthyroidism in boys.

Fibrous dysplasia may be monostatic or polyostotic. Occasionally it is monomelic, involving several bones in the same limb. Most, if not all, fibrous dysplastic lesions begin during the growth period. However, many silent lesions may not be detected until adulthood.

Schlumberger showed that the most common sites of involvement are the ribs, femur, tibia, maxilla, and calvarium.

Appearance on X-Ray

1. The characteristic picture is a lobulated or soap-bubble lesion eroding the cortex from within.
2. The lesion may appear cystic initially but the lobular and scalloped outlines are characteristic of the advanced lesion.
3. Pain is usually not a feature of this slow-growing process until pathologic fracture occurs.

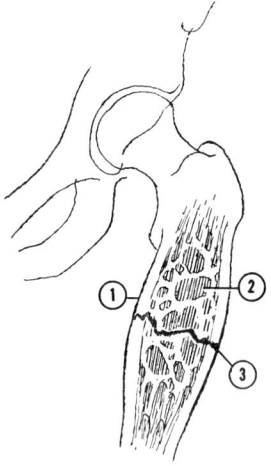

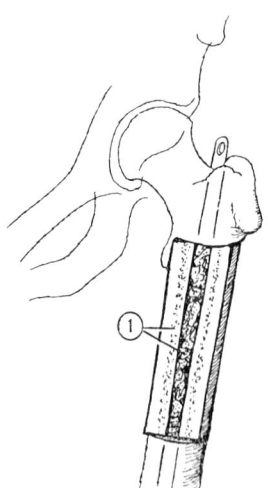

Management

Treatment is similar to that for other fragile bone problems, particularly osteogenesis imperfecta.

Intramedullary nail fixation should provide the structural strength necessary to prevent repeated fracture deformity.

1. Attempted excision of the lesion is usually ineffectual. Bone grafts are replaced entirely by the diseased tissue.

2. Fixation of involved bone should be similar to that for osteogenesis imperfecta. An expanding Bailey rod can be used to reinforce weight-bearing bones involved by fibrous dysplasia in a growing child.

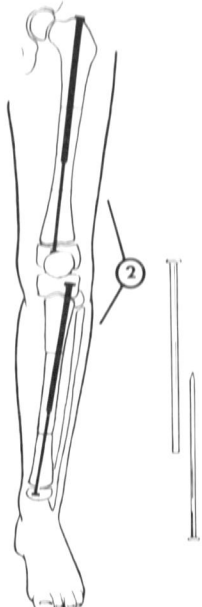

Shepherd's Crook Deformity in Fibrous Dysplasia

A frequent mechanical problem is a shepherd's crook deformity of the proximal femur. This gradually increases and produces severe crippling problems unless corrected.

This type of problem is characteristic of fibrous dysplasia and can be anticipated and prevented early in the management of the disease.

Zickel nail fixation can effectively prevent or correct this crippling deformity in children as young as 7 years.

Preoperative X-Ray

1. Fibrous dysplasia frequently may involve the entire femur.
2. The shaft becomes weakened and progressively deformed.
3. Repeated fractures add to the shepherd's crook deformity, or coxa vara, eventually crippling the victim.

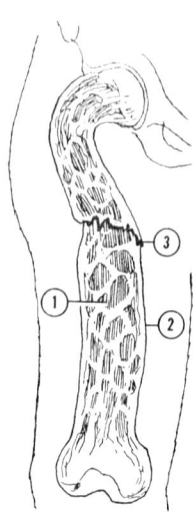

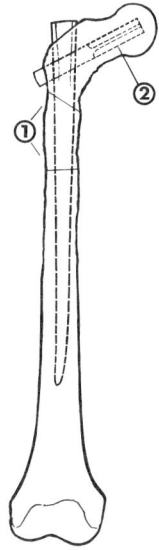

Postoperative X-Ray After Zickel Nail Fixation

1. The femur has been osteotomized to correct the coxa vara.
2. Internal fixation with the Zickel nail cut to fit the femur provides good immobilization of this severe problem.

CONGENITAL PSEUDOARTHROSIS

The most common congenital or developmental pseudoarthroses occur in the tibia and the clavicle.

The etiology and management of these two conditions are quite different and will be discussed separately.

CONGENITAL PSEUDOARTHROSIS OF THE TIBIA

REMARKS

Pseudoarthrosis may be congenital, or an anterolateral tibial angulation may be present at birth that later develops the defect. Frequently, pseudoarthrosis becomes manifest only after osteotomy to correct anterolateral angulation. Congenital tibial angulation should be treated by bracing rather than osteotomy in infants.

The other mode of presentation is a cystlike fibrous dysplasia in the tibia that eventually fractures and fails to heal. These congenital cysts of the tibia should be treated by curettage, bone grafting, and protection with a brace to prevent development of pseudoarthrosis.

The lesion of congenital pseudoarthrosis most often is a soft tissue neurofibroma or hamartoma that is locally invasive and that breaks down bone even after the pseudoarthrosis is thought to have healed. Recurrence must be anticipated until the patient is skeletally mature.

Treatment of the lesion should include excision of the soft tissue hamartoma and sclerotic bone along with rigid skeletal fixation and external orthotic support in order to prevent recurrence.

Long-term treatment by pulsing electromagnetic fields is proving useful as a supplement to prevent recurrence after surgery.

PATHOLOGIC FRACTURES

Preoperative X-Ray

1. Congenital pseudoarthrosis at the junction of the middle and lower thirds of the tibia.
2. Tapering of the fragments with anterolateral angulation is common.
3. Sclerosis of the bone ends is always present along with obliteration of the intramedullary canal.
4. Hamartoma of the surrounding soft tissue must be excised.

Preferred Method of Operation (Charnley Technique)

1. Excise sclerotic ends of the bone and thoroughly remove the surrounding fibrous hamartoma down to healthy soft tissue.
2. Pass a Steinmann pin through the medullary canal of the distal fragment, through the ankle and subtalar joint, and out through the os calcis.

Note: It may be possible to pass the nail through the anterior aspect of the lower end of the tibia and to traverse the neck of the talus, thereby avoiding penetration of the ankle joint.

3. Thread the pin into the medullary canal of the proximal fragment and drive the pin into the bone immediately below the tibial tubercle.

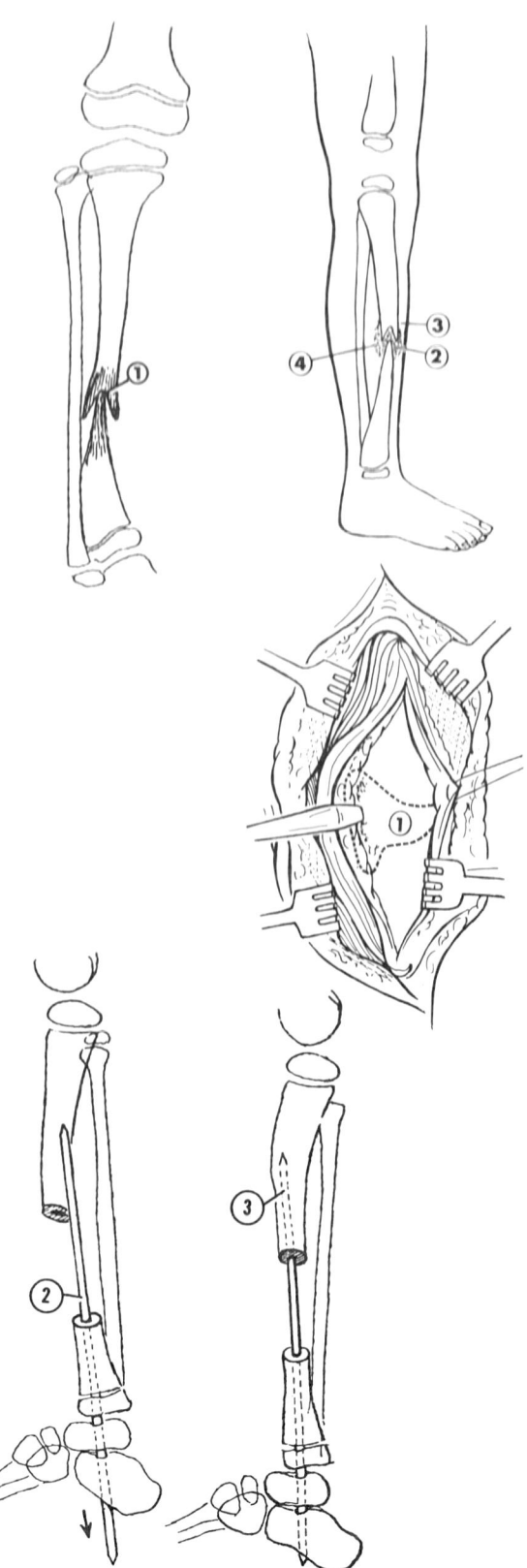

2107

Preferred Method of Operation (Charnley Technique) (Continued)

1. Pull the foot and the distal fragment downward and regain as much length as possible.
2. Place two tibial cortical grafts of appropriate length in the defect and tie them around the pin with catgut sutures.
3. Push the foot and the distal fragments upward; this impacts the grafts between the two tibial fragments.
4. Surround the entire site with cancellous bone slabs obtained from the ilium.
5. Cut the pin below the level of the skin.

Note: If the fibula is defective it should also be fixed with an intramedullary pin.

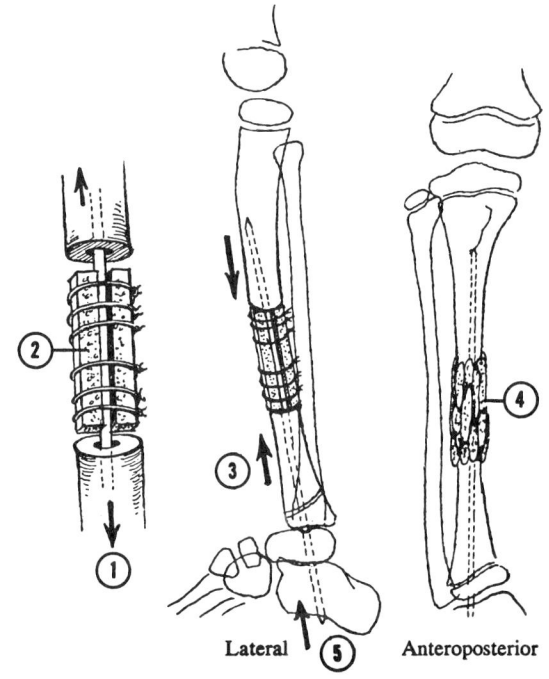
Lateral　　Anteroposterior

Immobilization

1. Apply a full-leg plaster cast from the groin to the toes.

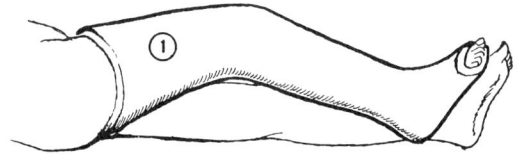

Postoperative Management

Allow the patient up on crutches with no weight bearing on the limb.

Change the plaster cast every six weeks.

Remove the pin when x-rays show good bone formation and consolidation at the site of the old defect, usually at the end of four to six months.

After removal of the pin, protect the limb with a long leg brace until remodeling is complete and a normal medullary canal in the tibia is reestablished.

Postoperative X-Ray

FOUR MONTHS AFTER OPERATION

1. Healing of the tibia and fibula is substantial and complete.
2. An intramedullary pin provides adequate protection from all shearing strains. It is now ready for removal.

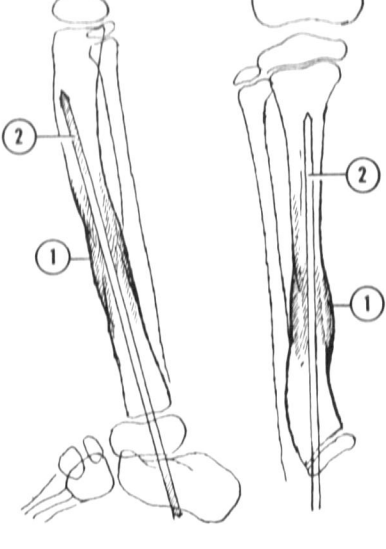

EIGHT MONTHS AFTER OPERATION

1. Remodeling is continuing.
2. The medullary canal in the tibia is reestablished.

Note: The limb frequently must be protected with at least a short leg orthosis until skeletal maturity is attained. Use of pulsed, inductively coupled electrical stimulation is also showing promise of success in resistant and difficult cases.

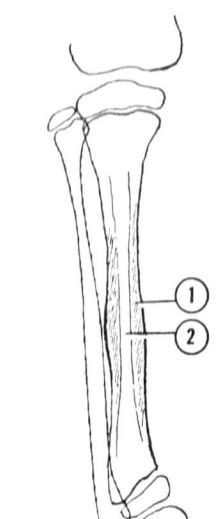

CONGENITAL PSEUDOARTHROSIS OF THE CLAVICLE

REMARKS

Congenital pseudoarthrosis of the clavicle is a rare condition with a very striking right-sided predominance. Because of its consistent location on the right side and in the midthird of the clavicle, Lloyd-Roberts has attributed it to excessive pressure from the subclavian artery, particularly when associated with an elevated first rib.

The diagnosis is usually made several months or years after birth. The most common finding is a lump or a prominent spike under the skin in the middle of the clavicle. Characteristically, pain is absent with pseudoarthrosis, in contrast to fracture or traumatic nonunion.

The condition from which congenital pseudoarthrosis must be differentiated is cleidocranial dysostosis, which frequently involves both clavicles as well as the skull bones.

Appearance on X-Ray

1. The deformity is consistent in the mid-third of the right clavicle.
2. The medial segment lies over and above the lateral segment.
3. No callus or reactive bone is evident.

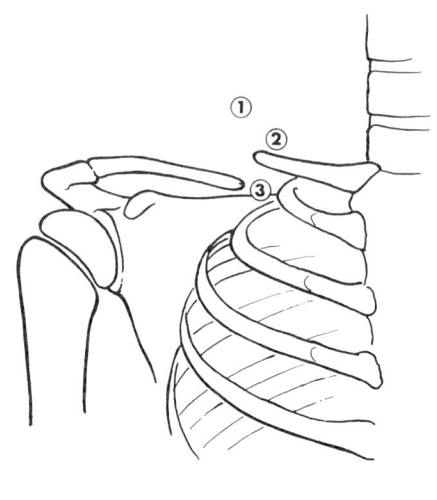

Management

Half of these cases are asymptomatic and need no treatment.

For the patient with discomfort or a very unsightly prominence, operative treatment may be indicated. This should include:

1. Excision of the cartilaginous cap at each end of the fragments and alignment of the fragments,
2. Bone grafting, and
3. Internal fixation with a Knowles pin inserted from posterior to anterior.

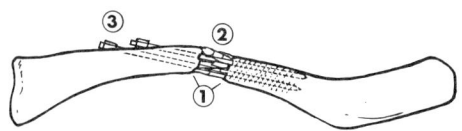

Note: A semitubular plate may also provide effective fixation (see page 534).

METAPHYSEAL CORTICAL DEFECT OR NONOSSIFYING FIBROMA

REMARKS

Metaphyseal cortical defect or nonossifying fibroma is a common fibrous deficiency that develops in children's bones and, over a period of two to five years, heals spontaneously.

Peterson and Fitzgerald have pointed out that these lesions usually become evident at about six years of age. Fractures, if they occur, appear on the average at about twelve years of age.

These lesions should be distinguished from solitary cysts, which are less likely to heal spontaneously. The metaphyseal cortical defect is eccentrically located in the cortex and frequently has a scalloped edge with surrounding sclerosis.

About 50 per cent of these lesions are in the femur, but on a percentage basis, the lesion most likely to fracture is located in the distal tibia or the humerus.

Microscopically, these lesions are similar to those of fibrous dysplasia, except for the absence of bone spicules in the fibrous tissue.

Appearance on X-Ray

1. The most common location is in the distal femur. The lesion is characteristically eccentric and surrounded by a sclerotic, scalloped margin.
2. The most common site of the fracture is the distal tibia. Fracture through a nonossifying fibroma may be distinguished from a bone cyst by the absence of a "fallen fragment sign." If the lesion were cystic, occasionally a small fracture fragment might be seen to have fallen into the cyst (see page 2112).

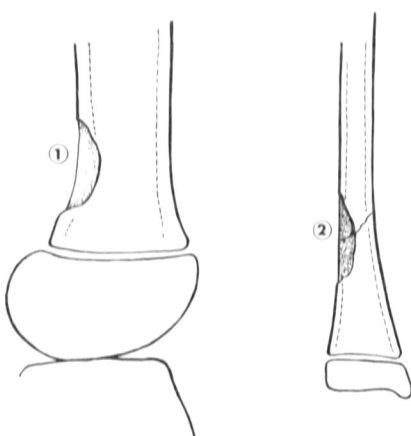

Management

These defects have such a characteristic radiographic appearance that biopsy is usually not necessary.

The fractures heal spontaneously and may also, in the process, obliterate the defect. However, for persistence of the lesion, particularly in active, young children, curettage and bone grafting may be warranted. Keep in mind that the lesion may recur even after operative treatment.

SOLITARY BONE CYST

REMARKS

Solitary bone cysts occur most typically in the proximal humerus, the proximal and distal ends of the femur, and the proximal tibia. They develop predominantly in boys between the ages of 3 and 19 years.

Aegerter and Kirkpatrick have designated them as posthematoma cysts, probably arising in a walled, liquified hematoma in spongy bone.

These lesions are commonly asymptomatic until fracture occurs.

Appearance on X-Ray

1. An oval radiolucent defect in the metaphysis.
2. A varying amount of bone separating the cyst from the metaphysis and the epiphysis.
3. A fracture line occurring through the thin cortex. Occasionally a small fragment drops into the cyst (fallen fragment sign).

Note: Fractures are likely to occur through the weak cystic wall. In 15 to 20 per cent of these lesions spontaneous obliteration follows fracture, but treatment should not be based on this chance happening.

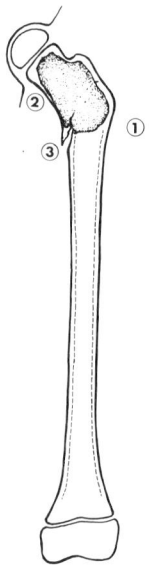

MANAGEMENT BY INJECTION

Scaglietti and coworkers have demonstrated that the isolated bone cysts contain fluid that is essentially a transudate. They have reasoned that with injection of a corticosteroid into the cyst cavity, the cystic fluid will be resorbed in the same manner as a transudate in a joint synovitis is resorbed.

Injection of methyl prednisolone acetate into the bone cyst appears to be a new and useful approach to obliterate the lesion without surgery.

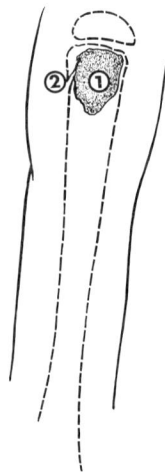

Preinjection X-Ray

1. A large cystic formation is evident in the upper third of the humerus.
2. A cortical fracture has occurred.

Technique of Injection

1. Two 18-gauge lumbar puncture type needles are injected using an obturator.

Note: If the wall of the cyst is thick, a cannulated needle mounted on a drill may be necessary.

2. Fluoroscopic control is important to ascertain the position of the needles.

3. The fluid is allowed to escape spontaneously through the needles.

4. Methyl prednisolone acetate is then injected; 40 to 80 mg are injected for a small cyst in a younger patient, but up to 200 mg. are injected for a larger cyst.

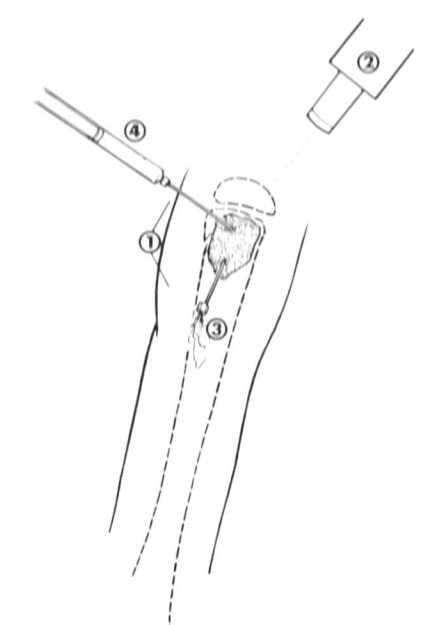

Postinjection X-Ray

1. At 4 months after injection of the cyst, the cavity is starting to fill with bone tissue.

2. At 15 months, the cyst is commonly obliterated.

Note: When the cyst involves a weight-bearing bone, the patient should protect it with crutches. If persistent areas are evident on follow-up x-ray, the injection should be repeated using doses of 40 to 80 mg. In older patients injection may have to be repeated several times since bone repair is slower.

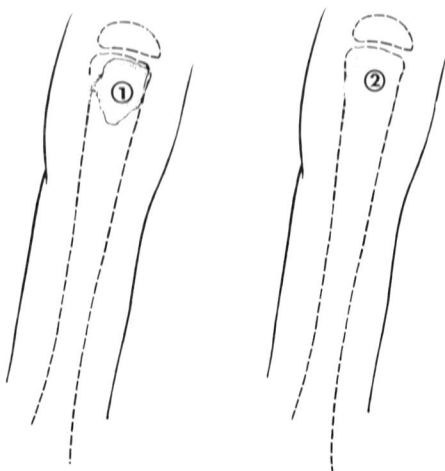

OPERATIVE REPAIR

Preoperative X-Ray

1. The cyst involves an extensive portion of the subtrochanteric area of the femur.
2. Slight expansion of the cortex is evident.
3. The fracture occurs through both cortices and produces slight varus deformity.

Note: Internal fixation is necessary because of the extensive involvement of the weight-bearing portion of the femur.

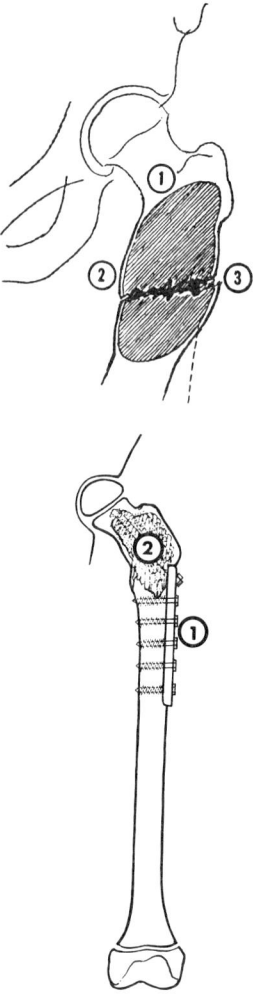

Postoperative X-Ray

1. The weakened subtrochanteric region has been protected by internal fixation using screws and plates.
2. Autogenous bone graft fills the cystic cavity.

Subsequent Treatment

The patient is kept on crutches and only partial weight bearing is allowed until the cyst fills in entirely.

Small persistent cystic areas can be injected postoperatively with methyl prednisolone.

ANEURYSMAL BONE CYST

REMARKS

This lesion is actually a cystic lesion of bone produced by flow of blood through a spongelike network of fibrous-walled channels of the bone marrow.

The lesion is found most often in the shafts of long bones, the flat bones, and the vertebrae.

The process has a propensity to lyse bone and expand the cortices outward. The periosteum tends to resist this expansion but eventually ruptures or fractures.

Although an aneurysmal bone cyst may present as a de novo lesion, Aegeter and coworkers have pointed out that it may also be secondary to other primary osseous lesions. Most commonly it is associated with unicameral bone cysts and giant cell tumors. Other associated lesions may include osteosarcoma, nonossifying fibroma, osteoblastoma, and hemangioma of bone.

Management of the lesion is usually by surgical curettage and bone grafting. The addition of cryotherapy may also help prevent recurrences, but this technique is still under investigation (see page 2122).

Preoperative X-Ray

Aneurysmal bone cyst of the femur.
1. Lesion is expansile and loculated.
2. Cortex is thin and attenuated.
3. There is a fracture through the cyst.

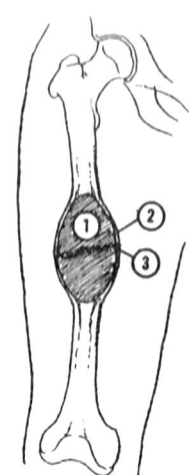

Fixation by Intramedullary Nailing

Note: Severe bleeding is likely with operative treatment of aneurysmal bone cysts. This problem and the recurrence rate of the condition can be diminished by the use of cryotherapy as described by Marcove and coworkers (see page 2122).

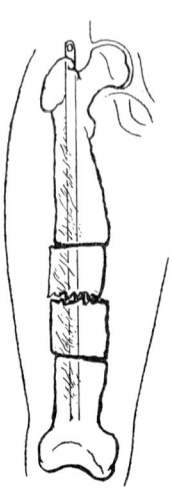

Benign and Malignant Bone Tumors and Tumor-Like Processes That Cause Pathologic Fracture

SOLITARY ENCHONDROMA

A solitary enchondroma is a circumscribed mass of cartilage cells occurring usually in the bones of the hands or feet. The lesion may occasionally develop at the ends of long bones or in the pelvis, but in these locations it is quite likely to behave as a chondrosarcoma.

There is no absolute means by which the clinician, the radiologist, or the pathologist can be certain that the cartilage lesion is an enchondroma rather than a chondrosarcoma. The diagnosis ultimately depends on the location and subsequent behavior of the cartilage cells.

In the bones of the hands and feet the lesion usually is eccentrically located but occasionally is centrally placed; it tends to distend the thin cortex, and the rarefied cystic area is usually demarcated by a thin zone of sclerotic bone.

In the large limb bones the lesions frequently undergo malignant transformation, whereas in lesions of the hands and feet this is indeed rare.

Fracture of the attenuated cortex may be the first indication of the lesion in the phalangeal, metacarpal, or metatarsal bones.

Always confirm the diagnosis by a biopsy.

Curettage and filling of the defect with cancellous bone chips or a solid bone graft is the treatment for lesions in the bones of the hands and feet.

For cartilage lesions in long bones, en bloc excision and graft replacement are indicated for presumed chondrosarcoma.

Marcove and coworkers have shown that cryotherapy is useful in managing the difficult problems of cartilage lesions in long bones or in flat bones that may be either enchondromas or low-grade chondrosarcomas (see page 2122).

Enchondroma

Preoperative X-Ray

Enchondroma of the phalanx.
1. Fracture through the attenuated cortex.
2. Distention of the shaft.
3. Thin sclerotic zone around lesion.

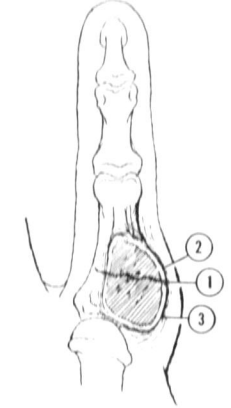

Postoperative X-Ray

1. Tumor has been curetted.
2. Defect has been packed with cancellous bone chips.

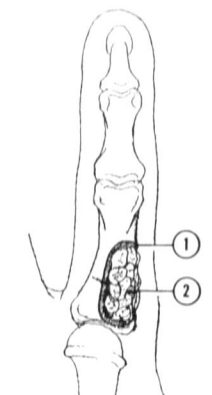

Preoperative X-Ray

Enchondroma of the metacarpal.
1. Distention of the entire shaft.
2. Distal and proximal articular surfaces are not involved.
3. Fracture through the thinned cortices.

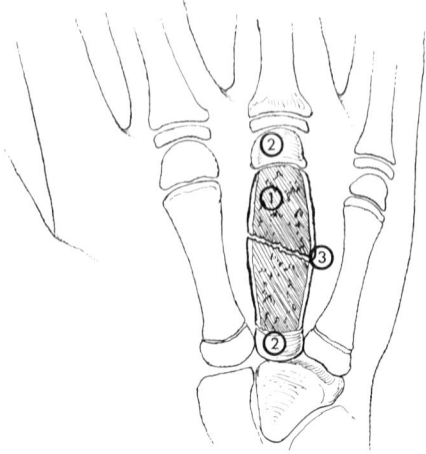

Postoperative X-Ray

1. Tibial graft replacing the resected metacarpal bone.
2. The distal articular cartilage and its subchondral bone have been preserved.

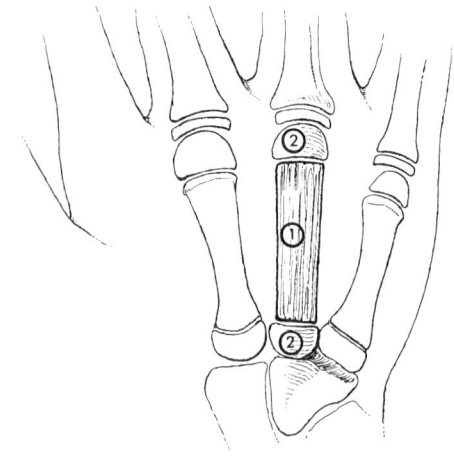

X-Ray Four Years After Resection of the Metacarpal Bone

1. The tibial graft is viable and has hypertrophied.
2. The distal articular cartilage has undergone necrosis.

Note: In spite of necrosis of the distal articular cartilage, this patient had 70 degrees of flexion at the metacarpophalangeal joint.

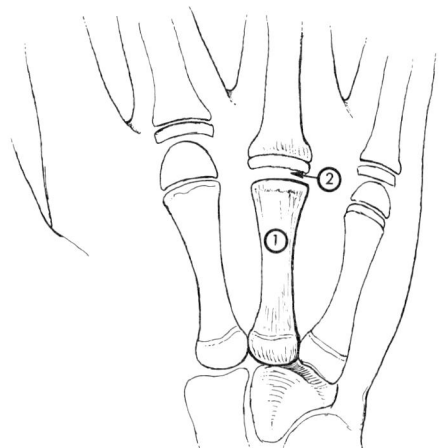

CHONDROSARCOMA

Preoperative X-Ray

1. A cartilaginous lesion in the distal femoral condyle. This location and the size of the tumor are consistent with a chondrosarcoma. After biopsy, the lesion should be treated by wide en bloc excision and, in this case, by replacement with a cadaver allograft.*
2. Fracture has occurred through the lesion.

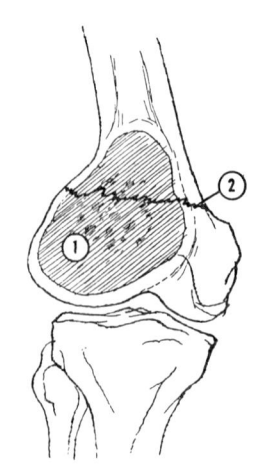

*Obtained from the Tissue Bank, Department of Surgery, University of Miami Medical Center, Miami, Florida 33101

X-Ray after Cadaver Allograft

1. The tumor has been completely resected en bloc.
2. A cadaver allograft has been fixed by transverse screws to the diaphysis.
3. Autogenous cancellous bone graft has been added to the junction between the host bone and the cadaver bone.

Note: The limb should be protected for four to six months with a brace or cast-brace device while the graft becomes solidly fixed to the host bone and ligaments.

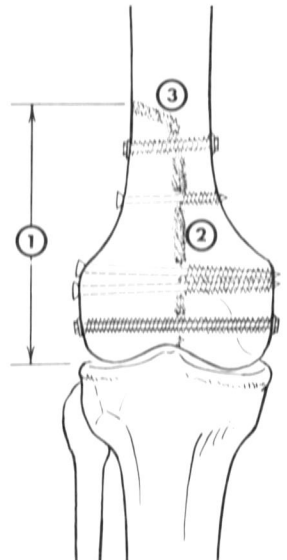

SOLITARY EOSINOPHILIC GRANULOMA OF BONE

REMARKS

This process falls into the category of histiocytosis, which includes Letterer-Siwe disease and Hand-Schuller-Christian disease, but has a considerably better prognosis than those conditions.

The osseous lesion results from a granulomatous proliferation of the intraosseous reticulum.

Flat bones, particularly the skull, the pelvis, and the vertebral bodies, are most frequently involved.

Lesions in the spine cause a characteristic vertebra plana or "coin-on-end" appearance from pronounced compression of the bodies. This may appear alarming, particularly in young children, in whom the lesion occurs most often. Nesbit and coworkers have shown that the usual course is spontaneous regression and partial reconstitution of the vertebral body. Rare cases of temporary paraparesis have been reported.

In the cyclindrical bones a lesion may occur in any location, but characteristically it is diaphyseal and erodes bone rapidly without producing initial reactive response. The radiographic appearance frequently mimics Ewing's sarcoma or metastatic neuroblastoma, both of which occur in a similar young age group. Because of this similarity, the lesion in the diaphyseal bone usually requires biopsy and curettage.

Appearance on X-Ray

Vertebral involvement

1. Vertebra plana is produced by eosinophilic granuloma in a young child.
2. The disc spaces are not involved.
3. There is usually no soft tissue swelling.

Note: This lesion is so characteristic that biopsy or treatment, other than brace protection, is usually not necessary.

4. The usual course is partial reconstitution which is similar to the growth in the uninvolved adjacent vertebral body. Slight scoliosis may occur.

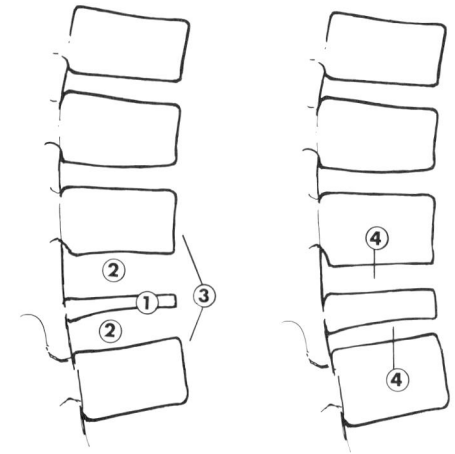

Cylindrical bone involvement

1. In the diaphysis the eosinophilic granuloma produces a lytic lesion and sometimes a small cortical fracture. This may appear quite similar to Ewing's sarcoma and usually requires biopsy.

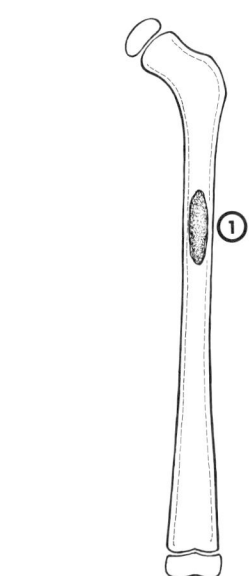

Management

Curettage in conjunction with the biopsy is usually effective in provoking a healing response of solitary eosinophilic granuloma. Protection of the weight-bearing bone for six to eight weeks after curettage is necessary during the healing process.

The patient should be followed closely, because multiple lesions may occasionally become evident and require further treatment. Fowles and Bobechko have pointed out that all patients with solitary eosinophilic granuloma of the bone improve regardless of the treatment they receive. This is a benign self-limiting process. Radiation treatment or other more vigorous therapy is not necessary and, moreover, may be hazardous.

GIANT CELL TUMOR (OSTEOCLASTOMA)

REMARKS

These tumors characteristically involve the metaphyseal and epiphyseal regions of long bones within the first decade after closure of the physes, i.e., at about age 15 to 25 years.

The tumor is slowly destructive, tends to recur, and, according to Aegerter, should always be considered a low-grade malignancy.

Osteoclastoma is prone to progress to a local aneurysmal bone cyst formation with pathologic fracture and extension into soft tissue. This tendency accounts for the sometimes dramatic and explosive behavior of an osteoclastoma. Lung metastases may also occasionally occur.

Osteoclastoma, which is a true tumor of osteoclasts, should be distinguished from a giant cell reactive process that is seen often in the metaphyseal and epiphyseal regions of bone. Differential diagnosis should also include aneurysmal bone cysts and brown tumors from hyperparathyroidism as well as reactive giant cell response to underlying malignancies such as osteosarcoma.

The diagnosis of osteoclastoma is one of exclusion after radiographic, laboratory, and microscopic studies have ruled out all other possibilities.

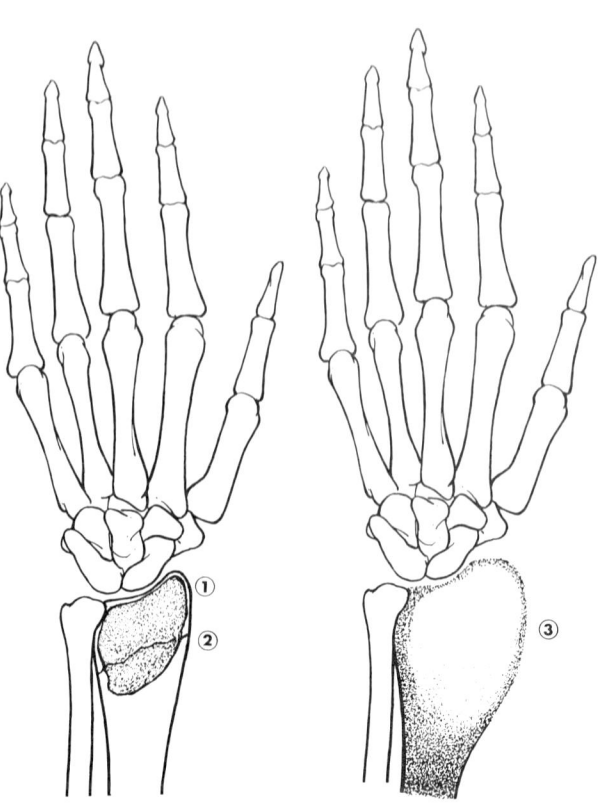

Appearance on X-Rays

1. Epiphyseal and metaphyseal eccentric location and expansion in the bone cortex.
2. Pathologic fracture through the cortex.
3. If an aneurysmal bone cyst is superimposed on the osteoclastoma, the lesion grows rapidly and appears to explode the bone.

Management

Giant cell tumors (osteoclastomas), although always considered potentially malignant, should be treated initially by local removal.

Curettage and bone graft, which have been recommended for small lesions with benign-appearing stroma, yield a recurrence rate approaching 50 per cent in many series.

More recently, Marcove and coworkers have demonstrated that cryotherapy considerably diminishes the recurrence rate as proven by "second look" biopsies.

European investigators, first Vidal and coworkers and more recently Persson and Wouters, have added to this concept by using methyl methacrylate to fill the cysts left after local removal.

These newer approaches have been effective in my experience and are worth employing cautiously for the treatment of difficult recurrent as well as of primary osteoclastomas.

Keep in mind that the tumor may occasionally metastasize to the lung. These metastatic lesions have proven to be extremely responsive to local pulmonary resection, as Goldenberg and coworkers have demonstrated.

TREATMENT BY CRYOTHERAPY AND METHYLMETHACRYLATE

Preoperative X-Ray

1. Giant cell tumor of the distal femur with pathologic fracture through the condyle.

Note: Attempted en bloc excision of this large tumor would require knee arthrodesis.

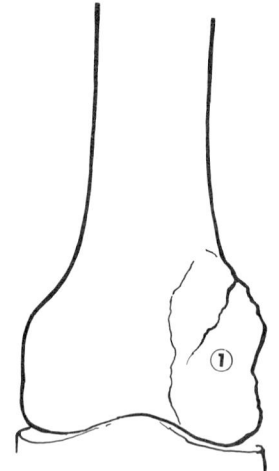

Technique of Cryotherapy (Marcove)

1. A pneumatic tourniquet is used to decrease bone bleeding and prevent the blood from acting as a barrier to achieve sufficient depth of freeze.

2. The lesion is approached anterolaterally and is completely and thoroughly curetted. Frozen sections are made to confirm the diagnosis of a giant cell tumor.

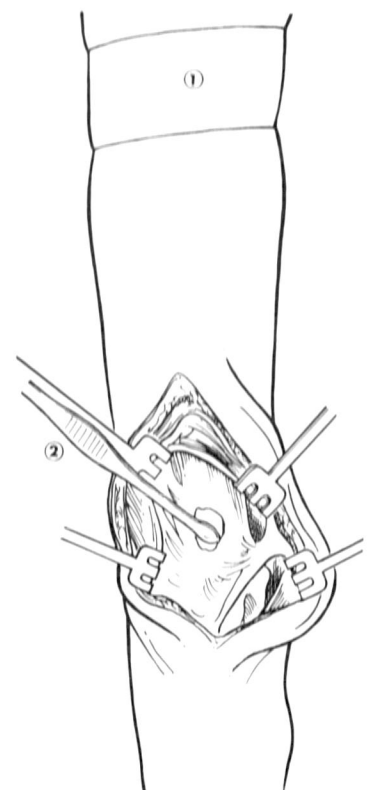

3. Through the opening into the cyst a funnel is inserted and sealed with Gelfoam. All areas of the cyst are covered with moist Gelfoam.

4. Liquid nitrogen is then poured into the cyst through the funnel to completely fill the bone cyst.

Note: During freezing the surrounding soft tissues should be protected by adequate mobilization and retraction as well as continuous lukewarm water irrigation. The temperature of the bone should be lowered to either $-60°C$ once or $-21°C$ three times to insure adequate cryonecrosis. Thermocouples should be used to confirm the bone temperature.

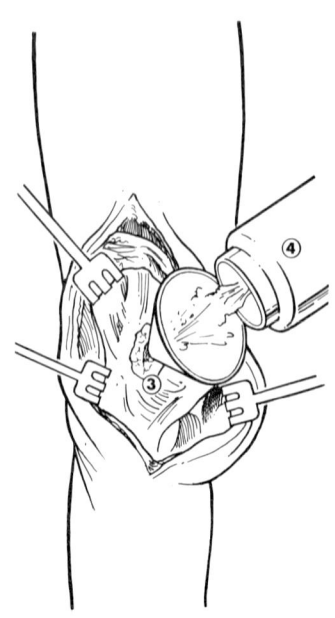

Technique of Cryotherapy (Marcove) (Continued)

1. After the tumor has been completely and thoroughly curetted, the cavity is packed completely with methyl methacrylate.

Note: Prophylactic antibodies should be used in conjunction with this combined cryotherapy treatment.

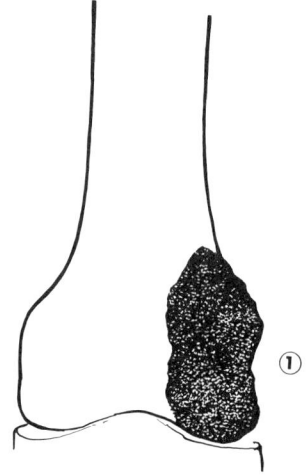

Subsequent Management

The limb is immobilized in a protective cast-brace postoperatively for three to six months.

X-rays are taken periodically to evaluate for evidence of recurrence. The bone immediately adjacent to the methyl methacrylate will become dense and sclerotic, but areas of osteolysis should cause one to suspect recurrence of the osteoclastoma. If in doubt, a second biopsy should be performed.

Curettage and cryotherapy can be repeated for recurrence, but occasionally amputation may be necessary and the patient should be forewarned of this possibility.

PRIMARY MALIGNANT BONE TUMORS

REMARKS

Pathologic fractures occur in the slower-growing primary malignant tumors, particularly the slower-growing osteosarcoma, chondrosarcoma, and reticulum cell sarcoma. Rapidly growing osteosarcomas, or Ewing's tumors, usually cause pain and systemic symptoms prior to pathologic fracture.

Adequate treatment requires ablation of the tumor, usually by amputation. For the slower-growing chondrosarcomas, wide en bloc resection and prosthetic replacement may be possible. This was the first indication for femoral prosthetic replacement reported by Austin Moore.

Fractures through radiosensitive lesions such as reticulum cell sarcoma or Ewing's tumor may be treated by radiation. However, Pritchard's recent studies from the Mayo Clinic experience showed the tendency for improved survival with surgical ablation of Ewing's tumor.

Osteogenic Sarcoma of the Osteolytic Type

Appearance on X-Ray

1. Marked destruction of bone with no new bone formation.
2. Fracture through the pathologic bone.

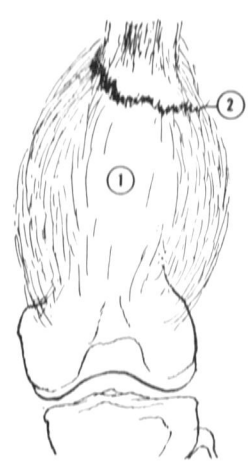

Management

1. The amputation should be done promptly, usually through the hip joint.
2. If the bone scan shows no evidence of tumor in the proximal femur, the amputation can be done at the high femoral level.

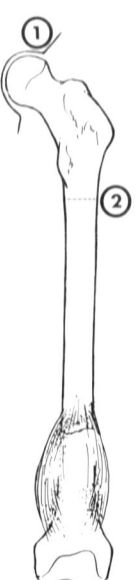

Chondrosarcoma

Appearance on X-Ray

1. Marked destruction of the upper end of the femur.
2. Fracture through the pathologic bone.

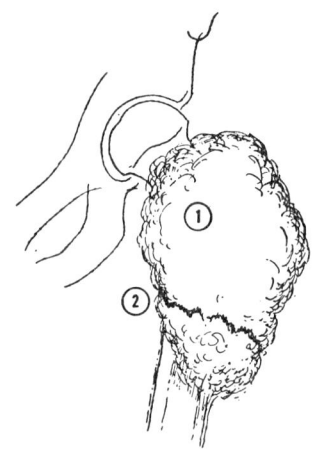

Management

1. If a wide en bloc resection of the chondrosarcoma is possible, a femoral prosthesis may be custom-made to replace the destroyed proximal femur.

Note: If adequate en bloc excision of the tumor is not possible, hip disarticulation is indicated.

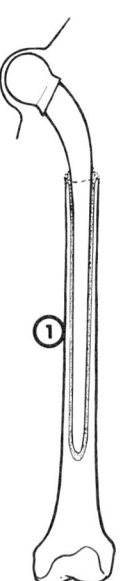

Reticulum Cell Sarcoma

Appearance on X-Ray

1. The tumor process is localized to the medullary canal.
2. A pathologic fracture has occurred through the cortex.

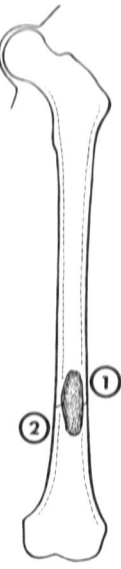

Management

1. The fracture has healed with external cast-brace immobilization.
2. The intramedullary tumor has responded to radiation therapy.

Note: Another biopsy should be done to determine if the radiation has completely eradicated the tumor. If tumor cells are still evident, an amputation should be performed. Sweet and coworkers have written a complete summary of the management and staging of reticulum cell sarcoma (histiocytic lymphoma of bone) and the indications for radiotherapy and chemotherapy.

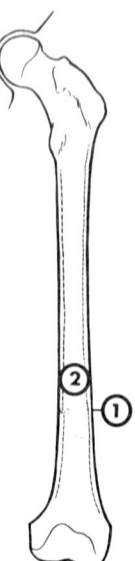

MULTIPLE MYELOMA (PLASMA CELL MYELOMA)

REMARKS

Plasma cell myeloma is a malignant neoplasm arising from the marrow reticulum and its derivatives.

Except for rare occasions, plasma cell myeloma occurs in patients older than 40 years. Flat bones with red marrow, and particularly the vertebral bodies, are most commonly involved.

The role of the plasma cells in producing serum globulins is abnormally altered by the myeloma, and death usually results from infection. Types of abnormal globulin produced by plasma cell myeloma vary from case to case. Protein electrophoresis commonly shows an abnormal peak between the beta and gamma elevations called the M (myeloma) protein.

Cryoglobulins are frequently produced by abnormal plasma cells and cause serum to precipitate when cooled. Bence Jones protein, a light chain globulin, may be formed by the plasma cells and excreted in the urine. Serum uric acid may be elevated owing to the breakdown of nucleic acid by the tumor. Amyloid is frequently deposited by leakage of the abnormal proteins out into collagenous tissue. The abnormal proteins, particularly the Bence Jones protein, deposit in the renal tubules and glomeruli and produce nephritis.

Despite the finding of characteristic protein abnormalities in the serum, diagnosis should be confirmed by marrow biopsy. Confusion with compression fractures associated with senescent osteoporosis is thereby avoided (see page 2089).

Of all the problems of plasma cell myeloma, the initial complaint is most often bone pain associated with fractures.

Spontaneous fractures of the vertebral bodies are best treated by a light, strong spinal brace.

Symptoms from long bone involvement can be significantly alleviated by rigid internal fixation.

The prognosis for plasma cell myeloma is similar to that for leukemia. Some patients die within a few months, but the average survival is two years. Some patients, however, can survive a good deal longer, as with chronic lymphocytic leukemia in older patients.

Like that for pathologic fractures associated with metastatic cancer, management of fractures from multiple myeloma should be guided by the current status of the patient rather than by preconceived notions about the length of survival.

Prereduction X-Ray

1. Spontaneous fracture of the femur.
2. Spontaneous fracture of the humerus.

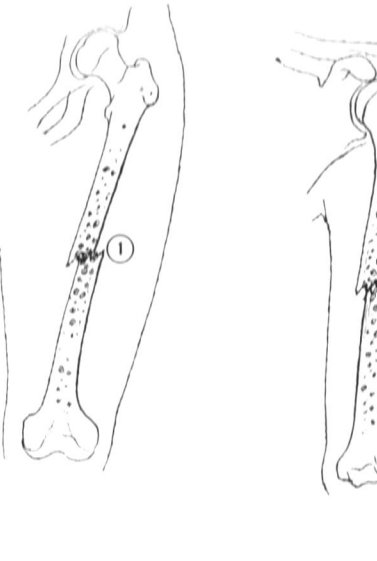

Postreduction X-Ray

1. Fracture is reduced and stabilized by an intramedullary nail.
2. Fracture is fixed by an intramedullary nail (Rush nail).

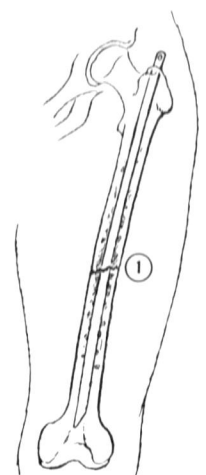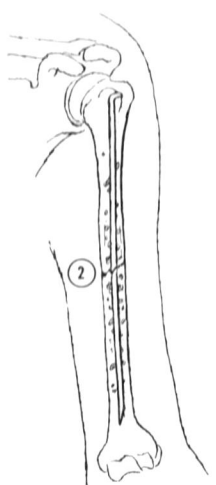

METASTATIC MALIGNANCY

REMARKS

Because of presumed poor prognosis, pathologic fractures from metastatic lesions have not always been effectively managed. Depending on the type of tumor, almost half of patients will live close to six months and 30 per cent will survive one year after pathologic fractures from metastases have occurred. Untreated, these fractures leave the patient bedridden and in pain.

The best approach is to treat the patient on the basis of current status rather than on some attempted prognosis of life expectancy.

Adequate internal fixation relieves pain that may be unresponsive to radiation treatment or chemotherapy. The patient may also occasionally regain walking ability.

The improved psychological and emotional outlook of a patient after adequate internal fixation of a pathologic fracture is also extremely beneficial.

The most common metastatic tumors causing pathologic fractures arise from the breast, lung, kidney, and colon.

The most common sites for pathologic fracture are the proximal femur and the hip. The most common site in the upper limb, similarly, is in the proximal half of the humerus.

In most instances, internal fixation is the treatment of choice. Frequently, the surgeon must be prepared to add to internal fixation with cryotherapy, methyl methacrylate, or supplemental internal fixation devices.

If postoperative radiation treatment is planned, it should include the ends of the nail or fixation device, which may have displaced cancer cells.

Types and Management of Pathologic Fractures from Metastatic Malignancies

1. The proximal femur is a common location for metastases, particularly from the breast.
2. Pathologic fractures in this area are best managed by replacement with a cemented Cathcart prosthesis.

Note: The cemented prosthesis is preferred owing to the high incidence of loosening after uncemented prosthetic replacement in pathologic fracture.

1. Pathologic fracture due to metastasis from breast carcinoma to the proximal femur.
2. Fixation with Zickel nail immobilizes the fracture. If necessary, methyl methacrylate may also be used to cement the nail in place.

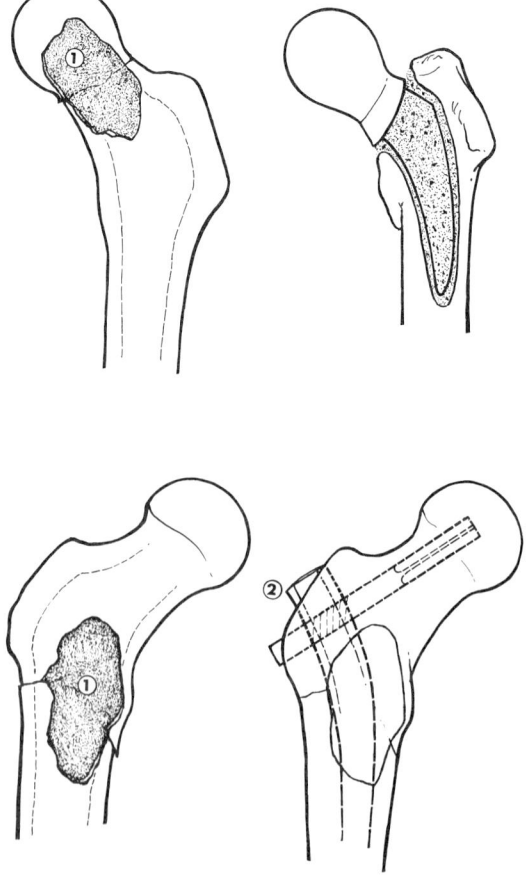

1. Pathologic fracture with metastatic melanoma to the distal femur.
2. Fixation is best accomplished by crossed Zickel nails.

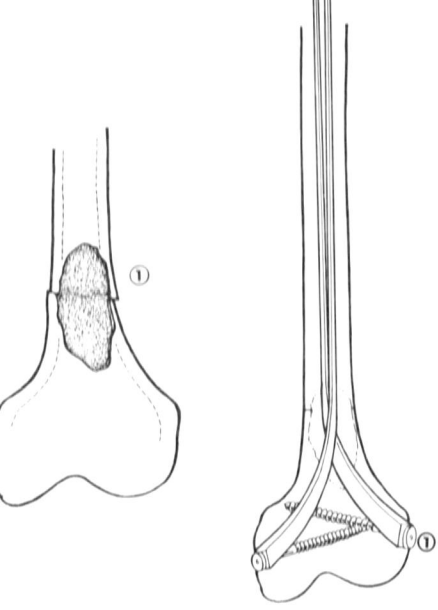

1. Metastatic lymphoma to the tibia.
2. Frequently the tibia can be best treated by external bracing or, if necessary,
3. Lottes nail fixation.

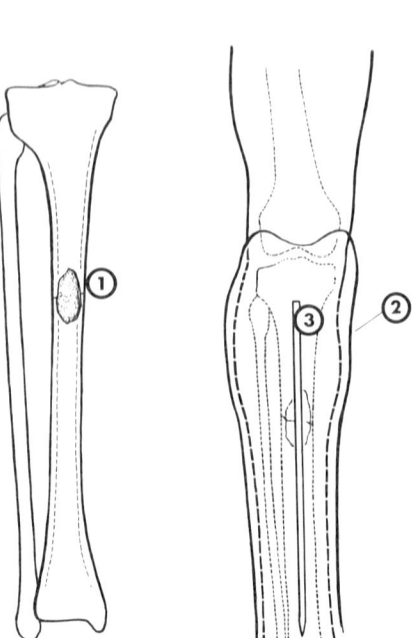

Types and Management of Pathologic Fractures from Metastatic Malignancies *(Continued)*

1. Pathologic fracture from metastatic breast carcinoma to the proximal humerus.
2. Adequate fixation is achieved by Kuntscher nail insertion.

1. Metastatic carcinoma may go to the distal humerus.
2. Fixation of the fracture is accomplished by crossed Rush pins and supplemental methyl methacrylate.

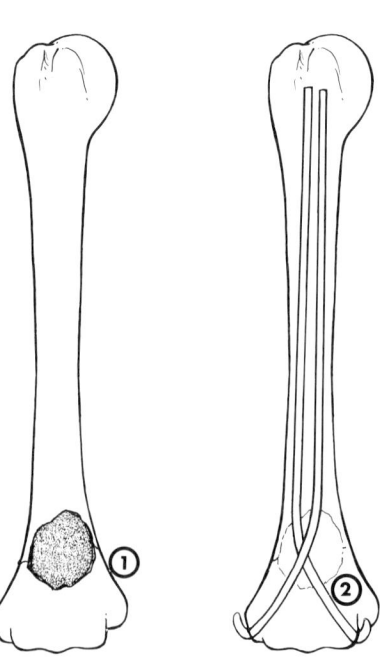

Prophylactic Fixation of Impending Pathologic Fracture

To avoid a fracture in a bone involved by metastatic tumor, Harrington and others have suggested the following criteria for prophylactic internal fixation.

1. A lytic lesion of 2.5 cm or involving 50 per cent of the diameter of the bone.
2. Involvement of the cortex of the bone.
3. A lesion from which a biopsy specimen has been removed.

Note: Lesions that remain persistently painful after radiation treatment also have a high incidence of fracture and should be treated prophylactically.

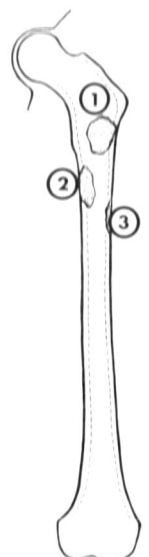

Preferred prophylactic treatment

1. Closed multiple Enders rods or similar intramedullary fixation is inserted under image-intensified fluoroscopy without opening the fracture site.

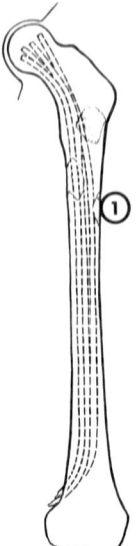

SUMMARY: PITFALLS AND COMPLICATIONS OF BIRTH FRACTURES AND PATHOLOGIC FRACTURES

Fractures evident at birth always unite. The major complication to avoid is overtreatment. It is also important to recognize any underlying congenital or developmental conditions, such as congenital pseudoarthroses or fragile bone disease, which may be contributing to the birth fracture.

Pathologic fractures in older patients result in general from underlying metabolic, developmental, or tumor processes weakening the bone. These demand alertness to the wide range of possible diagnoses. One should avoid treating any fracture routinely without inquiring into the possibility that altered bone structure has led to the fracture.

Osteoporosis, the most prevalent abnormality of bone structure, should be distinguished from other metabolic conditions causing similar weakening of bone. Treatment of the underlying metabolic skeletal aberration is as important as adequate management of the fracture.

Paget's disease, the second most common metabolic bone disease, can be managed medically to decrease the common complications of pathologic fracture and secondary deformity. Early recognition and treatment of Paget's disease with agents such as calcitonin considerably diminish the serious and potential complications from this common disorder. In the past, the management of pathologic fracture in Paget's disease has been complicated owing to failure of fixation, excessive blood loss, or immobilization hypocalcemia. These significant complications can be considerably diminished by an effective combination of medical and surgical management.

Developmental conditions such as osteogenesis imperfecta and fibrous dysplasia are common causes of pathologic fractures and crippling deformities. Recognizing the potential for these deformities is important in order to avoid significant lifelong complications. Internal fixation early in the disease process is especially important to prevent crippling deformities of weight-bearing bones. The use of an intramedullary device such as the Zickel nail or Bailey rod provides effective internal fixation and accommodates for growth.

Other developmental conditions such as bone cysts and fibrous cortical defects sometimes cause pathologic fractures. These conditions demand appreciation of their benign nature and distinction from the more aggressive bone-destroying processes. Pathologic fractures associated with solitary bone cysts may be difficult to manage and prone to recur. Prednisolone injection into the cyst appears to be an effective way of healing the bone lesion and preventing recurrent fracture.

Osteoclastoma is another cause of bone destruction and pathologic fracture that should be respected for its malignant potential. The similarities among osteoclastoma, giant cell tumor reaction (particularly that associated with underlying malignant processes), and aneurysmal bone cysts are important to keep in mind. New therapy, particularly cryotherapy and methyl methacrylate packing of the bone defect, provides effective means of avoiding recurrence of both the tumor and the pathologic fracture.

The possibility that any fracture may occasionally result from either a primary or a secondary malignancy in bone should always be considered before starting treatment. Ablation of the tumor is the chief concern with primary neoplasms. Adequate fracture fixation is the major objective in treating the pathologic fracture with metastasis.

Management of any pathologic fracture, from a metabolic, developmental, or tumor process, demands ingenuity and attention to all potential pitfalls and complications.

REFERENCES

Ahmadi, B., and Steel, H. H.: Congenital pseudarthrosis of the clavicle. Clin. Orthop., 126:130, 1977.
Andersen, K. S.: Congenital pseudarthrosis of the leg. J. Bone and Joint Surg., 58-A:657, 1976.
Anderson, J. T., and Dehner, L. P.: Osteolytic form of Paget's disease. J. Bone and Joint Surg., 43-A:994, 1976.
Barry, H. C.: Sarcoma in Paget's disease of bone in Australia. J. Bone and Joint Surg., 43-A:1122, 1976.
Bassett, C. A. L., Pilla, A. A., and Pawluk, R. J.: A non-operative salvage of surgically resistant pseudoarthroses and non-unions by pulsing electromagnetic fields. Clin. Orthop., 124:128, 1977.
Benson, D. R., Donaldson, D. H., and Millar, E. A.: The spine in osteogenesis imperfecta. J. Bone and Joint Surg., 60-A:925, 1978.
Biesecker, J. L., Marcove, R. C., Huvos, A. G., et al.: Aneurysmal bone cysts. Cancer, 62:615, 1970.
Charnley, J.: Congenital pseudoarthrosis of the tibia treated by the intramedullary nail. J. Bone and Joint Surg., 38-A:283, 1956.

REFERENCES

Connolly, J. F.: Shepherd's crook deformities of polyostotic fibrous dysplasia treated by osteotomy and Zickel nail fixation. Clin. Orthop., 123:22, 1977.

Douglass, H. O., Jr., Shukla, S. K., and Mindell, E.: Treatment of pathological fractures of long bones excluding those due to breast cancer. J. Bone and Joint Surg. 58-A:1055, 1976.

Dove, J.: Complete fractures of the femur in Paget's disease of bone. J. Bone and Joint Surg., 62-B:12, 1980.

Fowles, J. V., and Bobechko, W. P.: Solitary eosinophilic granuloma in bone. J. Bone and Joint Surg., 52-B:238, 1970.

Goldenberg, R. R., Campbell, C. J., and Bonfiglio, M.: Giant-cell tumor of bone. J. Bone and Joint Surg., 52-A:619, 1970.

Harrington, K. D.: The management of malignant pathologic fractures. *In* Instructional Course Lectures, American Academy of Orthopedic Surgeons, 26(16):147, 1977.

Khairi, M. R., and Johnston, C. C. Jr.: Treatment of Paget's disease of bone (osteitis deformans) with sodium etidronate (EHDP). Clin. Orthop., 127:94, 1977.

Krane, S. M.: Paget's disease of bone. Clin. Orthop., 127:24, 1977.

Levy, W. M., Miller, A. S., Bonakdarpour, A., et al.: Aneurysmal bone cyst secondary to other osseous lesions. Am. J. Clin. Pathol., 63:1, 1975.

Lindholm, T. S., Sevastikoglou, J. A., and Lindgren, U.: Interim report on treatment of osteoporotic patients with 1 alpha-hydroxyvitamin D_3 and calcium. Clin. Orthop., 135:232, 1978.

Lloyd-Roberts, G. C., Apley, A. G., and Owen, R.: Reflections upon the aetiology of congenital pseudoarthrosis of the clavicle. J. Bone and Joint Surg., 57-B:24, 1975.

Marafioti, R. L., and Westin, G. W.: Elongating intramedullary rods in the treatment of osteogenesis imperfecta. J. Bone and Joint Surg., 59-A:467, 1977.

Marcove, R. C., and Miller, T. R.: The treatment of primary and metastatic localized bone tumors by cryosurgery. Surg. Clin. North Am., 49:421, 1969.

Marcove, R. S., Weis, L. D., Vaghaiwalla, M. R., et al.: Cryosurgery in the treatment of giant cell tumors of bone. Clin. Orthop., 134:275, 1978.

Marshall, T. R., and Ling, J. T.: The brim sign. Am. J. Roentgenol., 90:1267, 1973.

Meyers, M. H., and Singer, F. R.: Osteotomy for tibia vara in Paget's disease under cover of calcitonin. J. Bone and Joint Surg., 60-A:810, 1978.

Nesbit, M. E., Kieffer, S., and D'Angio, G. J.: Reconstitution of vertebral height in histiocytosis X: a long-term follow-up. J. Bone and Joint Surg., 51-A:1360, 1969.

Persson, B. M., and Wouters, H. W.: Curettage and acrylic cementation in surgery of giant cell tumors of bone. Clin. Orthop., 120:125, 1976.

Peterson, H. A., and Fitzgerald, E. M.: Fractures through nonossifying fibromata in children. Minn. Med., 63:139, 1980.

Pritchard, D. J., Dahlin, D. C., Dauphine, R. T., et al.: Ewings' sarcoma. J. Bone and Joint Surg., 57-A:10, 1975.

Scaglietti, O., Marchetti, P. G., and Bartolozzi, P.: The effects of methylprednisolone acetate in the treatment of bone cysts. J. Bone and Joint Surg., 61-B:200, 1979.

Schlumberger, H. G.: Fibrous dysplasia of single bones (monostotic fibrous dysplasia). The Military Surgeon, 99:504, 1946.

Singer, F. R.: Human calcitonin treatment of Paget's disease of bone. Clin. Orthop., 127:86, 1977.

Singer, F. R., and Mills, B. G.: The etiology of Paget's disease of bone. Clin. Orthop., 127:37, 1977.

Sweet, D. L., Mass, D. P., Simon, M. A., et al.: Histiocytic lymphoma (reticulum-cell sarcoma) of bone. J. Bone and Joint Surg., 63-A:79, 1981.

REFERENCES

Zade, R. E., and Milgram, J. W.: Progression of Paget's disease in the tibia. J. Bone and Joint Surg., 58-A:876, 1976.

Zickel, R. E., Fietti, V. G. Jr., Lawsing, J. F. III, et al.: A new intramedullary fixation device for the distal third of the femur. Clin. Orthop., 125:85, 1977.

Zickel, R. E., and Mouradian, W. H.: Intramedullary fixation of pathological fractures and lesions of the subtrochanteric region of the femur. J. Bone and Joint Surg., 58-A: 1061, 1976.

MULTIPLE TRAUMA: EARLY MANAGEMENT IN THE EMERGENCY DEPARTMENT

IMMEDIATE TREATMENT PRINCIPLES

Place patient on multipurpose stretcher
Undress patient
Examine completely and reexamine frequently
(Initial examination and reexamination by same observer)
Establish priorities for further evaluation and immediate treatment
Resuscitate before moving

Insure adequate airway
Elevate chin (be alert to possible fracture of the cervical spine)
Pull tongue forward, clear secretions, insert nasopharyngeal airway
Intubate trachea if indicated

Stop obvious external hemorrhage
Use direct pressure (tourniquets rarely indicated)
Establish large-bore intravenous lines
Draw blood for crossmatch and analysis

Treat hemorrhagic shock
Administer balanced salt solution first, thereafter blood

Stabilize cervical spine
until fracture or neurologic deficit is ruled out

Monitor and record vital signs and ECG

Take an adequate history
This is vital!

EARLY EVALUATION AND MANAGEMENT (PERFORMED SIMULTANEOUSLY WITH IMMEDIATE TREATMENT)

Splint long-bone fractures

Catheterize bladder
Except if tear of posterior urethra is suspected by
- gross blood at the meatus
- patient's inability to void
- finding, on rectal examination, of a floating prostate

Perform urethrography
Monitor urine volume
Examine for hematuria

Insert CVP (central venous pressure) line at suitable site

Insert nasogastric tube and empty the stomach
Be alert to possible perforated esophagus

Obtain chest x-ray early

Give tetanus prophylaxis if indicated

Give antibiotics if indicated

Record fluids, drugs, and other therapy

Evaluate, record, and follow-up
- level of consciousness
- status of pupils
- function of cranial nerves
- motor power of extremities
- deep-tendon and plantar reflexes

The Committee on Trauma of the American College of Surgeons recognizes that the early management of the patient with multiple trauma will vary depending on facilities available and past experience of the physician. This poster sets forth some basic principles of management that are generally accepted. The following references are recommended for further study:

1. American College of Surgeons/Committee on Trauma: Early Care of the Injured Patient. Philadelphia, W.B. Saunders Company, 1976
2. Hospital Resources for Optimal Care of the Injured Patient. Bulletin of the American College of Surgeons, August, 1979
3. A Guide to Prophylaxis Against Tetanus in Wound Management. Bulletin of the American College of Surgeons, July, 1979

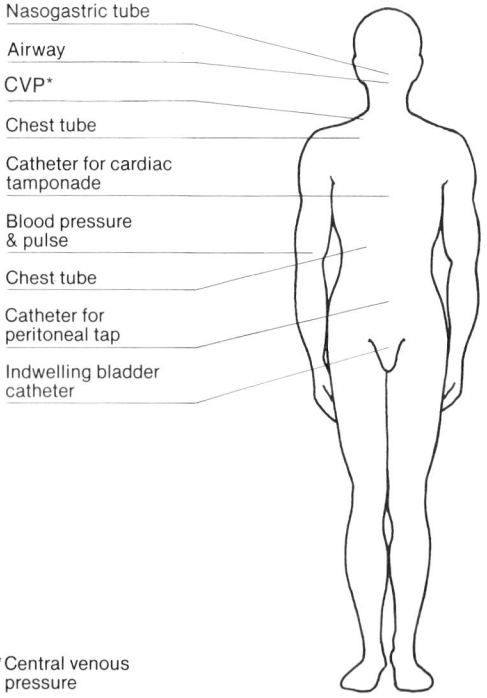

- Nasogastric tube
- Airway
- CVP*
- Chest tube
- Catheter for cardiac tamponade
- Blood pressure & pulse
- Chest tube
- Catheter for peritoneal tap
- Indwelling bladder catheter

*Central venous pressure

OTHER SPECIFIC PRINCIPLES

Thorax

Sucking wounds Seal with sterile, airtight dressing applied at the end of deep expiration

Hemothorax, pneumothorax, penetrating wounds Chest tubes required

Tension pneumothorax Relieve immediately with a needle inserted into pleural cavity, followed by insertion of chest tube
In case of massive airleak, consider ruptured bronchus

Flail chest with paradoxical respirations Probably requires endotracheal tube and ventilatory assistance

Ruptured thoracic aorta Associated with deceleration injuries
Fractured first rib may be a clue
Widened mediastinum seen on x-ray
Aortography required to exclude suspected findings

Ruptured diaphragm X-ray film shows intestines in chest

Cardiac tamponade Decreased blood pressure
Increased CVP (central venous pressure)
Distant heart sounds (chest x-ray may show no enlarged heart)
Treat immediately by pericardiocentesis

Abdomen

Signs of injury often present on physical examination
Peritoneal lavage may be indicated with equivocal findings
Suspect abdominal injury in patients with altered states of consciousness or unexplained hypotension

Gross or microscopic hematuria

Obtain intravenous pyelogram (IVP) and consider cystogram

Restlessness

Probably due to hypoxia or a full bladder

Distal pulse

A distal pulse does not exclude arterial injury

American College of Surgeons
Committee on Trauma
October, 1979

From: Committee on Trauma of the American College of Surgeons: Hospital resources for optimal care of the injured patient. Appendix D. Bull. Am. Coll. Surg., February 1980. Reprinted with permission.

TREATMENT PROTOCOL FOR PREHOSPITAL MANAGEMENT OF THE TRAUMA PATIENT

developed by the American College of Surgeons Committee on Trauma

Prehospital management of the severely injured patient frequently determines the final outcome; it is therefore essential that treatment protocols be established. Management of the severely injured patient begins with the evaluation and treatment by the Emergency Medical Technician-Ambulance (EMT-A), the EMT-Advanced, and the EMT-Paramedic, and continues until the patient is admitted to an appropriate facility.

Ideally, medical decision on categorization will have identified those institutions with the facilities and personnel to best manage patients with specific critical diseases and injuries. Where institutions are so identified, ambulances should bypass those facilities located closest to the accident and take the seriously injured patient directly to the identified center. Where distances are great or where such direct transport is not feasible, the patient should be taken to the closest facility for stabilization and then transferred to a more appropriate institution according to previously established categorization. Such a decision on need for transfer should rest with the physician.

Those dealing with the critically injured patient should routinely quickly evaluate the patient's condition and deal with the life-threatening injuries, followed by reevaluation for less obvious problems. This should be done rapidly so as not to delay the transport of such a patient.

Ambulance attendants should generally:

1. Perform patient triage with emphasis on the cardiorespiratory system, control of bleeding, state of consciousness, and evaluation of vital signs.
2. Contact the local communications center to establish medical control.
    a. Identify self, level of training, and the ambulance unit.
    b. Give patient's name, approximate age, sex, the nature of injury, vital signs, and state of consciousness.

Adapted from: Committee on Trauma of the American College of Surgeons: Hospital resources for optimal care of the injured patient. Appendix D. Bull. Am. Coll. Surg., February 1980. Reprinted with permission.

TREATMENT PROTOCOL FOR PREHOSPITAL MANAGEMENT OF TRAUMA PATIENT

  c. Request specific emergency needs upon arrival at the hospital. Identify specific items in history that may be useful to the physician at the hospital.
3. Where patient's condition is stable and no life-threatening conditions are present, alert the nearest hospital, giving the estimated time of arrival, and proceed there with the patient.

Prehospital Management

EVALUATION OF INJURY AND TRIAGE: PRIORITIES FOR TREATMENT, REGARDLESS OF INJURIES.

1. First priority:
   a. Airway and breathing difficulties.
   b. Cardiac arrest.
   c. Uncontrolled or suspected severe bleeding.
   d. Open chest or abdominal wounds.
   e. Severe shock.
   f. Severe head injuries.
   g. Severe medical problems.
2. Second priority:
   a. Burns.
   b. Major multiple fractures.
   c. Back injuries with or without spinal cord damage.
3. Lowest priority:
   a. Minor fractures or injuries.
   b. Obviously mortal wounds where death appears reasonably certain.

TREATMENT AT THE SCENE

The ABCs (Airway, Breathing, and Circulation) will be addressed for all trauma patients regardless of injury.

1. Airway and breathing difficulty. Note any signs of cyanosis, intercostal retraction, stridor, tachypnea, or other signs of respiratory distress.
   a. Restore the airway. (Remember that patient may have a neck injury.)
      (1) Extend the neck, tilt head backward.
      (2) Draw chin forward.
      (3) Clean out any foreign material in mouth or throat with fingers or suction.
   b. Institute artificial ventilation.
      (1) Mouth-to-mouth.
      (2) Mouth-to-nose or mouth-to-stoma.
      (3) By S-tube, ambu bag, or esophageal airway (where approved by medical control).
   c. For EMT-Advanced or Paramedic: Placement of an endotracheal tube as ordered by a physician.
2. Restore circulation.
   a. By external cardiac compression.
   b. For EMT-Advanced and Paramedic: Monitor electrocardiogram and defibrillate when necessary as ordered by a physician.
3. Administer oxygen.
   a. 100 per cent oxygen flow *except* in patients known to have chronic lung disease.
   b. In the latter case, use oxygen judiciously.
4. Maintain adequate ventilation and circulation.
   a. Resume CPR if necessary.
   b. EMT-Advanced and Paramedic: Monitor and defibrillate as necessary under medical control.
5. Control bleeding.
   a. External bleeding.
      (1) Direct pressure over wound (consider air splints).
      (2) Pressure points.
      (3) Use tourniquet as last resort.
   b. Internal bleeding (treat for shock).
      (1) If an extremity, apply pressure to injury.
      (2) If lower extremity of abdominal chest pelvic, consider MAST trousers.
      (3) Administer oxygen.
   c. Traumatic amputation.

TREATMENT PROTOCOL FOR PREHOSPITAL MANAGEMENT OF TRAUMA PATIENT

(1) Apply pressure dressing to injured.
(2) Use tourniquet as last resort.
(3) Wash dismembered part in normal saline or Ringer's lactate, place in moist sponge, and place in sterile plastic bag. Secure well, place on ice (if available), and transfer with patient.
(4) EMT-Advanced or Paramedic: Medication as ordered for pain (give IV).
(5) Start IV of Ringer's lactate solution with large-bore needle or catheter.

d. Impaled object.
(1) Cut clothing away from wound.
(2) Leave object in place. Support well with dressings to prevent movement and possible further damage.
(3) EMT-Advanced and Paramedic: Start IV of Ringer's lactate and give medication IV as ordered for pain.

6. Treat for shock.
a. Trendelenburg position.
b. MAST trousers.
c. Prevent loss of body heat.
d. EMT-Advanced and Paramedic: Start IV fluids using large-bore needle and Ringer's lactate solution.

7. Manage open chest injuries.
a. Open chest wounds.
(1) Maintain adequate airway and ventilate by whatever means are appropriate and necessary.
(2) Apply vaseline gauze, saran wrap, tape, etc. to seal open wound.
b. Flail chest.
(1) Maintain airway.
(2) Stabilize with sandbags with victim lying on his side if possible.
(3) EMT-Advanced and Paramedic: Endotracheal intubation when appropriate.
c. Treat for shock.
(1) Trendelenburg position.*
(2) MAST trousers may be contraindicated. Use with medical direction only.
(3) Note any cyanosis, intercostal retraction, stridor, tachypnea, or other signs of respiratory distress.
(4) Note any neck vein distention, any shifting of trachea, and any unstable portion of chest wall and treat as above.
(5) EMT-Advanced and Paramedic: Start IV fluids.

8. Manage abdominal injuries.
a. General.
(1) Note any wounds with evisceration. Handle only with wet sterile dressings.
(2) Do not put organs back into abdominal cavity.
(3) Cover any protruding organs with sterile moist gauze.
(4) Note any signs of contusions or abrasions on abdominal wall.
(5) Check for stab wounds, gunshot wounds.
(6) Check for abdominal tenderness.
b. Treat for shock.
(1) Trendelenburg position.*
(2) MAST trousers when not contraindicated.
(3) EMT-Advanced and Paramedic: Start IV fluids.
c. Pelvic injuries.
(1) Feel for areas of tenderness; look for discoloration, such as bruising and ecchymosis.
(2) Palpate pelvis for tenderness.
(3) Maintain in comfortable position. Keep nonambulatory.

*Trendelenburg position modified: patient supine with lower extremities elevated 45 degrees.

9. Manage major multiple fractures.
   a. Straighten severely angulated fractures.
   b. Do not attempt to *push* bones back under skin.
   c. Control bleeding.
   d. Immobilize joints above and below the fracture.
   e. Immobilize dislocated joints.
   f. Apply slight traction during splinting process.
   g. Splint firmly, but not enough to interfere with circulation.
   h. Apply traction splints or MAST trousers when appropriate.
   i. Check all pulses distal to injury before and after splinting.
   j. Apply sterile moist dressing over open wounds before splinting.
   k. In elbow and knee injuries, support well with pillows but do not splint.
   l. EMT-Advanced and Paramedic: IV should be started if fracture involves lower extremity.
10. Manage severe head injuries.
    a. Treat unconscious patient as if neck or spinal cord were injured. Use sandbags, cervical collar or short back board.
    b. Check and record:
       (1) Blood pressure.
       (2) Pulse.
       (3) Pupillary reaction.
       (4) Level of consciousness — AVPU.
          A — Alert
          V — Responds to vocal stimuli
          P — Responds to painful stimuli
          U — Unresponsive
       (5) Ability to move extremities.
       (6) Sensation level.
       (7) Ability to follow commands.
11. Burns — See Section A.
12. Manage back injuries.
    a. If injury to the spinal cord is present or suspected, extricate carefully using spine precautions.
    b. With any back injury, consider as possible cord injury or potential injury and use back board.
    c. Transport.

TRANSPORTATION
1. Destination.
   a. Uncomplicated trauma cases should be transported to the nearest hospital.
   b. All complicated trauma cases should be transported directly to the identified trauma hospital except in rural areas where distances are great. When the distance to such a center is too great, patients should be moved to the closest hospital for stabilization and treatment prior to transfer.
2. Treatment en route.
   a. Transport patient gently and efficiently.
   b. Monitor respiration and circulation — be prepared to support breathing and circulation as necessary.
   c. EMT-Advanced and Paramedic: Attach monitor and be prepared to defibrillate on order of physician when indicated.

BURNS

The management of burns depends on the appraisal of the severity of the injury. Burns may be divided into three levels.

CRITICAL BURNS
1. Burns complicated by respiratory tract injuries.
2. Partial-thickness burns of more than 20 per cent of the body surface.
3. Full-thickness burns of more than 10 per cent of the body surface.
4. Burns of the hands, feet, face, or genitalia.

5. Burns complicated by fractures or major soft-tissue injury.
6. Electrical burns.
7. Deep acid burns.

MODERATE BURNS

1. Partial-thickness burns of less than 20 per cent of the body surface.
2. Full-thickness burns of less than 2 per cent of the body surface, provided that the hands, feet, or genitalia are not involved.

MINOR BURNS

1. Partial-thickness burns of less than 15 per cent of the body surface.
2. Full-thickness burns of less than 2 per cent of the body surface that may be treated on an outpatient basis until the patient needs to be hospitalized for skin grafting.

In addition, the age and general physical condition of the patient may indicate that burns of smaller extent should be considered critical, i.e., patients over 50 or children 5 years of age or under.

Evaluation of Burn Injury

1. Depth and type of burn (electrical, chemical, flash).
2. Area of involvement (rule of 9s and anatomic area – mark on chart).
3. Pulmonary involvement, soft-tissue injury, and fractures.
4. Age, sex, general health of the patient.

Burn Management

Patients with burns in the critical category should be transferred to an identified burn center for their area.

PREHOSPITAL PROTOCOL

1. Initial assessment – assure airway, breathing, circulation and observe for subtle signs of respiratory tract burns, such as nasal and oropharyngeal burns and abnormal breathing sounds.
2. Administer oxygen by nasal cannula (4–6 liters/minute).
3. Remove clothing from burned areas, but do not remove any loose skin or tissue.
4. Observe for associated injuries – fractures, major soft tissue wounds.
5. Assess the extent of the burn (first, second, or third degree). Note type of burn (explosion, flame, hot liquids, electrical, or chemical).
6. Cover area with sterile sheets.
7. If burn is greater than 20 per cent of the body surface and an EMT-Advanced or Paramedic is aboard the ambulance, begin IV administration of Ringer's lactate solution through large-bore cannula on order of a physician. (Should not be started in a burned area.)
8. Obtain medical direction for instructions regarding:
   a. IV flow rate.
   b. Special instructions for respiratory distress.
   c. Special instructions for children with burns.
9. Transport to nearest qualified emergency room.

PRETRANSFER PROTOCOL

This is the treatment given at the local hospital prior to transfer to a burn center.

1. Patent airway. If patient has suffered burns of face or neck, insert oral airway or endotracheal tube to assure airway during transport.
2. Oxygen per nasal cannula as necessary. Remove all clothing and jewelry, especially rings.
3. Wrap patient in sterile sheets. *Do not* apply creams or ointments. *Do not* debride wound.
4. Administer Ringer's lactate or normal saline with large-bore needle (if

not already started in prehospital phase). IV should not be started in burned area. If a burned area must be used, a cutdown should be done.
5. Insert Foley catheter. Urine output should be closely monitored and maintained at approximately 30 ml/hour in adults.
6. If adult with over 30 per cent body burn, insert No. 18 nasogastric tube.
7. Keep patient NPO.
8. Administer pain medication as necessary IV. (IM medications are poorly absorbed and may be suddenly mobilized as tissue perfusion improves).

TRANSPORTATION

1. Consult with physician in burn unit prior to transfer.
2. Send adequate records.
3. Transport with adequately qualified personnel and equipment.

PNEUMATIC COUNTER-PRESSURE DEVICE

Theory

Just as leg elevation is effective in resuscitating simple fainting, and the G-suit is effective in preventing blackout from centrifugal force in high-performance aircraft, so pneumatic counter-pressure trousers can mobilize blood from the lower extremities and abdomen and return it to the heart-brain-lung circulation for temporary resuscitation without excessive crystalloid replacement. Since 80 per cent of blood is located in the capillary and venous circulation, approximately 30 per cent of cardiovascular volume can be mobilized and used.

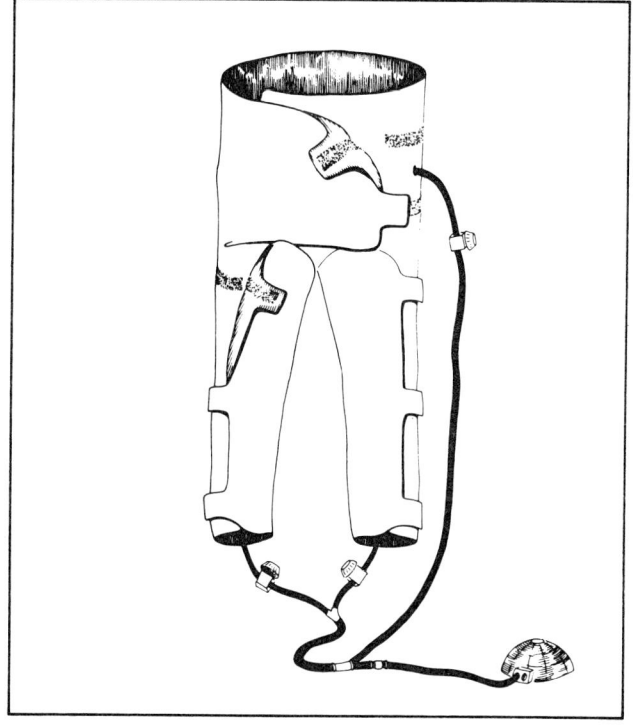

Indications

1. Systolic blood pressure below 100 when shocklike state exists. Hemorrhage control from fractured pelvis or intra-abdominal bleeding.
2. Stabilization of fractured pelvis or femur.

The material in this appendix is modified from Pneumatic Counter-Pressure Device, by Norman E. McSwain, Jr., M.D., F.A.C.S., published by the American College of Surgeons Committee on Trauma (Chicago, 1979). It is reprinted here with the kind permission of Dr. McSwain and the American College of Surgeons.

CAUTION

1. During later stages of pregnancy, only the leg segment is inflated.
2. Deflation must be done gradually and carefully. Rapid deflation can return the patient to shock.
3. Avoid applying air splints for more than two hours to swollen, fractured limbs, or compartmental syndromes may result.

Contraindications

Pulmonary edema.

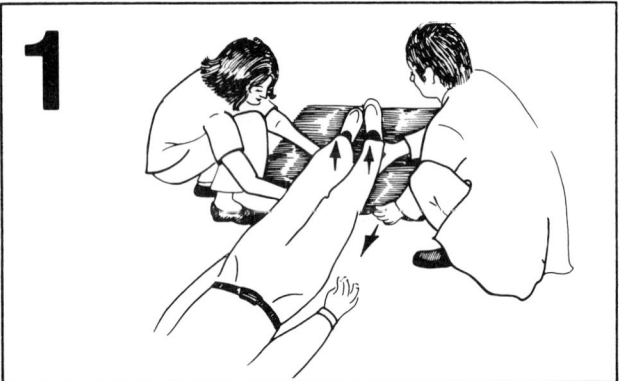

Application

1. Slide open trousers beneath raised feet.

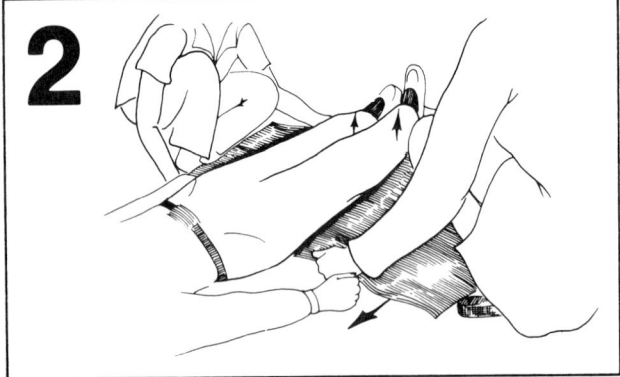

2. To the buttocks.

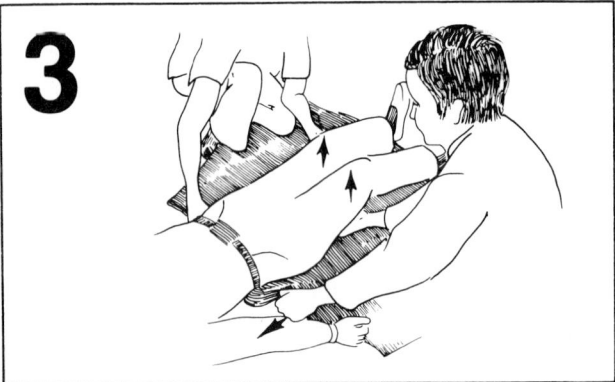

3. Elevate buttocks and bring trousers up to the rib cage.

4. Enclose left leg and close Velcro.

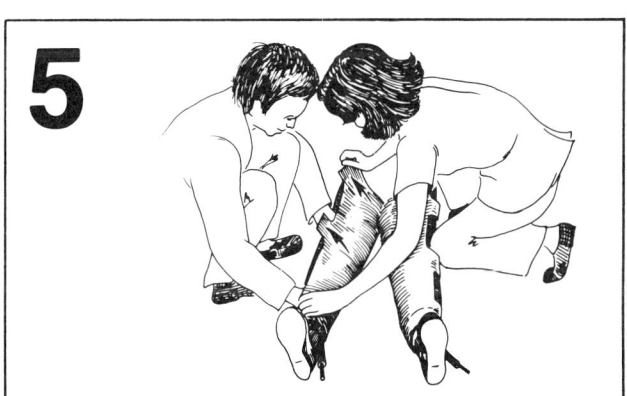

5. Enclose right leg and close Velcro.

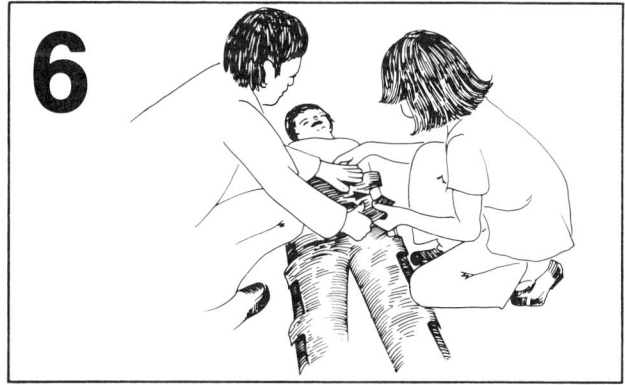

6. Enclose abdomen and close Velcro.

PNEUMATIC COUNTER-PRESSURE DEVICE

Application (Continued)

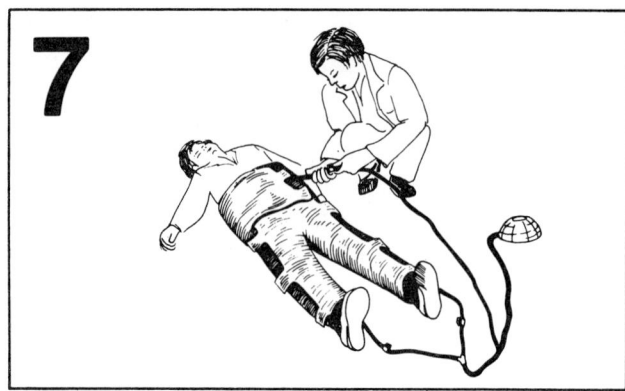

7. Open stopcocks.

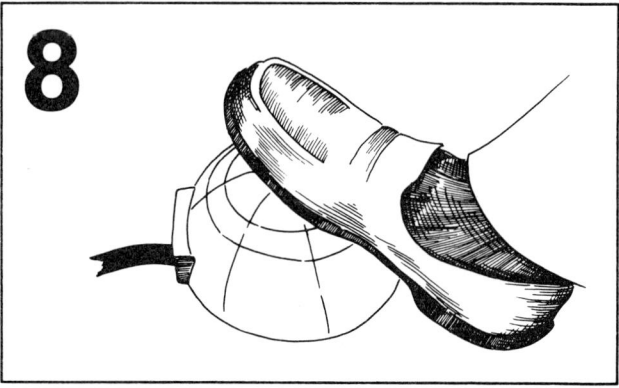

8. Inflate with foot pump.

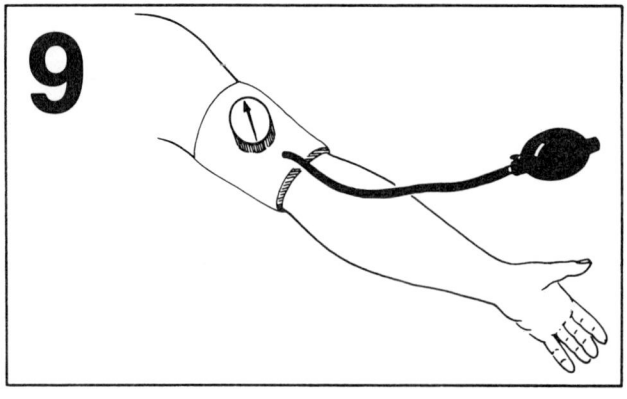

9. Check blood pressure. Stop inflation at 100 mm Hg.

10. Velcro straps, pop-off valves, or gauges prevent overinflation.

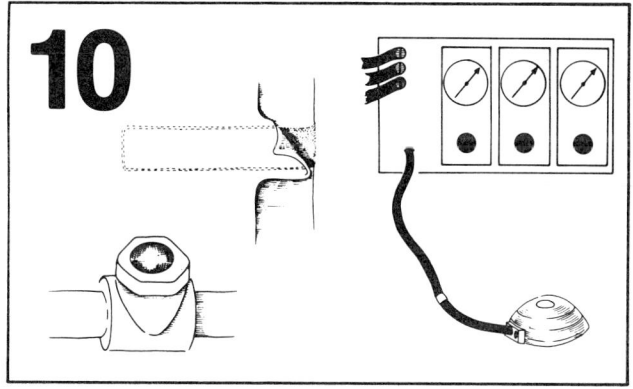

11. Close stopcocks.

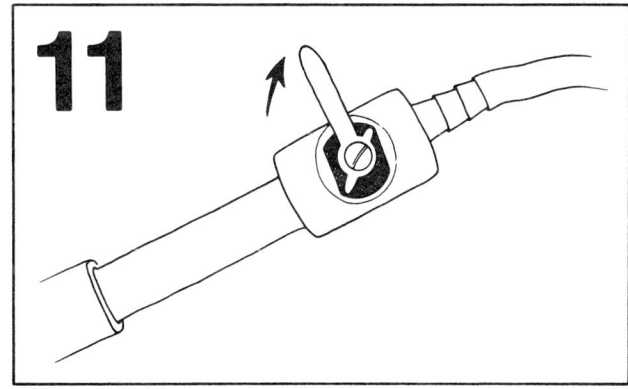

12. The device can be left in place fully inflated for two hours if necessary. If a longer period of inflation is necessary, alterations and additions should be considered.

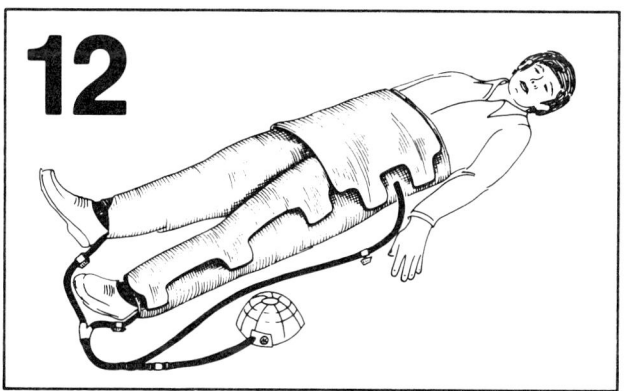

Gradual Deflation

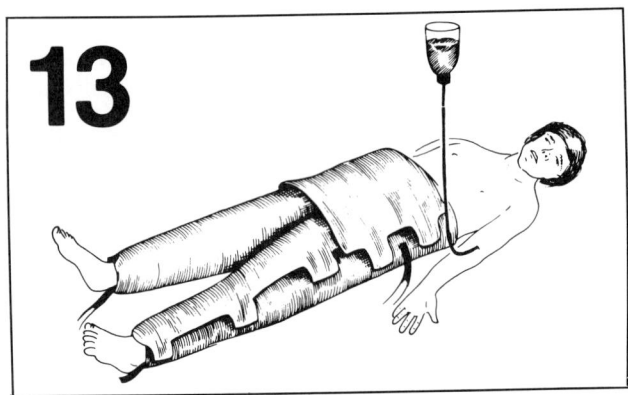

Warning: Rapid deflation can return patient to shock.
13. Intravenous lines are established and operating room is readied.

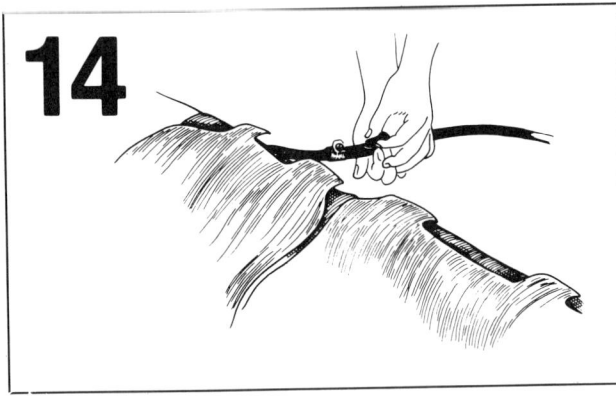

14. Open stopcock on abdominal section.

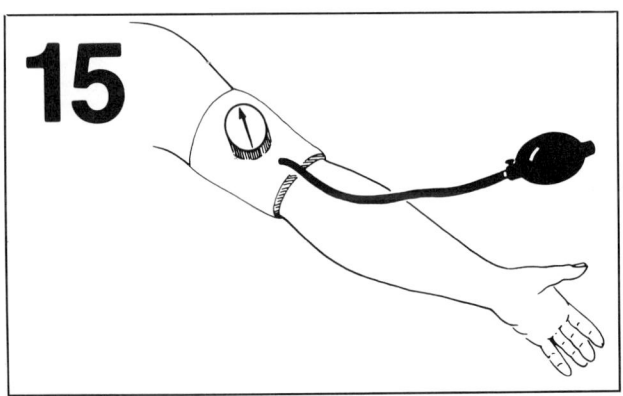

15. Stop deflation if blood pressure drops 5 mm Hg.

16. Administer intravenous fluid to restore blood pressure.

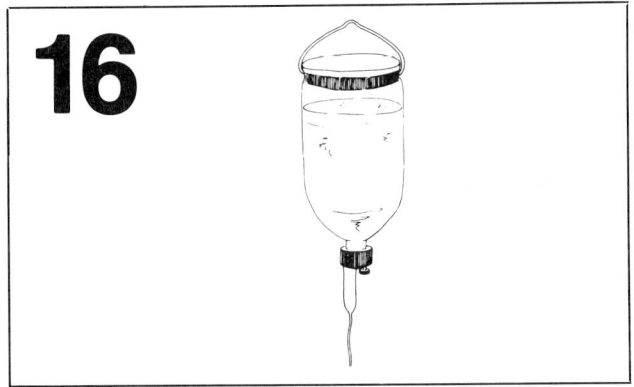

17. Deflation can continue while blood pressure is closely monitored. Patient can be taken to the operating room with the device inflated, if necessary.

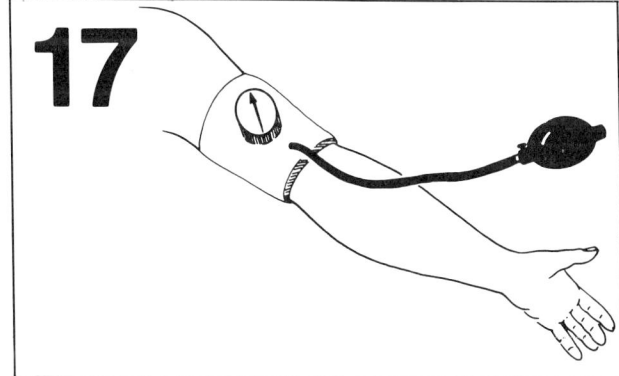

Summary

Application of the pneumatic compression device on the abdomen and legs transfers a significant volume of blood into the heart-brain-lung circulation. Although the lower extremities and abdomen may be partially deprived of blood supply, for this short period of time (less than two hours), no detrimental effect has been shown.

The major complication that has arisen with the application of a pneumatic compression device is its too rapid removal in the emergency room without proper volume replacement.

Deflation must be slow and gradual. Rapid deflation reduces the blood volume in the heart-brain-lung circulation and can return the patient to a shocklike state.

Important aspects during inflation, then, are monitoring of the blood pressure and inflating only as necessary to return the pressure to within acceptable limits. *On deflation, the hallmark again is blood pressure monitoring to prevent recurrence of shock.* Blood pressure is the single most important factor in the use of the pneumatic pressure device for treating patients in shock.

INDEX

Abscess, retroperitoneal, pelvic fractures and, 495
Acetabulum. See also *Hip joint*.
  development of, 1335
  dislocations and fracture-dislocations of, 1261–1364
  fractures of, 1335–1360
    bursting, 1348
      with displacement or comminution, 1351
      without displacement, 1349
    chronic hip dislocation with, 1313
    linear, 1337–1338
    pitfalls and complications of, 1361–1363
      chronic, 1362
    radiographic assessment of, 1272
    with chronic displacement of femoral head, 1359–1360
  injury of, mechanisms of, 1336
  inner wall of, fracture of, 1343–1347
    with intrapelvic protrusion of femoral head, 1345
  posterior, fractures of, 1339–1343
    comminuted, 1340
    types of, 1340
    with large fragment or posteriorly unstable hip, 1342
  rim of, fracture of, 1340
    hip dislocations with, 1266, 1283, 1285
    femoral shaft fracture, 1307
  superior dome of, fractures of, 1347–1359
    mechanism of, 1348
    operative fixation of, 1353
    with displacement or comminution, 1351
    with several fragments, 1358
    with single fragment, 1357
    without displacement, 1349
Acromioclavicular joint
  arthritis of, 555
  dislocation of, 547
    old, 554
  sprain of, 546
  subluxation of, 547
Acromioclavicular ligaments
  injury of, direct, 546
    indirect, 547
    mechanisms of, 546
  lesions of, 545–557
Acromioclavicular support, 550
Acromion, fractures of, 566
    and subcoracoid dislocation, 663
    retraction of greater tuberosity of humerus under, 695, 697

Adolescents
  epiphyseal or ligamentous knee injuries in, 1566
  fracture of clavicle in, 529
  fracture of tibial epiphysis in, 1890
  soft tissue repair of patellar instability in, 1675
  upper femoral epiphyseal separation in, 204–206
Adults. See also *Elderly*.
  avulsion fractures of tibial tuberosity in, 1659–1662
  compression fractures in, 10
  displaced fractures of ulna in, 934–937
  fracture of anatomic neck of humerus in, 716
  fracture of capitellum in, 778–781
    shear, 745
    types of, 779
  fracture of clavicle in, 529
  fracture of forearm bones in, epidemiology of, 896
    lower, 2-bone, 914
    upper, 2-bone, 908
  fracture of radial head and neck in, 858–869
  fracture of lower humerus in, 740
    reduction of, 770
  Monteggia fracture in, operative management of, 973–977
Age. See also *Children; Adults*
  and degenerative alterations of glenohumeral joint, 592
  and prognosis for physeal injuries, 153
Airway, in trauma patient, 2138, 2141
Ambulance, management of trauma patient in, 2140
Anaerobic infection, after open fractures, 129–132
Anconeus muscle, lateral, in Monteggia fracture, 973
Anesthesia
  for anterior cord syndrome, 355
  for fracture treatment, 114
  for reduction of posterior dislocation of elbow joint, 793
  for reduction of simple dislocation of metacarpophalangeal joint of thumb, 1178
  for reduction of 2-bone fractures of upper forearm, 909
  regional intravenous, for Colles' fracture, 1011
  for upper limb fractures, 114
Aneurysmal bone cyst, and pathologic fractures, 2114
Angular deformities, 51–54

i

INDEX

Ankle joint. See also specific parts.
  anatomy of, 1802–1806
  arthrodesis of. See *Arthrodesis, ankle*.
  bones of, 1803
  derotational osteotomy of, 1780
  diastasis of, and Maisonneuve fracture of proximal fibula, 1884
    transosseous screw fixation in, 1884
  dislocations of, 1916–1930
    anterior, 1918–1920
    lateral, 1921–1922
    posterior, 1916–1918
  flexion and extension of, widening of mortise with, 1803
  fracture-dislocations of, 1916–1922
    malunited, 1939–1946
    open, 1931–1938
    posterior, and vascular impairment, 1926
    irreducible, 1924
  fractures of, 1835–1886
    management of, 1841–1882
      based on classification and staging, 1843
    open, 1931–1938
      unstable, reduction and stabilization of, 1936
    pronation-abduction, 1837
      stages of, 1840
    pronation-dorsiflexion, differential diagnosis of, 1900
    pronation-external rotation, 1836, 1840
    supination-adduction, 1837
      stages of, 1839
    supination-external rotation, 1836
      stages of, 1839
    trimalleolar, gravity-assisted reduction of, 113
  injuries of, 1801–1949
    mechanisms of, 1802–1808
    pitfalls in managing, 1947–1948
    pronation-dorsiflexion, 1898–1915
      explosion, 1903
  instability of, anterior, 1830
    lateral, 1809, 1819, 1827
  ligaments of. See *Ligament(s), of ankle*.
  radiographic examination of, 103
  sprains of, 1801–1949
    acute, evaluation and management of, 1809–1834
    balancing exercises after, 1814, 1822, 1832
    grade I, 1812
    grade II, 1815
    grade III, 1816
      operative repair of, 1820
    initial evaluation of, 1809
    mechanisms of, 1806–1808
    selection of treatment for, 1812–1824
  varus deformity of, correction of, 255–256
Ankle mortise, 1802
  reduction and restoration of, 1842
  widening of, 1803, 1922
Ankylosis. See *Arthrodesis*.
Annular ligament, disruption of, in Monteggia fracture, 974
  reconstruction of, 975
Anterior cord syndrome, anterior decompression and cervical spine fusion in, 355–362
  bursting teardrop fractures of cervical spine and, 352–354
Antibiotics, in open fractures, 1754
Arch(es)
  carpal, proximal, disruption of, 1112–1113
  coracoacromial, rotator muscles under, 589
  longitudinal and transverse, of hand, 1054, 1139
  pelvic, 461
Arizona, University of, wrist arthroplasty, 1079
Arm. See also *Forearm*; and specific parts.
  arterial injuries in, diagnosis of, 828
  arterial thrombosis in, management of, 61
  fractures of, birth, 2083–2085
    intravenous regional anesthesia for, 114
  joint stiffness of, prevention of, 87
Arteriospasm, of brachial artery, 834
Artery(ies). See also *Blood vessels*.
  arm, injury of, diagnosis of, 828
    thrombosis of, management of, 61
  avulsion of, 59
  axillary, injury to, in glenohumeral dislocations, 642–644
  brachial, arteriospasm of, 834
    management of, in ischemia, 833
  dorsalis pedis, in posterior fracture-dislocation of ankle, 1926
  in pelvic fracture, 462, 483
  injury to, fracture management after, 69
  tibial shaft fractures and, 1793
  laceration of, 59
    common sites of, 63
    complete, from arterial avulsion, 59
    partial, 59
  ligamentum teres, in femoral neck fractures, 1418
  popliteal, in dislocation of knee, 1620
  thrombosis of, 60
    common sites for, 63
    in upper limb, management of, 61
Arthritis
  acromioclavicular, 555
  degenerative, ankle instability and, 1809, 1819, 1827
    hyperextension of cervical spine with, and central cord syndrome, 365–366
    of subtalar and tibiotalar joints, 2000–2004
  patellofemoral, chronic patellar dislocation or subluxation with, 1677
  post-traumatic, 93–95
    carpal, 1077, 1082
    common sites of, 94
    of hip joint, 1362
    treatment of, 95
  rheumatoid, with dislocation of atlas, 283
Arthrodesis
  ankle, 1883
    anterior, 1942
    compression, 1945
    for explosion fracture, 1911
    in malunited fracture-dislocations, 1941
  hip, DePalma, in malunited upper femoral epiphyseal slip, 215
  in old posterior glenohumeral dislocations, 636
  midtarsal, 2050
  subtalar and triple, after calcaneal fractures, 2030
  tibiotalar, 2001
  wrist, in chronic post-traumatic carpal arthritis, 1077, 1082

INDEX

Arthrography
  knee, 1559
  shoulder, 607
    in rotator cuff rupture, 647
  single-contrast, in knee injuries, 1559, 1567
Arthroplasty
  prosthetic. See *Prosthesis*.
  resectional, in fractures of head and neck of humerus, in glenohumeral dislocations, 661
  of elbow, for old unreduced dislocations, 844
Arthrotomy, of knee injuries, 1693
Articulations
  atlanto-axial, dislocation of, with fracture of odontoid, 288
  of clavicle, ligamentous injuries to, 545–565
  of lower cervical spine, 264
  of occiput, axis, and atlas, 263
Atlanto-axial joint
  anatomy of, after severe hyperflexion injury, 283
    normal, 283
  articulations of, dislocation of, with fracture of odontoid, 288
  dislocation of, traumatic forward, 282
  motion of, 265
  rotatory fixation of, 286
  subluxation of, rotatory, 286
    unilateral, 315–318
Atlanto-occipital joint, dislocations of, 306–309
  motion of, 265
Atlanto-odontoid fracture-dislocation, 331–333
Atlas
  articulations of, 263
  dislocation of
    posterior, with fracture of odontoid, 288
    traumatic forward, 319–325
      with fracture of odontoid, 288, 323–325
      without fracture of odontoid, 319–322
      with congenital or acquired odontoid abnormalities, 285
      with rheumatoid arthritis, 283
  fracture of, 310–311
    compression, 271
Atrophy, bone, 88–89
  muscle, and subluxation, 7
Avascular necrosis. See *Necrosis, avascular*.
Avulsion fractures, 12
  mallet finger with, 1214
  of cervical spine, 368
  of glenoid, with recurrent shoulder subluxation, 575
  of greater tuberosity of humerus, in glenohumeral dislocation, 652
  of iliac spine, 197
    anterior superior or inferior, 472
  of lesser trochanter, 1368
  of lesser tuberosity of humerus, 700
  of navicular bone, 2032
  of patella with dislocation, 1643
  of pelvis, 467, 472–474
  of thumb, 1182
  of tibial spine, 1609–1612
  of tibial tuberosity, 1617
    in adults, 1659–1662
  of tuberosity of ischium, 198, 473
Avulsion injuries
  and isolated posterior articular fracture of tibia, 1914–1915

Avulsion injuries (*Continued*)
  arterial, 59
  of apophysis of tibial tuberosity, 1612–1619
  of humeral epicondyle, 179–183
  of lumbosacral nerve root, 1291
  of patellar tendon, 1654–1658
Axillary artery, injury to, in glenohumeral dislocations, 642–644
Axillary nerve, 594
  injury to, in glenohumeral dislocations, 645
Axillary view, in acute posterior glenohumeral dislocation, 632
Axis, articulations of, 263
  odontoid process of. See *Odontoid process*.

Balancing exercises, after ankle sprain, 1814, 1822, 1832
Bandage, elastic, in grade I ankle sprains, 1813
  in tear of distal tibiofibular ligament, 1826
Barton's fracture, 1028–1032
  reverse, 1032
Barton's fracture-dislocation, 1028
  comminuted, 1029
Basilar fracture, of femoral neck, 1443–1444
Bayonet apposition, of femoral shaft fractures, 1486
Bennett's fracture, 1159–1163
Biceps tendon, graft of, in rotator cuff rupture, 649
  in irreducible fresh dislocation of glenohumeral joint, 625
Bicipital tendon, injury of, in fractures of upper humerus, 703
Bicipital tuberosity, in evaluation of rotational alignment of forearm, 892
Bicondylar fractures of tibia, 1714–1718
  fibula in, 1714
Bimalleolar fractures, 1872
  with lateral displacement of talus, 1873
  with medial displacement of talus, 1874
Binder, in fractures and dislocations of ribs, 504
Birth
  blood supply of femoral head and neck at, 1264
  distal femoral epiphyseal separation at, 220–221
  epiphyseal separation of lower humerus at, 184–185
  upper humeral epiphyseal seaparation at, 156–157
Birth fractures, 2081–2137
  causes of, 2087
  of arm, 2083–2085
  of clavicle, 2084
  of leg, 2085–2086
  of long bones, 2083–2087
  pitfalls and complications of, 2134–2135
Blair tibiotalar fusion, 2001
Bleeding, intrathoracic, 511
Blocker's shoulder, 92
Blood pressure, monitoring of, with pneumatic counter-pressure device, 2149
Blood supply
  changes in, femoral neck fractures with, 1417, 1421
  epiphyseal, and prognosis for physeal injuries, 154
  epiphyseal-metaphyseal, 145–147

iii

Blood supply (*Continued*)
  impairment of, in posterior ankle
      fracture-dislocations, 1926
    in supracondylar fracture of humerus, 831
  in bone, and fracture healing, 17–19
  in trauma patient, 2138, 2141
  of femoral head, 1263, 1418
    at birth, 1264
    at 3 years, 1265
    technetium-99m sulfur-colloid in evaluation
        of, 1452
  of femoral neck, 1263
    at birth, 1264
    at 3 years, 1265
  of scaphoid, 1060
  of talus, 1993
  of tibia, 1730
Blood vessels. See also *Artery(ies)*.
  femoral, in anterior hip dislocation, 1318
  injuries of
    direct, 827
    fractures and dislocations of elbow joint and,
        826–835
    fractures of clavicle and, 540
    fractures of lower humerus and, 747
    supracondylar fracture of humerus and, 831
  large, injuries to, 58
  near glenohumeral joint, 593–594
  of knee, 1622
  retinacular, in femoral neck fractures, 1417
Blood volume, restoration of, in shock, 80
Blount method, for distal radial and ulnar
      fractures, 985
  for fractures of mid-third of forearm, 995
  for fractures of proximal forearm, 1000
Böhler clamp, 2026
Böhler's angle, 2014
Bone
  aneurysmal cyst of, and pathologic fractures,
      2114
  circulation in, and fracture healing, 17–19
  decontamination of, 127
  diseased, compression fractures in, 11
  exposed, 1753
  fragments of, degree of displacement of, and
      healing, 27
  growth of, electrical stimulation of, 33, 494
      in nonunion of tibial shaft fractures, 1785
    stimulation of, 56–57
  healing of. See *Malunion; Nonunion;* and
      Union.
  ischemic necrosis of, 47–51
    common sites of, 48
    pathology of, 48
  loss of, with nonunion, 32
  Paget's disease of, and pathologic fractures,
      2092
  shortening of, 54–56
    examples of, 54
  solitary cyst of, and pathologic fractures, 2111
  solitary eosinophilic granuloma of, 2119
  Sudeck's acute atrophy of, 88–89
  tumors of, benign, and pathologic fracture,
      2116–2133
    malignant, and pathologic fractures, 2094,
        2116–2133
      primary, and pathologic fractures, 2124

Bone graft
  after cervical laminectomy, 372
  autogenous
    in tibial shaft fractures, 1762
      infected nonunion of, 42, 1791
      unstable nonunion of, 1786
    procedures for, 34, 43
  cancellous, application of, 35
    in segmented tibial shaft fractures, 1776
  iliac crest, 943
    in anterior cervical disc fusion, 391
    in anterior cord syndrome, 360
    in chronic acetabular disruption, 1360
    in displaced femoral neck fractures, 1439
    in nonunion of scaphoid, 1069
    in split-depression lateral tibial plateau
        fractures, 1711–1713
    in wiring of cervical vertebra dislocation, 343
  peg, 37
    in infected nonunion of tibia, 43
  plug, interbody, in anterior cervical spine
      fusion, 384
Bone peg grafts, 37
  in infected nonunion of tibia, 43
Bone plugs, interbody, in anterior cervical spine
    fusion, 384
Bone scan, in femoral neck fractures, 1423, 1452
Bosworth fracture, 1924
Boutonnière deformity, 75, 1149, 1156, 1217
  reverse, 1150
Brace, functional. See also *Cast-brace,
    functional*.
  sleeve, in fracture of ulna, 907
    in humeral shaft fractures, 721, 729
Brachial artery, arteriospasm of, 834
  management of, in ischemia, 833
Brachial plexus, injury to, in glenohumeral
    dislocations, 645
Breathing difficulty, in flail chest, 517
  in shock, 80
  in trauma patient, 2141
Brighton technique, of electrical osteogenesis, 33,
    1494, 1785
Brooks' technique of C1-C2 fusion, 321
Bryant traction, in distal femoral epiphyseal
    separation at birth, 221
  in femoral shaft fractures in children, 1506
  in subtrochanteric fractures, 1402
Buck's traction in intertrochanteric fracture,
    1374, 1376
Burns, prehospital management of, 2143
Bursting fractures. See *Compression fractures*.
Burwell and Charnley management of lateral
    malleolus fracture, 1851
Buttress plate, in Barton's fracture, 1029

Calcaneocuboid joint, fractures and
    fracture-dislocations of, 2045
Calcaneus
  fractures of, 2005–2030
    early mobilization after, 2018, 2021
    isolated, 2005–2011
      horizontal, 2009
      vertical, 2007
    joint depression type, 2013

INDEX

Calcaneus (*Continued*)
   fractures of, late complications of, 2027–2030
      management of, 2016–2027
      pathomechanics of, 2012
      tongue type, 2013, 2020
         displaced, 2025
      with implication of subtalar joint, 2011–216
   normal architecture of, 2012
   radiographic examination of, 104
Calcaneus traction, in comminuted fracture of inferior articular surface of tibia, 1909
Calcification, in tibial collateral ligament, 1579
Callus, excess, at site of fracture of clavicle, 540
   external or periosteal, formation of, 15
Campbell technique for old unreduced elbow joint dislocations, 841
Capitate bone
   anatomy of, 1115
   fracture of, 1115–1120
      dorsal perilunate dislocation with, 1101
      isolated, 1117
      mechanism of, 1116
      with carpal injuries, 1120
Capitate-scaphoid fracture, 1118
Capitellum, fracture of, 163–168
   in adult, 778–781
      types of, 779
      shear, 779
   in adults, 745
Capsule and capsular structures
   glenohumeral, 590–592
      injuries of, 587–683
   medial, of knee, and posterior cruciate tears, 1565
      operative repair of, 1571
   of interphalangeal joints of fingers, 1143
Carpal arch, proximal, disruption of, 1112–1113
Carpal bones. See also *Wrist*; and specific bones.
   anatomy of, 1052
   arthritis of, chronic post-traumatic, 1077, 1082
   dislocations and subluxations of, 1085
   fractures of, 1115–1129
   fractures and dislocations of, 1052–1058
      dorsal perilunate dislocation with, 1099–1102
      mechanisms of injury of, 1085
      normal relationships of, 1085
      stability of, 1057
Carpal tunnel, 1056
Carpal tunnel syndrome, 1131
Carpal tunnel view, of fracture of hook of hamate, 1125
Carpometacarpal joint(s)
   of fingers, 1190–1195
      dislocations of, 1191
      fracture-dislocations of, 1193
   of thumb
      dislocations of, unstable 1165–1168
      fracture-dislocation of, 1159–1163
      subluxation of, 1164–1165
      unstable, 1165–1168
Carpus. See also *Wrist*.
   dislocations and subluxations of, 1103–1114
   dislocation of metacarpal bones on, 1109–1110
   distal row of, disruption of, 1112–1113
   injuries of, fracture of capitate with, 1120
      neurologic complications of, 1130–1133
      pisiform fracture with, 1123

Carpus (*Continued*)
   proximal row of, disruption of, 1111
   scaphoid bone of. See *Scaphoid, carpal*.
Cartilages, costal, fractures and dislocations of, 506–508
Cast, plaster. See *Plaster cast*.
Cast wedging, in unstable tibial shaft fractures, 1746
Cast-brace, functional
   application of, 119
   in anterior cruciate ligament repair, 1596
   in anterolateral instability of knee, 1588
   in bicondylar and spinotuberosity fractures of tibia, 1717
   in displaced lateral tibial plateau fracture, 1705
   in femoral shaft fractures, 1460, 1467
      with tibial fracture, 1484
   in fracture of proximal radius, 925
   in fracture of radius, 905
   in grade III knee injuries, 1578
   in posterior cruciate ligament repair, 1602
   in subtrochanteric fractures, 1404
   in supracondylar fractures, 1515, 1520, 1524
   in 2-bone fractures of forearm, 912, 916, 944, 953
Cast-splint, in phalangeal or metacarpal fracture, 1157
Castle method, for infected open forearm fractures, 957
Cathcart prosthesis, in femoral neck fracture-dislocation, 1301
   in femoral neck fractures, 1425, 2095
Cauchoix and De Oliveira technique, for Barton's fracture, 1029
Caudal vertebra, chip of bone from, 377
Central cord syndrome, 275
   hyperextension of cervical spine with osteoarthritis and, 365–366
Cervical disc
   acute protrusion of, management of, 378–381
   collapsing, 376
   degenerative changes in, 377
   excision of, in anterior cervical spine fusion, 389
   exposure of, in anterior cervical spine fusion, 386
   injuries of, management of, 373–392
      radiographic features of, 376–378
   localization of, in anterior cervical spine fusion, 388
Cervical laminectomy, and cervical instability, 289
   posterior fusion following, 370–372
Cervical soft tissue, injuries of, management of, 373–392
Cervical spine
   anatomy of, 261–266
   contents of, 264
   dislocation of, backward, without disruption of osseous elements, 363–364
      management of, 303–305
      pitfalls of, 397–398
   emergency splinting of, 106, 291
   fracture-dislocations of
      hyperextension and compression, 366–369
      hyperflexion, 348–351
      management of, 303–305

INDEX

Cervical spine (*Continued*)
  fractures of
    bursting teardrop, and anterior cord syndrome, 352–354
    pitfalls of, 397–398
    radiographic examination of, 101
    simple compression, 345–348
  hyperextension of, with osteoarthritis, causing central cord syndrome, 365–366
  injuries of, 259–398
    emergency room treatment of, 292
    emergency treatment of, 290–302
    epidemiology of, 260
    extension, management of, 363–369
    flexion, management of, 345–362
    functional levels of, 395
    hyperflexion, 268–271
    indications for delayed surgery in, 305
    indications for immediate surgery in, 304
    lateral flexion, 281
    management of, goals of, 304
      rehabilitative, 393–396
    mechanisms of, 267–289
    radiographic evaluation of, 293–297
      in children, 296
    skull traction in, 298–302
    with sensory impairment, halo-pelvic hoop in, 302
  instability of, iatrogenic causes of, 289
  intervertebral disc of. See *Cervical disc.*
  lower, articulations of, 264
  motion of, 265–266
  subluxations of, management of, 303–305
    radiographic examination of, 101
  upper, injuries to, 282–289
    hyperextension-compression, 277
Cervical spine fusion
  anterior, bone graft in, 391
    interbody bone plugs in, 384
    in anterior cord syndrome, 355–362
    in traumatic forward dislocation of atlas, 320
  posterior, following laminectomies, 370–372
    in dislocation of cervical vertebra, 339–344
    indications for, 347
Cervical spinous processes, fracture of, 446
Cervical syndrome, chronic, management of, 382–392
Cervical vertebra(e)
  dislocation of, bilateral, 334–344
    open reduction, wiring, and posterior cervical fusion in, 339–344
    unilateral, 334–344
  hypermobile changes in, 378
  wiring of, 371
Cervicotrochanteric fractures, in children, 1447
Chance fracture, and visceral injury, 76
Charcot foot, 2050
Charnley technique, in compression arthrodesis of ankle, 1945
  in congenital pseudoarthrosis of tibia, 2107
Chauffeur's fracture, 926
Chest. See also *Thoracic cage.*
  bleeding in, 511
  flail. See *Flail chest.*
  major injuries to, management of, 501
  stove-in, 513–518
Chest wall, fracture of, and visceral injury, 76
  open wounds of, 512

Children. See also *Adolescents*; and *Infants*.
  adduction fractures of malleolus in, 251–252
  blood supply of femoral head and neck in, 1265
  cervical spine injuries in, radiographic evaluation of, 296
  cervicotrochanteric fractures in, 1447
  compression fractures in, 10
  congenital dislocation of radial head in, 972
  epiphyseal separation of lower humerus in, 185, 754
  femoral neck fractures in, 1444–1449
    and coxa vara deformity, 1455
  femoral shaft fractures in, 1501–1510
  fractures in, growth remodeling of, 988–991
  fractures of clavicle in, 528
  fractures of distal radius and ulna in, 982–986
  fractures of forearm in, 979–1002
    greenstick, 898
    open, 986–988
    upper, 998–1002
    with displacement, 991–996
  fractures of lower humerus in, 740
  fractures of radial head and neck in, 869
    operative reduction of, 873
  fracture of upper humeral epiphysis in, 716
  growth arrest in, and radioulnar joint disruption, 1043–1045
  growth remodeling of fracture deformities in, 988–991
  impacted fracture of proximal finger phalanx in, 1243
  intertrochanteric fractures in, 1390–1393, 1449
    displaced, 1392
    undisplaced, 1391
  Monteggia injury in, anterior, 964
    lateral, 968
    from adduction, 962
    unrecognized, 972
  older, distal femoral epiphyseal separation in, 221–222, 225–229
  soft tissue repair of patellar instability in, 1675
  subluxation of radial head in, 879–881
  subtrochanteric fractures in, 1402
  tibial spine injury in, 1611
  traumatic hip dislocation in, 1331–1334
  under 4, apophyseal separation of medial epicondyle of humerus in, 171
  under 9, acute upper femoral epiphyseal separation in, 201–202
  under 6, upper humeral epiphyseal separation in, 156–157
  upper humeral epiphyseal separation in, 158–160
  valgus deformities in, upper tibial metaphyseal fractures and, 1782
Chondrosarcoma, and pathologic fractures, 2118, 2126
Chrisman and Snook technique for reconstruction of lateral ankle ligaments, 1829
Circulation. See *Blood supply.*
Clamp, Böhler, 2026
Clavicle
  congenital pseudoarthrosis of, 2109
  excision of portion of, 542–544
  fractures of, 524–544
    birth, 2084
    closed reduction of, 528–532
    complete, 528

INDEX

Clavicle (*Continued*)
    fractures of, complications of, 537–544
        distal to and with disruption of
            coracoclavicular ligaments, 535
        fixation of, 534, 540
        mechanisms and classification of, 525–528
        nonunion of 41, 537
        open reduction of, 532–537
    fragmentation of, 543
    inner third of, fractures of, 527
    ligamentous injuries to articulations of, 545–565
    middle third of, fractures of, 525
    outer quarter of, nonunion of, 41
    outer third of, fractures of, 526
Clostridium, and myonecrosis, 130, 1755
Clostridium perfringens infection, 130
Clostridium tetani infections, 129
Coccyx, fracture of, with displacement, 477
"Cock robin" position, of atlanto-axial joint, 287
Codfish vertebrae, 2102
Collars, in cervical disc protrusion, 380
    Philadelphia, in fracture of atlas, 311
        in occipito-atlantal dislocation, 309
Collateral ligaments
    fibular, reattachment of, 1587
    of interphalangeal joint of thumb, rupture of, 1187
    of interphalangeal joints of fingers, 1143
    of metacarpophalangeal and interphalangeal joints, 1143
    radial, of metacarpophalangeal joint of thumb, injury to, 1185
    tibial, injury to, complications of, 1579–1581
        repair of, 1575
    ulnar, disruption of, complete, operative repair of, 1184
        in skier's thumb, 1181
Colles' fracture, 1009–1020
    malunion of, 1046
    nonunion of, 1049
    reduction of, 112
    with carpal scaphoid fracture, 1020
    with comminution, 1010, 1014
    types of, 1015
Comminuted fracture-dislocation, Barton's, 1029
Comminuted fractures, 11
    Colles', 1010, 1014
        types of, 1015
    of acetabular rim, hip dislocation with, 1286
        with fracture of femoral shaft, 1307
    of acetabulum, 1340, 1351
    of base of finger metacarpal, 1236
    of distal phalanx 1253
    of femoral neck, 1416
    of femoral shaft, 1466
        iatrogenic, 1467
    of greater trochanter, 1367
    of inferior articular surface of tibia, 1909–1914
    of medial cortex, 1372
    of patella, 1639–1642
        without displacement, 1632–1633, 1637
    of posterior acetabulum, 1340
    of radial head, with dislocation of distal radioulnar joint, 865
    of superior acetabular dome, 1351
    of surgical neck of humerus, 706

Comminuted fractures (*Continued*)
    of trapezium, 1128
    Smith's, 1024
Compartment syndromes, 64
    anterior, 66, 1713
    deep posterior, 67
    deformities from, 1795
    fasciotomy in, 68, 1794
    from skin traction, 68
    mechanism of, 64
    tibial shaft fractures and, 1793
Compression fractures, 10
    in diseased bone, 11
    of acetabulum, 1348
        with displacement or comminution, 1351
        without displacement, 1349
    of atlas, 271
    of cervical spine, 267, 270, 366–369
        simple, 345–348
        teardrop, and anterior cord syndrome, 352–354
    of humerus, 703
    of pelvis, 466
    of talus, 1959–1960, 1991–1992
    of thoracolumbar spine. See *Thoracolumbar spine, fractures of, compression.*
Compression plate
    drill guide for, 924, 931, 936
    fracture healing after, 16
    in displaced fractures of ulna, 935
    in forearm fractures, 918
        distal, 947
        nonunion of, 39
    in fracture of distal radius, 928
    in fracture of middle third of humerus, 732
    in fractures of proximal radius, 923
    in malunion of tibial shaft fracture, 1781
Compression screw. See *Screw, compression.*
Condyles
    femoral, displacement of, in supracondylar fractures, 1513, 1516
        fractures of, 1529–1536
    lateral, femoral, fractures of, 1529
        management of, 1530
        osteochondral, 1593
            management of, 1597
        of humeral epiphysis, fractures of, 163–168, 771–773
            with displacement and rotation, 165–168
            with displacement but without rotation, 164–165
        of lower humerus, fractures of, 744, 757. See also *Intercondylar T fractures, of lower humerus.*
        tibial. See *Tibial plateau fractures, lateral.*
    medial, femoral, fractures of, 1530
        management of, 1531
        of humeral epiphysis, fractures of, 773–776
            displaced, 774
        of distal end of proximal phalanx, fractures of, 1247
        of lower humerus, fractures of, 745
        tibial, fractures of, 1696–1718
            internal fixation in, 1707–1710
            unstable, 1708
Connolly technique for chronic anterior glenohumeral dislocations, 629

INDEX

Coracoacromial arch, rotator muscles under, 589
Coracoclavicular ligaments, disruption of, fracture of clavicle with, 535
Coracoid process, of scapula, fractures of, 566–567
    and subcoracoid dislocation, 663
Cord
    anterior, syndrome of, anterior decompression and cervical spine fusion in, 355–362
        bursting teardrop fractures of cervical spine and, 352–354
    central, syndrome of, 275
        hyperextension of cervical spine with osteoarthritis and, 365–366
    spinal, injury of, functional levels of, 395, 454–456
        rehabilitation after, 393–396
Coronoid process of radius
    fractures of, 876–879
        chip, 976
        posterior dislocation of elbow joint with, 807–809
        with displacement, 877
        with minimal displacement, 876
Corticosteroid, in solitary bone cyst, 2112
Cortisone, and pathologic fractures, 2098
Costal cartilages, fractures and dislocations of, 506–508
Costochondral joint, recurrent subluxation or dislocation of, 507–508
Coxa vara deformity, femoral neck fractures in children and, 1455
Crawford's criteria for stable impacted femoral neck fractures, 1427
Cruciate ligaments of knee, 1546
    anterior, 1546
        acute ruptures of, 1589–1598
        detachment of distal end of, repair of, 1594
        detachment of proximal end of, repair of, 1594
        injury of, mechanism of, 1590
            repair of, 1596
                indications for, 1593
        tear in, Lachman test for, 1556
    injuries to, 1548–1619
        operative repair of, 1573
    posterior, 1547
        acute tears of, 1599–1608
            and medial capsular tears, 1565
        injury of, mechanisms of, 1600, 1604
        operative repair of, 1600, 1606
        rupture of, direct blow to flexed knee and, 1603
Cryotherapy, in giant cell tumor, 2122
Cubitus valgus, supracondylar fracture and, 753
Cubitus varus, supracondylar fracture and, 750, 752
    typical, 749
Cuboid bone
    dislocation of, 2042
    fractures of, 2039–2044
        medial midtarsal dislocation with, 2046
        undisplaced, 2040
Cuneiform bone, dislocation of, 2043
    fractures of, 2039–2044
        undisplaced, 2040
Curbstone fracture, 1914–1915
Cyst, aneurysmal bone, and pathologic fractures, 2114

Cyst (*Continued*)
    fallen fragment sign in, 2112
    solitary bone, and pathologic fractures, 2111

Death, intertrochanteric fractures and, 1388
Debeyre repair of rotator cuff, 608
Debridement, wound, 127
    in open fractures of forearm, 954
Decompression, 4-compartment parafibular, 1794
Deltoid ligament, injuries of, 1824
    repair of, 1850
DePalma arthrodesis, of hip, in malunited upper femoral epiphyseal slip, 215
DeWald and Ray technique of applying halo-pelvic hoop, 302
Diabetes, midtarsal dislocation in, 2050
DIC phase, of shock, 78
Digitorum communis, dorsal expansion of, 1146
Dingley and Denham technique for pubic anterior hip dislocation, 1322
Dinner-fork deformity, 1010
Disc, intervertebral. See *Intervertebral disc.*
Disc distension test, 383
Dislocations
    definitions and causes of, 4–7
    direct, 5
    fracture with, 12
    indirect, 5
    management of, principles of, 1–141
    mechanisms producing, 5–7. See also specific types bones.
Disseminated intravascular coagulation phase, of shock, 78
Dorsal expansion, of digitorum communis, 1146
    shift of, 1147
Dorsal spinous processes, fracture of, 446
Dorsalis pedis artery, in posterior fracture-dislocation of ankle, 1926
Drainage tube, intrapleural, in flail chest, 516
    in tension pneumothorax, 510
Drawer sign
    anterior, ankle tests for, 1811, 1817
        knee, tests for, 1554, 1584
    posterior ankle, tests for, 1556
        knee, test for, in posterior cruciate ligament injury, 1604
Drill, for insertion of traction pins, 121
Drill guide, for dynamic compression plate, 924, 931, 936
Dunlop traction, in fractures of lower humerus, 766
Dunn and Hess technique for chronic acetabular disruption, 1360
Dura, compression of, without nerve root compression, 374
Dynamic compression plate. See *Compression plate.*
Dysplasia, fibrous, and pathologic fractures, 2104

Ecker, Latke, and Glazer reconstruction of patellar tendon, 1657
Elastic bandage, in grade I ankle sprains, 1813
    in tear of distal tibiofibular ligament, 1826
Elbow joint. See also specific parts.
    dislocations of, 756, 791–805
        and vascular injury, 828
        anterior, 795–797

Elbow joint (*Continued*)
  dislocations of, anterior, with fracture of olecranon, 815–818
    divergent, 803–805
      anteroposterior, 804
      medial-lateral, 804
    lateral, 797–800
    old unreduced, 839–847
      closed reduction of, 839
      open reduction of, 841
    posterior, 791–795
      uncomplicated, 792
      with fracture of coronoid process, 807–809
    recurrent, 837–838
    with fracture, 806–825
    with fracture of radial head, 809–815
  displacement of medial humeral epicondyle into, 174–178
  emergency splinting of, 108
  excision of, 845
  extension of, after humeral shaft fracture, 723
  flexion of, posterior Monteggia fracture with, 962
  fracture-dislocation of, transcondylar, 824–825
    with rupture of orbicular ligament, 821–823
  fractures and dislocations of, 739–885
    complications and pitfalls of, 883–885
    vascular and neural complications of, 826–836
  fractures of, sideswipe, 818–821
  fragment in, in avulsion of lateral humeral epicondyle, 180–183
  hyperextension of, and anterior Monteggia fracture, 899, 961
  instability of, fractures of lower humerus and, 747
  little leaguer's, 746, 777–778
  medial side of, in fractures of head and neck of radius, in children, 870
  motion of, loss of, fractures of lower humerus and, 747
  myositis ossificans in, traumatic, 91, 848–850
  normal, 756
  normal carrying angle of, 748
    variations of, 749
  nursemaid's, 879–881
  ossification centers of, 742
  resectional arthroplasty of, in old unreduced dislocations, 844
  stiffness of, prevention of, 86
  valgus deformity of, supracondylar fracture and, 753
  varus deformity of, supracondylar fracture and, 750, 752
  varus deformity of, typical, 749
Elderly
  femoral neck fracture in, 1407
    displaced, management of, 1424
  intertrochanteric fractures in, 1369
  osteoporosis in. See *Osteoporosis*.
  reduction of lower humeral fractures in, 770
Electrical osteogenesis, 33, 1494
  in nonunion of tibial shaft fracture, 1785
Elmelik repair of rotator cuff, 608
Elmslie-Trillot procedure, 1669, 1673
  in Osgood-Schlatter's syndrome, 1615
Embolism, fat. See *Fat embolism*.
Emergency room treatment, of cervical spine injuries, 292
  of multiple trauma, 2138–2139

Emergency splinting, 106
  of cervical spine, 106, 291
  of multiple fractures, 109
Emergency treatment
  of cervical spine injuries, 290–302
  of complications of rib fractures, 509–512
  of femoral shaft fractures, 1457
  prehospital, of trauma, 2140–2145
Enchondroma, solitary, and pathologic fractures, 2116
Ender's rod, in femoral shaft fracture with femoral neck fracture, 1482
  in intertrochanteric femoral fracture, 1376, 1379, 2096
Eosinophilic granuloma, solitary, of bone, 2119
Epicondyle, humeral. See *Humeral epicondyle*.
Epimysiotomy, in compartment syndromes, 1794
  in Volkmann's ischemic contracture, 66
Epiphyseal plates. See *Physis(es)*.
Epiphysis(es)
  circulation to, 145–147
    and prognosis for physeal injuries, 154
  injuries to, 143–258
    anatomic features of, 144–155
    management of, pitfalls in, 257–258
  of knee, injuries to, in adolescents, 1566
Epstein classification of hip dislocations, 1266
Epstein classification of hip fracture-dislocations, 1285, 1292–1297, 1312
Evans' technique for rotational alignment of forearm, 892
Exercises
  active, for hip, 137
  balancing, after ankle sprain, 1814, 1822, 1832
  flexion, for lumbar spinal injury, 136
  gravity, for shoulder, 139
  passive skateboard, for hip, 137
  passive stretching, for shoulder, 139
  quadriceps, 138
Explosion fracture, of inferior articular surface of tibia, 1909–1914
  ankle arthrodesis for, 1911
  pronation-dorsiflexion of ankle, management of, 1903
Extension block splint, in acute dorsal instability of interphalangeal joints of fingers, 1208
Extension fractures of lower humerus, 743
  management of, 758
Extensor apparatus, of knee joint, rupture of, 1649–1662

Facet joints, arthritic, injection of, 381–382
Fallen fragment sign, in bone cyst, 2112
Fascia, pretracheal, exposure of, in anterior cervical spine fusion, 385
  in anterior cord syndrome, 356
Fasciotomy
  in compartment syndromes, 68, 1794
  in ischemia of forearm, 833
  in Volkmann's ischemic contracture, 66
Fat embolism, 82–84
  diagnosis of, 83
  femoral shaft fractures and, 1479
  preventive treatment of, 83
Fatigue fractures
  of femoral neck, 1423
  of metatarsal bones, 2058
  of pelvis, 468
  of tibia, 1725

Fear sign, 1592, 1671
Feet. See *Foot.*
Femoral epiphysis
　distal, separation of, 219–233
　　at birth, 220–221
　　growth deformities following, 230–231
　　in older children, 221–222, 225–229
　　occult injuries and, 232–233
　　with backward displacement, 224–225
　　with irreducible displacement, 223
　proximal, separation of, 199–206
　　acute, in children under 9, 201–202
　　in adolescents, 204–206
　　in infants, 199–200
　　unreducible, 203
　slipped capital, 207–212
　　acute, 207–209
　　malunited, greater than 60°, 213–216
　　　involving both hips, 216
　　　involving one hip, 215
　　subacute or chronic, 210–212
　traumatic separation of, 1445
Femoral physis, lower, separation of, 150
　upper, separation of, 151
Femur
　condyles of. See *Condyles.*
　distal, fractures of, 1511–1536
　emergency splinting of, 109
　flexion and abduction of, pelvic injury with, 466
　flexion in neutral position of, pelvic injury with, 464
　fractures of, 1365–1540
　　gunshot, 1481
　　　.22-caliber, 134
　　delayed union of, 38
　　intertrochanteric. See *Intertrochanteric fractures.*
　　Paget's disease and, 2095
　　pitfalls of managing, 1537–1538
　　shotgun, 133, 1480
　　subtrochanteric. See *Subtrochanteric fractures.*
　　supracondylar. See *Supracondylar fractures, of femur.*
　　tibial shaft fractures with, 1796
　　trochanteric. See *Trochanter.*
　　unicondylar. See *Unicondylar fractures.*
　head of
　　avascular necrosis of, 1362
　　blood supply of, 1263, 1418
　　　at birth, 1264
　　　at 3 years, 1265
　　　technetium-99m sulfur-colloid in evaluation of, 1452
　　chronic displacement of, acetabular fracture with, 1359–1360
　　flattening of, 1420
　　fracture of, hip dislocation with, 1267, 1292–1297
　　　with fragment, 1293
　　in valgus, 1415
　　in varus, 1415
　　intrapelvic protrusion of, in fracture of inner acetabular wall, 1345
　　ischemic necrosis of, 48
　　prosthetic replacement of, 39
　　segmental collapse of, femoral neck fracture and, 1419
　　　femoral neck fracture reduction and, 1421

Femur (*Continued*)
　head of, segmental collapse of, nonunion of femoral neck fracture and, 1453
　head-neck relationships of, in subcapital fractures, 1414
　in osteogenesis imperfecta, 2102
　lateral rotation of, in subcapital fracture, 1410
　neck of
　　blood supply of, 1263
　　　at birth, 1264
　　　at 3 years, 1265
　　fracture-dislocations of, 1298–1305
　　fractures of, 1407–1455
　　　and ischemic necrosis, 48
　　　and segmental collapse of femoral head, 1419
　　　basilar, 1443–1444
　　　bone scan in, 1423, 1452
　　　collapse of posteroinferior cortex in, 1417
　　　complications of, 1449–1455
　　　delayed union of, 39
　　　displaced, management of, 1432
　　　　open reduction and posterior bone grafting of, 1439
　　　evaluation of patients for, 1422–1423
　　　femoral shaft fracture with, 1482
　　　hip dislocation with, 1298–1305
　　　in children, 1444–1449
　　　　and coxa vara deformity, 1455
　　　management of, 1424–1443
　　　mechanism of, 1408
　　　nonunion of, 39, 1418
　　　　and segmental collapse of femoral head, 1453
　　　old untreated, 1450
　　　reduction of, and segmental collapse of femoral head, 1421
　　　stable impacted, 1427
　　　subcapital. See *Subcapital fractures.*
　　　with circulatory changes, 1417, 1421
　　posterior comminution in, 1416
　　radiographic examination of, 103, 1422
　proximal
　　blood vessels of, in anterior hip dislocation, 1318
　　fractures of, 1366–1406
　　　90°-90° traction for, 122
　shepherd's crook deformity of, 21 ;5
　shaft of
　　fractures of, 1456–1510
　　　birth, 2085
　　　closed treatment of, 1460
　　　complications of, 1485
　　　comminuted, 1466
　　　　iatrogenic, 1467
　　　complications of, 1478–1500
　　　definitive treatment of, 1459–1478
　　　hip dislocations with, 1306–1309
　　　hip fracture with, 1307, 1481
　　　in children, 1501–1510
　　　internal fixation of, 1472
　　　　complications of, 1491
　　　supracondylar and distal, 1461
　　　3-dimensional biomechanics of, 1461
　　　torsional middle and proximal, 1464
　　　transverse, 1466
　　　　in children, 1504, 1507
　　　with tibial fracture, 1483
　　in supracondylar fractures, 1513, 1522

INDEX

Femur (*Continued*)
  in supracondylar fractures, overgrowth of, 57
  refractures of, 1460, 1488, 1491
Fibroma, nonossifying, and pathologic fractures, 2110
Fibrous dysplasia, and pathologic fractures, 2104
Fibula. See also *Tibia*.
  and tibial fracture deformity, 1728
  and tibial plateau fractures, 1699
  biomechanics of, 1726–1729
  dislocation of, 1924, 1926
  distal. See also *Ankle joint*.
    fracture of, rotational displacement of distal tibial epiphysis with, 1929–1930
  in bicondylar tibial fracture, 1714
  in tibial fractures, 1727
  proximal, Maisonneuve fracture of, 1884
  proximal to tibiofibular syndesmosis, fracture of, 1863, 1871
  shaft of, fractures of, 1797
  weight-bearing function of, 1727
Fibular bypass procedures, 1760
Fibular collateral ligament, reattachment of, 1587
Fibulotibial synostosis, 1760
Figure-of-eight harness, posterior, in fracture of clavicle, 528
Finger(s). See also specific bones and joints.
  carpometacarpal joints of, 1190–1195
    dislocations of, 1191
    fracture-dislocations of, 1193
  flexion of, abnormal, 1147
    normal, 1147
  fractures, dislocations, and fracture-dislocations of, 1190–1260
  interphalangeal joints of. See *Interphalangeal joints*.
  jammed, 1148–1152
    evaluation of, 1201
  mallet. See *Mallet finger deformity*.
  metacarpal bones of. See *Metacarpal bones, of fingers*.
  metacarpophalangeal joints of. See *Metacarpophalangeal joints*.
  normal, 1148
  phalangeal epiphyses of, distal, separation of, 195
    proximal and middle, separation of, 193–195
    separation of, 193–196
  phalanges of. See *Phalanx (phalanges), of fingers*.
Fingertip amputation, 1256
Fixation, incomplete, with nonunion, 31
  internal, 123
Flail chest, 513–518
  internal fixation of, 518
  management of, 516–518
    prehospital, 2142
Flat foot, after calcaneal fractures, 2017
Flexor profundus muscle, avulsion of, 1149, 1216
Floating knee, 1483
Flutter valve, in flail chest, 517
  in tension pneumothorax, 510
Foot. See also specific bones and joints.
  bones of. See also specific bones.
    fractures and fracture-dislocations of, 1951–2079
      pitfalls and complications of, 2078–2079
    Charcot, 2050

Foot (*Continued*)
  peroneal spastic flat, after calcaneal fracture, 2017
  posterior dislocation of, with posterior marginal fracture of tibia, 1887–1897
  stiffness of, after calcaneal fractures, 2017, 2029
Footballer's thigh, 92
Forceps, Weber's reduction, 1870, 1892
Forearm. See also specific bones; and *Radioulnar joints*.
  biomechanics of rotation and fracture reduction of, 888–896
  bones of, fracture of
    closed reduction and functional treatment of, 903–917
    complications and pitfalls of, 1003–1004
    direct, 896
    general considerations in treatment of, 901–902
    greenstick, 980
      in children, 898
    gunshot, 897, 955
    in adults, epidemiology of, 896
    in children, 979–1002
    indirect, 897
    mechanism of, 896–900
    nonunion of, compression plating for, 39
    open, in children, 986–988
    operative management of, 918–953
      indications for, 919
    plaster slabs for, 118
    torus, 980
  shafts of, fractures of, 887–1005
  distal, 2-bone fractures of, 944–948
    displaced, 914
    in adults, 914
    undisplaced, 914
  emergency splinting of, 108
  fracture deformities of, 894
  interosseous space of, 890
    effect of fractures on, 891
    narrowing of due to angulation, 894
  joints of. See *Radioulnar joints*.
  mid-third of, bones of, fractures of, greenstick, 996–998
    with displacement, in children, 991–996
  1-bone, 45, 957
  position of, in fractures of distal humerus, 761
  pronation and supination of, 890
    loss of, 891
  proximal, 2-bone fractures of, displaced, 909, 941–944
    in adults, 908
    in children, 998–1002
  rotation of, effect of fracture reduction on, 894
    evaluation of, 892
    in fractures of ulna with large defects, 938
  single-bone fractures of, radioulnar disruption in, 895
  2-bone fractures of
    open, management of, 954–958
    segmental, 949–953
  3-bone, 938–940
Fork deformity, 1010
Fracture
  clinical and radiographic features of, 100–105
  closed, 8
  complications of, 26–99

xi

Fracture (*Continued*)
　definitions of, 2–3
　distraction of, with nonunion, 32
　　with nonunion of tibia, 38
　fresh, internal fixation for, 123
　healing of. See also *Malunion; Nonunion;* and
　　Union.
　　circulation in bone and, 17–19
　　examples of, 14–17
　　functional rehabilitation during and after,
　　　135–141
　　local factors influencing, 27
　　rate of, conditions influencing, 21–25
　management of, principles of, 106–109
　mechanisms of injury in, 2–3. See also
　　specific bones.
　oblique, 9
　open. See *Open fractures.*
　reduction of, 110–114
　repair of, 13–20
　treatment of, complications of, 95–99
　　operative, pitfalls of, 98
　types of, 8–12
　with dislocation, 12
Fry exercise splint, 1346
Functional cast-brace. See *Cast-brace,*
　functional.
Functional sleeve, in fracture of ulna, 907
　in humeral shaft fractures, 721, 729
Fusion. See also *Arthrodesis.*
　cervical spine. See *Cervical spine fusion.*
　occipitocervical, in occipito-atlantal
　　dislocations, 307
　thoracolumbar spine, in flexion-rotation
　　fracture-dislocations, 426
　　spontaneous, 436

Gait, abnormalities of, after calcaneal fracture,
　2018
Galeazzi's fracture, resection of ulna in, 939
　rotational injury and, 898
Gangrene, gas, 130
　in open fractures, 129–132, 1755
Garden's classification of subcapital fractures,
　anteroposterior appearance and, 1412
　rotational instability and, 1410
Garden-spade deformity, 1021
Gardner-Wells traction, technique of applying,
　298
Gas gangrene, 130
　in open fractures, 129–132, 1755
Genu valgum, 1548
　femoral shaft fractures and, 1462, 1496
　pathologic results of, 1549
Genu varum, 1549
　femoral shaft fractures and, 1461, 1496
　pathologic results of, 1550
　supracondylar fractures and, 1519
Giant cell tumor, and pathologic fractures, 2121
Gilchrist stockinette. See *Velpeau sling.*
Glenohumeral joint
　anatomic features and mechanisms of injury of,
　　588–601
　arthrography of, 607
　　in rotator cuff rupture, 647
　degenerative alterations of, 592–593

Glenohumeral joint (*Continued*)
　dislocations of, 587–683
　　anterior, 4
　　　abduction and external rotation, 596
　　　immobilization of, 620
　　　old, 627–631
　　　　closed reduction of, 628
　　　　immobilization in, 629
　　　recurrent, immobilization in, 674
　　　　surgical repair in, 671
　　　reduction of, 618
　　　types of, 617
　　complications of, management of, 642–681
　　inferior, hyperabduction, 598, 606
　　irreducible fresh, 624–627
　　　surgical repair of, 625
　　management of, 616–641
　　　pitfalls of, 682–683
　　posterior
　　　acute, 632–635
　　　　immobilization of, 634
　　　　reduction of, 634
　　　adduction and internal rotation, 600
　　　old, 636–641
　　　　immobilization in, 640
　　　　operative reduction of, 637
　　　recurrent, 677
　　primary traumatic, and recurrent dislocation,
　　　669
　　recurrent, 668–681
　　　etiology of, 669
　　subcoracoid, and fracture of acromion, 663
　　　and fracture of coracoid process, 663
　　subluxation after, 607
　　voluntary, 681
　inferior fracture-subluxation of, 611–614
　injuries of, abduction and external rotation, 596
　　adduction and internal rotation (posterior
　　　lesions), 600
　　hyperabduction, 598, 606
　　mechanisms of, 595–601
　　ligaments and capsule of, 590–592
　　injuries of, 587–683
　muscles of, 589–590
　neurovascular structures near, 593–594
　normal motions of, 594–595
　sprains and subluxations of
　　abduction and external rotation, 596
　　acute anterior, 602–605
　　adduction and internal rotation, 600
　　hyperabduction, 598, 606
　　management of, 602–615
　　posterior, 614–615
　stiffness of, prevention of, 85
　subluxations of, 587–683
　　acute inferior or superior, 605–611
　　diffuse muscle atrophy and, 7
　　inferior, types of, 606
　　management of, pitfalls of, 682–683
　　recurrent anterior, 675
　　voluntary, 6, 681
Glenohumeral ligaments, 590–592
　anatomic variations in, and recurrent
　　glenohumeral dislocations, 669
　injuries of, 587–683
Glenohumeral synovial recesses, anatomic
　variations in, and recurrent glenohumeral
　dislocations, 669

INDEX

Glenoid cavity. See also *Glenohumeral joint.*
  fractures of, 570–582
    anterior, 571
      undisplaced, with separation of fragments, 574
    examples of, 574
    management of, 572–582
      nonoperative, 574
    posterior, 572, 579
      undisplaced, with separation of fragments, 574
    with recurrent dislocation, 575
  injury of, direct, 570
    indirect, 571
    mechanisms of, 570–572
Glenoplasty, in recurrent posterior glenohumeral dislocation repair, 678
Graft(s)
  biceps tendon, in rotator cuff rupture, 649
  bone. See *Bone graft.*
  dual onlay, 36
  inlay, 35
    sliding, 35
  skin, in open fractures, 1753
Graft bed, preparation of, in anterior cord syndrome, 359
Granuloma, solitary eosinophilic, of bone, 2119
Gravity method, for traumatic hip dislocation in children, 1332
  for trimalleolar fractures of ankle, 113
Greenstick fracture, 979
  of forearm bones, 980
    in children, 898
    mid-third of, 996–998
  of upper ulna, with dislocation of radial epiphysis, 969–972
Growth arrest, in children, and radioulnar joint disruption, 1043–1045
Growth deformities, after distal femoral epiphyseal fractures, 230–231
Growth remodeling, of fracture deformities, in children, 988–991
Gunshot. See also *Shotgun fractures.*
  and fracture, 132–134
  and fracture of femur, 1481
  and fracture of forearm bones, 897, 955
  and fractures of spine, 451–452
  and knee injury, 1694
  and thoracolumbar spinal injury, 415
  .22-caliber, and fracture of femur, 134
Gupta and Shravat technique for old unreduced posterior hip dislocation, 1311

Hagie pin, in displaced femoral neck fractures, 1441
Halo cast
  in central cord syndrome, 366
  in fracture of atlas, 311
  in fracture of neural arch of C2, 313
  in occipito-atlantal dislocation, 309
  in simple compression fractures of cervical spine, 347
  technique of applying, 301
Halo traction
  in cervical spine fracture-dislocation, 368
  in fracture of odontoid process, 332

Halo traction (*Continued*)
  in simple compression fractures of cervical spine, 346
  in traumatic forward dislocation of atlas, 320
  technique of applying, 299
Halo-pelvic hoop, technique of applying, in cervical injuries with sensory impairment, 302
Hamate bone, hook of, fracture of, 1124–1126
  mechanism of, 1124
Hand. See also specific bones and joints.
  anatomy of, 1138–1147
  fractures and dislocations of, 1137–1260
    pitfalls and complications of, 1258
  fractures of, closed management of, methods of, 1156–1157
  injuries of, management of, principles of, 1153–1157
  intrinsic-minus position of, 1147
  intrinsic-plus position of, 1144
  joint stiffness of, prevention of, 86
  ligaments of, 1138
    deep transverse, 1139
  longitudinal and transverse arches of, 1054, 1139
  muscles of, 1144–1147
  open wounds of, 1154
    crushing, 1154
  osseous components of, 1138
  tendons and joints of, injury of, mechanisms of, 1148–1152
Hand sling, in humeral shaft fractures, 720
Hand-shoulder disuse syndrome, in Colles' fracture, 1009, 1018
Hanging cast, in anatomic humeral neck fracture, 717
  in displaced fractures of anatomic and surgical humeral neck, 710
Hangman's fracture, 277, 312–314
Harness, posterior figure-of-eight, in fracture of clavicle, 528
Harralson and Boyd technique of reduction, 324
Harrington rods
  contraction (compression), in fixation of lumbar and thoracic spine, 420
    in hyperflexion fracture of thoracolumbar spine, 424
  distraction, in fixation of lumbar and thoracic spine, 420
    in flexion-rotation fracture-dislocation of thoracolumbar spine, 426
    in posterolateral decompression for neural deficit, 438
Haversian canal, disruption of, in tibial fractures, 1724
Heel, painful and tender, after calcaneal fractures, 2017, 2028
Hemarthrosis, of knee joint, acute traumatic, 1691–1692
Hemipelvis, upward dislocation of, 489–493
Hemiplegia, and inferior subluxation of glenohumeral joint, 600, 606
Hemothorax, 511
Henry's exposure
  in fracture of distal radius, 928
  in fractures of distal forearm, 944
  in posterior marginal fractures of tibia, 1893
  in segmental fractures of forearm, 950
Hindfoot, painful and tender, after calcaneal fractures, 2017, 2028

xiii

INDEX

Hip joint. See also specific parts.
  anatomy of, 1262–1267
  arthrodesis of, in malunited upper femoral epiphyseal slip, 215
  biomechanics of, 1421
  dislocations of, 1261–1364
    anterior, 1315–1330
      chronic, total hip replacement for, 1330
      fresh unreducible, 1323–1325
      obturator, mechanism of, 1316
        reduction of, 1319
      old unreduced, 1325–1330
      pubic, mechanism of, 1316
        reduction of, 1322
      typical deformity of, 1317
    chronic, with acetabular fracture, 1313
    chronic complications of, 1362
    femoral shaft fracture with, 1306–1309, 1481
    irreducible, operative approach to, 1277
    pitfalls and complications of, 1361–1363
    posterior, 1268–1314
      closed reduction of, 1273
      iliac, 1270
      ischial, 1271
      mechanism of, 1270
      old unreduced, 1309–1313
      recurrent traumatic, 1313–1314
      unreducible or incompletely reduced, 1276–1282
      with femoral head fracture, 1267, 1292–1297
      with femoral neck fracture, 1298–1305
      with fracture of acetabular rim, 1266, 1283, 1285
      with fracture of femoral shaft, 1306–1309
      with nerve injuries, 1290–1291
    radiographic assessment of, 1272
    traumatic, classification of, 1266
    in children, 1331–1334
  effusion in, and subluxation, 7
  exercises for muscles around, active, 137
    passive skateboard, 137
  fracture-dislocations of, 1261–1364
    posterior, 1282
      closed reduction of, 1273
      Epstein's types II, III, and IV, 1285
      Epstein's type V, 1292–1297
        old unreduced, reconstructive arthroplasty in, 1312
  fractures of, femoral shaft fracture with, 1307, 1481
    needs of patient in, 1370
  functional rehabilitation of, 137
  horseback rider's, 92
  injuries of, classification of, 1262–1267
  myositis ossificans of, 1363
  posterior exposure of, 1277
  redislocation and reduction of, 1280
  replacement of. See *Prosthesis, hip.*
  traumatic arthritis of, 1362
  unstable, with posterior acetabular fracture, 1342
Hippocratic method, for anterior dislocation of glenohumeral joint, 619
  for fracture of greater tuberosity of humerus, 654
  for old anterior glenohumeral dislocations, 628

Horseback rider's hip, 92
Hughston incision, 1571
Hughston technique, for posterior oblique and tibial collateral ligament repair, 1575
Hughston test, for posterolateral rotatory instability of knee, 1584
Humeral epicondyle
  lateral, avulsion of, 179–183
    with fragment in elbow joint, 180–183
    without fragment in elbow joint, 179–180
  medial
    apophyseal separation of, 169–178
      with gross displacement, 171–174
      with minimal displacement, 170
    displacement into elbow joint, 174–178
Humeral epiphysis
  lateral condyle of, fractures of, 163–168, 771–773
    with displacement and rotation, 165–168
    with displacement but without rotation, 164–165
  lower
    fractures of, 744
    separation of, 184–185, 754
      at birth, 184–185
      in childhood, 185, 754
      management of, 758
  medial condyle of, fractures of, 773–776
    displaced, 774
  separation of, diagnosis of, 757
  upper
    fracture of, in child, 716
    separation of, 156–162
      at birth and in children under 6, 156–157
      in children older than 6, 158–160
      unreducible, with severe displacement or dislocation, 160–162
Humerus. See also *Glenohumeral joint.*
  anatomic and surgical neck of, fractures of
    in glenohumeral dislocation, 659
    with displacement, 706–715
  anatomic neck of, fractures of, 715
    in adult, 716
  emergency splinting of, 108
  fractures of, 685–738
    and inferior subluxation of glenohumeral joint, 606
    complications and pitfalls of, 737
  greater tuberosity of
    fractures of, 695
      in glenohumeral dislocations, 652
      operative management of, 696
        indications for, 655
      with small fragment, 699
    type I and II fracture-dislocations of, 653
    type III fracture-dislocation of, 656
  head of
    avascular necrosis of, 705
    fracture of, in glenohumeral dislocations, 651, 659
    intrathoracic dislocation of, 664–667
  internal rotation of, marked, 633
    minimal, 633
  lesser tuberosity of, fracture of, 700
    with small fragment, 702
  lower
    condyles of, fractures of, 745

INDEX

Humerus (*Continued*)
  lower, condyles of, lateral, fractures of, 744, 757
    fractures of, 740–790
      complications of, 746–747
      correction of medial or lateral angulation in, 765
      extension, 743
        management of, 758
      flexion, 743
      in adults, 740
      in children, 740
      intercondylar T. See *Intercondylar T fractures, of lower humerus.*
      lateral (Dunlop) traction in, 766
      nonunion of, 747
      reduction of, 770
      supracondylar. See *Supracondylar fractures, of lower humerus.*
      torsional-varus deformity of, 724
      types of, 742
      undisplaced, 742
      with radial nerve injury, 732
  mid-third of, fracture of, 731
  shaft of, fractures of, 718–736
    birth, 2083
    delayed union or nonunion of, 40, 734–735
    in polytrauma, 727–733
    sideswipe, 818
    with marked displacement or angulation, 722–724
    with minimal or no displacement or angulation, 719–721
    with multiple long bone fractures, 730
    with radial nerve injury, 726–727
  surgical neck of, fracture of, comminuted, 706
  upper, fractures of, 686–717
    bending, 689
    direct, 689
    external torsional, 687
    indirect, 687
    internal torsional, 688
    management of, 690–702
    requiring no reduction, 691
    requiring reduction, 695
    undisplaced, 703
Hypercortisolism, and pathologic fractures, 2098
Hyperparathyroidism, and pathologic fractures, 2098
Hyperthermia, malignant, 81–82
Hypothenar muscles, 1145
Hypovolemic shock, 77–81
  anti-shock trousers for, 2146
  pelvic fractures and, 482
  treatment of, 2143

Iliac crest, bone grafting from, 943
Iliac spine, anterior superior or inferior, avulsion of, 472
  avulsion fracture of, 197
Iliopsoas muscle, in lesser trochanteric epiphyseal separation, 217
Immobilization, 115–124. See also specific methods.
  external, with internal fixation, 124
  fractures not requiring, 115
  fractures requiring, 116
  methods of, 116–124

Impaction fracture, 12
  and inadequate muscle function, with nonunion, 31
  of femoral neck, stable, 1427
  of humeral head, in glenohumeral dislocations, 651
  of proximal finger phalanx, in children, 1943
Incision
  Hughston, 1571
  in anterior cervical spine fusion, 385
  in anterior cord syndrome, 356
  in clavicular fractures, 533, 536
  in clavicular fragmentation, 543
  in intrathoracic dislocation of humeral head, 664
  in old glenohumeral dislocations, anterior, 630
    posterior, 637
  in rotator cuff repair, 608
  Leslie and Ryan, in recurrent anterior glenohumeral dislocation, 674
  Magnuson, in recurrent anterior glenohumeral dislocation, 671
  medial parapatellar, 1647
Infants
  fractures of clavicle in, 528
  intertrochanteric fractures in, 1390–1393, 1449
    displaced, 1392
    undisplaced, 1391
  posterior radial head dislocation in, 881–882
  upper femoral epiphyseal separation in, 199–200
  upper humeral epiphyseal separation in, 157
Infection, 57–58
  anaerobic, after open fractures, 129–132
  and fracture healing, 27
  and prognosis for physeal injuries, 154
  in femoral shaft fractures, 1489, 1492
    after interamedullary nailing, 1492
  in nonunion, 32, 42–46
  in nonunion of femur, after plating, 44
  in nonunion of radius, 1-bone-forearm treatment of, 45
  in nonunion of tibia, 42, 1790
  in tibia fracture, 58
    open, 1749
  intertrochanteric fractures and, 1389
  prevention of, in shock, 80
  talar fracture or fracture-dislocation and, 1999–2000
Infraspinatus muscle, in recurrent posterior glenohumeral dislocation repair, 678
Infraspinatus tendon, in chronic anterior glenohumeral dislocation repair, 629
Intercondylar T fractures
  of distal end of proximal phalanx of finger, 1247
  of lower humerus
    in adults, 746, 781–790
      management of, 782
      operative treatment of, 786
      types of, 782
Intercostal nerves, injection of, 503
Intermetacarpal ligaments, 1138
Interossei muscles, 1146
Interosseous membrane, in tibial fractures, 1727
Interosseous space of forearm, 890
  effect of fractures on, 891
  narrowing of due to angulation, 894
Interphalangeal joints, 1143
  capsule and collateral ligaments of, 1143

Interphalangeal joints (*Continued*)
  of fingers
    acute anterior instability or dislocation of, 1210
    acute dorsal instability of, 1208
    dislocation of, hyperextension, 1206
      lateral, 1204
    fracture-dislocations of, 1211
      with displaced fragment, 1212
    functional stability of, in jammed finger, 1203
    injuries to, 1200–1218
    proximal, anterior dislocation of, 1149
      chronic dorsal instability of, 1209
      lateral instability of, 1150
  of thumb, dislocation of, 1188
    injuries to, 1187–1189
    subluxation of, 1187
Intertrochanteric fractures, 1369–1387
  complications of, 1388–1390
  displaced, 1371
    operative management of, 1375
      position of patient for, 1378
    with comminution of medial cortex, 1372
  in infants and children, 1390–1393, 1449
    displaced, 1392
    undisplaced, 1391
  management of, 1373
  stable undisplaced, 1371
    management of, 1373
  types of and technical considerations in, 1371
  unstable, 1380
    with subtrochanteric component, 1381
  with subtrochanteric component, 1373, 1386, 1395
Intervertebral disc, 262. See also *Cervical disc.*
  bulging, 274
  detachment of, posterior dislocation following, 274
  hyperextension injuries of, 273
  separation of, 274
Intramedullary pin. See *Pins, intramedullary.*
Intrapleural drainage tube, in flail chest, 516
  in tension pneumothorax, 510
Intrinsic-minus position of hand, 1147
Intrinsic-plus position of hand, 1144
Inversion stress testing, of ankle, 1812, 1817
Irani technique, for femoral shaft fractures in children, 1501
Ischemia
  in arterial injury, 60
  muscle, decompression of, 1794
  supracondylar fractures of lower humerus and, 832, 835
    management of, 758, 832
  tibial shaft fractures and, 1793
  Volkman's, 66
Ischemic necrosis, 47–51
  common sites for, 48
  muscle, skin traction and, 68, 97
  pathology of, 48
Ischium, tuberosity of, avulsion of, 198, 473

Jammed finger, 1148–1152
  evaluation of, 1201
Jammed thumb, 1148, 1152
Jefferson's fracture, of atlas, 271, 310–311
Jerk test, 1558, 1584

Joint(s). See also specific joints.
  arthritic facet, injection of, 381–382
  stiffness of, 84–88
    prevention of, 85
Joint effusion, subluxation from, 7
Jones' fracture, 2066

Kirschner wire
  in Barton's fracture, 1030
  in Bennett's fracture, 1160
  in dislocations of carpometacarpal joints of fingers, 1192
  in displaced fragments of fractured scaphoid, 1093
  in fractures of head and neck of radius, 875
  in hand fractures, 1157
  in intercondylar T fractures of lower humerus, 789
  in oblique fracture of middle phalanx, 1252
Kleinert procedure for chronic dorsal subluxation of finger, 1209
Knee joint. See also specific parts.
  acute traumatic hemarthrosis of, 1691–1692
  anterolateral instability of, acute injuries and, 1582–1588
    mechanism of, 1583
    operative treatment of, 1585
    tests for, 1557, 1583
  aspiration of, 1692
  dislocations of, 1620–1630
    irreducible posterolateral, 1629
    lateral, 1627
    nonoperative treatment of, 1624
    operative repair of, 1626
    reduction of, 1623
  emergency splinting of, 109
  extended, injuries to, 1589–1598
  extensor apparatus of, rupture of, 1649–1662
  flexed
    in rupture of posterior cruciate ligament, 1603
    in supracondylar fractures, 1511, 1514, 1516, 1522
    injury to, 1552
      pathologic results of, 1552
  floating, 1483
  fracture-dislocations of, 1620–1630
    operative repair of, 1626
    unstable, 1626
  hyperextension of, in reduction of avulsion fracture of tibial spine, 1610
  injuries of, 1541–1722
    arthrography in, 1559, 1567
    femoral shaft fractures with, 1483
    gunshot, 1694
    hyperextension, 1550
    in adolescents, 1566
    open, 1693–1695
      contaminated, 1694
    pitfalls and complications of, 1719–1720
  ligaments of. See *Ligament(s), of knee.*
  manipulation of, after femoral shaft fractures, 1500
  motion of, in cast-brace, in femoral shaft fractures, 1463
  neurovascular anatomy of, 1622
  posterolateral rotatory instability of, test for, 1584

INDEX

Knee joint (*Continued*)
  post-traumatic ossification of, 91
  soft tissues of, anatomy of, 1542–1547
  stiffness of, femoral shaft fractures and, 1499
    prevention of, 86
  subluxation of, 6
  support structures of
    dynamic lateral, 1544
    dynamic medial, 1543
    posterior, 1545
    static lateral, 1544
    static medial, 1542
Knowles pins
  in displaced femoral neck fractures, 1441
  in femoral neck fracture with femoral shaft fracture, 1482
  in fractures of clavicle, 534, 540
  in intertrochanteric fractures, in infants and children, 1392
  in supracondylar fracture, 1525
  in undisplaced subcapital fractures, 1428, 1431
Kocher maneuver for anterior dislocation of glenohumeral joint, 619
Küntscher nail, in femoral shaft fractures, 1460, 1470
Kyphoscoliosis, 2103

Lachman test, for anterior cruciate tear, 1556
Laminectomy, and cervical instability, 289
  posterior cervical fusion following, 370–372
Laskin technique for unstable open ankle fractures, 1936
Lateral ligaments, of knee, operative repair of, 1601
Lauge-Hansen mechanistic classification of ankle fractures, 1835–1841
Learmonth, wound debridement of, 127
Leg. See also specific bones and joints.
  bones of. See also specific bones.
    birth fractures of, 2085–2086
  functional rehabilitation of, 138
  joint stiffness of, prevention of, 88
  lower, emergency splinting of, 109
Leslie and Ryan incision in recurrent anterior glenohumeral dislocation, 674
Ligament(s)
  acromioclavicular. See *Acromioclavicular ligaments*.
  and injuries to articulations of clavicle, 545–565
  annular, disruption of, in Monteggia fracture, 974
    reconstruction of, 975
  collateral. See *Collateral ligaments*.
  coracoclavicular, disruption of, fracture of clavicle with, 535
  deltoid, injuries of, 1824
    repair of, 1824
  glenohumeral, 590–592
    anatomic variations in, and recurrent glenohumeral dislocations, 669
    injuries of, 587–683
  injury to, and subluxation, 6
  intermetacarpal, 1138
  meniscofemoral and meniscotibial, repair of, 1574
  of ankle, 1805
    anterior, 1805

Ligament(s) (*Continued*)
  of ankle, injuries of, 1824–1834
    lateral, 1806
      reconstruction of, 1829
      recurrent instability of, 1827
      rupture of, 1816
        medial malleolar fracture with, 1861
    medial, 1806
    posterior, 1805
  of cervical spine, 262–264
  of hand, 1138
    deep transverse, 1139
  of knee
    anatomy of, 1542
    cruciate. See *Cruciate ligaments of knee*.
    injuries to, 1548–1619
      evaluation of, 1553–1560
        tests for, 1554
      in adolescents, 1566
      mechanism of, 1548
      vs. occult femoral epiphyseal injuries, 232
    lateral, operative repair of, 1601
    medial. See *Medial ligaments of knee*.
    posterior oblique, repair of, 1575
  of wrist, 1056
  orbicular, rupture of, 821–823
  posterior oblique and tibial collateral, repair of, 1575
  radial collateral, of metacarpophalangeal joint of thumb, injury to, 1185
  tibiofibular, anterior, in bimalleolar fractures, 1878
    distal, injuries to, 1883–1886
    tear of, 1826
Ligamentoplasty procedure, in ankle sprain, 1821
Ligamentum teres, artery of, in femoral neck fractures, 1418
Limb, lower. See *Leg*.
  upper. See *Arm*.
Lipscomb technique for acetabular fracture, 1345, 1351
Little leaguer's elbow, 746, 777–778
London management of scaphoid fractures, 1064
Loose cast syndrome, 96
Lottes nail
  in segmented tibial shaft fracture, 1767, 1772
    blind nailing, 1767
    open method of, 1772
  insertion of, 1769, 1774
  in unstable nonunion of tibial shaft fractures, 1788
Lumbar spine. See also *Thoracolumbar spine*.
  anatomy of, 401
  dislocations of, 399–458
    flexion-rotation, 429
    hyperextension-shear, 429
    management of, pitfalls of, 457–458
    reduction of, 430
    stabilization of, 432
    surgical treatment of, 430
    without fracture, 429–434
  flexion exercises for, 136
  fracture-dislocations of, 399–458
  fractures of, 399–458
    management of, pitfalls of, 457–458
  injuries of
    anatomic features and mechanisms of, 400–415

xvii

Lumbar spine (*Continued*)
  injuries of, evaluation of, 416–452
    initial, 417
  management of, 416–452
    methods of, 418–421
Lumbar spinous processes, fracture of, 448
Lumbar transverse processes, isolated fractures of, 445–446
Lumbar vertebrae, exposure of, in lumbar spine dislocation, 430
Lumbosacral nerve root avulsion, hip dislocation with, 1291
Lumbrical muscles, 1145
Lunate bone
  dislocations of, 1084–1102
    and proximal scaphoid dislocation, 1107
    and scaphoid dislocation, 1108
    chronic, with avascular necrosis, 1095–1096
    mechanism of, 1086
    volar, 1087–1094
      with scapholunate subluxation, 1091
  ischemic necrosis of, 50
  subluxations of, 1084–1102
Luxatio erecta, 622–624

Magnusson repair for recurrent anterior glenohumeral dislocation, 671
Magnusson wiring for transverse patellar fractures, 1637
Maisonneuve fracture of proximal fibula, 1884
Malgaigne fracture-dislocation, 489–493
Malignancy, metastatic, and pathologic fractures, 2129
Malignant bone tumors, and pathologic fractures, 2094, 2116–2133
  primary, and pathologic fractures, 2124
Malignant hyperthermia, 81–82
Malleolus(i)
  both, fractures of, 1872
    with lateral displacement of talus, 1873
    with medial displacement of talus, 1874
  fractures of, adduction, in children, 251–252
    stages of, 1838
  lateral, 1802
    fracture of, 1844
      irreducible, 1922–1928
      with lateral displacement, 1846
        nonoperative treatment of, 1852
        operative treatment of, 1847
      without lateral displacement, 1844
  medial, 1802
    fracture of, 1880, 1894
      fibular fracture proximal to tibiofibular syndesmosis with, 1866, 1869
      isolated, 1856
      with rupture of lateral ligament, 1861
Mallet finger deformity, 1148, 1213
  splint for, 1156
  tendon avulsions in, 1213
  with avulsion fracture, 1214
  without fracture, 1213
Malunion, 51–54
  of ankle fracture-dislocations, 1939–1946
  of distal radial fracture, 1045–1048
  of femoral shaft fractures, 1495
    after internal fixation, 1498
  of fractures of lower humerus, 747

Malunion (*Continued*)
  of talar fractures, 1997–1999
  of tibial shaft fractures, 1778–1793
  of upper femoral epiphyseal slips, greater than 60°, 213–216
    involving 1 hip, 215
    involving both hips, 216
  typical deformities of, 52
Maquet repair for chronic patellar subluxation or dislocation with patellofemoral arthritis, 1677
March fractures, 2058
MAST, 109, 483
  in femoral shaft fractures, 1457
Matson technique, of 4-compartment parafibular decompression, 1794
McLaughlin technique for old posterior glenohumeral dislocations, 637
Mechanisms of injury. See also specific injuries.
  in dislocation(s), 5–7
  in fracture(s), 2–3
Medial capsular structures of knee, and posterior cruciate tears, 1565
  operative repair of, 1571
Medial cortex, comminution of, 1372
Medial ligaments of knee
  injuries of
    examples of, 1564
    grade I, 1561
      management of, 1568
    grade II, 1562
      management of, 1569
    grade III, 1562
      surgical management of, 1570
      with instability in full extension, 1564
    grading of, 1561–1567
    management of, 1568–1578
    operative repair of, 1600
    pathologic results of, 1563
Median nerve, function of, in Colles' fracture, 1018
  in carpal injuries, 1131–1133
  injury of, in supracondyloid process fracture, 736
Medulla, of bone, circulation in, 18
Meniscofemoral ligaments, repair of, 1574
Meniscotibial ligaments, repair of, 1574
Meniscus, in weight bearing, 1697
  injury to, and anterior cruciate rupture, 1590
Metabolic disorders, and pathologic fractures, 2089–2099
Metacarpal bones
  of fingers
    base of, fracture of, 1236
    dislocation of, 1109–1110
    fifth, fracture-dislocation of, 1194
    fourth, fracture-dislocation of, 1193
      shaft of, fracture of, 1230
    fractures of, 1219–1238
      cast-splint immobilization in, 1157
    neck of, stable fracture of, 1221
      unstable fractures of, 1223
    normal anatomy of, 1221
    shaft of, fracture of, 1226
      displaced, 1227, 1232
      multiple displaced, 1231
      stable, 1226
      unstable, 1228
    third, shaft of, fracture of, 1230

INDEX

Metacarpal bones (*Continued*)
  of thumb
    base of, fractures of, 1168–1172
      stable, 1169
      unstable, 1171
    shaft of, fractures of, 1173–1176
      stable, 1173
      unstable, 1175
Metacarpal Ligaments, 1138
Metacarpophalangeal joints
  capsule and collateral ligaments of, 1143
  dislocation of, 1151
    complex, 1152
    mechanisms, of, 1151–1152
    simple, 1152
  of fingers, 1140
    dislocation of, complex, 1197
      simple, 1196
    fracture-dislocation of, 1199
    injuries of, 1195–1200
  of thumb, 1142
    dislocation of, complex, 1177
      simple, 1177
    injuries to, 1176–1186
    lateral instability of, 1151
    normal, 1177
Metaphyseal cortical defect, and pathologic fractures, 2110
Metaphysis, circulation to, 145–147
Metatarsal bones
  fifth base of, fractures of, 2064–2069
    proximal shaft of, fractures of, 2066
  fractures of, 2058–2069
    with displacement, 2060–2064
    without displacement, 2059–2060
  shaft of, fractures of, displaced, 2062
  tuberosity of, fracture of, 2065
Metatarsophalangeal joints, dislocations of, 2070–2072
  irreducible, 2072
Methylmethacrylate, in giant cell tumor, 2122
Midtarsal joint
  dislocations of, 2045–2050
    lateral swivel, 2047
    medial, with cuboid fracture, 2046
    medial swivel, 2046
    plantar, 2047
  fracture-dislocations of, 2045–2050
  fracture-subluxation of, 2041
  fusion of, 2050
  injuries to, 2042
  recurrent or persistent subluxation of, 2049
Military antishock trousers (MAST), 109, 483, 2146
  in femoral shaft fractures, 1457
Miller method for Colles' fracture, 1012
Mini-spica cast
  in femoral shaft fracture, 1470
  in Malgaigne fracture-dislocation, 492
  in subluxation of sacroiliac joint, 480
  in subtrochanteric fractures, 1404
Minnesota, University of, technique of posterolateral decompression for neural deficit, 437
Monteggia injury, 959–978
  anterior, 963
    from elbow hyperextension, 899, 961
    from torsional injury, 961
  in children, 964

Monteggia injury (*Continued*)
  closed reduction of, 963–969
  complications of, prevention and management of, 977–978
  direct, 963
  in adults, operative management of, 973–977
  in children, unrecognized, 972
  indirect, 961
  lateral, in children, 968
    from adduction, 962
  mechanisms of, 960–963
  posterior, 966
    with elbow flexion, 962
  torsional injury and, 900
Mortality, intertrochanteric fractures and, 1388
Motor innervation, in lower body, 403
Multangular bone, greater. See *Trapezium*.
  lesser, dislocation of, 1111–1112
Murray and Racz treatment of fat embolism, 84
Muscle(s)
  aconeus, in Monteggia fracture, 973
  anaerobic necrosis of. See *Myonecrosis, anaerobic.*
  compartment pressure of. See also *Compartment syndromes.*
    Whitesides' technique of measuring, 65
  diffuse atrophy of, subluxation from, 7
  flexor profundus, avulsion of, 1149, 1216
  glenohumeral, 589–590
  hypothenar, 1145
  iliapsoas, in lesser trochanteric epiphyseal separation, 217
  inadequate function of, and fracture impaction, with nonunion, 31
  interossei, 1146
  ischemic, decompression of, 1794
  ischemic necrosis of, skin traction and, 68, 97
  lumbrical, 1145
  of forearm, insertions of, 892
  of hand, 1144–1147
  of hip joint, active exercises for, 137
  of knee, anatomy of, 1542
  quadriceps, 1545
  thenar, 1145
Myelogram, in cervical spine injuries, 296
Myeloma, multiple, and pathologic fractures, 2090, 2128
Myonecrosis, anaerobic. See also *Gas Gangrene*.
  acute, treatment of, 132
  preventive treatment of, 131
  clostridial, 130, 1755
Myositis ossificans, fractures of lower humerus and, 747
  of hip joint, 1363
Myositis ossificans traumatica. See *Ossification, post-traumatic*.

Nail-plate, in subtrochanteric fractures, 1393
Nails. See *Pins*.
Navicular bone of tarsus
  fracture-dislocations of, 2031–2038
    chronic unrecognized, 2038
  fractures of, 2031–2038
    displaced, 2034
    management of, 2033–2038
    types of, 2031–2033
    undisplaced, 2034

INDEX

Necrosis
  avascular
    chronic lunate dislocation with, 1095–1096
    of femoral head, 1362
    of humeral head, 705
    of talus, 1993
  ischemic, 47–51
    common sites for, 48
    muscle, skin traction and, 68, 97
    pathology of, 48
  of muscle. See *Myonecrosis*.
Neer classification of supracondylar fractures, 1512
Neer prosthesis, in fractures of head and neck of humerus, 662
Nerve(s)
  axillary, 594
    injury to, in glenohumeral dislocations, 645
  functional levels of in spinal cord injury, 454–456
  in carpal injuries, 1130–1133
  injuries of, 74
    fracture of clavicle and, 540
    fractures and dislocations of elbow joint and, 836
    hip dislocations with, 1290–1291
    in fractures of lower humerus, 746
    in glenohumeral dislocations, 645–646
    in pelvic fracture, 462
    stretch, hip dislocations with, 1290
    treatment of fracture and, 97
  intercostal, injection of, 503
  median, function of, in Colles' fracture, 1018
    in carpal injuries, 1131–1133
    injury of, in supracondyloid process fracture, 736
  motor, to lower body, 403
  near glenohumeral joint, 593–594
  of knee, 1622
  peripheral, injuries to, sites of, 70
  peroneal, injuries of, hip dislocations with, 1290
  radial. See *Radial nerve*.
  sciatic, injuries of, hip dislocations with, 1290
  sensory, impairment of, in cervical spine injuries, 302
    to lower body, 403
  sural, in calcaneal fractures, 2028
  tibial, injuries of, hip dislocation with, 1290
  ulnar. See *Ulnar nerve*.
Nerve root
  compression of, clinical patterns of, 375–376
  eighth, compression of, 376
  in cervical spine injuries, 276
  lumbosacral, avulsion of, hip dislocation with, 1291
  seventh, compression of, 375
  sixth, compression of, 375
Neural arch of C2, fracture of, 312–314
Neurologic deficit, in compression fracture of thoracolumbar spine, 437
  in hyperflexion fractures of thoracolumbar vertebrae, 424
Neurologic signs in thoracolumbar spinal injuries, 404
  related to thoracolumbar spine anatomy, 402
Neurotrophy, diabetic, midtarsal dislocation in, 2050

Neurovascular structures. See *Blood vessels;* and *Nerve(s)*.
Neviaser technique for clavicular fixation, 534, 540
  for rotator cuff rupture with biceps graft, 649
Newborn. See *Birth;* and *Infants*.
Nightstick fracture, of ulna, 896
Nonunion, 19, 27–42
  clinical features of, 28
  incomplete fracture fixation with, 31
  infected, 32, 42–46
    of femur, after plating, 44
    of tibia, 42, 1790
    of tibial shaft fractures, 42, 1790
  management of, 30
    by electrical stimulation, 33, 1494, 1785
    by rigid fixation, 38
    operative, 33
  of distal radial fractures, 1045–1051
  of femoral neck fractures, with nonviable femoral head and segmental collapse, 1453
    with viable head, 1451
  of femoral shaft fractures, 38, 1493
  of forearm fractures, compression plating for, 39
  of fractures of clavicle, 41, 537
  of fractures of lower humerus, 747
  of humeral shaft, fractures of, 40, 734–735
  of scaphoid, 1068–1083
    bone grafting with radial styloidectomy in, 1069
    operation for, 37
  of talar fractures, 1997–1999
  of tibial shaft fractures, 35, 1778–1793
    diagnosis of, 1783
  radiographic features of, 29
  types of problems associated with, 31
Norwood technique for anterolateral instability of knee, 1585
Nursemaid's elbow, 879–881

Occipito-atlantal joint, dislocations of, 306–309
  motion of, 265
Occipitocervical fusion, in occipito-atlantal dislocations, 307
Occiput, articulations of, 263
Occiput-C1 dislocation, 282
Occiput-C1-C2 articulations, injuries peculiar to, 282–289
Ocular-palmar syndrome, in Colles' fracture, 1009, 1018
Odontoid process
  acquired abnormalities of, with dislocation of atlas, 285
  congenital abnormalities of, 326
    with dislocation of atlas, 285
  fractures of
    with dislocation, 288
    with displacement, 331–333
    without displacement, 287, 329
    traumatic forward dislocation with, 323–325
  lesions of, 326–327
    management of, 327
  superior subluxation of, 328–333

INDEX

Rehabilitation, after spinal cord injury, 393–396
   functional, 135–141
   in traumatic paraplegia, 453–456
Remodeling, after compression plating, 17
   growth, of fracture deformities, in children, 988–991
Respiration, assistance in, in shock, 80
   in flail chest, 517
   difficult, in trauma patient, 2141
Respiratory insufficiency, with fat embolism, 82
Reticulum cell sarcoma, and pathologic fractures, 2127
Retinacular blood vessels, in femoral neck fractures, 1417
Retroperitoneal abscess, pelvic fractures and, 495
Rheumatoid arthritis, with dislocation of atlas, 283
Ribs
   dislocations of, 502–505
   emergency splinting of, 107
   fractures of, 502–505
     complications of, emergency management of, 509–512
     double, 513–518
   lower, fractures and dislocations of, 505
   upper, fractures and dislocations of, 502–505
Ring, of Ranvier, 147
   pelvic, anterior segment of, double breaks in, 493–494
     single breaks in, 478–479
Riordan pin, in mallet finger, 1215
Robinson-Southwick method, of occipitocervical fusion, 307
   of posterior fusion following cervical laminectomies, 370–372
Rockwood technique of x-ray of sternoclavicular joint, 561
Rods. See also *Pins*.
   Ender's, in femoral shaft fracture with femoral neck fracture, 1482
     in intertrochanteric femoral fracture, 1376, 1379, 2096
   Harrington. See *Harrington rods*.
Rolando's intra-articular fracture, 1163
Rotator cuff, in irreducible fresh dislocation of glenohumeral head, 625
   rupture of, in glenohumeral dislocations, 646–651
   surgical repair of, 608
Rowland fixation technique for Colles' fracture, 1016
Rush pin, in displaced fractures of anatomic and surgical humeral neck, 714
   in lateral malleolus fracture, 1849
Russell traction, 122
   in femoral shaft fractures in children, 1508

Sacroiliac joint, subluxation of, 479–481
Sacrum, transverse fracture of, with displacement, 474–476
Sag test, 1556
Salvatori traction bow, 1906
Sarcoma, osteogenic, osteolytic type, 2125
   vs. post-traumatic ossification, 89
   reticulum cell, and pathologic fractures, 2127
Sarmiento and Laird screw fixation of medial femoral head fragment, 1295

Sarmiento method, for forearm fractures, 903–917
   for humeral shaft fractures, 721, 729
   for patellar-tendon-bearing cast, 1736
Scaphoid
   carpal
     blood supply of, 1060
     delayed union of, operation for, 37
     dislocation of, and dislocation of lunate, 1108
     fracture of, Colles' fracture with, 1020
     fractures of, 1059–1083
       dorsal, perilunate dislocation with, with displacement of fragments, 1100
         without displacement of fragments, 1099
       immobilization in, 1063
       rapidly healing, 1062
       recent, 1061–1067
         prognosis in, 1062
       stabilization of displaced fragments of, 1092
       subacute, 1067–1068
       unstable, displaced, or slowly healing, 1064
     mechanism of injury of, 1060
     nonunion of, 1068–1083
       bone grafting with radial styloidectomy in, 1069
       operation for, 37
     proximal, dislocation of, and dislocation of lunate, 1107
       ischemic necrosis of, 49
     radiographic examination of, 102
   tarsal. See *Navicular bone of tarsus*.
Scaphoid-capitate fracture syndrome, 1118
Scaphoid-scapholunate dissociation, rotatory subluxation of, 1103–1105
Scapholunate joint, dissociation of, 1087
   subluxation of, mechanisms of, 1087
   volar dislocation of lunate with, 1091
Scapula
   body of, fractures of, 566–567
   coracoid process of, fractures of, 566–567
     and subcoracoid dislocation, 663
   dislocation of, 583–584
   fractures of, 566–569
   glenoid fossa of. See *Glenoid cavity*.
   neck of, fractures of, 567–569
     with displacement, 568
   spine of, fractures of, 566–567
Scapulohumeral rhythm, 595
Schneider nail, in femoral shaft fractures, 1460, 1470
   operative technique for, 1474
Sciatic nerve, injuries of, hip dislocations with, 1290
Scoliosis, 2103
Scott repair for recurrent posterior glenohumeral dislocation, 678
Screw
   cancellous bone lag, in displaced talar neck fractures, 1971
     in isolated calcaneal fractures, 2010
   compression
     high-angle, in femoral neck fractures, 1434
       in intertrochanteric fractures, 1382
     in intertrochanteric fractures, 1377
     in medial malleolar fractures, 1860
     in unstable intertrochanteric fractures, 1386
   in internal fixation, 124
   in medial femoral head fragment, 1295
   in medial malleolar fractures, 1860

XXV

Screw (*Continued*)
  in radial styloid fracture, 1035
  in talar neck fracture, 1965
  small fragment, in fractures at base of thumb
      metacarpal, 1171
    in fractures of finger metacarpal, 1234
    in unstable fracture of shaft of thumb
      metacarpal, 1175
  transosseous, in ankle diastasis, 1884
Seat belt fracture, 413, 443–444
  and visceral injury, 76
Segmental fracture, 11
  of forearm bones, 949–953
  of tibial shaft, 1767–1777
Sensory innervation, impairment of, in cervical
      spine injuries, 302
  in lower body, 403
Sepsis, femoral shaft fractures and, 1479
  pelvic fracture and, 495
Sesamoid bones, of great toe, fractures of,
      2076–2077
Shenton's line, 1273
Shepherd's crook deformity in fibrous dysplasia,
      2105
Shirt-tackler's injury, 75
Shock, 77–81
  cardinal signs of, 79
  delayed femoral shaft fractures and, 1479
  development of, 77
  hypovolemic, pelvic fractures and, 482
  in trauma patient, 2142
  prevention and treatment of, 79, 106, 2143,
      2146
  spinal, 405
Shotgun fractures, 132–134
  of femur, 133, 1480
Shoulder
  blocker's, 92
  direct violence to, 690
  exercises for, gravity, 139
    passive stretching, 139
  functional rehabilitation of, 139
  radiographic examination of, 102, 607, 632,
      652, 676
Shoulder girdle. See also specific elements.
  fractures and dislocations of, 523–586
    pitfalls of, 585
Shoulder joint. See *Glenohumeral joint*.
Shumaker technique for clavicular
      fragmentation, 543
Skateboard exercises, passive, for hip injuries,
      137
Skeletal traction
  in acetabular wall fracture, 1345, 1351
  in anterior cord syndrome, 352
  in cervical spine fracture-dislocations, 349
  in displaced fractures of anatomic and surgical
      humeral neck, 711
  in explosion fracture of distal tibia, 1906, 1909
  in femoral shaft fractures, 1458, 1470, 1478
  in humeral shaft fractures, in polytrauma, 728
  in intercondylar T fractures of lower humerus,
      784
  in old unreduced hip dislocation, 1309
  in open fractures of forearm, 956
  in supracondylar fractures, 1518
  sites for, 121
Skier's thumb, 1181

Skin, grafting of, in open fractures, 1753
Skin traction, 121
  and compartment syndromes, 68
  and ischemic muscle necrosis, 68, 97
Skull traction, in cervical spine injuries, 298–302
Slabs, plaster, application of, 118
Sleeve, functional, in fracture of ulna, 907
  in humeral shaft fractures, 721, 729
Sling, hand, in humeral shaft fractures, 720
  pelvic, in Malgaigne fracture-dislocation, 491
  Velpeau. See *Velpeau sling*.
Slocum test, 1558
Smith's fracture, 1021–1028
  malunion of, 1046
  nonunion of, 1049
  with comminution, 1024
Smith's variations of normal carrying angle of
      elbow, 749
Soft tissue
  cervical, injuries of, management of, 373–392
  in repair of patellar instability, in children and
      adolescents, 1675
  of knee, anatomy of, 1542–1547
  severe damage of, and healing, 27
Soltanpur reduction for fractures of lower
      humerus, 770
Southwick fixation of intertrochanteric fractures,
      1382
Southwick high-angle compression hip screw, in
      femoral neck fractures, 1434
  in intertrochanteric fractures, 1382
Spak sling, in humeral shaft fracture, 720
Speed and Boyd reduction for fracture-dislocation
      of elbow joint, 822
Spica cast
  clavicular, in fractures of clavicle, 529
  in acute posterior glenohumeral dislocation, 635
  in femoral shaft fractures in children, 1501
  in fractures of clavicle, 529
  in posterior glenohumeral dislocations, old, 637
    recurrent, 680
  in traumatic hip dislocations in children, 1333
  pantaloon, in greater trochanter fractures, 1367
  thumb, in injuries to interphalangeal joint of
      thumb, 1188
    in skier's thumb, 1182
Spinal column. See *Spine*.
Spinal cord, injury of, functional levels of, 395,
      454–456
  rehabilitation after, 393–396
Spinal shock, 405
Spine. See also *Cervical spine; Lumbar spine;
      and Thoracic spine.*
  fracture of, and visceral injury, 77
  gunshot, 451–452
  functional rehabilitation of, 135
  hyperextension of, in cervical spine
      fracture-dislocations, 350
  in osteogenesis imperfecta, 2102
  of scapula, fractures of, 566–567
  of tibia, fractures of, 234–235
    avulsion, 1609–1612
    slightly displaced, 235
    with acute or chronic complete
      displacement, 236
  radiographic examination of, 104
  stabilization of, in backward dislocation of
      cervical spine, 364

INDEX

Spinotuberosity fractures of tibia, 1714–1718
    external, 1715
    internal, 1715
    lateral, 1708
Spinous processes, cervical and first dorsal, fracture of, 446
    isolated fractures of, 446–449
    lumbar, fracture of, 448
Spiral fracture, 10
Splint
    emergency, 106
        of cervical spine, 106, 291
        of multiple fractures, 109
    extension block, in acute dorsal instability of interphalangeal joints of fingers, 1208
    for mallet finger, 1156
    Fry exercise, 1346
    plaster, external, 117
    pneumatic compression, 2146
    sugar-tong, in Colles' fracture, 1012, 1017
        in Smith's fracture, 1027
Splint-cast, in phalangeal or metacarpal fracture, 1157
Spondylolisthesis, of sacrum, traumatic, 475
    stable, cast for, 442
Sprain. See specific joints.
Spring-loaded (Gardner-Wells) traction, technique of applying, 298
Steering wheel injury, 513–518
    management of, 514
Steinmann pins
    in Colles' fracture, 1017
    in fracture of olecranon, 816
    in open forearm fractures in children, 988
    in Smith's fracture, 1026
    in transcondylar fracture-dislocation of elbow joint, 825
    in unstable open ankle fracture, 1936
    in unstable tibial shaft fractures, 1745
Stellate fracture, of glenoid, 570
    management of, 572
Sternoclavicular joint
    dislocation of, 560
        anterior, 562
        anteroinferior, 559
        anterosuperior, 558
        mechanisms of, 558
        posterior, 563
        unreduced chronic, 564
    epiphyseal separation of, 560
    injuries of, 557–565
    sprain of, 559, 561
    subluxation of, 560, 562
        anterior, 4
Sternum, fractures of, 519–521
    with displacement, 520–521
Stimson technique, for anterior dislocation of glenohumeral joint, 618
    for dislocation or fracture-dislocation of hip, 1273
    for traumatic hip dislocation in children, 1332
Stove-in chest, 513–518
Straddle injury, of pelvis, 467
Strapping
    in dislocation of scapula, 584
    in fractures and dislocations of costal cartilages, 507
    in fractures and dislocations of ribs, 504

Strapping (*Continued*)
    in fractures of sternum, 520
    in recurrent subluxation or dislocation of costochondral joint, 508
Stress fractures. See *Fatigue fractures*.
Stress tests
    abduction and adduction, of knee, 1554
    of ankle, 1811
        inversion, 1812, 1817
    passive, of jammed finger, 1204
    varus, of knee, 1583
Styloid process of radius, fracture of, 1033–1035
    resection of, in nonunion of scaphoid, 1069
Styloidectomy, radial, in nonunion of scaphoid, 1069
Subcapital fractures. See also *Femur, neck of, fractures of*.
    classification of, anteroposterior appearance and, 1412
        rotational instability and, 1410
    complete, 1410, 1412
        with displacement, 1411, 1413
    displaced, 1410
    fracture line in, 1409
    head-neck relationships in, 1414
    impacted, management of, 1427
    incomplete, 1410, 1412
    malreduction of, 1415
    undisplaced, Knowles pin in, 1428, 1431
Subclavian approach to axillary artery injury, 644
Subcoracoid dislocation, 618
    and fracture of acromion, 663
    and fracture of coracoid process, 663
Subluxation. See also specific area.
    causes of, 6
    voluntary, 6
Subtalar joint
    arthritis of, 2000–2004
    arthrodesis of, after calcaneal fractures, 2030
    dislocation of, in talar neck fracture, 1953
        medial, 1981
        talar inversion injury and, 1957
    in calcaneal fractures, 2011–2016
    subluxation of, talar neck fracture with, 1953, 1962
Subtrochanteric fractures, 1393–1406
    nonoperative treatment of, 1401
    without intertrochanteric component, 1393
    reduction and Zickel nail fixation of, 1396
Sudeck's acute bone atrophy, 88–89
Sugar-tong splint, in Colles' fracture, 1012, 1017
    in Smith's fracture, 1027
Supracondylar fractures
    of femur
        operative reduction and internal fixation of, 1526
        torsional deformity with, 1518
        types of, 1512
        with displacement of condyles, 1513, 1516
        with fragmentation of femoral shaft, 1513, 1522
        with minimal displacement, 1512, 1514
    of lower humerus, 747–770
        and vascular injury, 828, 831
        diagnosis of, 756
        ischemia after, 832, 835
        management of, 758
        types of, 750

Supracondylar fractures (*Continued*)
　of lower humerus, typical deformity of, 750
　　with displacement, 743
　　with forward displacement, 768
　　with lateral tilt, 753
　　with medial displacement of distal fragment, 750
　　with medial tilt, 752
　　with posterior displacement, 751
　　without lateral displacement or angulation, 750
Supracondyloid process, fracture of, 736
Supraspinatus tendon, rupture of, arthrogram after, 608
Sural nerve, in calcaneal fractures, 2028
Sustentaculum, medial, in calcaneal fractures, 2021
Swan-neck deformity, 1150, 1209
Swanson replacement arthroplasty, 1073
　in chronic lunate dislocation, 1095
　in nonunion of scaphoid, 1073
　of radial head, 867
Synostosis, fibulotibial, 1760

T-condylar fractures. See *Intercondylar T fractures.*
Talectomy, 1999
Talocrural angle, 1842
Talonavicular joint, fractures and fracture-dislocations of, 2045
Talus. See also *Ankle joint.*
　anterior subluxation of, anterior marginal tibial fractures with, 1898–1908
　blood supply of, 1993
　body of, 1803
　　dislocation of, 1954
　　ischemic necrosis of, 50
　　undisplaced hyperextension fracture of, management of, 1960
　compression or mixed injuries of, 1959–1960, 1991–1992
　dislocations of, 1952–1992
　　total, 1983
　　upward, 1920–1921
　dome of, osteochondral fractures of, 1958, 1986
　eversion injuries of, 1958–1959, 1989–1991
　fracture-dislocations of, complications of, 1993–2004
　fractures of, 1952–1992
　　complications of, 1993–2004
　injuries of, hyperextension, 1952–1954, 1960–1976
　　hyperflexion, 1955, 1977–1979
　　inversion, 1956–1958, 1980–1989
　lateral displacement of, 1841
　　bimalleolar fractures with, 1873
　lateral process of, fractures of, 1974
　　displaced or unrecognized, 1976
　　hyperextension, 1954
　　osteochondral, 1818
　medial displacement of, bimalleolar fractures with, 1874
　neck of, fractures of
　　closed reduction and screw fixation in, 1965

Talus (*Continued*)
　neck of, fractures of, displaced, open reduction and screw fixation in, 1971
　　with dislocation of talar head or body, 1954, 1970
　　hyperextension, 1953
　　　management of, 1960
　　undisplaced, 1953
　　　management of, 1960
　　with subtalar subluxation, 1953, 1962
　normal healing of, 1995
　posterior displacement of, in posterior marginal fractures of tibia, 1888
　posterior process of, fracture of, 1977
Tarsal navicular bone. See *Navicular bone of tarsus.*
Tarsometatarsal joint
　anatomy of, 2051
　dislocations of, 2051–2057
　　direct, 2052
　　indirect, 2053
　　management of, 2054–2057
　　persistent or unrecognized, 2057
　fracture-dislocations of, 2051–2057
　　direct, 2052
　　indirect, 1053
　　management of, 2054–2057
Tarsus. See specific bones, e.g., *Navicular bone of tarsus.*
Teardrop fracture-dislocation, of cervical spine, 270
Technetium-99m sulfur-colloid, in evaluation of femoral head, 1452
Tendon(s)
　anterior tibial, in tarsometatarsal joint dislocation, 2056
　avulsions of, in mallet finger deformity, 1213
　biceps, graft of, in rotator cuff rupture, 649
　bicipital, injury of, in fractures of upper humerus, 703
　injuries to, 74–75
　of hand, injury of, mechanisms of, 1148–1152
　of knee, anatomy of, 1542
　patellar. See *Patellar tendon.*
　peroneal, in calcaneal fractures, 2017
　supraspinatus, rupture of, arthrogram after, 608
Tenosynovitis, peroneal, calcaneal fractures and, 2028
Tension pneumothorax, 509–510
Tetanus, after open fractures, 129–132
　clostridial, prophylaxis for, 130
Thenar muscles, 1145
Thigh, footballer's, 92
Thompson approach, for fracture of proximal forearm, 942
　for fractures of proximal radius, 922
Thoracic cage. See also specific elements.
　injuries to, 499–522
　　general considerations in, 500–501
　　management of, pitfalls of, 522
Thoracic spine. See also *Thoracolumbar spine.*
　dislocations of, 399–458
　　lateral, shearing, 449–451
　　management of, pitfalls of, 457–458
　fracture-dislocations of, 399–458
　fractures of, 399–458
　　management of, pitfalls of, 457–458

INDEX

Thoracic spine (*Continued*)
  hyperextension exercises for, 135
  injuries of
    anatomic features and mechanisms of, 400–415
    evaluation of, 416–452
      initial, 417
    management of, 416–452
      methods of, 418–421
      nonoperative postural reduction of, 418
      operative reduction and internal fixation of, 419
  normal anatomy of, 401
Thoracolumbar spinal fusion, in flexion-rotation fracture-dislocation, 426
  spontaneous, 436
Thoracolumbar spine. See also *Lumbar spine;* and *Thoracic spine.*
  emergency splinting of, 107
  fracture-dislocations of, flexion-rotation, 425–428
    hyperextension-shear, 439–442
  fractures of
    compression (bursting), 408, 436
      posterolateral decompression for neural deficit in, 437
      spontaneous fusion in, 436
      with osteoporosis, 435
    distraction (seat belt), 413, 443–444
    hyperflexion (wedge), 422–424
      with neurologic deficit, 424
      without neurologic deficit, 423
    unstable shear, 441
  injuries of
    compression, 408
      high-violence, 409
      low-violence, 409
    distraction, 413
    flexion-rotation, 409
    gunshot, 415
    hyperextension-shear, 411
    hyperflexion, 406
      stable, 407, 422
      unstable, 407, 422
    lateral bending, 414, 444–445
    lateral shearing, 414
    mechanisms of, 406–415
Thrombosis, arterial, 60
  common sites of, 63
  in upper limb, management of, 61
Thumb
  avulsion fracture of, 1182
  carpometacarpal joint of. See *Carpometacarpal joint, of thumb.*
  dislocations and fracture-dislocations of, 1158–1189
  interphalangeal joints of, dislocation of, 1188
    injuries to, 1187–1189
    subluxation of, 1187
  jammed, 1148–1152
  metacarpal bones of. See *Metacarpal bones, of thumb.*
  metacarpophalangeal joint of. See *Metacarpophalangeal joints.*
  skier's, 1181

Thumb spica cast, in injuries to interphalangeal joint of thumb, 1188
  in skier's thumb, 1182
Tibia
  condyles of, fractures of, 1696–1718
    internal fixation in, 1707–1710
    unstable, 1708
    lateral. See *Tibial plateau fractures, lateral.*
  congenital pseudoarthrosis of, 2106
  distal, fractures of, delayed union in, 1784
    internal rotation, 1902
    pronation-external rotation, 1901
  fractures of
    anterior marginal, with anterior subluxation of talus, 1898–1908
    bicondylar, 1714–1718
      fibula in, 1714
    fatigue, 1725
    femoral shaft fracture with, 1483
    fibula in, 1727
    infected, 58
    isolated articular, from avulsion injury, 1914–1915
    Paget's disease and, 2098
    posterior marginal
      avulsion injury and, 1914–1915
      operative reduction of, 1892–1896
      posterior dislocation of foot with, 1887–1897
      types and mechanisms of, 1888–1891
    spinotuberosity, 1714–1718
      external, 1715
      internal, 1715
      lateral, 1708
  inferior articular surface of, comminution of, 1909–1914
  ischemic necrosis of, 50
  posterior articular surface of, fixation of, 1870
  proximal, malunion of, 1782
  shaft of, fractures of, 1724–1748
    autogenous bone graft in, 1762
    biology of healing and management of, 1730–1740
    closed, 1749
    closed reduction of, 1733
    complications and pitfalls of, 1798–1799
    deformity of fibula in, 1728
    distraction of, 1766
    fibula and interosseous membrane in, 1727
    loose bone fragments in, 1758, 1765
    malunion and delayed union of, 1778–1793
    mechanisms and mechanics of, 1724–1726
    nonunion of, 35, 1778–1793
      diagnosis of, 1783
      infected, 42, 1790
      unstable, autogenous bone grafting in, 1786
      with fracture distraction, 38
    open, 1749–1766
      bone defects with, 1757–1764
      principles of management of, 1749–1751
    pitfalls of treating, 1764–1766
    problems in, 1767–1796
    segmental, 1767–1777
    shortening of, 1742
    3-dimensional management of, 1740–1744
    unstable, 1744–1748
    with femoral fractures, 1796

xxix

Tibia (*Continued*)
  spine of, fractures of, 234–235
    avulsion, 1609–1612
    slightly displaced, 235
    with acute or chronic complete displacement, 236
  tubercle of, avulsion of, 243–245
    types of, 243
  tuberosity of
    anterior displacement of, in chronic patellar subluxation or dislocation, 1677
    apophysis of, avulsion injuries of, 1612–1619
    avulsion fractures of, 1617
    in adults, 1659–1662
Tibia and fibula, fractures of, 1723–1800
  shafts of, fractures of, bilateral, 1743
Tibial collateral ligament, injury to, complications of, 1579–1581
  repair of, 1575
Tibial diaphysis, extruded fragments of, 1759
Tibial epiphysis
  distal
    fracture of, in adolescents, 1890
      two-fragment, in adolescents, 1896
    injuries of, 246–256
      and varus deformity, correction of, 255–256
      operative reduction and internal fixation in, 252–255
      types of, 247
    rotational displacement of, with or without fibular fracture, 1929–1930
  proximal, separation of, 237–242
    in adduction, abduction, and crushing injuries, 241–242
    in hyperextension injury, 238–240
Tibial metaphysis, upper, fractures of, and valgus deformities in children, 1782
Tibial nerve, injuries of, hip dislocation with, 1290
Tibial plateau fractures
  central-depression, 1704, 1706
  fibula and, 1699
  lateral, 1697
    displaced, closed reduction and cast-brace in, 1703–1707
    internal fixation in, 1707–1710
    split-depression, 1703, 1706
      bone grafting in, 1711–1713
    without fragmentation or depression, 1701–1702
  management of, 1700
Tibial tendon, anterior, in tarsometatarsal joint dislocation, 2056
Tibiocalcaneal fusion, 2000
Tibiofibular joint, proximal, dislocation of, 1688–1690
  types of, 1689
  subluxation of, 1688–1690
Tibiofibular ligament, anterior, in bimalleolar fractures, 1878
  distal, injuries to, 1883–1886
  tear of, 1825
Tibiofibular syndesmosis, fibular fracture and, 1863, 1871
  repair of, 1868
Tibiotalar contact, changes in, 1842

Tibiotalar joint, arthritis of, 2000–2004
  fusion of, 2001
Tight cast syndrome, 96
Toes
  fractures of, 2073–2077
    with displacement, 2074
    with minimal or no displacement, 2073–2074
  great, sesamoid bones of, fractures of, 2076–2077
  joint stiffness of, prevention of, 86
  phalanges of. See *Phalanx (phalanges), of toes*.
Torsion, and tibial fractures, biomechanics of, 1725
  internal, and ankle sprain, 1807
Torticollis, acute, 286
  in unilateral atlanto-axial subluxation, 315
Torus fracture, 979
  of forearm, 980
Tourniquet, in Colles' fracture, 1011
Traction
  balanced suspension apparatus for, 122
  Bryant, in distal femoral epiphyseal separation at birth, 221
  in femoral shaft fractures in children, 1506
  in subtrochanteric fractures, 1402
  Buck's, in intertrochanteric fracture, 1374, 1376
  cervical, in cervical disc protrusion, 379
  continuous, 120
    in reduction of fractures, 112
  excessive external torsion in, in femoral shaft fractures in children, 1509
  fixed, in distal radial and ulnar fractures in children, 984
    in fractures of mid-third of forearm, in children, 995
    in fractures of proximal forearm, 1000
  halo. See *Halo traction*.
  in reduction of fractures, 112
  lateral, in fractures of clavicle, 531
    in fractures of lower humerus, 766
  longitudinal, in dislocation of cervical vertebra, 337
  90°-90°, in proximal femoral fractures, 122
    in subtrochanteric fractures, 1403
  overhead, in cervical disc protrusion, 380
    in fractures of lower humerus, 763
  Quigley's, in lateral malleolus fracture, 1853
    in trimalleolar ankle fracture, 113
  Russell, 122
    in femoral shaft fractures in children, 1508
  skeletal. See *Skeletal traction*.
  skin, 121
    and compartment syndromes, 68
    and ischemic muscle necrosis, 97
  skull, in cervical spine injuries, 298–302
  spring-loaded (Gardner-Wells), technique of applying, 298
Traction bow, Salvatori, 1906
Traction pins, insertion of, 121
Transcervical fractures, in children, 1447
Transcondylar fractures, of lower humerus, management of, 758
Transverse fracture, 9
  of femoral shaft, 1466
    in children, 1504, 1507

INDEX

Transverse fracture (*Continued*)
  of humeral shaft, 732
  of patella, with separation of fragments, 1634–1639
  of sacrum, with displacement, 474–476
Transverse processes, lumbar, isolated fractures of, 445–446
Trapezium
  anatomy of, 1126
  fracture of, 1126–1129
    comminuted, 1128
    mechanism of, 1126
Trapezoid, dislocation of, 1111–1112
Trauma
  and arthritis. See *Arthritis, post-traumatic.*
  and prognosis for physeal injuries, 154
  multiple, early management of, 2138–2139
    humeral shaft fractures in, 727–733
    prehospital management of, 2140–2145
Trimalleolar fracture of ankle, gravity-assisted reduction of, 113, 1853
Triquetrum bone, fractures of, 1120–1121
  isolated, 1121
Trochanter
  greater, fracture of, 1366–1368
    slightly displaced, 1367
    undisplaced, 1366
  lesser, epiphyseal separation of, 217–218
    fracture of, 1368–1369
Trousers, military antishock, 109, 483
  in femoral shaft fractures, 1457
  pneumatic counter-pressure, 2146
Tumors, of bone, benign, and pathologic fracture, 2116–2133
  giant cell, and pathologic fractures, 2121
  malignant, and pathologic fractures, 2094, 2116–2133
  primary, and pathologic fractures, 2124
Turner-Warwick repositioning of fracture-dislocated prostate, 485

Ulna. See also *Forearm*; and *Radioulnar joints.*
  anterior displacement of, 818–821
  distal
    dislocations of, clinical appearance of, 1037
      dorsal, 1037
      manipulative reduction of, 1040
      traumatic, 1036–1042
      volar, 1038
    fractures of, in children, 982–986
    relationship to radius, 1037
    resection of, 939
    subluxation of, 1038
      hyperpronation, 1039
      traumatic, 1036–1042
  forward displacement of, 821–823
  fractures of, 906
    displaced, in adults, 934–937
    hyperextension, with anterior dislocation of radial epiphysis, 970
    in children, growth remodeling of, 988
    lateral angulation of, with lateral dislocation of radial epiphysis, 970
    medial angulation of, with medial fracture-separation of radial epiphysis, 971

Ulna (*Continued*)
  fractures of, nightstick, 896
    undisplaced, with anterior dislocation of radial epiphysis, 970
    with dislocation of radial head. See *Monteggia injury.*
    with large defects, 938–940
  infected nonunion of, 46
  and 1-bone-forearm, 45
  proximal, greenstick fractures of, with dislocation of radial epiphysis, 969–972
  radiographic examination of, 102
  relationship to distal radius, 1037
  resection of, in Galeazzi's fracture, 939
    in older adult, 1044
  shortening of, in younger patient, 1044
  subluxation of, with distal radial fracture, 1040
Ulnar collateral ligament, of metacarpophalangeal joint of thumb, disruption of, complete, operative repair of, 1184
  in skier's thumb, 1181
Ulnar nerve
  function of, in Colles' fracture, 1018
  in carpal injuries, 1130
  in displacement of radial humeral epicondyle into elbow joint, 174
  injury to, treatment of fracture and, 97
  progressive palsy of, fractures of lower humerus and, 747
Unicondylar fractures, 1529–1536
  in frontal plane, 1534
  management of, 1530
  operative reduction and internal fixation of, 1532
Union
  delayed, 19, 27–42
    clinical features of, 28
    management of, 30
      operative, 33
    of carpal scaphoid, 37
    of distal tibial fractures, 1784
    of femur, 38
    of humeral shaft fractures, 734–735
    of tibial shaft fractures, 1778–1793
    radiographic features of, 28
    sites of predilection for, 30
  diagnosis of, 104–105
  rate of, 20
University of Arizona wrist arthroplasty, 1079
University of Minnesota technique of posterolateral decompression for neural deficit, 437
Urethral injury, fracture-dislocation of pelvis with, stabilization of, 486
Urinary tract, injury to, pelvic fractures and, 484
Urologic injury, pelvic fractures and, 484

Valgus deformity
  fibular fracture and, 1726
  in femoral shaft fractures in children, 1510
  of femoral capital, 1415
  of knee, 1548
    femoral shaft fractures and, 1462, 1496
    pathologic results of, 1549
  of upper tibial metaphyseal fractures in children, 1782

XXXI

INDEX

Valve, flutter, in flail chest, 517
    in tension pneumothorax, 510
Varus deformity
    distal tibial epiphyseal injuries and, correction of, 255–256
    of ankle, correction of, 255–256
    of femoral capital, 1415
    of hip, femoral neck fractures in children and, 1455
    of knee, 1549
        femoral shaft fractures and, 1461, 1496
        pathologic results of, 1550
        supracondylar fractures and, 1519
    of tibia, 2098
    tibial fracture and, 1726
Vascular network. See *Blood vessels*.
Vascular space, expanded, phase of, of shock, 78
Vasoconstriction phase, of shock, 78
Vastus lateralis, 1545
Vastus medialis, 1545
Veins. See *Blood vessels*.
Velpeau sling
    in acromioclavicular dislocation, 554
    in acute anterior subluxation of glenohumeral joint, 602
    in anterior dislocation of glenohumeral joint, 620
    in inferior fracture-subluxation of glenohumeral joint, 612
    in rotator cuff repair, 611
    in upper humeral epiphyseal separation, 157
Vest, halo. See *Halo cast*.
Vertebrae
    caudal, chip of bone from, 377
    cervical. See *Cervical vertebrae*.
    codfish, 2102
    orientation of, in anterior cord syndrome, 358
    thoracolumbar, exposure of, in posterolateral decompression, 438
Vertebral bodies, anterior aspect of, exposure of, in anterior cord syndrome, 357
Vessels, blood. See *Blood vessels*.
Viscera, injuries to, complicating fractures, 76–77
Vital functions, measurement of, in shock, 80
Volar plate, in injuries to metacarpophalangeal joint of thumb, 1176
    in injuries to phalanges of fingers, 1150
Volkmann's ischemic contracture, 65
Voltz–University of Arizona wrist arthroplasty, 1079

Wagner apparatus, in femoral shaft fractures, 1479
    in malunion of femoral shaft fractures, 1499
Walk, abnormalities of, after calcaneal fracture, 2018
Weaver and Dunn repair of acromioclavicular dislocation, 552
Weber and Cech procedure in nonunion of fractures of clavicle, 538
Weber's reduction forceps, 1870, 1892

West Point view, for glenoid injuries with anterior subluxation, 676
Whirlpool therapy, in open tibial fractures, 1755
Whitesides' technique, of measurement of intracompartmental pressure, 65
Wire and wiring
    circumferential, in bicondylar and spinotuberosity fractures of tibia, 1716
    circumferential, in displaced tibial condylar fractures, 1709, 1712
    in femoral shaft fractures, 1477
    in tibial shaft fractures, 1731
    of lumbar and thoracic vertebrae, 421
    in internal fixation, 124
    Kirschner. See *Kirschner wire*.
    of cervical vertebra, 339–344, 371
    of greater tuberosity of humerus, 658
    tension-band, of patellar fractures, 1637
Wounds, open. See also *Open fractures*.
    closure of, 128
    crushing, of hand, 1154
    debridement of, 127
        in open fractures of forearm, 954
    in tibial shaft fractures, 1750
    multiple fractures of finger metacarpals with, 1232
    of chest wall, 512
    of hand, 1154
    of knee, 1693
    spontaneous intussusception in, 1751
Wrist
    anatomy of, 1052–1054
    arthrodesis of, in chronic post-traumatic carpal arthritis, 1077, 1082
    arthroplasty of, 1079
        in chronic post-traumatic carpal arthritis, 1077
    emergency splinting of, 108
    extension of, 1056
    flexion of, 1056
    fractures and dislocations of, 1007–1136
        complications and pitfalls of, 1134–1135
    motion of, mechanics of, 1054–1057
    normal, 1010
    radial deviation of, 1055
    standard x-ray views of, 1058
    ulnar deviation of, 1055
    volar and dorsal aspects of, 1053

X-ray examination of fractures, 100–105. See also *Radiographic assessment technique(s)*.

Yde classification of ankle fractures, 1835–1841

Zickel nail
    in subtrochanteric fractures, 1394, 2096
        procedure for, 1396
    in supracondylar fractures, 1526

6